A Clinician's Guide to Donation and Transplantation

Dianne LaPointe Rudow, DrNP, CCTC
Linda Ohler, RN, MSN, CCTC, FAAN
Teresa Shafer, RN, MSN, CPTC

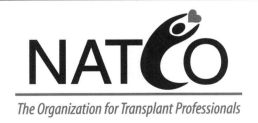

The Organization for Transplant Professionals

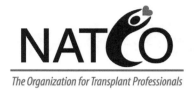

The Organization for Transplant Professionals

NATCO, The Organization for Transplant Professionals
P.O. Box 15384
Lenexa, KS 66285-5384
natco-info@goAMP.com
www.natco1.org

Copyright © 2006 by NATCO, The Organization for Transplant Professionals
ISBN 0-9624754-4-0

All rights reserved. No part of this publication may be reproduced, stored in a retrieval system or transmitted in any form or by any means, electronic, mechanical, photocopying, recording or otherwise, without written permission from NATCO, The Organization for Transplant Professionals. Printed in the United States of America.

Publisher: Applied Measurement Professionals, Inc.
             8310 Nieman Road
             Lenexa, KS 66214-1579

Book design by Applied Measurement Professionals, Inc.

A CLINICIAN'S GUIDE TO DONATION AND TRANSPLANTATION

Contents

Forward: A Clinicians Guide to Organ Donation and Transplantation		1
Front Bookends		5
1	The History of the Transplant Coordinator	7
	Teresa Shafer, RN, MSN, CPTC	
	NATCO Presidents	99
	Timelines	127
	Appendices	183
	Tables	239
	Figures	257
	Historical Photos	275
	References	305
	Back Bookends	319
2	Organ Allocation	321
	Walter Graham, Lin Johnson McGaw, RN, MEd, Kim Johnson, MS, Deanna C. Sampson, BS, JD, Cindy M. Sommers, Esq., Roger Brown, BS, CPTC	
3	General Medical Ethics – Organ Donation and Transplantation Snapshots	335
	Gloria J. Taylor, RN, MA, CPTC	
4	Multi-Cultural Considerations in Organ Donation and Transplantation	351
	Karen Garcia, MS, Clifton McClenney, MSM, Victoria Dent, BSW, Melissa Zinnerman, RN	
5	The Economics of Organ Donation and Transplantation	359
	G. Kent Holloway, MSF, Helen M. Hauff, RN, MBA, CCTC, CPTC	
6	The Gift of Tissue and Eye Donation	371
	Scott A. Brubaker, CTBS, Nancy Senst, RN, BSN, CPTC	
7	Kidney Transplantation	393
	Marilyn Rossman Bartucci, MSN, APRN, BC, CCTC	
8	Pancreas Transplantation	411
	Daniel C. Steen, RN, BA, Mary Beth Drangstveit, RN, BAN, CCTC	
9	Heart Transplantation	427
	Debi Dumas-Hicks, RN, BS, CCTC	
10	Lung Transplantation	441
	Tracy Evans-Walker, RN, BSN, CCTC	
11	Liver Transplantation	457
	Marian O'Rourke, RN, CCTC	
12	Intestinal Transplantation	481
	Laurel Williams, RN, MSN, CCTC, Deborah Andersen, RN, BSN, CCTC	

13	Islet Cell Transplantation	501
	Barbara DiMercurio, RN, BS	
14	The Ethics of Living Organ Donation	509
	Sheldon Zink, PhD, Stacey Wertlieb, MBe	
15	Living Lobar Lung Transplant Donors	521
	Ann M. Doyle, RN, CCRC	
16	Living Kidney Donors	527
	Catherine A. Garvey, RN, BA, CCTC	
17	The Living Liver Donor	535
	Dianne LaPointe Rudow, DrNP, CCTC	
18	Education and the Transplant Patient	549
	Marian Charlton, RN, CCTC, Kara Ventura, CPNP	
19	Long-term Complications Following Solid Organ Transplantation	559
	Jamie Blazek, FNP-C, MPH, CCTC, CCTN	
20	Infection in Solid Organ Transplant Recipients	573
	Meredith J. Aull, PharmD, Rudina Odeh-Ramadan, PharmD	
21	Transplant Immunology	605
	Linda Ohler, MSN, RN, CCTC, FAAN	
22	Pharmaceutical Care	613
	Steven Gabardi, PharmD, BCPS, Steven A. Baroletti, PharmD, BCPS, Lisa M. McDevitt, PharmD, BCPS, Sarah B. Saxer, PharmD, Fallon M. Vaughan, PharmD, Christin C. Rogers, PharmD	
23	Understanding Laboratory Values	651
	Sharon M. Augustine, RN, MS, CRNP, Suzanne Lanks, RN, MS, CRNP, Carol Wade, RN, MS, CRNP	
24	Women's Health After Transplant	673
	Lisa A. Coscia, RN, BSN, CCTC, Carolyn H. McGrory, RN, MS, John M. Davison, MD, Michael J. Moritz, MD, Vincent T. Armenti, MD, PhD	
25	Pediatric Transplantation	687
	Patricia Harren, DrNP, CPNP, CANP, CCTC	
26	Fundamentals of Successful Transplant Administration	695
	Tracy Giacoma, RN, MBA, MSN	
27	The Organ Donation Breakthrough Collaborative	711
	Teresa Shafer, RN, MSN, CPTC, Virginia McBride, RN, MPH, CPTC, Frank Zampiello, MD, John Chessare, MD, MPH, Dennis Wagner, MPA, Jade Perdue, MPA	
28	Clinical Diagnosis and Confirmatory Testing of Brain Death in Adults	747
	Eelco F. M. Wijdicks, MD	
29	Clinical Diagnosis and Confirmatory Testing of Brain Death in Children	771
	Stephen Ashwal, MD	

30	Requesting Organ Donation: Effective Communication	791

Teresa Shafer, RN, MSN, CPTC, Anne Kean, Laura A. Siminoff, PhD,
Rebecca Teagarden, BS, MA, Stacey Wertlieb, MBe, Meredith Wylie, BA, MA,
Sheldon Zink, PhD

31 Evaluation and Assessment of Organ Donors 805
Rebecca Menza, RN, MS, CPTC, P J Geraghty, REMT-P, BS, CPTC, CTBS

32 Adult Clinical Donor Care. 819
David J. Powner, MD, FCCP, FCCM, Kevin J. O'Connor, PA, MS, CPTC

33 Management of the Pediatric Organ Donor. 839
Thomas A. Nakagawa, MD, Steven S. Mou, MD

34 Surgical Recovery of Organs. 857
Tammie Peterson, RN, BSN, CPTC, Jennifer Johnson, RN, BSN, CPTC,
Amy Fleming, RN, BSN, CPTC, Mark Smith, CST, Marlon F. Levy, MD

35 Developing a Policy for Donation After Cardiac Death 867
Danielle L. Cornell, RN, BSN, CPTC, Charlie Alexander, RN, MSN, MBA, CPTC,
Karen Kennedy, RN, CPTC

36 Maximizing Organ Donation Opportunities Through Donation After
Cardiac Death 875
John Edwards, RN, RRT, CPTC, Patti Mulvania, RN, CEN, CPTC, Virginia Robertson,
Gweneth George, Richard Hasz, MFS, CPTC, Howard Nathan, CPTC,
Anthony D'Alessandro, MD

37 Organ Preservation. 891
Louise M. Jacobbi, CCTC, CPTC, Mitchell L. Henry, MD

38 The Vital Role of Medical Examiners and Coroners in Organ Transplantation . . . 903
Teresa J. Shafer, RN, MSN, CPTC, Lawrence L. Schkade, PhD, CCP,
Roger W. Evans, PhD, Kevin J. O'Connor, MS, PA, CPTC,
William Reitsma, RN, BSN, CPTC

General NATCO Resources 917

Index 919

Forward: A Clinician's Guide to Organ Donation and Transplantation

To accomplish great things, we must not only act but also dream, not only dream but also believe.
Anatole France, writer (1844-1924)

When one looks at where we began over a century ago and where we are today, the scientific evolution and our professional growth are truly amazing. Throughout each phase of development, a transplant coordinator has been influential in the progress of solid organ transplantation. Like no other publication, this comprehensive book captures the transplant coordinator's roles in the field of transplant. We all know of our physician partners who have pioneered transplantation; but finally all will know of the transplant coordinators who, with vision and perseverance, have made our profession what it is today.

Early transplant coordinators who cared for patients were "jacks-of-all-trades." Their focus was multifaceted: candidate selection, organ placement, organ preservation, immediate post transplant survival, management of rejection, patient education, and public awareness. A transplant coordinator may have managed more than one organ as well as all aspects of the procurement and transplantation process. Transplant coordinators were, and continue to be, individuals capable of multitasking in a complex healthcare environment.

As organ procurement organizations were established, the clinical and procurement roles became separated. Today's procurement coordinators are directly responsible for saving and changing lives. Whether by bold action or nuance, their actions ultimately determine whether or not organs are recovered. The procurement coordinator's practice is normally a solitary one – independent practitioners working with grieving families, critical care nurses, doctors, chaplains, transport personnel, medical examiners, police, district attorneys – basically anyone that walks into the donation and transplantation scenario. The procurement coordinator is in the eye of the storm.

Today's clinical coordinator may specialize in pre-transplant, post transplant, or living donor care. Typically, clinical transplant coordinators care for patients with one type of organ transplant; however as more combination transplants are being performed the coordinator needs expertise to care for combination and multi-visceral transplant recipients. As the complexity of care increases, more transplant centers are seeking the expertise of certified coordinators and those with specialized skills and advanced practice education such as nurse practitioners, clinical nurse specialists and physicians' assistants.

As the field has evolved and roles have changed, it has no longer been sufficient to understand the advances in the medical and nursing aspects of transplantation. The many challenges of transplant care require a multidisciplinary team approach to meet the needs of patients, families and the healthcare system. Transplant professionals must be well versed in all aspects of transplantation including public policy, patient advocacy, research, social work, psychiatry, and economics.

This book captures all facets of the field to provide transplant professionals with the tools to care for this complex and varied process. It is intended to provide a comprehensive review of all aspects of transplantation. NATCO's procurement and clinical transplant coordinator training courses were the first in 1983 and have remained a cornerstone in preparing coordinators to grasp the fundamentals. This textbook, the first of its kind, is developed by NATCO to compliment those courses and is another step in ensuring that practitioners are schooled in the science and art of transplant coordination. Each chapter has been developed and reviewed by nationally recognized experts and accomplished clinicians and will serve as an excellent resource for all practicing in the field of transplantation. It is a trip down memory lane; it is a proclamation of the impact transplant coordinators have had on the field; and it is a valuable tool for those studying for the transplant coordinator certification exam.

Dianne LaPointe Rudow, DrNP, CCTC
Linda Ohler, RN, MSN, CCTC, FAAN
Teresa Shafer, RN, MSN, CPTC
Editors

Book Dedication

That there be a better quality of life for patients with end-stage organ and tissue failure…and a respect for those who shared.

This book is dedicated to transplant coordinators throughout the world. To those who created the role, to those who continue to improve our practice and to the future coordinators who will benefit from the history of our professional growth. Virgil, an epic Roman poet (70 BC-19 BC once said, **"They can do all because they think they can."(1)** One would think he was describing a transplant coordinator.

>Virgil. Quotations Page. Available at: http://www.quotationspage.com/quotes/Virgil/. Date accessed: May 25, 2006.

Copy Editors
Rebecka Ryan, Aliso Viejo, CA
Katie Spiller, Encinitas, CA
Shani Zreik, Aliso Viejo, CA

Managing Editor
Christie Bowman, CAE, Lenexa, KS

Reviewers
Gregory Armstrong, Consultant, Brisbane, Australia
Carolyn Atkins, RN, BS, CCTC, Children's Medical Center Dallas, Dallas, TX
Wayne Babcock, RN, BSN, CPTC, California Transplant Donor Network, Modesto, CA
Mary Jane Badillo, BA, Tampa General Hospital, Tampa, FL
Robert Bray, PhD, Emory University School of Medicine, Atlanta, GA
Marian Charlton, RN, CCTC, New York Presbyterian Hospital, New York, NY
Gayl Chrysler, RN, MBA, American Red Cross, Woodbury, MN
Bernard Cohen, *retired*, Eurotransplant Director, The Netherlands
Carmen Cosio, MD, Baylor College of Medicine, Houston, TX
Ronald L. Dreffer, BS, CPTC, Musculoskeletal Transplant Foundation, Edison, NJ
Robert Duckworth, BS, CTBS, CPTC, St. Jude Medical, Incorporated, St. Paul, MN
John Edwards, BSN, RN, RRT, CPTC, Gift of Life Donor Program, Philadelphia, PA
Barbara A. Elick, RN, BSN, CPTC, CCTC, University of Minnesota & Fairview Health Services, Minneapolis, MN
Ron Ehrle, BSN, CPTC, LifeGift Organ Donation Center, Fort Worth, TX
Jan Finn, RN, MSN, CCRN, CPTC, Midwest Transplant Network, Westwood, KS
Vicki Fioravanti, RN, CCTC, Children's Mercy Hospital, Kansas City, MO
Steve Gabardi, PharmD, BCPS, Brigham & Women's Hospital/Northeastern University, Boston, MA
Patricia Harren, DrNP, CCTC, New York Presbyterian Medical Center, Center for Liver Disease & Transplant, New York, NY
Monica Horn, RN, CCRN, CCTC, Children's Hospital of Los Angeles, Los Angeles, CA
Louise M. Jacobbi, CPTC, CCTC, Organ Recovery Systems, Des Plaines, IL
Val Jeevanandum, MD, University of Chicago Hospitals, Chicago, IL
Linda L. Jones, RN, CCTC, CPTC, *retired*, Columbus, OH
David Kaufman, MD, St. Vincent's Hospital, Worchester, MA
Sherry LaForest, PharmD, University Hospital, Cleveland, OH
Dianne LaPointe Rudow, DrNP, CCTC, New York Presbyterian Medical Center, Center for Liver Disease & Transplant, New York, NY
Debbie Morgan, MSW, St. Barnabas Medical Center, Livingston, NJ
Howard Nathan, BS, CPTC, Gift of Life Donor Program, Philadelphia, PA
Linda Ohler, RN, MSN, CCTC, FAAN, Virginia Commonwealth University, Richmond, VA
Les Olson, BA, CPTC, SORS, LifeCenter Northwest Donor Network
Marian O'Rourke, RN, CCTC, Tulane Abdominal Transplant Institute, Tulane University Hospital & Clinic, New Orleans, LA
Jade Perdue, MPA, Department of Health & Human Services, HRSA, Rockville, MD
Michael G. Phillips, BHS, PA-C, CPTC, Life Connection of Ohio, Dayton, OH
Mark Reiner, PA, CPTC, Musculoskeletal Transplant Foundation, Edison, NJ
William Reitsma, RN, BSN, CPTC, New Jersey Organ & Tissue Sharing Network, Springfield, NJ
James Rodrigue, PhD, Beth Israel Deaconess Medical Center Boston, MA
Leo Roels, DonorAction, Belgium
Barbara Schanbacher, RN, BSN, CPTC, CCTC, *retired*, Iowa City, IA
Barbara Schulman, RN, CPTC, Transplant Consultant and Advisor, Los Angeles, CA
Nancy L. Senst, RN, BSN, CPTC, LifeSource, St. Paul, MN
Teresa Shafer, RN, MSN, CPTC, LifeGift Organ Donation Center, Fort Worth, TX
James W. Springer, BA, CPTC, LifeNet, Virginia Beach, VA
Paul Taylor, BS, CPTC, *retired*, Colorado
Janice Whaley, MPH, CTBS, CPTC, LifeGift Organ Donation Center, Houston, TX

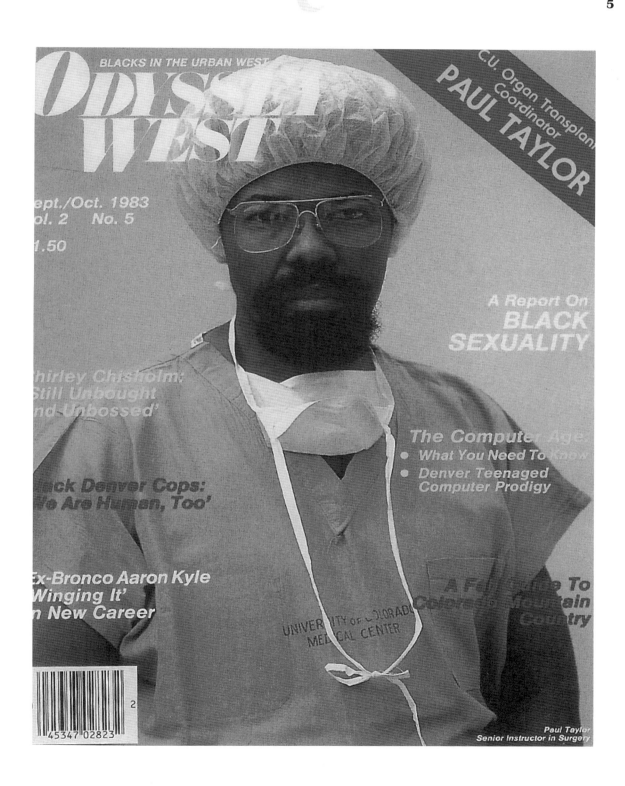

Chapter 1: THE HISTORY OF THE TRANSPLANT COORDINATOR

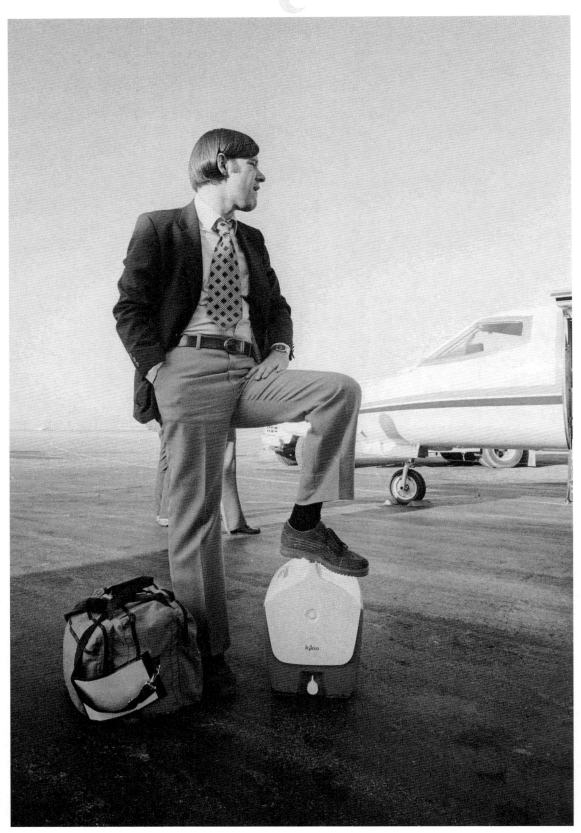

Section 1: Issues in Donation and Transplantation

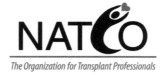

A CLINICIAN'S GUIDE TO DONATION AND TRANSPLANTATION

The History of the Transplant Coordinator

Teresa Shafer, RN, MSN, CPTC

A. Introduction to the Transplant Coordinator. 9
B. Early Events Leading up to the Modern Era of Transplantation. 11
C. Brain Death: Organ Recovery Before and After Brain Death Legislation 13
D. The Advent of Modern Organ Transplantation 17
    1. Kidney Transplantation 18
    2. Liver Transplantation 20
    3. Heart Transplantation 21
    4. Lung Transplantation 23
    5. Pancreas Transplantation 24
E. Birth of Transplant Coordination and the Transplant Coordinator 25
    1. Procurement Transplant Coordinators 26
    2. Clinical Transplant Coordinators 27
    3. Early Transplant Coordinators 28
    4. Birth of NATCO 41
F. National Organ Transplant Hearings 45
G. NATCO Annual Meetings 48
H. Training Courses for Clinical and Procurement Transplant Coordinators 48
I. Transplant Coordinators and Organ Sharing 53
    1. 24-ALERT System 55
    2. Extrarenal Transplant Programs (circa 1984) 61
    3. Transportation of Organs 63
J. Transplant Coordinator Research and Publications 64
    1. NATCO Newsletters 64
    2. *Progress in Transplantation* (formerly *Journal of Transplant Coordination*) 67
    3. Transplant Coordinators in the Press 68
K. 24-Hour-a-Day/7-Day-a-Week Dedication 70
L. Certification of Transplant Coordinators 74
    1. The American Board of Transplant Coordinators 76
    2. Transplant Coordinator Certification Statistics 77
    3. Coordinator Recertification 77

(outline continued, next page)

Photo, page 5: Paul Taylor, transplant coordinator. Odyssey West Photo courtesy of Blair-Caldwell African American Research Library. (Published with permission as originally seen—front cover of magazine.)

Photo, page 6: Brian Broznick, transplant coordinator. People Magazine Photo. ©Lynn Johnson/AURORA. (Published with permission as originally seen—in full page layout.)

M.	International Transplant Coordinators Organizations		78
	1.	Australasian Transplant Coordinators Association (ATCA)	78
	2.	European Transplant Coordinators Organization (ETCO)	78
	3.	United Kingdom Transplant Coordinators Association (UKTCA)	79
	4.	Japanese Transplant Coordinators Organization (JATCO)	81
	5.	Society of Transplant Coordinators Worldwide: Formation of the International Transplant Coordinators Society (ITCS)	84
N.	In Memoriam: Transplant Coordinator Pioneers		88
	1.	Billy G. Anderson, BA, CPTC	88
	2.	Brian A. Broznick, BS, CPTC	90
	3.	Gary Hall, BS, CPTC	92
	4.	Isao Tamaki	93
O.	Fast Forward: 2006 and Beyond		95
P.	NATCO Presidents		99
Q.	TimeLine of Transplantation and Transplant Coordinators		127
R.	Appendices: Testimony of Transplant Coordinators at NOTA Hearings		183
S.	Tables		239
T.	Figures		257
U.	Historical Photos		275
V.	References		305

A CLINICIAN'S GUIDE TO DONATION AND TRANSPLANTATION — Chapter 1

Introduction to the Transplant Coordinator

The worldwide system of transplantation could not exist as we know it today without the transplant coordinator. These unique, talented, and dedicated professionals make possible the recovery of organs in an expert, ethical and effective manner and coordinate the care of sick patients with end-stage organ failure who are awaiting transplantation and those who receive this miracle of life. They are the go-to, can-do, get-it-done glue and web that holds together the many disparate pieces of the complex process of transplantation. These words were written today, but they are essentially the same as appeared nearly three decades ago when another author stated that transplant coordinators are:

> "remarkable people who provide the glue that holds every transplantation together. They speak—with determination—of an idealistic objective: to assure a successful transplant for every person awaiting an organ or tissue. In other words, their goal is life. [They] are the operators of a vast, complex system held together by computers, long hours, and hard work. Careful cooperation is their stock-in-trade."[1]

The essential need for transplant coordinators has been noted by many, including Vincent et al,[2] who succinctly concluded that transplant coordinators were committed professionals who were critical to all endeavors in organ transplantation. "Coordinators tend to describe themselves as conduits through whom the system functions. But in many ways, they ... *are* the system."[3] The emergence of the transplant coordinator (a term used both for those professionals taking care of recipients and potential recipients and for the professionals who coordinate consent, donor management, and organ recovery) as a distinct profession had its roots in the early 1960s as transplantation programs began to develop. These individuals, creating the role as they worked, were often the jack-of-all-trades who performed the two tasks just described and many others. Individuals working in the departments of surgery, perfusion labs and dialysis units started to fill a unique role. Thomas Starzl, MD, renowned pioneer liver transplant surgeon, commented that procurement coordinators are "the unsung heroes of transplantation."[3]

Kootstra gets it right when he notes that European transplant coordinators, working in the style similar to US coordinators, did not start until the mid to late 1970s, and wrote:

> *The transplant coordinator is an American invention.* [emphasis added] It was recognized early in the US that paramedical personnel could be very supportive in the procurement of kidneys and successively in machine preservation and transplantation. In Europe, these procedures were kept in the hands of the doctors until in the mid-'70s. At the introduction in Europe initially doctors were recruited, later on paramedical personnel mainly from nursing staff [were] employed. Especially in the case of a multi organ donor (MOD), no team could currently do without a transplant coordinator.[4(p61)]

In this chapter, I attempt to weave together the milestones of transplantation (see Transplant Timeline) and intersperse the beginnings, development, and maturation of the newly emergent profession: the transplant coordinator. Transplant coordinators practice at the very heart of the robust and complex field of organ transplantation. They are the hub of the wheel that holds all the spokes together, caring for and bringing donors and recipients together. In so doing, they coordinate and collaborate with transplant surgeons, immunology specialists, attending and consulting physicians, nurses, hospital leaders, chaplains, social workers, and a host of others. Whatever needs attention in order to procure and transplant organs, the procurement transplant coordinator and the clinical transplant coordinator are the health care professionals who apply their specialized knowledge to the situation at hand and essentially make transplantation happen. Wearing many titles over the years, some of which are still used today, one sees glimpses of the evolution of the role in the title used (Table 1).

As early as 1980, and continuing through to today, published accounts of transplant coordinator roles may be found.[5-22] Tolboe[22] in 1980 describes the role of transplant coordinator in perhaps the first book chapter dedicated to that subject. The description of her role as a transplant coordinator was typical of transplant coordinator roles early on, structured in the all-inclusive, "do-it-all" mode:

"Primary responsibility for the smooth and integrated activity of this department is assumed by the transplant coordinators. Broadly, they are charged with the execution of duties in the following areas:
- Acquisition of both cadaveric and living donors for transplantation
- Organ preservation
- Patient education
- Inpatient, outpatient, and ambulatory care
- Review and supervision of transplant protocols
- Data collection and research activity
- Professional education
- Public education and public relations
- Administrative activities of the department[22(pp43-44)]

Before this time, the literature was devoid of descriptions of this new role. As Tolboe[22(p43)] noted:

Despite a relative diligent effort to identify, peruse, and utilize the available literature addressing the "role" of the transplant coordinator in this era of organ transplantation, one finds little discussion or information on the topic. There are some isolated accounts of dedicated individuals described non-critically, almost affectionately, as "ambulance chasers" endeavoring to recover usable organs for transplantation. These accounts are primarily public interest stories, altruistic in nature, but certainly reiterating the need for a general commitment to both the philosophy of and continued pressing need for organ donation.

In 1984, Howard Nathan of the North American Transplant Coordinator's Organization (NATCO) inquired into the history of transplant coordination when he sought information regarding the founding of NATCO.[23] Elick, in a most inclusive description of the transplant coordinator role, began her chapter with a definition of the transplant coordinator: "'Transplant coordinator,' broadly defined, has been the title given to persons who facilitate the transplant process—from donor identification and organ procurement to implantation and follow-up recipient care."[24(pp325-326)] Continuing through to today, authors continue to define the description and role of the transplant coordinator. "By definition, *coordination* means to work together harmoniously, to act together in a smooth, concerted manner. A transplant coordinator is a person who facilitates the transplant process. Implementation of the role varies among transplant programs and geographical areas; however, certain commonalities are shared by most transplant coordinators."[25(p17)]

Early in the profession, the practitioners developed a philosophy of transplant coordination that remains true even today (Table 2). The founders, the pioneers of the profession, set transplant coordinators' ideals and principles soundly, so much so that these principles continue to hold up today, even with the incredible amount of change that has occurred in the field of organ donation and transplantation.

Although numerous accounts of transplant coordination as a profession may now be found, a comprehensive look at the genesis of the field and the leaders who developed the field has not been compiled. Historical references to the transplant coordinator are made in some texts; however, they are made from the viewpoint of others such as immunologists and surgeons, invariably retaining that bias. One exception to this is Lee Gutkind's book, *Many Sleepless Nights*.[26] For four years, Gutkind immersed himself in transplantation and organ recovery at major transplant centers throughout the US and at Cambridge University in England. He did not limit himself solely to the viewpoints of surgeons and writes of his long hours spent with procurement coordinators such as Donald Denny, Brian Broznick, Bob Duckworth, Mike Callahan, Celia Wight, Sandy Bromberg and Marguerite Brown—and with clinical transplant coordinators Sandra Staschak and Joan Miller. The transplant coordinators' words and stories with Gutkind's framing are true to type. Gutkind characterizes *Many Sleepless Nights* as his most challenging and satisfying book. He "lived with people who traveled halfway around the world literally on the edge of death to transplant centers, hoping for miracles and jetted through the night" on organ donor recoveries. He confronted "the ethical, moral, scientific and humanistic viewpoints of organ transplantation through the eyes of the people most involved."[26]

As it is, any history is to some extent biased by the author and his or her audience, including the pieces selected for presentation. This account, this chapter, although extensive for its time, is by no means comprehensive. It is meant to recognize the accomplishments of transplant coordinators as a whole and in a generic sense, and also to portray some of the accomplishments of transplant coordinator pioneers and leaders, committing names and faces to print. However, it is not meant to recognize every individual who has practiced, indeed, only a small percentage of early practitioners are noted. I am optimistic in believing that this will be only the first of our profession's attempts at heralding some of the pioneers and leaders in our profession and that future such efforts will continue.

The information included here is based on numerous materials gathered from the literature, from the NATCO archives, the author's records, and interviews with transplant coordinators, many of whom are retired or are beginning to retire. Freely admitted, it is written from the bias of a former transplant coordinator. Further, this chapter has an American slant, although certain milestones in international transplant coordination are included, particularly in the Transplant Timeline, included herein. However, the chapter is not comprehensive but is a first effort in documenting the accomplishments of our colleagues. We should do more to document our history and recognize our colleagues. I hope that someone will continue this trend of documenting transplant coordinators' accomplishments and history and improve upon this particular effort.

Before continuing into the development of the transplant coordinator, a brief review of the history of dialysis, transplantation, brain death, and organ recovery follows. The brief narrative on transplant history included here is by no means inclusive. I would refer readers to two texts on the history of transplantation that I found truly excellent and presented in a chronological format: Nicholas Tilney's *Transplant: From Myth to Reality*[27] and Thomas Starzl's *Puzzle People*.[28]

I have included a transplant timeline at the end of this chapter, woven together from the many sources I reviewed in preparing to write this chapter and frame the transplant coordinator role in the history of transplantation (see Transplant Timeline). The timeline proved helpful in organizing the chapter, as it put into perspective the milestones in the history of transplantation and the natural evolution of the transplant coordinator's role. Although I am using the word "evolution" here in describing the development of the transplant coordinator role, readers should be aware that at some point the breakthrough of transplant coordinators coming into being was not just by chance, not just by evolution. *Specific individuals seized the moment and created their future—a future all transplant coordinators enjoy today.*

Early Events Leading Up to the Modern Era of Transplantation

The 13th century medieval story of Saints Cosmos and Damien tells of the act of transplanting the leg of a recently deceased Moor onto a devoted church member whose own leg was afflicted with gangrene. According to legend, the transplant was a success.[29,30] "For this deed, they are considered the patron saints of modern transplantation."[27(p9)] Given the scientific climate of the world during those times and the logical absurdity of the scenario, these accounts may have been more mythical than factual.[31]

The first reported use of a skin graft in a medical journal was in 1881. Although surgeons had known about skin grafts for at least 2000 years, a medical journal reports the first use of skin from a recently deceased person as a temporary graft. The patient was a man who was burned while leaning against a metal door when lightning struck.[32] The surgeon treating him took skin from a patient who had just died to be used as a temporary skin graft. Sir Winston Churchill described in 1930 the removal by an Irish surgeon of a 'shilling sized' part of his skin donated in 1898 to an officer friend and "this precious fragment was then grafted on to my friend's wound. It remains there to this day and did him lasting good in many ways. I for my part keep the scar as a souvenir."[33] While Churchill was most certainly mistaken about the retention of the small transplanted graft, he was not mistaken in his obvious pride in having donated and in his description of the gift as "precious."

Alexis Carrel pioneered the field of transplantation. "Carrel was born in Lyon, France, in 1873. While serving an internship in a hospital in Lyon in 1894, he was deeply affected by the assassination of the president of the French Republic, Sadi Carnot. Carnot's fatal knife wound had severed the portal vein, and the best surgeons in France were helpless to control the bleeding. Carrel observed correctly that if only surgeons could sew blood vessels together, this wound could have easily been closed and the patient saved. He left clinical medicine in 1901 and began a lifelong career in experimental vascular surgery."[35] He perfected the vascular anastomosis techniques (helping subsequent early researchers),[34] performed the first experimental (animal) kidney autotransplants with long-term survival, and conceived the idea of rejection by attributing the failure of experimental kidney allotransplant to what he termed "biological incompatibility."[36] Carrel was awarded the Nobel prize in 1912 in recognition of his work on vascular suture and the transplantation of blood vessels and organs. Several books chronicle his interesting life.[37,38]

Pioneering research by Vladimir Demikhov greatly advanced the field of experimental cardiac transplantation. His published works documented many experiments, including transplantation of the head, transplantation of halves of the body, and surgical combination of two animals with the creation of a single circulation. His initial work in cardiac transplantation involved canine heterotopic cardiac transplants to the inguinal region. His monograph reported a long series of 250 experimental efforts at transplanting a heterotopic intrathoracic cardiac graft. On June 30, 1946, Demikhov transplanted a heterotopic heart and lung; the animal survived for nine hours and 26 minutes. A subsequent experiment on a dog resulted in 25 days of survival, and the cause of death was probably dehiscence of the tracheobronchial suture line.[34] (See timeline for more on early transplant efforts.)

In the 1940s, Peter Brian Medawar, a British zoologist, reported using refrigerated skin as a temporary dressing to treat burns. Soon frozen skin was being used. Medawar was the first to demonstrate the immune origin of rejection. Building upon observations of the immune system dating back thousands of years, he used experimental skin transplants on animals to explain why burn victims from the bombing of civilians in England during World War II reject donated skin, why skin taken from one person and grafted onto another will not form a permanent graft. His work set the stage for the new field of transplantation biology.[32] He was to be honored throughout his life for his seminal work which marked the beginning of transplantation immunology, receiving a Nobel prize in 1960 and in 1965 being knighted by the Queen and thereafter being referred to as Sir Peter Medawar.

During the first half of the twentieth century, numerous experimental transplantations were done on animals, and isolated transplantations had been and were being increasingly performed in humans. It is important to understand the backdrop of the evolving field just before that time. The first practical dialysis machine was developed by Willem J. Kolff, MD, in the Netherlands in 1943 but could not be used for chronic long-term dialysis because it exhausted veins and arteries after only a few treatments. Beginning in 1943, Willem Kolff used dialysis on patients with kidney disease. His first patient was a 29-year-old woman whose vision was failing from the effects of hypertension and uremia. "The improvement with dialysis, particularly after removal of large amounts of water, was obvious: 'she was strikingly well and her mind was perfectly clear.' Her vision improved so that 'she could read the paper without any difficulty.' After twelve consecutive treatments, she died because she ran out of peripheral vessels to connect to the machine. At autopsy, both kidneys were shrunken and scarred." Kolff used dialysis on 17 persons, two of whom survived.[27(p146)]

Dialysis during these times was used to tide patients over during an acute but reversible bout of kidney failure until the kidneys could recover. "In these patients, surgical crosscuts to insert the plastic tubes from the machine into the blood vessels would start at the wrists, moving upward every few inches until the armpits were reached. When the arms were used up, the crosscuts would start at the feet and move to the groin. Once the leg vessels were exhausted, the string had played out and death would follow. Each crosscut could be used only two or three times."[28(p92)]

It wasn't until the development of the Scribner shunt in 1960 that the procedure became practical.[39-40] University of Washington nephrologist Dr. Belding Scribner developed a shunt whose Teflon components permitted semi-permanent access to a person's arteries. By using the shunt, each crosscut could provide a set of vessels that might be usable three times a week for many months or years.[28(p92)] The shunt greatly improved dialysis, and in 1966 the introduction of the arterio-venous fistula made chronic dialysis a reality.

The first long-term dialysis treatments began in 1960. The only two centers willing to provide dialysis in 1960 approached the problem differently. Both were in the United States, one in Seattle and the other one at the Brigham. The dialysis program in Seattle soon became overwhelmed with patients seeking help—not only those living locally, but also individuals from areas that did not offer such treatment. The financing of this effort was helped initially by a small grant from a private foundation, and the NIH [National Institutes of Health] offered modest support. Public fund drives became necessary. As sustaining even one patient cost thousands of dollars each year even at that time, the numbers of acceptances had to be limited. By the mid-1960s, physicians were arguing desperately against legislators, who denied any problem. "At the present time in the United States, there are no more than 50 to 100 patients on transplants plus chronic dialysis—yet in the last four years, since these techniques have become available, 10,000 or more ideal candidates have died in this country. For lack of the treatment, so obviously rigid selection of one sort or another must take place." The cries from patients and those trying to care for them became increasingly desperate.[27(pp149-150)]

Dr. Scribner helped open the first freestanding dialysis center in the world named the Seattle Artificial Kidney Center. Clyde Shields, an aircraft machinist for Boeing, became the first person to receive dialysis for chronic kidney failure at University Hospital in Seattle. For the first time in history, end-stage kidney disease was not a death sentence.[32] However, in 1961 and 1962, there were very few artificial kidneys available for chronic treatment. The problem was portrayed in *Life* magazine November 9, 1962, by pictures of a tribunal in Seattle deliberating which six patients among many candidates should be selected for entry into the only dialysis unit in the world designed for chronic care.[27(p92)] The cost of dialysis was a major obstacle for the patients. They were dialyzed if grants were available or if they could pay. Death Committees were established to make decisions regarding who received treatments. The End Stage Renal Disease Medicare Amendment in 1972, however, made it possible financially for patients to be treated by hemodialysis (see Timeline).

Brain Death: Organ Recovery before and after Brain Death Legislation

Brain death was described for the first time in 1959 in France. A group of neurosurgeons described a condition they termed "death of the nervous system." Seen in patients with structural brain lesions (usually traumatic), it was most likely to occur when the trauma had been complicated at a later time by respiratory arrest. These physicians noted that the state was characterized by persistent apneic coma, absent brainstem and tendon reflexes, and an electrically silent brain. The patients looked like cadavers, but had a regular pulse as long as artificial respiration was maintained. Disconnection from the ventilator produced no respiratory response. In 1959 Parisian neurophysiologists Molaret and Goulon published a much fuller account of what we now know as brain death, first terming it "coma dépassé" (a state beyond coma).[34,41,42]

Before the establishment and acceptance of brain death and brain death legislation, transplantation of kidneys began with removal of the kidneys from patients who had died as determined by a cessation of heart function, referred to as non-heart-beating donors, and only more recently donation-after-cardiac-death donors.

In the early 1960s, cadaveric donations were thought to be impractical and impossible. Living donors were the only available source of organs for transplantation. G. Melville Williams, MD, a pioneering transplant surgeon, recounts in a chapter on the history of transplantation[a] that the discovery of azathioprine (Imuran) was responsible for the burst of transplant activity in 1963, using living related donors in kidney transplantation. It soon became apparent to surgeons, however, that most patients had no appropriate living related donor. Kidneys from baboons and chimpanzees never functioned indefinitely; with early function being salutary in a majority of cases. Because of the unavailability of living-related donors, volunteer donors were sought, and kidneys were removed from inmates in the state penitentiaries.[43(p7)]

---

a. I would highly recommend that persons interested in this issue and during this time period read history texts discussing organ recovery in the era before brain death was medically, legally and/or socially recognized. The books I have previously mentioned are excellent.

Chapter 1: THE HISTORY OF THE TRANSPLANT COORDINATOR

At this time in Richmond, Virginia, David Hume transplanted one patient with a chimpanzee kidney which resulted in a two liter per hour diuresis and death. He quickly discussed the concept of cadaver donation with the medical examiner. Dr. Mann supported the concept of allowing the transplant team to remove organs from bodies he was authorized to examine in order to determine the cause of death. This aspect of law deserves emphasis, for it remains in place.

…therefore, in the early days in Richmond, family consent was generally considered unnecessary in these cases. However, most often the next of kin was informed of the potential use of the organs for transplantation and asked to consent. In instances in which the next of kin was unavailable or could not be found, the medical examiner empowered us to remove organs preliminary to his autopsy.

Having cleared the way for a source of cadaver organs, the next issue was declaring death prior to the death of the kidneys. Dr. Hume was fortunate to be associated with Dr. William Collins, the head of neurosurgery, who had strong feelings that patients having certain types of coma were in fact dead and should be removed from the respirator. I do not remember Dr. Collins specifying objective criteria for the determination of irreversible brain death, but in retrospect, all of the patients he judged to be brain-dead would have met modern criteria. Amazingly, all of us believed that a patient disconnected from the respirator was still alive until his heart stopped beating.

This belief led to a charade. The potential donor, invariably the victim of head trauma, would be pronounced hopelessly injured by Dr. Collins or a member of his staff. The injured person would then be moved to an operating room, still connected to mechanical ventilation. After appropriate preparation of the skin and application of drapes, the respirator was discontinued as the surgical team waited for the cessation of the heartbeat. Meanwhile, preparations were made in two other operating rooms for recipients, who would undergo skin preparation and draping, deferring the skin incision until word came from the donor room that the kidneys appeared normal.

When the heart stopped beating, a long midline incision was made. The left kidney was mobilized from behind the colon and rapidly excised. A 10-minute time frame was good, a 12-minute, average, and a 15-minute, slow. The cecum and right colon were then mobilized and the right kidney extracted, with the surgical team working from the aorta and vena cava to mobilization of the kidney and finally division of the ureter. Dr. Hume generally presided over a recipient requiring the left kidney. He was a meticulous surgeon, which was an interesting contrast to his flamboyant personality. He did not like to be 'assisted' very actively. He corrected my overly aggressive assistance at times by butting my head.[43(p7-8)]

The first organ procurement from heart-beating cadavers was by Guy Alexandre[44] (Leuven, Belgium) in 1963 and Jean Hamburger (France) in 1964. Five years before the 1968 publication of the Harvard committee's report concerning "irreversible coma" established a paradigm for defining death by neurologic criteria, in 1963, Dr. Alexandre, a Belgian surgeon, had not only adopted closely similar diagnostic criteria for brain death but also applied those criteria in performing the first organ transplant from a brain-dead donor. Machado provides an in-depth look into this first heart-beating, brain dead donor in his 2005 Neurology article[44], detailing the case along with the thinking at the time (which had been documented in the proceedings from a symposium), of how transplantation could be effected from individuals who had, what had been termed four years earlier, coma dépassé.

Alexandre had pursued a fellowship in surgical research at Harvard University under Murray's supervision in 1961 and 1962. He worked at the Peter Bent Brigham Hospital, directed by Francis D. Moore, and met Roy Calne for the first time in Boston, who was packing to return to England after completing a fellowship on Moore's service. After his fellowship, Alexandre returned to Belgium and immediately began the work to start a kidney transplantation program.[44]

On June 3, 1963, a patient with a severe head injury was brought to the emergency department of the Saint Pierre Hospital in Louvain, in profound coma. In spite of vigorous resuscitation procedures and the administration of vasopressors, and other drugs, the patient showed the clinical picture of coma dépassé.

At Alexandre's request, Jean Morelle, chair of the Department of Surgery, made "the most important decision of his career," allowing the removal of a kidney from that heart-beating patient. The graft functioned immediately after implant. The recipient, who had been maintained by peritoneal dialysis, died of sepsis—with his new kidney in place—on day 87.[44]

At a Ciba Symposium on Transplantation that took place in London in 1966, Alexandre made the following comments, detailing his brain death criteria, following a presentation given by Joseph Murray on "Organ Transplantation: The Practical Possibilities"[44,45]:

> To throw some fuel into the discussion, I would like to tell you what we consider as death when we have potential donors who have severe craniocerebral injuries. In nine cases we have used patients with head injuries, whose hearts had not stopped, to do kidney transplantations. Five conditions were always met in these nine cases: 1) complete bilateral mydriasis; 2) complete absence of reflexes, both natural and irresponsive to profound pain; 3) complete absence of spontaneous respiration, five minutes after mechanical respiration has been stopped; 4) falling blood pressure, necessitating increasing amounts of vasopressive drugs (either adrenaline or Neo-synephrine [phenylephrine hydrochloride]); 5) a flat EEG. All five conditions must be met before the removal of a kidney can be considered.[45]

Many of Alexandre's colleagues considered such actions ethically unacceptable. Calne remarked "Although Dr. Alexandre's criteria are medically persuasive, according to traditional definitions of death, he is, in fact, removing kidneys from live donors. I feel that if a patient has a heartbeat he cannot be regarded as a cadaver. Any modification of the means of diagnosing death to facilitate transplantation will cause the whole procedure to fall into disrepute."[27(p161), 44-45] Starzl also voiced similar concerns at the meeting: "I doubt if any of the members of our transplantation team could accept a person as being dead as long as there was a heart beat" over concern that the care of a trauma patient could be jeopardized by virtue of organ donor candidacy.[27(p161), 44-45] Dr. Starzl later noted that his fears were unfounded.[28(p148)]

Acceptance of brain death with subsequent recovery of kidneys was controversial among both the professional and lay public, with the widely quoted "You're dead when your doctor says you are," summarizing public ambivalence.[27(p161),46,47]

Often times during the early years of establishment of brain death, the organs were not removed until the heart had stopped. The kidneys were dissected free, the ventilator removed, and the kidneys removed after the heart had stopped beating.[4(p59)] As Tilney noted, however, practical considerations outweighed philosophy, and the results of transplantation from heart-beating cadavers compared favorably with the results for living donors, and the establishment of brain death as death became accepted in a relatively short time. In the 1960s, at Massachusetts General Hospital, a liver was recovered from a police officer whose heart was beating but whose brain was deemed dead. This seminal event led to the development of the concept of brain death as death, rather than the cessation of circulation, which previously defined death.[48]

The impetus for defining death on the basis of irreversible loss of total brain function was initiated by Beecher in 1968. A report of an ad hoc committee of Harvard Medical School examined the definition of brain death and published the first widely accepted guidelines for clinical management of the medically and ethically complex circumstances surrounding brain death. (Machado's earlier referenced article includes a table comparing Alexandre's initial brain death criteria to the later published and widely accepted Harvard criteria.)[44] Brain death was defined in terms of the entire brain: "…a person is dead if the entire brain is dead."[49-50] This definition has withstood biomedical advances in the past three decades.[51] Recognition of brain death as a legal means of pronouncing death has made available thousands of organs each year for organ transplantation.

The need for a uniform law governing organ donation was felt as the frequency of transplantation procedures increased in the early 1960s. It became apparent that a single, uniform statute was needed that could be adopted by all states. Although different states enacted their own cadaveric donation statutes, the provisions of these statutes varied widely. At that time, it was not clear whether a legal authorization signed in one state was effective if a death occurred elsewhere. It soon became clear that the legal confusion that resulted from these individualized laws was discouraging organ donation. As a result, physicians were sometimes reluctant to participate in organ donations for fear of possible legal liabilities.[52]

Chapter 1 — THE HISTORY OF THE TRANSPLANT COORDINATOR

In response to this proposal, the National Conference of Commissioners on Uniform State Laws formed a committee to draft a proposal for adoption by each state of legislation concerning the Uniform Anatomical Gift Act. This act has served as the medicolegal foundation for the growth of the field of transplantation, primarily in the area of cadaveric organ procurement.[51]

The Uniform Anatomical Gift Act, which established the legal framework for cadaveric organ donation, was passed in 1968. It was an important advance in organ procurement and was passed by all 50 states. It allowed individuals to make a decision regarding organ donation before death. By signing a uniform donor card, individuals could legally state their intent to be donors.

Kansas was the first state to adopt brain death laws in 1970.[53(p25),54] In 1974, the American Medical Association recognized brain death as a criterion for making the diagnosis of death. The American Medical Association resolved that "…death shall be determined by the clinical judgment of a physician using the necessary available and currently accepted criteria…" and that "…permanent and irreversible cessation of the function of the brain constitutes one of various criteria which can be used in the medical diagnosis of brain death."[49]

In 1975, the American Bar Association House of Delegates adopted the following definition of death: "For all legal purposes, a human body with irreversible cessation of total brain function, according to usual and customary standards of medical practice, shall be considered dead."[51,55]

In early transplant coordinator meetings, newsletters, and medical literature, the discussion of brain death, and the legal and ethical issues involved with it, were numerous and ever-present. The need to work within this framework and fully explore the practical associated issues required a new professional. There is no doubt that the development of brain death as death was a driving force in the need for and development of the organ procurement coordinator as a professional.

Dr. Norman Shumway died while I was writing this chapter. I had been speaking with Phyllis Weber about historical items of interest to include in this chapter when she mentioned his illness. Shortly after we spoke, he died, and one of Phyllis' staff forwarded an article appearing in the *New York Times* on February 11.[56] The *Times* article about Dr. Shumway included an interesting story about him, particularly as I was then writing the brain death section of this chapter. It clearly illustrated the difficulty transplant coordinators and surgeons had when working in organ donation and transplantation in the early days. This small piece of the article, nestled within the much larger article chronicling Dr. Shumway's substantial achievements, portrayed all too well the challenges they faced.

> Another barrier to heart transplants was a societal one. Even though Dr. Barnard's first donor was a brain-dead accident victim,[b] in the United States "there was a terrible furor about the brain death issue," Dr. Shumway said. In the late 1960s, Dr. John Hauser, the coroner of Santa Clara County, Calif., which included Stanford, sought criminal charges against Dr. Shumway for transplanting organs without an autopsy on the donor, an act that would have made transplantation impossible. The two men shouted at each other over the issue in Dr. Shumway's office, recalled Dr. Eugene Dong, then a transplant surgeon at Stanford and now a lawyer. But Louis P. Bergma, then the Santa Clara district attorney, did not file a criminal complaint, and the California Legislature soon resolved the conflict by adopting cessation of brain activity as a definition of death.[57]

In later years, after the "brain death" issue was settled, medical examiner and coroner problems remained, only the issue was not brain death, but forensic examination versus organ recovery. This was a challenge that transplant coordinators would fight to overcome. Numerous articles written by Teresa Shafer and her transplant coordinator colleagues and co-authors eventually proved to public policy analysts, legislators, and medical examiners that this was an issue that was, in fact, a nonissue: that death investigation and organ recovery were completely compatible and that organ donation could proceed without harming the death investigation.[58-63] The repercussions of particularly the first seminal publication on the issue in 1994 was reported throughout the world.[64-67] Like their colleague Dr. Shumway, Doctors Leonard Bailey and Richard Chinnock wrote in defense of the bold position put forward by the

---

b. Even though brain death laws had passed in South Africa, Dr. Barnard none the less took the donor off the ventilator in surgery, allowing the heart to stop on its own, rather than disconnecting the ventilator after the patient was pronounced brain dead, because of the prevailing societal and medical norms.

transplant coordinators, no doubt having lost many patients because of medical examiner denials of organ recovery in the face of an extreme shortage of donor hearts.[68]

The Advent of Modern Organ Transplantation

The modern era of transplantation was ushered in with kidney transplantation, the details of which are included below. Animal experimentation during the first half of the 20th century paved the way for human transplantation, beginning in earnest in the 1960s after the successful identical twin transplants that had been done to date (see Transplant Timeline). The operation perfected by Rene Küss in 1951 became the operation which was subsequently used by the successful twin cases in Boston and remains the standard kidney transplant procedure today[28(p89)] Toledo-Pareyra notes that surprisingly enough, Murray and his team were lucky enough to find other identical twins, one-to-two every year.[69-73] The critical question was how to overcome rejection and have success in non-identical-twin cases.[69]

In the early months of 1963, few programs in the United States existed. Only the Peter Bent Brigham in Boston (1954), Medical College of Virginia (MCV) in Richmond (1962, although an identical twin transplant was done in 1957), and the University of Colorado in Denver (1962) were consistently pursuing kidney transplantation.[69,70,74,75] Willard E. Goodwin had started the program at the University of California, Los Angeles (UCLA) in 1960, and along with David Hume (MCV) showed long-term commitment to developing renal transplantation.[76-78] From 1962 to 1964, the University of Colorado Transplant Program was the most active program in the world. It was here that Paul Taylor started his career in transplant coordination, working side-by-side with Dr. Starzl in starting a transplant program. Paul Taylor was on the team that performed the first human liver transplantation. Paul took care of the dogs in the dog lab and administered the first doses of 6-mercaptopurine when they had to be suspended in solution before administration. He coordinated donor procurements and kept meticulous records on the early patients who received transplants. Paul, one of the founders of NATCO, was an invaluable member of the Colorado team that would contribute so much to the field of transplantation.

In researching this chapter, I started by putting together a timeline which helped me to visualize the sequence of events leading up to the first transplantation. Getting to the beginning is not always easy because of the varying accounts of the past, but there were excellent books, chapters, journal articles, and newspaper articles to consult, all of which are included in the reference list. At first, I wanted to document the first of everything: the first transplant coordinator (first clinical and first procurement coordinators), and so on. Later, I found that documenting the firsts was not always possible and was not as important as getting started—documenting snippets of what is known and included in the texts mentioned as well as the NATCO archives. Because the field of transplant coordination has been somewhat poorly documented, it will be left to future authors to ferret out all of the "firsts," although a fair number of them are included herein.

There is plenty to find on the surgeons' side of transplantation. Our colleagues have done a better job of committing their history to paper. Other than the NATCO newsletters and Barbara Elick's account in the 1997 book *Organ and Tissue Donation for Transplantation*, few publications have thoroughly captured and documented our history. This chapter makes such an attempt, although, I confess in reading it after reviewing the NATCO newsletters, it falls somewhat short on that account. The early NATCO newsletters capture in details small and large the development of the transplant coordinator. None the less, it is a start, and I will leave it to future historians of transplant coordination to further document our work and our history.

As mentioned earlier, two books stand out that truly put transplant history in a readable and comprehensive manner. One is the recently published book by Nicholas Tilney, *Transplant: From Myth to Reality*,[27] and the other is Thomas Starzl's book, *The Puzzle People*.[28] Both of these books document the "firsts" with a more comprehensive view in Tilney's book, as it is specifically a text on the history of transplantation, while *Puzzle People* is written from a "memoirs" vantage. Starzl's book, framed as it is from the beginning and evolution of modern transplantation through one person's viewpoint (his), and laced throughout with personal stories and his own particular life events, is immensely readable. However, Tilney had nothing and Starzl had little to say about transplant coordinators, but for sheer readability and contextual framework of the beginning of the field of transplantation, these two are excellent resources. So, readers can skip the next four sections and read Tilney's detailed history of transplantation or continue reading here for a shorthand version of transplant history.

Kidney Transplantation

In 1902, Emerich Ullman performed the first successful experimental kidney transplantations with animals: autotransplantation of a dog kidney from its normal position to the vessels of the neck, which resulted in some urine flow. In 1902, dog-to-dog transplantations were performed by Alfred von Decastello. A dog-to-goat kidney transplantation was performed again by Ullman, who was surprised that it made urine for a time.[79(p1)] From 1905 to 1910, Unger performed more than 100 experimental kidney transplantations between animals. On December 10, 1910, Ernst Unger of Berlin, Germany transplanted a stillborn child's kidney to a baboon. The baboon died shortly after surgery but a postmortem examination revealed that the vascular anastomosis was successful. This success, and the new knowledge that monkeys and humans were serologically similar, led Unger to attempt, later in the same month, a monkey-to-human transplantation. The patient was a young girl dying of renal failure, and the kidney from a pig ape was sutured to the thigh vessels. No urine was produced. Unger's report concluded that there was a biochemical barrier to transplantation.[79(pp2-3)]

The first recorded human kidney transplant (animal kidney to human) was performed in 1906 by Mathieu Jaboulay in Lyon, France. After perfecting the suture methods of vascular repair, he transplanted the left kidney of a pig into the left elbow of a woman with nephritic syndrome. He transplanted organs into two patients in this manner, but both grafts failed. It was conceded by those involved that "although transplantation could be achieved by precise vascular anastomosis, and that the transfer of an organ to a distant site in the same animal did not appear to affect its function, kidneys—like skin grafts—survived only a few days when placed in a different animal."[27(p42)] The graft failed because of vascular thrombosis. (Ullman later claimed an earlier attempt in 1902—an attempt to transplant the kidney of a pig into the elbow of a young uremic woman which failed due to an inability to resolve the technical difficulties.)[80-82]

The first kidney transplantation between humans, in 1936, was unsuccessful. The recipient was a 26-year-old woman who was admitted in a uremic coma after swallowing mercury in a suicide attempt. Yu Yu Voronoy, a Russian surgeon, retrieved a kidney from a 60-year-old man who had died from a fracture at the base of the skull. He transplanted it on the recipient's right femoral vessels, the kidney was placed in a pouch in the groin and the ureter was brought out in the skin. Unknown to doctors at the time, there were mismatches in donor and recipient blood groups and the donor kidney worked poorly for two days and then failed. The recipient died a few days after transplantation. The autopsy revealed degenerative lesions of the tubules and glomeruli, but no vascular thrombosis. Voronoy tried four other such transplantations with cadaveric kidneys in the next few years, but they all failed.[36(pp80-81)]

In 1946, a young woman was admitted to Peter Bent Brigham Hospital in Boston. She was comatose and had been anuric for 10 days after an abortion caused septic shock and after she had received an incompatible blood transfusion. A kidney was removed from a cadaveric donor immediately after death and was transplanted on the humeral vessels in the recipient's cubital fossa. The kidney produced urine for only two days after transplantation; however, soon after the transplantation, the patient regained consciousness, natural diuresis was restored, and the transplanted kidney was removed. This may have been responsible for stimulating interest in kidney transplantation at Peter Bent Brigham Hospital.[36(p82),79(p4)]

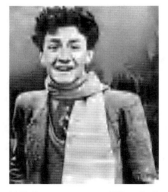

In the first use of a live related donor, a mother donated a kidney to her son. A 16-year-old roofer, Marius Renard, suffered a traumatic rupture of the right renal pedicle in a fall on December 18. A nephrectomy was performed. However, unknown at the time, he congenitally had but one kidney and anuria followed. The only possible solution was a transplantation that the mother as a donor proposed and insisted should be carried out. The kidney was transplanted at Necker Hospital in Paris, France by Louis Michon, Jean

(All photos courtesy of Kuss R, Bourget P, An Illustrated History of Organ Transplantation, 1992 Laboratories Sandoz, Rueil-Malmaison, France)

Vaysse, Nicolas Oeconomos, and Jean Hamburger on December 24, 1951. The graft functioned immediately following surgery, but it unfortunately ceased to function on the 22nd postoperative day. Marius died 10 days later due to the unavailability of hemodialysis. However, this event had a considerable impact on the scientific community. Surgical inspection of the graft revealed that immunological rejection, rather than stenosis or thrombosis of the renal artery, led to graft failure.36(p86),79(p4),83,84

Dr. Gabriel Richet, in a 1997 interview, remembers:

We had no chronic dialysis, not even a single artificial kidney. His mother insisted on giving one of her kidneys. As the blood groups were more or less compatible, within the limits of the knowledge of the day, we agreed to do it. The boy was transplanted on Christmas Eve, one week after the accident and I would like to show you the photograph to let you see how the family was happy. The patient is smiling and the mother too.

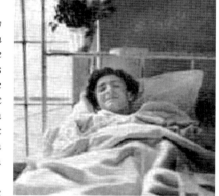

*Yes, on the 22nd day after the transplantation abruptly anuria reappeared. The kidney was hard and the surgeon looked at the kidney to make sure that there was no trouble in the renal artery but the patient died ten days later. This case raised wonderful emotion all over the world and we received a lot of letters and when the boy died, they cried at his funeral. There were many hundreds of flowers sent from different countries of Europe, even from Asia and certainly it was a very important [to] me. This transplantation had been the first one to be absolutely as perfect as the experiments in dogs by Dempster in England and Simonsen in Denmark. It was perfect because it was free of chronic uremia. There was no preexisting disease with circulation of the supposed nephrotoxins, no nephrological mishaps, no infection of the renal tract, thanks to our surgeons who anastomosed the ureter to the bladder of the boy. There was no stenosis of the renal artery. It was a true immunological rejection. We should have noticed the warning signs—minimal protein and a slight increase of the blood pressure. From a scientific point of view, it created another mind and John Merrill, who was interested and who had tried transplantation in chronic renal failure, was with Peter Medawar in London, and he flew across and it was the first time I met him and he became a friend.*85 (photos courtesy Novartis)

Kidney transplants were performed in Paris and Boston from 1950 to 1953 without immunosuppression and with only minor success. The first successful kidney transplant was performed on December 23, 1954 between identical twins at the Peter Bent Brigham Hospital in Boston by Joseph Murray and Hartwell Harrison. Dr. Murray shares the historic nature of this first successful transplant in his Nobel speech:

In the fall of 1954, Dr. Donald Miller of the US Public Health Service telephoned Dr. Merrill in order to refer a patient with severe renal disease. Moreover, Dr. Miller suggested there might be the opportunity for transplantation of a kidney because the patient had a healthy twin brother. Needless to say, the transplant team was interested in the possibility of transplanting a genetically compatible kidney. Cross skin grafting established genetic identity, renal disease was brought under control with medications and dialysis, and we were ready to apply our laboratory-tested surgical technique to man.

The only remaining problem was the ethical decision concerning the removal of a healthy organ from a normal person for the benefit of someone else. For the first time in medical history, a normal healthy person was to be subjected to a major surgical operation not for his own benefit. After many consultations with experienced physicians within and outside the Brigham and with clergy of all denominations, we felt it reasonable to offer the operations to the recipient, the donor and their family. We discussed in detail the preparations, anesthesia, operations, possible complications, and anticipated result.

At the conclusion of our last pre-operative discussion, the donor asked whether the hospital would be responsible for his health care for the rest of his life if he decided to donate his kidney. Dr. Harrison, the

(All photos courtesy of Kuss R, Bourget P, An Illustrated History of Organ Transplantation, 1992 Laboratories Sandoz, Rueil-Malmaison, France)

surgeon for the donor, said, "Of course not." But he immediately followed with the question, "Ronald, do you think anyone in this room would ever refuse to take care of you if you needed help?" Ronald paused, and then understood that his future depended upon our sense of professional responsibility rather than on legal assurances.

Once the patients and the team decided to proceed with the transplant, an extra professional burden falls on the surgeon performing the donor nephrectomy because his patient is expected to survive normally. In contrast, the surgeon performing the transplant is operating on a patient otherwise doomed to die, and the nephrologist caring for these critically ill patients cannot be faulted for failure to cure.

Post-operatively the transplanted kidney functioned immediately with a dramatic improvement in the patient's renal and cardiopulmonary status. This spectacular success was a clear demonstration that organ transplantation could be life-saving. In a way, it was spying into the future because we had achieved our long-term goal by bypassing, but not solving, the issue of biological incompatibility.[74]

This success was followed by subsequent attempts by Murray and Merrill that led to seven successful transplantations between identical twins in Boston. Most of the recipients of identical twin kidney grafts performed by Joseph Murray did well; some still have functioning kidneys more than 30 (perhaps now 40?) years after transplantation.

During 1963 and 1964, surgeons transplanted chimpanzee kidneys into 13 people; all died, but one lived for nine months. In the next 20 years, transplants with chimpanzee hearts and kidneys, and baboon hearts and livers—for a total of 28—were all tried, and all failed.[83]

The early 1960s were an optimistic time as all of the barriers, most notably the immunological barriers, had not yet been confronted. However, the attempts at cadaveric renal transplantation universally resulted in graft failure due to rejection. Kidney transplantation had to progress beyond just achieving success with living related donors. As can be seen in the Transplant Timeline, an explosion of "firsts" in transplantation marked the decade of the 1960s as organ transplantation began in earnest. Immunosuppressive and tissue typing advancements were made. In 1961, azathioprine became available for human use after the effectiveness of mercaptopurine was established in dog kidney transplants by Doctors Roy Calne and Charles Zukoski.

The first successful cadaveric kidney transplantation was performed in 1962, also by Hume and Murray, at Peter Bent Brigham Hospital in Massachusetts.[27(pp60-66),71,72] The first use of drugs exclusively for immunosuppression was not until 1962, when the first successful cadaveric kidney transplantation was performed by Dr. Murray at Peter Bent Brigham Hospital. Dr. Roy Calne and Dr. Murray used a combination of cortisone and azathioprine to immunosuppress the recipient and control rejection. The recipient had normal renal function for 21 months after transplantation.[36(p86),69,74,86] By 1963, prednisone and azathioprine were being used as a standard in immunosuppression, moving beyond the total body irradiation technique that had dismal outcomes in the early 1960s.[69,87]

Transplantation did indeed bloom in the 1960s as can be seen in the timeline. Transplant congresses were held, technical improvements in the transplant procedure and immunological monitoring gains were made, and improved preservation was accomplished most notably by Belzer and Collins. Organs were increasingly recovered from heart-beating cadaver donors in the '70s and finally, the introduction of cyclosporine in 1978 (trials) and combined with prednisone in 1980 led to significant gains in graft survival. The timeline is impressively detailed with the milestones made by the signature organ—the kidney—that made successful transplantation of other organs possible.

Liver Transplantation

After kidney transplantation, experimentation in canine transplant models closely followed in the mid-1950s. In 1955, C. Stuart Welch of Albany, New York, inserted an extra liver into the pelvis of a nonimmunosuppressed dog.[88,89] In 1956, Jack Cannon[90] of UCLA "wondered whether the liver might be an immunologically privileged organ and reported attempts at liver replacement in the orthotopic position, having removed the animal's own liver. However, there were no survivors from the operation." By the late 1950s and early 1960s, serious attempts at orthotopic liver transplantation in dogs were made independently by Dr. Francis Moore at the Peter Bent Brigham Hospital in Boston and Dr. Thomas Starzl at Northwestern University in Chicago.[27(pp201-202),91]

The first liver transplantation was performed by Dr. Thomas Starzl at the University of Colorado in Denver on March 11, 1963. The recipient, Bennie Solis, was a three-year-old boy with biliary atresia who had had multiple previous operations. The transplantation could not be completed because of a fatal hemorrhage from venous collaterals and an uncontrollable coagulopathy. The donor was another child who had died during an open-heart operation. Starzl writes extensively about this first transplantation in his memoirs[28(p168)] and notes, "Even for a team that had been fully prepared for technical vicissitudes by hundreds of animal operations, the exsanguination of this child was a terrible shock."[89(p12)]

Initial attempts were unsuccessful because of a combination of technical difficulties and the unavailability of effective means to prevent rejection. As increased experience was achieved, and with improvements in immunosuppression, prolonged liver recipient survivals were achieved. From 1963 to 1979, 170 patients underwent liver transplantation at the University of Colorado; 56 survived for one year, 25 for 13 to 22 years, and several remain alive with follow-ups of 17 to 31 years. In 1968, Roy Calne of Cambridge University founded the second liver transplantation program. As with renal grafts, the long-term survival rate after liver transplantation remained poor (18%-30% one-year patient survival) until the advent of cyclosporine.[92] The liver programs were suffering the same dismal results as were other transplant programs. In 1978, liver transplantation was not practiced with any regularity, and virtually all liver transplants were done in only two centers—Denver, Colorado and Cambridge, UK—and those procedures had an approximate 75% mortality rate. Starzl was invited to consider surgical chairmanships in several university departments as long as he did not pursue liver transplantation. "The drive and dedication of these two individuals alone kept the entire field going. Because of the enormity of the operative undertaking, the vast physiological changes to be overcome during placement of the organ, the functional complexity of the liver, and the persistently unsatisfactory results, little enthusiasm was manifested until others became convinced and joined the effort."[27(p202)]

The turning point is described by Starzl[89(p13)] in his chapter on the history of liver transplantation: "the frustration ended when cyclosporine became available for clinical use in 1979"[93] "and was combined with prednisone or lymphoid depletion in the first of the cyclosporine-based cocktails."[94] "Of our first 12 liver recipients treated with cyclosporine and prednisone in the first eight months of 1980, 11 lived for more than a year,"[95] "and seven were still alive over 12 years later." As the news was confirmed that a one-year patient survival rate of at least 70% was readily achievable, new liver programs proliferated worldwide.[89(p13)]

After FK506 was substituted for cyclosporine in 1989,[96] the one-year patient and liver graft survival rate increased again in the Pittsburgh experience,[97] an improvement similar to those experienced in multicenter trials in Europe. Liver transplantation success rates improved throughout the years, not only because of improved immunosuppression but also because of technical adjustments.[89(pp13-14),98-100]

Heart Transplantation

Alexis Carrel and Charles Guthrie reported transplantation of the heart and lungs while at the University of Chicago in 1905.[101] The heart of a small dog was transplanted into the neck of a larger one by anastomosing the caudal ends of the jugular vein and carotid artery to the aorta and pulmonary artery. The animal was not anticoagulated, and the experiment ended about two hours after circulation was established because of blood clot in the cavities of the transplanted heart. Carrel also reported in 1906 that he had transplanted the heart and lungs of a one-week-old cat into the neck of a larger cat.[102] The coronary circulation was immediately reestablished, and the "auricles began to beat. The lungs became red and after a few minutes effective pulsation of the ventricles appeared." Carrel stated that a phlegmon of the neck terminated this observation two days later.[103]

Vladimir Demikhov, the great Soviet researcher, described more than 20 different techniques for heart transplantation in 1950.[104] He also published descriptions of various techniques for heart and lung transplantation. He was even able to perform an orthotopic heart transplantation in a dog before the heart-lung machine was developed. He accomplished this by placing the donor heart above the dog's own heart, and then with a series of tubes and connections, he rerouted the blood from one heart to the other until he had the donor heart functioning in the appropriate position and the other heart removed. One of his dogs climbed the steps of the Kremlin on the sixth postoperative day but died shortly afterward of rejection.[103]

Richard Lower and Norman Shumway established the technique for heart transplantation as it is performed today.[105] Preservation of the cuff of recipient left and right atria with part of the atrial septum was described earlier by Brock[106] in England and Demikhov[107] in the Soviet Union, but it became popular only after Shumway and Lower reported it in their 1960 paper. Shumway stated:

> In 1958 when I started work at Stanford, the idea [cardiac transplantation] grew out of our local cooling experiments, since we had one hour of aortic cross-clamping during cardiopulmonary bypass. Accordingly we decided to remove the heart at the atrial level and then to suture it back into position. After several of these experiments, we found it would be easier to remove the heart of another dog and to do the actual allotransplant. Something like 20 to 30 experiments were performed before we had a survivor. All of this was done before chemical immune suppression was available.[103,108]

Dr. James Hardy performed the first heart transplant into a human (baboon to human) in 1964 at the University of Mississippi. The heart beat for 90 minutes before it stopped. "The recipient was a 68-year-old man with hypertension and severe coronary artery disease. The patient was actually moribund and had recently undergone an amputation for gangrene. The surgery team planned to use the heart of a young patient who was dying of irreversible brain damage. However, the prospective recipient became unstable before the donor was considered appropriate for heart removal. Therefore, it was decided to take the patient to the operating room and implant a chimpanzee heart. Although the transplantation was technically successful, the primate heart was too small to support the circulation, and it failed after two hours off cardiopulmonary bypass. It was concluded that 'this experience supports the scientific feasibility of heart transplantation in man.'"[35(p7),109]

"The operation 'precipitated intense ethical, moral, social, religious, financial, governmental and even legal concerns,' wrote Dr. Hardy. 'We had not transplanted merely a human heart, we had transplanted a subhuman heart.'"[110] Even some of his medical colleagues were critical. They said his nine years of work in the laboratory with animals were not adequate preparation for his bold move in the operating suite and that not enough was known about xenografts to warrant their use. Those first two operations (Hardy also performed the first human lung transplantation) in Mississippi—which were met with such dubious acceptance in the beginning—set the stage for all future heart and lung transplantations. They demonstrated that surgical techniques perfected in nine years of work on animals would work in humans. They proved that a transplanted lung would breathe and a transplanted heart would beat and support a blood pressure in a human host. Dr. Hardy said the operations "set in motion the inexorable process of human imagination and gradual acceptance which has evolved into our current almost casual attitude toward transplantation."[110]

The first human-to-human heart transplantation was performed on December 3, 1967 by Dr. Christian Barnard in the Groote Schuur Hospital in Cape Town, South Africa.[111,112] Dr. Barnard and his colleagues in South Africa transplanted the heart of a 24-year-old woman injured in a car accident into 54-year-old Louis Washkansky, who had severe coronary artery disease with myocardial infarctions. Barnard used techniques pioneered in the United States at Stanford University by Drs. Norman Shumway and Richard Lower. The recipient lived only 18 days, dying of pneumonia, but this transplantation was followed by a sudden flurry of increased interest in cardiac transplantation.[35(p7)] His donor, Denise Darvall, was very seriously injured in a car accident in Observatory, Cape Town. Denise's mother, who was also involved, died immediately. Denise had multiple injuries including a skull fracture and extensive head injuries. She could not be kept alive without mechanical assistance and was essentially brain dead. At 9 PM on the day of the accident, the resuscitation team stopped trying to revive Denise. After parental permission was obtained, Denise Darvall's heart went to the first human heart transplant recipient, Louis Washkansky, and her kidneys went to 10-year-old Jonathan van Wyk. In apartheid South Africa, that gave rise to some controversy, as the boy was black and Denise was white.[113] These events, involving people from different walks of life and circumstances in the dramatic milieu of organ donation and transplantation, of life ending and "beginning," would soon become commonplace. That this was the first was noteworthy. In truth, even today, one individual restoring life to others remains as dramatic as it was on December 3, 1967.

The field of heart transplantation exploded in 1968, with 109 cardiac transplantations done in 17 countries. Because graft survival statistics were low (approximately 22% one-year graft survival), this boom soon diminished and was revived only with the advent of cyclosporine in the late 1970s. The mean survival was only 29 days for the first 100 transplants, which dampened enthusiasm for the procedure, and by 1970, most institutions had abandoned it.[114,115]

By 1971, 146 of the first 170 heart transplant recipients were dead, and what had looked like a surgical miracle had turned into a disaster. Cardiac surgeons admitted defeat and called for a complete moratorium on heart transplants. Heart transplantation, which had been started with a worldwide flurry after Dr. Barnard's highly publicized cases, quickly slowed as the patients died. By the late 1970s, because of the poor results, few surgeons were attempting to do the operation, except for Dr. Norman Shumway.[34]

Shumway refused to honor the moratorium, spending the next decade building a team to conquer the scientific and procedural problems associated with the transplantation. He found ways to enlarge the pool of both donors and recipients, and he devised techniques to preserve hearts for transport before the transplantation.[116] His team found a way to spot rejection early, threading a catheter into the heart and removing a small piece of muscle for examination. Only if signs of rejection were present did it become necessary to administer the powerful immunosuppressants then used to stifle the body's defenses. In the 1970s, he and his team refined the operation, tackling the twin problems of rejection and the necessity for potentially dangerous drugs to suppress the immune system. Shumway pioneered the use of cyclosporine instead of traditional drugs, which made the operation much safer.[117] It wasn't until 1981 that the number of heart transplantations performed again reached greater than 100 per year. The 1980s witnessed routinely successful heart transplantation at a number of centers throughout the world.[35(p9)]

Lung Transplantation

Bronchial dehiscence plagued Demikhov's experiments in 1947. Haglin developed a method for reestablishing the bronchial circulation by vascular anastomosis.[118] The world's first lung transplantation was performed by Dr. James Hardy at the University of Mississippi in Jackson in 1963. The lung recipient was a 58-year-old prison inmate who was suffering from chronic infection, abscess, and atelectasis formation in his left lung. The donor lung came from a patient who died from a myocardial infarction. The patient survived for 18 days and maintained excellent arterial oxygen saturations for the first week after transplantation. Immunosuppressive therapy had not been developed and was not used in this first human lung transplantation.[119(p209)]

Dr. Denton Cooley performed the first clinical heart-lung transplantation in 1968. A patient with an atrioventricular canal defect received the heart and lungs of an anencephalic infant. The recipient survived for 14 hours before dying of respiratory insufficiency.[114,120] In 1969, Lillehei and colleagues[121] and in 1971, Christian Barnard[122] performed transplantations in patients with 8- and 23-day survivals, respectively. These early experiments, fueled by the optimism over heart transplants in the late '60s cooled until Shumway and colleagues performed the first successful transplantation. Both Lilliehei's and Barnard's patients were able to breathe spontaneously, providing helpful evidence that heart-lung denervation would not preclude patients' survival as it had in canine experiments.[35(pp10-11)] (see Transplant Timeline).

The first successful heart-lung transplantation was performed at Stanford University by Dr. Shumway and Dr. Bruce Reitz in 1981. A new clinical trial of heart-lung transplantation with the use of cyclosporine (approved by the Food and Drug Administration as an investigational drug) was approved by the Stanford institutional review board. The recipient, 45-year-old Mary Gohke, had end-stage pulmonary hypertension. The donor was brought to Stanford to minimize ischemic time. The patient was treated with cyclosporine and azathioprine for 14 days, and then azathioprine was discontinued and prednisone added. She was discharged from the hospital in good condition and did well for more than five years after transplantation.[35(pp10-11)] However, the early enthusiasm of the 1960s and early 1970s gave way to reality as most patients died soon after transplantation.

The growth of lung transplantation was slow because the eligibility criteria for lung transplant recipients were unclear, and despite clear improvement in function after transplantation, survival benefits were less clear. By 1978, 38 human lung transplantations had been performed. Bronchial disruption and the inability to differentiate infection from rejection appeared to be the major problems. Improved healing of the bronchial anastomosis was found after the introduction of cyclosporine. Additionally, limiting the length of the donor bronchus and extrinsic revascularization by wrapping the anastomosis with omentum led to advancements in anastomotic techniques. This culminated in a successful single-lung transplantation, a procedure pioneered by the Toronto Lung Transplant Group under the leadership of Joel Cooper and Griffith Pearson. In 1983, the Toronto Lung Transplant Group (consisting of Cooper, Pearson, and Patterson) accomplished long-term survival following a successful single-lung transplantation. The Toronto Lung Transplant Group used a technique of omentoplexy to reinforce the bronchial anastomosis. Subsequently, telescoping the bronchial anastomosis to a depth of one cartilaginous ring was shown to be equally effective, and thus omentopexy became unnecessary.[118]

Pancreas Transplantation

Experiments in pancreas transplantation began long before the discovery of insulin. The first recorded human pancreatic transplantation was performed 29 years before the isolation of insulin. Dr. Watson Williams transplanted two "brazil nut" sized chunks of freshly slaughtered sheep's pancreas to the abdominal wall of a 15-year-old boy at the Bristol Royal Infirmary in 1892. The recipient lived for three days.[123]

Animal experiments ultimately led to graft survival in the six-month range, thus inevitably human transplantation occurred next. Dr. Richard Lillehei and his surgical colleagues at the University of Minnesota were responsible for much of the early history of clinical pancreas transplantation.[124] In 1966, Dr. William Kelly and Dr. Richard Lillehei performed the first simultaneous kidney/pancreas transplant. They transplanted a duct ligated segmental graft simultaneous with a kidney in a uremic diabetic recipient who immediately became insulin independent. The graft functioned until the recipient died two months later of sepsis related to surgical complications.[124,125]

This team performed pancreas transplants in 13 more patients over the next seven years, nine of whom received concomitant renal grafts. The majority of the procedures involved placement of the whole gland and anastomosis of the adjacent duodenum surrounding the duct to the recipient small bowel. The return of the blood sugar to normal in several patients allowed reduction of cessation of the dose of insulin for periods of varying lengths. One graft functioned for a year. By 1977 data had accumulated [on] 57 grafts placed in 55 patients. Of these, only a single individual survived long-term.[126,127]

With this dismal record as background, and particularly when insulin could be given to temper the acute metabolic perturbations of diabetes, it was little wonder that transplantation of the pancreas was accepted more slowly than that of other organs. Other reasons for the relative lack of enthusiasm for the pancreatic procedure were obvious. The late sequellae of the disease often ravaged the potential recipients. The potential mortality from the transplant operation and its attendant treatment were of evident concern. Inflammation commonly developed in the new graft. Ductal leaks led to infection. Rejection was difficult to diagnose and control. Several of the immunosuppressive drugs worsened the existing diabetes. And in the same department of surgery as Lillehei, John Najarian and his associates were showing convincingly that renal transplant in insulin-controlled diabetics could be carried out with reasonable success and that complete control of blood sugar was not necessary for satisfactory kidney function. As a result, many physicians were unwilling to substitute the hazards of transplantation and immunosuppression for the more predictable dangers of insulin replacement.[27(p210)]

Following the introduction of cyclosporine and the improved methods to prevent leakage of pancreatic juice, improvements continued. In 1999, Dr. James Shapiro and Jonathan Lakey developed the Edmonton Protocol. Islet cell transplants were performed on patients who did not require other organ transplants and who had severe problems with type one diabetes. The new treatment method involved injecting islet cells from donor pancreata into a patient's portal vein in a nonsurgical procedure in combination with steroid-free antirejection drugs: sirolimus (Rapamune), tacrolimus (FK506 Prograf), and daclizimab (Zenapax). The cells migrated to the pancreas, where they produced insulin. The Edmonton group initially worked with seven patients, all of whom became insulin independent after the procedure. In September

2000, centers in the United States, Germany, Italy, and Switzerland began participating in the Immune Tolerance Network multicenter trial of the Edmonton Protocol.[128] Pancreas transplantation continues to evolve and has generally not enjoyed the success of the other solid-organ transplantations.

Birth of Transplant Coordination and the Transplant Coordinator

By March 1964, 342 non-twin kidney transplantations had been performed worldwide. The same group of physicians who recovered, preserved, and shared the organs were also responsible for the transplantation and postoperative care of the recipient. It soon became apparent that continuing in this mode would severely limit the number of donations and thus the number of transplantations performed.[129] Although surgeons were the pioneers who made organ transplantation technically possible, the creation of a system to support the myriad facets of transplantation and donation belonged to the coordinator.

Without this system, transplantation could not exist for the many who need an organ for a second chance at life. The hundreds of acts that must occur for a donor to be realized and the organ to be allocated and transplanted into a recipient who has been worked-up, put on the list and managed, can be overlooked when reading historical accounts of transplantation, which typically feature milestones of "firsts" in surgical and immunological accomplishments. By and large, it was the transplant coordinator who performed the majority of these hundreds of tasks.

Transplant coordinators began working in the United States in various capacities during the 1960s and in the United Kingdom, Belgium, and Germany in the mid-to-late 1970s[11] (*L. Roels, CPTC, written communication, May 30, 2006*), the Netherlands first appointed role was in 1979, [14(p.242),15,24(p.326)] Sweden and Australia in 1983,[15,16,24(p.326),130] (*G. Armstrong, RN, CPTC, written communication, April 27, 2006*), Spain in 1984,[9] and Japan in 1985 (*S. Hiraga, MD, written communication, May 24, 2006*). One report puts the official coordinator in Germany starting in the early 1980s (official appointment date often lagged behind actual starting time).[131] The first two transplant coordinators actually started working in Germany in 1979 in the cities of Hannover and Tübingen (see timeline). In 1986, full-time transplant coordinators began working in Singapore, where a subsequent increase in kidney transplantations was attributed in part to this position[12] (see Transplant Timeline).

The term "transplant coordinator" was likely coined by transplant surgeons who looked for people who could and would need to multi-task, would be asked to provide skills from several disciplines and to coordinate what was then a work-in-process. Although the term *transplant coordinator* was used early on in the United States, Amy Peele, NATCO president at the time, attended the second European Congress for Transplant Coordinators in Leiden, Holland. Peele noted that the term only began being used in Europe in 1978. A discussion was initiated by Drs. Cohen and Persijn, both of Leiden, of forming a transplant coordinators organization in Europe. Participants at the meeting agreed to form a European Transplant Coordinators Organization.[132]

Extraordinary relationships developed between transplant coordinators and surgeons/physicians in the early days of transplantation. They often saw more of each other than perhaps they did of their families. Their work depended on one another. This was true both in the procurement and recipient setting. Many of these collaborations were enduring, and their names became forever linked. Folkert O. Belzer, MD and Robert Hoffmann, BS, CPTC is one such example, and there are many more.

The 1960s were a very optimistic time for transplantation as can be seen by the many "firsts" in transplantation. Those who dedicated their lives to this work, assisting during the transplantation process, may not have had the title of transplant coordinator *yet*, but coordinators they were. They were the pioneers of our profession, making their way as they went. Their role was shaped by the needs of surgeons, patients, hospitals, the law, the coordinator's past medical background and education, and perhaps most importantly, the individual's own drive. More often than not, the early role was an all-inclusive, dual one as already outlined earlier in this chapter: performing both organ recovery and transplant recipient duties.

Procurement Transplant Coordinators

Organ recovery started as a hospital-based activity, typically located in the department of surgery at a major teaching institution. It was basically a procurement-driven activity developed in response to a surgeon's need to recover organs for his patients. The coordinator was not yet an identified transplant coordination professional. In fact, the coordination was accomplished by a combination of a surgeon and an operating room technician or nurse working together to respond to isolated occurrences of identified potential donors and recovering those organs for the patients in their own or nearby institutions who were in need of an organ transplant. Kidneys were removed after the donor's cardiac arrest.

In the early 1970s, following the adoption of brain death laws, expert staff were needed to wade through the myriad legal, ethical, and operational issues of recovering organs from heart-beating cadavers. It was a time-consuming process and one that surgeons were too busy and poorly suited to perform. Donor evaluation, management, and organ recovery became activities provided solely by clinical staff with administrative oversight provided by the department of surgery, or by a procurement director at the few existing independent organ procurement organizations (OPOs). The clinical staff working in transplantation often existed on the fringe of activities associated with busy surgical departments. During the 1960s and early 1970s, as the science of organ transplantation matured, a systematic approach to a more steady supply of organs was needed.

After transplantation became more common in the 1960s and early 1970s, staff was needed. Often, new appointments for these positions were the technicians working in the animal laboratories. They had to be available 24 hours per day, seven days a week to respond to the call that might result in an organ donor. Gary Hall, in an article on the "organ procurement system," illustrated the relationship of the transplant coordinator to various parties and entities involved in the donation and transplantation "universe" in an early (1985) NATCO newsletter.[133] Although the illustration is simplistic, in many ways, it could apply to coordination today. It is still the organ procurement coordinator who works with medical staff, nursing staff, transplant surgeons and physicians, administrators, social workers, and occasionally lawyers, to ensure that donation is effected legally, effectively, and ethically. The illustration below appeared with Mr. Hall's article and shows the transplant coordinator, in this case the procurement coordinator, at the hub of the wheel to which I referred in the beginning of this chapter.

**FIGURE 1.
THE ORGAN PROCUREMENT SYSTEM**

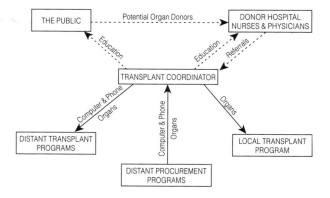

Fig. 1. Solid lines denote official communications link and responsibility (the official component); dashed lines represent unofficial lines of communications and/or ad hoc relationships (the unofficial component).

The first task of the procurement coordinator was to meet with the family of the potential donor to obtain permission to "harvest" (as it was commonly called) the kidneys. If permission was granted, the coordinator might remove lymph nodes at the donor's bedside, deliver them to the immunology laboratory, schedule the organ removal, assist in the surgery, and ultimately flush and cool the kidneys. The coordinator would then either place the kidneys on a portable perfusion pump or package them for transport to another destination. When the pump was used, the coordinator would monitor perfusate flow and electrolyte balances—sometimes with little sleep for a number of days—until the kidneys were transplanted. The coordinator usually accompanied kidneys on perfusion machines to their destination, often meeting the accepting center's transplant coordinator. Coordinators frequently conversed over the phone at odd hours of the night and met in airports after being awake for long hours. Because of this networking, coordinators grew familiar with each other's programs and developed friendships. By the time a small group of them met in Los Angeles in 1974, many of them already had long-standing professional relationships. [This "meeting" is covered in more depth under "Birth of NATCO".]

During those early surgical organ retrievals, transplant coordinators became managers, not by choice but by necessity. They were called on to coordinate multiple teams in removing organs, corneas, skin, bone and other tissues. Coordinators schooled in the organization of en bloc nephrectomies soon found themselves developing protocols to optimize removal of extrarenal organs. It became commonplace to coordinate the efforts of numerous surgical teams. In Europe, coordinators faced the additional challenge of dealing with the many different languages spoken by various surgical teams. Developing leadership skills often afforded the opportunity for experienced coordinators to move into management positions and direct overall efforts to increase organ and tissue donation.

Procurement coordinators were employed, for the most part, by the transplant programs that used the organs. But early on, the issues surrounding donors and their families were recognized as separate from those involving recipient care. Independent organ procurement agencies have now become the norm in the US.[134] Worldwide, however, many transplant programs continue to operate procurement protocols out of hospital-based programs[24(pp326-327)]

The next evolutionary step was characterized by the development of relationships with other hospitals and the establishment of formal agreements with these non-transplant institutions for the referral of potential donors.

Procurement coordinators were skilled in removing roadblocks. Indeed, a truth I learned early on in my career (or at least it seemed a truth to me), was that there was always someone or something that would be a roadblock to donation, in every donation, and that my job was to remove it. It happened time after time. Perhaps the "roadblock" was an individual (physician, nurse, or the third-cousin-once-removed) or was structural (flat tire on jet), but it was always something. Later in this chapter, stories told by coordinators outline such scenarios and illustrate the crucial role of the coordinator in obtaining the key ingredient for a life-saving transplant—an organ. No amount of surgical skill can be brought to bear in a transplant process unless an organ is donated.

Clinical Transplant Coordinators

Similarly, on the clinical side, the role of the clinical coordinator was ever-evolving. The first clinical transplant coordinators tended to be nurses working with dialysis patients or in the operating room. In the 1960s many of them began their careers in organ procurement but soon acquired the additional responsibility of maintaining the waiting list of potential recipients. The transplant coordinator was often the one who called patients in when a kidney became available.[24(p327)] Coordinators carried with them lists of their patients at all times with the patient's name, blood type, listing date, and, later, as the number of HLA antigens identified grew, any unacceptable antigens.

As transplantation flourished, clinical transplant coordinators were increasingly called on to manage the complicated care of patients, both in preparation for and after surgery. And because transplantation was a surgeon's domain, care of recipient patients was largely the responsibility of the watchful transplant coordinator who consulted a multitude of related specialists to provide ongoing post-transplant care. It was not uncommon for clinical coordinators to monitor and adjust immunosuppressive therapies, validate laboratory results, admit patients to hospitals for treatment of complications, and interpret clinical findings. Most of these coordinators were registered nurses with specialties in extended nursing roles. At that time, medical providers skilled in the art of caring for immunosuppressed patients were scarce, so clinical transplant coordinators were the reliable sleuths. Increasingly, their responsibilities began to center on recipients, rather than donors.

The increasing success of kidney transplantation launched successful efforts in transplantation of the pancreas, liver, and heart. As transplant numbers grew, clinical transplant coordinators were in demand to develop programs to accommodate these extrarenal patients. With the increased application of extrarenal transplantation, multiple organ recoveries became commonplace, programs multiplied, and more patients were transplanted.[135]

…By the early 1980s, many coordinators, especially in large programs, specialized in one organ subfield or perhaps even in one age group within one organ subfield. The degree of specialization and the number of clinical transplant coordinators within a given program became directly proportional to the number of transplants performed and the number of patients being followed.[136] In smaller programs, however, one coordinator often worked with both kidney and pancreas recipients, usually because they were transplanted simultaneously into one recipient. This also was the case with some heart and lung recipients.[24(pp327-328)]

Transplant coordinators were the key element that made possible the workup of multiple living donor candidates. They provided the vast majority of education to patients and monitored patients for signs and symptoms of rejection and infection.[24(p328)] In fact, when patients were called in to the transplant unit during the daytime, nighttime, or on weekends, it was usually the transplant coordinator who prioritized those calls, providing treatment and/or referral. The coordinators were also a valuable resource for physicians and surgeons as programs tweaked their protocols, attempting to increase graft survival rates.

In one of the most inclusive works written on the role of the clinical transplant coordinator, Donaldson[25] writes extensively about the educational background, experience, practice settings, teaching responsibilities, areas of expertise, on-call responsibilities, and orientation of the coordinator as well as the role of the coordinator in evaluation and listing of patients, education of patients, the decision process in listing patients, managing recipients' medications, and personal responsibility for preventing job stress and burn-out.

Early Transplant Coordinators

The field of transplantation required pioneering surgeons *and* coordinators. The illustrious accomplishments of surgeons and immunologists is documented in the accompanying timeline. However, to make the *system* work, a dedicated 24-hour, 7-days-a-week, 365-days-a-year professional was needed: a professional with responsibilities for both the donation and transplantation process who could coordinate donation from any hospital in a wide geographic area and who could follow patients from workup through transplantation through ad infinitum follow-up care. There were "no such animals," therefore, individuals poised to perform such duties seized the opportunity. In the early days, these individuals were often lab assistants, dialysis nurses, or other such non-physicians. Paul Taylor, Justine Willmert, Robert Hoffmann, Claire Day, Linda Jones, Stephen Kelley, Les Olson, Carolyn Atkins, Roger Smith, Phyllis Weber, Marguerite Brown, Joan Miller and many, many others paved the way.

During this time, possibly the first transplant coordinator began his career: Paul Taylor joined Dr. Starzl in Denver in 1962 and was one of the pivotal members of this pioneering transplant team. This was the way of many of the first transplant coordinators—working as laboratory assistants or nurse clinicians

A CLINICIAN'S GUIDE TO DONATION AND TRANSPLANTATION   *Chapter 1*

and quickly being consumed with the passion for the work and the thrill of being part of a small, intimate and pioneering "team." Paul quickly adapted to the unstructured, open-ended job that soon was to become a profession. When NATCO was formed in 1979, Paul was among the first officers of the organization, serving as historian.

From published articles, letters, resumés, and so on, the term transplant coordinator started to emerge. Maybe someone else can determine when those words were first uttered from someone's lips, but it is almost inconsequential since these early team members grew into the role and were performing the functions before we had a name for it.

There are certainly many more names than the ones that follow, but these are a sampling of some of the earliest coordinators who made significant contributions to the field. The information below is also not complete since some of it was taken from available printed sources in the NATCO archives, which are not all-inclusive of an individual's experience. A more inclusive biography of each of the Presidents of NATCO is included under that section. Further, the following chronicle of specific coordinators is not meant to be inclusive, but to provide a few of the names and contributions of early coordinators, providing readers with a timeline and sense of scope of practice in the field. *I will leave it to others to chronicle further the accomplishments of individual transplant coordinators.* Such endeavors are needed in our field.

- **Paul D. Taylor, BS, CPTC, 1962.** Paul D. Taylor was one such pioneer transplant coordinator who helped launch the field. He was hired by the University of Colorado and the Veterans Administration Medical Center in the research laboratories in 1962. He was promoted to senior instructor in surgery in 1969 at the University of Colorado, all of this while working with Dr. Thomas Starzl, pioneering the field of organ donation and transplantation. He was a member of the team that performed the world's first human liver transplantation in March 1963. Starzl noted that Paul had "also had been swept away by the transplant passion. He became a key player in all the laboratory studies. Now he would become an organ procurement officer whose task it was to visit hospitals throughout the region and identify victims of accidents or disease whose organs might still be useable."[28(p89)] Paul served as director of organ procurement from 1967 to 1987 at the University of Colorado and the Denver Veterans Administration Hospital. Paul Taylor moved to the University of Pittsburgh to continue his work in organ recovery and transplantation until his retirement on August 5, 1992, after 30 years in the field. In addition to his contributions to NATCO, Paul was a founding member of the American Society of Minority Health Care and Transplant Professionals (ASMHTP) and consulted in Europe, Canada, Japan and Holland. He was the first transplant coordinator to grace a magazine cover[137] (see face page of this chapter)! Paul received his A.S. from Garden City Community College in 1957 and his B.S. in Education at the University of Kansas in 1958 (*written communication, P. Taylor, BS, CPTC, January 26, 2006*).

- **Robert Gosnell, MBA, 1962.** (see NATCO Presidents for biography)

- **Robert M. Hoffmann, BS, CPTC, 1964.** Robert M. Hoffmann was hired by Folkert Belzer in 1964 as a research specialist in the Organ Preservation Laboratory and later became director of kidney procurement and preservation at the University of California, San Francisco. In 1975, he moved with Dr. Belzer to the University of Wisconsin, where he worked as a research associate in the Folkert Belzer Organ Preservation Laboratory, director of multi-organ procurement and preservation, and as director of the University of Wisconsin Organ Procurement Organization. He remained in Wisconsin until 2000, later relocating to the University of Florida at Shands as an organ procurement specialist and educator. Bob worked with Dr. Belzer in developing the Belzer kidney perfusion machine and the University of Wisconsin preservation solution also known as Viaspan. He published numerous book chapters and articles and lectured extensively throughout the United States and the world on organ preservation. By the time of this writing, Bob has recovered or been involved in the surgical removal of 4,452 kidneys, 1,966 livers, and 832 pancreata (*written communication, R. Hoffmann, BS, CPTC, April 2006*).

- **Justine G. Willmert, RN, 1965.** Justine G. Willmert worked in the operating room with Dr. John Najarian at the University of California, San Francisco. She moved to the University of Minnesota in 1967 and helped him set up the transplant program.[138] "Justine Willmert graduated from the Naeve Hospital School of Nursing. After four years as a transplant coordinator at UCSF she moved to Minnesota. For the last 12 years she has held the position of Transplant Coordinator Research Fellow at the University of Minnesota."[139] Justine was a true transplant coordinator pioneer on the clinical side, working on the first planning committee in setting up the first "organized' meeting of transplant coordinators in New York City [see Table 3] and for the subsequent meeting in Columbus [see Table 4]. In fact, Gerda Lipcamann couldn't attend the only planning meeting so Justine, Linda Jones, and Curtis Yeager put the program together. Justine is retired now and living in Phoenix, Arizona *(written communication, L. Jones, RN, CCTC, CPTC, May 2006)*.

- **Linda L. Jones, RN, CCTC, CPTC, 1965.** (see NATCO Presidents for biography)
- **Beth Cameron, RN, CCTC, 1954**. Beth Cameron worked at the Peter Bent Brigham Hospital in 1954 as a dialysis nurse when they did the first historic kidney transplant and then later went to University of Pennsylvania. Her name appears for the first time on the chart of the first University of Pennsylvania transplantation on February 19, 1966 (transplant was done February 10, 1966). She was probably a dialysis nurse then and later became a transplant coordinator but left Penn to go to Maine for a few years in the mid-1970s, returning to a coordinator position and then later as the lead coordinator and director from around 1980 until about 1999 (almost 20 years). She may have had the longest track record in dialysis/transplantation on the coordinator side—almost 45 years *(written communication, H. Nathan, BS, CPTC, February 6, 2006)*.
- **Claire Day, RN, CCTC, 1967**. "In 1967, Claire started the dialysis program at Shands Teaching Hospital in Gainesville, Florida. By 1974, she was the transplant coordinator basically focusing on the patient aspect of the program. Claire has worked with the education committee for the last several years."[140] The previous quote appeared in an early NATCO newsletter article about Claire. Claire worked in transplantation her entire career, served in numerous leadership capacities with NATCO and represented clinical coordinators in numerous other national venues. Day was on the original faculty for the clinical coordinator training course. She would remain a staple in NATCO's efforts to provide education to newcomers in the field and was the recipient of the NATCO/Novartis Award for her achievements in the field in 1997. She worked in the industry for more than 30 years, retiring only recently *(written communication, M. Reiner, PA, CPTC, June 2006)*.
- **Leslie C. Olson, BA, CPTC. 1968.** Leslie C. Olson started his career at the University of Minnesota, Minneapolis, becoming director of organ perfusion. From 1972 to 1978, he was director of organ procurement. From 1978 through 2001, Olson worked at the University of Miami Medical School as director of organ preservation, director of procurement, and as an adjunct assistant professor. He moved to LifeCenter Northwest, the OPO in Washington state in 2001, where he has performed the surgical recovery of abdominal organs for transplantation. During his career, Les has performed more than 6,000 cadaveric nephrectomies, 1,400 hepatectomies, 250 pancreatectomies, and 50 intestinal recoveries for transplantation.

  Les Olson has authored or coauthored more than 100 articles, abstracts, or book chapters and lectured extensively. He served on numerous committees for the United Network for Organ Sharing (UNOS), the Southeastern Organ Procurement Foundation (SEOPF), and various institutions and has been or is a member of numerous organizations, including transplant coordinator, organ preservation, and surgical associations. Mr. Olson was founder and member of the board of directors of the Kidney Foundation of South Florida as well as the Transplant Foundation of South Florida *(personal communication, L. Olson, BA, CPTC, April 21, 006)*.
- **Carolyn L. R. Atkins, RN, CCTC, 1969.** Carolyn L. R. Atkins has worked nearly her entire nursing career in transplantation. She started in 1969 as the renal transplant coordinator at the University of Texas Health Science Center, Parkland Memorial Hospital in Dallas. She was a post-transplant coordinator and director of nursing and held other positions at Dallas Nephrology Associates from 1985 to 1993. She worked at Children's Hospital of Dallas as a renal transplant coordinator from 1995 through 1998 and again from 2005 through the present. She worked from

2002 to 2005 at Medical City of Dallas as a clinical research nurse and also as a nephrology nurse consultant several times throughout her career.

Carolyn's career in transplantation cannot be separated from her nearly three decades of involvement, work, stewardship, and leadership of the National Kidney Foundation. She has chaired numerous committees and served in various officer capacities on the board of directors. Carolyn served on several NATCO committees, was chair of the strategic planning committee, and received the NATCO/Sandoz achievement award in 1993. She serves on the editorial board of *Progress in Transplantation*, has authored or coauthored numerous articles, primarily in nephrology and transplant-related journals, and she lectures extensively on transplantation and renal issues[140] (*written communication, C. Atkins, RN, CCTC, June 2006*).

- **Roger C. Smith, BA, 1969.** Roger C. Smith received a BA in microbiology from UCLA (1970) and in music from California State University (1972). He started working with Dr. Paul Terasaki in 1969 as a staff research associate and became a transplant coordinator in 1971. By 1974, Roger was appointed administrator of the Regional Organ Procurement Agency (ROPA) of Southern California and remained in that post until he left in 1994 to pursue other endeavors. He was the second NATCO newsletter editor, serving in that capacity from 1981 to 1982. Roger served in numerous leadership capacities in NATCO throughout his career, serving on the board of directors as treasurer from 1982 to 1984 and as chair of the ethics committee from 1987 to 1988 (*written communication, B. Schulman, RN, CPTC, May 25, 2006*).

- **Stephen E. Kelley, BS, CCTC, CPTC, 1969.** Stephen E. Kelley started working at the University of Iowa in 1969 before their first transplantation. Several of his first assignments were to conduct studies on various solutions for organ preservation. He then performed procedures involving kidney recovery and transplantation, working on the technique in the laboratory setting. In November 1969, the first renal transplantation was performed in Iowa and his job "solidified." Throughout his career, he has performed more than 3,000 nephrectomies, approximately 300 hepatectomies, and 100 pancreatectomies. He first assisted in more than 1,500 organ transplantations, doing the back-table preparation of the organ and performing the vascular anastamosis, and he has performed or assisted on more than 4,000 access procedures. Since 1973, he has served as instructor in microsurgery for surgery and urology residents in vascular access and cadaveric renal organ recoveries.

  Steve managed the transplant research laboratory and was an organ recovery coordinator for the University of Iowa and was promoted to director of organ recovery in 1981, while continuing to manage the laboratory. He left Iowa to start the transplant program at the Geisinger Clinic in Danville, Pa, where he was director of organ recovery. He moved to Denver in 2001, where he has worked as a surgical recovery specialist for the Colorado Organ Recovery System. Steve Kelley was one of the founding members of NATCO, served on its Multi-Organ and Tissue Sharing Committee, and, to this point, has worked for 37 years in the field of organ donation and transplantation. He has published or co-published nearly 60 articles, book chapters, abstracts, and posters (*written communication, S. Kelley, BS, CCTC, CPTC, May 5, 2006*).

- **Phyllis G. Weber, RN, CPTC, 1969.** Phyllis G. Weber was the first official head nurse at the Hospital of the University of Pennsylvania Transplant Unit. In 1976, she became transplant coordinator at Pacific Presbyterian Medical Center, where she remained until 1982. From 1983 to 1988, she was program director for the Northern California Transplant Bank, and in 1988 Phyllis Weber was named chief executive officer (CEO) at California Transplant Donor Network in San Francisco, where she remains until this day. Phyllis has served in numerous leadership capacities in the Association of Organ Procurement Organizations (AOPO), including serving as president from 1996 to 1997, UNOS, including terms on the board of directors from 1995 to 2000, a portion of that time serving as an officer—secretary. She received the 1999 AOPO/AIG Healthcare award. Phyllis Weber is one of three co-chairs of the 2005-2006 third US collaborative involving transplantation: Organ Transplant Breakthrough Collaborative National HHS initiative to increase transplantation (*written communication, P. Weber, RN, CPTC, June 2006*).

- **Joan Miller, RN, 1970.** Joan Miller was the first heart transplant coordinator in the world, starting at Stanford in 1970. After working in Florida and Southern California as an emergency room and OB/GYN nurse, Joan came to Stanford in 1963 where she worked on the cancer and metabolic research centers. She joined the Heart Transplant program at Stanford in the summer of 1970, originating the role of Heart Transplant Coordinator.

  Joan is a charter member of the International Society of Heart and Lung Transplantation and founded the nursing sessions of that society. She has contributed to nursing journals worldwide, written chapters for transplant nursing texts, presented at scientific sessions, served on the editorial board of a national nursing transplant journal, and lectured on heart and lung transplant extensively. She authored or co-authored several articles and served on the editorial board of the *Journal of Transplant Coordination* (now *Progress in Transplantation*) from 1998-2000.

  Over the years, her areas of expertise have expanded to include lung and pediatric transplant. Her favorite areas of nursing are teaching and she especially enjoys the one-on-one interaction with patients and their families.[141] Miller is currently Transplantation Nurse Educator in Adult and Pediatric Heart and Lung Transplantation *(written communication, J. Miller, RN, August 2006)*.

- **Leo Roels, CPTC, 1972.** For more than 25 years, Leo Roels was a procurement and clinical transplant coordinator for kidney, heart, liver, pancreas, and lung transplant programs at University Hospital GHB, Leuven and the Leuven Collaborative Group for Transplantation Donor Hospitals' Network. A pioneer in transplant coordination in Europe, Leo is a member of 13 professional transplant-related societies, editor and associate editor of transplant journals, author or coauthor of more than 45 articles and book chapters, has given invited lectures in more than 20 countries, and has lectured or provided session chairmanship in international congresses throughout the world. His background is like that of many early coordinators, having graduated with a bachelor's degree in chemistry from the Rega School, Catholic University in Leuven, Belgium. He was instrumental in crafting presumed consent legislation in 1986 as a consultant to the Ministry of Health in Belgium. Like many of his colleagues in the United States, Mr. Roels was the transplant coordinator who did it all: procurement, clinical recipient coordination, organ retrieval system development, crafting of legislation favorable to organ donation, public education, research, and teaching. He was president of the European Transplant Coordinators Organization (ETCO) from 1993 to 1997. Leo moved from his transplant coordinator position in Leuven to Donor Action in 1999, and became managing director in 2001. The Donor Action program is a quality management program designed to maximize a hospital's donation potential by focusing on hospital processes in the donation process *(written communication, L. Roels, CPTC, April 21, 2006)*.

- **Patricia Gamberg, RN, FNP, CCTC, 1973.** Patricia Gamberg obtained her nursing degree at Presbyterian Hospital in Pittsburgh, Pennsylvania and worked at Stanford Hospital at Stanford University Medical Center on the cancer research unit and the general clinical research unit, later joining the cardiac transplant program in 1973. She helped to develop the protocols and teaching manual used in the Stanford program. Pat was instrumental in the development of the credentialing program for transplant coordinators and has served as a resource and mentor for transplant programs throughout the country.[141] Gamberg taught at the NATCO Clinical Training Course in 1985 and at the time was the Nurse Educator for transplantation in the Department of Cardiovascular Surgery, Stanford University Medical Center, Stanford, California. She continues in her present position at Stanford on the Cardiac Transplant Team and throughout the years has continued to lecture and advance the field, authoring or co-authoring numerous articles on transplantation.

- **Robert Duckworth, BS, CTBS, CPTC, 1973.** Robert Duckworth started in 1973 working in the transplant service in the Department of Surgery at the University of Mississippi. This was where the historic first human lung transplantation took place in 1963 and the first heart transplantation (chimpanzee to human) took place in 1964. He moved to the Nashville Transplant Program in 1977, to the Pittsburgh Transplant Foundation in 1983, to the Nebraska Organ Retrieval System in 1985, Southwest Organ Bank in Galveston in 1991, to the University of Nebraska in 1995, and in 1998 changed directions somewhat, leaving the transplant coordinator role to work as a specialist for St. Jude Medical Center. He has had an extremely well rounded coordinator career, working in that capacity for 25 years.

Bob may hold the record as a faculty member on the NATCO Procurement Introductory Course, teaching at the first one held in 1982 through 1990—nine years! His contributions to the introductory course were substantial, since in the early days of the Procurement and Clinical training courses, the entire course was prepared for and administered by practicing coordinators in the field. There was no management association to help in this regard. Transplant coordinators like Bob squeezed yet one more responsibility into their busy roles. He was the chair of the Procurement Examination Committee and served on the American Board of Transplant Coordinators (ABTC), now the American Board for Transplant Certification, for nine years, as well as serving on various NATCO committees *(written communication, R. Duckworth, BS, CTBS, CPTC, May 20, 2006).*

- **Geraldine M. Rasmussen, RN, 1973.** Geraldine Rasmussen was the procurement transplant coordinator for the New York—New Jersey Transplant Program when it began in 1973 and later was executive administrator for the New York Regional Transplant Program from 1978 to 1988.[142]
- **Donald W. Denny, MSW, 1974.** Don Denny was one of transplant coordination's most influential pioneers. He was one of the primary drivers in pushing coordinators to maximize organ donation from each donor by placing every organ possible, including extra-renal organs. He was one of the few who developed the 24-ALERT system, making possible more organized extrarenal organ sharing. Don Denny was sought by policy makers and reporters alike for information on the nation's organ donation and transplantation system. His career personified the independent practice-based profession of transplant coordination. His name graced the covers and articles of numerous pieces in both lay and professional publications.

"Don Denny was the first procurement coordinator here in Philadelphia—May of 1974 for Delaware Valley Transplant Program (KIDNEY-1); followed by Steve Sammut in 1976, and me in 1978. We were all called **transplant coordinators**, and it was a separate independent organization from the hospitals started by the transplant surgeons in December 1972" *(written communication, H. Nathan, BS, CPTC, February 6, 2006).*

Don Denny knew what needed to be done to build a competent organ donation and recovery system, as evidenced by his writings and testimony at the National Organ Transplant Hearings. He was the director of the Procurement and Transplant Foundation at the University of Pittsburgh. He was a key witness at the National Organ Transplant Hearings in 1983. His testimony and interaction with Senator Al Gore, the presiding chair of the hearings, and others, was precise and informed. Indeed, he called for many of the reforms and actions that ultimately were adopted and/or occurred in the United States in the next 20 years (see testimony in Appendix). As one reads Denny's testimony, it is apparent that he had a clear view of the industry and where it needed to be in order to maximize the number of lives saved in this country. It is also clear that he was an expert and spoke from his position as a transplant coordinator:

> My name is Donald W. Denny. I am the Director of Organ Procurement for the Transplant Foundation at the University of Pittsburgh. I am also a member of the North American Transplant Coordinators Organization (NATCO), a professional association of the transplant and organ procurement coordinators from the United States, Canada and several foreign countries. My testimony today will primarily reflect my personal experience, attitudes and values. I am also designated as the official representative of NATCO at these hearings, but when expressing the point of view of this association of over 350 transplant professionals, the context of my remarks will identify my position as a spokesman.[143]

Donald Denny received the NATCO/Sandoz achievement award in 1985.

- **Barbara Schulman, RN, CPTC, 1974.** (see NATCO Presidents for biography)
- **Barbara Schanbacher, RN, BSN, CPTC, CCTC, 1974.** (see NATCO Presidents for biography)
- **Marilyn R. Bartucci, MSN, APRN, BC, CCTC, 1974.** Marilyn Bartucci began her career in transplantation as a staff nurse in the transplant unit in 1974 and assistant head nurse in 1975 at the University Hospitals of Cleveland in Cleveland, Ohio. In 1978 she became the clinical nurse specialist for the renal transplant program. At the same time she served as a clinical instructor in

nursing at Case Western Reserve University, Frances Payne Bolton School of Nursing beginning in 1979. She was promoted to the head nurse manager of the transplant center at The University Hospitals in 1986 and to administrative director in 1998. She received her BSN from Marquette University in Milwaukee, Wisconsin and an MSN from Case Western University in Cleveland, Ohio in 1979.[144] Marilyn served in numerous leadership capacities in NATCO throughout her career, including the board of directors, and while working as a clinician and transplant administrator, participated in numerous research projects. She has written 37 articles in refereed journals and 15 book chapters, most as first author, on the clinical care of transplant recipients, immunology, and organ donation. Marilyn is currently scientific affairs manager for immunology with Astellas Pharma US, Inc.

- **Shawney Fine, RN, 1974.** Shawney Fine started work with Dr. Paul Terasaki in 1974 as a transplant coordinator with ROPA in Los Angeles, California.[145]
- **Bill G. Anderson, BS, CPTC, 1974** (see In Memoriam section for biography)
- **Ronald L. Dreffer, BS, CPTC, 1975.** (see NATCO Presidents for biography)
- **Michael G. Phillips, BHS, PA-C, CPTC, 1975.** Michael G. Phillips started his career in organ recovery in 1975 as a transplant coordinator for Duke University Medical Center. Before that, he had worked as a radiologic technologist and physician's assistant. Mike was possibly the first formally trained physician assistant in organ procurement. He soon became chief of organ procurement and tissue donation and in 1981 moved to Birmingham, Alabama to take the assistant director position at the Alabama Organ Center. In January 1987 he became the director. He remained director of the Alabama Organ Center until July 10, 1996, and in June 1998, became CEO of Life Connection of Ohio, Dayton and Toledo offices. Phillips was later in 1999 named president and CEO of Life Connection, where he continues to work today. Phillips has chaired and served on dozens of committees for NATCO, SEOPF, UNOS, AOPO, the National Kidney Foundation, the International Society for Organ Preservation, Duke University, North Carolina, and governmental agencies. He was deeply involved in many significant achievements and milestones in each of these organizations.

  Mike Phillips is a prolific author, with more than 60 book chapters, articles in scientific journals and newsletters, abstracts, and clinical training handbooks and manuals, most as first author. His contributions in education are substantive, with numerous training manuals produced as well as holding numerous faculty appointments at the University of Alabama and the Medical College of Ohio. In May 1973 he received his bachelor of health science degree from Duke University School of Medicine. He is president and CEO of the Foundation for the Human Donation Science Graduate Certificate Program at the Medical College of Ohio, the first collegiate program to teach transplant coordination. He designed the curriculum in conjunction with the Dean of Allied Health (*written communication, M. Phillips, BHS, PA-C, CPTC, April 2006*).
- **James W. Springer, BA, CPTC, 1975.** James W. Springer began his career as a kidney procurement and preservation technician in the department of organ procurement and preservation at Midwest Organ Bank in Kansas City, Missouri. He moved to Denver, Colorado in 1987 as executive director of Colorado Organ Recovery Systems, and in 1999 entered transplantation industry work, first with National Disease Research Interchange, and in 2001 with St. Jude Medical as an OPO specialist. Jim served on numerous UNOS and NATCO committees throughout his career, taught at NATCO's procurement training course, was chairman of the ABTC examination committee from 1989 to 1992, and served on the UNOS board of directors as a regional councilor from 1999 to 2001 (*written communication, J. Springer, BA, CPTC, February 2006*).
- **Gloria Horns, RN, 1975.** Gloria Horns was actually involved in the field of transplantation before 1975 because she worked as a staff nurse in the transplantation unit at the Peter Bent Brigham Hospital in Boston after her graduation from Skidmore College in Saratoga Springs, New York, where she obtained her degree in nursing. While she was in Boston, she was asked to participate in the certificate program in health policy at Harvard's School of Public Health. Gloria left the Peter Bent Brigham Hospital and worked for two years as the study coordinator of the transplant registrar

with the New England Organ Bank. She managed the Kidney Transplant Histocompatibility Study, which was a nationwide collaborative study of the National Institutes of Health for the New England region. In 1976, Gloria went to San Francisco, assuming the position of transplant coordinator/clinical specialist with the transplant service at the University Hospital, where she coordinated the care of approximately 1200 patients in different stages of transplantation. While working at the University full time, Gloria received her law degree.[146]

- **Winifred B. Mack, RN, BSN, MPA, 1976.** (see NATCO Presidents for biography)
- **Herbert E. Teachey, MBA, CPTC, 1976.** Herbert E. Teachey started at the Medical College of Virginia (MCV) as the administrator for the transplant program, laboratory, and dialysis unit. At that time, the surgeons, residents, or others talked to families, requesting consent. In a short period, Teachey was called and asked if he could request consent from a family that looked like their loved one might be a good donor. Very shortly, Teachey's role morphed into a transplant coordinator role. He hired an assistant and promoted her as administrative assistant. His assistant basically ran the office and he was free to do transplant coordinator work, which was much more exciting! He excelled at making transportation arrangements, which was fortuitous since MCV at the time did more long-distance procurements than any other transplant program in the country (see last page of this chapter for a full-page photo of Teachey in *Raytheon Magazine* in 1985, doing exactly that). Teachey worked at MCV for 13 years, until 1989.

During the time at MCV, Teachey was very active with NATCO, chairing and later co-chairing the Multiorgan Committee. He worked with Don Denny and Brian Broznick in creating and running 24-ALERT. He and Brian wrote the algorithms for organ placement, and Rick Sheppeck did the programming. In remembering the development of 24-ALERT, Teachey recalled that he didn't know when writing the algorithm for heart placement that as someone's medical condition worsened, the number should increase. Therefore, he did it vice versa, thus the reason for status 1 hearts being the sickest. Since Brian Broznick wrote the liver algorithms, status 4 livers were the sickest! Rick Sheppeck, a medical student, and Teachey worked all day, so they generally conferred at night, while creating 24-ALERT, the extrarenal organ sharing system in the United States for many years before UNOS. Herbert Teachey served in several NATCO roles and was part of that early group of transplant coordinators who shaped the face of transplant coordination.

Teachey moved from MCV to accept a position with Sandoz Pharmaceuticals in 1989 where he worked with OPOs to improve organ recovery efficiency and increase rates of procurement. In 1993, he started the Mid-South Tissue Bank in Memphis, Tennessee, and in 1996 he moved to Regeneration Technologies, where he assisted tissue banks in improving recovery efficiency. He remained at Regeneration Technologies until 2001. Mr. Teachey received his bachelor's degree in psychology from the College of William and Mary and his master's degree in business administration from Virginia Commonwealth University. Herbert Teachey now resides in England with his wife but has plans to return to the states in two years *(oral communication, H. Teachey, MBA, CPTC, June 2006)*.

- **Mark R. Reiner, PA, CPTC, 1976.** (see NATCO Presidents for biography)
- **Kate Hume, RN, MSN, 1976.** (see NATCO Presidents for biography)
- **Meredith (Mikki) A. Masteller, RN, BSN, CPTC, 1976.** Mikki Masteller was a transplant coordinator at the University of California, San Diego. She received a bachelor of science in nursing from the University of Minnesota in 1968. Mikki was the first coeditor of the NATCO newsletter, her coeditor being her colleague Julie Hall. The two coeditors produced the first two issues of the newsletter in 1980 after the formation of NATCO. In 1981 Roger Smith became editor. Mastellar served on numerous NATCO committees throughout the years, primarily in chair and co-chair capacities.[144(p14)]
- **Anita L. Principe, RN, MPA, CCTC, CPTC 1976.** (see NATCO Presidents for biography)
- **Faye D. Davis, BA, MSN, 1977.** Faye Davis began her career in organ procurement in 1977 as a procurement transplant coordinator at the Medical College of Georgia and was promoted to associate director in September 1978. In October 1979, she moved to the New England Organ Bank

Chapter 1: THE HISTORY OF THE TRANSPLANT COORDINATOR

in Boston to take the position of director of organ donation. In January 1983 she took the position of director of organ procurement at the Washington Organ Bank and in June 1983 as the director of organ procurement at the Washington Hospital Center. In 1986, she was director of procurement at The Methodist Hospital in Houston, Texas. Faye Davis was the first executive director hired for the New York Regional Transplant Program, in 1988, one of the largest OPOs in the country. (Editor's note: I know of no other individual who has served in a senior leadership capacity, such as the executive director or director of procurement, of six different OPOs during her career.)

Faye Davis organized and was founder of the very first Procurement Training Course that was held at the Rolling Ridge Conference Center in North Andover, Massachusetts in 1982 and served on the faculty of the NATCO Training Courses, both procurement and clinical, for many years. She served on numerous NATCO committees and lectured throughout the United States. She authored many publications, including book chapters and lectured extensively on transplantation, organ procurement and the grieving family. Davis was an early developer of organ recovery systems throughout service areas; systems that included creating hospital contracts, donor referral systems, death record reviews and professional and public education, during the late 1970s and early 1980s. She was acknowledged by her peers throughout her career and was the first recipient of the NATCO-Sandoz Achievement Award in 1984 for lifetime achievement.[142,147]

- **Howard M. Nathan, BS, CPTC, 1978.** Howard M. Nathan joined Gift of Life (formerly Delaware Valley Transplant Program) in 1978 as a transplant coordinator and became executive director in 1984. His title was changed to president and CEO in 1999. He is immediate past president of the Coalition on Donation and has served on the UNOS board of directors for three terms, serving as an officer, treasurer, and region two counselor. Nathan is a past president of AOPO and serves or has served on numerous other national and state organizations, including the American Society for Bioethics and Humanities (formerly known as the American Association of Bioethics), Musculoskeletal Transplant Foundation, Medical Board of Trustees, National Kidney Foundation-US Transplant Games Committee, NATCO, The James Redford Institute for Transplant Awareness, American Red Cross Blood Services (Penn Jersey Region), and Governor's Organ Donation Advisory Committee for the Commonwealth of Pennsylvania, among others. In 1999, he served as a consultant to the National Academy of Sciences' Institute of Medicine and testified before the US House of Representatives and the House of Commons, Ottawa, Canada on organ and tissue donation issues.

  A visible figure in the field of transplantation, Nathan is a regular presenter at both regional and national organ procurement, transplantation and other medical/health care conferences, and he has published more than 85 scientific papers and abstracts. He was presented with The Belzer Award for outstanding abstract at the 4th International Society for Organ Sharing Congress in 1997. He is consulted frequently by members of the media and has appeared on national TV news and talk programs, including *ABC News, CBS News, CNN, Fox Cable News, the Phil Donahue Show, Morton Downey Jr,* and *Geraldo*. In 1996 Nathan received the Caring for Kids Award, presented by Bell Atlantic Corporation, on behalf of his work with St. Christopher's Hospital for Children, Philadelphia, Pennsylvania. He also received the AOPO Outstanding Achievement Award for 1996, was honored by the National Kidney Foundation of the Delaware Valley in 1994, and received the NATCO Achievement Award, Advancing the Science of Immunology and Expanding the Promise of Transplantation, in August 1992.

  Nathan is a graduate of Juniata College, Huntingdon, Pennsylvania, where he received his bachelor of science degree in biology. He has also done graduate work in public health at the University of Pittsburgh. Before joining Gift of Life, he was a research specialist in microbiology and electron microscopy at The Wistar Institute, Philadelphia, Pennsylvania (*written communication, H. Nathan, BS, CPTC, May 2006*).

- **Brian A. Broznick, BS, CPTC, 1978.** (see In Memoriam section for biography)

- **Jane A. Warmbrodt, M.A., 1978.** Jane Warmbrodt introduced hospital development as an integral component of the procurement transplant coordinator's role while working at Midwest Organ Bank in Kansas City. She worked from 1978 to 1988 at Midwest Organ Bank in Kansas City, Missouri as the Director of Professional Services and Marketing. Jane was on the strategic planning committee that helped design ABTC and was a member of the first Board of Governors of the American Board of Transplant Coordinators. She served on the Board of Directors of the American Council on Transplantation, on the faculty of the NATCO Training Course in North Andover, Massachusetts and was an appointee on the Surgeon General's Workshop on Increasing Organ Donation. Jane received the NATCO/Sandoz Achievement Award in 1986. She left Midwest Organ Bank in 1988 to work at Sandoz Pharmaceuticals as a Professional Marketing Specialist and Business Unit Leader where she worked with organ procurement organizations. After leaving Sandoz in 1991, Warmbrodt served as a management consultant. She received a BA in marketing from the University of Arkansas in Fayetville, Arkansas and an MA in administration from Webster University in Kansas City, Missouri *(written communication, J. Warmbrodt, August 2006)*.

- ***Betty (Irwin) C. Crandall, RN, MS, 1978***. Betty (Irwin) Crandall started her career in transplantation as a clinical nurse specialist in renal transplantation at The Johns Hopkins Hospital in Baltimore, Maryland,[148] and remained in that position for 10 years, through 1988. From there she served as Clinical Director and later Director of Nursing at CVPH Medical Center in Plattsburgh, New York, and in 1997 returned to a transplantation focus at Sentara Norfolk General Hospital, Sentara Healthcare in Norfolk, Virginia as Operating Center Manager in 1997, as Operating Center Manager, Transplant/CVT Research in early 1998, and in August, 1998 as Director of Cardiac/Vascular/Transplant Clinical Specialty Services through the present.

  Crandall taught at the NATCO Clinical Training Course in 1985. She has chaired the UNOS Transplant Administrator's Committee, served on the Board of Directors of the National Kidney Foundation of the Virginias, and served as a reviewer for *Nursing Economics (written communication, B. Crandall, August, 2006)*.

- ***Amy S. Peele, RN, CPTC, 1978***. (see NATCO Presidents for biography)
- ***Barbara A. Elick, RN, BSN, CPTC, CCTC, 1978***. (see NATCO Presidents for biography)
- ***Mary Anne (House) Park, RN, MSN, CTBS, CPTC**, 1979*. Mary Ann House "has been senior surgical transplant coordinator for three and one half years at the Medical College of Georgia dealing strictly in organ procurement. Mary Anne was secretary of NATCO in 1981-1982."[174] Mary Anne (House) Park started her career in organ procurement in 1969 at the Medical College of Georgia and was promoted to administrator of the program in February 1983, where she remained until 1995. Mary Anne was involved in all facets of NATCO's development and the advancement of the profession, chairing or serving on the Education Committee, Members' Education Subcommittee, Membership Committee, Training and Development Committee, Research Committee, Publications Committee, Standards of Practice Subcommittee, Communications Committee, Newsletter Committee, and Quality Assurance Committee. She has authored or coauthored 30 book chapters, articles, and abstracts.

  Most notable was her role as an educator for those entering or in the profession. Mary Anne held numerous roles, including chairperson, on multiple education committees for most of the major transplant organizations including NATCO, AOPO, UNOS, SEOPF, and AATB. Mary Anne gave more than 1,500 lectures throughout her career in organ procurement. She also served as historian of NATCO from 1981 to 1982 and was the newsletter editor from 1982 to 1989.

  House left her imprint on the profession with her untiring devotion to education and advancement of transplant coordinator professionals. She left the field on September 16, 1996 and is currently the director of clinical research services in the Department of Surgery at the Medical College of Georgia *(written communication, M. Park, RN, MSN, CTBS, CPTC, May 2006)*.

- ***Celia Wight, RN, 1980.*** Celia Wight is included here as a representative of European coordinators. From England, she is well known throughout the European community. Wight was appointed as an operating room nurse at Addenbrooke's Hospital in Cambridge, United Kingdom in 1972, where she became involved in non-heart-beating donor cases. In 1980 she was asked to join the transplant team as the transplant coordinator at Addenbrooke's Hospital. From 1980 to 1986 she was regional transplant coordinator for the East Anglican Regional Health Authority based at

Chapter 1: THE HISTORY OF THE TRANSPLANT COORDINATOR

both Addenbrooke's and Papworth Hospitals, and from 1986 to 1990 as senior regional transplant coordinator for the same hospitals. In addition, from 1990 to 1992 she worked as transplant manager at Addenbrooke's Hospital. She left Addenbrooke's Hospital to work from 1992 to 1994 in the Netherlands as the international coordinator for the European Donor Hospital Education Programme, a communication skills awareness program based at the Eurotransplant Foundation in Leiden, The Netherlands. From 1998 to 2003, she served as manager of the Donor Action Foundation, a donor hospital development program.

Celia has had numerous achievements and has been involved with transplant coordinators and leaders worldwide. She was a founder and first president of the United Kingdom Transplant Coordinators Association (UKTCA), second President of the European Transplant Coordinators Organization (ETCO), and was a member of NATCO, the British Transplantation Society, European Liver Club, and the European Society for Organ Transplantation. Wight has authored over 70 articles, most as first author, and has lectured extensively throughout the world. She made numerous media appearances over the years, advised on television shows on donation and transplantation, and has been profiled in several magazines. In nearly all ways, her early years closely paralleled those of her American colleagues. She is now retired and living in Canada with her husband (*written communication, C. Wight, RN, CPTC, May 30, 2006*).

Names from the first NATCO newsletters, workshops, and meeting brochures from 1979 through 1981 provide a glimpse of the early practitioners in the field, those who worked in the profession through its early, formative years. This list is not meant to be inclusive of everyone who worked in the field at that time, but gives readers a glimpse of some of the early practitioners who were drawn to this work, and in varying degrees helped shape the field of transplant coordination. The names are taken with the information available from their appearance in the newsletter or meeting brochure *at the time*. Many of the names readers will recognize are listed for an organization with which they are least known. Coordinators did move throughout the years, to advance their career or start new programs.

Transplant Coordinators Named in NATCO Newsletters and Meeting Brochures, 1979–1981

Vicki Aslanian, Upstate Medical Center, Syracuse, NY
Patricia L. Barber, FNP, University of Illinois Medical Center, Chicago, IL
Lois Bartell, RN, Transplant Coordinator, University of Minnesota, Minneapolis, MN
SSgt. J.B. Burris, Wilford Hall USAF Medical Center, TX
Nicole Bertinshaw, Foothills Hospital, Calgary, Canada
Marcia Blech, BS, MA, Cleveland Clinic Foundation, Cleveland Heights, OH
John Bleifuss, Washington state
Caroline Buszta, RN
Virginia "Ginny" Callanen, RN, BSN, MS, Transplant Coordinator, New England Organ Bank, Boston, MA
Elizabeth Cameron, RN
Bill Cantirino, State University of New York (SUNY) at Stony Brook, NY
Carlos Castaneda
Carol Christiansen
Mel Cohen, Director, Metro Organ Retrieval and Exchange, Toronto, Ontario, Canada
John Collins
Patricia Conway, RN
Alice Curtis, RN
Shelley Daltz, Transplant Coordinator
Faye Davis, RN, MSN, Inter-Hospital Organ Bank, (later, New England Organ Bank), Boston, MA
Claire Day, RN, Adult Transplant Coordinator, Shands Teaching Hospital, Gainesville, FL
Eileen DeMayo, RN, Los Angeles, CA
John Dennis
Don Denny, MSW, Director of Organ Procurement, Transplant Organ Procurement Foundation of Western Pennsylvania, Pittsburgh, PA
Chris De Voe, RN
Paul Deutsch
Ronald Dreffer, BS, Transplant Coordinator, University of Cincinnati Medical Center, Cincinnati, OH
Rosemary Dresser

Robert Duckworth, Transplant Coordinator, Nashville Transplant Program, Nashville, TN

Barbara Elick, RN, Southwest Organ Bank, Dallas, TX (later from the University of Minnesota)

Jacqueline Elkin, RN, Washington University School of Medicine, St. Louis, MO

Daniel Ferree, SEOPF, Richmond, VA

Lea Emmett, SUNY Downstate Medical Center, Brooklyn, NY

Mary Ann Farnsworth, RN, Coordinator, Kidney Donor Program, Division of Urology, University of Oregon Health Science Center, Portland, OR

Susan Fischer, RN, University of Oregon, Portland, OR

Tracy Fleeter, RN

Charles Foxworth

Pat Garrison, Transplant Coordinator, Phoenix Transplant Coordination Service, Good Samaritan Hospital, Phoenix, AZ

Cyrena Gilman, RN, Riley Hospital for Children, Indianapolis, IN

Barbara Giordano, RN, Newark Beth Israel Medical Center, Newark, NJ

Christine Gladden, RN

Robert Gosnell, Director of Administration and Organ Recovery, South Texas Organ Bank, San Antonio, TX

Toni Greenslade, RN, BSN, Nurse Clinician, Renal Transplant Program, Children's Memorial Hospital, Chicago, IL

Cecil H. Gunter, Northwest Kidney Center, Seattle, WA

Tom Hagan, Preservation Technologist, Phoenix Renal Transplant Center, Phoenix, AZ

Steve Haid, Washington University School of Medicine, St. Louis, MO

Julie Hall, UCSD Medical Center, San Diego, CA

Arthur Harrell, MA, Delaware Valley Transplant Program, Philadelphia, PA

Robert Hoffmann, Transplant Specialist, University of Wisconsin, Madison, WI

Susan Hopper, RN, MSN, Transplant Coordinator, UCSF, San Francisco, CA

Mary Ann House, RN, MSN, Medical College of Georgia, GA

Kate Hume, RN, MSN, Renal Transplant Clinical Specialist, Northwestern Memorial Hospital, Chicago, IL

Louise Jacobbi, Clinical Research Associate, Louisiana State University Medical Center, Shreveport, LA

Linda L. Jones, Ohio State University, Columbus, OH

Carol Kaczarczyk, RN, New England Organ Bank

Diane Kaschak, Albert Einstein Medical Center, Philadelphia, PA

Stephen Kelley, Organ Recovery Coordinator, University of Iowa, Department of Surgery, Iowa City, IA

Kristen Koser, RN, Transplant Coordinator, University of Iowa Hospitals, Iowa City, IA

Mathew J. Korten, Delaware Valley Transplant Program

Jo Leslie, PA, Transplant Coordinator, Greater Baltimore Organ Procurement and Preservation Center, Baltimore, MD

Carol Lieberman, RN, Portland, OR

Gerda Lipcaman, Transplant Coordinator, Organ Procurement Agency of Michigan, Ann Arbor, MI

Joanne van Looven, Florida Hospital, Organ Transplant, Orlando, FL

Louise L. Loring, Heart Transplant Coordinator, University of Wisconsin

Judith Lucier, RN, New England Organ Bank, Boston, MA

Judith Lutton, University of Texas MC, Surgery Renal Transplant, San Antonio, TX

Winnie Mack, RN, BSN, SUNY at Stony Brook, NY

Marge Maeser, RN, Washington University, St. Louis, MO

Ann Martin, RN, Transplant Coordinator, Medical College of Virginia, Richmond, VA

Micki Masteller, UCSD Medical Center, San Diego, CA

O'Neill Mathews, RN, BS, Organ Procurement Coordinator, Nashville Transplant Program, Nashville, TN

Burton Mattice, Miami Valley Hospital, Dayton, OH

Robert K. McAtee, South Texas Organ Bank, San Antonio, TX

Gwen McNalt, University of Illinois, Chicago, IL

Rita Menard, RN

Michael Merriman, PA, Transplant Coordinator, Bowman Gray School of Medicine, Winston-Salem, NC

Judy Messinger, BS, Organ Procurement Agency of NW Ohio, Maumee, OH

Richard Metz, Transplant Coordinator, Phoenix, AZ

Douglas Miller, University of Wisconsin, Madison, WI

Howard Nathan, transplant coordinator, Delaware Valley Transplant Program, Philadelphia, PA

Chapter 1
THE HISTORY OF THE TRANSPLANT COORDINATOR

Deborah Nelson, RN
Mary Jane Nevin, RN, Northwestern, Chicago, IL
Dave Mainous, Transplant Coordinator, Indiana Medical Center & Veterans Administration Center, Indianapolis, IN
Les Olson, Transplant Coordinator and Director of Preservation, University of Miami Medical School, Jackson Memorial Medical Center, Miami, FL
Glenda Payne, RN
Amy Peele, RN, Transplant Coordinator, University of Chicago Hospitals and Clinics, Chicago, IL
Patricia A. Prekup, Transplant Coordinator, Phoenix, AZ
Diane Prindle, Organ Recovery, Inc, Cleveland, OH
Geraldine Rasmussen, New York Regional Transplant Program, NY
Jane Reed, Midwest Organ Bank, Kansas City, MO
Mark Reiner, PA, Nashville Transplant Program, Nashville, TN
Sylvia Rodgers, RN, Procurement Coordinator, Atlanta Regional OPA, Atlanta, GA
Kathy Rudd, Mayo Clinic, Rochester, MN
Stephen M. Sammut, MA, Executive Director, Delaware Valley Transplant Program
John Sampson, NY Hospital Cornell Medical Center, New York, NY
Barbara Schanbacher, RN, BSN, University Hospital and Clinics, Iowa City, IA
Anne Schefiliti, RN, SEOPF, Richmond, VA
Barbara Schulman, RN, Transplant Coordinator, ROPA of Southern California, CA
Ewing von Schmittow, PA, Director of Organ Procurement, Nashville Transplant Program, Nashville, TN
Barbara Self, RN, Transplant Coordinator, Los Angeles, CA
Marge Severeid, Mayo Clinic, Rochester, MN
Mary Ann Sherman, RN, Heart Transplant Coordinator, Arizona Health Sciences Center, Tucson, AZ
Cheryl Shimek, RN
Michael Sicuro, Preservation Technician, Loyola University Medical Center, Maywood, IL
Tracy Siegler
Luke Skelley, Nashville Organ Donor Program, Nashville, TN
Penny Smith
Roger C. Smith, Administrator/Transplant Coordinator, ROPA of Southern California, CA
Laurie Ruse Sophie, RN, Transplant Clinical Specialist, University of Chicago Hospital and Clinics, Chicago, IL
Jim Springer, Midwest Organ Bank, Kansas City, MO
Bruce Sutphin
Sally Taber, St. Mary's Hospital, Portsmouth, England
Herb Teachey, Medical College of Virginia, Richmond, VA
Paul Taylor, Transplant Coordinator, University of Colorado MC, Denver, CO
Thomas Threlkeld, Transplant Coordinator, University of Kentucky Medical Center, Lexington, KY
Donna Tomky, RN, Nurse Practitioner/Pre-Transplant Coordinator, Chicago, IL
Gail Tyndall, RN
Maxine Uniewski
E. Jane Van Hook, RN, Transplant Coordinator, University of Minnesota, Minneapolis, MN
Ivy Vincent, University of Texas Medical School, Department of Surgery, Houston, TX
Jos Vroeman
Julie Wade, RN, Yuba City, CA
Howell Warner, Nashville Transplant Program
Jane Waskerwitz, RN, University of Michigan Renal Clinic, Ann Arbor, MI
J.D. Waters, Transplant Coordinator, Southwest Organ Bank, Dallas, TX
Lisa Watson, RN, Shands Hospital, Gainesville, FL
Phyllis G. Weber, RN, Northern California Transplant Bank, San Francisco, CA
Bruce White, BS, Transplant Coordinator, Maine Medical Center, Portland, ME
Daniel Williams
Justine Willmert, Transplant Coordinator, University of Minnesota, Minneapolis, MN
Curtis Yeager, Howard University, Washington, DC
Emi Yoshihara, ROPA of Southern California, Los Angeles, CA
Ken Youngstein
Dominick Zangari, BS, New England Organ Bank, Boston, MA

Birth of NATCO

"No one should work alone, as one needs others with whom to share ideas."[149]

"The administrative council, with the benefit of the dedicated efforts and recommendations of the program committee, voted and finalized the excellent program that will be presented in June. Our determinations were motivated directly toward seeking to answer the challenges facing the coordinator of today. We analyzed, reasoned, and reached the conclusions, which we believe will achieve these goals. The team who prepared the 1980 conference…considered various aspects of transplantation coordination, striving to enhance the professional skills of the men and women whose critical awareness will be beckoned by the on-call demands of the telephone."[149]

Transplant coordinators needed one another. Through trial and error throughout the late 1960s and 1970s, they found other colleagues from whom they could learn but also with whom they could network in order to create a means of sharing organs from one donor across the country with patients at other centers. NATCO grew out of the need for coordinators to accomplish what needed to be accomplished to help build the US donation and transplantation system as well as to define their profession. They were living it, day-to-day. They lived it together, working and talking to one another 24/7, at the same time creating a framework for their practice. Ron Dreffer's presidential address details an occurrence a decade earlier which led to the formation of NATCO—"Ten years ago a great debate occurred among three southern California coordinators, Barb Schulman, Roger Smith and Shawney Fine, regarding a difficult legal point concerning a potential donor referral. Dr. Thomas Berne, a transplant surgeon at the University of Southern California, entered into the discussion. He wondered how many other coordinators are dealing with this very same issue in the United States. Dr. Berne stated: 'You really should start a national transplant coordinators organization.' With that came the birth of NATCO."[150]

This account was shared by Barbara Schulman in an earlier NATCO newsletter[23] as well as during an interview she gave for the NATCO 30-year anniversary.[151] She recounts that discussion and then further carries forward the story. After the conversation between the ROPA coordinators that day, the next day they met with ROPA Director, Paul Terasaki, PhD, and received his approval to dispatch a letter to the 110 transplant centers in the country. The letter queried the centers about interest in having a meeting in Los Angeles. Forty-four transplant coordinators responded to the transplant coordinator meeting invitation and 25 arrived in Los Angeles from across the country for the two-day meeting. "We became acquainted, discussed ROPA's original legal question and many, many other coordinators' medical, legal, religious, financial and social issues. We found meeting each other to be most productive, informative, (job description and background varied greatly) and of great value."[23] The group planned a fall meeting (August) to be held in New York City in conjunction with the International Transplant Society meeting.

True to the intial plan, the first formal meeting of transplant coordinators convened at the New York Blood Center on August 19 and 20, 1976 (Figure 1, Table 3). Twenty-five coordinators attended the transplant coordinators workshop. Organizers of the meeting were Geraldine Rasmussen (NY), Justine Willmert (MN), and John Bleifuss (WA). There was, as reported in the NATCO newsletter, an "excellent scientific program, good camaraderie, and worthwhile sharing of experiences."[23] (See photos for two pictures from that historic meeting.)

It would be nearly two years before the next organized meeting of coordinators was held. The second such meeting was held on April 6 and 7, 1978 in Columbus, Ohio, as coordinators continued to define their field (Table 4). The organizers of this meeting were Gerda Lipcaman (MI), Linda Jones (OH), Justine Willmert (MN), and Curtis Yeager (DC). There were "fabulous concurrent organ procurement, preservation and nursing sessions."[23]

The third organized coordinators meeting, the last to be held before coordinators officially formed their society—NATCO—was held in Chicago on May 30 and 31, 1979 at the Holiday Inn, Chicago City Center. It was at this meeting that various options of joining existing organizations or remaining independent were presented and discussed. A vote was taken and it was unanimous that the coordinators decided to formalize as an independent organization.[23] The first officers were elected at this meeting (Table 5). A photo of the first officers is included in the photo section.

President's Message

It's a ....It's a ....
It's an Organization!!!!!!

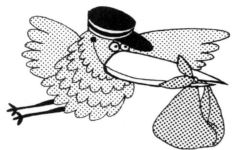

Name: NATCO
Date: Wednesday, May 30, 1979
Time: 14:00 hrs.
Place: Chicago, Illinois

The birth was painless, only the gestation seemed to take forever. The arduous struggle between those that wished its birth and those that did not has been resolved.

But, like all acts of nature it could not be stopped. Despite the negatives, the hurdles, the delays, the problems, NATCO was born and from its onset came the display of determination, that it was here to stay.

Congratulations came pouring in from other transplant professional organizations, from officers and members alike, such as the International Society of Transplantation and the American Society of Transplant Surgeons.

Giants in our field greeted us, told us they needed and wanted us and offered their support with great encouragement. Men like Dr. Thomas Berne, who conceived the very idea and Drs. John Najarian, Thomas Starzl, Paul I. Terasaki, Felix Rapaport, Jeremiah Turcotte and Frederick Merkel welcomed us.

The first few months were not easy. So much to be established, organized and planned, and yet what a pleasure. Imagine the opportunities I have had as your president this first year. Nothing to tear down, only to build up; particularly with the fresh, exuberant pride and enthusiasm all members have exhibited. Committees have been established, chairpersons have volunteered and work has begun.

What a super organization to lead! What an advantage! What members! If I sound like a proud parent, I am, for involvement has come from all aspects of our profession as transplant coordinators. You all bring a wealth of talent and experience to NATCO, the administrators, the nurses, the perfusion technicians, the procurement personnel - an organization of organizers.

Responsibility with optimism, is to move forward positively and to act. This year will see NATCO uniting transplant coordinators dedicated to promoting the highest professional standards for the optimum care of the patient. Great emphasis will be on study, discussion and exchange of information. Cooperation with other professional organizations, hospitals, universities and governmental agencies will be encouraged.

My goal as NATCO president is to improve the quality of performance in each area of coordination activity.

It is with a sense of extreme pride and joy that I share with you the birth and growth progress of NATCO and I respectfully invite all transplant coordinators to join this vital group. Your suggestions, recommendations and needs will be our plans for the future.

Barbara Schulman, R.N.
President

The preceding and the following articles, from the very first issue of the NATCO Newsletter, confirm the formation of NATCO and give the election results:

Meet Your Officers

In this most important year of NATCO, it is your elected officers who will direct the future of this organization.

President Barbara Schulman is a graduate of New York University, Bellevue School of Nursing. She served three years as a First Lieutenant in the US Army Nurse Corps. Returning to civilian life she held several nursing positions before joining the Regional Organ Procurement Agency of Southern California in 1974.

President-elect Kate Hume received a B.S. in Nursing from Bowling Green State University and has just completed her M.S. in Medical-Surgical Nursing. In 1975 she began working at Northwestern Memorial Hospital in Chicago. One year later Kate accepted her present position as a Nurse Clinician for their transplant program.

Secretary Barbara Schanbacher obtained her B.S. in Nursing from the University of Iowa. She spent several years as Head Nurse before advancing to her current position. Barbara is now the Coordinator of the Transplantation Services at the University Hospital and Clinics in Iowa City.

Treasurer Bob Gosnell has both a B.S. and a B.S.H.A. from South West Texas State and will receive his MBA soon. Bob spent his last ten years in the Air Force with the Wilford Hall USAF Medical Center Transplant Unit. During that time he was Supervisor of Organ Preservation and Research. In 1976 he accepted his present position as the Director of Administration and Organ Recovery for the South Texas Organ Bank, Inc.

Parliamentarian Paul Taylor is a graduate of the University of Kansas with a B.S. degree in education. He spent several years as a laboratory technician and coordinator for the Organ Transplant Program at the University of Colorado Medical Center.

Director of Public Relations, Winifred Mack, has a B.S. in Nursing and is now enrolled in the Masters program at C.W. Post College. She was a hemodialysis staff nurse for several years before becoming a transplant coordinator in 1976 for the Nassau County Medical Center. Then in 1978 her position changed to Transplant Coordinator for the University Hospital S.U.N.Y. Stonybrook, New York.

Historian Justine Willmert graduated from the Naeve Hospital School of Nursing. After four years as a Transplant Coordinator at UCSF she moved to Minnesota. For the last twelve years she has held the position of Transplant Coordinator Research Fellow at the University of Minnesota.[140]

Five of the seven names listed in this article would at some point be president of NATCO: Barbara Schulman, Kate Hume, Barbara Schanbacher, Bob Gosnell, and Winifred Mack. Additionally at this meeting, a newsletter was established, committees were formed, and communication lines between coordinators were encouraged. The president's message on page one of NATCO's first newsletter captures the excitement of the event of forming a society in Chicago:

> The first official NATCO meeting was held in Boston in conjunction with the International Transplantation Society. The scientific meeting was interesting, the social hours exciting and continuing friendships were established. The name—NATCO—and the logo created by artist Warren Joseph Smith were adopted at a spirited business meeting.[22]

NATCO's logo was not changed again until 2003, when "The Organization for Transplant Professionals" was added to recognize the diversity of professionals in NATCO's membership.

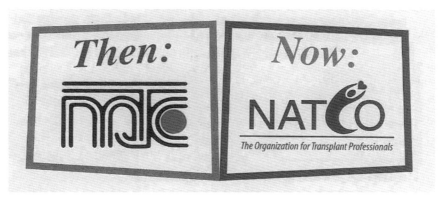

Chapter 1: THE HISTORY OF THE TRANSPLANT COORDINATOR

There was no shortage of leaders to form the transplant coordinators' professional society or to frame and advance this new profession. They were self-directed and driven to this job to make a difference, thriving in the challenging working conditions and the newness of the field. As early as the third newsletter, a column titled "Call for Leadership" was included: "A professional organization needs strong leadership and representation to be effective and accomplish its goals and dreams. The Nominations and Elections Committee cordially invites NATCO members to run for office."[152] Committees were where the work was done for this new profession; indeed, that much has not changed. They were busy building their roles and the profession. For a listing of all committees and committee chairs and members for the first three years of NATCO, see Figures 2 through 4.

Barbara Schulman, RN, NATCO's first president, was instrumental in building the organization and has remained active and a member of the organization through present day. Her remarks, delivered at NATCO's 30th annual meeting on July 31, 2005, are included below in their entirety. They shed light on her remarkable involvement in the organization she helped found:

CHOOSE LIFE
Barbara Schulman, RN, CPTC

Choose Life is a Jewish tenet that has served me well. First as a child, during WWII, in Nazi occupied Belgium, when my parents changed my name, hid me in a Catholic orphanage and saved me from certain death by their unselfish decision.

Choose Life influenced my desire to become a nurse. Choose Life guided me when considering a career in transplantation in 1974. The concepts were new, challenging, difficult, inviting.

My past OR experience was the reason Dr. Paul Terasaki hired me to join Shawney Fine, then a dialysis nurse. Our assignment—to create a Regional Organ Procurement Agency (ROPA) located in the UCLA Tissue Typing lab that would supply kidneys to the many Transplant Centers in Los Angeles. Our task—to develop a program that would enlist the 300 community hospitals in Southern California to notify us of potential brain death cases… and we would do the rest. Our direction—to teach that it was "a matter of death and life" rather than "life and death."

Shawney and I have remained friends and today she and her husband, Dr. Richard Fine, President of the American Transplant Society (ATS) send their congratulations and utmost admiration for NATCO's accomplishments.

In 1975, when we were discussing upcoming brain death legislation in California, Dr. Thomas Berne, a transplant surgeon passing our office remarked, "I wonder how many other coordinators in the country are discussing that very subject right now. You really should start a professional organization." We thought that was brilliant, somewhere to go for all the answers—Amazing! Thirty years later, we still have more questions than answers.

Dr. Terasaki was providing tissue typing analysis and transplant results to a good many kidney transplant centers in the country by sending out monthly reports. We asked to include a letter of invitation with our job description. Forty-four people responded and 25 arrived in Los Angeles for a first meeting in early 1976 that would be followed by a larger meeting that August in New York City.

We assigned committees to plan yearly meetings that took place in Columbus, San Antonio and Chicago. Not much happened in between. We had, however, become caring colleagues. We knew we could call on anyone 24/7, anywhere in the country to discuss the tough issues.

In 1979, I was asked to review and report the organization's future options. We had invitations to affiliate with many organizations, even the then Society of Transplantation. The doctors stated we could attend their meetings but not the dinner/dance. That cinched it. We voted unanimously to remain independent. Think about it—if we had only been asked to the dance?

We chose a name and commissioned a logo. Julie Hall and Mikki Masteller of UCSD were co-editors of the newsletter and as such, authored the dedication statement that still inspires us today. I was elected President and our first official NATCO Convention was held on June 27 and 28, 1980 in Boston.

The site was especially significant, in that, Boston was the city in which the first long-term, successful solid organ transplant, a renal transplant between identical twins, was performed by Dr. Joseph Murray 25 years earlier. He lectured to us there on the State of the Art. In 1990, he received a Nobel Prize in Medicine for his triumph in transplantation.

Kate Hume from Chicago was the second President. The meeting in June of 1981 had David Sutherland discussing transplantation progress with the pancreas, Tom Starzl, the liver, John Pennock from Stanford, the heart and even Robert Jarvik on the development of the Artificial Heart. We were well on our way, dealing with current relevant interesting topics such as scientific writing, immunosuppressive strategies, time management principles and professional standards for transplant coordinators.

Robert Gosnell was a part of NATCO since its inception and he became President in 1981. His extensive experience in procurement and preservation matters with the organ transplant team in the US Air Force and then as a civilian, had great influence on us. The meeting in his San Antonio hometown had coordinator visitors from Holland, England, France and Germany.

NATCO had begun to establish an international presence and became the model for all future transplant coordinators' organizations in the world. Professionally, NATCO has experienced much.

Personally, I became a recipient's wife and a donor's mother. My husband, J. Brin had an irreversible Interstitial Nephritis reaction as a result of the drug Augmentin and required dialysis. Our four adult daughters and one son all volunteered to donate.

More than five years ago, on April 28, 2000 at Johns Hopkins Hospital, Dr. Lloyd Ratner performed a laparoscopic nephrectomy on my daughter Jessica. Dr. Robert Montgomery was J's surgeon. The donor, Jessica, and her 17-month-old daughter, Abby, and J, the recipient, are well today. J., who delivered the first lecture on legal aspects of transplantation at the 1980 Boston meeting.

I found being familiar with the nuances of transplantation to be the most helpful tool for my family, and it became the reason I joined the University of Southern California's (USC) transplant team, under the direction of Dr. Rick Selby, as a community transplant liaison and ombudsman. I've expanded the transplant coordinators' role yet another notch.

Today, I still help patients to Choose Life by arranging for the Gifts of Life.

Thank you.[153]

National Organ Transplant Hearings

Leading up to the organ transplant hearings in Washington, DC in 1983, organ procurement activities were being rapidly organized across the country. Organ transplantation's visibility was at an all-time high. The first National Organ Donor Awareness Week was pronounced for April 24 through 30, 1983 (Figure 5). Organ procurement and transplantation became much more developed during the 1970s, although the graft and patient survival rates remained disappointing by today's standards. After cyclosporine was developed, the field expanded dramatically with transplant centers and OPOs being created throughout the country. There were numerous stories in the press that consisted of pleas from families of dying loved ones for an organ, the dramatic nature of the surgeons' and transplant coordinators' jobs, allegations of profiting from transplantation of organs from foreign nationals, brain death, fairness of allocation, and so

Chapter 1 — THE HISTORY OF THE TRANSPLANT COORDINATOR

on. A young senator from Tennessee held hearings on the issue—Albert Gore, Jr, destined to become Vice President of the United States (Figure 6).

Seven days of hearings were held before two committees.[154-157] Four transplant coordinators testified, representing transplant coordinators throughout the country. Most have likely never read their testimony. Bernard Reams, Jr JD, PhD, professor of law and director of the law library at Washington University in St. Louis, compiled a legislative history of Public Law Number 98-507, and in the three-volume set, included the oral and written testimony of all witnesses during the nearly year period over which the hearings were held.[158] I highly recommend it, because it gives one a glimpse into the history of the field, the challenges faced by coordinators, surgeons, recipients, and others. The coordinator testimony was superb, revealing everything that was right and fine with our field and our colleagues. The transplant coordinator testimony and panel interactions were an integral part of the hearings. The testimony, prepared statements, and interaction with other panelists at the hearings of Donald Denny, Winifred Mack, and Amy Peele are included in the Appendix in their entirety. Gary Hall, an organ procurement coordinator at the University of Tennessee in Memphis, also testified at the hearings on behalf of his program.

Don Denny's testimony predicted and called for many of the improvements in organ donation that we now enjoy. In reading his testimony in the context of other testimony given by multiple professionals, he was bold, informed, and precise in his requests and challenges. His expertise was obvious and was rooted in his practice—which was running an organ procurement organization. Transplant coordinators reading his testimony will be proud of how he represented not only the profession of transplant coordination but also for the improvements he called for in the field of transplantation.

Denny was prescient in his call for collaboration, noting that they could not get the job done alone and calling in his testimony for a national task force, composed of leaders from government, medicine, organ procurement, and interested lay groups to tackle the problems impacting the recovery of organs for transplantation. "It is time that the transplant professionals in this country recognize that they need to involve their colleagues in the medical profession. The neurosurgeons, the neurologists, the critical care medicine physicians, the emergency physicians, the pediatricians should be members of such a task force. They are the physicians who will recognize donors. They are the people who need to be convinced that it is important to work with us. The critical care nurses are by far our most vital ally. They, too, should be involved in a national task force. This task force should be given the charge of coming up with solutions for developing and improving the system nationwide."[143]

As the national co-chair of the 2003 to 2005 national Organ Donation Breakthrough Collaborative, I would say that Denny's words calling for collaboration with other health care professionals ring as true today as they did on that 13th day of April, 1983. He also called for state and national requirements for hospitals to have policies and procedures on brain death, the need for more extensive coverage of regions of the country not served by organ procurement programs, identifying and referring potential donors, to have the Health Care Financing Administration (now CMS) provide financial incentives to those hospitals where the donors and kidneys were recovered, better public and professional education, and drew attention to the "need for better statistical information" on the number and types of donors, contributing to the ultimate crafting of what we now know as the scientific registry of donors and recipients. All of Denny's calls to action were ultimately fulfilled by industry and government.

Denny, Peele, and Mack all spoke of 24-ALERT and the need to maximize the number of organs placed from each donor. In these hearings, this was the transplant coordinator's issue. They spoke eloquently and at length about organ allocation.

> NATCO has also been a major force for the sharing of extrarenal organs. The major system used by procurement personnel to locate recipients for available extrarenal organs is sponsored by NATCO. At this time, approximately 17 transplant centers are involved in extrarenal organ transplantation in the United States and Canada. This number will become swollen during the next several months when at least five additional centers will inaugurate heart transplant programs and another six centers will begin transplanting livers. Last year, NATCO recognized the problem faced by organ procurement personnel in locating suitable recipients for extrarenal organs, which may become available in local community hospitals. The UNOS computer system has great utility in helping to distribute kidneys, but is much less effective in the area of extrarenal organ sharing."[143]

(See Appendix 1 for original transcripts of testimony given by transplant coordinators on extrarenal organ sharing and the need to maximize organ placement.)

Peele called for establishment of an office that very soon after passage of the law came into being—the Division of Organ Transplantation, part of the Public Health Service. "Because of conflicting views and programs developing under federal auspices, I support an office within the Public Health Service to coordinate federal organ and tissue transplantation policies."[159] All three coordinators testifying on behalf of NATCO, Don Denny, Amy Peele, and Winifred Mack, were speaking from their knowledge, expertise, and in-the-trenches view of the field they, along with their transplant coordinator and surgeon colleagues, were helping to develop. The transplant coordinator witnesses made an indelible impression during the hearings. Following the hearings and the passage of the National Organ Transplant Act, HHS Secretary Margaret Heckler named a council, the American Council on Transplantation, to advise her on improving the nation's organ donation and transplantation network. Three of the 25 members were transplant coordinators: Don Denny, Ron Dreffer and Jane Warmbrodt.

The testimony is a fascinating depiction of the birth of the US Organ Procurement and Transplant Network (OPTN). Many of the reforms that were called for by various witnesses came to fruition while others were but ripples in a pond. Charles and Marilyn Fiske, parents of Jamie Fiske, the little girl who received a liver transplant after the first national plea for an organ was made, changed the course of transplantation and gave ethicists and transplant professionals cause for debate that continues today in allocation of organs. Charles Fiske, a Boston University School of Medicine administrator, conducted a desperate media campaign and persuaded the American Academy of Pediatrics to allow him to make a plea before 1000 academy members at their annual meeting in New York City.

Another child, 13-month-old Brandon Hall, and his mother were also at the hearings where his mother testified. His mother was testifying on April 13, when, dramatically, they received a call during the hearings that a liver had been found for him. Brandon Hall ultimately received two livers but died May 12, 1983 (Figure 7). Don Denny's testimony provided in the Appendix refers to the fact that Brandon Hall and his mother were flying back to Memphis for his liver transplant, which was made possible, in part, by the NATCO 24-ALERT system.

NATCO Annual Meetings

The first annual meeting held under the official NATCO name (5th annual transplant coordinator meeting in the United States)[c] was held in Boston in 1980 at the Copley Plaza Hotel. It was the 25th anniversary of the first successful kidney transplant and Dr. Joseph E. Murray, professor of surgery and chief of the Division of Plastic Surgery at Harvard Medical School and surgeon who performed the first successful kidney transplant, gave the keynote address on Friday, June 27. The topics covered at that first meeting[160] of the newly organized NATCO reveal the breadth of the coordinators' roles—topics that are still discussed today. They were:

- A Medical Examiner's Perspective on Organ Retrieval
- The Neurosurgeon's Approach to Ethical Issues in Transplantation
- Psychosocial Implications of Living Related and Cadaveric Organ Donation
- Development of Education Materials Workshop
- Management of the Pediatric Transplant Patient
- Fiscal Issues Relating to Transplant Services
- Organ Preservation Troubleshooting
- Short- and Long-Term Complications of Transplantation
- Management of Hypertension in the Transplant Patient
- Methods for Determining Regional Procurement Potential and Planning Procurement Strategy
- Dynamics of Organ Preservation
- Management of the Cadaver Organ Donor
- Update on Preservation Research
- Patients Speak Out
- Legal Responsibilities Relating to Coordinator Matters
- Organ Procurement—In-Service Approach for Success
- Infectious Disease in the Transplant Patient
- Multidisciplinary Approach to Recipient Education

Annual meetings have continued to be held every year since the beginning of NATCO. The first meeting held in Boston is actually termed the 5th annual meeting since four transplant coordinator meetings had already been held. Every coordinator can remember their first annual meeting and can recall at least one role model from the leaders at the meeting. Annual meetings are organized by NATCO members, a program chair, and include expert speakers for the current topics of the day. For a list of where each annual meeting was held since 1980, see the Transplant Timeline.

Training Courses for Clinical and Procurement Transplant Coordinators

As coordinators continued to network, lean on one another, and develop their profession, they developed training courses for new practitioners. Many of the pioneers in the field mentioned earlier in this chapter were the instructors for the course. The tradition has continued to this time, in 2006, with NATCO presidents selecting training course co-chairs who are responsible for everything from selecting faculty for the course to determining curriculum needs.

By the time NATCO held its first training course for new coordinators in 1982, transplant coordinators had emerged as a profession over the previous 20 years and had their own professional society for three

---

c. NATCO meetings have been numbered from the very first meeting that occurred in Los Angeles in 1975. Although NATCO was created on Wednesday, May 30, 1979 in Chicago, the first official organized meeting in Boston is now actually termed the 5th Annual NATCO meeting. All other meeting numbers have followed that convention through to the present day, with NATCO to have its 32nd Annual Meeting in New York City, August 12-15, 2007.

A CLINICIAN'S GUIDE TO DONATION AND TRANSPLANTATION   Chapter 1

years. Many accomplishments would be forthcoming, but the first order of business had to be training new practitioners. Who could train them? The answer could only be those who were practicing and had developed the field. These courses had terrific clinical and professional content; however, their added value could not be denied. In many ways, they felt like a sorority or fraternity house during pledge week. Close quarters and a full week of training by coordinators in the field fostered friendships and lasting professional contacts. The first training course, one for procurement coordinators, was held on October 17 through 22, 1982 at the Rolling Ridge Conference Center in North Andover, Massachusetts. The course curriculum was developed by 50 coordinators, physicians, and others interested in organ transplantation.

Five-Day Course on Procurement

An intensive five-day procurement course will be offered on October 17-22 at North Andover, Massachusetts.

The course curriculum was planned by more than fifty coordinators, physicians and others interested in organ transplantation. The subject matter for the course has been selected to foster a common background of knowledge and skill amongst Transplant Coordinators, which will promote increased organ donation, uniform high standards in organ procurement, preservation, and distribution, and accelerate the inter-regional sharing of cadaveric organs and tissues.

The curriculum will consist of twenty-one hours of core didactic material and nine hours of clinical opportunities to be selected by the participants. A comprehensive course syllabus consisting of summaries, references, and reprints will be provided for each student.

Many members of NATCO have been involved with designing the course, and the organization highly endorses the work that has been achieved. The course will be integrated into NATCO's education committee, and the intention of that committee is that the course be offered yearly in varying locations throughout the United States. All newcomers to the field of procurement are encouraged to participate in the course. A brochure and registration form may be obtained by contacting Faye D. Davis, New England Organ Bank, Box 235, Boston MA.[161]

Faye Davis was the inspiration and a large part of the drive behind this first procurement training course. She remained intimately tied to the course throughout the rest of her career in organ recovery. She earned the respect of her peers (Figure 8) and was recipient of the very first NATCO/Sandoz Achievement Award for career accomplishments in 1984.

Articles describing the 1984 procurement and clinical training courses, in many ways, could have been written today as several topics and organizational details are the same. The following articles described both courses in the NATCO newsletter:

A TRAINING COURSE ON PROCUREMENT FOR TRANSPLANT COORDINATORS

The purpose of the course is to provide introductory instruction to Transplant Coordinators in the procurement of organs and tissues for clinical allotransplantation. The course was developed as a response to the ever-increasing need for cadaveric organs and tissues. The subject matter has been selected to foster a common background of knowledge and skills amongst Transplant Coordinators, which will promote increased organ donation, uniform high standards in organ procurement, preservation, and distribution, and accelerate the inter-regional exchange of cadaveric organs.

The curriculum is presented in lectures, workshops, small group discussions, and visits to hospitals. Faculty membership is drawn from experienced transplant coordinators, physicians, and other professionals with an interest in organ and tissue procurement, preservation, and distribution for clinical transplantation. The high faculty to student ratio will permit ample opportunity to answer questions and to review unfamiliar concepts according to the needs of individual students. It is recognized that participants will have diverse backgrounds, and the teaching methods will be sufficiently flexible to accommodate special needs for instruction.

Chapter 1: THE HISTORY OF THE TRANSPLANT COORDINATOR

The major topics that will be covered include:

History of organ procurement and transplantation

Independent organ procurement agencies vs. hospital based programs

Identification and management of the multiple donor

Professional education

Public education and public relations

Declaration of brain death

Obtaining permission for organ donation

Legal issues in organ donation

Histocompatibility and the transplant coordinator

Development of a procurement program in a hospital and in a region

Preservation and transportation of organs for transplantation

Professional ethics for the transplant coordinator

Psychological factors of organ procurement

Career opportunities for the transplant coordinator

The role of the transplant coordinator

Organ sharing

The multiple organ donor—surgical considerations

Special emphasis is placed on student participation in exercise designed to promote confidence and ability in interpersonal transactions. The skilled transplant coordinator guides and comforts a family considering permission for organ donation, negotiates adroitly with the hospital program, and persuasively interest physicians in participating in such a program. These skills will be learned and practiced in the conferences and workshops under the tutelage of senior transplant coordinators and transplant surgeons.[162]

A TRAINING COURSE ON CLINICAL CARE OF THE TRANSPLANT PATIENT

The purpose of this course is to provide in-depth basic instruction to the clinical transplant coordinator and nurse in the overall health care of the transplant recipient and family. The course was developed as a response to the ever increasing numbers of transplant recipients in need of specialized care. The subject matter has been selected to foster a core knowledge and skills level amongst clinical care transplant coordinators and nurses which will promote uniform high standards of care for the transplant recipient. This quality of care is designed to ultimately promote the overall well-being of the patient population we serve.

The curriculum is presented in lectures, workshops, small group discussions. Faculty membership is drawn from experienced clinical care transplant coordinators, nurses, physicians, and other health care professionals with an interest in the care of the transplant recipient. A high faculty to student ratio will permit ample opportunity to answer questions and review unfamiliar concepts according to the needs of the individual student. It is recognized that students will have diverse backgrounds, and the teaching methods will be sufficiently flexible to accommodate special needs for instruction.

A CLINICIAN'S GUIDE TO DONATION AND TRANSPLANTATION

The major topics that will be discussed include:

History of Transplantation
Overview of Organ Procurement and the Role of the Procurement Coordinator
Overview of the Role of the Clinical Transplant Coordinator
ESRD—Overview of Etiology and Treatment Options
Histocompatibility
Identification and Work-up of the Potential Recipient
Living Related Donors
Extra Renal Transplantation—(Heart, Lung, Liver, Pancreas)
Peri-operative Care of the Transplant Patient
Immunobiology I—Immunosuppression and Blood Transfusions
Immunobiology II—Rejection Therapy
Infectious Complications of Transplantation
The Non-Compliant Patient
Post Transplant Complications I—Short Term
Post Transplant Complications II—Long Term
Post Transplant Follow-up I—Short Term
Post Transplant Follow-up II—Long Term
Pediatric Transplantation
Psychosocial Aspects of Transplantation
Legal Consideration of the Clinical Coordinator Role
Patient Education—Materials and Methods
Ethical Issues in Patient Care
Time Management and Priority Setting
Expanding Horizons for the Clinical Coordinator
Stress Management

Special emphasis is placed on student participation in workshop format as well as in exercises designed to promote confidence and ability in interpersonal transactions. The skilled transplant coordinator and nurse works with physicians, dialysis units and hospital personnel in a team effort to identify the potential transplant recipient. The coordinator works closely with the potential transplant recipient in accomplishing a pre-transplant work-up. The coordinator works with families to help identify living related donors, where the situation is appropriate. The coordinator is responsible for patient and family education both pre and post transplant. The coordinator is responsible for patient follow-up, and also systems development, to accomplish follow-up as part of the health care team. These skills will be learned and practiced in the conferences and workshops under the tutelage of experienced physicians, clinical care coordinators and nurses.[163]

The first procurement training course was held in North Andover, Massachusetts at a 38-acre retreat composed of rolling hills and lakefront and the 40-room Georgian estate in October 1982. Numerous pictures of this first historic course appear in the photo section at the end of this chapter. Following this first training course, the following article appeared in the NATCO newsletter:

A FIRST FOR ORGAN PROCUREMENT

This October a five-day training course on Organ Procurement was held in North Andover, Massachusetts. The Rolling Ridge Conference Center of North Andover and the New England Organ Bank of Boston provided a warm, New England style atmosphere.

Back to nature…this unique conference center (an old mansion converted into a conference center) was just the ideal site to relax and admire the beautiful autumn trees full of bright and brilliant colors. The mansion was full of New England charm—there were wood burning fireplaces throughout the main floor, and each window gave a fantastic view of the trees, the rolling hills and the lake. The food was good, considering no red meat was served.

The training course was a great success. The course curriculum was planned by 50 coordinators, physicians and members of NATCO. The subject matter provided a concrete background of knowledge and skills shared amongst transplant coordinators. A course syllabus was given to each participant that compiled a number of references, reprints and summaries. Some handouts and brochures were also available. Students found themselves at great ease, talking with other coordinators—small groups were often sites at the end of a period, at break time and during dinner.

Most evident to me was the great feeling of togetherness created and shared by the transplant coordinators, the visiting doctors, and other interested persons that pooled their knowledge, skills and expertise in a unified and a professional manner. This, I felt, made, or added to, an ideal atmosphere for each student. The Thursday night hayride and lobster dinner highlighted New England in the fall. A couple of fun-filled hours on an old-fashioned hayride brought us closer together in the brisk night air. Lobster and steamers graced the dinner table. Thanks to Faye Davis, who gave a quick and easy lesson in eating lobster, the dinner was a success. The evening was then completed by a dance—music from the '50s and '70s. We had a great time!

To Faye Davis and the staff of the New England Organ Bank and to the staff at Rolling Ridge Conference Center, thanks for the warm New England hospitality. You made it all possible! Ivy Vincent, University of Texas, Houston[164]

The training courses have become a rite of passage for coordinators. Perhaps the most important aspect of the meeting is the networking and information sharing. Whether reading early articles like the one above from a NATCO newsletter or hearing participants' comments today, nearly 25 years later, there can be no doubt that the training courses are a formative event in coordinators' careers—particularly of those who stay. I went to the training course in Rolling Ridge the third time it was held—in 1985. There were several other women in the room I was sleeping in—we had bunk beds. I was where I wanted to be—with other new recruits and colleagues. There were approximately 45 people in our class. We received a 2.5-inch-thick three-ring binder full of materials for the course, which had the NATCO logo and the words "A Training Course for Procurement and Transplant Coordinators" on it. The binder was full, and the topics covered in the procurement course included history of transplantation, philosophy of transplant coordination, donor evaluation, management and recovery, hospital development, histocompatibility, organ allocation (in which the NATCO 24-ALERT was taught), bone, skin, and eye procurement, financial management, professional education, stress management, public education and time management. It was a remarkably diverse course and was spread over *seven days*. We had time to bond and to absorb the material. As I was preparing to write this chapter, I pulled out the old binder for the first time in over two decades! In the inside pocket, I found a letter from one of my roommates. That letter captures the intense feelings many of us carried coming into the profession:

Dear Teresa,

Enclosed is our list of "winners" from our awards presentation at Rolling Ridge. It sure was a lot of fun wasn't it? My mind has drifted back there time and time again this week. When the time finally came to leave Rolling Ridge, I felt myself not wanting to leave. Funny thing—I couldn't stand the place the first few days being there. I hated saying goodbye to all those wonderful people and cried a lot on the bus going back to the airport and during the (following) week. Around Wednesday I hit bottom and called you, Jean, Chuck McCluskey, and Amy.

I saw our administrator on Monday and focused on the job responsibilities and qualifications for coordinators. I really opened her eyes but also learned that a new doctor has been appointed interim director of our program. So, tomorrow I'm off to see him too. Right now I'm fighting for a full-time position and salary as an organ procurement coordinator. There is no such position at the "_____

A CLINICIAN'S GUIDE TO DONATION AND TRANSPLANTATION

___" Medical Center yet—three of us "so called" coordinators do the procurement as an on-call thing, so it's a lot of convincing. I'm giving them one year to get this going then I'm considering relocating. But, I've never wanted anything more than this and am so anxious to get going (written communication, procurement course participant to Teresa Shafer, November 3, 1985).

The experience portrayed in this letter was shared by many coordinators in the early days who were drawn to the passion of the field, fighting for the position and ready to commit heart and soul. I could not have imagined writing this chapter 21 years into the future and am therefore glad that I did not discard the letter since it so aptly demonstrates the sense of dedication and commitment of individuals entering the profession. The person who wrote it is no longer in the field. Married with children, it was probably hard to sustain the kind of drive evidenced in the letter with the lifestyle required of a coordinator. Now, in 2006, partially because of the nursing shortage, we no longer have registered nurses and other qualified applicants bashing in the door to get in, but it was not so in the beginning...

The Clinical Coordinators Course was held at Seven Springs Ski Resort that November. I also attended that class since my job early on was like that of most coordinators: performing both recipient coordination and donor procurement. From the beginning, I wanted solely to work in an organ procurement capacity, however, and soon got my wish when the hospital hired a recipient transplant coordinator. In other parts of the world, transplant coordinator training courses continue to prepare practitioners for the transplant coordinator profession.[165-171]

Transplant Coordinators and Organ Sharing

Transplant coordinators were ingenious in the methods they used to procure and share organs. In the early to mid 1960s, they were working through the complexities of sharing kidneys from non-heart-beating donors when the preservation science was still being learned. After recovering kidneys, if both could not be used, they were calling other programs to see if they had a use for the other kidney. There was no organized sharing system because it was before SEOPF or UNOS. Bob Hoffmann, a transplant coordinator who started in 1964 (see Early Pioneers section), recalls they could drive 400 to 500 miles with a machine to do a recovery, but were often woozy when they got there. "That's a long way!" The preservation machines were not truly portable and had to be transported in a truck or van to the donor recovery site.

In talking to Bob about the photos of early preservation machines, I told him that I had found online a story written by Dr. Belzer about the possibility of being crushed by one of these machines during transport. Bob immediately said he remembered the incident well. Bob Hoffmann's comments follow those of Dr. Belzer's below:

> In August 1967, a middle-aged man with amyloidosis presented with renal failure, but because of his systemic disease, he had not been considered suitable for dialysis or for kidney transplantation. I had just harvested a kidney, which was placed on the preservation circuit in the laboratory. I worked alone in San Francisco at this time; Najarian had left for Minnesota, and Dr. Sam Kountz would not arrive until several months later. I discussed the option to accept this kidney with the patient; he accepted. The transplant was performed with a total preservation time of 17 hours. The kidney functioned immediately, although not perfectly, and hypothermic perfusion preservation of a human kidney had become a reality.[172]

> We were still unsure of human kidney tolerance to hypothermic preservation and, consequently, wanted to begin perfusion preservation immediately after harvesting the kidney in the donor hospital. However, we did not have a machine that was sufficiently portable to carry to the donor hospital. An unattended laundry cart was found in the hospital corridor one night and was immediately requisitioned for use in our laboratory. With the expertise of Chester Truman from the instrument shop at Moffin Hospital, the laboratory perfusion equipment was modified to fit onto this cart. It was a wonderful machine to behold because everything moved. The membrane oxygenator, one of the first built by the Waters Company, consisted of a silastic envelope in which the fluid was oxygenated. This moved with a rocking motion. The pulsatile pump, organ

chamber, and arterial and venous reservoirs were all made in the laboratory but functioned surprisingly well. It took two or three people to move the machine, and with a rented Avis truck and a forklift we were able to travel to any hospital in the vicinity. The first few times we used this perfusion machine, one of our procurement technicians, Ken Steeper, would drive the truck, while Bob Hoffmann and I sat in the back, supporting and steadying the perfusion machine with our feet. Subsequently, we decided to secure the machine with ropes tied to the truck, which was a fortunate idea. On one of the trips we had to stop suddenly to avoid an accident. The ropes held the machine, but the force of the stop caused the steel frame of the perfusion cart to bend. Had this happened on one of our previous runs, Bob and I would undoubtedly have been crushed by the machine![173]

Bob remembers that he and Dr. Belzer had been loading the machine onto the Avis truck one time and an old man was watching them said, "*I am watching you guys and you are not doing it right. That is not going to work. If you have to brake, those are not going to hold.*" They were going to Stanford. They did have to brake and fortunately the sage advice had spared them since they were not sitting where they normally would have sat.

Bob also remembers that on returning to San Francisco, Dr. Belzer complained about how dangerous the Avis truck and transportation setup was and that someone was going to get hurt, which was overheard by a kidney recipient. Soon, funds were raised by the patient and a van was purchased for transport—a van with a raised roof, cables for securing the preservation machine, a portable generator and a nice seat in the back for the coordinator to sit on. "*It was beautiful. Soon everyone was coming to look at it and then they got one.*" Multiple pictures of these kidney vans can be seen in the photo section. The Avis rental truck experience endured by Bob Hoffmann and Fred Belzer enabled others to benefit (*oral communication, R. Hoffmann, BS, CPTC, June 2, 2006)!*

Surgeons and their laboratory assistants were at the forefront of these early transplantation attempts. G. Melville Williams remembers the early surgical years:

> Although the pathophysiology of antibody mediated rejection was established, this did little for the Medical College of Virginia (MCV) transplant program, which was supported entirely by an NIH grant which paid for hemodialysis. This fixed the number of patients waiting for cadaveric grafts. We had binding commitments to our transplant patients to sustain life, which meant that patients rejecting kidneys comprised an increasing proportion of our recipient pool on hemodialysis. All too often we could not use perfect kidneys because our recipients had antibodies cytotoxic for donor lymphocytes. This dreadful wastage of organs could be corrected if there were greater numbers of recipients. Since there was no way to pay for this, we offered the organs to other centers. These cooperating centers would send us kidneys they could not use. Even better, we could send serum from our immunized patients to other centers, so that they could do a cross-match and send us organs they could not use but we could on the basis of serological testing. Thus kidney sharing began as a way to salvage transplant programs and prevent the wastage of organs. It was borne of necessity.

> The concept was accepted readily by Dr. Bernard Amos of Duke, who saw to it that the typing labs of co-operating centers were on the same page. The idea caught on rapidly. The rationale was simple; the larger the pool of donors and recipients, the greater the chance of successful matching of donor and recipient. When payment for dialysis through Medicare came into being, large dialysis units were established, and, sharing to be able to transplant at all, soon turned into sharing for the best histocompatibility as the HLA system was discovered. However, the benefits of remote cross-matches and tissue matching never reached early expectations. All too often a donor site negative cross-match became positive when performed at the host center, resulting in a wasted effort, and, even worse, a wasted kidney on many occasions. Those of us in the Southeast who started and systematized organ sharing were distressed because as many as 28 percent of kidneys recovered were never transplanted despite well-intentioned efforts. This was particularly true for non-blood group O kidneys because O type kidneys were all too often transplanted into

non-O recipients, leaving behind immunized blood group O patients on dialysis (G.M. Williams, MD, written communication, October 2005).

Kidney sharing was later accomplished through the Southeastern Procurement Foundation (SEOPF), but in those early years, extrarenal organ sharing had been implemented and accomplished by transplant coordinators through NATCO. The coordinators developed a system for transplant programs to list their patients awaiting extrarenal transplantation. Coordinators called the 1-800-DONORALERT hotline and printed lists of patients.

I clearly remember, as a new organ procurement coordinator, being proud knowing that the organ sharing system in the United States for hearts, livers—extrarenal organs—was developed and run by transplant coordinators. I remember making those calls into 24-ALERT and getting recipient information. The coordinators who developed and ran this system were my role models, my colleagues! I suspect that few of today's coordinators realize that the first organized sharing system for extrarenal organs was developed, implemented, and operated by transplant coordinators. This was pre-UNOS. As always, the coordinators had a need and blazed their own trails.

24-ALERT System

In September 1982, NATCO inaugurated the 24-ALERT System[d] which provided transplant coordinators with immediate knowledge of potential extrarenal organ recipients. It became operational on April 4, 1983. NATCO spread the word about the readiness and operation of 24-ALERT throughout the medical industry, and its availability was reported widely in scientific journals and the media.[174-180] In its first three years of operation, 24-ALERT was responsible for the successful recovery of more than 700 livers, 600 hearts, and 22 heart-lung blocks.

In 1985, the following article detailing 24-ALERT first appeared in the NATCO newsletter:

The need for extrarenal organs (hearts, heart-lungs, livers, lungs and pancreas) for clinical transplantation is increasing. Approximately 17 extrarenal transplant centers are now active in the US and Canada. None is able to provide sufficient numbers of extrarenal organs from local donors to satisfy center transplant needs fully. A large pool of potential donors is available, however, through collaboration with the approximately 120 renal procurement programs in North America, which generate more than 2,500 kidney donors annually. The development of surgical techniques for successful multi-organ retrieval has encouraged many renal procurement programs to consider cooperation with geographically distant centers in the recovery of extrarenal organs.

Successful intercenter collaboration requires detailed communication of extrarenal organ needs to the renal procurement programs. Since extrarenal donor requirements change frequently, the need for an economical communications system that could be easily updated and be readily accessible by procurement personnel 24 hours a day was recognized by the North American Transplant Coordinators Organization (NATCO). The UNOS computer system, which has proven to be of great value for distribution of donor kidneys, was determined to be of less utility for this purpose because of cost, inability to access the system without a computer terminal (e.g., in a donor hospital), limited use among organ procurement programs in the US and complete lack of use in Canada.

---

d. Members of the NATCO Multiorgan Procurement Committee Ad Hoc Study Group to develop 24-ALERT were Herb Teachy, Medical College of Virginia, chairman; Don Denny, University of Pittsburgh, secretary; Anita Principe and Peter Kuemmel, Montefiore Medical Center, New York; Judy Dickens and Miriam Zamble, St. Louis University Hospital; Bill Vaughn, Aetna Insurance Company; Mike Phillips, University of Alabama; Bob Grant, Greater Baltimore Organ Procurement and Perfusion Center (GBOPPC), Baltimore; Gary Hall, University of Tennessee; Louise Loring, Baptist Hospital, Birmingham; Tom Hagen, Phoenix Transplant Center; Ron Dreffer, University of Cincinnati; Mel Cohen, Multiple Organ Retrieval and Exchange (MORE) Program, Toronto, Ontario, Canada; Michael Bloch, University Hospital, London, Ontario, Canada; Mitch Goldman, International Society for Heart Transplant; Steve Sammut, Delaware Valley Transplant Program, Philadelphia; and E. Jane Van Hook, University of Minnesota.

Chapter 1: THE HISTORY OF THE TRANSPLANT COORDINATOR

On September 23, 1982, NATCO inaugurated a recorded telephone message system to disseminate information concerning extrarenal organ donor needs to procurement programs throughout the US and Canada. Accessed easily from any telephone 24 hours-a-day, the recorded message details the extrarenal organs sought by each participating center, the donor criteria and the donor referral phone number of the extrarenal center's organ procurement program. Updated p.r.n (generally every day), the system is provided at no cost to all renal and extrarenal procurement programs. Named the NATCO 24-ALERT SYSTEM; from its mnemonic telephone number, the service has been utilized by 15 extrarenal transplant centers to list organ donor needs during the first five months of its availability. During this same interval, 72 extrarenal organs were recovered by 10 of these extrarenal centers in collaboration with 48 kidney procurement programs as a direct result of information secured from the 24-ALERT System.[181]

Articles about 24-ALERT abounded in scientific journals, magazines, newspapers, newsletters, and other printed materials (Figure 9). The NATCO archives contains dozens of them. The media was fascinated with the role of the coordinator, and they got it right, as evidenced by this excerpt:

"If a call to the 24-Alert computer should result in a match with one of Teachey's waiting recipients, his goal is to respond as immediately as is humanly possible. He can't waste valuable time. If Virginia should turn down the offered tissue, it must be done quickly in order for other centers to have an opportunity to evaluate the organ donor. But when the team elects to "go," it sets a complex machine in motion.

For all the technology and medical expertise that are brought to bear in this operation, the most sensitive moments involved in any gift of living tissues are those when the donor's family is asked for their consent. For this man who administers a budget of $1.5 million annually and has participated in hundreds of procedures, all that had gone before is as nothing. Each instance of contact with the people who must grapple with the decision of whether to extend their lost loved one's life in a fellow human is as new as his first experience, and medical science becomes irrelevant. No case is ever easy. But Teachey brings a unique awareness of the human spirit with him. And in every case, the family's wishes are honored absolutely and without question.

Herb Teachey doesn't persuade a donor's family to make a decision so much as he opens up their awareness to an option they may not have considered. He introduced the idea of providing a spark of good from the tragedy of loss. And when he unlocks the generosity that makes humankind unique among living creatures, the people who must make the decision can take comfort in the quiet awareness that they have, in a sense memorialized their loved one through an act of kindness. The questions surrounding organ transplantation will undoubtedly be argued for centuries but Teachey and the families he reaches are touched by a process that transcends the controversy and goes to the very center of the human sprit. In the end, their feelings tell them they have done the right thing.

Teachey describes MCV's team as "fast and good" in an area of medical practice where just being good is not enough. Speed is vital in several areas. First, the center must preserve its long-term reputation for reaching a decision on an offered organ without delay; Teachey strives for five minutes.[e] Then it cannot afford to blunder on the transportation and coordination—an entire discipline in itself."[182]

See back cover of this chapter for full page photo of Teachey that appeared in *Raytheon Magazine* in 1985.)

Bob Duckworth wrote an article for the 30th anniversary NATCO newsletter on the history of 24-ALERT:

---

e. Author's note: My administrative assistant proofed this manuscript and her notes in the margin, next to the five minute quote from Herb Teachey says, "Is this right? 5 minutes???" Maybe they were good old days, after all...

24-Alert Organ Sharing System

By Bob Duckworth, BS, Consultant, St. Jude Medical, Inc., Bellevue, NE

"This is the NATCO 24-Alert Organ Sharing System…" Many a long night started out with those words. 24-Alert was a system started by NATCO and several multi-organ (or "extra-renal" in that day's parlance) transplant centers in the early 1980s to help locate available organ donors for their waiting non-renal transplant recipients. At the time, the computer sharing systems available had very limited or no extra-renal listing capabilities, and something had to be done. [Renal sharing was handled by the SEOPF (Southeastern Organ Procurement Foundation) and UNOS was a fledgling voluntary organization.]

24-Alert started out as a humble answering machine in the offices of "TOPF", the Transplant Organ Procurement Foundation at the University of Pittsburgh (later the Pittsburgh Transplant Foundation) in the early 1980s. TOPF coordinators would receive listing information from transplant centers via phone and would simply record messages describing the needed organs and pertinent recipient parameters on an answering machine tape to which anyone could dial in and listen. The idea was that the coordinator could call from the donor ICU, listen to the recording and then contact the appropriate centers with waiting patients. This worked very well until the number of transplant centers and recipients listed simply got to be too numerous and difficult to manage. Toward the end of the tape version of the system, recordings could run 20-30 minutes.

The problem was there wasn't any way to stratify the listings to the donor that one might have. If you had the misfortune to have a blood type "AB" donor, you had to sit and listen to the complete recording to be certain that no "AB" recipients were hiding at the end of the recording.

This was not very efficient, and as today, transplantation could be a bit stressful. It was hard to hang on the phone listening to 24-Alert, manage your donor, AND fight off the transplant surgeons all at the same time. "When are we going to the operating room?!"

Efforts to find a better system began. Personal computers were just becoming available in those days, and the thought was that this would be a really great way to deal with what was still a small effort to list several dozen individuals waiting for a transplant. The only problem was that there wasn't a good method of accessing this data while in the ICU managing a donor. None of us wanted to lug a computer terminal around with us.

Enter VOTAN, a cutting edge company in what was then the "Silicon Rut", the forerunner of the Silicon Valley of California. VOTAN had a new system that was capable of operating a personal computer by voice command. Boy, was it ever expensive! Remember, these were the early days and big money and little function were the watchwords of personal computing.

NATCO began to raise funds to purchase the necessary hardware, and those of us at TOPF began to scratch our heads trying to figure out how to make all of this work. Remember, we were entering the digital age armed with our extensive knowledge of the use of analog telephone answering machines and donor management.

Enter Rick Sheppeck, a Pittsburgh medical student who moonlighted as our whipping boy at TOPF. Professing to have some knowledge of computer programming, Sheppeck proceeded to write the code to run the new, improved digital 24-Alert system. Of course, he wrote it in the cutting-edge computer language of that day, K & R "C". He did this while going to medical school, working with us at night, and I think he had a local garage band at that time, as well. Needless-to-say, he slept just about as much as we did in those days.

Now the NATCO 24-Alert system was state-of-the-art. Callers would go through a "brief" training routine to teach the machine to recognize their voice and then could answer questions, enter donor data, and respond to prompts by speaking. Recipient waiting lists would be sorted by organ needed, blood type and weight parameters and matched recipient results were audible output spoken by Sheppeck's recorded voice from the computer. It was the cat's pajamas. Mind you it wasn't particularly pretty to listen to, but it worked.

Even more important, the coordinators at TOPF could input recipient data by typing it into the database. No more two-hour, 5:30 p.m. recording sessions in the guts of Scaife Hall to update the system for the evening's donor onslaught. (Yes, donors always happened at night back then too.) Recipient data could be updated without lengthy off-line sessions.

24-Alert went through several iterations of VOTAN speech-recognition hardware, each improving its function and utility to the transplant community. Finally in 1986, with the advent of UNOS as a national contractor/sharing system, NATCO transferred 24-Alert to UNOS, and the last chapter in the history of the NATCO 24-Alert System was cast into time. (See Figures 10 and 11; see photo of UNOS President, G. Melville Williams, presenting UNOS Resolution to Steve Haid, President, NATCO.)

NATCO leadership was significant to the success of the 24-Alert system in all of its forms. The Pittsburgh personnel who maintained and operated the system on a daily basis were also critical to its success. NATCO led the way to better organ sharing and service to waiting patients as it should, and as it does, today.[183]

The following testimonial appeared in a 1984 NATCO newsletter from a coordinator in the field:

24-ALERT—HOW IT WORKS FOR ME AND ALL OF US!

"A long time ago" I used to receive calls (during business hours) from Herb Teachey of MCV and John Kiernan from NYCP to inform our program of an urgent need usually for one of their patients who needed a heart transplant. Most often those phone calls were directed to larger volume organ procurement agencies and population centers just due to percentages for procurement. Once the heart was procured, I'd receive a phone call back from those centers (usually during business hours the following day) informing me that there was no longer a need. In addition to those calls every month since early 1981, our program received a list of all the patients awaiting liver transplants at the University of Pittsburgh.

That "a long time ago" was just last August! Literally hundreds of phone calls might have taken place in order to procure just one heart. It was soon evident that a system was needed 24 hours a day to organize these procurement requests, especially since more centers were planning to perform extra-renal organ transplants. The coordinators saw that need and developed that system through NATCO's Multi-Organ Procurement Committee. Hence the birth of NATCO's 24-ALERT on Sept. 23, 1982. In this article I hope to show the ease in which 24-ALERT can be utilized and how it helps make the coordinator's job more effective, professional, and efficient.

Getting to Info. The idea is simple—24-hour access to needs of the patients waiting for extra-renal transplantation in the US and Canada for all organ procurement coordinators and it is as close as your nearest telephone. From our program at the DVTP telephone access is very important since we have six organ procurement coordinators on call covering 143 hospitals in a 250 mile radius. A portable computer terminal for each of us would be costly and possibly unreliable since it would sit in the back of a car in heat, cold, and bumpy roads. In practice once I have identified a donor, I will then dial 24-ALERT to determine what organs are needed before approaching a family for consent. Usually this is done from the ICU. When I dial 24-ALERT, I hear a description of the organs needed, the size and body weight, the blood type, whether a crossmatch is necessary, other data such as main stem bronchus diameter for lung transplants, when the patient needs to be transported to the recipient center, and of course the contact person and phone number. In addition the most important entry about the transplant patient is the priority status. Priority 1 represents patients with extremely urgent need. Priority 2 are patients hospitalized but stable. Priority 3 represents patients at home waiting for a transplant.

This enables the organ procurement coordinator to select which appropriate extra-renal center to call.

The Contact. With donor information at hand, I usually make a preliminary phone call to the target recipient center to discuss the donor information and most importantly whether the recipient transplant center will be available for harvest at the time the donor will be available for harvest. Finding out about time delays now increases the success of the organ procurement. Once final lab studies have been completed and the donor is approved, I then make my final approach to the family for extra-renal organ donations. Prior to this final discussion, only general discussion on organ donation is my routine.

Because of 24-ALERT our program during a three-week period in July and August, retrieved five multi-organ donors with three different transplant centers. As the number of extra-renal organ transplant centers grows and the needs of those recipients increase, the organ procurement coordinator will be routinely performing multiorgan procurement harvests. The 24-ALERT systems will continue to update and watch those needs because we the coordinators will see to its ongoing development. Howard M. Nathan, Delaware Valley Transplant Program, Philadelphia[184]

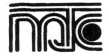

NATCO
North
American
Transplant
Coordinators
Organization

4 April 1983

Dear NATCO Member:

We, the Executive Council, are proud to announce to our members our newest accomplishment, 800-24-DONOR. This is a national donor referral number sponsored by NATCO and available 24 hours per day for professionals who have questions or problems regarding a donor. They will be referred to the appropriate center listed. 800-24-DONOR is in effect as of today, April 4, 1983.

Along with 412-24-ALERT, it is temporarily based out of the University of Pittsburgh. If you have any further questions, please contact your Executive Council or any of the coordinators at the University of Pittsburgh.

Sincerely yours,

Winnie Mack

Winnie Mack
President

Chapter 1: THE HISTORY OF THE TRANSPLANT COORDINATOR

The NATCO archives contain dozens of letters and other various correspondence regarding 24-ALERT. It was a vital, functional program belonging to coordinators and making it possible for them to save more lives. There were regular updates in every NATCO newsletter with the numbers of organs shared. Ron Dreffer, in his closing remarks at the ninth annual NATCO meeting in Minneapolis, listing all of NATCO's accomplishments that year, included, "And, our *own pride and joy*, NATCO 24-ALERT: 213 livers, 136 hearts, six heart/lungs."[185]

Coordinators did whatever it took to make sure the organ was transplanted. The logistical details of such arrangements can often lead to an entire evening between friends, sharing such war stories. Pumping kidneys in the early days required extended travel time for coordinators who were often already exhausted from handling the donor case for 24 to 48 hours. Jim Springer remembers:

> One most memorable case involved the proverbial "hop, skip, and a jump" from Kansas City to San Antonio. Back in the '70s, we used a company plane to fly kidneys to most destinations in the Midwest region. I had a case where one kidney was going to Little Rock, the other to San Antonio. We flew in bad weather to Little Rock and transferred one kidney to their preservation machine, only to discover the weather deteriorated so badly (fog, storms, etc) that we could not proceed. After checking with the USAF and finding they were also grounded, the FBO operator said it was too bad we couldn't get to Texarkana since one of their planes was stuck there due to the Little Rock weather. Being industrious (and stupid) coordinators, we checked with the Arkansas Highway Patrol about the possibility of getting help with the 150 mile trip to Texarkana where I could then catch the private plane to San Antonio. They agreed and I was pleased to think that I could get an hour or two of sleep in the patrol car as we traveled through Arkansas since I had already been up overnight (we used to routinely handle the cases from start to finish in those days). But no, no, no—it turns out the patrol cars were restricted to certain regions or counties, so I had to transfer from one car to another to another about every 20 minutes… forget the sleep. Then we arrived at the uncontrolled airport in Texarkana where the pilot was eager to get into the air because of course… the weather was getting worse and worse. We climbed into the plane, fought through some lousy weather and communication issues with ATC and, finally, arrived in San Antonio… only to find the airport at bare minimums. With a little luck, and perhaps a bit of illegal dipping below minimums to find the airport runway strobe lights, we landed, and I successfully transferred the kidney to the OPO staff. Then off to the usual uncomfortable airport seat for five hours before a commercial flight back to KC. Another day's (or two) work in the glory days of procurement coordination (*written communication, J. Springer, BA, CPTC, February 9, 2006*)!

Ken Richardson, at the time a procurement coordinator at Jewish Hospital in Kentucky at the time, remembers:

> It was early 1981 (I remember because I had recently married). I had completed the recovery of two kidneys from a 22 y/o WM SP MVA. The recovery took place at a small community hospital in Kentucky. The patient had an elevated serum creatinine, but I knew he was dehydrated. Long story short, I had trouble placing the kidneys, and the SEOPF Kidney Center suggested I take them to Dr. George Abuna in Kuwait City. I was waiting on a call back from ROPA in LA. They were interested in one kidney but it was taking time to find the recipient. I couldn't wait any longer so I left one kidney on ice, in case ROPA wanted it. I took the other kidney, on the pump, to Kuwait. It was quite an experience.
>
> I took a charter plane from Louisville, KY to New York City. It was a Thursday. Kuwait Airlines, coincidentally, had a regular flight between NYC and Kuwait City, leaving Thursday and returning on Sunday. They held the plane for me. I had no luggage other than the pump, three backup batteries, a hand pump, extra ice, and sterile supplies in the event I had to take the kidney off the pump. I had no change of clothes, not even a toothbrush.
>
> By the time the kidney was placed, I had already been up for 24 hours. The flight from NYC to Kuwait City took 14 hours (stopover in London, England). When I arrived in Kuwait City it was dark. I had no idea what day it was. Staff from the hospital met me at the plane and took me

straight to the hospital, bypassing customs. At the hospital, the cassette was transferred from my Waters portable to a base unit. I was taken to the Sheraton Hotel where I collapsed into bed. The next day, a driver took me around to clear up any customs issues and I got a tour of the hospital and the city. This was a Saturday. I was still very confused due to lack of sleep, but on Sunday I got on a plane and returned to NYC via London. The movie was Star Wars (the original now called episode IV, A New Hope).

It was an amazing adventure but one I never wanted to repeat. I have never been so exhausted and jet-lagged. To the best of my knowledge, the recipient did well. It was hard to get follow-up. ROPA didn't take the other kidney so I could have taken both to Kuwait City. It is something I won't forget *(written communication, K. E. Richardson, MBA, February 6, 2006)*.

Many coordinators have had the experience of an organ being dropped on the operating room floor. Both Paul Taylor and Jim Springer recall the effects of dropping organs and the subsequent function in the recipient. Paul Taylor remembers doing this in the dog laboratory and transplanting the organ after the drop. He recalled discussing with Dr. Starzl that this was bound to happen and that they should study it in the lab to show if there would be any ill effects. Jim recalled:

> ... a story about the positive effect of dropping kidneys on the OR floor. We had an opportunity in the mid-'70s to transplant kidneys from the same donor into two twins who had the same kidney disease. We felt this could be a great case to write up as we could compare the post-transplant function and rejection episodes to see if the kidneys followed the same course. The first transplant was done and we moved to the second patient when the surgeon (note: it was the surgeon, not the coordinator!) was moving the kidney from the Waters preservation machine to the basin when he accidentally dropped it on the floor (a preview of ER and television programming yet to come!). After a few choice words cutting through the silent OR, the surgeon examined the kidney carefully, asked for antibiotic solutions, and proceeded. The best part of this story is that the kidney that was dropped functioned like a champ immediately, while the other had a period of ATN and delayed function" *(written communication, J. Springer, BA, CPTC, February 9, 2006)*!

It has happened that organs have been dropped, although such events are exceedingly rare. The few instances that happened in the early days normally revolved around the kidney being placed in the bag and the bag having a defective heat seal, thus, a hole, in the bottom of the bag. For this reason, coordinators do such transfers now over the basin. If the bag has a hole in the bottom, the worst that could happen is for it to enter the basin.

H. Keith Johnson, MD, in his chapter on the development of OPOs, correctly opines that everyone has their stories. "During these early days of transplantation, retrieval of the organ for transplant proved to be as much of an adventure as the transplant itself. Every program that was active during this era accumulated its own mythology regarding the donation process. The kidney that spilled out of the cooler onto the floor of the resident's car was subsequently rinsed off with saline and transplanted without postoperative problems. A Stewart Preservation machine was impounded (kidney and all) in a secluded hanger at the Chicago airport until a bomb squad could examine and proclaim its safety."[129(p48)]

Extrarenal Transplant Programs (circa 1984)

One could imagine that it was not so difficult getting through the list with the few extrarenal programs there were in the early days of transplant coordination. A 1984 NATCO newsletter contained the list of extrarenal transplant programs:

Hearts
    USA
Stanford University, Stanford, CA
Medical College of Virginia, Richmond, VA
University of Minnesota, Minneapolis, MN
University of Arizona, Tucson, AZ

Texas Heart Institute, Houston, TX
University of St. Louis, St. Louis, MO
University of Alabama, Birmingham, Alabama
Methodist Hospital of Indiana, Indianapolis, IN
Columbia Presbyterian Medical Center, NYC, NY
Johns Hopkins University, Baltimore, MD
University of Pittsburgh, Pittsburgh, PA

Canada
University of Western Ontario, London, Ontario
Institute of Cardiologie, Montreal, Quebec
Notre Dame Hospital, Montreal, Quebec

Livers
USA
University of Tennessee, Memphis, TN
University of Minnesota, Minneapolis, MN
New England Deaconess Hospital, Boston, MA
Massachusetts General Hospital, Boston, MA
Yale University, New Haven, CT
University of California, Sacramento, CA
University of California, San Diego, CA
Louisiana State University, Shreveport, LA
Good Samaritan Hospital, Phoenix, AZ
University of Pittsburgh, Pittsburgh, PA

Canada
University of Western Ontario, London, Ontario

Heart-Lungs
USA
Johns Hopkins University, Baltimore, MD
Stanford University, Stanford CA
Texas Heart Institute, Houston, TX
University of Pittsburgh, Pittsburgh, PA

Canada
University of Western Ontario, London, Ontario

Pancreas
USA
University of Minnesota, Minneapolis, MN
Mount Carmel Hospital, Detroit, MI
University of Cincinnati, Cincinnati, OH
Louisiana State University, Shreveport, LA
University of Miami, Miami, FL
University of Pittsburgh, Pittsburgh, PA
University of Wisconsin, Madison, WI

Canada
University of Western Ontario, London, Ontario[186]

Transportation of Organs

Flight attendants and other airline personnel were often involved in the drama of shipping kidneys across the country in the early days. The following "Captain's Announcement" was published in a 1983 NATCO newsletter:

CAPTAIN'S ANNOUNCEMENT

A captain's announcement regarding
    two special passengers:
In case you are curious about
    all the commotion
In front of the plane, as
    We got into motion
We've got two guests, who
    are traveling first class.
They've got special lunches. They're
    carried in glass,
They're living creatures, with no
    eyes, ears or nose.
They look like they're scared,
    lying flat and exposed.
They're glad to be with us, glad
    they are alive
And the greatest thing is
    that today before five
They will enter the bodies of
    two human beings.
As a gift from a donor
    neither has ever seen
After years of dialysis, pain
    and frustration,
Two people today will have
    the elation—of
Living a normal Life!
So we welcome those life
    saving guests on board
With this donor's gift—our
    spirits have soared
Among all the wonderful people
    we please
Our priority passengers today
    are these
    Two Kidneys!

    Tom Scanlon
    Washington, D.C.
    Eastern Flight #190
    11-10-82
    12:30 p.m.[187]

Chapter 1: THE HISTORY OF THE TRANSPLANT COORDINATOR

Procurement coordinators faced many challenges in arranging for transportation of organs. They continue to face and overcome challenges as this story of a more recent vintage demonstrates. Joe Nespral, who now works in San Antonio, but previously worked in Puerto Rico, has an incredible story of what must be a record-breaking ischemic time on a heart transplant as well as a mode of transport larger than normal:

I think it was in 1995, I was trying to place a pediatric heart from a donor at the Childrens Hospital in San Juan, Puerto Rico. After multiple attempts to place this heart had failed due to prolonged ischemic times because of the distances around the country, I made the offer to Loma Linda thinking that there was no way they would accept. When they responded that they would accept, but needed some time to make flight arrangements I was shocked. The Loma Linda coordinator called me back stating that they needed more time to figure out the flight arrangements because the Lear jet they usually use could not make the flight without stopping for fuel. Since they were willing to push the ischemic time due to the distance, they could not add any more time having to fuel up. So after a while she called me back saying that they might have found a solution to flying non-stop from California to Puerto Rico. They were working on chartering either a DC9 or Boeing 727. We set up an operating room time for about 15 hours later and waited. Finally, Dr. Bailey arrived with an assistant and his coordinator on that big jet flying non-stop for approximately 11 plus hours. We went to the operating room after formal introductions were made to all of the hospital administrators and chiefs of staff who had come to welcome the famous Dr. Bailey. The baby heart was beautiful. Dr. Bailey recovered and packed it and took the time to personally thank everyone in the operating room, maintaining his cool. The follow up was that they had successfully transplanted the heart with a record 12 plus hours ischemic time. Unfortunately the recipient died days later, but the heart was working perfectly; the patient died from other complications —not from the donor heart (*written communication, J. Nespral, MD, CPTC, June 18, 2006*).

Transplant Coordinator Research and Publications

NATCO Newsletters

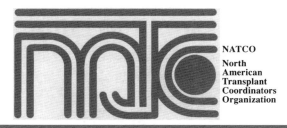

Dedication:
That there be a better quality of life for the thousands of patients with end-stage organ failure...and a respect for those who shared.

NATCO
North American Transplant Coordinators Organization

Newsletter Volume 1, Number 1
To provide a forum for the exchange of information relating to all fazes of transplantation.

The image above shows the masthead for the first newsletter.[188] NATCO was to retain this look for many, many years, until the masthead was revised in 2003. There was one thing that did change before the next newsletter and that was that "*fazes* of transplantation" changed to "*phases* of transplantation"! Number 2 of volume 1 was appropriately changed.[189]

NATCO, as detailed in its first newsletter, was "born" at 2 PM on Wednesday, May 30, 1979 in Chicago, Illinois. The return address on the newsletter:

NATCO
North
American
Transplant
Coordinators
Organization

Newsletter

C/O ROPA
1000 Veteran Avenue
Los Angeles, California 90024

The NATCO newsletters open the door to understanding how the transplant coordinator role developed over the years. Fortunately, the central office kept historical copies of all of the newsletters, dating back to the first in 1980. Newsletters were forthcoming immediately after the formation of NATCO in 1979. Julie Hall and Mikki Masteller of the UCSD Medical Center were the first editors in 1980, followed by Roger Smith at the Regional Organ Procurement Agency in Los Angeles from 1981 to 1982, and later by Mary Ann House at the Medical College of Georgia in Augusta from 1983 to 1990. The early editors did it all, because NATCO did not have a management firm with a home office location until many years later. Indeed, the return address on the newsletter was the address of the OPO or transplant center at which the editors worked. The editor's personalities at times peaked through the scientific and organizational content, making it all the more interesting.

The NATCO newsletter's role in rapid development of the profession cannot be understated. It was where everyone came to keep in touch. Notices were sent out, written inquiries served as modern day listservs (albeit, months slower), and articles, meeting announcements, and job openings were posted. Opinions flowed freely, and by reading those early newsletters, one can see how driven and talented this new group of professionals was. A 1980 article in *Dialysis and Transplantation* noted that NATCO's "lively newsletter" went to more than 500 coordinators, transplant surgeons, nephrologists, and immunologists.[1]

The newsletter topics revealed that transplant coordinators had pressing needs, both operationally in their day-to-day jobs and professionally, in their quest to increase their knowledge base. In that first newsletter, there were articles titled "Having Problems Finding a Home for Kidneys?" Robert Gosnell, South Texas Organ Bank, San Antonio, Texas and "Dealing with the Families of Renal Donors" by Dave Mainous, transplant coordinator at Indiana Medical Center and Veterans Administration Center in Indianapolis. In "The Perils of Organ Transportation," Robert K. McAtee, of South Texas Organ Bank in San Antonio describes a kidney cassette rupturing at 24,000 feet and his backup plan of having the flight attendant don mask and gloves and assist in packaging the kidney, using the extra plasmanate and sterile bags he carried for just such an emergency. "Have Solution—Will Travel" is an article by Louise Loring, heart transplant coordinator from the University of Wisconsin, who relates an organ offer from Dave Mainous for an "A" blood group heart, wanting to know how soon they could get there. In her article she talks about the age limit for cardiac donors being 35 years old for women and 40 years old for men![188]

There were six committee reports in the first NATCO newsletter in 1980: Ethics Committee, Legal Committee, Scientific Committee, Education Committee, Membership Committee for Procurement Personnel, and Membership Committee for the Transplant Nursing Professional. These transplant coordinators got busy, immediately after the first meeting where NATCO was officially formed.

Excerpts from NATCO committee reports in the first NATCO newsletter follow:

From Ethics: "Integrity must be the foundation on which we build respectability among our colleagues and the public." Chairperson: Cecil Gunter, Northwest Kidney Center, Seattle.

From Legal: "Currently, some 20 states have a 'Brain Death Law', and a number of others have proposals in consideration. This revolution has brought about a substantial increase in the use of cadaveric tissue and organs for transplant." Chairperson: Michael L. Merriman, PA, Transplant Coordinator, Bowman Gray School of Medicine, Winston-Salem, North Carolina.

From Scientific: "The immediate goals of this committee will be to work in conjunction with the Program Committee to help maintain a wide variety and high quality of scientific presentations at our meetings." Steve Haid, Washington University School of Medicine, Department of Surgery, St. Louis, MO.

From Education: "One of the greatest challenges we face as members of NATCO, is in the area of education. A large share of our activity on a day to day basis directed toward education, specifically, to patients, professionals and the lay public." Barbara Schanbacher, RN, Transplant Coordinator, University of Iowa Hospitals, Iowa City, IA.

From Membership, Transplant Nurses: "There are times of happiness and sadness in our everyday dealings with transplant nursing. However, nothing is more comforting to realize through exposure to other transplant programs that we are not alone in the trials and tribulations in the care of the transplant patient." Linda L. Jones, RN, Ohio State University Hospital, Columbus, OH.[190]

From Membership, Procurement: "As chairman of the membership committee for the professional procurement personnel, I would like to encourage you to become a member and support the activities of NATCO. As an administrator of an organ procurement agency, I am excited by the formation of NATCO as a formal group and feel that it will meet the needs of a variety of occupational titles in the field of transplantation that have been neglected.

I was part of the original formation of this group when one of our surgeons suggested a potential need for transplant coordinators to meet with each other from all over the country and exchange ideas either formally or informally. What was gleaned from the first steering meeting of 35 individuals was that everyone had a different educational background and each one, although having this general title of Transplant Coordinator, had quite unique occupations within this particular title.

I have attended each of the early workshops that have been organized and watched as this original group of 35 expanded to over 200. I have also had the pleasure of meeting and sharing ideas with so many of the people I talk with on the telephone in my daily routine from around the country and formed lasting friendships with many of them in this past four years.

NATCO was formed by both nursing and non-nursing personnel in the field of transplantation and is unique because it seems to bridge the wide gap that has existed for so long between dialysis and transplantation. I think as a group this gap will disappear and form a very cohesive union that will undoubtedly benefit the one person we are all working for, the ESRD patient." Chairperson: Roger C. Smith Jr. ROPA of Southern California, Los Angeles, CA.

There is no doubt that the spirit of the coordinator is evident from the very first newsletter. The content of these newsletters captured the very essence of their jobs. They were clearing new ground. These were individuals who were venturing forth into hospitals without transplant programs, reviewing patients who might be candidates for donation, educating nurses and physicians about the need for organ donation, brain death, the legal requirements for consent, and everything else needed to create a dynamic system of surveillance, referral, and recovery of organs from potential donors.

The newsletter was a place for problem solving. Throughout the newsletters, coordinators posted pieces about problems they had encountered and solved, or inquired about whether or not someone else had yet dealt with an issue they were facing. The following article is a good example of a coordinator sharing his ingenuity in ensuring that a kidney was not discarded. It was in the very first issue of the newsletter:

The Perils of Organ Transportation

What would you do if you were transporting a kidney by air from your home base and as the aircraft ascends to its proper altitude, the bubble trap on the cassette ruptures?

Well, it happened to me while en route to Augusta, Georgia with a very good kidney. My first reaction was complete helplessness. 24,000 feet in the air and the perfusate was running all over the transport module and the seat. Then I realized that in my travel bag were four (4) sterile bags and a 240 cc bottle of plasmanate for just this kind of emergency.

This backup procedure is as follows:

(1) Turn the machine off, get the flight attendant to help you and instruct him/her to put on cap, mask and sterile gloves. (2) Open the sterilization bag and have the flight attendant remove the sterile plastic bag. (3) Place half the plasmanate in the first bag. (4) Put on sterile gloves, disconnect kidney from the cassette and place it in the bag with the plasmanate and tie it with heavy silk, or tie the upper part of the plastic bag. (5) Put plasmanate in the second bag and place the first bag inside the second one and tie it securely. Place the bagged kidney in the ice compartment of the transporter. If you have two kidneys on the machine the same procedure can be followed. I hope this type of incident will never happen to you, but one never knows what can happen while in flight.

Robert K. McAtee
Supervisor of Organ Preservation
South Texas Organ Bank, Inc.
San Antonio, Texas 78228 [191]

Bob McAtee's was a nice story to include here for several reasons:
- It was in the very first issue of the newsletter, a newsletter that took off immediately in the spirit of the life these early coordinators lived—improvising and making it happen.
- It illustrates the point that coordinators have always been ingenious in problem-solving complicated logistics.
- It demonstrates that the newsletter was a meeting place for coordinators to share ideas.
- It serves as a reminder to 21st century coordinators of how far we have come in having a more systematic existence in our jobs.
- It shows us that flight attendants are certainly less flexible in their willingness to take on new job duties today than they were in the old days!

Progress in Transplantation (formerly Journal of Transplant Coordination)

Since the beginning, transplant coordinators have been an integral part of transplant teams worldwide, in the scientific arena as well as the procurement and clinical setting. Their names have appeared as authors and coauthors of historic articles in major journals attesting to their contributions to transplant advancement. [24(p330)] A basic tenet of a profession is that its practice is based on research and that practice is improved through research. Transplant coordinators published their research in other transplant, medical, and nursing journals before the establishment of their own scientific journal in 1991. Talk of a journal had been ongoing for some time; however, the cost considerations were formidable. The NATCO board of directors nonetheless made the commitment to fund a journal for transplant coordinators. Barbara Elick, NATCO president in 1990, was the driving force behind the journal and was the founding editor. Gayl Chrysler and Anita Principe were assistant editors (for more about Barbara Elick, see NATCO Presidents).

The Journal's focus was, and has remained, international in scope and facilitates communication between all disciplines of transplantation. The content ranges in scope from scientific research to clinical application of that research and case studies. The first issue of the journal presented such topics as state-of-the-art information on organ and tissue donation among minorities, a literature review of infectious disease transmission through organ and tissue transplantation, donor coordination activities, tissue banking, other ethical issues, and pertinent legislation affecting the transplant community. The second issue of the journal featured the proceedings from the Division of Transplantation's first annual meeting.

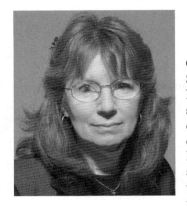

Linda Ohler, Editor, 1994

The next major change came in 1994 when Linda Ohler, RN, MSN, CCTC, was named editor-in-chief. Linda remains in that position today. She was recently recognized as a Fellow of the American Academy of Nursing and has spent the past decade building the journal's reputation and soliciting manuscripts from throughout the industry. Gayl Chrysler stayed on and Teresa Shafer was added as an associate editor. Coordinators have continued to publish their research and have been helped in this regard as Linda and others have consistently offered writing and publishing classes at NATCO annual meetings. The journal was published three times a year until 1996 when it was increased to four times per year, where it has remained. The quality of manuscripts has increased over the years. It was indexed in 1997. The journal publishes a broad range of peer-reviewed clinical and procurement articles and profession-oriented material for transplant professionals. The journal seeks to provide content that is relevant to and reflective of the growing diversity of the professional transplant community. It also welcomes letters to the editor, case studies in procurement and clinical aspects, clinical practice papers, original research, quality assurance guidelines, and special reports on professional, educational, economic, ethical, and medical-legal issues.

In 2000, the name of the journal was changed to *Progress in Transplantation*, to reflect the broader nature of its contributing authors and to appeal to a broader readership. As stated earlier, the journal has had an international reach. In 1999, other transplant coordinator societies were given the opportunity to formally specify *Progress in Transplantation* as the scientific journal for their membership. *Progress in Transplantation* is now the official publication of NATCO, The Organization for Transplant Professionals; Australasian Transplant Co-ordinators Association; Society for Transplant Social Workers; and is endorsed by the Association for Nurses Endorsing Transplantation; Canadian Association of Transplantation; International Transplant Coordinators Society, Japan Transplant Coordinators Organization, United Kingdom Transplant Coordinators' Association, and North American Liver Transplant Social Workers.

Transplant Coordinators in the Press

Transplant coordinators, particularly procurement coordinators, were often in local, national, and international press (Figure 12). Their job was dramatic and required expertise that only a handful of people in the world possessed. They knew the system since they helped create it, and they were adept at wading through the morass of legal, ethical, clinical, and logistical issues involved in donor referral, consent, clinical management, and coordination of operative recovery by multiple teams. Further, on the recipient side of transplant coordination, the transplant coordinators negotiated the same, often thorny issues in the transplant evaluation, preparation for the operation, education, and the post-operative follow-up care.

Coordinators were a favorite subject of the media and no more so than during the mid-1980s after the success of cyclosporine spurred clinical activity in all areas of transplantation. In a May 2, 1983 issue of *People* magazine, a picture of Brian Broznick, procurement coordinator for the University of Pittsburgh, standing on the airport tarmac, with his foot on a cooler, staring off into the distance with a Lear jet in the background, covers the entire page with the title on the adjacent page, "The Desperate Hunt for Life." The article begins:

A CLINICIAN'S GUIDE TO DONATION AND TRANSPLANTATION

Last Dec. 7 organ procurement coordinator Brian Broznick was driving home from a TV studio in Pittsburgh, where he had just appeared on an evening talk show, when his electronic beeper alerted him to an urgent call: A liver, 559 miles away in Nashville, Tenn., was available for transplant. Broznick, 31, rushed home to set in motion an elaborate plan that cost $65,000 and eventually involved dozens of doctors, nurses and medical technicians. Twenty-four hours later a dying man had a new liver. Broznick helped save his life.

In the two years since he joined the University of Pittsburgh Transplant Foundation, the nation's largest and busiest transplant center, Broznick has retrieved hundreds of organs. But most of his work involved livers. Ninety percent of the nation's liver transplants are performed in Pittsburgh, since Dr. Thomas Starzl—who pioneered the surgery in Colorado in 1963—joined the Pittsburgh staff in 1981. Last year alone, the foundation's three organ procurers obtained 80 livers for the surgeons, and Broznick, who was involved in more than half of the procurements, proved himself indispensable to the phenomenal process of organ transplants. "I play a major role in what goes on," he says. "All of us who do this work are a tightly knit group."[192]

The article takes the reader through one scenario, from start to finish of Broznick's job in coordinating a liver recovery and allocation of the organ to a waiting recipient. Further quotes from this article point to the coordinator's expertise, the demanding nature of the job, and the unquestioned commitment of those working in the field:

- Some 300 organ procurement coordinators around the country belong to NATCO, and through it match donors of livers, kidneys, pancreases, hearts, lungs and corneas to recipients whose lives can be saved or transformed by these organs.
- Broznick must travel more than 100,000 miles a year in pursuit of available livers. The work is physically exhausting—he's on call 24 hours a day, seven days a week—and emotionally draining.
- He sometimes spends hours with the donor family to explain the need for organs. "I really *live* this job," he says. "People depend on me for their very life."
- His schedule leaves little time for family pleasure—holiday dinners and movie dates with his wife are often interrupted by Broznick's beeper.
- The hardest part of his job is encouraging reluctant families to donate their relatives' organs. If a potential donor is within 150 miles of Pittsburgh, Brian approaches the family himself. Otherwise, they will be approached by an organ procurer in their own region. "I try to get the family to discuss their feelings, to vent their grief. If I have to sit with them for 10 hours, that's fine."[192]
- In the last paragraph of the article, the author writes "For that unexpected new life, Lessley [the recipient] knows he can thank the generosity of Victor Brock and his parents." The article then concludes with the following, and last, sentence "And, of course, the dedication of Brian Broznick." [emphasis added][192]

Later that year, on August 29, 1983, the cover of *Newsweek* magazine depicted the cover story: "The Replaceable Body: How Transplants Save Lives."[193] This article, like the *People* magazine article, begins with the coordinator and the tremendous commitment he lives:

At 10:30 a.m. the phone rings on the desk of Donald W. Denny, coordinator of organ transplants at the University of Pittsburgh School of Medicine. The caller on the other end, Burt Mattice, Denny's counterpart at Miami Valley Hospital in Dayton, Ohio, wants to know if surgeons at Pittsburgh can use the liver of a local five-year-old boy who has been struck by a car, suffering irreversible brain injury. He has been pronounced legally dead, but is being maintained on a mechanical respirator. Denny knows that 1,100 miles away in San Antonio, Texas, another five-year-old boy is dying of an incurable liver disease and has been waiting for just such a donor. Denny goes into action, triggering a precisely timed plan for saving the child's life.

Denny alerts the parents of the San Antonio boy and they immediately arrange to fly with their son to Pittsburgh. Then Denny, Dr. Thomas Starzl, the country's leading liver transplant surgeon, and a surgical assistant, Dr. Shin Yang, take a hospital van to Allegheny County Airport where they board a chartered jet for Dayton. Arriving at the Dayton hospital, the surgeons don scrub suits and perform a two-hour operation to remove the dead child's liver. Denny, meanwhile, calls Starzl's team at Pittsburgh Children's Hospital and signals them to start removing the San Antonio boy's diseased liver the minute he arrives.

After removing the donor liver in Dayton, Starzl chills the organ with a salt solution and places it in an Igloo picnic cooler for the return trip to Pittsburgh. On the plane back, Starzl, Denny and Shin relax with a few beers. When they arrive at Children's Hospital, their patient is fully prepped and, over the next four hours, Starzl and surgeon Byers Shaw install the new liver. A week later their young patient is doing fine."[193]

And, like the *People* magazine article, the *Newsweek* article contains many quotes revealing of a coordinator's commitment, professional responsibilities, and outlook on life:

For Donald Denny, 48, it was a routine day's work. So far, this year has been even busier than last when he and his associate, Brian Broznick, 30, traveled 77,000 miles to obtain 102 kidneys, 80 livers, 22 hearts, and three sets of hearts and lungs for transplantation. "Calls come in at 2 in the morning, on Christmas Day," says Denny. "I had to leave before dinner on my daughter's 16th birthday. And transplant coordinators at many of the nation's 156 medical centers where such surgery is performed are leading similarly hectic lives."[193]

The October 1984 issue of *American Way* ran an article, "The Gift of Life," with the subheading: "From the relatively young science of organ transplantation has emerged a new breed of professional: the transplant coordinator, who is charged with matching donor organs with recipients."[194] Amy Peele, transplant coordinator for Rush-Presbyterian-St. Luke's Medical Center in Chicago, was the subject of the article. Herbert Teachey, transplant coordinator for the Medical College of Virginia (MCV), and a private pilot himself, was in two publications concerning jet transportation and transplantation. *Raytheon Magazine* featured Teachey in a several page article. The full page photo of Teachey is included at the end of this chapter. In the article, he remarked that it was fair to say that MCV pioneered long distance organ transplantation in 1977.[195] Paul Taylor, transplant coordinator for the University of Colorado graced the cover of *Odyssey West*[137] and was also featured in an *Ebony* article the following year.[196]

The "bookends" of this chapter are the full page photos of transplant coordinators that were run as a full page photo in the magazine in which they appeared.

24-Hour-a-Day/7-Day-a-Week Dedication

Many staff who hired on to this exciting new job, soon to become a lifelong career for many, in the early days clearly remember the siren call of the exciting work, the autonomous practice in a new profession. Collaborative practice with surgeons, and the idea of working in small, elite teams with the noble goal of saving lives was irresistible. It was irresistible, whether one's background was as a registered nurse, laboratory technician, physician's assistant, dialysis technician, or other health care-related background. This was a new field of practice: it offered to the practitioner the opportunity for creative and flexible practice as well as a truly equal place on a team that included transplant physicians and surgeons. That the "trade-off" was often long and unpredictable work hours was one many were more than willing to take.

The field has become much more organized and has adopted the trappings of mature organizations (executive management, human resources, communications and marketing staff, improved staffing schedules, etc). But transplant coordinators from the early days remember small and intimate organizational meetings or journal club meetings over wine with colleagues and surgeons. The rules were few, and the work was exciting, fulfilling, exhausting, and ultimately, "defining" of the profession.

Transplant coordinators work hard. The industry struggles today to retain qualified staff. The "excitement" of the job; the novel, trailblazing aspect of the field has waned over the years as the field has matured. Early articles about the role of the transplant coordinator were uniform in their assessment of their work environment.

Clearly, the work of the transplant coordinator is not for everyone: Inherent in these rare people is a willingness to work—work extremely hard—with their counterparts all over the world. The 24-hour availability factor in their job description winnows out the faint-hearted. Sophisticated computer systems link transplant centers, carrying information from state to state and country to country, searching out the right donor, the right organ, the properly matched recipient; but in the end, it is people who must make the system work. The coordinators' efforts are concentrated on putting all transplantable tissue to good use; they are acutely aware of the need of the patient and the generosity of the donor.[1]

The job demanded time and ultimate commitment in order to build the profession and overcome challenges in practice, many of which have already been covered. Our job was unique, thus there was plenty of room for creative thinking. I entered the field in 1985—eager to get in. Coming from a critical care background, this role seemed a dream one—autonomous clinical practice in close collaboration with other coordinator and physician colleagues on a team! Hospital nursing on the other hand, was well defined, structured, and predictable. Even though I had advanced into administrative positions in critical care, I clearly remember pushing and making it happen to become a full-time transplant coordinator. From the ground up, I was part of a small team that built a hospital-based OPO. The excitement of working autonomously and collaborating with transplant surgeons, nurses, and executives in multiple hospitals throughout a defined service area was new and exciting. I thought it was an ideal job for a critical care nurse and gladly left my position as assistant director of critical care to begin a completely new career—that of a transplant coordinator. Dr. Starzl, in his book *The Puzzle People*, speaks of Paul Taylor, being swept away by the transplant passion, when he spoke about him moving into an "organ procurement officer" position. It was that way for many of us. It was a phenomenon I was to observe over and over throughout my career. As organ donation and transplantation became mainstream, however, fewer coordinators have had to enter this way—fighting their way in sometimes—and have had shorter tenures. We are now in a position of trying to recruit individuals into this position that may not have the same appeal as it once did.

Working 24 to 36 hours was routine, and 48-hour marathon shifts were not uncommon. The 48-hour stints would happen when there were several cases or one's partner was out of town. We joked about it (Figure 13), and it led to an incredible closeness between coordinators and the colleagues they talked to day and night. Only coordinators could do our job. There was no staffing agency to call for the next shift. When potential donors presented themselves, the window of opportunity was small, and the task had to be accomplished right then and there or that opportunity was lost forever. Because there were times of no activity, these opportunities could not be missed. This was a time in my life when I was single and dating. I met my future husband while I was a coordinator; so he knew what he was getting into. The job was exciting and was interesting to others—a great topic of conversation at "social gatherings." I am sure that if truthful, most coordinators would say that a small piece of them identified with "Chip Masters, Organ Courier."[f]

Bob Duckworth, who started in 1973, gives a more realistic viewpoint of family life and of the long, long work hours:

Life on the Cutting Edge of Medicine or
Why your spouse is mad at you all of the time.

I have to tell you that a career in transplantation is a mixed blessing. On one hand, we all had opportunities that we would have never had in other fields of medicine.

---

f. Chip Masters was a fictional character occurring in a comedy skit on an NBC program—"Friday Night"—somewhat along the lines of "Saturday Night Live." Actor Dave Thomas parodied Richard Harris in Camelot costume playing a liver patient strapped to a gurney needing a liver transplant. Actor Buck Henry played the father of the potential donor—(a young woman who was brain dead) and who was asked to donate her organs, and the star, Steve Guttenberg, played an organ procurement coordinator. When we meet Chip Masters, Organ Courier, he is on a date with a highly paid glamorous fashion model (of course), played by Candace Bergen. He is in a lab coat (typical braggadocio, of course!) and has his cooler with him at the restaurant. His antics in some cases cut close to the bone and in others parodied the dramatic nature of our jobs …running through an x-ray machine with a cooler with a dog showing interest in the cooler to the distaste of the airport screeners, implying MD "status" with the family, informing the potential liver recipient that a liver has been found, and all with a super-cool, super-confident shtick.

Chapter 1: THE HISTORY OF THE TRANSPLANT COORDINATOR

On the other hand, some of us exacted a terrible toll on our personal lives and those we loved who made up that life. I can only tell you of my experiences. Others will perhaps speak of theirs, though they may well choose to leave these memories buried. Maybe that is the wisest course.

I was fortunate to have entered this field six months out of undergraduate school. This was of value, as I knew of no other adult life aside from that of the transplantation service. My spouse and I simply grew as a married couple thinking that being on call, working 48 hours straight, and all that went with having a job as the principal factor in a life together was "normal". Only as we matured and had other experiences with our life did it become apparent that we weren't like "normal" people; people who could plan, do, and live in an 8-to-5 world.

Still we adapted and made the best of what the "job" dealt us. Children came, grew and did the things that children do in a normal life. The only issue was that "daddy" wasn't always there. Daddy was at work much of the time. I'm told that I made the important events, though to be truthful, I can't remember all of them. Seems sleep-deprivation might have had something to do with that. More about that later as we move forward. I do remember flying off just hours after my second child was born. My chief-of-service took care of my wife post-partum and she was understanding. At least she said she understood.

My family adapted marvelously to the task of transplantation. The kids were pretty normal; my spouse was a key player in the communication nexus that became our house. She could be counted on to relay current information to surgeons, other transplant coordinators from all over the country, and as I recall, even posted a few cases for us in the O.R. 24-hours-a-day, she answered the phone and told people what was happening with the current case. She was an integral part of the team even though she never left the ground or scrubbed a single case. My colleagues were her colleagues as well. We went to meetings together where she became known to those with whom I worked and called friends and fellow sufferers. In short, she was the best partner I could have, and the process and job became ingrained in our lives together.

Others weren't so lucky. Human relationships are frail and difficult at best. Transplantation is a demanding profession. Many of my colleagues' relationships didn't survive the requirements of a career in this field. I don't know how the divorce rates among transplanters compare to that of the general (normal?) public, but I can only surmise that they are much higher. Those experiences happily (and sadly) belong to others.

Sleep:

I quickly learned that sleep is the most important commodity that anyone in transplantation can possess. There was never enough. This is true for all of us; there were and still are, no exceptions. The lack of sleep is a constant in medicine, but that lack is much more acute in transplantation.

We lived in a "normal" 8-to-5 world. Meaning those with whom we needed to interact to "run" the business of transplantation—administrators, vendors, businesses outside the hospital, educators, etc.—all worked normal hours. We were forced to work these hours as well to make certain that our services ran smoothly and that we could accomplish all the myriad issues that were necessary to operate organ recovery programs

Transplantation runs on the exact reverse of this schedule i.e. we worked quite literally from 5-to-8 in our clinical practices. Donors were "declared" on afternoon/evening rounds typically. The operating rooms were pretty much off-limits to us during the daylight hours. Couldn't interfere with the "day" schedule with trivialities such as organ recovery procedures. The surgeons we worked with had "normal" practices that required them to be in the clinic or office during the daylight hours. We all put on our transplantation suits as the sun went down. We were off to take care of the donors and get the organs our patient required to live. Off into a darkening sky to a faraway place to meet in a strange operating room to participate in a rather strange act—organ recovery.

A CLINICIAN'S GUIDE TO DONATION AND TRANSPLANTATION

We slept on the airplanes, we slept in the ambulances taking us into the hospitals, and we slept in the OR lounges waiting for our rooms to turn. Falling asleep in the OR wasn't unheard of. One surgeon I worked with was famous for his ability to sleep almost never. He would however sleep whenever and wherever he could and was adept at finding cubbyholes in which to sleep wherever he went. We took his example to heart.

In my 25 years in the field, I guesstimate that I missed about five year's worth of sleep. A damn long time to be awake in my opinion. I've been "out" now for eight years and seem to have almost regulated my sleep patterns to normal periods.

There is hope for the reformed transplanter.
(written communication, R. Duckworth, BS, CTBS, CPTC, January 20, 2006)

Although in the early days the hours might have been longer because there were fewer people in the field, there were also fewer rules with which to contend. I remember when the donor chart was only two pages long—one actual sheet of paper, printed front and back! In fact, in an early NATCO newsletter, there is a call for OPOs to provide "uniform and complete donor data and to adopt the same donor form."[197] This should sound very familiar to today's practitioners as well since we continue as an industry to promote a uniform donor chart. There was a sample form from Delaware Valley Transplant Program in the newsletter that other OPOs could have had printed inexpensively. The form was one page, front and back. Today, the donor chart itself is, at a minimum, 30 pages long!

The endurance needed by a coordinator is not only for working long hours, but also for emotional strength. It is the transplant coordinator who stands between the grief of a family in loss and the possibility of a life-saving transplantation. All coordinators have their own stories about sharing intimate moments with families during the consent process, and although they appreciate the positive outcomes of such contact, they also know that the experiences are often quite draining.

In one consent situation, the young 17-year-old daughter of parents going through a nasty divorce became a potential donor following a sudden accident. The mother wanted to donate, but the father found out and was staunchly opposed to donation—primarily due to the mother's wishes to do so. As a coordinator trying to work through this type of family situation, I was finally facing the following two comments and positions by the parents. The father was saying, "If you proceed with the donation, I will contact my lawyer," and the mother said "if you don't proceed with donation, I will contact my lawyer." Our legal advisor was contemplating the positions of acts of commission versus acts of omission when the younger sister settled the issue. She bravely stood up and addressed both parents, saying her sister had told her she wanted to be an organ donor if anything had ever happened. With that brave statement, the father realized he was wrong, and the donation proceeded (written communication, J. Springer, BA, CPTC, February 9, 2006).

This story is not as dramatic as many consent situations that continue to occur every day somewhere in the country. That is one thing that has not changed over the years—there is nearly always drama, tension, and conflict to overcome in these situations, but at the same time, unbelievable fulfillment, as transplant coordinators know that they are privileged to share such intimate moments with incredible donor families.

Clinical Transplant Coordinators take their work home with them. Like the procurement coordinator, they roll 24 hours a day, taking calls at home from patients who are waiting for an organ, who are post-transplant, or from their family members. They educate patients and families and manage disease processes before and after transplantation. They also share intimate moments with people at the best—and worst—of times in their lives. They frequently advocate for patients during the acceptance committee meetings, offering insight into patients' motivations and ability to successfully handle the transplant scenario. It is the transplant coordinator who normally spends more time with the potential recipient, recipient and their family.

Chapter 1 — THE HISTORY OF THE TRANSPLANT COORDINATOR

Transplant recipients remember their transplant coordinators. They share pictures of their child who has now had his first school day, prom, graduation and wedding. These patients are enormously grateful, and the rewards for the clinical transplant coordinator are hard to measure. They connect with their coordinator so much so that they are often upset when the coordinator quits or leaves the transplant center. "Some patients feel that being a coordinator is almost like being a nun. There is no quitting—it is a lifetime avocation" *(oral communication, former clinical transplant coordinator, September 2006)!*

This opportunity for saving lives and making human connections is one that all transplant coordinators enjoy. Clinical transplant coordinators also have to have a certain toughness to carry the patient through the experience. I enjoyed Gutkind's book because he chose stories from the hundreds of vignettes he observed during his four years of following transplant teams that poignantly points to the sometimes frustrating bond existing between transplant coordinators, potential recipients, recipients, and their families. The following excerpt from *Many Sleepless Nights*,[26] relays two stories involving Sandra Staschak, Senior Transplant Coordinator at the University of Pittsburgh.

> But patients are not always appreciative, especially as the wait for a donor organ goes on and on; they often become very angry and they will frequently vent their anger on the social worker or most especially the coordinator, rather than the surgeons, with whom they have cast their fate. Staschak tells of one woman, the mother of a teenage son waiting for a transplant, who "blew up" one day at the outpatient clinic. "She just went crazy, screaming and yelling at me that we were letting her son die. She came back to my office later and apologized, but before she did that she went shopping in a supermarket, got angry with another shopper and punched him."
>
> Unfortunately, patients can only see their own case, they feel themselves declining on a daily basis, and they always think that they are the sickest person; they can't even imagine that there could possibly be anybody sicker than they are. I myself would probably do the same thing. If I've got ascites [swelling in the abdomen], and I was itching like crazy…"How can you tell me there is anybody sicker?" But in reality, I know we have to take the whole list into consideration.
>
> "What makes you mad, however—it's so terribly frustrating—is when you are trying to help a patient, *trying to help them live a little longer,* and no matter how much they complain and how sick they are, they simply will not take one measure of responsibility for themselves."
>
> Later that day, at the outpatient clinic, Sandee Staschak confronted a yellow-faced woman in her early thirties, in a lightweight denim jacket.
>
> "Where were you Saturday afternoon?"
>
> "I was in my apartment."
>
> "You were *not* in your apartment. I called you up. There was a liver for you. There was a donor that matched. You keep complaining you've been waiting so long and here, we had a liver in your blood type and size, and I called you in. But you weren't there."
>
> "…And then I got the police to dispatch a car, so someone could knock on your door. So I know that you weren't home. We can't help you here unless you cooperate with us," said Sandee, staring at the woman, nodding vigorously, sighing deeply, tears welling up in her round blue eyes, "So how about it?"
>
> The woman received her liver transplant soon after.[26(pp205-207)]

Certification of Transplant Coordinators

During the early 1990s, the field of transplant coordination grew exponentially as the proliferation of transplantation centers and OPOs was made possible by the success achieved with the introduction of better immunosuppressive regimens. In 1985, NATCO established the Credentialing Task Force, chaired by Louise Jacobbi. This eight-person task force drew from experts within the now diversified field of transplant coordination. Procurement coordinators, perfusion technicians, hospital development personnel, clinical transplant coordinators, kidney placement specialists, public education personnel, administrators, and others who worked in the field were loosely termed transplant coordinators. In 1986, the NATCO membership voted to establish a national certification program.

This task force investigated various methods of certification used by other allied health professionals in America. They were challenged with developing a testing process that was valid, one that would be recognized by other professionals in the country. Eventually, a two-tiered system was decided upon: two tests would be offered, one for procurement coordinators and one for clinical coordinators. There would be no grandfathering of coordinators currently practicing in the field. Each practitioner would have to pass the examination if they so chose, to establish recognition of their own expertise.

In 1986 and 1987, the NATCO board of directors launched national certification with the funding of the first job analysis survey.[g] The task force was expanded. Each person on the task force, representing different expertise in the field, drew in four-to-five other such experts each in their field of expertise, expanding the core group to approximately 32 individuals. Other specialists were sought to provide input into the process of developing such a certification examination. The task force consulted those for whom we provide services: trauma surgeons, neurosurgeons, transplant surgeons, and hospital and OPO administrators. From this group of experts, questions were developed to send to the transplant coordinator industry.

The transplant industry was then asked to weigh each task as to its relative importance and frequency. These questions composed the first job analysis survey. The survey was designed to determine what it was that the transplant coordinator professional did in order that a test could later be developed, appropriately weighted, and testing expertise for those tasks within the scope of practice of the transplant coordinator.

The survey was sent to all transplant coordinators, to 1200 transplant surgeons and physicians, and to OPO administrators. This first job analysis survey was sent to many in the field of transplantation. Clinical and Procurement Advisory Committee meetings were held to lend expertise to the development of the test matrix and questions.

In July 1988, the American Board of Transplant Coordinators (ABTC) was incorporated as a separate body from NATCO. The first examinations were held with test fees of $250 per candidate, and in 1989, NATCO was awarded a $66,000 federal grant to maintain the certification program.

Certification is the formal recognition of practitioners who have met the eligibility requirements, and who have demonstrated knowledge of information for safe and effective practice in the discipline of transplant coordination. The intent of the entry-level certification program is to provide assurance to health care consumers that a certified practitioner has successfully completed an examination assessing knowledge, experience, and skills required for entry level and safe, effective practice in the disciplines of transplant coordination.

Promoting "standards of practice" and certification of coordinators assures the public and health care consumers that practice within the discipline is performed by competent professionals. A certification or credentialing program promotes the establishment of excellence in the discipline of transplant coordination.

The certification process establishes group identity and promotes common goals:
1. Defined standards of practice
2. Encouragement of educational endeavors
3. Advancement of credentialed practitioners
4. Advancement of the discipline of transplant coordination

Responsibility for certification includes providing a program that adequately and fairly evaluates the knowledge, skills, and practice of an individual for safe and effective practice and providing credentials to those practitioners who meet the required level of competence.

---

g. This was the first job analysis, funded and conducted by NATCO in 1986 and 1987. However, certainly previous job classifications were shared at the dawn of the first meetings of coordinators in 1976 when they began to meet and shared job descriptions, and later, when Claire Day, noting that there was no such requirement for a transplant coordinator in the ESRD regulation, in 1981 wrote the Office of Standards and Certification, Health Standards and Quality Bureau in Baltimore. She and co-workers forwarded a paper stating the intent and qualifications of including the critical role of transplant coordinator in the regulation (see Figure 14).

Chapter 1 — THE HISTORY OF THE TRANSPLANT COORDINATOR

The American Board of Transplant Coordinators

The American Board of Transplant Coordinators (ABTC), now the American Board for Transplant Certification, was organized in 1987 as the national certification board to promote competency, safeguard high quality performance, and promote adherence to standards of practice in transplant coordination (Table 6). The ABTC provides a process of certification for health care professionals practicing in the field of transplantation. The ABTC, through its credentialing efforts, has provided the means to promote national standards to evaluate professionalism of transplant coordinators. The formation, function, and organization of the ABTC was initiated by an appointed presidential task force of NATCO, the professional society of transplant coordination. The findings and recommendations of this task force were approved by the professional society with the understanding that the ABTC, when incorporated, would function independently as the credentialing body for the profession of transplant coordination.

The creation of ABTC was modeled after the guidelines of the National Commission for Health Certifying Agencies and is an independent, nonprofit, voluntary certification organization. The ABTC is composed of recognized transplant specialists whose primary purpose is to credential professionals in accordance with the *Standards of Practice* as set forth by the profession for transplant coordinators.

The ABTC has specific purposes and has had numerous accomplishments (Table 7). The ABTC does not define requirements for hiring practices in any transplant or organ procurement facility nor does the ABTC define who shall or shall not practice in any category of transplant coordination. This has been defined by the job analyses, which resulted in the *Standards of Practice* published by NATCO. The ABTC has the ability to confirm credentials of practitioners for employers and agencies that reimburse for services of practitioners.

Candidates for Certification

Number of coordinators taking and passing the certification examination each year:

Year	Procurement (CPTC)	Clinical (CCTC)	Total
1988	179	131	310
1989	143	114	257
1990	96	93	189
1991	101	94	195
1992	107	119	226
1993	117	92	209
1994	115	105	220
1995	71	96	167
1996	75	94	169
1997	97	108	205
1998	105	90	195
1999	92	110	202
2000	95	111	206
2001	64	21	85
2002	82	72	154
2003	84	76	160
2004	70	75	145
2005	78	89	167

The ABTC offers examinations for certification in transplant coordination to individual practitioners. Candidates are notified of their performance on examinations and are issued certification in accordance with predetermined requirements. Examination items and content are composed and/or reviewed by expert members of the profession. These experts comprise the ABTC Procurement and Clinical Examination Committees with participation by invited medical specialists and outside test development experts.

Each ABTC examination is based on a national job analysis. The results of the analysis define the domains of clinical transplant and procurement/preservation practice by identifying the actual job-related knowledge required of transplant coordinators in the field. The examination tests whether a transplant coordinator has the job-related knowledge necessary to function in the role of transplant coordinator. Because a transplant coordinator must be able to interpret and analyze clinical data and apply knowledge to synthesize, evaluate and modify care based upon clients' needs, the questions require three levels of cognitive process: (1) recall, (2) application, and (3) analysis.

A CLINICIAN'S GUIDE TO DONATION AND TRANSPLANTATION

ABTC certification may be obtained in clinical and/or procurement transplant coordination, and achievement of this credential will be designated by:

- Certified Clinical Transplant Coordinator (CCTC)
- Certified Procurement/Preservation Transplant Coordinator (CPTC)

A candidate who has met all the requirements and has successfully passed the examination(s) of the ABTC in the area of procurement/preservation and/or clinical transplantation will be issued a certificate by the ABTC. This certificate will be issued by the Board of Governors and will attest to the qualifications of the transplant coordinator in the area of procurement or clinical transplant coordination.

Transplant Coordinator Certification Statistics:

The first administration of the certified procurement/preservation transplant coordinator examination and the certified clinical transplant coordinator examination took place on July 9, 1988 in Orlando, Florida in conjunction with the NATCO annual meeting. Testing was offered in only one location and one time per year from 1988 to 1990. In 1991, the examination was administered for the first time in more than one location: Chicago, Illinois and in Halifax, Nova Scotia, Canada. In 1992, the examination was administered in three locations: Los Angeles, California; Washington, DC; and Kansas City, Missouri. In 1993, the examination was also offered in three locations: Seattle, Washington; Chicago, Illinois; and Washington, DC. In September 2001, the first computer-based examination was offered. ABTC now offers computer-based exams across the country.

The fact that test volumes are decreasing may be attributed, paradoxically, to both attrition with failure to recruit and retain new staff long enough for them to sit for the exam as well as staff retention of those coordinators who are staying with the job longer than two years.

Coordinator Recertification

The ABTC requires CPTCs and CCTCs to recertify by continuing education every three years. The first group of certificants to recertify passed the examination in 1988 and were required to recertify in 1991. The number of individuals who have been recertified (1991-2005) are shown in the adjacent chart.

Candidates Recertification

Number of coordinators recertifying per year

Year	Procurement (CPTC)	Clinical (CCTC)	Total
1991	107	83	190
1992	76	73	149
1993	45	57	102
1994	133	121	254
1995	114	135	249
1996	97	103	200
1997	158	142	300
1998	108	166	264
1999	105	136	241
2000	163	190	353
2001	126	187	313
2002	112	178	290
2003	164	224	388
2004	106	143	249
2005	88	174	262

(as of February 21, 2006)

The intent of recertification is to provide assurance that a certified practitioner has maintained competency in the practice of transplant coordination. The method and procedures used for recertification may be either continuing education or reexamination. Ongoing evaluation of certification is in accordance with furthering the profession, strengthening the ability of the individuals and in the best interest of the public. Recertification will be granted by the board only to members who fulfill the requirements of recertification either through reexamination or continuing education.

Credentials are a profession's way of saying that this individual has exhibited certain minimum levels of expertise in his or her field. Maintenance of credentials is the challenge facing all professions where it is possible to test for expertise in one's field. Nursing, medicine, and other allied health professions face the

Chapter 1: THE HISTORY OF THE TRANSPLANT COORDINATOR

Total Number of Certified Transplant Coordinators			
Year	Procurement (CPTC)	Clinical (CCTC)	Total
1988	179	131	300
1989	322	245	567
1990	418	338	756
1991	448	384	832
1992	488	461	949
1993	548	520	1068
1994	585	540	1125
1995	590	585	1175
1996	605	627	1232
1997	615	682	1297
1998	540	544	1084
1999	570	466	1036
2000	513	459	972
2001	626	570	1196
2002	630	710	1340
2003	625	715	1340
2004	611	796	1407
2005	618	812	1430

challenge of determining how to measure whether or not an individual maintains such expertise. Transplant coordinators, like physicians and nurses in other specialties, currently may recertify by retesting *or* by providing documentation of attendance at educational symposiums approved by the ABTC for continuing education units.

The first round of recertification by either examination or documentation of appropriate continuing education occurred in 1991. To keep the test matrix appropriate for the expertise of the professional it is testing, the job analysis survey should be repeated every five years. ABTC is currently in the process of completing a job analysis survey. From this survey, the test will be modified to be current with the practice of transplant coordinator professionals. Frequency and relative importance of tasks may shift over time in this young profession. This second job analysis survey was sent to all transplant coordinators because expert practitioners should drive further development of the test matrix. The profession is now defined enough that the survey was not sent to persons outside the field of transplant coordination such as transplant surgeons and physicians.

Whether or not the accumulation of continuing education credits will remain sufficient for recertification for professionals in the future is questionable. We will continue to monitor the progress and adequacy of ABTCs testing compared with other professions.

As of February 21, 2006, there are currently 618 procurement coordinators (CPTC) and 812 clinical transplant coordinators (CCTCs) in the United States and abroad. People are surprised when they hear these numbers. They are low and speak to the desperate need to educate and train more coordinators. Organ procurement organizations and transplant centers alike are having difficulty staffing their facilities with these highly specialized, expert practitioners.

International Transplant Coordinators Organizations

Estimates of when the position of transplant coordinator developed in other countries are included earlier in this chapter and in the accompanying timetable. This section provides a little history about transplant coordinator societies other than NATCO around the world (Table 8).

Australasian Transplant Coordinators Association (ATCA)

See the Transplant Timeline for ATCA milestones.

European Transplant Coordinators Organization (ETCO)

To substitute for what surely will be a forthcoming historical text on transplant coordinators in Europe, I will insert here an article that appeared in a 1983 NATCO newsletter, detailing the proceedings of the Second European Congress for Transplant Coordinators on October 1, 1982:

A CLINICIAN'S GUIDE TO DONATION AND TRANSPLANTATION Chapter 1

Second European Congress for Transplant Coordinators

On October 1, 1982, the Eurotransplant Foundation hosted the Second European Congress for Transplant Coordinators in Leiden, Holland. A major portion of the program explored the role of the transplant coordinator in various parts of the world. There were over 100 participants, who represented a variety of professional disciplines involved in transplantation throughout Europe.

The morning session began with Sally Taber from the United Kingdom providing an overview of the various transplant coordinators' roles in Europe. This subject was extensively discussed at the European Dialysis and Transplant Nurses Association Meeting (EDTNA) in Madrid on September 6-9, 1982. In Europe the term "transplant coordinator" has only been in existence since 1978. These positions are filled with a variety of different types of personnel, with a great range of duties and responsibilities. However, all have the intention of procuring more kidneys.

Next, Amy S. Peele discussed the role of the transplant coordinator in the United States. She reviewed the government's support of the ESRD program, the types of roles transplant coordinators assume in the US and various mythologies incorporated in increase[ing] organ donation throughout the country, i.e. the CDC approach.

Physicians from Germany, France and Scandinavia, followed, sharing their experiences in the development of the role of the transplant coordinator in their countries. The French government has allocated funds for seven positions in organ procurement, which are currently being filled. In Germany, the position is being considered. In Scandinavia, there are no transplant coordinators as of yet; however, 85% of their transplants are from cadavers. In Holland, there are four transplant coordinators, one nurse and three MDs. The implementation of the coordinator's role in Holland has resulted in a 30% increase in the retrieval rate.

One of the concerns which received great attention was the subject of which professional qualifications were necessary to fill a coordinator's position. The majority of transplant coordinators in Europe are doctors. The final consensus was that education was not the major concern; more important is the personal ability to create a productive program.

The afternoon session was initiated by Laura Sophie, who discussed the intensive care nurses' perceptions of cadaver organ procurement. She pointed out how important the ICU nurse is in donor referrals, and outlined the referral process and the key players involved in each step. During the remainder of the afternoon, such topics as the increased interest and activity in multiorgan procurement and the use of the triple lumen catheter in donor procurement were discussed.

Cold storage was discussed by Dr. Opelz from Heidelberg. His comments supported cold storage up to 48 hours over machine preservation. Dr. Famulari from Rome discussed kidneys perfused longer than 40 hours and reported a graft survival rate slightly lower than normal results. Doctors Cohen and Persijn, both from Leiden, initiated the discussion which explored the formation of a Transplant Coordinator's Organization in Europe. Participants at this meeting agreed to organize a European Transplant Coordinator's Organization (ETCO). ETCO will look to NATCO for some guidance and support during its development.

In summary, the meeting was very productive and informative, and the hospitality exhibited by the Eurotransplant Foundation was outstanding.[198]

See also the Transplant Timeline for ETCO milestones.

United Kingdom Transplant Coordinators Association (UKTCA)

Celia Wight, one of the early English transplant coordinators, agreed to submit a short piece on the beginnings of the UKTCA. Celia had earlier written an account of the beginning of the UKTCA, but expanded upon it further, providing names of early transplant coordinators in the United Kingdom (UK):

One thing that is not always recognized is the role Sally Taber played in the development of transplant coordination in the UK. She was head nurse on the Renal Ward at Addenbrooke's

Hospital Cambridge (AHC) and was asked (or persuaded) by the Department of Health (DOH) to sponsor a fairly brief fact-finding trip to certain transplant centers in the US circa 1979 and report back to the DOH. Her report was very positive, and the DOH acknowledged it favorably but did nothing! In 1979 to 1980, Sally left Cambridge and was appointed as a transplant coordinator by Professor Maurice Slapack in his renal transplant unit at St. Mary's Hospital, Portsmouth, England. She was the first "officially named transplant coordinator" in the UK and, historically unusual, had never previously been involved in organ donation. Sally was only involved with transplantation patients as head nurse on the renal transplantation ward. She married quite soon after her appointment in Portsmouth and I believe did not stay longer than a year. She was not replaced for some time.

Since the 1970s I worked in the operating room at Addenbrooke's Hospital Cambridge (AHC) and knew of Sally, but our professional paths never crossed. In my time in the operating room I became the "unofficial transplant coordinator" for non-heart-beating kidney donation—mainly with the anesthesia department. In the 1970s, Dr. Roy Calne started the first liver transplant unit in Europe at AHC and I became involved in the rather dismal start of liver transplantation as an operating room nurse. As the liver transplantation program grew, the coordination became chaotic. At that time, AHC was the only liver transplant program in Europe and had no problem with donors. Roy Calne, who knew Starzl well and the infrastructure in both Denver and Pittsburgh, found money from somewhere and asked me if I would become the transplant coordinator for AHC. Knowing nothing about the job, I gaily said "yes!" The year was 1980. I did overlap for some months with Sally Taber and it seems rather unfair that I became viewed as the first UK transplant coordinator when it was really Sally. She helped me a lot, but the big difference was that AHC was a multiorgan transplantation center and closely attached to Papworth Hospital where heart transplantation was restarted in the UK following the almost worldwide moratorium. All the heart surgeons had trained in the US and knew only too well the value of a full time transplant coordinator, so my job was extended to include Papworth. Incidentally, I went about three times to Pittsburgh to "learn the ropes" and cannot praise or thank Dr. Starzl enough for the time he spent in making sure I had good background training.

Now I carry on with the previously written information: Those involved in the very beginning were Sally Taber, Bill Essex with Paul McMaster in Birmingham (ex RAF), myself (ex OR nurse) and to some extent Jim Colbert at the renal transplant center in Liverpool. Jim was an ex-renal technician and never quite saw the role of the transplant coordinator like the majority of us—but in the beginning he definitely wanted to be involved. Both Sally and I went to a NATCO meeting circa 1981 and it must have been on Bill's suggestion in 1982 or 1983 that we (three out of the four of us) get together for regular meetings. I believe we did so in the beginning as a self-help group. I think that we had the vision as to where transplant coordinators in the UK should fit into the scheme of things initially based on the US model. At that time the vast majority of US transplant coordinators were like us—hospital based. The independent OPO system was either about to come in vogue or was in its infancy. Our small group decided that we would form an organization and that I would be chair. As more transplant coordinators were appointed, without exception, they all wanted to join and contribute to the association. The US transplant coordinators were very generous, providing all their literature which we brought home and rewrote for the UKTCA, as seemed appropriate at the time. I do remember how cocky I must have appeared, given zero experience, but somehow or other it worked, as we did manage to start the association.

As always, politics at the time were interesting. In some ways we were treated as a joke but even so, the "old" UKTS (UK Transplant Service, equivalent to UNOS) was very keen that we associate ourselves with them (remember we had little idea of what we were doing or how to do it). The main UKTS person we dealt with initially was the founder of the blood transfusion service. Somehow or other we took the small amount of funds they could provide and avoided the offer to combine forces. Naive as we were, we realized or hoped that transplant coordinators would eventually become a professional voice, and we did not want to immediately trust and/or

A CLINICIAN'S GUIDE TO DONATION AND TRANSPLANTATION

commit to any existing organizations. The greatest early help came from Sandoz (now Novartis). Sandoz provided real help, practical advice, availability, training, and access to all UK Sandoz resources. Very importantly for the UKTCA, Sandoz provided funds to produce literature about organ donation and transplantation and the UKTCA. The success of UKTCA to Sandoz is obvious! But we could never have really started without them.

The next big thing for the UKTCA was the Ben Hardwick story. Ben was a beautiful toddler with biliary atresia who needed a liver transplant and became a major media story in the UK. At that time, I was chair of UKTCA as well as a transplant coordinator in Cambridge. Due to the all very coincidental events of the Ben Hardwick story and its associated press interest, along with the fact that I was the local transplant coordinator as well as chair of the UKTCA at the time, I was afforded the opportunity to speak publicly many times of the transplant coordinator's role in organ donation. From this time on, the DHS could no longer ignore us, and the UKTCA chair was gradually invited to sit on all appropriate DOH committees, etc. In fact the DHS was eventually very helpful to the UKTCA.

There was important UK medical support at the time: Roy Calne and Ross Taylor, renal surgeon in Newcastle (I have no memory of initial help/support from the British Transplant Society) followed by multiorgan transplant surgeons. Renal-only transplant centers were initially not really interested in transplant coordinators or the UKTCA. Looking back, the real catalyst for the appointment of transplant coordinators was the advent of multiorgan donation, and the development of professional relationships with the intensive care unit. I would say that in the beginning we were trying to create a visible, respected and *accepted* platform for transplant coordinators and the UKTCA. My memories of the early days are of a happy and dedicated small group of transplant coordinators with a common objective, which probably included survival and professional status. Later transplant coordinators had to deal with the future issues that came with a larger membership and a recognized position in the transplant community (*written communication, C. Wight, RN, CPTC, April 25, 2006*).

Japanese Transplant Coordinators Organization (JATCO)

The Japanese Transplant Coordinators Organization was founded on September 6, 1991, six years after the first transplant coordinator starting working in Japan in 1985. Seigo Hiraga, MD, writes to Teresa Shafer:

As to the matter of your inquiry, your information is right as JATCO was established on September 6, 1991 with the agreement and general assembly. Before establishing JATCO, you know, we attended the NATCO meeting for learning from your organization, and I met you on the first time at the welcome party for new participants and you played the role for new members. At that time I was entrusted to research on transplant coordinator from Japan Ministry of Health and Welfare and I participated in the NATCO meeting with Isao Tamaki, Osamu Kato, and Mitsutoshi Yuasa (they may be called founding members of JATCO including me). Mr. Isao Tamaki was the first president of JATCO.

Seigo Hiraga, MD had the role of researching, promoting, and establishing the transplant network and transplant coordinator profession in Japan. He recommended Mr. Isao Tamaki as the first president of JATCO and advised JATCO, serving for a couple of terms himself. Dr. Hiraga has remained a member of an advisory committee to support JATCO.

In 1985, Dr. Hiraga, a 1968 graduate of the Tokyo Medical and Dental University majoring in urology, accepted a position as associate professor at Tokai University School of Medicine, Department of Transplantation and Kidney Center with the recommendation of Dean Professor Kyoichiro Ochiai, Saitama Medical School and Professor Hiroyuki Oshima, Tokyo Medical and Dental University. This move resulted in his deep involvement in the transplantation field, the development of a transplant network and the development of transplant coordination in Japan. In 1986, Seigo Hiraga spent two months during the summer at the Karolinska Institute Huddinge Hospital with Professor Carl-Gustav Groth. It was here that he met his first transplant coordinator: Ms. Ann-Christine Croon. He knew that such a profession also existed in Western countries. From the beginning, Dr. Hiraga was interested in the transplant coordinator

Chapter 1 — THE HISTORY OF THE TRANSPLANT COORDINATOR

role because he had realized its importance when a kidney donor first appeared in his own hospital at Tokai University.

In 1989, Dr. Hiraga visited Dallas through the Japan-North America Medical Exchange Foundation (JANAMEF) in Japan. He was charged with investigating the status of transplant coordinators in the United States and was also interested in looking at the transplant network system (UNOS) and how it worked in regions of the country. Even though he stayed a short four months, he studied and learned a great deal about transplant coordinators and the organ donation and transplantation system in the United States. Dr. Hiraga chose Dallas to visit because he had come to know Dr. Pedro Vergne-Marini, a physician at Methodist Medical Center in Dallas who was involved in a transplantation with a patient of Dr. Hiraga's who had end-stage renal disease. He met many transplant surgeons, transplant coordinators, and associated transplant professionals, and observed and participated in approximately 100 transplant surgeries as he was certified by the Educational Commission for Foreign Medical Graduates. Staying at Methodist Medical Center, he also visited Baylor University Medical Center, meeting Dr. Goran Klintmalm and Southwest Organ Bank where he met Stephen Haid, executive director and Suzanne Lane Conrad, CPTC.

Seigo Hiraga learned a great deal from these contacts and on his return to Japan, was requested to give a lecture of the report by the JANAMEF. At the time of the lecture, Dr. Sadayoshi Kitagawa, director of the Health Ministry research group for "social problems in organ transplantation in Japan" attended and Dr. Hiraga was added to his research organization. In August 1991, Dr. Hiraga, along with three transplant coordinators, Isao Tamaki, Osamu Kato and Mitsutoshi Yuasa, attended the 16th annual NATCO meeting in Halifax, Nova Scotia, where "we talked about JATCO and observed NATCO." Following the meeting, on September 6, 1991, JATCO was established. In 1993, Dr. Hiraga was invited to the 8th ETCO and ESOT meeting in Rhodes, Greece, by Leo Roels. Paraphrasing Dr. Hiraga's communication to me,

> I heard that you suggested to Leo to invite me. I was able to spend a truly pleasant and unforgettable time with you and Don [my husband], Greg Armstrong and Sally Tan. Do you remember that I invited you to Japan at that time? I had already had an idea while in Greece that I wanted to invite you next year to Japan since, although it was not known at the time, I had been entrusted by the Ministry to chair the transplant coordinators research group. On August 29, 1994, the International Transplant Coordinators Meeting was held in Kyoto during the 15th World Congress of the Transplantation Society. Professor Kazuo Ota at Tokyo Womens Medical University was the Chairman of the Congress. He was supportive of holding the ITCM meeting. At that time, I was able to meet all of you again and also to meet Dr. Groth, Ms. Croon and the Karolinska group, and Dr. Klintmalm from Dallas. It was a very nice time even though the weather was incredibly hot and humid. With this, and what I have written below, I believe I have written most of the memory I have of the beginnings of and my enthusiastic support for, establishment of transplant coordinators, JATCO, ITCM, ITCS, and the organ transplant network system in Japan. I trust you to make use of this description or not, and I hope this has been helpful.

> In January, 1985, the 18th Clinical Conference for Renal Transplantation was held in Sendai, Japan. Dr. Yoshio Taguchi, chairman and associate professor of Tohoku University, organized the conference. Mr. Paul Taylor, transplant coordinator at the University of Colorado was an invited speaker. Many Japanese surgeons studied in Dr. Thomas Starzl's department in Denver, arranged by Dr. Iwatsuki from Japan. Dr. Starzl, having an open mind, allowed this relationship to continue after moving to Pittsburgh. Professor Hiroshi Takagi, a surgeon at Nagoya University communicated with Dr. Starzl's program and arranged to invite Paul Taylor to Japan.[h] This could have been the first time the Japanese coordinators encountered a "real" transplant coordinator, and it was at this time that the "bud" was born. About that time, the transplant field in Japan noticed the profession of the transplant coordinator in Western countries. Compared to the US, the Japanese social state of mind in regards to transplant medicine lagged far behind. "As you know, we could perform only kidney transplants in Japan."

---

h. Paul was later invited to Japan again in 1994, along with Teresa Shafer, Leo Roels, Greg Armstrong, and Sue Falvey; each was the president, with the exception of Armstrong, of their society at that time.

Isao Tamaki, Osamu Kato, Mitsutoshi Yuasa, perhaps Sachiko Zama and several others attended this seminal lecture by Paul Taylor, the American transplant coordinator. After the conference, the necessity of researching the need of and the role for transplant coordinators in Japan became apparent and the activities needed to advance the establishment of transplant coordinators were discussed.

In January 1987, the first Transplant Coordinators Conference was held at the Second Red Cross Hospital in Nagoya. Professor Takagi managed the first meeting for transplant coordinators in Nagoya where Osamu Kato was working as a transplant coordinator. Fifteen to 20 individuals attended the meeting. Later, when the first International Transplant Coordinators meeting was held in Kyoto, I (Dr. Hiraga) invited Professor Takagi to be the honorary president and give the keynote address.

In February 1988, the second Japanese Transplant Coordinators Conference was held in Nagoya. Dr. Guido Persijn, director of Eurotransplant was the invited speaker. In 1989, the third Japanese transplant coordinators meeting was held in Nagoya with the invited speakers being Barbara Schulman, a NATCO coordinator and Gene Pierce, executive director of UNOS. About that time, Mitsutoshi Yuasa, RN, was perhaps the first Japanese transplant coordinator who started attending NATCO meetings.

In 1990, the Japan Ministry of Health and Welfare drew up a budget for 19 transplant coordinators for the first time; 10 of which were coordinators that had been appointed at the 14 renal transplant centers which were part of the transplant system of the Ministry of Health and Welfare. Isao Tamaki and Osamu Kato were among these coordinators. Centers were set up in respective kidney transplant hospitals; only kidney transplantation was possible at that time.

Around this time the Ministry organized a research group for establishing a social system of organ transplantation in Japan, and the transplant coordinator was one of the subjects of the research group. Professor Hiroshi Takagi was the chairman of the research group for the transplant coordinator and I was a member of his group. Later, in 1991, the Ministry drew up a budget for an additional 10 transplant coordinators, making a total of 29 coordinators.

On September 9, 1991, JATCO was formed and the first meeting was held in Ebisu, Tokyo. The second transplant coordinators training course was also held in Ebisu. Mr. Isao Tamaki was elected as the first president. I am unclear about the number of participants at this first official JATCO meeting; however, the number of initial members were 98, consisting of the 29 "official transplant coordinators," others serving in a similar capacity, transplant doctors, and others. Isao Tamaki, a transplant coordinator whose office was in Tokyo, was ultimately elected three times as JATCO president, serving from September 1991 to September 1997. The second president of JATCO was Osamu Kato, a coordinator from Nagoya.

In April 1995, just before the passage of the Organ Transplant Act[i] the new transplant network, Japan Kidney Transplant Network (JKTNW), was reorganized. JKTNW consisted of five "block" centers. The Transplant Coordinators Committee was created, and I was a member of the committee. We held the employment examination and accepted Isao Tamaki, Osamu Kato, and Sachiko Zama as the first JKTNW coordinators, who also soon became members of the JKTNW Transplant Coordinators Committee. In Osaka, Mitsutoshi Yuasa, Setsuko Konaka, and others belonged to the Osaka Kidney Bank and moved to one of the block centers; however, I am a little unclear on the exact organization of their programs as Osaka is far from the Tokyo area.

At the end of 1995, 15 JKTNW coordinators, who were full-time transplant coordinators, and 49 local coordinators, most of whom were part-time, were appointed in respective prefectures. The classification of full-time versus part-time was probably due to financial considerations, since a subsidy was provided by the Ministry of Health and local government, half and half in the case of local coordinators.

Keeping pace with establishing the kidney (organ) transplant network, the new Organ Transplant Act was proposed and passed in June 1997 and was enforced in October 1997. At the same time, the JKTNW was reorganized to Japan Organ Transplant Network (JOTNW) which consisted of

---

i. The Japan Organ Transplant Act is a very strict act permitting organ donation from brain-dead patients in very narrow circumstances (previously discussed elsewhere in this chapter) and kidney and cornea donation from donation-after-cardiac-death donors

seven block centers and one subcenter in the Okinawa prefecture. The first cardiac, liver, and kidney transplantation under the new Act was performed on February 28, 1999, coincidentially at the same time that Greg Armstrong, Australian transplant coordinator, had been invited to Mishima, Japan. We introduced Greg to local customs and sights and met Isao Tamaki in Tokyo in order that we could discuss transplant coordination. All of the transplant coordinators in JKTNW moved to JOTNW.

After Professor Takagi, I became chairman of the research group for the development of transplant coordinators in Japan. I chaired the committee between 1993 and 1999, during the time the Japan Organ Transplant Law passed in 1997. The Japan Organ Transplant Network (JOTNW) was founded and the first case of organ transplantation from a brain-dead donor was performed during that time. During my time as chairman, with the support of Dr. Takagi and surgeons who recommended me, I arranged to have the first International Transplant Coordinators meeting in Kyoto, from which the International Transplant Coordinators Society was born. Dr. Sadayoshi Kitagawa, a former high official in the Ministry of Health and the chief organizer of the entire research program surrounding the social problems of organ transplantation in Japan, was also a strong supporter of my endeavors in developing a strong system of transplant coordinators.

Through the foreign invitation program in the Foundation, and as chairman, I was able to invite you (Teresa Shafer) and Leo Roels, to Japan in 1998 and Greg Armstrong the following year. Through the same program, Marlene Abe, the third generation Japanese-American transplant coordinator working for the Regional Organ Procurement Agency (ROPA) in Los Angeles, spoke to the aforementioned research group, and I attended three NATCO annual meetings and one ETCO meeting in Rhodes, in all as a regular member of those societies. These meetings were instrumental in our development of the transplant coordinator system in Japan (written communication, S. Hiraga, May 29, 2006).

Society of Transplant Coordinators Worldwide: Formation of the International Transplant Coordinators Society (ITCS)

Just as coordinators networked and shared ideas and ways to do the job, so they did internationally as countries throughout the world set up transplant programs. Invariably one of the first and most important pieces to have in place, along with the surgeon, was the transplant coordinator.

Perhaps a forerunner to the International Transplant Coordinators Society, which is discussed at length below, was the meeting held on April 13, 1983 at the University of Limburg, Masstricht, Netherlands. The International Congress on Organ Procurement (ICOP) placed the following invitation in the NATCO newsletter for transplant coordinators to attend an international transplant coordinator forum at the ICOP Transplant Coordinators Meeting:

International Congress on Organ Procurement
April 13, 1983: Masstricht, Netherlands
Attention: Transplant Coordinators

Transplant Coordinators are cordially invited to attend the ICOP Transplant Coordinators Meeting, which will be held in conjunction with the International Congress on Organ Procurement.

An international transplant coordinator forum is invited to discuss the following topics:
- The organization of organ procurement programs
- Donor cards; are they useful?
- Who points the finger? Identification of potential donors.
- Education, procurement and preservation; one job?
- Are transplant coordinators to be employed by an organ exchange organization?
- Donor management.

---

j. The representative carrying the bill was Taro Nakayama, MD, the former Foreign Minister.

- Neonatal organ donors.
- Non heart beating donors.
- Training of transplant coordinators.

Coordinators, who are interested in presenting a paper on one of these subjects, are requested to contact the ICOP congress secretariat.

The ICOP Transplant Coordinators Meeting will be held prior to the International Congress on Organ Procurement on Wednesday, April 13, 1983, from 13.30 hours to 17.30 hours at the University of Limburg Main Building, 53 Tongersesstraat, Masstricht, Netherlands. Registration at 13.00 hours, free of charge.

J.A. van der Vliet, MD
Congress Secretary, ICOP

J.P.A.M. Vroeman, MD
Member Organizing Committee ICOP[199]

The transplant coordinators' practice and profession was built not only on their education and clinical work but also on sharing and networking. US coordinators, speaking with their international colleagues, formed lasting friendships and soon learned that their profession was little different from country to country. The US, having first developed the transplant coordinator role and profession, has been visited often by transplant coordinators and surgeons from around the world as they searched for professionals with common goals who could help them establish their position. Job descriptions and protocols for donor management, immunosuppression and patient care were freely shared. US coordinators were often invited to lecture abroad and were given opportunities to visit countries they otherwise never would have visited. I was fortunate enough to travel to Japan twice, Greece, Australia, and Canada, giving lectures and providing consultation. Many other NATCO presidents and experienced coordinators have also had these same experiences.

The first International Transplant Coordinators meeting was held on August 29, 1994, immediately in advance of the formation of The International Transplant Coordinators Society on August 31, 1994. Dr. Seigo Hiraga, president of the organizing committee for that first meeting, gave the welcome address, which was included in the meeting syllabus (see welcome address, below). It seemed appropriate that one of the first coordinators in the world, if not the first coordinator, Paul Taylor, was a cochair of the first panel of the meeting. The other US speaker that day was Teresa Shafer, who also chaired the next panel. The rest of the international speakers represent many of the leaders and founders of the transplant coordinator profession in their respective countries: Leo Roels, Greg Armstrong, Sue Falvey, president of the UKTCA at the time, Sally Tan, Osamu Kato, Tom Karbe, Haken Gabel, Celia White and others (see meeting syllabus in Table 9; also Figure 15).

The formation of the society was sealed in Kyoto, Japan, in a bar at the Prince Takaragaike Hotel. Dr. Seigo Hiraga (Japan), Leo Roels (Belgium), Greg Armstrong (Australia), Sally Tan (Singapore), and Teresa Shafer (US) met that night (see photo of founding members in Photo section). They talked about the need for an international transplant coordinators group that would provide structure and a common ground for coordinators to gather as an international group, much as the Transplantation Society provided the same for surgeons and physicians. The officers were formed from this small group, with Seigo Hiraga, MD as president, Greg Armstrong, vice president, Sally Tan, treasurer, Leo Roels, scientific program director, and Teresa Shafer as treasurer. The group immediately went to work attempting to fulfill the goals of the society.

The goals of the society:
- foster communication and collaboration among transplant coordinators individually as well as with national and international associations or societies interested in the field of transplantation, transplant coordination, and related subjects,
- provide professional education to its membership with a goal of enhancing the profession of the transplant coordinator. The education may take the form of a biennial meeting with the

presentation of abstracts, formation of specific education meetings, or endorsement of existing educational programs of transplant coordinator societies and/or organizations,
- promote research and provide a forum for the presentation or research finding on organ and tissue donation, procurement and transplantation, and
- provide its membership and the general public information on an international level concerning organ and tissue donation and the benefits of organ and tissue transplantation.

The membership brochure was entitled "International Transplant Coordinators Society: The Society for Transplant Coordinators World-Wide." The ITCS has held six international meetings since its inception in 1994, usually in conjunction with the Society for Organ Sharing (SOS) or The Transplantation Society (TTS). The SOS is now called the International Society of Organ Donation and Preservation (ISODP). Coordinators have attended, presented their research and advanced the practice of transplant coordination worldwide. The meetings have been held in:

ITCS Meetings:

1994	Kyoto, Japan	1st ITCS Meeting	*(with 15th Intl Cong of TTS)*
1995	Paris, France	2nd ITCS Meeting	(with SOS)
1997	Washington, DC	3rd ITCS Meeting	*(with SOS)*
1999	Maastricht, Netherlands	4th ITCS Meeting	*(with SOS)*
2001	Nagoya, Japan	5th ITCS Meeting	*(with SOS)*
2003	Warsaw, Poland	6th ITCS Meeting	*(with ISODP)*
2005	Gramado, Brazil	7th ITCS Meeting	*(with ISODP)*

ITCS Workshops:

1999—Singapore

Before the formation of the International Transplant Coordinators Society (ITCS), there was no international body, no umbrella organization, to access expertise in transplant coordination topics *around the globe*. The ITCS was formed in order to create a structure that could respond to transplant coordination issues at international meetings, a structure similar to what The Transplantation Society provides for physicians, surgeons, immunologists and other related specialties.

The ITCS is a society of transplant coordinators, both *clinical* and *procurement*, who provide a major portion of the infrastructure in which organ or tissue donation and transplantation occur. The ITCS provides a transplant coordinator organization capable of developing coordinator meetings and topics within an international setting. Transplant coordinators are the professionals who can best address the issues facing the field of transplant coordination and, further, transplant coordinators should do and report the research, which builds the science upon which this profession is based.

Given its umbrella-like and complementary character, the ITCS is supportive of and encourages membership in transplant coordinators' own national societies, such as the Australasian Transplant Coordinators Association, the European Transplant Coordinators Organization, the Japanese Transplant Coordinators Organization, the North American Transplant Coordinators Organization, the United Kingdom Transplant Coordinators Association, and other national transplant coordinators organizations.[200]

Dr. Seigo Hiraga, first president of the ITCS, evidences in his welcome address to the first International Transplant Coordinators meeting, the need for such a gathering:

A CLINICIAN'S GUIDE TO DONATION AND TRANSPLANTATION

International Transplant Coordinators Meeting
August 29, 1994
WELCOME ADDRESS

On behalf of the local Organizing Committee, I would like to extend our sincere appreciation and warmest welcome to all the participants in the International Transplant Coordinators Meeting, which is being held in Kyoto August 29, 1994.

The roles of transplant coordinators have become increasingly important in the professional field, and it is no exaggeration to say that transplant coordinators are key persons in promoting advancement of transplant medicine. Transplant coordinators, although active in their respective countries and in regional areas such as the North American Transplant Coordinators Organization, the European Transplant Coordinators Organization, the Australasian Transplant Coordinators Association, and the Japan Transplant Coordinators Organization, have never had the opportunity worldwide to gather together in the same place, and at the same time, to communicate with each other. This event will be extremely important for widening knowledge, improving professional quality, and contributing to the educational aspects of transplantation.

Our professional work is dedicated to helping suffering patients. The meaning of our discipline should be explained in a common language with the common heart of "a gift of life". This meeting is the first international opportunity for transplant coordinators, and for anyone related to or interested in transplant coordination, to present details on our activities, to share ideas, experiences, and problems, and to get to know each other.

I am convinced this meeting will be valuable and useful in the future activities of transplant coordinators and allied health personnel, and I hope our society will grow and expand in the future. I want to express my appreciation to the Transplant Society and the Local Organizing Committee of the 15th World Congress of the Transplant Society for their generous support for this first International Transplant Coordinators Meeting in Japan.

Last but not least, I sincerely hope every participant will develop strong bonds of friendship and understanding through the meeting. Indeed, Kyoto is one of the world's most historic, and beautiful, and fantastic cities, well worth your attendance. To all, enjoy yourselves to your heart's content!

Seigo Hiraga, M.D., Ph.D.
President
Local Organizing Committee
International Transplant Coordinators Meeting[201]

Transplant coordinator colleagues from around the world have more in common than not. Consider this story, from Greg Armstrong, from Brisbane, Australia…it sounds much like the stories shared earlier in this chapter from American coordinators.

> We had a liver donor in Christchurch, New Zealand and to save on charter costs we went from Brisbane to Sydney by commercial airline and then caught an international flight to Auckland, New Zealand. We had a small charter plane waiting for us there and it flew us down to Christchurch. We did the donor and caught a taxi out to Christchurch airport where we caught the early morning international flight back to Brisbane—total round trip—approx 5000 miles—total time 11 hours (written communication, G. Armstrong, January 23, 2006)!

Chapter 1: THE HISTORY OF THE TRANSPLANT COORDINATOR

In Memoriam: Transplant Coordinator Pioneers

Our profession, now approaching 45 years in existence, has seen some of its earliest members depart. Three individuals in particular were pioneers in the field and contributed greatly to the development and practice of the field of transplant coordination, and they did it on their own terms…not as "helpers," "assistants," or anything of the kind. They were *transplant coordinators*. I have fond memories of all of these gentlemen and many could say more about them.

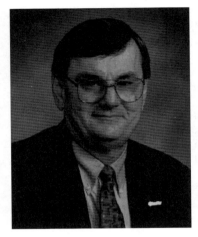

Billy G. Anderson, BA, CPTC
1952—2002

At the very first meeting I attended, a SEOPF meeting in Raleigh Durham, NC, I felt fortunate to tag along with a large group of coordinators to dinner. As usual, it was a raucous affair—laughter, story-telling, and jokes. It was my first time to meet Bill Anderson. He picked up the tab for the entire table—at least 20 people. I was soon to learn it was a common trait of this boisterous crowd in the early days to do exactly that. Bill talked a lot and had plans for the future. Also at that first meeting in 1985, I met H. M. Lee, MD, the accomplished transplant surgeon from Medical College of Virginia. I am not sure why we were on the subject of Bill, but Dr. Lee confided in me that Bill thought he was going to build a tissue "empire". Indeed, that is exactly what Bill did. He grew a company he founded, Virginia Beach-based LifeNet, into an $85 million company with over 350 employees and tissue distribution programs worldwide. I have often thought of Dr. Lee's comment over the years when I think of Bill. Bill was bold, went for broke, and accomplished everything he set out to do. And, as his long-time associate, Helen Leslie-Bottenfield notes below, he was a restless character. What a nice description that is of Bill. He died on May 21, 2002, of injuries sustained in a car crash in North Carolina.[203]

Bill Anderson was a pioneer in the field of organ and tissue donation and a gentleman who would help anyone in need. He spent his life helping people, and when he left this world on May 21, 2002, he was able to fulfill his life's work by becoming an organ and tissue donor.

Bill's commitment to the organization he founded in 1982 and to organ and tissue donation were his passions. To so many, Bill was an anonymous champion for all of the unknown recipients and for the families of donors. He strived continuously in his scientific quest to develop new and improved allograft tissue implants—always thinking of the patient who would ultimately receive the gift.

During two decades as the CEO of LifeNet, Bill Anderson created and built a nonprofit organization that serves patients all across the United States and throughout the world.

Through Bill's vision and compassion, his company touched numerous families, whose members now live fuller lives through organ and tissue donation and transplantation.

A native of Statesville, NC, Anderson earned a degree in biology from Wake Forest. He spent a year at Southern College of Optometry in Memphis before becoming director of organ procurement at Wake Forest's Bowman Gray School of Medicine.

Anderson quickly warmed to the work and decided it would be his life's mission.

In 1976, Anderson brought his newfound passion to Norfolk, and became head of the Eastern Virginia Renal Transplant Program at then Norfolk General Hospital. In 1980, Bill Anderson established the

---

k. Throughout the development of the transplant coordinator role, coordinators recognized their unique role and professional status as an autonomous one. The transplant coordinator worked collaboratively with transplant surgeons, social workers, nurses, dieticians, and others in the field of transplantation. Only once, in reading the voluminous historical transplant coordinator references did I see the word "assistant," in an opinion piece that history has fortunately shown to have been a very singular and minority position.."[202]

Eastern Virginia Transplant Program, through which they continued to manage organ donation and education.

In 1982, responding to an ever-increasing need for human tissue, Anderson formed and incorporated the Eastern Virginia Tissue Bank, which went on to become LifeNet.

Anderson urged LifeNet to experiment with new processing and storage techniques and helped refine the complex logistics of matching donors and recipients. He also spearheaded the push for education, both of the general donor public and of the professionals in the field.

His passion for serving others permeated everything that Bill stood for. He was passionate about the need to support organ procurement and transplantation by protecting the integrity of the donation process. True to his and his organization's mission, Bill Anderson became an organ and tissue donor on May 21, 2002. His mission of service continues.

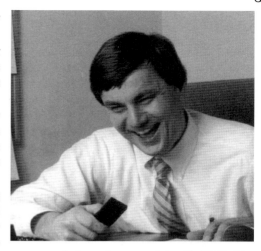

Bill is survived by his wife Darleen, one son Brandon and his wife Ilana, his daughter Brittany, and many LifeNet "family" members who all miss him terribly. The true measure of this man's greatness lies in the lives of the many people he touched so profoundly. A colleague of Bill's stated, "It is clear to me that heroes still exist and are among us...poised and ready to respond as the situation demands. Bill was [and will always be] just such a hero" *(written communication, LifeNet, April 27, 2006)*.

Helen Leslie-Bottenfield, his chief operating officer and right arm, has had a long involvement in transplant coordination. In what became an extraordinary partnership for our field, Helen and Bill worked together for more than 22 years. Helen remembers...

I started working with Bill in early 1980. He and I met over two long days of coffee, doughnuts and a Kidney Foundation exhibit at a local Health Fair. I was volunteering, and he was there representing the local transplant center. Two days later Bill called and asked me if I'd like to work as a part time organ procurement coordinator. I stumbled all over myself saying yes. Problem was, Bill's idea of part-time was about 70 hours a week! In less than two months, I quit my other part time teaching job and jumped into this field forever. Bill was an incredible mentor and friend whom I was blessed to work beside for over 22 years. He taught by example and never asked me to do anything he wouldn't do himself. We ate many late night, early morning meals at Denny's as we talked about life and death that we saw on a daily basis. Bill never lost his awe about the gift of organ/tissue donation. Likewise, he maintained the highest level of personal and professional integrity in the donation process. Bill was a restless character who never stopped looking for ways to make us all better at every aspect of our work. He was a true advocate for those patients waiting for a transplant, and he would fight anything or anyone who tried to pose a barrier to donation. Of all the difficult decisions that had to be made after Bill's tragic accident, Bill's wife, Darleen said the one about donation was a simple one. In the end, it was actually Bill's designated decision on his driver's license that we used. He would have expected no less. Although traumatic injuries to some organs precluded donation, Bill donated his heart, liver, kidneys, corneas, and all tissue. He would have been so pleased to know the legacy of life that he was able to give. I was the lucky one, because I knew the man beneath the loud voice. I knew how passionately he lived and loved and I am a better person for having walked a while with a giant like Bill. Thanks for allowing me to share (written communication, H. Leslie-Bottenfield, February 14, 2006).

(All photos courtesy of LifeNet.)

THE HISTORY OF THE TRANSPLANT COORDINATOR

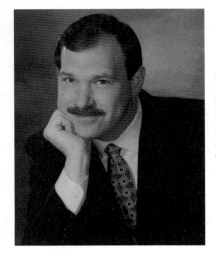

Brian A. Broznick, BS, CPTC
1952—2003

I wasn't sure how to start this paragraph about Brian Broznick. Fortunately for me, this is the day of the Internet, and in reading the numerous articles about Brian on the Internet, this quote from the *Pittsburgh Gazette* says most eloquently what I just wrote about Bill Anderson, that is, that *transplant coordinator* leaders did it on their own terms…not as "helpers," "assistants," or anything of the kind. The quote follows:

> A time existed in Pittsburgh's history when the economy rested more on brawn than brain. Although intellectual capital was always an underlying local strength, futurists would not have dreamed that the city would one day become a world leader in organ transplantation. That this extraordinary development occurred *was not just due* to the decision of some hugely talented physicians to practice here. It took administrators and visionaries and people with unbounded faith and enthusiasm. **To a significant extent, it took Brian A. Broznick.**[204] (emphasis added)

The italicized print above says what was said in the very first paragraph of this chapter—that the field of transplantation could not have been developed as it has been without transplant coordinators. Brian was one of those coordinators. He was quiet, unassuming, …and *driven*. The *Post-Gazette* put it in a wonderful way: "He was able to balance personal compassion with a sense of administrative fairness, and his integrity won him great respect among transplant professionals. Above all, he was an apostle for the cause of organ transplantation."[204]

Brian Broznick was president and CEO of the Center for Organ Recovery and Education (CORE) in Pittsburgh, Pennsylvania, when he died of pancreatic cancer on November 2, 2003. He was 51. He grew up on Pittsburgh's south side, where he graduated from South Side Catholic High School. He attended Duquesne University, graduating with a biology degree.

He then went to work running an ambulance service for a local funeral home. One day, while driving CORE's founder to the airport to drop off a kidney, Mr. Broznick learned about the opportunities in organ procurement. In 1978, he took a job tending to and transporting donated kidneys. He later became senior organ procurement coordinator, and in 1985 was named chief executive.[205]

Broznick was a passionate advocate of organ and tissue donation for the past 25 years. He began his career in procurement in 1978 as a chief renal perfusionist at CORE, and served as senior organ procurement coordinator before being named to head the OPO in 1985. It is estimated that more than 300,000 people in western Pennsylvania, West Virginia, and a small portion of New York received life-saving transplants during his stewardship.[206]

Mr. Broznick initiated programs at CORE that have served as models for other organ procurement organizations nationwide, including routine referral of all acute-care hospital deaths and first-person consent for organ donation.[207] His influence on organ donation issues had a national reach. He was a force behind the passage in 1994 of Pennsylvania Act 102, which required hospitals to notify recovery groups about all deaths—which had the effect of encouraging donations. Other parties around the country used the law as a guide in framing their own regulations.[205]

In a tribute to Broznick, the Association of Organ Procurement Organizations (AOPO) executive committee observed: "Brian was a dear friend to many in the OPO community, as well as a mentor, role model, and colleague. He led by example, and the accomplishments and contributions of CORE under his direction made a significant difference in community approaches and understanding of organ donation."[207]

Broznick's name was added to the AOPO Memorial Fund "to honor the memory of members of the OPO and others whose commitment to maintaining the public trust regarding organ and tissue donation was clearly evidenced in their professional careers and personal life." He joins Bill Anderson, the former CEO of LifeNet, the OPO covering most of the state of Virginia, who was killed in

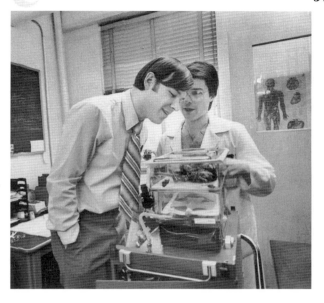

a car accident in May 2002. The fund was developed for three uses: (1) to provide annual scholarship(s) to donor family member(s) for travel to the National Donor Ceremony; (2) to provide annual scholarship(s) to assist OPO employees in pursuing formal training or experience in quality improvement; and (3) to support local fund(s) established to memorialize OPO employees for significant contributions to advancing the public's trust with organ and tissue donation. Brian was unique in many ways.

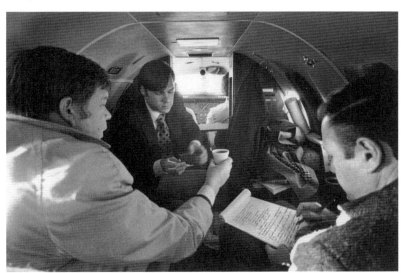

Brian Broznick in plane, facing camera.

He married Susan Stuart, who had worked at CORE since 1987, starting as an organ procurement coordinator, eventually rising to assistant as his number two. Five years before his death, Susan left a promising career at CORE for personal reasons. Susan and Brian wanted to marry and didn't feel it was fair to employees if they both kept working there. Susan returned to CORE after his death and succeeded her late husband as president. In a newspaper interview she stated, "It's an honor to work for an organization like CORE, and it's an honor to carry on the legacy that I think Brian has built in this service area," she said. "When Brian became ill, we talked about it, and he discussed it with me—would I be interested in going back to CORE? There wasn't a moment's hesitation."[208]

(All photos courtesy of Susan Stuart and/or CORE.)

THE HISTORY OF THE TRANSPLANT COORDINATOR

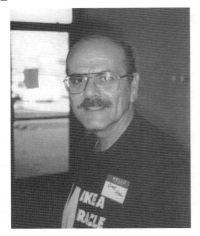

Gary Hall, BS, CPTC
1943—2001

Gary worked for Mid-South Transplant Foundation for 18 years; first as a coordinator and then as director of procurement. Gary passed away in December 2001.

Gary Hall began his career in organ procurement during the infancy of transplantation in the 1970s. He was an individual who had a true passion for donation and he loved his job. During the 1980s, Gary's vision for the role of organ recovery coordinators was instrumental in the development of the NATCO introductory course that has grown during the past 20 years and is today part of the training for all individuals entering the industry.

Gary was a dedicated employee of Mid-South Transplant Foundation for 18 years, where his career gave him many opportunities. In the early 1980s, when insurance companies viewed liver transplantation as experimental, Gary testified in front of the US Congress about the need for insurance coverage for liver recipients. He also served on many committees at the local, regional, and national level and was a respected member of the organ procurement community.

Because of health problems, Gary became disabled in 1998. He was preceded in death by his wife of many years, Cheryl. They have three children, Stephanie, Adam, and Alexander all of the Memphis area (*written communication, J. Shipman, March 20, 2006*).

(*photo courtesy of Judy Shipman*)

Isao Tamaki
1954—2004

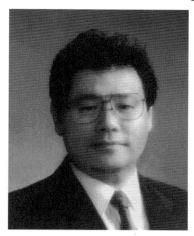

Isao Tamaki was the first JATCO President and was re-elected, holding the position for six years. He pioneered the transplant coordinator role in Japan.

Isao Tamaki started working in the field of transplantation in 1977, like so many other beginners, in the laboratory. Mr. Etsuo Sakurai, a donor coordinator in Japan and a former colleague of Mr. Tamaki while at Hachioji Medical Center, Tokyo Medical University, remembers that Isao started work in experimental transplantation in 1977. His background work, before he became an "official" transplant coordinator, was in experimental transplant immunology and experimental organ perfusion. Isao had a master of agriculture degree, graduating from the Graduate School of Tokyo, University of Agriculture. Isao officially started work as a full-time transplant coordinator in 1985.

Isao left a family—a wife and four children. His oldest, Shintaro, will graduate from Tokyo Medical University, where Isao worked. His second son, Yuuki, a 20-year-old student at Azabu Veterinary Medical University remembers that his father mostly wanted to become a veterinary surgeon from Kaoru when he was younger. His daughters, Mai and Yui, twins, are in high school. A scholarship was established to assist with the significant educational expenses of the children.

To understand the history of Japanese transplant coordinators and the huge challenges they faced due to the Japanese society's longstanding problem with brain death, the reader will benefit from reading the history of JATCO discussed earlier in this chapter. I marveled at the wonderful spirit of the transplant coordinators I met on my first trip to Japan as have several other American and European transplant coordinators who have traveled to Japan, lecturing and attempting to move donation and transplantation forward in that country. Japanese transplant surgeons and coordinators have struggled since the beginning of transplantation in Japan without the ability to recover organs from brain-dead donors. There were no brain death laws—the government would not approve the laws (see earlier discussion on brain death). It is hard to imagine being a transplant coordinator in a country where brain death laws were forbidden. Isao Tamaki was a terrific example of the boundless enthusiasm I encountered in every Japanese transplant coordinator. They were all bent on making a difference and improving their country's organ donation and transplantation system.

Dr. Hiraga pays Isao Tamaki the greatest tribute when he says of him: "He lived in the age of convulsion [turmoil] in organ transplantation in Japan and dedicated his life to the dawn of transplant medicine in Japan. He was loved by all the persons who contacted with him, and I believe he was a real transplant coordinator" *(written communication, S. Hiraga, MD, May 29, 2006)*.

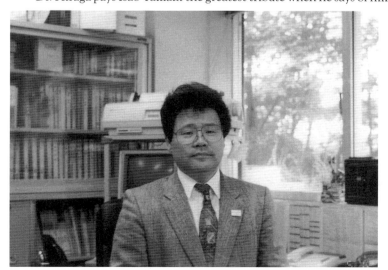

I would like to share a personal story about Isao that is more lighthearted, but truly conveys the enthusiasm of a Japanese transplant coordinator. At the time it was a little hair-raising, but I treasure this experience my husband and I shared with Isao Tamaki. We had just taken

Chapter 1 **THE HISTORY OF THE TRANSPLANT COORDINATOR**

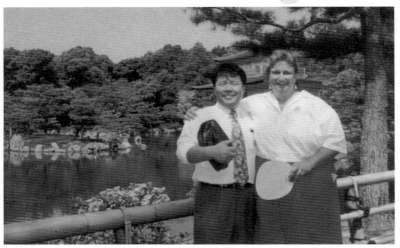

1994 photo of Isao Tamaki, President, Japanese Transplant Coordinators Organization, JATCO, and Teresa Shafer, President, NATCO. Taken in Kyoto in front of a Kyoto shrine during the 15th International Transplant Congress of the Transplantation Society.

our first trip to Japan during the 15th International Transplant Congress in Japan in 1994. We were in Japan for a week and were busy every moment, seeing the sights and meeting transplant coordinators and surgeons from Japan. Dr. Seigo Hiraga was our amiable and excellent host. All good things come to an end and so it came that it was time for us to return home. Isao had volunteered to take us to the Tokyo's Narita airport to catch our flight home to Fort Worth, Texas. We stopped at a Japanese shrine—quickly—and then piled back into his car for the drive to the airport. The traffic was unbelievable. Tokyo. Rush hour. Two fire engines were coming up behind us on the stalled freeway, and the cars somehow parted, allowing the trucks to go through. Isao did not miss a beat when he smiled and reached under his seat pulling out an emergency light like those used on emergency vehicles, and slipped in directly behind the fire engines. "Kidney car!" he exclaimed. "There are only two of these in Japan!" On went the lights and we followed the fire engines through the traffic snarl, reaching Narita in good time. If you have ever seen David Letterman's face when someone does something with gusto and a little strange, maybe that's what my husband, Don, and I looked like. Like Dr. Hiraga, I believe he was a real transplant coordinator, too. You can't get much closer to Chip Masters than the Japanese Kidney Car experience we had with Isao Tamaki!

Isao Tamaki was a terrific ambassador for organ donation as the first president of JATCO. It was a great honor to know Isao. He was smart, dedicated and a role model for all of the young and enthusiastic transplant coordinators following him into the position.

(first two photos courtesy of Seigo Hiraga, MD, third photo from NATCO Archives)

A CLINICIAN'S GUIDE TO DONATION AND TRANSPLANTATION

Fast Forward: 2006 and Beyond

Today's OPOs and transplant centers benefit from the application of standard business practices and increased resource application that began well after transplant coordinators and surgeons had pioneered and established the field. To a large degree the feeling of opening a new field of practice, of pioneering a new profession, is gone, of course, because organ donation and transplantation are indeed mainstream. OPOs and transplant centers are staffed by senior managers who remember the "old days" and the sacrifices and commitments they made to work in the field. Those days and that environment are gone now, and in its place are the growing pains of adapting the transplant coordinator function to mainstream organizational business practices. These growing pains are often acute as OPOs and transplant centers struggle to structure and restructure the transplant coordinator job in order to retain new recruits entering the field. The transplant coordinator of earlier times, whose job was broad and inclusive, is, in most parts of the country, no more. Instead, in order to get the work done, the job has been broken up into its elemental pieces, with intensive training in each section.

Hospital development, public education, family requesting, donor management, and operative recovery, in some OPOs, have evolved into five different positions: marketing staff to manage the hospital's donation system, educational specialists to conduct public education activities, requestor/family support staff, often bilingual, who are skilled in bereavement scenarios and in obtaining consent for donation, donor management specialists who manage the donors in the intensive care unit, and finally operating room technicians who are skilled in coordinating the activities of several operative teams and organ perfusion.

Similarly, clinical coordinators have become specialized in various ways, depending on the size and complexity of the transplant program, into transplant referral and evaluation coordinators, pre-transplant and post-transplant coordinators and living donor work-up coordinators. Transplant coordinators rotate through each of these positions on a schedule in some centers.

I probably feel as G. Melville Williams, MD, felt when he lamented the splitting of the transplant coordinator job into two jobs: one for procurement and one for clinical (only now, each of these jobs have been split into many more pieces!):

> History is useful only when we can determine whether we have lost a golden kernel from the past in the modernization process. Certainly legislation and OPO infrastructure have expanded organ donation. Every small hospital knows its responsibility and how to reach transplant networks. The organ procurement coordinators are better in obtaining consent for organ donation than physicians without experience in talking to grieving families. Yet, putting myself in their place, it must be a sad and demanding profession. The stress and long hours of caring for the potential donor and attending to the needs of sad and sometimes bitter loved ones takes a toll and results in turnover. Organ procurement coordinators just "burn out."
>
> The problem may be overspecialization. The recovery coordinator rarely sees the sparkle return to a recipient who has undergone successful transplant. If they do, it is in relation to a "media event." The surgeon is witness to transplant miracles daily and wants more. Yet he or she rarely deals with the truly hard emotions related to the recovery of organs he uses. Our fellows never discuss organ donation with families and would just feel uncomfortable doing so. To them, organs are wonderful, living "things," not part of Mr. Jones, the family breadwinner killed by a stray bullet. It is important to ask ourselves if something is missing. Should our recovery coordinators spend one month each year in the hospital on the wards and in the follow-up clinic? Should our fellows be called to the intensive care units to meet with the families and learn from the coordinators the *meaning* of organ donation? Is dealing more and more with less and less the way to go?[43(p12)]

I must confess, this is the way I feel about the coordinator position becoming more and more subdivided and insular. We shall see what the future holds for the transplant coordinator. I feel secure in knowing, however, that the pioneers founded the profession on solid ground and that there is a huge crop of new, fresh, dedicated and talented procurement and clinical transplant coordinators ready to carry the field forward. They will save lives and in so doing, will leave their mark on history.

Chapter 1: THE HISTORY OF THE TRANSPLANT COORDINATOR

The dramatic nature of the gift exchange makes the transplant coordinator's job, whether it be procurement or clinical, one of the best jobs in the world. People search for meaning in much that they do. Transplant coordinators do not have to search—it is in front of them every day as they go to work. I don't particularly believe in fate, none the less, there are times when one definitely feels a higher power must have been involved in our work. Transplant coordinators are often surprised themselves, just when they think they have seen everything, as this next story will confirm:

It's 1996 at the Children's Hospital San Juan, Puerto Rico. A pediatric donor heart has been accepted by Tampa General. This was the first time they were going to pass the four-hour ischemic time mark and were very nervous about it. Additionally, this was the first heart we had placed from Puerto Rico. We set the operating room time, the Tampa team arrived, it's a beautiful heart, they leave, the ambulance ride back to the airport is on time, everything's cool. Then 20 minutes later I get the call from the coordinator saying that they were about to board the plane, the jet's front tire was flat and they were going to lose the heart. I said " What's the problem? Change the tire and go!" What I didn't realize was that it takes several hours to fix a jet flat tire. Obviously everybody was bummed out—the child in Tampa was very sick and would not get transplanted this day. Believe it or not, several hours earlier while in the PICU, the pediatrician gave me a heads up on another potential donor that had just arrived in the same unit. Well, several hours later after completing the donor and being up for over 24 hours, the referral on the other child came in. The pediatrician said that they had declared the child brain dead and the parents wanted to donate. When I went in to obtain consent from the parents and finally got around to looking at the patients chart, I noticed that this child was about the same size as the previous donor from whom we had just lost the heart. My adrenalin started pumping again, I'm now running on fumes, and low and behold ... it couldn't be, this kid had the same blood type. I ran the heart list and guess who was at the top of the list? Yep, the same kid from Tampa General. After the cardiology consult cleared the heart, I called Tampa General with the offer, they were stunned—same size and ABO. They were desperate because the kid was hanging on by a thread. They accepted, we set the operating room time, they arrived and recovered the heart and rushed back to Tampa and transplanted it. Happy ending, the kid made it and was released several days later. I guess it was meant to be for that kid, two exact donor hearts, same size, same ABO, within 24 hours, after losing the first one, from, of all things, a flat tire. I'm exhausted from just thinking about those back to back cases... (written communication, J. Nespral, MD, CPTC, June 19, 2006).

I tried to weave this string of historical events, coordinator recollections, and personal comments into a profile worthy of those individuals who founded the transplant coordinator profession. Most of us like to read "stories." It makes the world real, tangible, touchable. I apologize for the many omissions that necessarily occur when writing a history covering nearly 45 years. My intent was to capture the spirit and art as well as the development and science of transplant coordination.

Such spirit includes the sense of affinity career coordinators have for their colleagues and the profession. Felix Rapaport, MD, includes a quote attributed to John Marquis Converse, MD, his mentor, in Rapaport's chapter on "The Life and Times of a Transplant Immunosurgeon" that seems perfectly suited for "career" coordinators: "...How fortunate, indeed, are those who meet the right person at the right time!"[209(p351)] Transplant coordinator founders and pioneers have invariably had such opportune meetings since many of them profiled in this chapter have served, knowingly and unknowingly, as role models and mentors to those who followed in their footsteps.

If truthful, most coordinators entering the field until only the most recent of times will acknowledge that they were drawn to the drama of life from death and the ability to make a difference in the world. We all have our stories and perhaps someone will one day put together a collection of those stories. My fondest memories at NATCO meetings have always been of listening to the "war" stories of fellow coordinators—clinical and procurement alike. Stories linked to practice make learning easy. I have also noticed that transplant coordinator stories from international colleagues mirror our own.

In his remarks prepared for this chapter, G. Melville Williams, MD notes that:

There is danger that we forget our humanitarian obligations. This is particularly true for surgeons who used to care for donors, obtain consent, take out organs and transplant them. Currently, transplant surgeons rarely ask for consent to recover organs. We treat organs more and more like a hip prosthesis which costs so much and must be put in right. It is you, the coordinators in the field, that bear the immense responsibility for dignified, compassionate efforts in organ recovery and in the ever enlarging follow-up clinics. I hope the stories I related above will keep the human side of transplantation green. Everyone in the field has his own accounts of meaningful events. No one needs to tell you the best thing you can do for a grieving family is optimal utilization of their loved ones organs *(written communication, G. M. Williams, MD, October 2005) [emphasis added]*.

I have drawn on remarks by Dr. Williams because of his own remarkable contributions to the field of transplantation and his clear regard for the transplant coordinator. He need not worry about transplant coordinators losing their humanitarian side, or, of them ever growing casual about their responsibility for unflagging and compassionate efforts in working with donor families and transplant recipients. It is, quite simply, the heart and soul of their job.

With that said, I will close with one more transplant coordinator story and a letter from a donor family member, ending this history, with all of its likely imperfections, on a true note. The true note? How transplant coordinators feel about donor families and/or their transplant recipient patients (in the case of a clinical transplant coordinator) and how recipients and donor family members feel about their transplant coordinators.

My favorite donor family story, one that would help a coordinator get out of bed for yet another donor after just completing one: In one of our first donor family recognition ceremonies, a mother of a young high school boy who had died suddenly in a traffic accident talked about her experience with donation. She began by outlining all of the pain and things that went wrong at the hospital—the tremendous stress, sadness, poor communication, anger, confusion—everything that added up to a description of her two-day hospital experience as a solid, black tapestry—as black and dark as anyone could imagine. Then, turning to the organ donation experience, she talked about how it finally allowed her and her family to take control of something at the hospital and to find some reason or solace in this senseless death. She slowly and emotionally described her overall memory of the death of her son as that of a very dark and black tapestry... all with a very slender, but bright, sliver of gold that weaved its way through that darkness—the gold representing the control and meaning they applied to this terrible day. I often thought of that picture when thinking of how difficult our jobs were at times—it kept me from quitting as there were other families to support and black days to color" (written communication, J. Springer, February 9, 2006).

Letter from donor family member:

Dear Jamie,

I don't know if I told you before, but thank you for being so awesome to me and my family. That week was such a big, awful nightmare and one big blur; there isn't much I remember about it. But I do remember that just when I was ready to rip both my brother's and sister's heads off, you were there for me to vent to. I felt really alone with Bill having his wife there and Nancy having all of her local buddies, but you were like an old friend that I had known forever. I guess what I am trying to say is you really went above and beyond, and I will never forget that. I also wanted to say thank you for being there for my mom when we couldn't. I'm so glad she wasn't alone. You respected her even when she wasn't really there anymore. There have been many times since her passing when I had been mad at her for even moving to Texas, because if she hadn't she would have never died there. But there again it is a miracle that God thought my mom to be so special he took her in a way that she'd be able to live on by helping others. I also wanted you to know that yes, organ donation does offer comfort on the really hard days.

Chapter 1 — THE HISTORY OF THE TRANSPLANT COORDINATOR

But all the special gestures that you and your organization do really help on those days that it felt like everyone had already forgotten about her. I just hope that one day I can be there and do for someone what you have done for us. I will never forget and always consider you a friend.

Sincerely,
Melissa[1]

Acknowledgments

I thank Lydia Stoner and Karla Diaz, LifeGift, for their assistance with this chapter. I would also like to recognize the excellent work of previous authors on the subject of transplant coordinators, including Barbara Elick, Claire Day, Celia Wight, Michael Phillips, Terri Donaldson and Nancy Tolboe.

I extend thank you's to those who lent materials, photos, and/or text for the chapter, including Christie Bowman and Dede Panjada for the NATCO archives, Barbara Schulman, first NATCO president, Paul Taylor, retired (30-year transplant coordinator!), Michael Phillips, Howard Nathan, Susan Stuart (wife of the late Brian Broznick), Helen Leslie-Bottenfield, Bob Duckworth, Jim Springer, Phyllis Weber, Seigo Hiraga (Japan), Ken Richardson, Greg Armstrong (Australia), Leo Roels, (Belgium), Bernard Cohen (the Netherlands), Bob Hoffmann, Linda Jones, and Karen Risk. I thank them as well for their frequent encouragement and e-mails. A double thank-you is in order for Leo Roels of Belgium, who must have responded to (a conservative estimate) over 50 e-mail requests for more information and fact-checking.

I thank the reviewers of the chapter, including Greg Armstrong, Bernard Cohen, Ron Dreffer, Bob Duckworth, Ron Ehrle, Barbara Elick, Louise Jacobbi, Linda Jones, Jamie Mazella, Howard Nathan, Mary Anne (House) Park, Michael Phillips, Mark Reiner, Leo Roels, Dianne LaPointe Rudow, Barbara Schanbacher, Barbara Schulman, Nancy Senst, Jolie (Savas) Slaton, Jim Springer, and Paul Taylor.

---

1. Author's note: (written communication, Melissa, donor family member to Jamie Mazzella, procurement transplant coordinator, June 2006, reprinted with permission.) Names of other family members changed. OPO name deleted since letters like these come to coordinators in all OPOs. This just happens to be a beautiful letter I had access to while writing this chapter.

NATCO Presidents

NATCO's presidents have shaped NATCO and were shaped by NATCO as much as any individuals could be by a professional society. The emergent profession of transplant coordinators was provided shelter and structure when NATCO was formed in 1976. The presidents over the years came from many different backgrounds, but all nurtured a fierce desire to legitimize the profession, further bolster the coordinator's knowledge base and autonomy, and underpin the transplant coordinator's practice with research and science.

Barbara Schulman, RN, CPTC
1979-1980
1st President

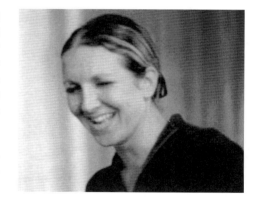

Barbara Schulman is a graduate of the New York University, Bellevue School of Nursing and was a first lieutenant in the United States Army Nurse Corps for four years. She was a senior transplant coordinator for the Regional Organ Procurement Agency (ROPA) of Southern California located at UCLA from 1974 to 1992. She was a senior donor development coordinator for the American Red Cross Tissue Services from 1995 to 1997.

She was one of NATCO's founders while at ROPA, then located in the Paul I. Terasaki Tissue Typing Laboratory at the University of California, Los Angeles, in September 1975. She was elected first president of NATCO on May 30, 1979 in Chicago, Illinois and as such helped establish the NATCO name, first logo, and dedication. During her presidency, the first newsletter was produced and the Public Relations, Ethics, Legal, Scientific and Education Committees were created. On June 27 and 28, 1980, she presided at the conference in Boston, Massachusetts prior to the VIII International Congress of the Transplantation Society.

Ms. Schulman was a founding member of the board of governors of the American Board of Transplant Coordinators. She was on the committee that developed and wrote the first certification exam and was also chairman of its Judiciary Committee.

Ms. Schulman was an original board member in Pittsburgh, Pennsylvania of the Transplant Recipient International Organization (TRIO) and a founder of and advisor to their Los Angeles chapter. She lectured extensively on a variety of critical issues regarding transplantation throughout the United States and has guest lectured in Singapore, Japan, and Nova Scotia and has served as a consultant to the California Medical Association committee on transplantation.

She served as the University of Southern California's kidney/pancreas transplant liaison, expert and advisor to dialysis center patients, staff and nephrologists in Southern California, from 2000 to 2006. She has experience as an operating room, field, family service, distribution, donor hospital development, and recipient coordinator. She is married to J. Brin Schulman, Esq. Ms. Schulman presently is a legal nurse consultant in transplantation matters.

Chapter 1 — **THE HISTORY OF THE TRANSPLANT COORDINATOR**

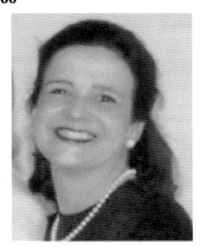

Kate Hume, RN, MSN
1980-1981
2nd President

Kate Hume received a bachelor of science degree in nursing from Bowling Green State University and completed her master's degree in medical-surgical nursing. In 1975 she began working at Northwestern Memorial Hospital in Chicago. One year later Kate accepted the position as a nurse clinician for their transplant program.

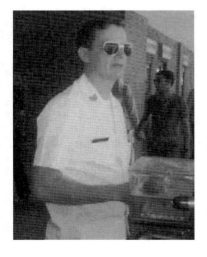

Robert Gosnell, MBA
1981-1982
3rd President

Robert Gosnell joined the Air Force in 1954 and became a surgical technician in 1960. He began working in the transplant research laboratory in Wilford Hall, San Antonio in 1961. One of the original procurement coordinators, he began his career in typical fashion during those early times, starting in the dog lab, experimenting with organ recovery and transplantation techniques and organ preservation. He worked on the transplant team, participating in the first kidney transplantation in San Antonio in 1961, and he performed extensive research in organ preservation and organ recovery techniques throughout his career at Wilford Hall and South Texas Organ Bank.

Mr. Gosnell was the founder of South Texas Organ Bank. He retired from the Air Force in 1977, and continued working as executive director of South Texas Organ Bank until his retirement in 1985.

The third president of NATCO, Mr. Gosnell remembers well all the first organizational coordinator meetings, including the first informal gathering in Los Angeles. He was one of the original procurement coordinators, using his experience, along with his colleagues, to shape the newly emergent profession of transplant coordinator. Mr. Gosnell traveled to Belgium in 1985, later hosting European transplant coordinator and physician visitors at his home when the NATCO annual meeting was held in San Antonio in1985. He published in *Urology*. Robert Gosnell received his bachelor's degree in business and his master's degree in business administration from Southwestern State University.

Winifred B. Mack, RN, BSN, MPA
1982-1983
4th President

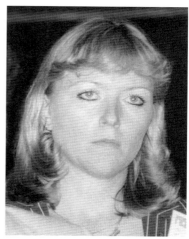

Winnie Mack is presently deputy executive director/chief operating officer for the North Shore Long Island Jewish Health System at Southside Hospital in Bay Shore, Long Island, New York. She has held many administrative positions since leaving the transplant program at Stony Brook University Hospital in Long Island in 1985. She was the first transplant coordinator on Long Island (1975-1985), working on a federal grant for the Nassau Community Medical Center, then for the New York/New Jersey Transplant Program, and ultimately at Stony Brook.

Winnie is a graduate of Nassau Community College and received her AAS degree in 1970. She continued her education at Long Island University and completed BSN and MPA degrees. Her thesis was a video on education in organ procurement, which had been used for education in the Long Island area, where she was responsible for organ procurement.

She was one of NATCO's founders while working at Stony Brook University Hospital. She was elected the first director of public relations (1979-1980), president elect (1981-1982), president (1982-1983), and immediate past president (1983-1984) of NATCO. She testified in 1983 before Senator Al Gore, representing NATCO at the congressional hearings on liver transplantation. She contributed to the publication *Model for a Regional Collaborative Retrieval Program* in collaboration with Joel Sherlock, MD published in *Transplant Proceedings* (Vol. 11, No. 2, June 1979).

Winnie was one of the founding members of The New York Transplant Society. She participated on the Advisory Committee for Transplant led by C. Everett Koop, Surgeon General. She has served as a board member for the Nassau Community College Clinical Technology Program and as a member and committee chair for the operating room on the Nassau/Suffolk Hospital Council Shared Services. She maintains her membership in the Association of Operating Room Nurses and New York Organization of Nurse Executives nursing organizations.

Winnie's clinical experience has been diverse, including work in the operating room, medical-surgical nursing units, maternity services, and dialysis. While working in dialysis, she was given the opportunity to pilot the federal grant on organ procurement.

Winnie is married to William S. Mack, a detective in the Nassau County Police department, and has a son, Patrick.

Chapter 1 — **THE HISTORY OF THE TRANSPLANT COORDINATOR**

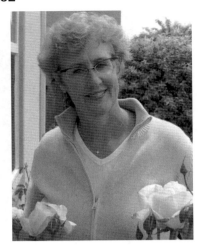

Amy S. Peele, RN, CPTC
1983-1984
5th President

Amy Peele enjoyed a 20 year career in transplantation. She is most proud of the part she played, during her tenure as president of NATCO, in passing the National Transplant Act and elevating the specialty of transplant coordinator to a true profession.

After graduating from South Chicago Community School of Nursing, she was employed at the University of Chicago and worked as a clinical and procurement coordinator for four and a half years. In 1982, she joined the staff of Rush Presbyterian St. Luke's Medical Center in Chicago, and in 1984 she was appointed director of their organ procurement program. While there, she worked with an orthopedic oncologist to create the first sterile bone bank in Chicago. During that same year, she was invited to be part of an American medical delegation that went to China to help educate local professionals in the areas of nephrology and transplantation.

Soon thereafter, Amy was recruited by the University of California, San Francisco, to be a clinical and procurement coordinator for their program, which averaged 250 kidney transplantations annually. She created a position at the university as a transplant liaison, to develop outreach programs in order to maintain and increase patient referrals. In this role, she initiated systems for assessing the success of the university's various programs, developed a referral database, and interacted directly with referring physicians, insurers, organ procurement organizations, and pharmaceutical companies.

She served as president of NATCO from 1983 to 1984 and, during that period, was called on multiple occasions to testify before both the Senate and the House of Representatives in Washington, DC in support of the National Transplant Act, which was passed and realized funding within one year. This legislation created the Division of Organ Transplantation and provided funding for the establishment of the United Network for Organ Sharing as the official transplant organization. She was also invited to participate on a task force with then Surgeon General C. Everett Koop that created a national organization, the American Council of Transplantation.

Amy also spent three years working with Sandoz Pharmaceuticals as an organ procurement organization development specialist. In this role, she assisted the organ procurement organizations in the Western region of the country in developing strategic plans that would maximize organ and tissue donation. Along with Jane Warmbrodt, she created a training program for hospital development, which has since been implemented throughout the country. She was part of the faculty for NATCO's procurement and clinical training programs, and she was on the original American Board of Transplant Coordinators and participated in the committee that developed and wrote the first certification exam.

Amy spent the last years of her career in the managed care arena, where she designed and conducted a Centers of Excellence process for Health Plan of the Redwoods and established their technology assessment unit. She joined Kaiser Permanente as manager of their National Transplant Network that coordinated transplant care for all of their 7.5 million members.

Among her many published articles and chapters in the area of transplantation, she has written for *Nursing Clinics of North America* and the textbook *Comprehensive Nephrology Nursing*.

Amy is now living in Marin County with her husband and teenage daughter and son, working as a writer of murder mysteries. Wouldn't you know, her first mystery killed off a transplant surgeon. She is also writing a compelling memoir titled *Aunt Mary's Guide to Raising Children the Old Fashioned Way*.

Ronald L. Dreffer, BS, CPTC
1984-1985
6th President

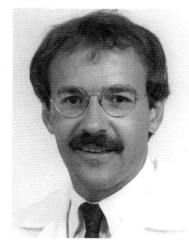

Ronald Dreffer is a graduate of the US Naval Medical Corps serving in Vietnam. He attended the University of Cincinnati, where he received a bachelor of science degree in biology.

Mr. Dreffer began his career in the field of transplantation, organ procurement, preservation, and research in 1975. He was the executive director of the Ohio Valley LifeCenter in Cincinnati, which served three transplant centers: The Christ Hospital, University of Cincinnati Hospital and Medical Center, and Children's Hospital Medical Center.

Mr. Dreffer has been an active member of NATCO since 1979, chairing a number of committees and serving as faculty for annual meetings. He was on the faculty for the first Introductory Training Course for Organ Procurement Coordinators. He served as NATCO president in 1984-1985. In 1985 he was chosen to serve as a member and committee chairman of the National Task Force on Organ Transplantation.

He was an active board member of the American Council on Transplantation, United Network for Organ Sharing, National Association of Patients on Hemodialysis and Transplantation, Association of Organ Procurement Organizations, and the International Congress on Ethics, Justice, and Commerce in Transplantation.

Mr. Dreffer was a member and committee chairman of the South-Eastern Organ Procurement Foundation, Hastings Center for Bio-Medical Ethics, Kidney Foundation of Greater Cincinnati, and the Surgeon General's Workshop on Increasing Organ Donation. He was a consultant for Sandoz Pharmaceuticals, Kentucky Organ Donor Affiliates, Maryland Organ Procurement Center, and The Partnership for Organ Donation. He has appeared on the *Phil Donahue* and *Today* shows and has made numerous appearances and lectures regarding organ and tissue donation, procurement, preservation, transplantation and ethics.

Additionally, Mr. Dreffer has published professional and research papers on biomedical aspects of organ and tissue procurement, preservation, and ethics. He resides in Cincinnati, Ohio and is married to Margaret S. Dreffer, RN, ET, and they have two daughters, Amy Lynn and Caryn Anne.

Mark R. Reiner, PA, CPTC
1985-1986
7th President

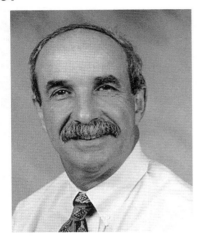

Mark Reiner began his career in the field of transplantation in 1976 as an organ procurement coordinator. He served as the executive director of LifeQuest organ procurement organization from 1979 through 1986; as vice president of Muskuloskeletal Foundation from 1986 to 1989; as executive director of Golden State Donor Services from 1989 through 1991, and as executive director of Transplant Resource Center of Maryland from 1991 to 1992. Currently, Mr. Reiner is a senior regional director for the Musculoskeletal Transplant Foundation. He resides in Atlanta, Georgia.

Mr. Reiner has been active with numerous professional organizations on a national level and an active NATCO member since 1980. Having chaired several committees, he assisted in the preparation of NATCO testimony to various legislative and governmental bodies including the Task Force on Organ Transplantation and twice to the Institute of Medicine on donation after cardiac death. Mr. Reiner was on the first faculty for the Introductory Training Course for Organ Procurement Coordinators.

Elected NATCO president in 1985, Mr. Reiner was involved in the formation of the United Network for Organ Sharing (UNOS). He led the negotiations, which led to the inclusion of the NATCO 24-ALERT organ sharing system and the 24-DONOR telephone hotline by UNOS. He served on the first UNOS board of directors representing transplant coordinators.

In 1999, he was presented with the NATCO-Novartis Achievement Award for his work and efforts in the field of transplantation. He served on the board of directors and as chairman of the American Board of Transplant Coordinators and was instrumental in the development of a computer-based certification exam for transplant coordinators. Additionally, he served on the National Donor Family Council Executive Committee of the National Kidney Foundation.

Stephen D. Haid, MS, CPTC
1986-1987
8th President

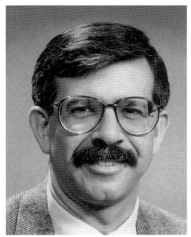

Steve Haid began his career in organ procurement in 1974 at Washington University School of Medicine in St. Louis, Missouri. He worked as an organ procurement coordinator and supervisor of a special surgical unit designed specifically for organ recovery procedures. He moved to Dallas, Texas in 1982 as the manager of organ recovery services for Southwest Organ Bank, and he became the executive director in 1987. He was concurrently executive director of Organ Recovery Systems, Inc., which was a management company for multiple organ recovery companies in four states.

Mr. Haid joined NATCO in 1975 and was a member for more than 20 years. He chaired nine committees and subcommittees and served on numerous others. He served as a member of the editorial board of the NATCO *Journal of Transplant Coordination* for seven years and was a faculty member of the Training Course on Procurement for Transplant Coordinators in 1983. Mr. Haid served as NATCO's president in 1986 and 1987. A memorable event during his term was the transfer of NATCO 24-ALERT (the association's system used to match donor organs with waiting recipients) to the United Network for Organ Sharing (UNOS). In 1987, he presented written testimony, on behalf of NATCO, to the Energy and Commerce Committee, United States House of Representatives on the reauthorization of the National Organ Transplant Act.

In addition to his NATCO involvement, Mr. Haid assumed leadership roles in several other transplant-related organizations, including the American Council on Transplantation, the Coalition on Donation, the Texas Transplantation Society, UNOS, and several others. He served on the editorial board of *Nephrology News and Issues* from 1991 to 1997. As a board member of the American Board of Transplant Coordinators, Mr. Haid helped develop the certification process for procurement and transplant coordinators. He served as president of the Association of Organ Procurement Organizations (AOPO) in 1992 and 1993 and led that organization in its first strategic planning. During his term, he testified, on behalf of AOPO, before the US House of Representatives Subcommittee on Health and the Environment, Committee on Energy and Commerce, regarding the reauthorization of the National Organ Transplant Act.

Mr. Haid received a bachelor's degree in biology at the University of Missouri, St. Louis, and his master of science degree in health care administration at Texas Woman's University, Denton, Texas. He has authored 25 published articles and book chapters and has presented more than 30 abstracts and presentations throughout the United States.

Chapter 1 — THE HISTORY OF THE TRANSPLANT COORDINATOR

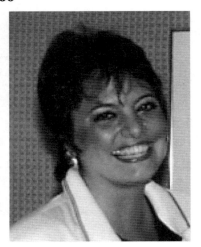

Anita L. Principe, RN, MPA, CCTC, CPTC
1987-1988
9th President

Anita L. Principe, RN, MPA, CCTC, CPTC, administrative director for Transplant Services at Montefiore Medical Center, Bronx, NY, a pioneer in organ transplantation, was one of the first to coordinate a multiorgan transplant program in the New York area. Ms. Principe was also one of the first in the country to establish a hospital-based organ procurement program for a large network of university and community-based hospitals in the New York metropolitan area.

She was a founding member of NATCO. As president, Ms. Principe led a national effort to establish uniform professional standards of practice for clinical and procurement transplant coordination and initiated the first national certification examination for credentialing transplant coordinators. Ms. Principe was the first associate editor for the *Journal of Transplant Coordination*.

As a founding member of the American Board of Transplant Coordinators, the national academic certification board for transplant coordinators, she served as its first vice chairman and succeeded as its chairman of the board of governors.

Ms. Principe served on the first board of directors of the United Network for Organ Sharing (UNOS) and has been appointed to numerous UNOS committees including the Scientific Advisory Committee, Membership and Professional Standards Committee, and the Transplant Administrators Committee.

Ms. Principe currently serves on the board of directors of the New York Organ Donor Network, Inc. She has participated in the Greater New York Hospital Association organ donor initiative and led the first New York State Organ and Tissue Donation Awareness Campaign. She was a member of the Surgeon General's Workshop on Increasing Organ Donation and an advisor to the End Stage Renal Disease Program Study Committee and Transplant Issues Sub-Committee of the Institute of Medicine National Academy of Sciences.

She has dedicated 30 years to the field and received a "Lifetime Achievement Award," established by the Transplant Recipient International Organization. She is the first recipient of this award, which was named "The Anita Principe Award" in her honor.

Barbara Schanbacher, RN, BSN, CCTC, CPTC
1988-1989
10th President

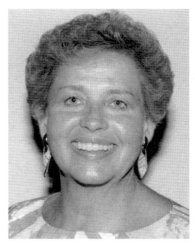

Barbara Schanbacher graduated from the University of Iowa College of Nursing with a BSN in nursing. She began her career as a staff nurse on a general surgery unit that housed cardio/thoracic, neurosurgery, gynecology, urology and general surgery patients. Three years later, she was appointed head nurse in that unit, a position she held until Dr. Robert Corry asked her to become the university's first transplant coordinator in 1974. With no prior knowledge of transplantation, she created her own job description. While reading a transplantation journal, she learned about the University of Minnesota's world-renowned transplant program and their coordinator, Justine Wilmert. Barb called Justine, traveled to Minneapolis to visit her program, and maintains that friendship to this day. In early 1976, Barbara Schulman and others from Dr. Terasaki's program at the University of California, Los Angeles invited 25 transplant coordinators from around the country to discuss the need for a formal venue for coordinators to share experiences and learn about this relatively new specialty. From that first meeting, NATCO was ultimately born. Barb Schanbacher was elected to the first board of directors and served in many capacities through the years, the last as president in 1988 and 1989. Schanbacher served on several boards of directors: the United Network for Organ Sharing, American Council on Transplantation, and the Kidney Foundation of Iowa. A sentinel event in the history of transplant coordination was the development of the credentialing process for transplant coordinators. She assumed a leadership position in the development of the American Board of Transplant Coordinators as the first chairperson of the Clinical Examination Committee. She served on the faculty of the NATCO education courses for many years.

From a personal standpoint, Barb cites the most valuable facet of her career as the life-long friendships she has enjoyed during her 30 years in the field. In the old days, organ sharing was conducted by friends calling friends, so close relationships evolved into deep lasting friendships. The sharing of common experiences has bonded transplant coordinators like no other profession.

THE HISTORY OF THE TRANSPLANT COORDINATOR

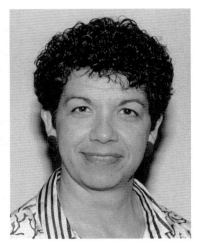

Louise M. Jacobbi, CCTC, CPTC
1989-1990
11th President

Louise M. Jacobbi, CCTC, CPTC is currently the president of Saturn Management Services and the director of new business for Organ Recovery Systems, Inc. She is a founding director of the Legacy Donor Foundation, a group dedicated solely to educating the public about the need for organ donation. The scope of her consulting work for Saturn Management reaches into the biotech, transplant, organ and tissue recovery communities and government agencies.

She served as the executive director of the Louisiana Organ Procurement Agency from 1990 to 1999. Before that, she was instructor in surgery at the Louisiana State University School of Medicine, Shreveport, and a clinical research associate at Tulane University. She began her career in transplantation in New York in 1962 at the University of Buffalo, doing research in the new discipline of transplant immunology. Ms. Jacobbi assisted in the founding of four organ recovery agencies and served as the director of two of them. She also assisted in the development of three histocompatibility laboratories, serving as a director/supervisor in all.

Ms. Jacobbi was one of the original group who conceived of and secured a grant from the Health Resources and Services Administration (HRSA) to implement the American Board of Transplant Coordinators, and she also served as the first board chair. During this same time, she served on the board of directors for the United Network for Organ Sharing, chairing and serving on several committees. She is board-certified as both a clinical and a procurement coordinator and recently received Emeritus status. Ms. Jacobbi currently is a director on the board of the American Liver Foundation and has chaired their Public Policy Committee for seven years. In 2001 she received their Humanitarian of the Year award. She served on the public policy committee of the National Kidney Foundation and served as treasurer of the Foundation for the Advancement of Transplantation and Immunogenetics. She served on the Association of Organ Procurement Organizations Standards and Accreditation Committee and on the Advisory Council of the National Institutes of Health (NIH) for the National Institute for Allergy and Infectious Diseases. She has been the principal investigator on several studies funded by grants from NIH and HRSA, which focused on increasing organ donation and credentialing of allied health professionals in transplantation. Over the years she has served on the Institute of Medicine and Surgeon General's advisory committees on transplantation and donation.

In 1987 she received the Sandoz/NATCO Achievement Award, in 1990 the Outstanding Technologist Award from the American Society of Histocompatibility and Immunogenetics, and in 1997 the AOPO Excellence in Management Award and the UpJohn/ SEOPF Award.

She has worked in transplantation and donation for more than 40 years, is widely published in the field, and has been an invited lecturer on those topics on three continents.

Barbara A. Elick, RN, BSN, CCTC, CPTC
1990-1991
12th President

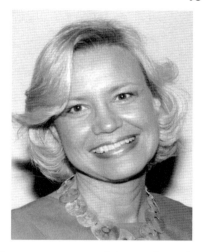

Barbara Elick currently serves as administrative director, of Transplant Services, University of Minnesota and Fairview Health Services. A transplant professional for more than 27 years, Barb Elick has worked in organ procurement and clinical transplantation in one of the oldest and largest transplant programs in the country, the University of Minnesota. With the merger of a community-based hospital system in 1996 (Fairview Health Services) and the academic health center–based hospital of the University of Minnesota, there was an opportunity to structure a partnership creating Transplant Services. As administrator of the newly created partnership of eight specialty transplant programs (heart, intestine, islet, kidney, liver, lung, pancreas, and living donors) at Fairview-University Medical Center, and faculty in the Department of Surgery at the University of Minnesota, Ms. Elick's responsibilities include business and strategic planning for the transplant service line.

After working as procurement coordinator with the Southwest Organ Bank and clinical coordinator at University of Texas Health Sciences Center in Dallas in the 1970s, she moved to the University of Minnesota in 1980 to work with the newly formed pancreas transplantation program alongside director David E. R. Sutherland, MD, PhD. She helped create additional extrarenal transplant services in the 1990s with stellar leaders Nancy L. Ascher, MD (liver), Ron Ferguson, MD and Chip Bolman, MD (heart), and Marshall Hertz, MD (lung). Growing under the tutelage of Richard L. Simmons, MD, PhD, and director John S. Najarian, MD, the program today performs 500 transplants yearly, maintaining its recognized leadership in the field. Ms. Elick was the driving force behind creation of *The Transplant Center*, a comprehensive ambulatory care facility providing pre-transplant and post-transplant care to recipients and donors of organ transplants and creating the Living Donor Program as an independent service. She led development of the Transplant Patient Assistance Fund and the Roberta Simmons Memorial Fund to assist living donors and conduct research on living donation. Recently, she collaborated with the University of Minnesota Academic Health Center and the National Kidney Foundation in co-hosting the 2004 Transplant Games, dedicated to the celebration of 50 years of transplantation.

Ms. Elick was instrumental in the development of the American Board of Transplant Coordinators and participated as both board and committee member for the United Network for Organ Sharing. Ms. Elick was a participant in the Surgeon General's Workshop on Donation and Transplantation in 1991 and was the contract officer and principal investigator of the Health Care Financing Administration and Division of Organ Transplantation grant titled, "Transplant Coordinator Professional Profile and Minority Education and Recruitment." In 1993, she was recognized by the Howard University Transplant and Dialysis Center for contributions as an advocate for minority participation in the field of nursing and transplant coordination. Ms. Elick was founding editor of the *Journal of Transplant Coordination* and has authored more than 60 publications on transplantation.

Her contributions to NATCO were accomplished with the help and support of a number of bright and thoughtful colleagues, and numerous dedicated committee leaders and members. Those "in cahoots" included life-long friends and NATCO past presidents Anita Principe (New York), Barb Schanbacher (Iowa), and Louise Jacobbi (Louisiana).

THE HISTORY OF THE TRANSPLANT COORDINATOR

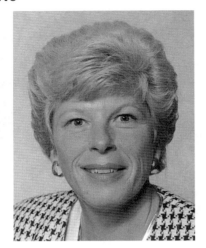

Linda L. Jones, RN, CCTC, CPTC
1991-1992
13th President

Linda Jones, retired chief executive officer of Lifeline of Ohio Organ Procurement Organization (LOOP), is currently the program director of the "Lives Worth Saving Program," Nisonger Center, The Ohio State University. She also serves as the primary investigator of LOOP's Health Resources and Services Administration (HRSA) grant to evaluate the effectiveness of a statewide donor registry. Ms. Jones was the senior clinical transplant coordinator at The Ohio State University Medical Center (OSUMC) from 1968 to 1981. From 1981 to 1983, she was the head nurse of the blood bank at OSUMC. She returned to transplantation in 1983 as the senior transplant coordinator for transplantation and procurement until 1985 when she and Ronald Ferguson, MD, founded LOOP. Ms. Jones was the co-director of LOOP from 1985 to 1992, became the chief executive officer in 1992 and held that position until retirement in 2003. She has spent more than 31 years in the transplantation and donation field and is extremely proud of being a part of the evolution of transplantation and organ recovery.

Ms. Jones is a graduate of Akron General School of Nursing affiliated, at the time, with Akron University. She spent her first seven years of her nursing career in the operating room, public health, and intensive care. It was while working in the intensive care unit at OSUMC that she was recruited to become a part of the OSUMC Transplant Program, a decision she will never regret.

Ms. Jones was a presenter in 1976 at the first gathering of clinical/procurement professionals in New York City and in 1978 hosted the first official meeting of these professionals in Columbus, Ohio. During her years in transplantation/organ recovery nationally she has chaired and served on numerous NATCO, UNOS, and AOPO committees. She served as NATCO's first parliamentarian, and after serving on the NATCO board as councilor at large, secretary and president-elect, she became the NATCO president in 1991. During her tenure as NATCO's president, two major accomplishments were the implementation of NATCO's first Transplant Institute and the formation of the International Transplant Coordinator Ad Hoc Committee. She has continued her NATCO activities, serving most recently on the Silver Anniversary Task Force.

Ms. Jones served on the UNOS Foreign Relations, Education, and Ad hoc, Membership and Standard, Pediatric, and Organ Procurement Organization committees during 1989 through 2003. During 1992 and 1993, she served on the UNOS board of directors and executive committee. During 1987 through 2003, she served on AOPO's Member Data Acquisition, Nominating, Membership, Ad hoc Special Projects, Data and Information Management, Ad Hoc Legislative, and Standards and Accreditation Committees. In 1993 she was program co-chair and became a member of the AOPO board and served as its secretary. From 1998 through 2002, her great interest and expertise was spent serving and chairing AOPO's Standards and Accreditation Committee. She became AOPO's first Emeritus member upon retirement in 2003.

Ms. Jones has lectured and presented nationally on various transplantation and organ recovery topics and has several publications. She is the recipient of the NATCO-Novartis Achievement award, the AIG Healthcare/AOPO Excellence in Leadership award, and the National Kidney Foundation of Ohio Governor's award. She was a finalist as the entrepreneur of the year for Business Leadership, Master Category in 2002. She worked diligently as the chair of the Ohio Second Chance Trust Fund Advisory Committee, which is appointed by the governor of Ohio from 2001 to 2002, and was instrumental in the implementation of Ohio's first person consent donor registry.

Ms. Jones is a wife to Jim Jones, retired athletic director of The Ohio State University, proud mother of Lynnae MaGinn and Bill Jones, and proudest grandmother of two granddaughters.

Lisa R. Kory, RN, BSN, CPTC
1992-1993
14th President

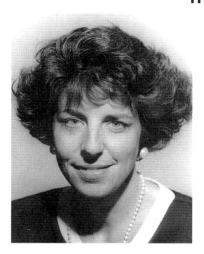

Lisa Kory received her bachelor of science degree in nursing from Indiana University in 1980. Lisa worked as a staff nurse in Indianapolis in critical care units and later as an oncology clinical specialist in Palo Alto, California. She began her career in organ donation and transplantation in 1986 as a clinical transplant coordinator for the University of California San Francisco Medical Center. In 1988, she joined the California Transplant Donor Network as a transplant coordinator, soon becoming a senior transplant coordinator. She worked there until 1994 and then moved to Washington, DC to assume the position of executive director of Transplant Recipients International Organization (TRIO).

Ms. Kory served on the NATCO board of directors from 1990 to 1994. She was a member of the procurement credentialing committee from 1988 to 1994, and served on various other committees, including the Education, Ethics, and Fund Raising committees.

She served on the United Network for Organ Sharing Board of Directors from 1992 to 1994 and has also served on various UNOS committees, including the Executive committee, Organ Procurement and Distribution committee, and the Patient Affairs committee from 1993 to 1994. A member of the American Society of Minority Health and Transplant Professionals, she served on its board of directors from 1995 to 1997. Ms. Kory is a member of the American Association of Critical Care Nurses and the American Nephrology Nurses Association.

Lisa lives with her husband, Kenneth Moritsugu, MD, Deputy Surgeon General of the United States, and their daughter, in suburban Virginia.

THE HISTORY OF THE TRANSPLANT COORDINATOR

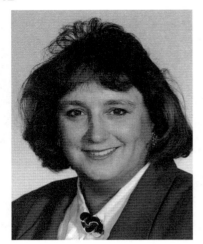

Teresa J. Shafer, RN, MSN, CPTC
1993-1994
15th President

Teresa Shafer is currently the executive vice president and chief operating officer of LifeGift Organ Donation Center, an organ procurement organization in Texas with offices and service areas in and around Houston, Fort Worth, Lubbock, and Amarillo, Texas. She oversees operations for organ and tissue recovery in 109 Texas counties, a population of 7.6 million people. A registered nurse, board certified in organ procurement, Teresa Shafer has been a leader in the field of transplantation, beginning her career in transplantation in 1985 as one of the principals who launched a hospital-based organ procurement organization at Harris Methodist Fort Worth in Fort Worth, Texas, termed Tarrant County Organ Donor Program. Before that, she had served in various staff and leadership positions in critical care nursing in Los Angeles, California; Champaign, Illinois; and Fort Worth, Texas.

Shafer received her bachelor of science degree in nursing cum laude in 1977 from Indiana State University in Terre Haute and her master of science degree in nursing cum laude from the University of Texas at Austin in 1980.

Ms. Shafer served as president of NATCO from 1993 to 1994, a time when she was busy conducting research and publishing in the area of medical examiner and coroner issues in organ transplantation. Her presidency allowed her to give a larger stage to the issue and began a steady movement toward the elimination of lives lost due to medical examiner and coroner denials of organ recovery. During her presidency, she appointed a new editor for *Progress in Transplantation* and became associate editor of the publication. A new publisher for the scientific journal was soon identified and hired. In 1994, she received the Association of Organ Procurement Organization's (AOPO/Sandoz) Excellence in Management award, in 1996, the NATCO/Sandoz Achievement Award, and in 2005, the Association of Organ Procurement President's Award. Most recently, Shafer was named chair of the ABTC Procurement Job Analysis Committee in 2006.

As president and past-president of NATCO, Shafer served as a board member for the United Network for Organ Sharing (UNOS). She served on numerous UNOS committees over the years and was instrumental, with UNOS, in creating new language in the Centers for Disease Control's Morbidity and Mortality Weekly Report providing guidance for transplant surgeons in using organs from donors with identified at-risk behavior. She received the AOPO President's Award in 1995 for significant and sustained contributions to the mission of AOPO. Shafer has been a member of numerous local, state, national, and international boards and committees and received a "Great Women of Texas" award for leadership and career accomplishments in 2001 from the Fort Worth Business Press and JP Morgan Chase.

A prolific author, Shafer has conducted research, managed several grants, including a $1.1 million US Department of Health and Human Services grant in 1999, and she has written more than 60 articles, book chapters, and abstracts, nearly all as first author. She won the J. Kent Trinkle Texas Transplantation Society Best Abstract award three times in 1997, 2003, and 2005. She is associate editor of *Progress in Transplantation* and a reviewer for several other transplantation and medical journals. Shafer was an invited researcher to Japan where she received a research grant from the Japan Human Science Promotion Foundation, consulting on Japan's organ donation system and brain death legislation in 1998. She has also consulted in Canada on organ recovery system structures and has lectured extensively throughout the country and the world. Shafer is a founding member of the International Transplant Coordinators Society.

Finally, from 2003 to 2005, Shafer served as national co-chair of US Department of Health and Human Services Organ Donation Breakthrough Collaborative, a national effort to increase organ donation and save the lives of thousands of additional transplant patients each year. For the first time ever, organ donation increased nearly 20% in the United States.

Teresa was raised on a farm in rural central Illinois and moved to Texas in 1980. She is married to Donald George Akagi and lives in Fort Worth, Texas.

A CLINICIAN'S GUIDE TO DONATION AND TRANSPLANTATION

Christine J. Gilmore, RN, BSN, CCTC
1994-1995
16th President

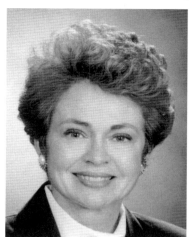

Education
Indiana State University, Terre Haute, Ind, OSII, 2005
Indiana State University, Terre Haute, Ind, BSN, 1984
Indiana University/Purdue University, Indianapolis, Ind ADN, 1971

Licensure: Registered Nurse, Indiana

Career Activities
(1971-74) Chief Transplant Nurse/Critical Care Nurse; Supervisor and Coordinator of Renal Nursing Services, Methodist Hospital, Ind.
(1979-1982) Director of Nursing Services; Critical Care Nurse, Vermillion Hospital, Ind.
(1984-1988) Manager, Transplant Center; Renal/Liver Transplant Clinical Coordinator, Methodist Hospital, Ind.
(1988-2000) Administrative Director, Transplant Center, Clarian Health Partners, Ind.
(2000) First attempted retirement.
(2001-2004) Director, Research, Prof. Education and Family Services, Indiana Organ Procurement Organization, Inc.
(2004) Second attempted retirement.
(2004-present) Health Careers Teacher, Fountain and Warren Co. High Schools, Attica, Ind.

Career/Professional Society Activities
Board Member, Secretary of the Corporation, Indiana Organ Procurement Organization
Board Member, Executive Committee Member, United Network for Organ Sharing
President, Board Member, Operations Chair, Patient Care Services Chair, North American Transplant Coordinator Organization
Member, Sigma Theta Tau Nursing Honorary Society
Delegate, Indiana State Nurses Association
Board Member. National Kidney Foundation of Ind.
Past President, Central Indiana NKF Chapter
Founding Committee Member, "Indiana Gift of Life Run"
Member, International Nurses Society
Member, American Nephrology Nurses
Member, Indiana Governor's Task Force on Organ Procurement and Transplantation
Founding Member, Indiana Tissue and Organs United for Caring Hoosiers
Representative, American Heart Association Speaker's Bureau

Volunteer Activities, Hobbies and Interests
Historic Preservation and Restoration; Docent, Attica Historic Village
Reading; Founder, Attica Book Club
Health and Society; Parish Nurse
Traveling
Anything and everything with husband, children, and grandchildren

Chapter 1: THE HISTORY OF THE TRANSPLANT COORDINATOR

NATCO Memories

From my first meeting in 1986 in Colorado, to the much anticipated 30-year anniversary, NATCO has offered me the opportunities of networking, education, legislative change-making, celebration, and fun. Highlights for me include taking the first NATCO credentialing exam in Orlando in 1988; the fantastic annual meetings; the challenging and very gratifying committee and board work; the development of the introductory courses, professional workshops, and the Transplant Institute; the affiliation with other transplant organizations and members; the creation of the member newsletter; and our organization's development of standards of practice and code of ethics. It has been a true privilege and honor to share with my colleagues the wonderful evolution of our transplant science.

Married to Thomas S. Gilmore and lives in Attica, Indiana. They have four wonderful children and seven grandchildren.

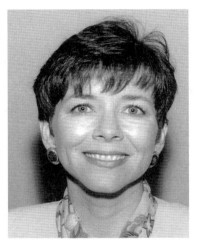

Suzanne Lane Conrad, RN, MS, CPTC
1995-1996
17th President

Suzanne Conrad is chief executive officer for Iowa Donor Network, a position she has held for nine years. Before coming to Iowa, she worked for Southwest Organ Bank (now Southwest Transplant Alliance) for 12 years in various hospital development and professional education management positions. In her tenure there, she established the organization's full-time, full-service marketing department.

In addition to on-the-job experience, Ms. Conrad currently serves on the Health and Human Services Secretary's Advisory Committee on Transplantation and the Advisory Committee to the Gift of Life Institute, Philadelphia, Pennsylvania. She is also current co-chair of the Legislative and Regulatory Affairs Committee of the Association of Organ Procurement Organizations (AOPO). Ms. Conrad also currently serves as treasurer of the National Kidney Foundation of Iowa. Before serving as president, she was NATCO's treasurer and chaired many of its organizational committees over the years. She is a past member of the executive committee of the National Kidney Foundation's National Donor Family Council and the LifeNet board of directors. Ms. Conrad has served two terms on the board of the United Network for Organ Sharing (UNOS), one as its treasurer and is a current member of the UNOS/Organ Procurement and Transplantation Network's Liver and Intestine Transplantation Committee. She has also served on the Scientific Registry of Transplant Recipients Scientific Advisory Committee. Ms. Conrad has served on the editorial boards of *Progress in Transplantation* and *Transplant Chronicles*.

A graduate of the University of Massachusetts, Lowell, she holds a bachelor of science degree in nursing. Ms. Conrad earned a master's degree in healthcare administration from Texas Woman's University in 1992. In February 2005, Ms. Conrad donated a kidney to a dear friend and Iowa Donor Network board member.

Frances M. Hoffman, RN, MSN, NP, CCTC
1996–1997
18th President

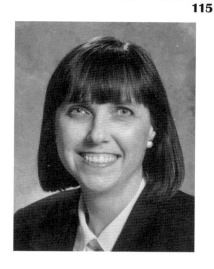

Frances Hoffman is the director of transplant and cardiovascular midlevel provider services at Abbott Northwestern Hospital in Minneapolis, Minnesota, where her areas of responsibility include the heart and kidney transplant programs, and midlevel providers in the cardiovascular services division. She joined the staff of Abbott Northwestern in 1984, as a clinical nurse specialist in cardiovascular surgery. She was involved with initiation of the heart transplant and mechanical assist programs in 1985, when her activities included both clinical care of patients and organ procurement. Although her administrative responsibilities have increased over the years, she remains involved in direct patient care.

Ms. Hoffman received her bachelors degree in nursing from the College of St. Scholastica in Duluth, Minnesota, and completed her master's degree in nursing with a focus on nursing education and the clinical nurse specialist role at the University of Minnesota. Twenty years later, she returned to the University of Minnesota to complete the acute care nurse practitioner program, and became ANCC certified in 2001.

A member of NATCO since 1986, Ms. Hoffman served in many roles starting as a faculty member of the Introductory Course for Transplant Coordinators. She became clinical course consultant, and served from 1990 to 1992. She began her term on the board of directors as councilor at large in 1993, and subsequently served as treasurer, and then as president from 1996 to 1997. After serving as immediate past president, she returned to the introductory course for a second term as clinical course consultant, and later cochaired the NATCO annual meeting in 2004. She has been a member of the editorial board for *Progress in Transplantation* since 1994. Ms. Hoffman has also served in leadership positions within the International Society for Heart and Lung Transplantation where she has chaired the nursing council and served on the board of directors, and in the United Network for Organ Sharing where she served on the board of directors, the Executive Committee, and the Thoracic Organ Transplantation Committee. She has published and spoken widely in the field of transplantation. In 2000, Ms. Hoffman received the NATCO–Novartis Achievement Award.

Chapter 1: THE HISTORY OF THE TRANSPLANT COORDINATOR

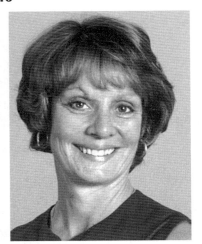

Laurel Williams, RN, MSN, CCTC
1997-1998
19th President

Laurie Williams is currently the manager of the liver and intestinal coordinators for the organ transplant program at the University of Nebraska Medical Center in Omaha, where she began working in 1985. She received her bachelor of science in nursing from the University of Michigan School of Nursing and her master's degree in nursing at Wayne State University School of Nursing in Detroit with the focus on children and adolescents.

Ms. Williams was awarded the NATCO/Novartis Achievement Award, which is one of the highest honors bestowed by NATCO. The award was established to recognize significant achievement within NATCO and the fields of donation and transplantation. She is also the editor-in chief of *Transplant Chronicles*, a quarterly newsletter for transplant recipients with the goal of bringing timely education and support to recipients, helping them to maintain and maximize their health and quality of life.

Ms. Williams served as president of NATCO from 1997 to 1998 and Immediate past president from 1998 to 1999. She has published and spoken widely on the subject of liver and intestinal transplantation.

A CLINICIAN'S GUIDE TO DONATION AND TRANSPLANTATION

Mary Ann M. Palumbi, RN, BS, CCTC
1998-1999
20th President

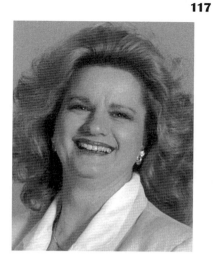

Mary Ann Palumbi has been active in the field of transplantation since June 1980. She began her career at Presbyterian University Hospital (UPMC) as the first clinical coordinator for the renal transplant program. During this same period, she functioned as both organ procurement coordinator as well as a clinical transplant coordinator. She was recruited to Allegheny General Hospital in 1986 to oversee the development of a multiorgan transplant center. She continues in this administrative position serving as the senior director of transplantation services at Allegheny General Hospital in Pittsburgh, Pennsylvania.

In the past 25 years, she has presented more than 500 professional presentations on organ donation and transplantation, most recently dealing with the economic aspects of transplantation. She has more than 25 professional publications, including two book chapters. She was a contributing editor for *Nursing Core Curriculum on Organ Donation and Transplantation*, produced through the United Network for Organ Sharing and distributed to all college-and hospital-based nursing programs throughout the country.

An active member of NATCO since 1980, she has chaired a number of committees, including serving as co-chair of the NATCO Introductory Course for more than eight years. She served on the board of directors as a councilor at large for three years, then as president. Other professional activities include director, board of directors, United Network for Organ Sharing (1999-2000); vice-president, board of directors, National Kidney Foundation of Western Pennsylvania (1986-1988); and director, board of directors, The Center for Organ Recovery (a regional organ procurement organization), from 1996 to the present.

In 2001, Ms. Palumbi was the first member of NATCO to be appointed by then Secretary of Health and Human Services, Donna Shalala, to the Advisory Committee on Transplantation. This committee was established to oversee transplant policy through the Organ Procurement and Transplantation Network.

Her current responsibilities include senior administrative, clinical development, and fiscal responsibilities for multiorgan transplant programs; the histocompatibility laboratory; Mechanical Heart Services; and the Center for Bloodless Medicine and Surgery. She is also responsible for evaluation of and participation in all managed care contracts for these departments; development and follow-up of all quality improvement projects for all departments; and preparation and review of all regulatory agencies protocols and policies, and implementation of processes to meet these standards.

THE HISTORY OF THE TRANSPLANT COORDINATOR

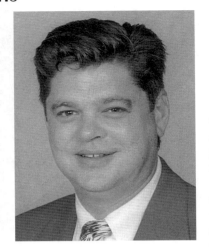

Bruce Nicely, RN, CPTC
1999-2000
21st President

The presidency of NATCO during its 25th anniversary year was exciting and an important personal and professional challenge. As is always the case with a successful organization, we had the participation of many outstanding individuals who generously gave their time and talent for the betterment of our profession.

We focused on updating NATCO's image during the silver anniversary year, and we used the time to reflect on and remember important milestones. The society's logo and support materials were all updated, bringing an exciting, fresh look to the emblem designed to capture our dynamic membership and functions. NATCO's flagship publication—*The Journal of Transplant Coordination*—was changed to *Progress in Transplantation*, another accomplishment to reflect the broadening, rapidly growing number and type of professionals involved in care of donors, donor families, and recipients.

NATCO reached out to other transplant organizations in an effort to become the major resource for perspectives from those closest to the miracle of transplantation. Tens of thousands of miles and lots of hotel rooms helped us accomplish our mission. Tremendous effort was given to improving and expanding NATCO's educational offerings for professionals, with much success. NATCO courses became the hallmark for education of both new and seasoned transplant professionals.

It was and will always be a distinct honor and privilege to have held the office of president of NATCO. I fondly recall the 1500 e-mails I received during my tenure, which I equate to real interest in the organization among its membership. I think often and remember warmly the friendship and partnership with the late Pam Gale, NATCO's associate executive director. Applied Measurement Professionals linked with NATCO always to make a topnotch professional society. Executive Office staff members Dede Gish Panjada, Executive Director; Christie Bowman, Association Manager; and Cheri Jones, Meeting Manager, worked long, hard hours to help NATCO succeed.

The NATCO presidency was a proud, yet humbling experience for me. I sincerely hope our paths cross again. In closing, I thank all NATCO members who allowed me the honor of serving as their leader. To all current and future members, God bless you for your work. The work—and you—are very special.

A CLINICIAN'S GUIDE TO DONATION AND TRANSPLANTATION

Jeffrey S. Mitoff, RN, BSN, CPTC
2000-2001
22nd President

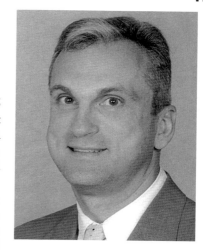

Jeff Mitoff received a BS in microbiology and nursing in 1985 from Ohio State University. Following graduation, he took his first job as a nurse in the surgical intensive care unit at a downtown trauma center in Columbus, Ohio. It was in this position that Mr. Mitoff developed his clinical skills along with becoming acquainted with the process of organ donation.

Mr. Mitoff remembers the opportunity that led to his work in organ recovery: "Working one day with an organ donor case, Linda Jones came in as the coordinator. She mentioned to me that she was in the process of increasing staff at LifeLine of Ohio and asked if I might be interested in such a position. I had always been impressed at the professionalism of the LifeLine of Ohio staff and jumped at the opportunity. I was hired as a procurement coordinator and began a long journey in this field in 1987."

"I remember how different it was with the whole process back then. I can remember calling on the phone and getting the computer-generated match run and hand writing it down, you had to write fast or go through the whole list again because there was no way of pausing the voice. I can remember getting the first fax machine in our office, the kind with the curly roll paper. The first cell phone that was bigger and heavier than a laptop computer; the first computers in the office with the green neon letters on a black screen."

Mr. Mitoff worked 10 years at LifeLine of Ohio before relocating to Phoenix, Arizona to take a position as the procurement director for Donor Network of Arizona, where he worked for three years. He moved to the clinical side of transplantation coordination when in 2000, he started at the new Mayo Clinical Hospital in Phoenix. During the first year, while they performed only 16 kidney transplants, all of them living related, they were able to focus their efforts on building the list. Mr. Mitoff worked for Mayo Clinic Hospital in Phoenix for four years and during his last year there, 75 kidney transplantations were performed.

In 2004, Mr. Mitoff once again transitioned, this time to the transplantation industry side, when he was recruited by AirNet, an airline specializing in express transportation, its goal being expansion of the shipping of organs in a more timely manner.

Mr. Mitoff has been a NATCO member since the very beginning of his career in 1987, serving as co-chair of the annual meeting in Boston in 1995, serving on the board of directors as councilor at large in 1997, and president in 2000. During his year as president of NATCO, the first hospital development training course was held. Additionally, the Education Task Force was established to review the content of the Introductory Course. This lead to the development of the patient simulations and now to the online education task force, which is working on developing an online exam preparation.

THE HISTORY OF THE TRANSPLANT COORDINATOR

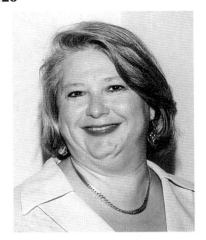

Judy S. Graham, MS, CS, CPHQ, CPTC
2001-2002
23rd President

Judy Graham has 26 years of nursing experience, receiving her first degrees from Washington School of Practical Nursing and East Central College in Union, Missouri. After several years of bedside nursing in the Trauma Surgical Critical Care Unit at St. Louis University Medical Center, she moved to New York City. There she received her BSN (1992) and MS (1996) degrees as a critical care clinical nurse specialist with additional postgraduate studies in research, critical thinking, and adult education at Columbia University School of Nursing and Barnard Teachers College. For six years, Ms. Graham used her critical care skills to manage organ donors and obtaining consent for donation as a transplant coordinator.

In 1996 she became the quality systems manager and corporate compliance officer at the New York Organ Donor Network, where she developed and implemented an organization-wide quality and compliance program. During this time, Ms. Graham taught multiple aspects of the organ donation process at two national forums, served as president of NATCO and on the board of directors for the Organ Procurement Transplant Network/United Network of Organ Sharing. Since 2002, Judy has devoted her time to quality and performance improvement in the acute care hospital setting, first as a performance improvement specialist for the oncology, digestive diseases, vascular diseases, organ and stem cell transplant service lines at New York-Presbyterian Hospital. Presently, Ms. Graham is responsible for quality, patient safety, and compliance with performance improvement initiatives at the New York-Presbyterian Healthcare System. As well as serving as liaison to the system's 48 facilities that span the continuum from ambulatory care networks to acute care hospitals, and to long-term care institutions, she is a regular quality assurance performance improvement consultant at Shepton Mallet Treatment Centre, Somerset, UK. There she promotes the best of practices of a US academic medical center and hospital system while maintaining standards required of an Independent Sector Treatment Centre in the UK National Health Service.

Barry S. Friedman, RN, MBA, CPTC
2002-2003
24th President

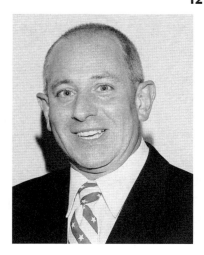

Barry Friedman's career in solid-organ transplantation began in 1984 as a staff nurse at Barnes Hospital St. Louis, Missouri, in the cardiothoracic intensive care unit, which included heart transplantation patients. He attended Southern Illinois University and graduated with a bachelor's degree in nursing in 1984 and attended Southern Illinois University for an MBA with a minor in health care administration in 1998. In 1986 he officially became an organ procurement coordinator with Mid-America Transplant Services in St Louis, Missouri. He continued his career as a procurement coordinator until 1991, and then began his career as a pediatric clinical transplant coordinator at SSM Cardinal Glennon Children's Hospital in St. Louis, Missouri. His scope as a clinical coordinator included heart, liver, and kidney transplants and he soon became the administrative director of the pediatric solid-organ transplant program at Cardinal Glennon.

In March 2003, Barry accepted a position at Children's Medical Center in Dallas Texas, as the administrative director of solid-organ transplantation, where he is responsible for the heart, liver, kidney, and intestinal transplantation programs.

Barry has been an active member of the US Air Force Reserves as a flight nurse and served in Iraq during Operation Iraqi Freedom as director of operations for aeromedical services in a remote location in the Middle East. He is currently a Major.

Barry is married to Shelley Friedman and has two daughters, Erin who is a junior at St. Louis University and Paige who is a senior in high school at Core Jesu Academy in St. Louis. Barry enjoys watching professional sports and enjoys his daily visits to the health club at 5:30 AM, where he works out for one hour. Barry and his family enjoy vacations centered on the beach.

His professional activities have also included being on the board of directors of NATCO. He has also been involved with the United Network of Organ Sharing (UNOS) as a member of their board of directors.

THE HISTORY OF THE TRANSPLANT COORDINATOR

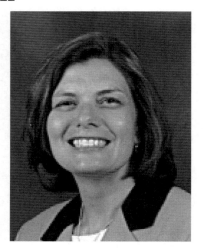

Nancy L. Senst, RN, CPTC
2003-2004
25th President

Nancy Senst is a graduate of St. Joseph's Hospital School of Nursing, Marshfield, Wisconsin and completed her bachelor's degree in nursing at Edgewood College, Madison, Wisconsin. After working as a pediatric and adult intensive care nurse in Wisconsin and Minnesota, Nancy joined the field of organ and tissue donation in 1989. During her career, she worked as a procurement, education, and hospital development coordinator with LifeSource, the organ procurement organization based in St. Paul, Minnesota. She continues to work at LifeSource as their tissue project manager. Early in her donation career, colleagues encouraged her to join and participate in NATCO. She worked with many NATCO committees as a member and chair, and later joined the board of directors as councilor-at-large and then president.

In her year as president, the world celebrated the 50th year of transplantation. For NATCO, donation and transplantation had a year of positive growth and development. Education programs continued to be strong. The annual meeting in San Francisco was one of the most highly attended ever. Throughout the year, more than 850 people participated in NATCO education programs. A request for proposal was developed to revamp the entire hospital development course, which would once again put NATCO in the education forefront.

2003-2004 was a year of increased collaboration with other professional organizations. The Coordinator Committee became a standing committee within the UNOS structure, for the first time grants from the Health Resources and Services Administration (HRSA) were presented at the annual meeting, joint education was sponsored and designed with International Transplant Nurses Society (ITNS), ATC, National Kidney Foundation, and ISOP. NATCO started a whole new visibility through these programs and exhibits at other professional meetings.

During that year, HRSA brought forth an Organ Breakthrough Collaborative. NATCO proudly participated in the Expert Learning Panels and the Leadership Coordinating Council. Donation increased an amazing 10%.

Publications within NATCO continued to thrive. *Progress in Transplantation* saw an increase in continuing education enrollments, the number of submitted manuscripts continued to grow rapidly, and more than 2,000 professionals now subscribed. The *In Touch* newsletter was updated, and each issue was sponsored by a corporate colleague. The Professional Practice Core Competencies created in 2002 received copyright notification from the Library of Congress.

Technology was increasingly important to the field. After a request for proposal (RFP) process, NATCO moved to a new Internet service provider so that abstracts could be submitted on line and members could vote, register for meetings, and search the NATCO directory electronically. Resource councils through various list servs were set up with nearly 600 members participating. NATCO also heard from its members electronically, 632 members took time to complete a membership survey that will help guide the organization in the future.

Two more RFPs set the stage for NATCO's future that year. A consultant was hired to review our management company, Applied Measurement Professionals, and review the organization overall. Through the membership survey, NATCO clearly heard that members wanted a stronger voice in Washington, DC. A new firm was hired, and we are now walking the Hill with purpose and speaking with one voice.

Ms. Senst's dedication to donors, their families, and the recipients, who continue to wait for a second chance at life, guided her, the NATCO Board and Committee chairs through a year of growth, change, and success.

Dianne LaPointe Rudow, DrNP, CCTC
2004-2005
26th President

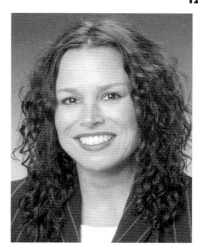

Dianne LaPointe Rudow is presently the senior transplant coordinator and clinical director of living donor liver transplant and outpatient service at the Center for Liver Disease and Transplant at New York Presbyterian Hospital. She is an assistant professor of clinical nursing at Columbia University, serves on the Editorial Board of *Progress in Transplantation*, and provides consulting services to various transplant nursing education companies.

She was one of the first individuals in the United States to graduate with a doctorate of nursing practice (DrNP) from Columbia University in 2005. Additional education includes 1996: Adelphi University School of Nursing Adult Nurse Practitioner-Post Master's Certificate Program; 1991: Hunter-Bellevue School of Nursing Master of Science in Nursing; 1987: Hunter-Bellevue School of Nursing Bachelor of Science in Nursing.

NATCO's accomplishments during Dr. LaPointe Rudow's term include partnering with the American Society of Transplant Surgeons at the Transplant Institute, preserving NATCO's history by spearheading the development of and co-editing the first transplant and procurement textbook, *A Clinician's Guide to Donation and Transplantation*, appointing an Online Education Task Force to make the NATCO Introductory Education Course content accessible to all transplant professionals, and presiding over NATCO's 30th anniversary annual meeting in July 2005 in Atlanta.

Dr. LaPointe Rudow is a member of the OPTN/UNOS board of directors and serves on the policy advisory group of OPTN/UNOS Executive Committee. She also serves on the board of directors of the UNOS Foundation. She has served on the membership committee of the American Society of Transplantation and on the clinical advisory committee for the New York Center for Liver Transplantation.

Dr. LaPointe Rudow has lectured on all aspects of transplantation, participates as a content expert at consensus conferences, has published extensively on living donor liver transplantation, and heads the Independent Donor Advocate Team at New York Presbyterian Hospital, Center for Liver Disease and Transplantation in New York.

THE HISTORY OF THE TRANSPLANT COORDINATOR

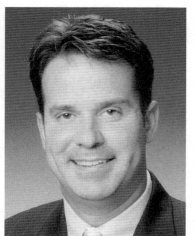

Charles E. Alexander, RN, MSN, MBA, CPTC
2005-2006
27th President

Mr. Alexander has been active in the field of transplantation since 1995. He began his career at Transplant Resource Center of Maryland as an operating room perfusionist, later assuming the role of organ recovery coordinator. In 1999 Alexander started the first Hospital Development Department for Transplant Resource Center, later becoming the manager of hospital development. In 2003 Mr. Alexander became the director of clinical and hospital services. In April of 2004, Mr. Alexander was promoted to president and chief executive officer of the organization.

In the past 10 years, he has presented more than 200 professional presentations on organ and tissue donation and transplantation. He has published in several professional publications, including case studies in organ donor management, the use of Airway Pressure Release Ventilation modes of ventilation in organ donors, continuous venovenous hemodialysis, and donation after cardiac death.

An active member of NATCO since 1996, he has chaired a number of committees, including the NATCO Introductory Course, Membership and Public Policy committees. He served on the board of directors from 2003 to 2006, as secretary for two years, president-elect and then as president. Mr. Alexander served on the United Network for Organ Sharing board of directors in 2005 and 2006, was vice-chair of the UNOS Organ Procurement Organization Committee, and served in various information technology groups. Mr. Alexander is a member of the Maryland Organization for Nurse Executives and the Greater Baltimore Healthcare Committee and has served on several committees of the Association of Organ Procurement Organizations (AOPO).

Mr. Alexander's prior clinical experiences include working as a registered nurse in the medical intensive care unit at The Johns Hopkins Hospital (two years) and in the trauma resuscitation unit at the R. Adams Cowley Shock Trauma Center in Baltimore, Maryland (six years). He has earned a BS degree from the School of Marketing and Economics at Towson University, a BSN from Villa Julie College, a master's degree in nursing from The Johns Hopkins University, and an MBA from The Johns Hopkins University, each in the Baltimore area.

Marian O'Rourke, RN, CCTC
2006-2007
28th President

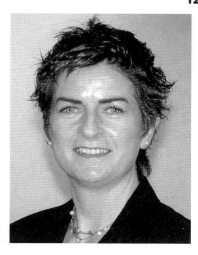

Ms. O'Rourke graduated from the Limerick Regional School of Nursing, Limerick, Ireland in 1987 and after a brief period working in Ireland, she moved to London and specialized in intensive care nursing for five years. In 1991, she moved to New York and began her career in solid-organ transplantation at the Recanati/Miller Transplantation Institute at the Mount Sinai Medical Center. Ms. O'Rourke was a liver transplant coordinator for five years and in 1997 became the senior clinical coordinator for the adult liver transplant program. In 1998, she helped establish an intestinal transplant program and an adult living donor liver transplant program. In January 2004, she joined the Tulane Abdominal Transplant Institute as the director of transplant administration at Tulane University Hospital and Clinic in New Orleans, Louisiana.

Ms. O'Rourke has been an active member of NATCO, The Organization for Transplant Professionals since 1992. She served on the research committee for many years and was the clinical co-chair of the 2002 NATCO annual meeting in Washington, DC. She has served on the NATCO board of directors since 2002 initially as councilor at large, secretary, president elect and president. Ms. O'Rourke is the first non-American president of NATCO.

Ms. O'Rourke has also been an active member of UNOS/OPTN and served two terms on the Data Advisory Committee. She also served as an at-large member of the UNOS/OPTN Transplant Coordinators Committee from 2003 to 2006. Ms. O'Rourke served as the NATCO chair of the 2005 American Transplant Congress Nursing Pre-Symposia sponsored by NATCO and the International Transplant Nurses Society. In 2006, she became an associate member of AST.

In the past 15 years, Ms. O'Rourke has presented at numerous national and international transplantation meetings on a wide variety of topics and has published on a number of different aspects of transplantation, including living liver donation, liver transplantation in methadone-dependent patients, and recovery of delayed type hypersensitivity after liver transplantation.

Ms. O'Rourke is an avid supporter of the transplant center's role in education and awareness efforts to promote organ donation and speaks on the topic frequently both locally and nationally.

Chapter 1 — **THE HISTORY OF THE TRANSPLANT COORDINATOR**

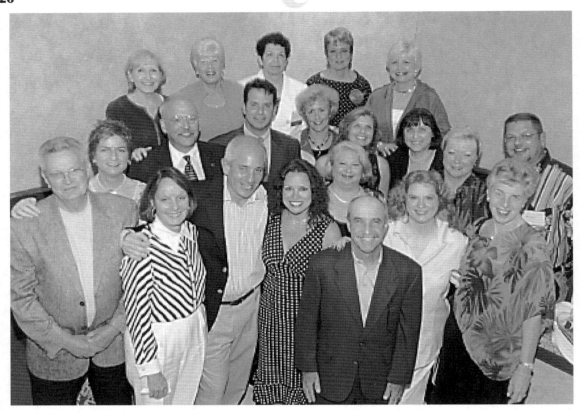

2005 NATCO Annual Meeting: Past President's Reception

First Semicircle:

Laurel Williams, 97-98
Barry Friedman, 02-03
Dianne Lapointe Rudow, 04-05
Judy Graham, 01-02
Mark Reiner, 85-86
Mary Ann Palumbi, 98-99
Lisa Kory, 92-93

Second Semicircle:

Robert Gosnell, 81-82
Marian O'Rourke, 06-07
Ron Dreffer, 84-85
Charles Alexander, 05-06
Amy Peele, 83-84
Nancy Senst, 03-04
Frances Hoffman, 96-97
Winifred Mack, 82-83
Bruce Nicely, 99-2000

Third Semicircle

Barbara Schulman, 79-80
Linda Jones, 92-93
Louise Jacobbi, 89-90
Anita Princie, 87-88
Barbara Elick, 90-91

Missing in Action(!):

Kate Hume, 80-81
Steve Haid, 86-87
Barb Schanbacher, 88-89
Teresa Shafer, 93-94
Christine Gilmore, 94-95
Suzanne Conrad, 95-96
Jeff Mitoff, 00-01

A CLINICIAN'S GUIDE TO DONATION AND TRANSPLANTATION

When	What	Who	Where
Fourth Century BC	Chinese text describes switching of hearts: Chinese texts describe a surgeon who switches the hearts of 2 soldiers; these accounts say that both patients survived. Faced with one soldier displaying a strong spirit but a weak will, the other the reverse—allegedly anesthetized them both with wine, performed thoracotomies, and exchanged their hearts to cure the disequilibrium in their energies. This is the first known description of a body-to-body transfer.[27(p7),31]	Tsin Yue-Jen, Chinese surgeon	China
Third Century AD	According to Christian mythology, described in Jacopo da Varagine's Leggenda Aura in 348 CE. The twin brothers Saints Cosmos and Damian replace a gangrenous leg of a Roman deacon Justinian with a leg from a recently buried Ethiopian Moor. This is the first description of a new concept: the body of a dead person can help a living person.[27(p7),29,30,32]	Saints Cosmos and Damian, Christian surgeons	Turkey
1628	Human circulatory system documented: William Harvey publishes breakthrough work on the human circulatory system. He validated his work by dissecting the bodies of his father and his sister. Until the mid-19th century, bodies from the gallows were the only legal source of bodies for study and research in Great Britain; grave robbers supplied medical schools with bodies. Exercitatio Anatomica de Motu Cordis et Sanguinis in Animalibus (An Anatomical Exercise on the Motion of the Heart and Blood in Animals)[32,210]	William Harvey	Great Britain
1667	First transfusion of blood: The discovery of blood circulation leads to experiments in blood transfusion. Blood from a lamb was administered to a 15-year-old boy who suffered from high fevers. In 1668, after several people had died following transfusions, authorities in France and Great Britain, where most of the deaths had occurred, prohibited any more experiments.[29(p20),210]	Jean-Baptiste Denys, French physician	France
1682	First bone transplant recorded when a defect in a Russian soldier's head is filled with a piece of dog skull. This anecdotal case was recorded in church history because the patient was excommunicated. Two years later, he requested that the transplant be removed so that he could return to the good graces of the church.[27(p13-14),31]	Job van Meeneren, Dutch physician	Netherlands
1778	Use of the term transplantation for the first time. Hunter implanted rooster spurs onto the comb of the rooster and later implanted human cadaver teeth onto the same comb before finally transplanting teeth from a human cadaver to a live human recipient. He attributed the success to "the disposition displayed by all living substance to unite when in contact with another substance, even if circulation is transported inside one of them.[82(p16),211]	John Hunter, Scottish surgeon *Known as the father of British "Scientific surgery"*	St. Georges Hospital London, England

Chapter 1 — THE HISTORY OF THE TRANSPLANT COORDINATOR

When	What	Who	Where
1816	Eight xenotransfusion experiments performed between animals of different species. Leacock concluded that donor and recipient should be the same species. He also recommended human to human transfusion. Leacock defended his dissertation, On the Transfusion of Blood in Extreme Cases of Haemorrhage, in 1816. He advocated the transfusion of human blood as treatment for hemorrhage, but also for "deficiency of blood."[211-213]	John Henry Leacock, physician	Edinburgh, Scotland
1818	First human-to-human blood transfusion. Transfusion of 4 ounces of blood from a man to his wife, replacing the blood she just lost during childbirth—the first well-documented case of person-to-person blood transfusion. Ten other women suffering from similar blood loss receive transfusions, which help half of them.[32,211,214-215]	James Blundell, MD British obstetrician	England
1831	Frankenstein published. Book describes a morally and physically superior creature constructed parts from graveyards and electrically revitalized; this creature turns to violence only when his fictional creator rejects him. This is the first positive and negative depiction—in literature and "media"—of the use of organs and parts from dead people.[27(p6),32]	Mary Wollstonecraft Shelley	England
1861	Term "dialysis" first used. Demonstration that a semipermeable membrane of parchment coated with a soluble protein, albumin, would allow diffusion of crystalloids—low-molecular-weight salts in solution—from high to low concentrations, but not colloids—large nondissolved protein particles in suspension. He also showed that urea, one of the body's waste products that is normally filtered from the serum into the urine by the kidney, could traverse the membrane into a surrounding water bath. Fifty years would pass before medical applicability of this concept is demonstrated.[27(p145),216]	Thomas Graham, Scottish professor of chemistry	Anderson's University Glasgow, Scotland
1868	Recognition that bone marrow is the source of blood cells. Neumann discovered the presence of nucleated red blood cells in bone marrow sap of humans and rabbits obtained by squeezing bones. He was the first to conclude that blood formation was a continuous process, occuring during postnatal life. In subsequent studies, he proved that leukocytes are also formed in the bone marrow. Anticipating the future, Neumann postulated a common stem cell for all hematopoietic cells. His colleagues and contemporary investigators ridiculed and vehemently opposed his ideas.[217(p294),218,219]	Ernst Neumann, cytologist, pathologist, hematologist	Königsberg, Prussia, Germany
1878	First successful human-to-human bone transplant: This operation, which used bone from a cadaver, remained unusual because there was no way to process and preserve human tissues.[32]		

When	What	Who	Where
1881	First reported use of skin graft: Although surgeons have known about skin grafts for at least 2000 years, a medical journal reports the first use of skin from a recently deceased person as a temporary graft. The patient is a man who was burned while leaning again a metal door when lightning struck.[32]		
1896	First attempts at bone marrow transplant. First attempts to use bone marrow as treatment for leukemia; patients receive the marrow orally after meals, but it has no effect. In the next few years, intravenous injections of bone marrow to treat aplastic anemia have some success.[31]		
1892	First recorded human pancreatic transplantation performed—29 years before the isolation of insulin. Dr. Watson Williams transplanted 2 "brazil nut"–sized chunks of freshly slaughtered sheep's pancreas to the abdominal wall of a 15-year-old boy at the Bristol Royal Infirmary. The recipient lived for 3 days.[123(p152),220]	Watson Williams, MD	Bristol Royal Infirmary, Bristol, England
1901	Blood groups O, A, B, and AB discovered. German scientist Dr. Karl Landsteiner classifies blood into 3 groups (A, B and O), and his colleagues adds a fourth (AB). All people fall into one of these groups, and by 1907 doctors realize that blood transfusions must be between people from the same group.[32,221]	Karl Landsteiner, MD *(Received Nobel Prize in 1930)*	Germany
1902	Technique discovered for connecting blood vessels. French surgeon Alexis Carrel develops surgical techniques for sewing arteries and veins that are used in organ transplantation and other surgical procedures today. He also demonstrated techniques for preserving blood vessels and organs in cold storage.[27(pp36-37),36(pp77-79),82(p28),222]	Alexis Carrel, MD	France
1902	First successful experimental kidney transplantations were performed with animals. Autotransplantation of a dog kidney from its normal position to the vessels of the neck resulted in some urine flow. Dog-to-goat kidney transplant passed a little urine for a while.[31,79(p1),81,82(p27),223]	Emerich Ullmann, MD	Vienna Medical School, Vienna, Austria
1902	Dog-to-dog kidney transplants.[79(p1),224]	Alfred von Decastello	2nd Medical Clinical, Vienna, Austria
1905	First reported heart transplantation was performed by transplanting a smaller dog heart into the neck of a larger dog by anastomosing the caudal ends of the jugular vein and carotid artery to the aorta and pulmonary artery. This transplanted heart survived for about 2 hours. The animal was not anticoagulated, and the experiment ended because of blood clot in the cavities of the transplanted heart.[101,114(p194)]	Alexis Carrell, MD, and Charles Guthrie, physiologist	University of Chicago Medical Center, Chicago, Illinois

Chapter 1 — THE HISTORY OF THE TRANSPLANT COORDINATOR

When	What	Who	Where
1905 December 7	First successful corneal transplant: Alois Glogar was a day laborer from a small town in the Czech Republic who had been blinded in both eyes a year earlier while slaking lime. Around the same time, an 11-year-old boy named Karl Brauer was brought to Zirm's clinic due to an accident that left metal pieces in his eyes. When attempts to save Brauer's eyes were unsuccessful, Zirm enucleated them and saved the corneas for transplantation into Glogar's. Although complications affected one eye, the other remained clear, allowing Glogar to return to work. [225(p275),226-232]	Eduard Zirm, MD	Olmutz, Moldavia
1905	First rabbit kidney grafted into human. French surgeon M. Princteau through a nephrotomy grafts pieces of a rabbit kidney into a 16-year-old with kidney failure; the patient dies 2 weeks later. [128]	M. Princeteau, MD French surgeon	France
1905	Development of "en-bloc" transplantation of two kidneys with their excretory apparatus, essentially used in the cat. They also perfused the kidney with Locke's solution prior to reimplantation, the principle of which is still used today. [82(p28)]	Alexis Carrell, MD and Charles Guthrie, physiologist	University of Chicago Medical Center, Chicago, Illinois
1906 January 24	First documented human kidney transplantation from animal to human. Transplantation of left kidney of pig into the left elbow of a woman suffering from nephritic syndrome. The graft failed because of vascular thrombosis. On April 9, he tries a similar procedure with a goat kidney. These events are often reported as the first true xenotransplantation experiments and even as the first attempts at organ transplantation. At the time, these procedures were termed heterotransplantation of heterografts. Dr Jaboulay was the teacher of Alexis Carrell. [36(p76),79(p2),80,82(p32),211,233]	Mathieu Jaboulay, MD	The Lyon School, Lyon, France
1908 February 6	Carrell performed a successful autotransplantation of a kidney in a dog with, for the first time, long-term graft survival. The circulation was interrupted for only 30 minutes. Four hours after the operation, the animal drank and walked around. on February 19, the right kidney was removed. Diuresis was normal. In March, 1909, the dog gave birth to 11 puppies and another 3 puppies in December of the same year. In July 1910, the animal, in excellent health, died suddenly from small intestinal obstruction due to ileus. At autopsy, the kidney was strictly normal in term of its appearance. [36(p78), 92(p29)]	Alexis Carrel, MD (*Received the 1912 Nobel Prize in medicine.*)	Department of Experimental Surgery, the Rockefeller Institute, New York City, United States
1908	Successful transplantation of a lower limb between two fox terriers. Carrell had many visitors to his laboratory and one of them remarked: "During my visit, I saw another black dog walking around there days after being transplanted with a white foreleg and, next to it, a yellow dog transplanted with a white limb 6 days previously, hopping along gaily, with a fully viable transplanted limb, because of the dressing." [82(p30)]	Alexis Carrel, MD (*Received the 1912 Nobel Prize in medicine.*)	Department of Experimental Surgery, the Rockefeller Institute, New York City, United States

When	What	Who	Where
1905–1910	Ernst Unger performed more than 100 experimental kidneys transplantations between animals.[79(p2)]	Ernst Unger, MD Berlin surgeon	Berlin, Germany
1908	First knee transplant. Erich Lexer (Germany) transplants knee-joint from a cadaver donor. Outcome unsuccessful.[32,235,236]	Erich Lexer, MD	Germany
1909	Transplant of en-bloc kidneys from a Borneo macaque monkey into a young girl with chronic nephritis in a preterminal condition. A small amount of urine is produced but the girl dies 32 hours after transplantation.[27(p219),36(p80),237]	Ernst Unger, MD	Berlin, Germany
1910 December 10	Transplantation of stillborn child's kidney grafted to baboon. Baboon died 18 hours after the operation but postmortem examination revealed vascular anastomosis was successful. This success, and the new knowledge that monkey and humans were serologically similar, led Unger to attempt, later in the same month, a monkey-to-human transplantation. The patient was a young girl dying of renal failure, and the kidney from a pig ape was sutured to the thigh vessels. No urine was produced. Unger's report concluded that there was a biochemical barrier to transplantation.[79(p3), 82(p33)]	Ernst Unger, MD	Berlin, Germany
1913	Japanese monkey kidney is transplanted into a young girl suffering from mercury poisoning nephritis; it produces a small amount of urine, but the girl dies 60 hours after transplantation.[36(p80),82(p33),238]	Schonstadt French surgeon	France
1913	First artificial kidney developed. To keep blood from clotting, it uses anticoagulant substances taken from leeches. This machine achieves dialysis—a word coined in 1861—on animals, but it is never tried on humans. They used hirudin, produced from leeches obtained from Parisian barbers, as an anticoagulant. Animal blood was passed from an arterial cannula through celloidin tubes that were contained in a glass "jacket." The glass jacket was filled with saline or artificial serum. They coined the term "artificial kidney." Blood was returned into the vein of the animal via another cannula. The inventors wrote: "this apparatus might be applied to human beings suffering from certain toxic states, especially if due to kidney damage, in the hope of tiding a patient over a dangerous chemical emergency." The apparatus was never used to treat a patient.[27(p.145),32,216,239-241]	John Jacob Abel (first professor of pharmacy at Johns Hopkins University School of Medicine) and colleagues: Leonard C. Rowntree, Benjamin B. Turner	Johns Hopkins University School of Medicine, Baltimore, Md
1920 June 12	Testicular and Ovarian Xenotransplantation. Slices of ape testicles transplanted into the scrotum. Dr. Alexis Carrel had taught his young friend, an ingenious and skillful surgeon, the technique of transplanting. By 1930, Voronoff had done 500 of what he referred to as "homografts," or a transplantation of a sister species. He soon began transplanting primate	Serge Voronoff, MD Russian-born surgeon	Collége de France, Paris, France

Chapter 1 — **THE HISTORY OF THE TRANSPLANT COORDINATOR**

When	What	Who	Where
	ovaries into women struggling with menopause. Voronoff even implanted a human ovary into an ape named Nora and attempted an unsuccessful artificial insemination. By the time of his death in 1951, Voronoff had transplanted ape tissues into 2000 patients. These attempts were discredited when others could not repeat the results – basically the grafts were destroyed within days of implantation.27(pp30-35),211,242-244		
1922	Discovery of Insulin therapy. The discovery of insulin was one of the most revolutionary moments in medicine. Though it took some time to work out proper dosages and to develop manufacturing processes to make enough insulin of consistent strength and purity, the introduction of insulin seemed literally like a miracle. One year the disease was an automatic death sentence; the next, people—even children—had hopes of living full and productive lives with the disease. Estimates show that more than 15 million diabetics are living today who would have died at an early age without insulin.27(p.207-209),245-247	Frederick G. Banting, MD Charles H. Best (medical student) (In 1923, the Nobel Prize was awarded to Banting and John James McLeod, MD, a professor of physiology for the discovery.)	University of Toronto, Toronto, Canada
1923	Lamb kidney transplanted into a patient afflicted by mercury poisoning. The patient lived for 9 days after the surgery.211,248	Harold Neuhof, MD	Mount Sinai Hospital, New York City
1923–1963	Cessation of Xenotransplantation-1923-1963: There is a 40-year gap before the next experiments involving xenotransplantation. This loss of interest in the field resulted from scientists' inability to discover and solve the issues of immunosuppression. This failure is epitomized by the conclusion Jaboulay came to after his experiments: "heterografts [xenografts] probably create conditions that promote blood coagulation, which is avoided by autografts."211		
1924	First attempt at human pancreas transplantation. Pybus tries to transplant human cadaveric pancreas tissue in an attempt to cure diabetes, but the grafts are rejected because of lack of immunosuppression.245	Charles Pybus, MD English surgeon	England
1925	First dialysis of human. Dr Haas performs dialyses on a patient with acute renal failure for the first time. Although the therapeutic approach is correct, the patients die because the results achieved are not yet sufficient. (Dialyzed 2 humans after preliminary trials with dogs.)27(p145),31,249	Georg Haas, MD	Giessen, Germany
1935	First organ perfusion machine. It was in France that Lindbergh and noted French surgeon Dr Alexis Carrel continued the work they had begun earlier on an "artificial heart"—a perfusion pump to keep organs alive outside the body by providing them with necessary blood and air under normothermic conditions. In collaboration with Lindbergh, he devised a machine for supplying a sterile respiratory system to organs removed from the body, Lindbergh having solved the mechanical problems involved. He discussed this aspect of his work and its implications in his book The Culture of Organs.250-252	Alexis Carrel, MD, and Charles Lindbergh, pioneering aviator	Paris, France

A CLINICIAN'S GUIDE TO DONATION AND TRANSPLANTATION — Chapter 1

When	What	Who	Where
1936	First kidney transplantation between humans (unsuccessful). The recipient was a 26-year-old woman who was admitted in a uremic coma after swallowing mercury in a suicide attempt. Voronoy retrieved a kidney from a 60-year-old man who had died from a fracture at the base of the skull and grafted it to vessels in her right groin. Unknown to doctors at the time, there were mismatches in donor and recipient blood groups (donor was B, recipient was O) and the donor kidney worked poorly for 2 days and then failed. The patient died 4 days following transplantation. Voronoy went on to transplant stored kidneys taken from cadavers 9 to 20 days previously. None functioned. In 1950, he reported on the results of 5 cadaveric kidney transplants.[27(p43-44),36(p76),82(p36),253-256]	Yu Yu Voronoy, MD Russian surgeon	Kherson, Ukraine, Russia
1943	First practical dialysis machine developed. It used more than 30 yards of cellophane tubing. Modified versions of this machine achieved some success in the 1950s for patients with acute kidney failure who needed temporary assistance until their own kidneys recovered. 17 patients were dialyzed, 2 recovered. Patients with chronic kidney failure cannot receive dialysis because the machine exhausts veins and arteries and only a few treatments are possible.[27(p144-147),31]	Willem Kolff, MD, and associates	Netherlands
1943	Demonstrated that skin allograft rejection in humans was an immunological process.[27(p110),258,258]	Peter B. Medawar, MA, D.S.c. zoologist, Thomas Gibson, MD, plastic surgeon	England
1944	First to demonstrate the immune origin of rejection. Confirmed the observations and conclusions of Gibson and Medawar in well-controlled rabbit experiments. Building upon observations of the immune system dating back thousands of years, Peter Medawar uses experimental skin transplants on animals to explain why burn victims from the bombing of civilians in England during World War II reject donated skin. His work sets the stage for a new field, transplantation biology. Medawar discovers that animal embryos exposed to foreign tissues do not reject the tissues and concludes that rejection of a transplant is based on immunological factors.[27(p109-124),32,257,259,260]	Sir Peter B. Medawar, MA, D.S.c., British zoologist *(Received Nobel Prize in 1960 with Dr Frank Macfarlane Burnet of the University of Melbourne in Australia. Medawar was knighted in 1965.)*	Oxford, England
mid-1940s	First successful heart-lung transplantation in animal (dog) experiments. In all, Demikhov subjected 67 dogs to replacement of both heart and lungs. Although many died on the operating room table or within 24 hours of operation, 8 survived more than 48 hours, with 2 animals surviving 5 and 6 days, respectively. Demikhov's experiments proved that from a technical surgical point of view, the operation was feasible. One of his dogs climbed the steps of the Kremlin on the sixth postoperative day but died shortly afterwards of rejection.[35(pp4-5),103,261(p91)]	Vladimir P. Demikhov, MD	Soviet Union
1944 December 15	The first eye bank in the United States, The National Eye Bank, opens in New York City. Corneas can be stored there for up to 6 days, allowing more flexibility in helping the long list of people waiting for sight-restoring surgery.[32,262]	R. Townley Paton, MD founder	New York City

Chapter 1 — THE HISTORY OF THE TRANSPLANT COORDINATOR

When	What	Who	Where
1947	First U.S. human kidney transplant – used as a temporary measure. Young woman admitted to Peter Bent Brigham Hospital in Boston. She was comatose and had been anuric for 10 days after an abortion caused septic shock and after she had received an incompatible blood transfusion. Kidney removed from a cadaveric donor immediately after death was transplanted on the major artery and vein in the recipient's cubital fossa. Kidney produced urine for only 2 days after transplantation; however, soon after the transplantation, the patient regained consciousness, natural diuresis was restored, and the transplanted kidney was removed. The healthy kidney had sustained the patient during an acute episode of renal failure.[27(pp53-55), 36(p82),79(p4),82(p38),263(p15)]	Charles Hufnagel, MD, Ernest Landsteiner, MD, David M. Hume, MD	Peter Bent Brigham Hospital, Boston, Mass
1948	Introduction of the terminology "histocompatibility genes" to describe a special class of dominant genes determining the outcome of allogeneic transplants.[82(p48)]	George D. Snell, PhD	The Jackson Laboratory, Bar Harbor, Maine
1948	Described single dominant histocompatibility locus (later called H-2) in mouse, analogous to the human leukocyte antigen (HLA) system used today for tissue matching. (George Snell received the Nobel Prize in Medicine with Baruj Benacerraf, Jean Dausset for their discoveries concerning "genetically determined structures on the cell surface that regulate immunological reactions".)[257,264]	Peter Gorer, MD, George D. Snell, PhD	Gorer – Department of Immunobiology, Guy's Hospital, King's College, London, UK Snell – The Jackson Laboratory, Bar Harbor, Maine
1949	First Bone Bank established—first to process and store bone and tissue.[32]	US Naval Hospital	Bethesda, Md
1950	First successful whole lung transplantation in animals. Use of operative approach similar to that of today with performance of a venous anastomosis using a cuff of left atrium.[265(p209),266]	Henry Métras	France
1950 June 17	In Chicago, a surgically excised ("free") kidney allograft was transplanted to the normal anatomic location in a recipient whose own kidney was removed—44-year-old Mrs Howard Tucker, from Jasper, Ind, who had polycystic kidney disease. The kidney came from a woman the same age, physical size, and blood type as Mrs Tucker; forty-five minutes after the donor's death (due to liver disease), the operation began. Under the watchful eyes of visiting surgeons and doctors, and with a camera crew in the operating room, Dr Richard Lawler went on to complete the transplantation. At the 6th month the kidney was destroyed, but Mrs Tucker went on to live for 5 more years with her polycystic kidney, passing away on April 30, 1955. This was the only transplant surgery ever performed at Little Company of Mary Hospital. Claims of allograft function were controversial.[27(p47-48),82(p38),257,267,268]	Richard H. Lawler, MD Raymond Murphy, MD James West, MD; the superintendent of the hospital Mother Mary Dunston Kelleher, who gave her permission for the surgery to commence.	Little Company of Mary Hospital, Evergreen Park (Chicago land area), Illinois

A CLINICIAN'S GUIDE TO DONATION AND TRANSPLANTATION

When	What	Who	Where
1950–1953	Kidney transplantations performed without immunosuppression, in Paris, France and Boston, Mass. Cortisone-like medications were used to suppress the human body's immune system, resulting in some success with kidney transplantation. The Boston cases were published in 1955: 9 cadaveric or surgically removed kidneys were transplanted, 8 to the thighs and 1 to the normal anatomic location of recipients with kidney failure. One thigh kidney functioned for 5 months. The French teams preferred the retroperitoneal iliac abdominal implantation.35(p86-82),76,79(p6),82(p51)	Jean Hamburger, MD, and René Küss, MD (Paris), and David M. Hume, MD, and John P. Merrill, MD (Boston)	Necker Hospital, Paris, France Peter Bent Brigham Hospital Boston, Mass
1950's	First kidney donors were from postmortem donors, from hydrocephalic children who had one kidney taken out for drainage of cerebral fluid via the ureter (Matson procedure) or from relatives, although rare. (First living related transplant is in December 1952 when a mother gives a kidney to her son.)4(pp57-58)		
1951	Renal transplantation operation perfected and performed. This operation was subsequently used by the successful twin cases in Boston and remains the standard procedure for kidney transplantation today.28(p89)	René Küss, MD	Paris, France
1951 January 12	First case of organ sharing and preservation. A person sentenced to death, was decapitated by the guillotine. Both kidneys were procured on the spot and one was flushed with plasma, the other with "serum de Ringer." One kidney was transplanted by Dubost and Oeconomos in Hospital Necker, the other in either the same hospital or somewhere else by Servelle and Rougeule. The ischemia times were very short by current standards: 1 hour 50 minutes and 3 hours 20 minutes, respectively. Both kidneys developed function, but the patients died at day 17 and 20. Also, an early example of non-heart-beating donation.4(p58),82(pp39-40),269,270	Transplanted by 2 teams: Charles Dubost, MD, Nicolas Oeconomos, MD, and Marceau Servelle, MD, J. Rougeulle, MD	Necker Hospital, Paris, France
1951 January	First transplant from living donor. After the January 12 transplants from the donor mentioned above, Küss transplanted a kidney into a 44 year old woman with advanced renal failure. The kidney was removed from therapeutic reasons after a Matson's procedure for hydrocephalus, in whihc the ureter acted as a drainage tract. The kidney was placed in the iliac fossa. Urine resulted after removal of vacular clamps, but remained minimal. 30 days post-transplant she developed severe hematuria and died several days later.37(pp83-84),271	René Küss, MD J. Teinturier, MD P. Milliez, MD	Paris, France
1951 March	First patient to receive dialysis prior to transplantation. A 37-year-old boiler repairman with end stage glomerulonephritis was transferred from the Peter Bent Brigham Hospital in Boston after being dialyzed to Springfield, Massachusetts in March 1951. Ten days later, upon the patient's return to his home hospital, surgeon James Scola grafted a kidney removed from a living donor with cancer of the ureter, joining the renal artery to a large artery in the upper abdomen of the recipient. Because the graft did not function intially, the patient was transferred back to Boston for dialysis before dying of rejection after five weeks.27(p55),36(p84),82(p43):272	James V. Scola, MD	Springfield, Mass

Chapter 1

135

Chapter 1   THE HISTORY OF THE TRANSPLANT COORDINATOR

When	What	Who	Where
1952 December 24	First Living Related Kidney transplantation. A 16-year-old roofer, Marius Renard, ruptured his solitary kidney in a fall on December 18. Anuria followed and it became apparent he had been born with only one kidney. The only possible solution was a transplantation that the mother proposed and insisted should be carried out. The graft was placed in the iliac region, according to the technique developed the previous year in Paris. It functioned immediately after surgery, but unfortunately ceased to function on the 22nd postoperative day. Marious died 10 days later owing to the unavailability of hemodialysis. However, this event had a considerable impact on the scientific community. Surgical inspection of the graft revealed that immunological rejection, rather than stenosis or thrombosis of the renal artery, led to graft failure.27(pp49-50),36(p86),79(p2),92(pp93-94),83-85,273	Louis Michon, MD Jean Hamburger, MD Nicolas Oeconomos, MD Jean Vaysse, MD	Hospital Necker, Paris, France
Early to mid 1950s	Simple Cold Storage of Organs. Simple hypothermia had been used for years to preserve human tissues.(Hyatt) This technique was applied to organs in the early 1950's for whole organ storage. (Bogardus and Schlosser) It was recognized that cooling could be achieved with vascular flushing with an electrolyte solution, (Pegg and Calne) but intially no great significance was attached to the precise composition of the flush solution. The assumption was that the preservation was due to rapid cooling and the removal of blood from the vascular system. One such solution used in 1967 was perfudex (Brunius).274-277	G.M. Bogardus and R.J. Schlosser, D.E. Pegg and R.Y. Calne, U. Brunius	Cambridge, England Göteberg, Sweden
1953	Reported the use of lymphoid cells to transfer immunity to skin grafts and other tissues in the mouse. Showed the strong association of acquired tolerance with hematolymphopoietic chimerism. This article is widely considered to be the bedrock of modern transplantation immunology.82(p48),257,258	Rupert E. Billingham, PhD Leslie Brent, PhD Sir Peter B. Medawar, MA, D.Sc, OM, CH	England
1953	First successful surgery using heart-lung bypass: Cecelia Bavolek became the first to successfully undergo open heart bypass surgery, with a machine totally supporting her heart and lung functions. The machine, developed by Dr John Heysham Gibbon in Philadelphia, paves the way for more effective heart surgery techniques including transplantation.27(p167),32	John Heysham Gibbon, MD	Philadelphia, Pa
1954 February 12	First International Conference on Transplantation. It attracted a small band of pioneers (fewer than 50 participants) who literally defined the scope of the field and raised almost all of the fundamental questions that continue to occupy transplant professional today.287(p135-136),209(p363)	John M. Converse, MD chair and organizer	Barbizon Plaza Hotel, New York City
1954 December 23	First successful kidney transplantation in humans. A kidney transplant between 23-year-old identical twins, Richard and Ronald Herrick, Richard who is dying of advanced glomerulonephritis. The kidney is implanted using the Parisian techique in the iliac position with implantation of the ureter into the bladder. After 90 minutes ischemic time, the kidney	Joseph E. Murray, MD, and Hartwell Harrison, MD (Dr Murray received Nobel Prize in 1990.)	Peter Bent Brigham Hospital, Boston, Mass

A CLINICIAN'S GUIDE TO DONATION AND TRANSPLANTATION

When	What	Who	Where
	functioned immediately and the blood urea level rapidly returned to normal. Due to persistent hypertension, the patient's own kidneys were removed at 6 months post-transplant. He returned to work adn lef a normal life, later marrying his nurse. This is the first successful—defined as lasting more than 6 months—organ transplantation in recorded history. Both twins do well and lead productive lives—demonstrating, among other things, that living donation can be made without serious psychological or physiological problems.27(60-67),32,36(pp86-87),71,72,74,79(p2),82(p45)		
1955	First heart valve and artery transplantations. The first successful transplantations of a human heart valve and an artery for a femoral bypass procedure were performed. Dr Murray uses the main aortic valve of a male victim of an automobile accident to perform the world's first heart valve transplantation on a patient with a severely leaking aortic valve. The transplanted valve functioned well for more than 8 years.31,83,279	Gordon Murray, MD	Toronto, Ontario
1955	First experimental liver transplantation, using an additional liver and transplanting it into the pelvis or right paravertebral gutter in nonimmunosuppressed dogs.88,89(p1)	C. Stuart Welch, MD	Albany, NY
1956	First orthotopic liver transplant in dog.89(p1)	Jack A. Cannon, MD	University of California, Los Angeles
1956	First bone marrow transplantation using related donor: Dr E. Donnall Thomas performs the first successful bone marrow transplantation that results in long-term survival of the patient. In 1957, he publishes a report of his work, which shows complete remission of leukemia by treating patients with total body irradiation followed by an infusion of marrow from an identical twin.280-281	E. Donnall Thomas, MD *(Received Nobel Prize in 1990.)*	Mary Imogene Basset Hospital, Cooperstown, NY
1958	First kidney transplantation in humans using immunosuppression. Young woman admitted to hospital with anuria after her solitary kidney had been removed because of life-threatening hemorrhage. She had been kept alive for several days with hemodialysis but it was impossible to continue. Before transplantation, she received 600 rads total body irradiation, considered to be sublethal. A kidney that was removed after a Matson's operation became available and was transplanted into the woman's thigh. The ureter was brought out into the skin. She was kept in a sterile environment and received bone marrow from 11 different donors, including several of her brothers in the hope of obtaining a crossed acceptance to oe of the bone marrow donors or any other person. Her postoperative course was complicated by leukopenia and she eventually died of a massive hemorrhage. Similar transplantations had the same dismal results using very high doses of irradiation.36(pp87-88),82(p51)	Joseph E. Murray, MD *(Received Nobel Prize in 1990)*	Peter Bent Brigham Hospital, Boston, Mass

Chapter 1 — THE HISTORY OF THE TRANSPLANT COORDINATOR

When	What	Who	Where
1958	Discovery of first HLA antigen. French physician Jean Dausset describes the first leukocyte antigen, MAC (now know as HLA-A2). The discovery allows for tissue matching beyond blood types.[282]	Jean G.P.J. Dausset, MD (*Receives Nobel Prize in 1980*)	Immuno-haematology Laboratory at the National Blood Transfusion Centre, Paris, France
1959 January 24	First successful kidney transplantation between non-identical (dizygotic/fraternal) twins. The recipient, John Riteris, was a 26-year-old man with end-stage renal disease due to glomerulonephritis and pyelonephritis. He received 2 doses (250 and 200 rads) of irradiation 1 week apart. His brother, Andrew Riteris, was irradiated before surgery to donate a kidney to his brother. The kidney was placed in the iliac region, with implantation of the ureter into the bladder. After several days of acute tubular necrosis (ATN), the kidney graft started to function. A few months after transplantation, he had a rejection episode successfully treated with steroids and low doses of total body irradiation. He lived a normal life over many years without receiving any other immunosuppression. before dying 27 years later after heart surgery. The brothers did not talk in donor-donee language. His brother recounts, "the only reference he [John] made to it was in an inscription in a book he gave me one week before his death, 27 years later. The inscription read: 'To Andrew – Thanks for the second drink.'"[27(p72),36(p76,88),283]	Joseph E. Murray, MD	Peter Bent Brigham Hospital, Boston, Mass
1959 June	Second successful kidney transplantation between non-identical (dizygotic/fraternal) twins – this time in Paris. 37-year-old man with ESRD who received 460 rads of irradiataion in two sessions pre-transplant. Normal renal function restored, he led a normal life, dying 26 years later of bladder cancer.[27(p73),36(p89),284]	Jean Hamburger, MD	Necker Hospital Paris, France
1959	Group of neurosurgeons described a condition they termed "death of the nervous system." Seen in patients with structural brain lesions (usually traumatic) and was most likely to occur when the trauma had been complicated at a later time by respiratory arrest. Characterized by persistent apneic coma, absent brainstem and tendon reflexes, and an electrically silent brain. The patient looked like cadavers, but had a regular pulse as long as artificial respiration owes maintained. Disconnection from ventilator produced no respiratory response.[44,285-286]	Pierre Wertheimer, MD Michel Jouvet, MD J. Descotes, MD	Lyon, France
1959	The Landmark "Le Coma Dépassé". Much fuller account of brain death first termed "coma dépassé" (a state beyond coma) described in article detailing 23 cases from the Claude Bernard Hospital – a coma associated with complete lack of cognitive and vegetative functons which went well beyond the deepest comas so far described. It is best translated as "irreversible or irretrievable coma". (The title of the Harvard Report in 1968 became "Irreversible Coma",	Parisian neurophysiologists P. Mollaret, MD, and M. Goulon, MD	Claude Bernard Hospital Paris, France

A CLINICIAN'S GUIDE TO DONATION AND TRANSPLANTATION

When	What	Who	Where
	although the committee members resonsible for the report were not aware of this document). The paper distinguished coma dépassé from other types of comatose states and brought a comprehensive clinical and EEG description together with the observations of diabetes insipidus, vascular collapse, and neurogenic pulmonary edema, all major derangement facing modern neurointensivists and neurosurgeons. It took more than 15 years before it became known in the United Kingdom and the United States.[41,42,44]		
1959–1962	First attempts at immunosuppression for organ transplants were with total body irradiation. In Boston, 12 cases were treated this way, but with only 1 long-term survival in a man receiving his transplant from his nonidentical twin. In Paris, similar success was also obtained with sibling grafts. New approaches were needed to prevent the body from fighting off a "foreign" donor kidney when an identical twin donor was not available. These isolated kidney survivals gave hope that success might be obtained in nontwin cases.[27(p67-75),79(p5),287-289]	Joseph E. Murray, MD John P. Merrill, MD and Jean Hamburger, MD	Peter Bent Brigham Hospital, Boston, Mass and Necker Hospital, Paris, France
1959	Drug-induced immunological tolerance: In rabbits given bovine serum albumin (BSA) while also being treated with the drug 6-mercaptopurine (6-MP), 6-MP suppressed the antibody response to BSA and rendered the animals tolerant to the foreign protein; the experiments were driven by the hypothesis that the proliferating immunocytes of an expanding antigen-specific clone would be selectively vulnerable to antimetabolite drug therapy.[27(p75-76),258,290]	Robert Schwartz, MD William Dameshek, MD Boston hematologists	Boston, Mass
1959	Independently demonstrated a 6-mercaptopurine dose-related prolongation of skin allograft survival in rabbits.[257,291,292]	Robert Schwartz, MD William Dameshek, MD and William Meeker, Richard Condie	Boston, Mass and Minneapolis, Minn
1959	Use of chemical Immunosuppression in animals. Effectiveness of 6-mercaptopurine established in canine transplants independently by 2 teams.[82(58),293-294]	Roy Calne, MD Charles Zukoski, MD HM Lee, MD David M. Hume, MD	St. Mary's Hospital, London, England Medical College of Virginia (MCV), Richmond, Va
1960 January	First successful kidney transplant between nontwin siblings. 36-year-old male recipient with renal carcinoma received kidney from 42-year-old sister. He was irradiated for immunosuppression. He died 4 and one half months later of disseminated liver metastasis.[36(pp76,90),295]	René Küss, MD	Foch Hospital Surenes, France
1960	First long-term dialysis treatment. Creation of external arteriovenous shunt, a device to connect the circulation of the patient to the tubing of the machine as needed. Clyde Shields, an aircraft	Belding H. Scribner, MD, nephrologist	University of Washington, Seattle

Chapter 1 — **THE HISTORY OF THE TRANSPLANT COORDINATOR**

When	What	Who	Where
	machinist for Boeing, becomes the first person to receive dialysis for chronic kidney failure at University Hospital in Seattle. Creation of the shunt whose Teflon components permit semipermanent access to a person's arteries allow Shields to live for another 11 years. For the first time in history, end-stage kidney disease is not a death sentence. A couple of years later, Dr Scribner helped open the first free-standing dialysis center in the world named the Seattle Artificial Kidney Center.[27(p149),31,39,40]		
1960s	Tissue typing advancements. Better techniques for matching donor and recipient blood and tissue types, as well as improvements in preserving cadaveric (from recently deceased donors) kidneys, were developed.[32]		
1960	Drs Richard Lower and Norman Shumway outlined the fudamental of current cardiac transplantation techniques in animal experiments.[296]	Richard R. Lower, MD Norman E. Shumway, MD	Stanford University Palo Alto, Calif
1961	First use of the term xenotransplantation to refer to interspecies transplantation.[211]	Peter Gorer, MD London geneticist	Department of Immunobiology, Guy's Hospital, King's College, London, UK
1961	Azathioprine, or, Imuran (An imidazole derivative of 6-mercaptopurine, BW-322) dramatically extends graft survival in dog kidney transplants.[276(p.76-78),79(p5),297]	Sir Roy Y. Calne, MD Guy P.J. Alexandre, MD Joseph E. Murray, MD	Peter Bent Brigham Hospital, Boston, Mass
1962	Immunosuppressive advancement. Imuran (azathioprine) became available for human use after effectiveness of 6-mercaptopurine was established in dog kidney transplants. Use of prednisolone with Imuran occurred intermittently but became standard regimen by 1963.[27(p.76),79(p5),87,128]	developed by Gertrude B. Elion and George H. Hitchings, PhD (Both received Nobel Prize in 1988)	Burroughs Welcome Laboratory Tuckahoe, New York
1962 March 27	Renal Transplant Program started at the Denver Veterans Administration Hospital with their first transplant being an identical twin transplant case on March 27. Later, on November 24, a mother-to-son transplant was performed, this patient receiving combination therapy of irradiation, Imuran and prednisone.[28(pp91-94)]	Thomas E. Starzl, MD Robert Brittain, MD Bill Waddell, MD Oliver Stonington, MD	Denver Veterans Administration Hospital Denver, Colo
1962 April	First successful cadaveric kidney transplant. Immunosuppression used—azathioprine and actinomycin C. The graft functioned for more than a year (21 months), an absolute record at that time.[31,36(pp76,92),69,74,79(p5),87]	Joseph E. Murray, MD	Peter Bent Brigham Hospital Boston, Mass

A CLINICIAN'S GUIDE TO DONATION AND TRANSPLANTATION

When	What	Who	Where
1962 October	Renal Transplant Program started at Medical College of Virginia. Dr David Hume left the Peter Bent Brigham Hospital and started the kidney transplant program at MCV. He employed whole body irradiation, prednisone, and a "sterile room" patterned after the success of this approach in early experimental bone marrow transplants. Imuran was used when experiments in dogs demonstrated a wider therapeutic margin than irradiation. In October 1962, the first cadaver kidney transplant took place. Although 1962 is designated as the formal starting point for the kidney program, it should be noted that Dr Hume performed a kidney transplant between twins involving a living donor in 1957.[28(p76),36(p92),298]	David M. Hume, MD	Medical College of Virginia Richmond, Va
1962 October	Hume performed the second successful cadaveric kidney transplant, using similar immunosuppressive regime to Murray in April. As with Murray's case, this kidney kept the recipient off dialysis for about 1 year. The success of those 2 transplants (Murray's and Hume's) significantly encouraged cadaveric kidney transplantations.[36(p92)]	David M. Hume, MD	Medical College of Virginia Richmond, Va
1962-1968	First US transplant coordinators begin work, often beginning as transplant assistants, either in dog or perfusion labs, or in the case of clinical coordinators, as nurses working with dialysis patients or in the operating room.	Paul Taylor (Colo); Justine Willmert, RN (Minn); Beth Cameron, RN (Mass, Pa); Robert Gosnell (Tex); Robert Hoffmann (Wis); Claire Day, RN (Fla); Linda Jones, RN (Ohio); Les Olsen (Minn); Stephen Kelley (Iowa); Roger Smith (Calif); Phyllis Weber, RN (Pa, Calif); and many others	Denver, Colo; Minneapolis, Minn; San Antonio, Tex; Madison, Wis; Gainesville, Fla; Columbus, Ohio; Iowa City, Iowa; Philadelphia, Pa; San Francisco, Calif
Early months of 1963	Only three transplant centers in United States consistently pursuing kidney transplantation: Peter Bent Brigham Hospital (Murray and Merrill), Medical College of Virginia (Hume), University of Colorado (Starzl).[69,74]	Joseph E. Murray, MD David M. Hume, MD Thomas E. Starzl, MD	Boston, Mass Richmond, Va Denver, Colo
1963 March 1	First human liver transplant. The recipient, Bennie Solis, was a 3-year-old boy with biliary atresia who had had multiple previous operations. The transplantation could not be completed because of a fatal hemorrhage from venous collaterals and an uncontrollable coagulopathy. The donor was another child who had died during an open heart operation.[28(pp.96-100),8 9(pp11-12),91(p102),99]	Thomas E. Starzl, MD	University of Colorado, Denver, Colo

Chapter 1

141

Chapter 1 — THE HISTORY OF THE TRANSPLANT COORDINATOR

When	What	Who	Where
1963	Description of world's first 3 attempts at orthotopic liver transplantation in humans (March 1, May 5, and June 24, 1963), with maximum survival of 21 days.[99,240]	Thomas E. Starzl, MD	University of Colorado, Denver, Colo
1963	First human lung transplant. The recipient, John Russell, was a 58-year-old man, serving a life sentence in prison, who presented with a squamous carcinoma of the left lung. The donor lung came from a patient who had died after myocardial infarction. The recipient maintained excellent arterial saturations for the first week post-transplant and survived for 18 days before dying of multiorgan failure.[27(180-183),36(p209),299]	James D. Hardy, MD	University of Mississippi, Jackson, Miss
1963	Xenotransplantation of chimpanzee kidneys to patients with chronic renal failure with maximum survival of 9 months. The patient who survived 9 months was a 23-year-old woman who received a chimpanzee kidney on January 13th. She died 9 months later due only to an acute electrolyte imbalance. This is the longest survival ever recorded for any xenotransplantation.[211,257,300]	Keith Reemtsma, MD	Tulane University, New Orleans, La
1963–1964	Primate organs transplanted into humans: Surgeons transplant chimpanzee kidneys into 13 people; all die, but one lives for 9 months. In the next 20 years, transplantations of chimpanzee hearts and kidneys and baboon hearts and livers—for a total of 28—are all tried, and all fail.[6(p3),32,118,211]	Various surgeons, most in United States, including Keith Reemtsma, MD (New Orleans), Thomas E. Starzl, MD (Denver), Claude Hitchings, MD (Minneapolis, Minn, 2/16/1963); one in France, one in Rome	United States, France, Italy
1963	Xenotransplantation of baboon kidneys to 6 human recipients with life-supporting function of 6 to 60 days.[257,301]	Thomas E. Starzl, MD	University of Colorado, Denver, Colo
1963	Hyperacute rejection of ABO incompatible kidneys described. Rejection attributed to antigraft antibodies (host isoagglutinins); recommendations made to prevent this complication.[257,302]	Thomas E. Starzl, MD	University of Colorado, Denver, Colo
1963	Report of world's first prolonged engraftment of human allogeneic bone marrow. Dr Mathe tried a radical treatment to save a 26-year-old man dying of acute leukemia—the total replacement of bone marrow. A massive dose of total body irradiation was delivered to suppress the young man's immunological defenses and then marrow extracted from his father, mother, sister, and 3 brothers was injected. The patient became violently ill, but he recovered and was released from the hospital. He died without leukemia recurrence after 20 months, probably from complications of graft-versus-host disease.[193(p42),257]	Georges Mathe, MD	Institute of Oncology and Immunology, Villejuif, France

A CLINICIAN'S GUIDE TO DONATION AND TRANSPLANTATION — Chapter 1

When	What	Who	Where
1963 September	The Washington Congress. First transplantation congress is initiated by the U.S. National Academy of Science and its National Research Council—the first meeting to compare results. The results remained dismal with a failure rate during the first three months following transplantation of 45% in living related donor transplantations and fully 85% of cadaveric transplantations. At that time, a total of 244 transplantations had been performed in the world, including 28 between monozygotic twins. Starzl's and Marchioro's data from Colorado, however, caused a sensation: 27 successive transplants over 10 months with 25 from living donors and 2 cadaveric kidneys (which never functioned). In the 25 kidneys from living donors, 90% achieved immediate diuresis and 18 of the recipients (75%) were alive with good renal function. This was a record at the time. Among those in attendance: Medawar, Amos, Teraski, immunologists and teams from the US: Brigham (Murray and Merrill) and Massachussetts General (Russell) in Boston, Richmond (Hume), Denver (Starzl and Marchioro), Los Angeles (Goodwin) and Cleveland (Kolff and Poutasse); Great Britain: London hospitals – Jammersmith (Schakman), St Mary's (Peart, Porter), Westminster (Calne), and Leeds (Parsons) and Edinbrugh (Woodruff); France, from Paris: Necker (Hamburger and Antoine) and Roch (Küss and Poisson). Other centers in the process of forming or just getting started in the U.S. Montreal and Brussels, were not represented.[87(pp58-61)]	Attended by all of the (less than 30) American, French, English and Scottish physicians, surgeons and immunologists interested in transplantation.	"A small overheated room of the rather ancient building of the National Institute of Health" Washington, DC
1963 June 3	First organ procurement from brain dead, heart beating donor. A patient with a severe head injury was brought to the emergency department in profound coma. In spite of vigorous resuscitation procedures and the administration of vasopressors and other drugs, the patient showed the clinical picture of "coma depassé". At Alexandre's request, Jean Morelle, chair of the department of surgery, made "the most important decision of his career," allowing the removal of a kidney from that heart-beating patient. The graft functioned immediately after implant. The recipient, who had been maintained by peritoneal dialysis, died of sepsis – with his new kidney in place–on day 87.[44]	Guy P.J. Alexandre, MD	Saint Pierre Hospital Leuven, Belgium
1963–1964	First organ procurements from heart-beating cadavers in Europe by Guy Alexandre (Leuven, Belgium) in 1963 and Jean Hamburger (France) in 1964. The organs were not removed, however, until the heart had stopped. The kidneys were dissected free, the ventilator removed, and the kidneys removed after the heart had stopped beating.[4(p59)]	Guy P.J. Alexandre, MD Jean Hamburger, MD	Leuven, Belgium Paris, France
1964	First heart transplanted into a man. Heart of a chimpanzee transplanted into the chest of a dying man, 68-year-old Boyd Rush. The heart beat 90 minutes before it stopped.[114(p197),115,303]	James D. Hardy, MD	University of Mississippi Medical Center, Jackson

Chapter 1 — **THE HISTORY OF THE TRANSPLANT COORDINATOR**

When	What	Who	Where
1964	First hand transplant is attempted in Ecuador. Patient is given what by modern standards would be primitive immunosuppressive agents. Graft is rejected within 2 weeks. Little testing or follow-up to allow for appropriate gain of information from experience.[355(p309)]		Ecuador
1964	Recognition that positive cross-matching (cytotoxic crossmatch) leads to hyperacute rejection. The supreme contribution of tissue typing proved to be the antibody test developed by Terasaki to measure tissue antigens. The antibodies he used, which kill white blood cells, are not normally present in the blood. He described how these antibodies, if present in the recipient and directed against the cells of the donor, can cause destruction of a transplanted kidney within minutes (hyperacute rejection). His recommendation that a crossmatch be done is still carried out before every transplantation in the world.[28(p123),304]	Paul I. Terasaki, PhD	University of California Los Angeles (UCLA) Immunogenetics Center Los Angeles, Calif
1964	First prospective trial of HLA matching for donor selection, begun in 1964. Reported on in 1966.[275,305]	Paul I. Terasaki, PhD, Thomas E. Starzl, MD	Los Angeles, Calif Denver, Colo
1969 June 27	Several transplant centers began to share kidneys as a means of extending kidney survival, after the discovery that kidney graft survival increased with matching. With this experience, the Kidney Disease and Control (KDC) Agency of the Public Health Service awarded 7 contracts to transplant centers throughout the United States. Purpose: Development of an organ procurement and sharing network to prove the feasibility of procuring kidneys in one place and preserving, matching, and transporting them in a viable condition for transplantation.[306(p1),307(p101)]	Grant awarded to Medical College of Virginia Principal Investigator: David M. Hume, MD Grant manager: James Pierce, MD	Membership of the contract: MCV, Duke Univesity, University of North Carolina, Georgetown University, Johns Hopkis University, University of Maryland, University of Virginia, Emory University and Danville Memorial Hospital United States
1965	First long-term survival (up to 9 months) of heart allografts in any species (in this case, dogs); azathioprine-based immunosuppression was guided by electrocardiogram voltage changes, especially R-wave diminution.[257,308]	Richard R. Lower, MD Norman E. Shumway, MD	Stanford University Hospital, Palo Alto, Calif
1965	Reemtsma distinguishes the terms heterograft and xenograft: heterograft "designates grafts along the lines of species, genus, and family" whereas xenograft refers to "transplants between individuals of greater genetic disparity."[211]	Keith Reemtsma, MD	Tulane University, New Orleans, La

A CLINICIAN'S GUIDE TO DONATION AND TRANSPLANTATION Chapter 1

When	What	Who	Where
1965	Early organ preservation accomplished with a biologic fluid such as whole blood. In the beginning researchers took their cue from physiologic studies and assumed that the best approach would be normothermic perfusion with blood. The major problem with this approach proved to be the instability of the formed elements and progressive vascular obstruction, and, as a result, blood as a perfusate was abandoned in favor of acellular perfusates.[252(p101)]	Arthur L. Humphries, MD	Medical College of Georgia, Augusta, Georgia
1965	First >1-year survival after liver replacement in any species (mongrel dogs) with recognition of the liver's unusual ability to induce tolerance under a 3- to 4-month course of azathioprine, or in this canine model after only a few perioperative injections of antilymphocyte serum or antilymphocyte globulin.[257,311]	Thomas E. Starzl, MD	University of Colorado, Denver, Colo
1966 March 8-11	Criteria proposed for removal of organs from heart-beating donors that were similar to the Harvard criteria that would be proposed 5 years later. Criteria proposed by Belgian surgeon at a Ciba Symposium where he reported he had applied his diagnostic criteria for brain death already – performing the first organ transplant from a brain dead donor. His remarks were controversial at the time.[28(pp.145-149),44,45]	Guy P.J. Alexandre, MD (Leuven, Belgium)	Ciba Foundation House, London, England
1966	Demonstration that the onset of hyperacute rejection becomes faster as the zoological classifications of recipient and donor grow more distant.[211,313-314]	Robert J. Perper, MD John S. Najarian, MD	University of Minnesota, Minneapolis
1966 December	First successful human pancreas transplantation. The 31-year-old recipient had uncontrolled diabetes and kidney failure. Transplantation of a duct-ligated segmental graft simultaneous with a kidney in a uremic diabetic recipient who immediately became insulin independent. The graft functioned until the recipient died 4 and one half months later (requiring only 2 injections of insulin during that time), of sepsis related to surgical complications. The team had earlier done the first human pancreas transplant only the month before in November on a 28 year old woman suffering from diabetes since age 9.[87(p94),124(p122),125]	Richard C. Lillehei, MD William D. Kelly, MD	University of Minnesota Medical Center, Minneapolis
1967	Creation of Eurotransplant. Professor Dr Jon J. van Rood founded Eurotransplant to allow central registration of all patients who were waiting for a donor organ; the aim was and is to increase the chance of finding a good match between the donors' and the recipients' tissue groups. One of Eurotransplant's most important tasks, therefore, was the registration of patients who qualify for transplantation. The Eurotransplant International Foundation is responsible for the mediation and allocation of organ donation procedures in Austria, Belgium, Germany, Luxembourg, the Netherlands, and Slovenia. In this international collaborative framework, the participants include all transplant hospitals, tissue-typing laboratories, and hospitals where organ donations take place.[4(p56),315-316]	Jon J. VanRood, MD	Blood Bank, University Hospital Leiden, The Netherlands

Chapter 1 — THE HISTORY OF THE TRANSPLANT COORDINATOR

When	What	Who	Where
1967	ALG (antilymphocyte globulin) used clinically for the first time; the "antibody induction" as an adjunct to azathioprine and prednisone in kidney recipients was similar to the strategy employed today with monoclonal antibodies.[257,317]	Thomas E. Starzl, MD	University of Colorado, Denver
1967	First successful liver transplantation. Dr Thomas Starzl of the University of Colorado Hospital performs the first successful liver transplantation due to improved immunosuppression. The child died of recurrent hepatoma 13 months following transplantation. Subsequently, the first report of prolonged survival (4 of 7 patients) after orthotopic liver transplantation, performed between July 1967 and March 1968 in Denver.[34,318]	Thomas E. Starzl, MD	University of Colorado Hospital, Denver, Colorado
1967 December 3	First successful heart transplantion. On December 3, 1967, South African surgeon Christiaan Barnard conducted the first heart transplantation on 53-year-old Lewis Washkansky. The surgery was a success. A young woman, Denise Darvall, had been struck by a car and suffered severe brain damage. Her father did not hesitate when approached for permission to donate her organs. On 3 December 1967, the team emerged from 9 hours of operating and suddenly international attention was focused on Groote Schuur Hospital. Eighteen days after the operation, Washkansky died of double pneumonia. His new heart beat strongly to the end. The original theatre where this transplantation was performed has been turned into a museum in honor of these pioneers of medicine, and to the first heart donor and recipient.[35(p7),111-113,319]	Christiaan N. Barnard, MD	Groote Shuur Hospital, Cape Town, South Africa
1967 December 6	First US heart transplantation. Three days after Christiaan Barnard's heart transplantation in South Africa, the first American heart transplantation was performed in a 17-day-old baby with Ebstein's anomaly. The donor was a 2-day-old neonate who was anencephalic. The recipient died from metabolic and respiratory acidosis within 7 hours of procedure.[35(p7),320]	Adrian Kantrowitz, MD	Maimonides Medical Center, Brooklyn, New York
1967	First simultaneous kidney/pancreas transplantation in the world.[31]	Richard C. Lillehei, MD	University of Minnesota Medical Center, Minneapolis
1967 August	Development of kidney preservation. The basic technique for organ preservation by continuous, relatively low pressure, perfusion at hypothermic temperatures (6° – 12°C) with cryoprecipitated plasma, which was a method for removing aggregated lipid that otherwise tended to accumulate in cooled plasma and obstruct circulation. Belzer remembers: "In August 1967, a middle-aged man with amyloidosis presented with renal failure, but because of his systemic disease, he had not been considered suitable for dialysis or for kidney transplantation. I had just harvested a kidney, which was placed on the preservation circuit in the laboratory. I worked alone in San	Folkert O. Belzer, MD	University of California San Francisco (UCSF) Medical Center San Francisco, Calif

A CLINICIAN'S GUIDE TO DONATION AND TRANSPLANTATION

When	What	Who	Where
	Francisco at this time; Najarian had left for Minnesota, and Dr Sam Kountz would not arrive until several months later. I discussed the option to accept this kidney with the patient; he accepted. The transplant was performed with a total preservation time of 17 hours. The kidney functioned immediately, although not perfectly, and hypothermic perfusion preservation of a human kidney had become a reality."[172,173,321,322]		
1968 January 6	Second U.S. Heart Transplant. The Stanford team, the most active of all the transplantation groups and responsible for many developments in transplantation patient care, does its first heart transplantation which is the second one done in the United States and the fourth heart transplantation in the world. Recipient: Mike Kasperak, 53 years old, suffering from chronic myocarditis. The donor is a 43 year old woman with a cerebral hemorrhage.[35(p8),82(p118)]	Norman E. Shumway, MD	Stanford University Hospital, Palo Alto, Calif
1968	First clinical heart-lung transplant. A 2-month-old patient with an atrioventricular canal defect is transplanted with the heart/lungs of an anencephalic infant donor. The recipient survived for 14 hours before dying of respiratory insufficiency.[114(p198),120]	Denton A. Cooley, MD	St. Luke's Episcopal Hospital, Houston, Tex
1968	First successful bone marrow transplantation. Performed in a child with severe immunodeficiency.[217(p300),323]	Robert A. Good, MD	University of Minnesota, Minneapolis
1968	First attempted pig heart transplantation. Dr Ross attempts to transplant a pig heart into a patient, but the heart ceases functioning in minutes.[324]	Donald N. Ross, MD	National Heart Hospital, London, England
Before 1968	Non–heart-beating organ recovery. Before 1968, the steps to donation began with discontinuing the ventilator. During the 5 to 10 minutes before the heart stopped and death was pronounced, the organs to be transplanted were variably damaged by oxygen starvation and the gradually failing and ultimately absent circulation.[28(pp148-149),44,45]		U.S. and Europe (with exceptions of the heart-beating recoveries by Guy Alexandre,1963 and Jean Hamburger, 1964, mentioned earlier in 1963-1964)
1968	U.S.: First definition of brain death based on neurological criteria: the Harvard Ad Hoc Committee report. This legal reform made possible procurement of organs from heart-beating cadavers. Public support for this report, which advocated acceptance of brain death, was overwhelming. Amended in 1969.[50]	Ad Hoc Committee of the Harvard Medical School to Examine the Definition of Brain Death	Harvard Medical School, Boston, Mass

Chapter 1 — THE HISTORY OF THE TRANSPLANT COORDINATOR

When	What	Who	Where
1968	First organ procurement organization established: New England Organ Bank in Boston. Paul Russell, MD, gave this account of the history of the development of the OPO: "The need for cooperation among hospitals and transplantation programs became very clear for the fist time on Sunday morning in 1967. Dr. Francis moore telephoned me to say that he had heard of the tragic shooting of a police officer in Boston. The policeman had been taken to Massachusetts General Hospital (MGH) with a head wound, and radio reports said that the officer was not expected to recover. Dr. Moore asked me to speak to the officer's family and explain that there was a patient at the Peter Bent Brigham Hospital who needed a new liver. I spoke to his wife and obtained permission to procure the liver. Dr. Anthony Monaco, then Chief Resident in Surgery at MGH, led the effort to remove the liver and deliver to the Brigham as part of the first liver transplant procedure in New England. In conversations a few weeks later, all agreed that similar siutations would arise again. As cadaveric donors were being used somewhat more frequently with the recent clarification of brain death by the Harvard criteria, it seemed that the need for this kind of combined effort would grow."[307(p130)]	Benjamin Barnes, MD, Administrator, Paul Russell, MD, Chairman of the Board New England Organ Bank (first name for organization was Interhospital Organ Bank)	New England Organ Bank Boston, Mass
1968 August 31	World's first quadruple organ donor. A 20-year-old Texas woman, Nelva Lou Hernandez, is brain dead after a gunshot wound to the head. In what became a nationwide sensation, DeBakey's team transplanted her heart, a lung and both kidneys into waiting recipients. Her corneas were also harvested. The surgeon said he believed the three-and-a-half hour operation was the greatest number of organs ever transplanted from a single donor. Her photo and a photo of the surgeons involved is on the front page of the Houston Chronicle. William C. Carroll, a 50-year-old Scottsdale, Ariz. industrial worker, received the heart. William J. Whaley, 39, of Fort Lauderdale, Fla, received the lung. Thomas A. Stevenson, 24, of Houston got one kidney. And William G. Kaiser, 41, the other. It was Kaiser's second kidney transplant. The first came from a 15-year-old Conroe boy killed in a car accident, a boy whose heart was also transplanted by Cooley.[32,82(p119),326]	Michael E. DeBakey, MD	The Methodist Hospital, Houston, Texas
1968	Uniform Anatomical Gift Act, the first legislative proposal addressing organ donation, is drafted. The Uniform Anatomical Gift Act establishes the Uniform Organ Donor Card as a legal document in all 50 states, making it possible for anyone 18 years or older to legally donate his or her organs upon death. This Act also banned the sale of organs and tissues. It was revised in 1987.[32,325]	National Conference of Commissioners on Uniform State Laws	United States
1968 February	France – "Collection of organs for therapeutic purposes in an operating room, already performed for years, was finally authorized. In April of the same year, the Jeanneney circular was released which defined brain death and authorized organ removal in subjects dying under such conditions."[82(p65)]	French Ministry of Social Affairs decree	France

When	What	Who	Where
1968 November 14	First single lung transplantation. Recipient, Aloïs Vereeken, is a 21-year-old sandblaster with pulmonary silicosis, receives a right lung transplant. Treated with azathioprene, prednisolone and ALG, by 3 months, his lung had reached 80% of normal function. He survived a few days out of the hospital and at autopsy, his lungs showed minimal signs of rejection.[27(p183),327]	Frits Derom, MD	Ghent University Hospital, Ghent, Belgium
1969	First partial larynx transplantation: A Belgian doctor performs a subtotal transplantation of a larynx, but the patient dies without speaking.[324,328]	Paul Kluyskens, MD Severin Ringoir, MD	Ghent University Hospital, Ghent, Belgium
1969 June 3	First pancreas transplantation with long-term survival.[257,329]	Richard C. Lillehei, MD, and William D. Kelly, MD	University of Minnesota Medical Center, Minneapolis, Minn
1969	Kidney disease and control was placed under the aegis of the Public Health Services, of the Department of Health, Education and Welfare.[53(p25)]	Public Health Service, US government	United States
1969	The Southeastern Regional Organ Procurement Program is formed as a membership and scientific organization: the Southeastern Organ Procurement Foundation (SEOPF). Founded by Dr David Hume of the Medical College of Virginia in cooperation with Dr Bernard Amos of Duke University. They organized SEOPF after determining that tissue typing would provide increased graft survival for kidney recipients if good matches could be obtained. It implemented a computer-matching system in December 1969.[306(p1),330,331(p1)]	David M. Hume, MD D. Bernard Amos, MD	Medical College of Virginia, Richmond, Va . Duke University, Durham, NC
1969	Simple Cold Storage of Kidneys demonstrated effective. A seminal paper was published in 1969 by Geoffrey Collins, MD, working in Dr Paul Terasaki's laboratory. In this study, dog kidneys were successfully preserved for 30 hours by simple cold storage after vascular flushout with a solution containing a high concentration of potassium and glucose. These kidneys regained immediate function following autotransplantation. Because of the simplicity of this method, it was rapidly adopted by many clinical transplant centers throughout the world. For the next 2 decades, very little was added to clinical preservation. Most studies that appeared during that period attempted to credit or discredit both preservation methods.[173,252(p101),332]	Geoffrey Collins, MD	United States
1969	Establishment of France Transplant.[333]	Jean B. G. J. Dausset, MD Founder and President	Paris, France
1970	Discovery of the fungus that lead to cyclosporine, in samples of soil from Wisconsin and the Hardangger Vidda (fjord) in Norway. A tradition established as part of a program set up in 1957 to search for new antibiotic drugs from fungal metabolites was for Sandoz employees on business trips and holidays to take plastic bags with them for collecting soil samples that were catalogued	B. Thiel (workers at Sandoz)	Basle, Switzerland

Chapter 1 — **THE HISTORY OF THE TRANSPLANT COORDINATOR**

When	What	Who	Where
	and later screened. In March 1970 in the Microbiology Department at Sandoz Ltd (Basel), a Swiss pharmaceutical company, the fungus Tolypocladium inflatum Gams was isolated by B. Thiele from 2 soil samples, the first from Wisconsin in the United States and the second from the Hardanger Vidda in Norway. These soil samples had been collected by Sandoz employees.[334]		
1970	Kansas became the first state to enact brain death legislation equating brain death with death. At the end of 1989, all states except South Dakota had either a brain death statute or a state supreme court decision endorsing the concept.[53(p23),54(p25)]	Kansas state government	Kansas
1970	First experimental islet cell transplantation in 1970. Approximately 500 isolated islet cells were transplanted intraperitoneally in diabetic rats, with subsequent long-term amelioration of diabetes. Following these findings, Kemp described a newer method of implantation, by intraportal injection and embolization of islet cells into the liver. This technique improved control of diabetes much more quickly than intraperitoneal transplantation.[92,123(p.154),335]	Paul E. Lacy, MD David W. Scharp, MD Walter F. Ballinger, MD Charles B. Kemp, MD	Barnes-Jewish Hospital, St. Louis, Mo
1970–1971	Unexpectedly, long survival was achieved at a high rate and about equally at all levels of HLA mismatch, using live donor and cadaveric kidneys. However, the best function, histological appearance of allografts, and survival, as well as least dependence on immunosuppression, was with zero-HLA mismatched kidney allografts.[257,336,337]	M. Ray Mickey Paul Terasaki, PhD Thomas E. Starzl, MD	Los Angeles, Calif Denver, Colo
1971	By 1971, all states had adopted the Uniform Anatomical Gift Act (UAGA) relatively similar to the draft put forth in 1963, by the Commissioners on Uniform State Laws.	State Legislatures	United States
1972	Discovery of cyclosporine: Cyclosporine was first isolated from 2 strains of Fungi Imperfecti from soil samples by the Department of Microbiology at Sandoz in Basle as an antifungal agent of limited activity.[28(p.210-214),338(p179)]	Workers at Sandoz	Basle, Switzerland
1972	Federal law – End Stage Renal Disease Act. Social Security Ammendments of 1972 (PL 92603), passed to pay for dialysis treatments. Law paves the way for Medicare coverage of renal dialysis and kidney transplantations. Medicare's End-Stage Renal Disease Program is enacted, providing funding for all people needing kidney dialysis—the first, and still only, national coverage for the treatment of a specific disease. A major factor prompting government action is media coverage of local committees that decide who receives dialysis and life, and who is left to die.[27(pp.149-155),31,54(p.25)]	US Congress	United States
1973	First Bone Marrow Registry established – the Anthony Nolan Trust, by his mother, Shirley Nolan. The trust was initially set up to find a donor for Anthony Nolan who died from Wiscott-Aldrich Syndrome after failure to find a compatible bone marrow donor. Following this, Jeffrey McCulloch on behalf of a consortium, including the American association of Blood Banks, the	Shirley Nolan	England

When	What	Who	Where
1973	American Red Cross and the Council of Community Blood Centers, established the National Marrow Donor Program (NMDP) in Minneapolis in 1986 and in 1988 the World Marrow Donor Association (WMDA) was established by Jan van Rood and colleagues. For her work with the Trust, Shirley was presented to the Queen in 1992 and awarded an OBE in 1999.[217(p302),339-341]		
1973	First successful bone marrow transplant from unrelated donor. Marrow from a person in Denmark is transplanted into a 5-year-old with severe combined immunodeficiency disease known as bubble boy syndrome. A few successful previous bone marrow transplantations had all involved related donors. The patient receives multiple infusions of marrow and, after he receives the seventh transplant, hematological function becomes normal.[31,280,342]		Memorial Sloan-Kettering Cancer Center in New York City
1974	World's first islet cell transplantation: The procedure works for only a short time before the patient's immune system destroys the new cells.[128,343]	David E. R. Sutherland, MD, PhD	University of Minnesota, Minneapolis
Mid-1970s	European Transplant Coordinators— the concept of transplant coordinator begins, as it did in the United States. First European transplant coordinators begin work, often beginning as transplant assistants, either as nurses working with dialysis patients or in the operating room or in perfusion laboratories. (*written communication, L. Roels, April 2006*)	Sally Taber (UK), Bernd Heigel, Christl Schulz (Germany), Leo Roels, CPTC Betty Vanhaelewijck (Belgium)	Netherlands, United Kingdom, Germany, Belgium
1975	South-Eastern Organ Procurement Foundation was incorporated with 18 members in a 6-state area.[306(p1),331(p1)]	Gene Pierce Executive Director	Richmond, Va
1975 Fall	Great debate among 3 Regional Organ Procurement Agency of Southern California transplant coordinators (Shawney Fine, Roger Smith, and Barbara Schulman) regarding a difficult legal point concerning a potential donor referral. Enter Thomas Berne, a transplant surgeon at the University of Southern California—he joins the discussion, offers advice and then says, "I wonder how many other coordinators are dealing with this very issue in the US today? You really should start a national transplant coordinators organization!" What a fabulous idea, we thought.[23(p6)]	Shawney Fine, RN Roger Smith Barbara Schulman, RN transplant coordinators	Regional Organ Procurement Agency of Southern California, Los Angeles, Calif
1975 Fall (the next day)	The three Regional Organ Procurement Agency transplant coordinators discussed the subject of the previous day with agency director Paul Terasaki, PhD and received his approval to dispatch a letter to the 110 U.S. transplant centers requesting interest in a meeting to be held in Los Angeles. A job description was sent with the letter.[23(p6),153]	Shawney Fine, RN Roger Smith, BA Barbara Schulman, RN, CPTC and Paul I. Terasaki, PhD	Regional Organ Procurement Agency of Southern California, Los Angeles, Calif

Chapter 1 — THE HISTORY OF THE TRANSPLANT COORDINATOR

When	What	Who	Where
1976	**First Annual Meeting of Transplant Coordinators** Forty-four transplant coordinators responded to the transplant coordinator meeting invitation and 24 arrive in Los Angeles from across the United States for 2-day meeting. "We became acquainted, discussed [Regional Organ Procurement Agency's] ROPA's original legal question and many, many other coordinators' medical, legal, religious, financial, and social issues. Found meeting each other to be most productive informative (job description and background varied greatly), and of great value." The group planned a fall meeting (August) to be held in New York City in conjunction with the International Transplant Society meeting.[23](p6),153	Meeting Planners: Shawney Fine, RN Roger Smith, BA Barbara Schulman, RN	Los Angeles, CA
1976 August 19-20	**Second Annual Meeting of Transplant Coordinators** First *formal* meeting of Transplant Coordinators! Transplant Coordinators Workshop. Twenty-five coordinators attend. Excellent scientific program, good camaraderie, worth-while sharing of experiences. (This meeting is technically the second meeting ever of US transplant coordinators. It is the first organized meeting with an agenda. See Figure 1 and Table 3: Transplant Coordinators Workshop Brochure, 1976).[153,344]	Organizers for the meeting: Geraldine M. Rasmussen, RN (NY), Justine G. J. Willmert, RN (Minn) John Bleifuss (Wash)	New York City, NY
1976	Discovery of immunsuppressive properties of cyclosporine. Isolated from the fungus Beauveria nivea, cyclosporine is shown to be immunosuppressive—a watershed for both solid-organ and bone marrow transplantation. It is the first immunosuppressive drug that allowed selective immunoregulation of T cells without excessive toxic effects.[38](pp210-214),[240,294,299](p179),[345-347]	Jean-Francois Borel, PhD Swiss biochemist	Basle, Switzerland
1976	First organ procurement organization founded in Canada— in Toronto. The sole transplant coordinator was involved in the procurement and distribution of 64 kidneys in the first year.[348]		Toronto, Ontario, Canada
1976 December 22	"Loi Caillavet" passed in France, first European country with an organ procurement law that is based on the principle of presumed consent. Law number 76-1181.[349,350](p199-200)	French Legislature	Paris, France
1977	South-Eastern Organ Procurement Foundation (SEOPF) implements the first computer-based organ matching system, dubbed the "United Network for Organ Sharing." This enabled "non-SEOPF" transplant centers to use the computer system for registering potential kidney recipients and sharing kidneys. The registration fee was $200.[306](p1),[307](p131),351		Richmond, Va
1978	First living-related pancreas transplantation. The transplant functioned for 84 months.[257,343]	David E. R. Sutherland, MD, PhD	University of Minnesota Medical Center, Minneapolis

A CLINICIAN'S GUIDE TO DONATION AND TRANSPLANTATION   Chapter 1

When	What	Who	Where
1978	United Kingdom Transplant Service formed in order to provide 2 major services: the national tissue typing laboratory and the organ matching and distribution system.[352]		United Kingdom
1978	Successful clinical application of DR matching.[353]	Alan Ting, PhD Peter J. Morris, MD	Nuffield Dept. of Surgery, John Radcliffe Hospital, Oxford, U.K.
1978 May	First clinical use of cyclosporine—human trials in Cambridge, beginning in the late spring of 1978.[28(pp210-214),93,294,334,354]	Sir Roy Y. Calne, MD	Addenbrooke's Hospital Cambridge, England
1978 April 6-7	**Third Meeting of Transplant Coordinators** "Fabulous concurrent organ procurement, preservation and nursing sessions."[23(p2)] (see table 4)	Meeting planners: Gerda Lipcaman (Michigan), Linda L. Jones, RN (Ohio), Curtis Yeager (Washington, DC)	Columbus, Ohio
1979 May 30-31	**Fourth Meeting of Transplant Coordinators** Fourth Meeting of Transplant Coordinators Meeting in Chicago. After various options of joining existing organizations or remaining independent were presented and discussed, a unanimous vote to formalize as an independent organization was registered. A newsletter was established, committees formed, and communication lines between coordinators encouraged. $25.00 per year dues. The brochure, for the first time, lists on the cover: North American Transplant Coordinators Organization.[23(p6),355] (see table 5)	First officers: President, Barbara Schulman, RN; President-Elect, Kate Hume, RN; Secretary, Barbara Schanbacher, RN; Treasurer Robert Gosnell; Parliamentarian, Paul Taylor; Historian, Justine Willmert, RN	Chicago, IL
1979 May 30	NATCO—"born" at 14:00 hours on Wednesday, May 30, 1979.[139]		
1979	First transplant coordinators start in Germany. (written communication, L. Roels, September 2006	Heiner Smit, RN Bernd Heigel, RN	Chicago, Ill University Hospital Dept. of Surgery Tübingen, Germany University Hospital Dept. of Surgery Hannover, Germany
1979	First NATCO newsletter issued and dedication statement formed by co-editors: That there be a better quality of life for the thousands of end-stage organ failure patients...... and a respect for those who shared.[149]	Julie Hall, RN Meredith A. (Mikki) Mastellar, RN, BSN First Editors	University of California San Diego Organ Procurement Organization

Chapter 1 **THE HISTORY OF THE TRANSPLANT COORDINATOR**

When	What	Who	Where
1979	First living-related pancreas transplantation.[259,343]	David E. R. Sutherland, MD, PhD	University of Minnesota, Minneapolis
1979	First full-time transplant coordinator position established in the Netherlands and later that year in the United Kingdom.[11,14(p.242),15,24(p326)]	Daan van der Vliet, MD, PhD, The Netherlands Sally Taber, MA, RN, SCM, MHSM, United Kingdom	The Netherlands United Kingdom
1980	Use of cyclosporine combined with prednisone to prevent rejection and avoid the early side effects of high-dose cyclosporine.[94,257]	Thomas E. Starzl, MD	University of Colorado, Denver, Colo
1980 June 27-28	**Fifth Annual NATCO Meeting** *President: Barbara Schulman, RN* First official NATCO (Fifth Annual gathering of US Transplant Coordinators) meeting in Boston in conjunction with the International Transplantation Society meeting. Interesting scientific meeting, exciting social hours, and continuing friendships established. Adoption of name and first bylaws proposed by Paul Taylor (Colorado), logo created by artist Warren Joseph Smith at "spirited" business meeting. Kate Hume is program chair.[23(p6)]	First NATCO President (1979–1980): Barbara Schulman, RN	Boston, Mass
1980	Canadian Association of Transplantation formed (it is a transplant coordinators organization).[24(p326),348]		Canada
1980	Establishment of neurological criteria for determination of death, expanding on Harvard Criteria. Proposes a uniform definition of death act.[51,356]	President's Commission for Study of Ethical Problems in Medicine & Biomedical Research	Boston, Mass
1980–1982	More transplant coordinator begin work in other German cities. *(written communication, L. Roels, September 2006)*	Christi Schulz, RN 1980 Karl Wagner, MD 1981 Hans Penke, RN 1982	University Hospital "Grosshadern" Munich, Germany University Hospital "Steglitz" West Berlin, Germany University Hospital Bonn, Germany

When	What	Who	Where
1981	First call for research papers in a NATCO newsletter: Transplant coordinators put a call out in the NATCO newsletter asking all of its members whether or not they had published or participated in research. The goal was to put such papers into a NATCO resource manual and make it available to fellow practitioners.[351]	Patricia L. Barber, RN, FNP, CCTC transplant coordinator	University of Illinois Medical Center, Department of Surgery, Chicago, Ill
1981 June 7-8	**Sixth Annual NATCO Meeting** *President: Kate Hume, RN, MSN* NATCO 6th annual meeting expanded to 2.5 days. NATCO history for this meeting and subsequent NATCO events and meetings are fully recorded in the historian book established by Faye Davis.[23(p6)]	Second NATCO President (1980–1981): Kate Hume, RN, MSN	Chicago, Ill
1981	Uniform Determination of Death Act recommended for adoption by all 50 states. Federal law recognizes brain death. A presidential commission (UDDA) under President Ronald Reagan refines the concept of brain death in 1980 and proposes a "Uniform Declaration of Death Act," which followed the Harvard Ad Hoc Committee on Irreversible Coma. Adopted by 43 states. The model bill states that an individual who has sustained either (1) irreversible cessation of circulatory and respiratory functions or (2) irreversible cessation of all functions of the entire brain, including the brain stem, is dead.[32,51]		United States
1981	First Publication of Transplant Coordinator Role. When the role of the transplant coordinator is not mentioned as part of the end-stage renal disease regulations. Claire Day, RN, contacts the Office of Standards and Certification, Health Standards and Quality Bureau in Baltimore. She and coworkers forward a paper stating the intent and qualifications of including the critical role of the transplant coordinator in the regulation to the office. (See Figure 14 in appendix)[5]	Claire Day, RN, CCTC Cy Gilman, RN, Mark R. Reiner, PA, CPTC transplant coordinators	Shands Hospital, University of Florida, Gainesville
1981	World's first successful combined heart and lung transplant. The donor for the procedure was brought to the transplantation center to minimize the ischemic time. The recipient was 45-year-old advertising executive Mary Gohlke, who lived 5 more years and wrote a book about her experience.[26,32,35(p11),358,359]	Bruce A. Reitz, MD Norman Shumway, MD	Stanford University Hospital, Palo Alto, Calif
1981	First mention of a transplant-coordinator-authored article mentioned in NATCO newsletter. An early feature of NATCO newsletters was "Articles of Interest from the Scientific Studies" Committee. Invariably, the articles summarized were authored by their colleague surgeons, physicians, immunologists, etc. The article by a transplant coordinator: Sophie LR. Meeting the Immunologic Challenge of Transplant Nursing. Heart and Lung Vol. 9, No.4: 690-694, July-August, 1980. (Certainly other articles were likely published before then by coordinators, but this was the first one featured in a NATCO newsletter.)[360]	Laurie Ruse Sophie, RN, transplant clinical specialist	University of Chicago Hospital and Clinics, Chicago, Ill

When	What	Who	Where
1981	First use of monoclonal antibodies (muromonab OKT3) in humans.[361,362]	A. Benedict Cosimi, MD	Massachusetts General Hospital, Boston, Mass
1982 May 26-29	**Seventh Annual NATCO Meeting** *President: Robert Gosnell, MBA*	Third NATCO President (1981-1982): Robert Gosnell, MBA	San Antonio, Tex
1982 August 24	First meeting to develop the 24-Alert Organ Acquisition System. The 24-hour alert was a recorded informational telephone service providing coordinators with a current list of urgently needed extra renal organs at participating transplant centers throughout the United States and Canada. The service provided a detailed recorded listing of heart, liver, lung and pancreas needs by center, including donor ABO, size, age requirements, and referral numbers. It was available 24 hours a day, was confidential and up-to-date.[355(p10)]	Herbert E. Teachey, MBA, CPTC, Chair (Donald W. Denny, MSW, later added as Co-Chair) NATCO Mult-Organ Procurement Committee (see article for lst of committee members)	Stouffers National Center, Crystal City, Virginia, VA
1982	First articles appearing in NATCO newsletter published by a procurement transplant coordinator. The 2 articles written by procurement coordinators: 1. Hoffmann RM, Mackety AA, Glass NR, Belzer FO. A method for salvaging vasospastic cadaver kidneys. *Dialysis and Transplantation.* 1981;10(12):991-998. 2. Taylor PD. Liver transplantation. *American Journal of Nursing.* 1981;9(19):1672-1673.[363]	Robert M. Hoffmann, BS, CPTC Paul D. Taylor, BS, CPTC	University of Colorado, Denver (Taylor) and University of Wisconsin, Madison (Hoffmann)
1982 October 17-22	NATCO holds the first "training course," then the Procurement Self-Education Course, which would eventually become the Introductory Education Course.[355]	Faye D. Davis, RN, MSN Organizer for meeting	Rolling Ridge Conference Center, North Andover, Mass
1982	First permanent artificial heart: Jarvik 7 transplanted into Barney Clark, a 61-year-old retired dentist. Clark is forced to remain inactive because the heart is kept beating by an external compressor attached to the implant by hoses. Clark lives 112 days.[279,364]	William C. DeVries, MD	Salt Lake City, Utah
1982	First transplant coordinator appointed in Australia—in Sydney. Victoria, Australia follows in 1985, and the first coordinator in Queensland is appointed in 1987. (*written communication*, G. Armstrong, CPTC, May 2006)	Elizabeth Yeo, RN	Sydney, Australia

When	What	Who	Where
1982 October 1	Second European Congress for Transplant Coordinators hosted by Eurotransplant Foundation. Roles of transpalnt coordinators in various parts of the world discussed. Fromation of a European Transplant Coordinators Organization is discussed.[198]	Speakers: Sally Taber, RN, Amy Peele, RN, CPTC, Laura Ruse Sophie, RN, Bernard Cohen, PhD, Guido Perseijn, MD, Gerhard Opelz, MD	Leiden, The Netherlands
1982–1983	United Kingdom Transplant Coordinators Association (UKTCA) formed. (written communication, C. Wight, RN, May 2006)	Celia Wight, RN first chairman	United Kingdom
1982	The South-Eastern Organ procurement Foundation and the United Network for Organ Sharing (UNOS) created "The Kidney Center" because of the complexity of sharing kidneys over a large portion of the country. The Kidney Center was staffed 24 hours a day with personnel who could run the computer and locate recipients for kidneys and other organs, arrange kidney transportation, maintain and update registry files for those who requested it, and attempt to locate organs through the UNOS/STAT system for patients who were critically ill.[306(p1),331(p1)]	Gene Pierce Executive Director	Southeastern Organ Procurement Foundation (SEOPF) Richmond, Va
1982	New editor for NATCO newsletter. Mary Anne House would serve as editor through 1989.[365]	Mary Ann House, RN, MSN, CTBS, CPTC, senior surgical transplant coordinator	Medical College of Georgia, Augusta
1982 June 1	Approval of Austrian presumed consent law "Krankenanstaltengesetz 62a" on June 18, 1982.[350(p132),366]	Austrian Legislature	Austria
1983 March 18	European Transplant Coordinators Organization (ETCO) established. 24(p329).[165]	by: Bernard Cohen, PhD (chairman, The Netherlands), Rutger Jan Ploeg (secretary, The Netherlands), Celia Wight (UK), Antonio Famulari (Italy), Bernd Heigel (Germany)	Amsterdam, The Netherlands
1983 April 13	First meeting of European Transplant Coordinators Organization		Maastricht, The Netherlands
1983 November 23	First European Transplant Coordinators Organization (ETCO) Congress, in conjunction with European Society of Organ Transplantation Congress	Bernard Cohen, PhD, ETCO President 1983–1985 (First ETCO president)	Zurich, Switzerland

When	What	Who	Where
1983 June 29 – July 2	**Eighth Annual NATCO Meeting** *President: Winifred B. Mack, RN, BSN, MPA*	Fourth NATCO President (1982–1983): Winifred B. Mack, RN, BSN, MPA	New York, NY
1983	First transplant coordinators appointed in Sweden.[15,16,24(p329),367]	Ann Christin Coon (Stockholm) Marie Omnell-Persson (Malmoe)	Stockholm, Sweden Malmoe, Sweden
1983	French government allocated funds for 7 organ procurement transplant coordinators.[131]	French government	France
1983 April 13, 14, and 27, July 29, October 17, November 7, 9, 1983 (and February 9, 1984)	Senate Hearings on National Organ Transplant Act. Transplant coordinators testify to House and Senate Committees during National Transplant Hearings, the hearings that led to the passage of the National Organ Transplant Act. (See Appendix 1 for transplant coordinator testimony.)[158]	Senator Al Gore presiding. Transplant coordinator witnesses: Donald W. Denny, MSW (Pa), Gary Hall, BS, CPTC (Tenn) Winifred B. Mack, RN, BSN, MPA (NY), Amy S. Peele, RN, CPTC (Illinois)	Washington, DC
1983 April 24-30	First Declaration of National Organ Donor Awareness Week by Congress. Senate Joint Resolution 78, to authorize and request the President to issue the proclamation. (See Figure 2.)	First session of the 98th Congress	Washington, DC
1983	NATCO develops the NATCO/Sandoz Achievement Award (now the NATCO/Novartis Achievement Award) to honor its own members.[355]	First Achievement Award is given to Faye D. Davis, RN, in 1984	United States
1983 June 7, 8, 9	Surgeon General's Workshop on Solid Organ Procurement for Transplantation. The Honorable C. Everett Koop holds workshop. 49 healthcare and transplant professionals, policy analysts, ethicists, media and members of the public are included on the panel.[368,369]	Three transplant coordinators are on the panel: Donald W. Denny, MSW, Winifred B. Mack, RN, BSN, MPA (representing NATCO) and Jane Van Hook, RN (representing AACN)	Project HOPE Health Sciences Education Center, Millwood, Va

A CLINICIAN'S GUIDE TO DONATION AND TRANSPLANTATION

When	What	Who	Where
1983	First successful (long term) single lung transplant. (first successful transplant since Derom achieved success in 1968 whose with a patient who survived 10 months). Dr. Cooper transplants 58-year-old Tom Hall, who suffers from pulmonary fibrosis. Hall lives for more than six years before dying of kidney failure.[207,370]	Joel D. Cooper, MD	Toronto General Hospital, Canada
1983	The first NATCO Clinical Self-Education Course is offered.[355]		
1983 April 4	24-Alert System (1-800-24-DONOR line) becomes operational. (see extensive discussion in chapter text. Also refer to appendix with transplant coordinator testimony of Denny, Mack and Peele, referencing the operational 24 ALERT for the first time, a few days after it goes live.)[143,159,174,184,355]	Program written by Herbert E. Teachey, MBA, CPTC, Brian A. Broznick, BS, CPTC, Donald W. Denny, MSW, Richard Sheppeck, BS	Pittsburgh, Pa
1983 November	Cyclosporine introduced. Food and Drug Administration approves the immunosuppressive cyclosporine for general use in United States. Its ability to improve graft and survival rates heralds a new era for kidney, liver, and heart transplantation.[334,351]	Food and Drug Administration	United States
1983	First multivisceral transplantation.[259]		Children's Hosptial of Pittsburgh Pittsburgh, Pa
1983 May 2	Brian Broznick, procurement transplant coordinator for the University of Pittsburgh School of Medicine, is featured in a full page photo in People magazine, his interview embodying the essence of what it is to be a procurement transplant coordinator.[192,371]	Brian A. Broznick, BS, CPTC	University of Pittsburgh School of Medicine Pittsburgh, Pa
1983	Paul Taylor is on the front cover of Odyssey West Magazine. "Colorado University Organ Transplant Coordinator." (see photos in Appendix)[137,372]	Paul D. Taylor, BS, CPTC	University of Colorado, Denver, Colo
1983 August 29	Don Denny, director of organ procurement for the University of Pittsburgh School of Medicine and Burt Mattice, procurement transplant coordinator for the Miami Valley OPO, appear in the first paragraph and throughout the article in a cover story in Newsweek.[193,372]	Donald W. Denny, MSW Burton J. Mattice, MBA, CPTC	Pittsburgh, Pa Dayton, Ohio
1984 April	More transplant coordinators are featured in national magazines. Paul Taylor is featured in Ebony magazine: "Savings Lives Through Transplants." Other coordinators are featured in Life, The New York Times, Nursing 84. In 1985 the trend would continue with Herb Teachey in Professional Pilot and Raytheon Magazine, and Amy Peele in the October issue of American Airlines In-flight magazine.[112,182,185,194-196,372]	Paul D. Taylor, BS, CPTC (Colo), Herbert E. Teachey, MBA, CPTC (Va), Amy S. Peele, RN, CPTC (Ill)	United States

Chapter 1 — THE HISTORY OF THE TRANSPLANT COORDINATOR

When	What	Who	Where
1984 August 26-31	Ninth Annual NATCO Meeting President: Amy S. Peele, RN, CPTC NATCO/Sandoz Achievement Award: Faye D. Davis, RN, MSN	Fifth NATCO President (1983–1984): Amy S. Peele, RN, CPTC	Minneapolis, Minn
1984	First NATCO training and development course for clinical transplant coordinators.[355]		Baltimore, Md
After 1983	First appointed transplant coordinator position in Germany.[9,131]		Germany
1984	Deutsche Stiftung Organtransplantation founded. (Germany's equivalent of UNOS)[131]		Neu-Isenburg Germany
1984	National Organ Transplant Act (Public Law 98-507) passed. Authorizes establishment of an Organ Procurement and Transplant Network to provide a central registry linking donors and potential recipients, authorizes financial support for organ procurement organizations, and prohibits the buying and selling of organs. [S.B. 2048. Title: A bill to provide for the establishment of a Task Force in Organ Procurement and Transplantation and an Organ Procurement and Transplantation Registry, and for other purposes. 10/19/1984.[158,291(p.2),351,373]	Sponsor: Senator Orrin G. Hatch of Utah (introduced 11/3/1983) Eight Cosponsors US Congress	United States
1984	Organ Procurement and Transplant Network (OPTN) established. (due to National Organ Transplant Act) Guaranteed, among other things, fairness in the distribution of donated organs. The United Network for Organ Sharing (UNOS) of Richmond, Virginia, subsequently receives the contract with the Federal government to oversee the OPTN. This same federal law also forbids the sale of organs and tissues. UNOS separates from the South-Eastern Organ Procurement Foundation and is incorporated as a nonprofit member organization.[31,48,291(p.2),351,373]	Organ Procurement Transplant Network	United States
1984	Certification of organ procurement organizations required by the Health Care and Finance Administration for the first time. (Due to National Organ Transplant Act) Certification required that organ procurement organizations meet specific performance standards.[158,322,374(p22)]	Health Care and Finance Administration	United States
1984	The first statistics generated from the 1-800-24-DONOR line are given: 213 liver, 136 heart, 6 heart/lung.[355]	NATCO 24-ALERT	United States
1984 Fall	Fall Statistics: livers 308, hearts 222, heart-lungs 9. Eight-channel operating system delivered and programmed enabling NATCO 24-ALERT to handle up to 8 calls simultaneously and have better voice quality. "The new systems will also be faster than the single channel system currently in use and probably be compatible with terminals already available at many transplant centers so that hard copies can be made." (NATCO fall 1984 newsletter)[355]	NATCO 24-ALERT	United States

When	What	Who	Where
1984 February 14	First heart-liver transplantation. Stormie Jones undergoes the world's first heart and liver transplant on Feb. 14. She is the first to undergo heart and liver transplantation for familial hypercholesterolemia and helps to define the underlying defects associated with this disease. She dies almost 7 years later, in November of 1990, of cardiac rejection.28(p329-332),128,371,375,376	Thomas E. Starzl, MD	Children's Hospital of Pittsburgh, Pittsburgh, Pa
1984 October 26	"Baby Fae," a 12-day-old girl born with a hypoplastic heart, receives baboon heart transplant. After initial improvement, inexorable rejection develops when her red blood cells clump together, obstructing microcirculation throughout her body. She died 20 days after her transplant on November 15, 1984.27(p217),377(p407),378	Leonard L. Bailey, MD	Loma Linda University Medical Center, Loma Linda, Calif
1984	Second Procurement Training Course (termed First NATCO Introductory Education Course) is held.355	Faye D. Davis, RN, MSN Chairperson	Rolling Ridge Conference Center, North Andover, Mass
1984 May 30	First organizational meeting of the United Network for Organ Sharing held. The meeting was attended by various transplant programs, organ procurement agencies, and histocompatibility labs. The proposed bylaws were discussed and adopted by those attending. A slate of officers was prepared by the steering committee: G. Melville Williams, MD, president; Oscar Salvatierra, MD, San Francisco, vice president; H. Keith Johnson, MD, Nashville, secretary; Charles B. Carpenter, Boston, treasurer. Mr Gene Pierce was appointed executive director until such a time as a permanent director could be found. 379	John McDonald, MD, representing the steering committee, presided over the meeting.	Chicago, Ill
1984	First transplant coordinator appears in Spain in Catalonia.9,13		Catalonia, Spain
1984	Association of Organ Procurement Organizations is formed.	H. Keith Johnson, MD Nashville, Tenn first president	Washington, DC
1985 July 21-25	**10th Annual NATCO Meeting** *President: Ronald L. Dreffer, BS, CPTC* NATCO/Sandoz Achievement Award: Donald W. Denny, MSW	Sixth NATCO President (1984–1985): Ronald L. Dreffer, BS, CPTC	Hotel del Coronado, San Diego, Calif
1985	Task force to study accreditation of transplant coordinators established by NATCO board of directors at annual meeting.355	Louise M. Jacobbi, CCTC, CPTC (drove the process to create credentialing for transplant coordinators) Barbara Schanbacher is the clinical co-chair and Bob Duckworth, the procurement co-chair)	San Diego, Calif

Chapter 1 THE HISTORY OF THE TRANSPLANT COORDINATOR

When	What	Who	Where
1986	First (former) transplant coordinator to serve on United Network for Organ Sharing (UNOS) board of directors.	Howard M. Nathan, BS, CPTC, executive director, Delaware Valley Transplant Program, and president, Association of Organ Procurement Organizations	Delaware Valley Transplant Program, Philadelphia, Pa
1985	NATCO membership at 552 with 120 clinical coordinators and 242 procurement coordinators.[355]	North American Transplant Coordinators Organization	United States
1985	NATCO begins to influence legislation with a strong united voice for transplant coordinators.[355]	North American Transplant Coordinators Organization	Washington, DC
1985 February 11-12 (first meeting)	American Council on Transplantation appointed by DHHS Secretary Margaret Heckler to advise on how to improve the U.S. system of organ donation and transplantation. The panel, set up under legislation signed by President Reagan last October, must report to Congress and Secretary Heckler within seven months on the use of drugs to prevent the patient's body from rejecting a transplanted organ. It must issue its final report within a year. The law establishes a program for grants to organizations that arrange for transplant organs to be donated. The program is financed for a total of $25 million over three years. The legislation also calls for establishing a network to match donor organs to prospective recipients. Three transplant coordinators of 25 member-panel members are named to the panel.[380]	Donald W. Denny, MSW Ronald L. Dreffer, BS, CPTC Jane A. Warmbrodt, M.A.	Arlington, VA
1985	Extrarenal organ sharing becomes computerized through NATCO. The 24-Alert system was put on the computer in 1985. Prior to that, it functioned with two answering machines in the TOPF offices at the University of Pittsburgh. The South-Eastern Organ Procurement Foundation also had an operational organ sharing system at this time for kidneys.[355]	Donald W. Denny, MSW, Brian A. Broznick, BS, CPTC, Herbert E. Teachey, MBA, CPTC, organ procurement coordinators, Rick Sheppeck, medical student	Computer system maintained at University of Pittsburgh
1985 November	Fourth European Transplant Coordinators Organization (ETCO) Congress, jointly with European Society of Organ Transplantation Congress.	Bernard Cohen, PhD The Netherlands ETCO President 1983–1985 (First ETCO president)	Munich, Germany
1986	Full-time transplant coordinators start working in Singapore.[12,24(p326)]	Sally (Tan) Kong first transplant coordinator	Singapore

A CLINICIAN'S GUIDE TO DONATION AND TRANSPLANTATION

Chapter 1

When	What	Who	Where
1986	PL99509 – the Omnibus Budget Reconciliation Act of 1986. Required Request Law. In an attempt to increase organ donation, law requires all hospitals to establish protocols for offering families of deceased patients the option of organ donation.[32]	US Congress	President Ronald Reagan signs Omnibus Budget Reconciliation Act.
1986	OPO Consolidation and Service Area Designation. PL99509 – the Omnibus Budget Reconciliation Act of 1986. Mandates that all organ procurement organizations (OPOs) and transplant centers become members of the national Organ Procurement and Transplant Network (OPTN). This historic development, coupled with federal regulation for OPO certification, forced the merger and elimination of many of the nation's OPOs. More than 30% of the OPOs consolidated. Each OPO was granted a specific service area for which it was responsible for educational activities, organ procurement, and organ distribution.[374(p22)]	US Congress	President Ronald Reagan signs Omnibus Budget Reconciliation Act.
1986 June 13	Approval of Belgian transplant law (presumed consent)[350(p133),381]	Wivina Demeester, Minister of Health and Social Affairs	Belgium
1986 June 29– July 2	**11th Annual NATCO Meeting** President: *Mark R. Reiner, PA, CPTC* NATCO/*Sandoz Achievement Award: Jane Warmbrodt, MA*	Seventh NATCO President (1985–1986): Mark R. Reiner, PA, CPTC	Denver, Colo
1986 March	Cumulative report of organs placed through 24-ALERT: livers 917, hearts 853, heart-lungs 46, tissue donors 46, lungs 3.[355]	NATCO 24-ALERT	United States
1986	NATCO submits a grant for funds to create a certification examination for transplant coordinators and the idea of the American Board of Transplant Coordinators (ABTC) is born. ABTC's purposes are to: (1) Implement educational and competency standards established by NATCO, (2) Define and certify transplant coordinators as a profession, (3) Credential practitioners in transplant coordination, (4) Maintain a registry of credentialed transplant practitioners, and (5) Promote continuing growth of the field of transplant coordination.	Louise M. Jacobbi, CCTC, CPTC, Chair (Louise drove the process to create credentialing for transplant coordinators) Barbara Schanbacher is the clinical cochair and Bob Duckworth, the procurement chair)	United States
1986	Standards of practice for clinical and procurement transplant coordinators developed by NATCO.[355]	Barbara Schanbacher, RN, BSN, CPTC, CCTC, Howard Adams, RN, PhD	United States

Chapter 1 — THE HISTORY OF THE TRANSPLANT COORDINATOR

When	What	Who	Where
1986	Organ Procurement and Transplant Network is established and United Network for Organ Sharing wins initial federal contract to operate it.[306(p.2),334(p.2),351]	G. Melville Williams, MD first president	Richmond, Va
1986 December 5	United Network for Organ Sharing (UNOS) adopts and assumes operations of NATCO's 24-ALERT voice-activated computer organ-sharing system on December 5.[355]	Stephen D. Haid, MS, CPTC, NATCO president gives 24-Alert to UNOS	Richmond, Va
1986	First successful double lung transplantation. Dr Cooper transplants a double lung into Ann Harrison, who suffers from emphysema. Harrison lives until 2001, when she dies of a brain aneurysm. This was the first successful double lung transplant since Derom.[279,383]	Joel D. Cooper, MD	Toronto General Hospital, Canada
1987	South-Eastern Organ Procurement Foundation (SEOPF) and United Network for Organ Sharing (UNOS) separate, with SEOPF signing over to UNOS the Organ Center computer facility, office space, and personnel.[306(p3)]	SEOPF UNOS	Richmond, Va
1987	Plan proposed in 1987 for allocation of cadaveric kidneys and accepted for national organ distribution. Mandatory sharing of 6 antigen match kidneys begins.[257,383]	Thomas E. Starzl, MD	University of Pittsburgh, Pa
1987	First Japanese transplant coordinators meeting. Invited speaker: Paul D. Taylor, BS, CPTC, transplant coordinator. 24 participants. *(written communication, S. Hiraga, MD, June 2006)*	Professor Hiroshi Takagi, MD, Meeting organizer	Second Red Cross Hospital in Nagoya, Japan
1987 June 28–July 2	**12th Annual NATCO Meeting** *President: Stephen D. Haid, MS, CPTC* NATCO/Sandoz Achievement Award: Louise Jacobbi, CCTC, CPTC	Eighth NATCO President (1986–1987): Stephen D. Haid, MS, CPTC	Philadelphia, Pa
1987 November	First successful intestinal transplantation. Tabatha Foster, a three-and-one-half-year-old child, whose intestines were lost shortly after birth due to a mid-gut volvulus, underwent the same multivisceral transplantation developed in dogs nearly 3 decades before. She recovered promptly from the difficult operation and was able to eat for the first time in her life. It was the first demonstration that transplantation of a complete intestine from a cadaver donor might be feasible. She survived for more than 6 months, and was sustained with enteral feeding until death from a B-cell lymphoma (posttransplant lymphoproliferative disorder).[28(p306),384(p172),385,386]	Thomas E. Starzl, MD	Children's Hospital of Pittsburgh, Pa
1987 November	Fifth European Transplant Coordinators Organization (ETCO) Congress, jointly with European Society of Organ Transplantation.	Celia Wight, RN United Kingdom ETCO president 1987–1991 (Second ETCO president)	Gothenburg, Sweden

When	What	Who	Where
1987	Australasian Transplant Coordinators Association (ATCA) is named and formed (later, legally incorporated in 1990). Founding members: Greg Armstrong, Graham Kidd, Sally Gordon, Elizabeth Yeo, Michael McBride, Glenda Balderson, Bet Martyn, Geoff Scully, Maxine Morand, Trevor Wedding. (written communication, G. Armstrong, CPTC, May 2006)	Bet Martyn first president	Sydney, Australia
1987	First meeting of Australian and New Zealand Transplant Coordinators. (written communication, G. Armstrong, CPTC, May 2006)	Elizabeth Yeo, RN Program Chair	Sydney, Australia
1987	First living heart donor – First "domino" transplantation. Clinton House, whose lungs had been damaged by cystic fibrosis, received the heart and lungs of a man who had died in a car accident. The heart-and-lung unit offered a better prognosis than the lungs alone.) Then, House's heart was transplanted into John Couch, a patient with congestive heart failure.[312,387]	Bruce A. Reitz, MD (William A. Baumgartner, MD	John's Hopkins Medical Center Baltimore, Md
1988 July 17–21	**13th Annual NATCO Meeting** Anita L. Principe, RN, MPA, CPTC, CCTC NATCO/Sandoz Achievement Award: Mary Anne House, RN, MSN	Ninth NATCO President (1987–1988): Anita L. Principe, RN, MPA, CPTC, CCTC	Orlando, Fla
1988	First certification examination for clinical and procurement transplant coordinators is offered by American Board of Transplant Coordinators (ABTC).[355]	300 transplant coordinators take and pass the exam (179 procurement, 131 clinical)	Orlando, Fla
1988	Extended preservation of the liver described with University of Wisconsin (UW) solution. Belzer felt the first generation of preservation solutions did not pay sufficient attention to controlling cell swelling. His group designed a new solution containing optimized concentrations of the impermeant solutes, lactobionate and raffinose, to control cell volume, and 5% hydroxyethyl starch to prevent extracellular edema. Folkert Belzer remembers: "A patient with end-stage liver disease was transferred from the intensive care unit of one of our referring hospitals to our intensive care unit. A liver became available in Texas, and because the recipient required a number of diagnostic procedures, the transplant was scheduled for 8:00 AM the next morning. The liver was successfully transplanted after 20 hours of preservation; the recipient was extubated the next day and transferred to the transplant unit on the second postoperative day with excellent liver functions and, as of this writing, is alive and well today. Elective and scheduled liver transplantation became a reality and we continue to perform this operation on a scheduled basis unless the recipient's condition requires an emergency liver transplantation."[173,259,322(p102),388,389]	Folkert O. Belzer, MD	University of Wisconsin, Madison

Chapter 1 — THE HISTORY OF THE TRANSPLANT COORDINATOR

When	What	Who	Where
1988	First sciatic nerve transplantation: Nine-year-old Matthew Beech, who had his sciatic nerve destroyed in a water-skiing accident, receives sciatic nerve from a 16-year-old female who died of a hemorrhage. Two years after the surgery, Beech could feel pinpricks on the sole of his foot for the first time since the accident, showing that the axons had grown through the graft and down the nerves to the sole of the foot.[259]	Alan R. Hudson, MD, and Susan E. Mackinnon, MD	University of Toronto, Toronto, Canada
1988	NATCO hires Applied Management Professionals (AMP) Management Services to act as its executive office headquarters.[355]	Deidre Gish Panjeda, AMP employee, becomes executive director of NATCO	Lenexa, Kan
1988 March 31,	Medicare Conditions of Participation for Hospitals published. A hospital may continue to participate in Medicare and Medicaid only if it establishes written protocols to identify potential organ donors that: (1) assure that families of potential donors are made aware that they have an option to donate organs or tissue and an option to decline to donate; (2) encourage discretion and sensitivity with respect to the circumstances, views, and beliefs of families of potential donors; and (3) require that an organ procurement agency be notified of potential donors.	Health Care Financing Administration	Baltimore, Md
1988 February	Second Japanese transplant coordinators conference. Invited speaker: Guido Persijn, MD, PhD, director, Eurotransplant. (written communication, S. Hiraga, MD, June 2006)		Nagoya, Japan
1988	First successful liver-bowel transplantation: Liver and 6 m (20 ft) of bowel transplanted into 41-year-old Doris Wells, who had been unable to eat or drink after having her small bowel removed due to superior mesenteric artery thrombosis from antithrombie III deficiency in 1987. During that time, she was fed intravenously through a device, which she was hooked up to for 8 to 12 hours each night. Following the transplant, mild rejection and graft-versus-host-disease developed during the early post operative period, but were easily treated with augmented immunosuppresion.[259,390]	David R. Grant, MD	University Hospital of London Health Sciences Centre in London, Ontario
1988	First split-liver transplantation performed. Two patients in the same hospital receive a liver transplant, when one donated organ is cut in half.[89,351,391]	Rudolf Pichlmayr, MD	Klinik fur Abdominal und Transplantations-chirurgie, Medizinische Hochschule, Hannover, Germany
1989 January	Australian and New Zealand Organ Donor Registry proposed by the Australasian Transplant Coordinators Association (ATCA). The registry contains demographic and clinical details on all organ donors in Australia and New Zealand donors. The registry is jointly established with Australian and New Zealand Dialysis and Transplant Registry and continues through the present day. (written communication, G. Armstrong, CPTC, May 2006)	Proposed by Greg Armstrong, RN, CPTC, transplant coordinator and other ATCA members.	Australia

When	What	Who	Where
1989	First combination heart, liver, and kidney transplantation: Surgeons transplant a heart, liver, and kidney into a 26-year-old woman. She survives for 4 months.[279]		Presbyterian Hospital in Pittsburgh, Pa
1989 July 9-13	**14th Annual NATCO Meeting** *President: Barbara Schanbacher, RN, BSN, CPTC, CCTC* *NATCO/Sandoz Achievement Award: Barbara Schulman, RN, CPTC*	10th NATCO President (1988–1989): Barbara Schanbacher, RN, BSN, CPTC, CCTC	Washington, DC
1989	World's first successful living donor liver transplantation, from a mother to son.[392-393]	Russell W. Strong, MD	Princess Alexandra Hospital, Woolloongabba, Brisbane, Australia
1989	Demonstrated superiority of tacrolimus to cyclosporine in preventing allograft rejection; intestinal transplantation emerged as a clinical reality.[96,240]	Thomas E. Starzl, MD	University of Pittsburgh, Pittsburgh, Pa
1989	First successful transplantation of total cadaveric small bowel.[257,394]	Olivier Goulet, MD	Paris, France
1989	Third Japanese transplant coordinators conference. Invited speakers: Barbara Schulman, RN, CPTC, transplant coordinator and Gene Pierce, United Network for Organ Sharing (written communication, S. Hiraga, MD, June 2006)		Nagoya, Japan
1989 November	Sixth European Transplant Coordinators Organization (ETCO) Congress, in conjunction with European Society of Organ Transplantation Congress.	Celia Wight, RN United Kingdom ETCO president 1987–1991 (Second ETCO president)	Barcelona, Spain
1989	Australian Transplant Coordinators Association establishes Australian and New Zealand extra-renal organ allocation protocols—the system remains in use with minor modifications. (written communication, G. Armstrong, CPTC, May 2006)	Australian Transplant Coordinators Organization	Australia
1989 August 11-15	**15th Annual NATCO Meeting** *President: Louise M. Jacobbi, AA, CPTC, CCTC* *NATCO/Sandoz Achievement Award: Suzanne B. Dutton, RN, CCTC*	11th NATCO President (1989–1990): Louise M. Jacobbi, AA, CPTC, CCTC	San Francisco, Calif
1990	World's first successful living-related lung transplantation: The lobe of one lung, from the mother, is transplanted into a 12-year-old girl.[279,395]	Vaughn A. Starnes, MD	Stanford University Hospital, Palo Alto, Calif

Chapter 1 — THE HISTORY OF THE TRANSPLANT COORDINATOR

When	What	Who	Where
1990	The first documented patient to achieve insulin-independence. The duration of insulin independence was brief.[123(p162),396]	David W. Scharp, MD	St. Louis, Mo
1990	The first issue of the Journal of Transplant Coordination (now Progress in Transplantation) is published. Barb Elick is the first editor. The profession's scientific journal allows its practitioners to publish research in the field of transplantation and transplant coordination in a journal dedicated to their practice. (First published by Munksgaard in Copenhagen, Denmark.)[355]	Barbara A. Elick, RN, BSN, CPTC, editor	Minneapolis, Minn
1990	The Japan Ministry of Health and Welfare authorized a budget for 19 transplant coordinators. Around this time, the Ministry organized a research group for establishing a social system of organ transplantation in Japan. The transplant coordinator was one of the subjects of the research. The budget was realized with the proposal of this group. (written communication, S. Hiraga, MD, June 2006)	Professor Hiroshi Takagi, MD, chairman, and Seigo Hiraga, MD, member of the transplant coordinator section of the research group	Tokyo, Japan
1991	The Japan Ministry of Health and Welfare authorized adding funds for 10 additional transplant coordinators to the budget. (written communication, S. Hiraga, MD, June 2006)		Tokyo, Japan
1991 September 9	Japanese Transplant Coordinators Organization (JATCO) formed. First JATCO meeting held. Founding members: Isao Tamaki, Osamu Kato, Mitsutoshi Yuasa, and Seigo Hiraga, MD. There were 98 initial members of JATCO, members consisting of transplant doctors and transplant coordinators, mainly the 29 "official" transplant coordinators authorized by the Ministry of Health and Welfare. (personal communication, S. Hiraga, MD, June 2006)	JATCO First President: Isao Tamaki, MS, transplant coordinator	Tokyo, Ebisu Japan
1991 September	Second Japanese transplant coordinator training course performed. (At the same meeting as the first meeting of the Japanese Transplant Coordinators Organization specified above.) (written communication, S. Hiraga, MD, June 2006)		Tokyo, Ebisu Japan
1991	First nonphysician United Network for Organ Sharing (UNOS) regional councillor elected to serve on UNOS board of directors—former transplant coordinator.	Howard M. Nathan, BS, CPTC, executive director, Delaware Valley Transplant Program, and president, Association of Organ Procurement Organizations	Delaware Valley Transplant Program, Philadelphia, Pa
1991 August 11-15	**16th Annual NATCO Meeting** *President: Barbara A. Elick, RN, BSN, CPTC, CCTC* *NATCO/Sandoz Achievement Award: James Springer, CPTC*	12th NATCO President (1990–1991): Barbara A. Elick, RN, BSN, CPTC, CCTC	Halifax, Nova Scotia

A CLINICIAN'S GUIDE TO DONATION AND TRANSPLANTATION — Chapter 1

When	What	Who	Where
1991 August 11-15	First (and only) NATCO meeting outside the United States.	Barbara A. Elick, RN, BSN, CPTC, CCTC NATCO president	Halifax, Nova Scotia
1991	NATCO's president participates in a White House reception held by First Lady Barbara Bush in honor of organ and tissue donor awareness week. "The Bushes have a personal involvement in the donor program. Their daughter, Robin, was an eye donor upon her death several years ago."[355]	Barbara A. Elick, RN, BSN, CPTC, CCTC NATCO president	White House, Washington, DC
1991	NATCO testifies at 2 public hearings. The first is sponsored by the Food and Drug Administration (FDA) and was held to solicit information and views of interested persons on the need to expand the federal regulation of organ and tissue transplantation to prevent the transmission of HIV from an organ and tissue donor to recipients. The second was sponsored by the Transplant Consensus Group, which was formed as a result of the FDA's Public Hearing on Human Organ and Tissue Donation.[355]		
1991	NATCO hires its first legislative consultant through Nursing Economics and continued in the following years.[355]	Carmella Bocchino, RN, (1991–1993), Kathleen Smith, RN (1994–1998), Eileen Meier, RN (1999–2004)	Washington, DC
1991 April 1	United Kingdom Transplant (UKT) established. UKT replaced the United Kingdom Transplant Service, operated by a regional health authority. UKT roots date back to 1971, when the decision was first made to distribute kidneys on a national basis. The primary service of the UKT is to assist the clinical practice of organ transplantation in the UK by distributing organs in the most effective manner.[352]		United Kingdom
1991	First successful human islet cell transplantation achieving insulin independence, using a repeatable techniqiue.[123(p162),397]	Garth L. Warnock, MD, Norman Kneteman, MD, Ray Rajotte, PhD	University of Alberta in Edmonton, Canada
1991 October	Seventh European Transplant Coordinators Organization (ETCO) Congress, in conjunction with European Society of Organ Transplantation Congress.	Jean-Jacques Colpart, ETCO president 1991–1993 (Third ETCO president)	Maastricht, The Netherlands
1992	First xenotransplant bone marrow (and kidney) transplant from nonhuman primate: Researchers transplant baboon bone marrow and a kidney into a patient. The patient dies 26 days later of an infection.[128]	University of Pittsburgh researchers	University of Pittsburgh, Pittsburgh, Pa

Chapter 1 — **THE HISTORY OF THE TRANSPLANT COORDINATOR**

When	What	Who	Where
1992 June	Baboon liver transplanted into man, afflicted with hepatitis C, dying of liver failure. Survival was 70 days.[89(p19),398]	Thomas E. Starzl, MD	University of Pittsburgh, Pittsburgh, Pa
1992 August 16-20	**17th Annual NATCO Meeting** *President: Linda L. Jones, RN, CPTC, CCTC* *NATCO/Sandoz Achievement Award: Howard M. Nathan, BS, CPTC*	13th NATCO President (1991–1992): Linda L. Jones, RN, CPTC, CCTC	Kansas City, Mo
1992	First pig liver transplants: Doctors at Duke University use pig liver as a "bridge" to keep 2 women alive while awaiting liver transplants. In one patient, the liver is kept outside the body and hooked to the liver arteries—she survives long enough to receive a human liver. In the other, the pig liver is implanted beside her own liver and she lives for 32 hours.[399]	Ravi S. Chari, MD	Duke University, Durham, NC
1992	NATCO develops Code of Ethics for Transplant Coordinators. Distributes to all members.[355]		United States
1992	Chimerism was discovered in organ transplant recipients, allowing allograft acceptance to be explained.[257,400]	Thomas E. Starzl, MD	University of Pittsburgh, Pittsburgh, Pa
1992	First unrelated, living donor pancreas transplantation.[343]	David E. R. Sutherland, MD, PhD	University of Minnesota, Minneapolis
1993 August 15-18	**18th Annual NATCO Meeting** *President: Lisa R. Kory, RN, BSN, CPTC* *NATCO/Sandoz Achievement Award: Carolyn Atkins, RN, CCTC*	14th NATCO President (1992–1993): Lisa R. Kory, RN, BSN, CPTC	Seattle, Wash
1993	Number of Transplant Coordinators in Europe and United States: Austria, 5; Belgium, 14; France, 87; West Germany, 28; Netherlands, 7; Spain, 86; Sweden, 10; Switzerland, 7; United Kingdom, 52. United States >2000 (estimate based on the fact that there were 1068 certified transplant coordinators in the United States at that time and not all are certified.)[252,401] *(oral communication, C. Bowman, March 2006)*		
1993 October	Ninth European Transplant Coordinators Organization (ETCO) Congress, in conjunction with European Society of Organ Transplantation Congress. Invited lecturer Teresa J. Shafer, RN, MSN, CPTC, NATCO president.	Leo Roels, CPTC, ETCO president 1993–1997 (Fourth ETCO president)	Rhodes, Greece

A CLINICIAN'S GUIDE TO DONATION AND TRANSPLANTATION

When	What	Who	Where
1993	First successful living-related lung lobes transplantation (one from each of recipient's parents), University of Southern California.[387]	Vaughn A. Starnes, MD	University of Southern California Medical Center, Los Angeles
1994 August 14-17	**19th Annual NATCO Meeting** President: *Teresa J. Shafer, RN, MSN, CPTC* NATCO/Sandoz Achievement Award: Robert Duckworth, CPTC	15th NATCO President (1993–1994): Teresa J. Shafer, RN, MSN, CPTC	New Orleans, La
1994	Elimination of medical examiner organ recovery denials proposed. Journal of the American Medical Association publishes seminal paper authored by NATCO members that, for the first time, documents the extent of the loss of life due to medical examiner denials of organ recovery. It openly calls for ZERO medical examiner denials throughout the country. It was reported widely throughout US and overseas press.[58,64-67]	Teresa J. Shafer, RN, MSN, CPTC, Lawrence L. Schkade, PhD, Howell E. Warner, BA, CPTC, Mark Eakin, PhD, Kevin O'Connor, PA, CPTC, James W. Springer, BS, CPTC, Timothy Jankiewicz, RN, CPTC, William Reitsma, RN, BSN, CPTC, Janet Steele, RN, CPTC, Karyn Keen-Denton, RN, CPTC	LifeGift Organ Donation Center Fort Worth, Tex
1994	Food and Drug Administration approves the immunosuppressive tacrolimus, which advances understanding of the human rejection response.[343]		United States
1994	New Editor of Journal of Transplant Coordination appointed.[355]	Linda Ohler, RN, MSN, CCTC	Fairfax, Va
1994	NATCO develops policy statements on Health Care Reform and Directed Donation.[355]		United States
1994	"The Nicholas Effect." Nicholas Green was killed by car bandits in Italy in October 1994. Reg Green, his father, remembers: "When our family— my wife Maggie, our 4-year-old Eleanor and I—drove through Messina, Sicily, to our hotel in the early hours of the morning one day last September, I felt I had never been in a bleaker place. We didn't know a soul, the streets were deserted, and we were leaving at the hospital our 7-year-old son in a deep and dreadful coma. I remember the hushed room and the physicians standing in a small group, hesitant to ask crass questions about organ donation. As it happens, we were able to relieve them of the thankless task. We looked at each other. "Now that he's gone, shouldn't we give the organs?'" one of us	Nicholas Green	Messina, Sicily

Chapter 1: THE HISTORY OF THE TRANSPLANT COORDINATOR

When	What	Who	Where
	asked. "Yes," the other replied. And that was all there was to it." Since that time, organ donation in Italy has dramatically increased and schools, hospitals, and all manner of historical sites have been named for the young boy and donation in Italy has dramatically increased. It is called "The Nicholas Effect."[403,404]		
1994 August 29	First International Transplant Coordinators Society (ITCS) meeting. Transplant coordinators throughout the world speak. For list of speakers and topics, see Table 8. (Held with 15th International Congress of the Transplantation Society)	Seigo Hiraga, MD (president)	Kyoto, Japan
1994 August 31	International Transplant Coordinators Society (ITCS) formed. The immediate goals of the society are to foster communication and collaboration among transplant coordinators individually as well as with national and international associations or societies interested in the field of transplantation, transplant coordination and related subjects, provide professional education to its membership through various meetings and activities, promote research, and advance the field of transplantation and transplant coordination.[200]	Siego Hiraga, MD, president; Greg Armstrong, RN, CPTC, vice president; Sally (Tan) Kong, secretary; Leo Roels, BS, CPTC, scientific program director; Teresa Shafer, RN, MSN, CPTC, treasurer	Prince Takaragaike Hotel, Kyoto, Japan
1995	Food and Drug Administration approves mycophenolate mofetil, a new immunosuppressant that substantially reduces the incidence of organ rejection following transplantation.[402]	Food and Drug Administration	United States
1995	NATCO sends written support to U.S. House of Representatives Durbin and AOPO, supporting an insert with tax return forms promoting organ donation.[355]	Christine J. Gilmore, RN, BSN, CCTC NATCO President	Washington, DC
1995 August 14	Transplantation of all abdominal organs: In order to transplant a new kidney, pancreas, stomach, liver, large and small bowel, and one iliac artery, doctors remove all abdominal organs from a patient, Leonardo Cioce, with Gardner's syndrome. The operation, 36 hours in length, is successful and the patient returns to Italy seven months following his transplant.[128,405,406]	Andreas G. Tzakis, MD	University of Miami School of Medicine Miami, Fla
1995	NATCO submits comments on proposed policy published in Federal Register regarding insurance coverage of transplantations.[355]	Mary Ann Palumbi, RN, BS, CCTC NATCO President	United States
1995	NATCO submits response to the proposed rule-making regulations regarding the Organ Procurement Transplant Network.[355]	Mary Ann Palumbi, RN, BS, CCTC NATCO President	United States

A CLINICIAN'S GUIDE TO DONATION AND TRANSPLANTATION

Chapter 1

When	What	Who	Where
1995	NATCO endorses National Kidney Foundations' Donor Family Bill of Rights.[355]		United States
1995	First International Non-Heart-Beating Donor Workshop, with approval of the 4 'Maastricht NHBD Categories' and the 10-minute dead donor rule.[407]	Gauke Kootstra, MD	Maastricht The Netherlands
1995 July 30 – August 2	**20th Annual NATCO Meeting** *President: Christine J. Gilmore, RN, BSN, CCTC* NATCO/Sandoz Achievement Award: Mary Ann Palumbi, RN, BS, CCTC	16th NATCO President (1994–1995): Christine J. Gilmore, RN, BSN, CCTC	Boston, Mass
1995	First laparoscopic live-donor nephrectomy—in which the live donor's kidney is removed through a site a bit larger than a silver dollar. Using sharp-edged hollow cylinders, the team removed a kidney from Baltimore resident Larry Butts through an incision a few inches wide. They then transplanted the kidney into Butts's wife, Chestina, in renal failure due to diabetic nephropathy.[408,409]	Lloyd E. Ratner, MD, and Louis Kavoussi, MD	Johns Hopkins Bayview Medical Center Baltimore, Md
1995	75 transplant coordinators employed in United Kingdom.[410]		United Kingdom
1995	Ninth European Transplant Coordinators Organization (ETCO) Congress, in conjunction with European Society of Organ Transplantation Congress. Invited lecture by Suzanne Lane-Conrad, incoming NATCO president.	Leo Roels, CPTC, ETCO president 1993-1997 (Fourth ETCO president)	Vienna, Austria
1995	National Donor Family Study established in 1995—ongoing evaluation of donor families perceptions and experiences of organ donation. Undertaken every 2 years. Geoffrey Scully *(personal communication, G. Armstrong, RN, CPTC, May 2006)*	Greg Armstrong, RN, CPTC,	Australia
1995	Second International Transplant Coordinators Society (ITCS) meeting. *(Held with the Society for Organ Sharing meeting)*		Paris, France
1996	NATCO conducts the Inaugural Education Needs Assessment Survey of its membership. Future educational offerings will be based on this survey.[355]		United States
1996 August 4-7	**21st Annual NATCO Meeting** *President: Suzanne Lane Conrad, RN, MS, CPTC* NATCO/Sandoz Achievement Award: Teresa J. Shafer, RN, MSN, CPTC	17th NATCO President (1995–1996): Suzanne Lane Conrad, RN, MS, CPTC	San Diego, Calif
1996	Transplant Coordinator Process and Outcome Standards of Practice are published.[355]	NATCO North American Transplant Coordinators Organization	United States

Chapter 1 **THE HISTORY OF THE TRANSPLANT COORDINATOR**

When	What	Who	Where
1997 July 27-30	**22nd Annual NATCO Meeting** President: Frances M. Hoffmann, RN, MSN, NP, CCTC NATCO/Sandoz Achievement Award: Claire Day, RN, BSN, CCTC	18th NATCO President (1996–1997): Frances M. Hoffmann, RN, MSN, NP, CCTC	Minneapolis, Minn
1997	Written and verbal testimony on "non–heart-beating-donors" is presented by NATCO before the US Senate.[355]		
1997 June	Japanese Organ Transplant Law passed with brain death provisions after decades of social opposition. A bill introduced by 14 parliament members including Radayoshi Morii, is introduced in April, 1994, approximately 2 years after the report of the Prime Minister's Ad Hoc Committee on Brain Death and Organ Transplantation. After 2 years, it is abandoned. In December 1996, another bill is introduced and after much debate, opposition and 2 amendments, the law is passed both houses of the Diet in June 1997 and became effective October 16, 1997. The law establishes a regulation for 2 kinds of death, and required donors to consent in writing both to organ donation and to testing for brain death, leading to concerns that organ donation will continue to be impeded in Japan.[411-414]	Japanese Diet	Japan
1997	Venezuelan National Transplant Organization founded.[415]		Venezuela
1997	10th European Transplant Coordinators Organization (ETCO) Congress, in conjunction with European Society of Organ Transplantation Congress.	Leo Roels, CPTC, ETCO president 1993-1997 (Fourth ETCO president)	Budapest, Hungary
1997	Third International Transplant Coordinators Society (ITCS) meeting. *(Held with the Society for Organ meeting)*		Washington, DC
1998	Only 5 transplant centers in India have transplant coordinators. (Out of a total of 28 kidney, 6 heart, 6 liver programs)[416]		India
1988 August 9-12	**23rd Annual NATCO Meeting** President: Laurel Williams, RN, MSN, NP, CCTC NATCO/Novartis Achievement Award: Barbara Schanbacher, RN, BSN, CCTC, CPTC	19th NATCO President (1997–1998): Lauren Williams, RN, MSN, NP, CCTC	New York, NY
1998	Routine Notification. Federal regulations are enacted to increase organ and tissue donation by requiring hospitals to notify the designated organ procurement organization of all deaths and imminent deaths. HCFA's Hospital Conditions of Participation.[31,32]	Health Care Financing Administration	United States

A CLINICIAN'S GUIDE TO DONATION AND TRANSPLANTATION

Chapter 1

When	What	Who	Where
1998	First total larynx transplant. Performed on 40-year-old Timothy Heidler, whose larynx was destroyed 20 years before in a motorcycle accident. Three days after the surgery, Heidler is able to speak for the first time since the accident.[259,417]	Marshall Strome, MD	Cleveland Clinic Cleveland, Ohio
1998	Establishment of the Donor Action Foundation. Celia Wight (Cambridge, UK) appointed as first manager of the Foundation with offices in Leiden and subsequently in Cambridge (UK). (*written communication, C. Wight, RN, CPTC, May 2006*)	Eurotransplant (The Netherlands), Organizacion Nacional de Trasplantes (Spain), Partnership for Organ Donation (USA)	Leiden The Netherlands
1998	First successful live-donor partial pancreas transplantation.[128]	David E. R. Sutherland, MD, PhD	University of Minnesota, Minneapolis
1998 September 23	First successful hand transplant. New Zealander Clint Hallam receives hand transplant in Lyon, France. Hallam had lost his right hand in a sawing accident while in prison years earlier. International team of physicians led by Dr. Jean-Michel Dubernard performs the thirteen-hour operation.[418(p.309),419-421]	Jean-Michel Dubernard, MD and Earl Owen, MD	Lyon, France
1998	NATCO begins offering 1-hour education workshops using videoconferencing technology.[355]		United States
1999 July 24-28	**24th Annual NATCO Meeting** *President: Mary Ann M. Palumbi, RN, BSN, CCTC* *NATCO/Novartis Achievement Award: Mark Reiner, CPTC*	20th NATCO President (1998–1999): Mary Ann M. Palumbi, RN, BSN, CCTC	Albuquerque, NM
1999	The Edmonton Protocol developed. Islet cell transplants are performed on patients who do not require other organ transplants (eg, kidney) but who have had severe problems with diabetes (type 1). The new treatment method involves injecting islet cells from donor pancreases into a patient's portal vein in a nonsurgical procedure in combination with steroid-free antirejection drugs. Lakey and Shapiro from Rajotte's group in Edmonton obtained insulin independence in 7 consecutive patients using islets from multiple donors. Paper published in the New England Journal of Medicine.[123(p162),128,422,423]	James M. Shapiro, MD, and Jonathan R. Lakey, PhD	University of Alberta Edmonton, Canada
1999	Organ Donor Leave Act legislation is passed, enabling federal employees who choose to become living organ donors to receive paid leave.[402]	US Congress	United States
1999	NATCO develops and offers the first Advanced Hospital Development Course at the request of the Association of Organ Procurement Organizations.[355]		

175

Chapter 1 — **THE HISTORY OF THE TRANSPLANT COORDINATOR**

When	What	Who	Where
1999 April	Critical Care Nurse, with a circulation of approximately 80,000 devotes entire April issue to organ donation and transplantation. Many transplant coordinators are authors in this issue which is entirely dedicated to organ donation and transplantation.[424]	Franki Chablewski; RN, MS Education Specialist, UNOS Co-editor of CCN issue	United States
1999	Fourth International Transplant Coordinators Society (ITCS) meeting. *(Held with the Society for Organ Sharing meeting.)*		Maastricht, The Netherlands
1999	Food and Drug Administration approves sirolimus, a new immunosuppressant used to prevent organ rejection in kidney transplant recipients.[402]	Food and Drug Administration	United States
1999	NATCO's scientific journal changes its name from *Journal of Transplant Coordination* to *Progress in Transplantation*.[355]	Linda Ohler, RN, MSN, CCTC, editor, leads this change	United States
1999	Already pioneered in Japan and performed in France and Belgium, the first US kidney transplant across immunological and blood group barriers is performed through a process of desensitization via plasmapheresis and intravenous immunoglobulin. This enables transplantations to occur between donors and recipients of different blood types.[402]		United States
1999	NATCO presents testimony to Senate and House Committees and meets with Senator Frist and Representatives Billirakis and Bliley regarding support of the National Organ Transplant Act (NOTA) Reauthorization Bill.[355]		United States
1999	International Transplant Coordinators Society (ITCS) Workshop held in Singapore.	Sally Kong, RN organizer	Singapore
1999	New procedure to enable kidney transplantation: High PRA rescue (high panel reactive antibody rescue) developed. The procedure involves plasmapheresis, in which patients are connected to a machine that removes their blood, separates the serum containing the antibodies, returns the red and white cells and platelets, and replaces the serum with a protein solution. Patients are also treated with 3 antirejection drugs.[128]		University of Maryland Medical Center, Baltimore, Md
1999	NATCO offers first Advanced Hospital Development Course at the request of the Association of Organ Procurement Organizations.[355]		United States
1999	First US hand transplantation. The surgical process, a joint project of the University of Louisville, the Kleinert, Kutz and Associates Hand Care Center and the Jewish Hospital, occurred Sunday afternoon at the hospital. The surgeons attached a donor hand, wrist, and portion of a forearm to a 37-year-old man. The patient, Matthew David Scott of Absecon, NJ, lost his hand in a 1995 firecracker accident.[425,426]	Warren C. Breidenback, MD, lead surgeon	United States

A CLINICIAN'S GUIDE TO DONATION AND TRANSPLANTATION

When	What	Who	Where
2000	NATCO endorses H.R. 5464: "Organ Coordinator Improvement Act" introduced by Congressman Inslee, which would provide grant monies to organ procurement organizations.[355]		United States
2000 August 5-9	**25th Annual NATCO Meeting** President: Bruce Nicely, RN, CPTC *NATCO/Novartis Achievement Award: Frances M. Hoffmann, RN, MSN, NP, CCTC*	21st NATCO President (1999–2000): Bruce Nicely, RN, CPTC	Orlando, Fla
2000	Two new programs aimed at increasing the donor pool become available. In paired exchange, 2 incompatible living donor recipient pairs exchange kidney donors so that each recipient can undergo transplantation. Live donor list exchange allows an incompatible donor to provide a kidney for a patient on the list awaiting a deceased donor kidney. In return, the incompatible recipient receives an allocation priority for the next available deceased donor kidney.[402]		United States
2000 January 12	First double-hand transplantation. A 50-member surgical team led by Jean-Michel Dubernard performs the world's first double hand transplantation in Lyon, France. The procedure takes 17 hours. The patient, Denis Chatelier, is a 33-year-old man whose hands were blown off when a homemade model rocket exploded prematurely. His operation is the first in a series of 5 double hand transplants that France will use to determine whether the transplantation of limbs and other external multitissue organs will become commonplace there.[419,427,428]	Jean-Michel Dubernard, MD	Lyon, France
2000	First womb transplantation: Uterus of a 46-year-old is transplanted into a 26-year-old woman. The uterus produces 2 menstrual periods before it fails after 3 months and has to be removed.[242,429]	Wafa Fageeh, MD	King Fahad Hospital and Research Centre in Jeddah, Saudi Arabia
2001	NATCO offers the Medical/Behavioral History Interviewing Workshop in conjunction with the Transplant Institute.[355]		United States
2001 July 15-18	**26th Annual NATCO Meeting** President: Jeffrey S. Mitoff, RN, BSN, CPTC *NATCO/Novartis Achievement Award: Linda Jones, RN, CPTC, CCTC*	22nd NATCO President (2000–2001): Jeffrey S. Mitoff, RN, BSN, CPTC	Long Beach, Calif
2001	For the first time, the number of living organ donors (6528) exceeds the number of deceased donors (6081) in the United States. With the widespread use of laparoscopic kidney donor surgery, improved success with living donor liver transplantations, more family members, friends, and even strangers are donating organs while alive. Hospitals and doctors become more liberal with policies toward living donors and the waiting lists and patients dying on the list grows.[32,351]		United States

Chapter 1 — THE HISTORY OF THE TRANSPLANT COORDINATOR

When	What	Who	Where
2001	Transplant Coordination program started at the University Hospital of Caracas, a 1200-bed teaching hospital with a service area of about 1.5 million inhabitants. Following the introduction of a transplant coordinator, donation increased substantially.[430]	University Hospital of Caracas	Caracas, Venezuela
2001	Fifth International Transplant Coordinators Society (ITCS) meeting. (Held with the Society for Organ Sharing meeting.)		Nagoya, Japan
2002 July 28-31	**27th Annual NATCO Meeting** *President: Judy M. Graham, MS, CS, CPHQ, CPTC* *NATCO/Novartis Achievement Award: Linda Ohler, RN, MSN, CCTC*	23rd NATCO President (2001–2002): Judy M. Graham, MS, CS, CPHQ, CPTC	Washington, DC
2002	NATCO publishes the *Core Competencies for Clinical Transplant Coordinators and Procurement Transplant Coordinators*.[355]		United States
2003 July 27-30	**28th Annual NATCO Meeting** *President: Barry S. Friedman, RN, BSN, MBA, CPTC* *NATCO/Novartis Achievement Award: Laurie Williams, RN, MSN, CCTC*	24th NATCO President (2002–2003): Barry S. Friedman, RN, BSN, MBA, CPTC	New Orleans, La
2003 October	National Organ Donation Breakthrough Collaborative launched under stewardship of Department of Health and Human Services Secretary Tommy Thompson. Most successful project in history of organ donation: 19% increase in organ donation in 2 years following introduction of collaborative, a greater than 600% improvement over the previous decade. Program is initiated to spread best known practices in organ donation to the nation's largest hospitals to achieve organ donation rates of 75% or higher. Goals of the collaborative: (1) Conversion rate 75%, (2) Timely Notification Rate 100%, (3) Referral Rate 100%, (4) Effective Requestor Rate 100%, and (5) ZERO, Medical Examiner Denials of Organ Recovery.[431,432]	National cochairs: Teresa J. Shafer, RN, MSN, CPTC, LifeGift Organ Donation Center, (Tex) John Chessare, MD, MPH, Boston Medical Center, (Mass) Program Director: Dennis Wagner, US Department of Health and Human Services	Washington, DC
2003	NATCO adds "The Organization for Transplant Professionals" to its moniker to recognize the diversity of professionals in NATCO's membership.[355]		United States
2003	The transplant waiting list grew to more than 80,000 candidates, with the expectation that it will reach 100,000 candidates by 2010.[402]		United States
2003	Sixth International Transplant Coordinators Society (ITCS) meeting. (Held with the International Society for Organ Donation and Preservation meeting.)		Warsaw, Poland
2003	First tongue transplantation: A 14-hour procedure was performed on a 42-year-old man suffering from a malignant tumor affecting his tongue and jaw.[259,433]	Christian Kermer, MD, Franz Watzinger, MD	Vienna's General Hospital, Austria

A CLINICIAN'S GUIDE TO DONATION AND TRANSPLANTATION

When	What	Who	Where
2003 August	Seminal paper published in New England Journal of Medicine on potential US donor pool "Estimating the Number of Potential Organ Donors in the United States" Several authors are NATCO members, former transplant coordinators. Study finds that "Lack of consent to a request for donation was the primary cause of the gap between the number of potential donors and the number of actual donors. Since potential and actual donors are highly concentrated in larger hospitals, resources invested to improve the process of obtaining consent in larger hospitals should maximize the rate of organ recovery. The performance of organ-procurement organizations can be assessed objectively through the comparison of the number of actual donors with the number of potential donors in the given service area."[434]	Ellen Sheehy, Suzanne L. Conrad, Lori E. Brigham, Richard Luskin, Phyllis G. Weber, Mark Eakin, Lawrence L. Schkade, Larry L. Hunsicker	Falls Church, Virginia Association of Organ Procurement Organization
2004 August 1-4	**29th Annual NATCO Meeting** President: *Nancy L. Senst, RN, BSN, CPTC* NATCO/Novartis Achievement Award: Lisa Kory, RN, BSN, CPTC	25th NATCO President (2003–2004): Nancy L. Senst, RN, BSN, CPTC	San Francisco, Calif
2004	NATCO's Resource Council listservs open a door for information sharing among transplant and procurement practitioners around the world.[355]		United States
2004 August	First ankle transplantation. The ankle of a 17-year-old boy (who had died in a car accident) is transplanted into Silvano Bordon, a 48-year-old rally driver, who had lost mobility of his foot in an accident in 1991.[259]	Sandro Giannini, MD	Italy
2004	Turkey: 50 certified transplant coordinators and assistants at organ/tissue procurement agencies and transplantation centers throughout the country.[435]		Turkey
2004	*50th Anniversary of First Successful Kidney Transplantation:* One-and 5-year survival rates for transplanted organs continue to increase. HLA matching improves this survival by at most 10%, and researchers continue to search for still-unknown components of the immune system that define immune rejection. A growing list of immunosuppressive drugs continues to bind strangers together in their ability to help each other. But the Holy Grail of immunosuppression—preventing organ rejection without negative side effects—remains elusive.[32]		Peter Bent Brigham Hospital, Boston, Mass
2005 January 19	First living donor islet transplantation: A team of surgeons at the Kyoto University Hospital in Japan, under the supervision of Dr James Shapiro (see 1999: The Edmonton Protocol), took islet cells from the pancreas of a 56-year-old woman and transplanted them into the liver of her 27-year-old diabetic daughter. The transplanted cells began producing insulin within minutes. The patient achieved insulin independence on February 10, 2005.[436]		Kyoto University Hospital Kyoto, Japan

Chapter 1

179

Chapter 1 — THE HISTORY OF THE TRANSPLANT COORDINATOR

When	What	Who	Where
2005 July 31 – August 3	**30th Annual NATCO Meeting** President: Dianne LapointeRudow, DrNP, CCT NATCO/Sandoz Achievement Award: David Powner, MD	26th NATCO President (2004–2005): Dianne Lapointe Rudow, DrNP, CCTC	Atlanta, Ga
2005	A total of 256 transplant centers in the United States.[355]		United States
2005	NATCO celebrates its 30-year anniversary. Special commemorative computer disks with interviews of transplant coordinators is given to meeting participants. Old footage of transplant coordinators is used as well as interviews with current leaders in the field. A Past President's reception is held and 23 of the past 30 presidents attend.[355]	Dianne Lapointe Rudow, DrNP, CCTC is president for the 30th annual meeting	Atlanta, Ga
2005 November 27	World's first successful partial face transplantation. Recipient is a 38-year-old French woman who had lost her nose, lips, and chin after being savaged by a dog.[437,438]	Team led by Professor Bernard Devauchelle, MD, and Professor Jean Michel Dubernard, MD	Amiens, France
2005 May 15	Altruistic donor makes possible the first "domino" 3-way kidney transplantation. Before the surgeries, transplant specialists searched their waiting list of recipients for the best possible "matches" for kidney donors and discovered that a domino-effect could be achieved by including an altruistic nondirected living donor who was willing to give his kidney to anyone who needed it.[439,440]		Johns Hopkins Comprehensive Transplant Center, Baltimore, Md
2005 June 27	Seventh International Transplant Coordinators Society (ITCS) meeting. *(Held with the International Society for Organ Donation and Preservation meeting.)*		Gramado, Brazil
2005 May	First "Collaborative" National Learning Congress. The Organ Donation Breakthrough Collaborative concludes in May 2005 with the National Learning Congress. The collaborative resulted in dramatic improvement in conversion rates in 2004 and 2005, resulting in the largest increase in organ donation in more than a decade. Joint effort involved organ procurement organizations and hospitals along with leadership of national organizations throughout the healthcare and transplantation industry.[432]	Teresa J. Shafer, RN, MSN, CPTC (Fort Worth, Tex) and John Chessare, MD, MPH (Boston, Mass), cochairs. Dennis Wagner, MPA, director	Pittsburgh, Pa
2005 September	Organ Transplant Breakthrough Collaborative is launched. The Transplant Collaborative adds the third "estate" to the collaborative methodology: transplant centers. Transplant centers join organ procurement organizations and donor hospitals in attempting to increase the organ yield from 3.0 organs per donor transplanted o 3.75 organs per donor transplanted.	Phyllis G. Weber, RN, CPTC, (Calif) Anthony D'Allesandro, MD (Wis) and	Los Angeles, CA

A CLINICIAN'S GUIDE TO DONATION AND TRANSPLANTATION

When	What	Who	Where
		Michael Moncure, MD, (Kansas) cochairs. Dennis Wagner, MPA (Washington DC) and Kevin O'Connor, PA, CPTC (Penn) codirectors	
2005 April	NATCO leadership participated in leadership group of Donation After Cardiac Death Consensus Conference.	Charlie Alexander, RN, MSN, MBA, CPTC NATCO President	Philadelphia, Pa
2005	Transplant Hospital CMS Conditions of Participation require that each transplant program must have a certified clinical transplant coordinator (CCTC). NATCO had commented on regulation, met with CMS on regulations and testified at the Department of Health and Human Services Secretary's Advisory Council on Transplantation.	Centers for Medicare and Medicaid Services (CMS)	Baltimore, Md
2005	NATCO past president moderates panel at Congressional hearing regarding Medicare coverage for immunosuppressive medications.	Dianne Lapointe Rudow, DrNP, CCTC	Washington, DC
2006	NATCO participates in a transplantation roundtable "Fly-In" for Capitol Hill visits and hearing regarding appropriation of $5 million to fund the Organ Donation and Recovery Improvement Act of 2004. This was the first concerted effort of the transplant community to work together on legislative initiatives.	Dianne Lapointe Rudow, DrNP, CCTC	Washington, DC
2006 August 26-30	**31st Annual NATCO Meeting** *President: Charlie Alexander, RN, MSN, MBA, CPTC* *NATCO/Sandoz Achievement Award: Suzanne Lane Conrad, RN, MS, CPTC*	27th NATCO President (2005–2006): Charlie Alexander, RN, MSN, MBA, CPTC	Chicago, Ill
2006 February 20	Successful removal of a heart that had been transplanted into a 12-year-old girl, Hannah Clark, after her own once-failing heart had recovered and was keeping her alive by itself. The girl's own heart was left in her body during the "piggy-back" transplantation in 1996. The girl began to reject the transplanted organ in 2006, and surgeons removed it. Her own heart had repaired itself.[441]	Magdi Yacoub, MD and Victor Tsang, MD	Great Ormond Street Hospital, London, England
2006 April	Critical Care Nurse, with a circulation of approximately 80,000 devotes entire April issue to organ donation and transplantation. Many NATCO members are authors for the articles in this issue, dedicated entirely to organ donation and transplantation.[442]	Franki Chablewski, RN, MS Education Specialist, UNOS Co-editor of CCN issue	United States

Chapter 1 — THE HISTORY OF THE TRANSPLANT COORDINATOR

When	What	Who	Where
2006	NATCO produces first textbook on organ procurement and clinical care of the recipient.	Editors: Dianne LaPointe Rudow, DrNP, CCTC; Linda Ohler, RN, MSN, CCTC, FAAN; Teresa Shafer, RN, MSN, CPTC	United States
2007 August 6-9	**32nd Annual NATCO Meeting** *President: Marian O'Rourke, RN, CCTC*	28th NATCO President (2006–2007): Marian O'Rourke, RN, CCTC	New York, NY

Appendices

Appendix 1:
    National Organ Transplant Hearings
    Schedule of Witnesses

Appendix 2:
    National Organ Transplant Hearings
    Testimony of Don Denny, Director of Organ Procurement, University of Pittsburgh
    April 13, 1983

Appendix 3:
    National Organ Transplant Hearings
    Testimony of Winifred Mack, President, NATCO
    April 27, 1983

Appendix 4:
    National Organ Transplant Hearings
    Testimony of Amy Peele, President, NATCO
    October 17, 1983
    November 7, 1983

Chapter 1 — THE HISTORY OF THE TRANSPLANT COORDINATOR

Appendix 1, 1983 National Organ Transplant Hearings

HEARINGS
BEFORE THE
SUBCOMMITTEE ON INVESTIGATIONS AND OVERSIGHTS
OF THE
COMMITTEE ON SCIENCE AND TECHNOLOGY
U.S. HOUSE OF REPRESENTATIVES
NINETY-EIGHTH CONGRESS
FIRST SESSION

APRIL 13, 14, 27, 1983

WITNESSES

April 13, 1983:
- Hon. Harold E. Ford, a Representative in Congress from the State of Tennessee
- Billie Hall, with son, Brandon Hall;
  - Capt. John H. Broderick, with daughter, Adriane;
  - James Williams, M.D., associate professor of surgery, University of Tennessee College of Medicine, Memphis, Tenn.; and
  - **Gary Hall, transplant coordinator, University of Tennessee College of Medicine, Memphis, Tenn.**
- Norman Shumway, M.D., professor of surgery, Stanford University School of Medicine, Stanford, Calif.;
  - Thomas E. Starzl, M.D., professor of surgery, University of Pittsburgh School of Medicine, Pittsburgh, Pa.; and
  - G. Melville Williams, M.D., professor of surgery, Johns Hopkins Hospital, Baltimore, Md.
- **Donald W. Denny, director of organ procurement, transplantation office, University of Pittsburgh School of Medicine, Pittsburgh, Pa.;**
  - William W. Pfaff, M.D., past president, South-East Organ Procurement Foundation, University of Florida College of Medicine, department of surgery, and
  - Raymond Coleman, founding president, donor alert, Warwick, R.I.

April 14, 1983:
- Hon, Joe Moakley, a Representative in the Congress from the State of Massachusetts
- Charles and Marilyn Fiske, and daughter Jamie, liver transplant patient;
  - Michele Jones, kidney transplant recipient;
  - David Ogden, M.D., professor of medicine, chief, renal section, University of Arizona Health Science Center; and
  - Thelma King Thiel, vice chairman and Executive Director, American Liver Foundation
- Alexander Morgan Capron, Executive Director, President's Commission for the Study of Ethical Problems in Medicine and Biomedical and Behavioral Research;
  - Dr. James Childress, professor of religious studies, University of Virginia; and
  - Dr. Robert M. Veatch, professor of medical Ethics, senior research scholar, Kennedy Institute of Ethics, Georgetown University

Appendix 1, 1983 National Organ Transplant Hearings

David Wiecking, M.D., office of the chief medical examiner, Richmond, Va.;
- Roger W. Evans research scientist, health and population study center, Battelle Institute, Seattle, Wash.; and
- John McCabe, legal counsel, National Conference of Commissioners on Uniform State Laws, Chicago, IL

<u>April 27, 1983</u>:
- Edward N. Brandt, Jr., M.D., Assistant Secretary for Health, Department of Health and Human Services
- C. Everett Koop, M.D., Surgeon General, U.S. Public Health Service
- Carolyne K. Davis, Administrator, Health Care Financing Administration; accompanied by Dr. Donald Young
- John F. Beary, III, M.D., Acting Assistant Secretary of Defense [health affairs], Department of Defense; accompanied by Alexander Rodriquez, M.D., medical director, O-Champus; and Robert L. Gilliat, Esq., Assistant General Counsel [manpower and health affairs], Department of Defense
- Hon. Dale Bumpers, a U.S. Senator from the State of Arkansas
- Dr. H. David Banta, M.D., Assistant Director for Health and Life Sciences, Office of Technology Assessment
- Kenneth W. Sell, M.D., Ph. D., American Association of Tissue Banks
- Peter Safar, M.D., university professor and director of resuscitation research center, University of Pittsburgh
- Dr. Richard A. Rettig, professor and chairman, department of social sciences, Illinois Institute if Technology
- Dr. Jeffrey M. Prottas, visiting professor, center for health policy analysis and research, Florence Heller Graduate School, Brandeis University
- **Winifred B. Mack, president, North American Transplant Coordinators Organization, SUNY at Stony Brook**

Appendix 1, 1983 National Organ Transplant Hearings

HEARINGS
BEFORE THE
SUBCOMMITTEE ON
INVESTIGATIONS AND OVERSIGHTS
OF THE
COMMITTEE ON
SCIENCE AND TECHNOLOGY
U.S. HOUSE OF REPRESENTATIVES
NINETY-EIGHTH CONGRESS
FIRST SESSION

NOVEMBER 7, 9, 1983

WITNESSES

November 7, 1983:

    Peter Ivanovich, M.D., Department of Medicine, Northwestern University;
  Ernest T. Bauer, chairperson, Patient Action Committee, End Stage Renal Disease Network 23;
  Barbara Lindsay, member, ESRD Network 23; and Warren Reich, professor of bioethics, director, Division of Health and Humanities, Department of Community and Family Medicine, Georgetown University.

    Nicholas J. Feduska, M.D., chairman, Committee on Organ Sharing and Preservation, American Society of Transplant Surgeons;
  Amy S. Peele, president, North American Transplant Coordinators Organization;
  John C. McDonald, M.D., president, Southeastern Organ Procurement Foundation;
  Paul I. Terasaki, M.D., director, Southern California Regional Organ Procurement Agency;
  Henry Krakauer, M.D., National Institute of Allergy and Infectious Diseases, National Institutes of Health.

    Jimmy Light, M.D., director, Organ Procurement and Transplantation, Washington Hospital Center;
  G. Baird Helfrich, M.D., director, Division of Transplantation, Georgetown University Hospital;
  Said A. Karmi, professor of surgery and urology and co-director, George Washington University Transplant Service; and
  George E. Schreiner, M.D., professor of medicine and director, Nephrology Division, Georgetown University Hospital.

November 9, 1983:

    Peter Dobrovitz, kidney recipient, Rochester, N.Y.; John Newmann, president, National Association of Patients on Hemodialysis and Transplantation, New York, N.Y.;
  Ira Griefer, M.D., medical director, National Kidney Foundation; and
  Mary Ann Engebretsen, Miami, Fla., accompanied by her daughter, Trine.

    Marvin Brams, M.D., Department of Urban Affairs and Public Policy, University of Delaware, Newark, Del.;
  H. Barry Jacobs, M.D., medical director, International Kidney Exchange. Ltd., Reston, Va; and
  Oscar Salvatierra, Jr., M.D., president, American Society of Transplant Surgeons.

    George J. Annas, J.D., M.P.H., Utley Professor of Health Law, Boston University Schools of Medicine and Public Health, Boston, Mass.;

Appendix 1, 1983 National Organ Transplant Hearings

Barry Brenner, Harvard University Medical School, Brigham and Women's Hospital, Boston, Mass.;

Robert Veatch, Ph.D., professor of medical ethics, Kennedy Institute of Ethics, Georgetown University, Washington, D.C.;

Arthur L. Caplan, associate for the humanities, the Hastings Center, Hastings-on-Hudson, New York; and

Samuel Gorovitz, Department of Philosophy, University of Maryland, College Park, Md.

Appendix 1, 1983 National Organ Transplant Hearings

HEARINGS
BEFORE THE
SUBCOMMITTEE ON
HEALTH AND THE ENVIRONMENT
OF THE
COMMITTEE ON
ENERGY AND COMMERCE
U.S. HOUSE OF REPRESENTATIVES
NINETY-EIGHTH CONGRESS
FIRST SESSION

JULY 29, OCTOBER 17, 31, 1983

WITNESSES

July 29, 1983:
- Gore, Hon, Albert, Jr., a Representative in Congress from the State of Tennessee
- Richardson, Mr. and Mrs. James, Charlotte, N.C
- Montgomery, Deborah, Cincinnati, Ohio
- White, Raymond, D., Brentwood, Tenn.
- Walden, Hope, on behalf of American Liver Foundation
- Turpin, Marian, Baltimore, Md
- Salvatierra, Oscar K., M.D., president, American Society of Transplant Surgeons
- Belzer, Folkert, M.D., professor and chairman, Department of Surgery, University of Wisconsin
- Prottas, Dr. Jeffrey M., senior research associate, Health Policy Center, Brandeis University
- Young, James, M.D., vice president and medical director, Blue Cross and\ Blue Shield of Massachusetts, Inc.
- Evans, Roger W., Ph.D., research scientist, Health and Population Study Center, Battelle Human Affairs Research Centers
- Stenholm, Hon. Charles W., a Representative in Congress from the State of Texas
- Glickman, Hon. Dan, a Representative in Congress from the State of Kansas
- Marriott, Hon. Dan, a Representative in Congress from the State of Utah.
- Greater Cincinnati Hospital Council
- Congressional Budget Office

October 17, 1983
- Gore, Hon, Albert, Jr., a Representative in Congress from the State of Tennessee
- Brandt, Edward N., Jr., Assistant Secretary for Health, Office of Assistant Secretary for Health, Department of Health and Human Services
- Davis, Carolyne K., Ph.D., Administrator, Health Care Financing Administration, Office of Assistant Secretary for Health, Department of Health and Human Services
- Salvatierra, Oscar K., M.D., president, American Society of Transplant Surgeons
- Peele, Amy S., president, North American Transplant Coordinators Organization

Appendix 1, 1983 National Organ Transplant Hearings

Carter, Charles, M.D., vice president, Southeastern Organ Procurement Foundation
Johnson, Keith, M.D., president, Association of Independent Organ Procurement Agencies
Starzl, Thomas E., M.D., Ph.D., professor of surgery, University of Pittsburgh
Jacobs, Barry, M.D., medical director, International Kidney Exchange, Ltd
Friedlaender, Gary E., M.D., interim president, American Council on Transplantation

October 31, 1983:

Towers, Bernard, M.D., Ch.B., professor of anatomy, pediatrics and psychiatry, and cochairman, UCLA Program in Medicine, Law and Human Values
Ettenger, Robert B., M.D., president, American Society of Transplant Physicians
Salvatierra, Oscar K., M.D., president, American Society of Transplant Surgeons
Terasaki Paul I., Ph.D., president, The Transplant Society
Mendez, Robert, M.D., Urological Consultants Medical Group, Inc
Berne, Thomas V., M.D., chief, Renal Transplant Unit, Department of Surgery, Los Angeles County USC Medical Center
Greco, Maria, co president, Orange County Chapter, American Liver Foundation
Memel, Robert, president, Southern California Chapter, American Liver Foundation

Material submitted for the record by:
American Heart Association
American Heart Association/Greater Los Angeles Affiliate, Inc
American Liver Foundation: Brochure, Transplants A Gift of Life, Questions and Answers About the Organ Donor Program and Statement
American Society of Transplant Physicians, Statement
American Society of Transplant Surgeons: Letter, dated October 6, 1983, from Oscar Salvatierra to C. Everett Koop re supportive position of congressional legislation recently introduced;
Letter, dated October 13, 1983, from cardiac transplant program at Stanford University to Oscar Salvatierra re need of legislation to organ transplantation.
Blue Cross and Blue Shield Association
Gorovitz, Samuel
International Kidney Exchange, Ltd., letter, dated October 19, 1983, from Dr. Jacobs to Chairman Waxman and Congressman Albert Gore, Jr., re: answers to question of appropriate psychiatric or psychological evaluations of all health, living donors
Juvenile Diabetes Foundation International
National Kidney Foundation
Northern California Transplant Bank
Skeen, Hon. Joe, a Representative in Congress from the State of New Mexico

Appendix 1, 1983 National Organ Transplant Hearings

HEARINGS
BEFORE THE
SUBCOMMITTEE ON HEALTH
OF THE
COMMITTEE ON
COMMITTEE ON WAYS AND MEANS
NINETY-EIGHTH CONGRESS
SECOND SESSION

FEBRUARY 9, 1984

WITNESSES

Department of Health and Human Services:
Edward N. Brandt. Jr.. M.D., Assistant Secretary for Health
Carolyne K. Davis, Ph.D., Administrator, Health Care Financing Administration

---

American Association of Tissue Banks, Robert E. Stevenson, Ph.D.
American Liver Foundation, Gail Rempell
American Medical Association, James E. Davis, M.D., Leonard D. Fenninger, M.D., and Harry N. Peterson
American Society of Transplant Surgeons:
    Oscar Salvatierra, M.D.
    Norman Shumway, M.D.
    Thomas Starzl, M.D.
Barnes, Benjamin A., M.D., New England Organ Bank, Inc.
Davis, James E., M.D., American Medical Association
Eye Bank Association of America, A.H. Snyder, Jr
Fenninger, Leonard D., M.D., American Medical Association
Gore, Hon. Albert, Jr., a Representative in Congress from the State of Tennessee
Heck, Ellen, University of Texas Health and Science Center of Dallas
Karsten, Glen W., The Living Bank International
Living Bank International, Glen W. Karsten
Madigan, Hon. Edward R., a Representative in Congress from the State of Illinois
National Kidney Foundation, David A. Ogden, M.D.
New England Organ Bank, Inc., Benjamin A. Barnes, M.D.
North American Transplant Coordinator's Organization, Amy S. Peele
Ogden, David A., M.D., National Kidney Foundation
Peele, Amy S., North American Transplant Coordinator's Organization
Peterson, Harry N., American Medical Association
Rempell, Gail, American Liver Foundation
Salvatierra, Oscar, M.D., University of California at San Francisco, American Society of Transplant Surgeons
Shumway, Norman, M.D., Stanford University, American Society of Transplant Surgeons

Appendix 1, 1983 National Organ Transplant Hearings

Snyder, A.H., Jr., Eye Bank Association of America
Stanford University, Norman Shumway, M.D.
Starzl, Thomas, M.D., University of Pittsburgh, American Society of Transplant Surgeons
Stevenson, Robert E., Ph.D., American Association of Tissue Banks
University of California at San Francisco, Oscar Salvatierra, M.D.
University of Pittsburgh, Thomas Starzl, M.D.
University of Texas Health Science Center at Dallas, Ellen Heck
Walgren. Hon. Doug, a Representative in Congress from the State of Pennsylvania
Waxman, Hon. Henry A., a Representative in Congress from the State of California, and Chairman, Subcommittee on Health and the Environment, Committee on Energy and Commerce

Material submitted for the record by:
Abernathy, Y.T., Eye Bank Association of America, Southeast Region, letter
American Academy of Pediatrics, Paul F. Wehrle, M.D., letter
American Association of Nephrology Nurses and Technicians, Mary Baker, letter
American Burn Association, Charles R. Baxter, M.D., statement
American Council on Transplantation, Gary B. Friedlaender, M.D., letter and statement
Arizona Kidney Foundation, James F. Pfenning, letter
Baker, Mary, American Association of Nephrology Nurses and Technicians, letter
Baxter, Charles R., M.D., American Burn Association, statement
Blue Cross and Blue Shield Association, Mary Nell Lehnhard, letter and statement
Braine, Hayden G., M.D., Johns Hopkins Oncology Center, letter
Dobrovitz, Peter, Rochester, N.Y., statement
East Tennessee Eye Bank, David G. Gerkin, M.D., letter
Eye Bank Association of America, Southeast Region, Y.T. Abernathy, letter
Eye-Bank for Sight Restoration, Inc., Mary Jane O'Neil, statement
Friedlaender, Gary B., M.D., American Council on Transplantation, letter and statement
Gerkin, David G., M.D., East Tennessee Eye Bank, letter
Goldbeck, Willis B., Washington Business Group on Health, statement
Johns Hopkins Oncology Center:
    Hayden G. Braine, M.D., letter
    Albert H. Owens, Jr., M.D., letter
Juvenile Diabetes Foundation International, Jason S. Robert, letter
Lehnhard, Mary Nell, Blue Cross and Blue Shield Association, letter and statement
National Association of Patients on Hemodialysis and Transplantation, Inc., statement
O'Neil, Mary Jane, Eye-Bank for Sight Restoration, Inc., statement
Owens, Albert H., Jr., M.D., Johns Hopkins Oncology Center letter
Pfenning, James F., Arizona Kidney Foundation, letter
Phoenix Transplant Center, Good Samaritan Medical Center, B. A. VanderWerf, M.D., Ph.D., letter
Roberts, Jason S., Juvenile Diabetes Foundation International, letter
Vander Werf, B.A., M.D., Ph.D., Phoenix Transplant Center, Good Samaritan Medical Center, letter
Washington Business Group on Health, Willis B. Goldbeck, statement
Wehrle, Paul F., M.D., American Academy of Pediatrics, letter

Appendix 2, 1983 National Organ Transplant Hearings, D. Denny Testimony

Testimony, Prepared Statements, and Testimony Interaction
With Other Panelists at NOTA Hearings:

Donald Denny
Winifred Mack
Amy Peele

STATEMENT OF DONALD W. DENNY
DIRECTOR OF ORGAN PROCUREMENT
TRANSPLANTATION OFFICE
UNIVERSITY OF PITTSBURGH SCHOOL OF MEDICINE

Mr. DENNY. Mr. Chairman, members of the subcommittee, I thank you for conducting these hearings today. The subject of organ procurement and distribution for transplantation is of national concern.

Despite the headlines that you perhaps have seen, and despite some of the comments that I have heard here today, I would like to indicate at the outset that I believe there is in effect today in this country an effective system for the procurement of vital organs for transplantation. It is not a random process.

The process is not an easy one. The system is not a perfect one. We have heard that there are this year approximately 2,500 post-mortem organ donors, but yet all studies indicate that this is anywhere from one-tenth to one-third of the potential donors from whom organs could be recovered.

The recovery of organs for transplantation is a three-tier process. In trying to understand where the problems lie behind the shortage of organs, behind the fact that we are now recovering so few of the organs from all of the potential donors, I would like very briefly to outline this three-tier process. The three tiers are, in short, the organ procurement programs in this Nation; the physicians and nurses at the acute care hospitals in the United States; and third, all of us, the general public, those of us who inevitably will die, those of us who will succumb at one time or another, and who could be potential vital organ donors.

The first tier, the organ procurement programs in this country:

There is a nationwide regionalized system for the recovery of organs for transplantation. There are in the United States approximately 110 organ procurement programs. These 110 programs have been established over the past several years primarily to serve the need for the recovery of kidneys for transplantation. In recent years with the development of extra-renal—that is, organs other than kidneys—transplantation, these 110 organ procurement programs have been challenged to recover hearts, livers, heart-lungs, pancreas, and so forth, as well as kidneys from their donors.

The 110 organ procurement programs in this country today are, in large part, run by and made effective by the organ procurement professionals, non-physicians like myself, most of whom belong to a nationwide association of coordinators, the North American Transplant Coordinators Organization. Over 360 of us in this country labor to provide organ donation education of physicians and nurses, as well as the public. We are also available generally to receive the referrals of donors, to evaluate donors, and to assist on the scene in donor hospitals in making possible the necessary clinical, medicolegal, and psychological adjustments which are necessary to recover the organs for transplantation.

The 110 organ procurement programs and their associated organ procurement coordinators struggle to provide professional education, to doctors and nursed especially. In my area, I speak over 120 times a year to medical staffs in acute care hospitals, to critical care nurses in intensive care units and emergency rooms, trying to help them understand the importance of recovering organs for transplantation, conveying

A CLINICIAN'S GUIDE TO DONATION AND TRANSPLANTATION

Appendix 2, 1983 National Organ Transplant Hearings, D. Denny Testimony

to them who donors are, helping them understand how to manage these donors so that vital organ function can be sustained, helping them understand the psychology of the donation process in dealing with grieving families.

But it is not just a matter of information giving, unfortunately. We are all besieged by sources of information. We are all besieged by demands to pay attention to urgent needs. Maybe this is especially true of physicians and nurses.

Information giving is frequently not enough—helping a doctor understand that there is a need for organs, who donors may be and what the process is. Sometimes the challenge is to excite them, to make them feel it as we feel it. And sometimes we despair because we are unable, through information giving or through challenging their feelings of caring for dying patients; we are unable to secure their cooperation.

The dissemination of information of physicians and nurses carried out by 110 organ procurement programs in this country has been spotty in some areas. We have received referrals of donors and calls from physicians as far away as the west coast who have called Pittsburgh to ask who donors are, what should they do because they think they have a donor in the hospital, and they are unaware of their own local organ procurement programs in these other areas of the country. It is a tremendous job to try to educate and sustain interest among physicians and nurses in organ donation when their primary concern is caring for living patients, patients who are ill of other diseases.

Because of the apparent lack of a uniform method to educate physicians and nurses in this country today, because of the apparent holes in our educational system, the North American Transplant Coordinators Organization recently established a 24-hour information and referral service for doctors and nurses throughout the country. An 800 number, so it is a toll-free call, is available to physicians and nurses anywhere in the Nation who are not aware of who donors may be or do not know how to contact their own local procurement program. This 800 number is a mnemonic number that is easy to remember, 800-24-DONOR. You pick up the phone and dial 800-24-DONOR.

Mr. GORE. How recently was this established?

Mr. DENNY. This was established 10 days ago. Our struggle now is to acquaint physicians and nurses throughout the country with the availability of this number. Let me stress that this 800 number is not meant to supplant of 24-hour referral numbers in place at the 110 procurement programs; Instead [it's] for a doctor who does not [know] who to call in his own area and, believe me, there are many of them.

The organ procurement programs, going further into my brief look at this three-tier process, also, in addition to providing education, provide the manpower and the technology for the recovery of organs for transplantation. Surgeons, physicians, and paraprofessionals like myself are available 24 hours a day, around the clock, throughout this country, to recover organs for transplant. Every organ procurement program has as one of its major goals the recovery of kidney for transplantation for the nearly 6,000 people who are now waiting for renal transplantation in this country.

Additionally, however, the organ procurement programs collaborate to a great degree in the recovery of extra-renal, non-kidney, organs for transplantation. Cooperation between these 110 organ procurement programs has developed dramatically over the past 2 years. Witness the fact that the University of Pittsburgh, which has a very large waiting list for liver and heart transplant patients, now works collaboratively with other organ procurement programs around the country in recovering two-thirds of the livers that we transplant and three-fourths of the hearts that we transplant. In other words, our own area, within 140 miles of Pittsburgh, which is the geographic region that our organ procurement program covers directly, isn't sufficient to provide the organs for transplantation that we need, especially in the area of livers and hearts.

Through the collaboration of other organ procurement programs, we have flown as far west as Oklahoma City and Fargo, N. Dakota, and as far south as Houston and Miami to recover organs for transplantation through the good efforts of organ procurement professionals in those areas.

Yet, I have to admit before this committee this morning that, although we have collaborated with almost 50 of the 110 organ procurement programs in this Nation recovering extra-renal organs, there are still many of these programs that do not call us when they have kidney donors, and do not give us an opportunity to recover livers or hearts from their donors.

Chapter 1: THE HISTORY OF THE TRANSPLANT COORDINATOR

Appendix 2, 1983 National Organ Transplant Hearings, D. Denny Testimony

The system is developing. One of the reasons that we don't receive collaboration from all of the organ procurement programs is that they are in need also of education. They need also to understand that working with us in recovering hearts and livers is not going to compromise their kidneys which they need desperately for transplantation locally.

In addition to organ procurement education, and procurement services, organ procurement programs are actively involved in the distribution of organs for transplantation. In the case of kidneys—you shall hear from Dr. Pfaff in a few minutes—there is a computer system which is an excellent means of locating suitable recipients nationwide for transplantation of kidneys. When we have kidneys available in the Pittsburgh area that we are unable to transplant among our patients, the computer will print out for us a list of suitably matched recipients throughout the country.

The computer system has limitations, however. In the distribution of extra-renal organs, a somewhat different system has been utilized to supplement it. The computer is a fixed-base operation. A terminal is located in my office, but there is no terminal in the community hospital where I may have a donor. What do I do at 2 o'clock in the morning when a donor is identified in a community hospital 100 miles from Pittsburgh and I am preparing to sit down and talk with grieving family to suggest that they donate organs? I need to know immediately where a suitable recipient for the heart or liver may be. In the case of kidneys, we can wait until the organs have been removed and access the terminal when we get back after the donor surgery. In the case of hearts and livers, we need to know where the recipients are before we remove the organs because of the very limited preservation times that we have for these organs.

I can't access a terminal at 2 o'clock in the morning from 100 miles away from my office. Instead, what we have now is a 24-hour telephone system, also established by the North American Transplant Coordinators Organization, a telephone system which is contrived to provide information concerning the needs for hearts, livers, heart-lungs, and other extra-renal organs to organ procurement professionals around the country. Twenty-four hours a day, if we access a central telephone number, we are informed through a recorded message of what organs are needed from Stanford, Calif., to Pittsburgh, from New York City to Virginia to Memphis, Tenn.

Fifteen extra-renal transplant centers now cooperate and list their extra-renal organ donor needs on this 24-Alert System. The calling coordinator or physician will be told the blood type, the size of the donor that is sought, the distance that the transplant center is willing to fly, the telephone number to call if a donor is available. The caller is also informed of the potential recipient's medical condition, that is, the degree of urgency for transplantation.

Brandon Hall today is flying back to Memphis for his liver transplant. This liver transplant was made possible by the fact that the organ procurement coordinator in Virginia who recognized the donor called the 24-Alert telephone number and was informed through this service that the University of Tennessee had an urgent need for a pediatric donor liver of a given size and blood type for Brandon Hall. He copied down the phone number and gave them a call.

This system doesn't sound very sophisticated. Computers sound so much more high-tech, don't they, than phones and recorded answering services? But this system works. It is effective. It is available to all of us, and it has made possible in the last 6 months the transplantation of 48 livers at 5 centers, and 25 hearts at 9 centers.

Going on briefly in my description of the three-tier system, the second tier are the health professionals, the doctors and the nurses in this country, who are in a position to recognize suitable donors to provide the organs for transplantation. I have been an organ procurement professional for the past 9 years. I am glad to say that the physicians and nurses in this country, by and large, support organ donation. Unfortunately, however, verbal support isn't sufficient. We also have to have their active support. Unfortunately also, it is accurate to say that many physicians and nurses do not collaborate with us in recovering organs for transplantation.

Ignorance, apathy, indifference, they all play a part. But perhaps the biggest problem is the medicolegal problem—physicians and nurses who fear that if they cooperate in the recovery of organs for transplantation, they will be vulnerable to litigation. We live in a litigious society, and physicians especially know how damaging nuisance lawsuits can be. As a result, they oftentimes practice defensively.

Appendix 2, 1983 National Organ Transplant Hearings, D. Denny Testimony

Their patients are not waiting for transplant, and our requests that they help us sometimes fall on deaf ears because of their fear of medicolegal vulnerability.

Brain death is a central issue related to organ donation. You can't escape it. By definition, all donors are victims of brain death. They are medically and legally dead because their brains are dead. They are no longer thinking, feeling, willing, reflexive people. Artificially their hearts and their respiratory systems continue to function, and this is what allows the viability of the organs to be preserved until they are removed and chilled.

Physicians are especially concerned about the public's acceptance of brain death. Thirty-five States now have passed statutes recognizing that brain death, is death. Fifteen States do not have laws defining brain death, but in those 15 States, common law or appellate court decisions allow the recovery of organs for transplantation following pronouncement of death on the basis of brain death.

But despite legal support, doctors and nurses often fear that the public does not accept brain death and do not cooperate with us. Less than 1 percent of all the deaths that occur in this country occur under the circumstances of brain death and among the population that is within the right age frame to be a donor.

In my mind, the health professionals, the doctors, and the nurses in this country, are the weak link between the first tier, the organ procurement programs, and the third tier, the lay public. In my experience in the Pittsburgh area and in Pennsylvania generally, approximately one out of five families says no to organ donation; but four out of five families who are approached and offered the opportunity, say yes. These figures are not duplicated in many other racial, and educational factors influence whether or not members of the public will say yes to organ donation at the time of death.

The American public, however, does have a big heart. One of the gratifying aspects of my job is that I deal with these grieving families and see firsthand the value that it provides the grieving family to be told that the organs from their loved one now sustain life in two, three, four, or five other patients.

In my experience, only 1 out of 10 families of a brain dead victim initiates the request to donate. Most families at the time of death are too overcome with their own grief to remember the need for organs. I am not concerned by the fact that the National Kidney Foundation poll recently found the only 40 percent of the white population and 20 percent of the black population would be willing to donate organs of their loved ones at the time of death. We don't want to believe that we are going to die. We don't want to believe that our loved ones are going to die. As a result, when we are asked—not at the time of death, but at the time of life—whether or not we would donate, of course we say no. It is too scary to even consider that these people might die. At the time of death, as I said, only 1 out of 10 families initiates the request to donate. But 8 of those 10 families, in my experience, do donate if they are offered the opportunity.

The problem comes, again at the medical professional level, the need for physicians and nurses to adequately explain brain death to the families and to offer donation. It is so difficult sometimes for doctors and nurses, who themselves grieve when they lose a patient, to sit down and try to explain to a family that their loved one in the intensive care unit is dead. It is especially difficult because this patient does not look dead. He is, remember, a victim of brain death. Artificially, his heart and his lungs are continuing to function.

To try to explain to a family that this brain-dead victim who looks as though he is alive and merely comatose is really dead is difficult for the physicians, and sometimes they shirk it. Sometimes they shirk it because of their own grief, their own pain, the assault on their integrity which they are experiencing because of the death. Sometimes it is so much easier for a physician to distance himself from the family.

The American public is hungry for information about organ donation. Thousands and thousands of donor cards are distributed by our program and other programs around the country, but it is not enough. We need more public education, not only with regard to organ donation, but with regard to brain death as well. It is time that we stopped hiding brain death and talked about it openly. It is time the medical profession talked about it openly.

Public education in the past has been primarily aimed at the people who already are convinced that organ donation is a good thing. Public education is largely directed toward white middle-class America.

Chapter 1 — THE HISTORY OF THE TRANSPLANT COORDINATOR

Appendix 2, 1983 National Organ Transplant Hearings, D. Denny Testimony

We need public educational efforts which are directed toward population subgroups, Spanish Americans, black Americans, Americans from the Mediterranean Basin, and so on. These groups do donate with the same high frequency as the white middle-class public does.

Physicians and nurses are consumers of the media, and they generally follow and do not lead public donation. If we educate the public, we will also indeed be educating the medical professionals. If they feel that the public is comfortable with brain death and with organ donation, they will be much more likely to collaborate with us.

I have five recommendations. First of all, it is time that the transplant professionals in this country recognize that they can't do the job alone. There is a need for a national task force to be composed of leaders from government, medicine, organ procurement, and interested lay groups to tackle the problems impeding the recovery of organs for transplantation. It is time that the transplant professionals in this country recognize that they need to involve their colleagues in the medical profession. The neurosurgeons, the neurologists, the critical care medicine physicians, the emergency physicians, the pediatricians should be members of such a task force. They are the physicians who will recognize donors. They are the people who need to be convicted that it is important to work with us. The critical care nurses are by far our most vital ally. They, too, should be involved in a national task force. This task force should be given the charge of coming up with solutions for developing and improving the system nationwide.

My second recommendation derives from the fact that every hospital in this country must be certified to function, must be certified on several levels. Departments of health in the various States have the responsibility of certifying hospitals in their States. The Joint Commission for the Accreditation of Hospitals also provides accreditation of hospitals on a national level.

There should be developed for accreditation two requirements either on the State or on the national level. The first requirement should be that there be a policy and an operational protocol for the determination of brain death. Second, there should be a requirement for certification that every hospital established a policy and a protocol for recognizing potential donors and referring donors for the nearest organ procurement program.

Doctors refer donors. Hospitals don't refer donors, but if the hospitals have the rules and the regulations, the doctors may be made more willing to comply, to cooperate.

My third recommendation: there should be a financial incentive program established by the Health Care Finance Administration, which has the responsibility of funding kidney transplantation. A financial incentive would reward hospitals at which donors are identified and from whom organs are recovered.

It is well known that kidney transplantation is much more cost effective than is hemodialysis or peritoneal dialysis for the treatment of end-stage renal failure patients.

This country, and you and I as taxpayers, have an incentive in seeing more people transplanted, if only because it costs less. It makes good sense to me to recommend that the Health Care Finance Administration provide a financial incentive to those hospitals from which kidneys are recovered. Since almost every postmortem kidney donor is also a potential postmortem extrarenal donor, this will increase the number of extra-renal donors, this will increase the number of extra-renal organs available.

My fourth recommendation is that there is a need for strengthening public and professional education. Public education has been tried in many forms on the local level, for example, health fairs, talks to school groups. These kinds of local educational efforts, to my mind, are not effective.

What is effective is use of the national media, not only to provide information about donation and brain death, but to excite people. We have to inform, but we have to motivate, as well. We have to touch their feelings. There is much more work that we could do in public education. I would like to see the American Advertising Council take on a campaign in this country to help educate Americans about organ donation.

Finally, there is a need for statistical information. As we have heard today, we have to talk in general figures, because nobody really knows how many potential donors there are in this country, for instance. Nobody really knows how many potential donors are referred. Nobody really knows how many end-stage renal disease patients there are in this country. Nobody really knows how many potential recipients of

Appendix 2, 1983 National Organ Transplant Hearings, D. Denny Testimony

extra-renal organs there are. One vital question, I think, needs to be addressed, and that is how many potential pediatric donors are there between the ages of 6 months and 5 years?

The need for pediatric liver donors between six months and five is tremendous. We have a waiting list over 35 children in this age bracket who are waiting for liver transplants. I know, we all know that many of them will die because we will not find organs for them. We may be faced with the fact that there are not enough potential pediatric donors in the Nation to meet the needs of all of these youngsters.

Again, let me congratulate this subcommittee, Chairman Gore, members of the subcommittee, for your interests, for your efforts in spotlighting the accomplishments and the problems and the goals that we strive for as the future unfolds for us in what is a very promising time for transplantation. Thank you.

[The prepared statement of Mr. Donald W. Denny follows:]

PREPARED STATEMENT OF DONALD W. DENNY

My name is Donald W. Denny. I am the Director of Organ Procurement for the Transplant Foundation at the University of Pittsburgh. I am also a member of the North American Transplant Coordinators Organization (NATCO), a professional association of the transplant and organ procurement coordinators from the United States, Canada and several foreign countries. My testimony today will primarily reflect my personal experience, attitudes and values. I am also designated as the official representative of NATCO at these hearings, but when expressing the point of view of this association of over 350 transplant professionals, the context of my remarks will identify my position as a spokesman.

I wish to express my appreciation to the Chairman and members of this Subcommittee for conducting these hearings into the subject of post mortem vital organ procurement and distribution for transplantation. I have been closely involved in organ procurement for the past nine years, have participated in the organization of and have administered two organ procurement programs. I believe that the subject of these hearings is a health care crisis, which requires broad national attention and the problem-solving efforts of individuals, organization and government.

Recent advance is transplantation surgery and immunology now provide the opportunity for additional years of life and health to many Americans who in the past were doomed to an existence supported by a machine, as in the case of victims of end-stage kidney disease, or were cut down by death prematurely, as in the case of people suffering from end-stage heart and liver disease. Other witnesses before this Subcommittee will provide substantive information to support my contention that medical science has moved beyond the frontier in organ transplantation, has, indeed, reached a fertile high ground and needs but the active support and investment of this nation to establish a living monument to the value of human life and the spirit of brotherhood: the giving of life, one to another, on a large scale through organ transplantation. My focus today will be with one obstacle impending realization of this bright promise: the shortage of human organ for transplantation that exists now and, unless nationwide efforts are undertaken, will increase tomorrow.

The shortage of organs for transplantation is not a new problem. My colleagues and I have worked for years to overcome the fact that the demand for port mortem kidneys has long exceeded the supply. The number of post mortem kidneys transplanted in the United States has remained relatively stable for several years, despite the fact that the national waiting list has continued to grow annually. The shortage of kidneys for transplantation has received relatively little attention, largely because renal transplantation is not a form of transplant therapy, which is often an alternative to death. We have, fortunately, the artificial kidney machine which can sustain life for most end-stage renal disease (ESRD) patients who elect to wait for a transplant, as well as those patients who do not wish to consider or are unsuitable for transplantation. The undeniable facts that a real kidney, a transplanted kidney, provides a better quality of life for ESRD patients and that renal transplantation is more cost-effective per patient life-year than the artificial kidney have not been sufficient to cause the national sense of urgency which underlies these hearings.

Chapter 1 — THE HISTORY OF THE TRANSPLANT COORDINATOR

Appendix 2, 1983 National Organ Transplant Hearings, D. Denny Testimony

Without intending to diminish the meaning and the importance of this Subcommittee's purpose today, I must lament, however, the fact that recent publicity concerning the need for a liver transplant for a handful of patients at two or three transplant centers (including my own) has outweighed the silent suffering of many thousands of patients waiting for a kidney transplant at 150 transplant hospitals over the past decade in moving the conscience of this nation.

Yet, it is undeniable that liver and heart transplant candidates, unlike kidney transplant patients, have only one other option: death. I cannot blame the media or the public for being more profoundly stirred by a picture of one sad-eyed dying child waiting and hoping for a liver donor than by cold statistics which represent the plight of faceless thousands of ESRD patients. We who spend our professional lives seeking donors of extrarenal organs (i.e., organs other than kidneys) have also been vulnerable to the poignancy of the individual child's desperate need. And when such a patient dies because an organ is not found in time, we also feel a crushing sense of sadness and failure. But we also feel something else, something the public generally does not, namely frustration and anger. The reason is that we know that many more organs are needlessly wasted than are recovered for transplantation. We know that the shortage of organs at this time is not due to a lack of technology, manpower, knowledge of funding, as much as it is due to ignorance, inertia, selfishness and parochialism.

We know, in short, that despite what one reads in the newspaper, there is a system in place in this country for the recovery of organs for transplantation, but that this system does not work as effectively as possible because of the lack of individual and institutional commitment to the recovery of organs for transplantation.

From February 1981, through February 1983, 126 post mortem livers were transplanted at the University Health Center of Pittsburgh. During this same period, 44 adults and 27 children died before we found a suitable organ for them. During this same interval, 41 patients received heart transplants at our Center, but 8 other patients succumbed to heart failure before we could transplant them. The success of liver and heart transplantation today is encouraging many more institutions to establish programs for the transplantation of these organs in order to meet the needs of increasing numbers of potential recipients. The problem promises to become worse.

I need to define some limitations in order to express fully the nature of the problem. The post mortem recovery of vital organs for transplantation is limited by the circumstances of death, donor age, donor medical history, qualify of organ function and temporal restrictions. Because vital organs are very vulnerable to lack of oxygenated blood at normal body temperature, we are unable to consider as donors of vital organs any individual whose death is determined b the traditional criteria, i.e., irreversible cessation of heart and lung functions. Organ death occurs within minutes of cessation of the circulation. Vital organ procurement is limited to patients who are medically and legally dead, but whose heart and lung functions are artificially maintained with mechanical ventilation and intravenous hydration until the organs are surgically removed and chilled. In practice this means that organ donors must be victims of brain death, i.e., patients who have suffered catastrophic, irreversible and complete cessation of integrated brain function as the result of trauma, stroke, brain tumor and/or oxygen deprivation. The brain death syndrome by definition always includes destruction of brain stem function, among the sequelae of which is the total inability to breath spontaneously. Forty years ago before the development of the mechanical ventilator, which is used to take over respiratory functions for patients who have difficultly breathing or cannot breath spontaneously, death of the brain resulted in cessation of breathing and, secondarily, heart failure when the heart muscle died due to lack of oxygen. Use of the mechanical ventilator has intruded upon this natural sequence of events and physicians have had to develop new operational criteria for determining when death has occurred in patients suffering from total and irreparable brain destruction. Pronouncement of death after determination of brain death is a commonplace event in the United States and is sanctioned by either statute or common law in all 50 states. Organ donation is not the primary or even secondary rationale for accepting brain death as death of the individual, but it is a necessary precondition for organ retrieval for transplantation.

A CLINICIAN'S GUIDE TO DONATION AND TRANSPLANTATION

Appendix 2, 1983 National Organ Transplant Hearings, D. Denny Testimony

Another limitation to donation is donor age. The inevitable consequences of aging, including vascular disease and the slow loss of optimum organ function, limits chronological age acceptable for donors. Kidneys are generally accepted from donors

up to their mid-50s and sometime beyond. Liver donors are rarely considered beyond age 45; while heart donors are carefully evaluated if they are 35 and are seldom accepted beyond 40. Minimum age limits are also a factor. Kidney donors must generally be one year or older. Liver donors can be accepted from age 6 months and up, however. Heart donors are seldom less than age 15.

Other factors which can contraindicate organ donation include: previous disease involving the organ considered for donation, infection, cancer (except primary brain tumors) and acute injury to the organs due to trauma, oxygen deprivation and persistent periods of low blood pressure.

How many patients in this country's hospitals are victims of brain death and have suitable organs for transplantation? Again, no one really knows. Retrospective studies of hospital Charts of patients dying in hospitals suggest between 0.77% and 3.5% of hospitalized patients are acceptable as kidney donors.[1-3] The difference in the conclusions is due to variations in acceptable criteria between investigators. (The percentage of potential donors in these studies which actually did provide organs for transplantation ranged from 17.0% to 19.03%.[2,3] Since only patients who die in hospitals may be considered for vital organ donation, it is important to consider that only 38% to 60% of the deaths in this country occur in hospitals.[1-3] Assuming that half of the annual deaths in the United States occur in hospitals (which may be generous, since statistics on hospital deaths include patients who are dead on arrival and who expire in the Emergency Department soon after arrival), how many in-hospital deaths occur? In 1981, the last year for which statistics are available, there were a total of 1,987,512 deaths in this country (4), of which 50% is 993,756. Multiplying this figure by the above cited percentages of in-hospital deaths which would have been acceptable kidney donors, yields as estimated range of potential donors I the United States of 7,652 to 34,781. Because the age criteria for liver and heart donors is less liberal than for kidney donors, the potential number of extrarenal donors is undoubtedly fewer than is indicated by this range.

How many donors annually yield vital organs for transplantation in the United States? One way of determining an approximation is by looking at the number of post mortem kidney transplants yearly. In 1981, the last year for which I have firm figures, there were 3,427 post mortem kidneys transplanted in this country. Since each donor yields two kidneys, dividing this number by two results in a figure of 1,713 donors. However, since there is approximately 25% wastage of donor kidneys (as a result of surgical error, unexpected anomalies, no suitably matched recipients available), the total number of <u>available</u> kidneys during 1981 was approximate number of donors in that year. In other words, we are now recovering organs, at best, from fewer than one out of every three possible donors.

This figure does not represent the total number of potential donors referred to organ procurement programs. Organ donation is a voluntary activity in this country requiring consent of the nearest next-of-kin (a practical necessity for all organ procurement programs even when a donor has signed a donor card or other document allowing recovery of organs after death). Organ donation is unacceptable to some families and a percentage of prospective donors is lost for this reason. My experience is that approximately one out of five prospective donors referred to us does not yield organs for want of family consent. This figure varies around the country according to cultural, racial and educational characteristics of the population. Black families, for instance, are much less likely to donate than white families for reasons which are not understood. The number of families which not to donate is, however, somewhat larger, since an unknown number of potential donors are recognized by physicians, who approach the families and are refused, and never inform the local organ procurement program of their efforts.

I value the fact that organ donation in this country is a voluntary, altruistic act determined by the values of the people concerned. National polls have indicated, however, that 70% and more of the people in this country regard organ donation favorably and would be willing to donate a family member's organs at the time of death.[5,6] I would be against legislation which would make donation either compulsory or subject to financial reward. Another option exists, one which is in practice in a few European countries, which is to assume that consent of the individual has been given for post mortem organ donation at

Appendix 2, 1983 National Organ Transplant Hearings, D. Denny Testimony

the time of his death unless a document signed by the individual indicating opposition to donation is presented when he expires. Given the litigious climate of this country and the vulnerability of the medical profession in particular to nuisance suits, I doubt that this option is realistic. Even if such a system were legal, I am sure that surviving next-of-kin would also be asked to consent to recovery of the organs, even as they are now.

Obviously, one means of increasing the numbers of organs donated would be to enhance the willingness of families to donate through educational programs. Educational efforts directed at the lay public have been an important component of many organ procurement programs' efforts for the past decade. Many approaches have been tried: professional advertising technique (billboards, radio and television public service announcements, ads in newspapers and magazines), didactic presentation to students, churches and service clubs and news and feature stories released to the print and electronics media. While I am sure that these efforts have had an impact (some more than others), I am unaware of any reliable studies which can document the effectiveness of public education efforts tried thus far. I am personally biased in favor of the effectiveness of the free educational opportunities afforded by the media, although I have tried all the options cited above at one time or another. News and feature stories focusing on people with whom the public can identify reach the largest audience, have more emotional impact and require less financial investment than costly billboards, public service announcements, health fairs in shopping centers or classroom talks. Stories about patients waiting for transplantation, about patients who have been successfully transplanted, about individual donors and their families' feelings regarding donation have great human appeal. The media becomes quickly jaded, however, and one must constantly seek new "angles" with which to interest the press.

Until recently, kidney donation and transplantation have been the primary thrust of public education for most procurement programs. One indication of the effectiveness of these efforts is greater frequency with which the public is willing to donate kidneys as opposed to livers and hearts. The heart, of course, is a special case in view of the great symbolic and emotional investment traditionally associated with this simplest of all the vital organs. On the other hand, very little emotional attachment to the liver exists for most of us, and yet many families who are very willing to donate their family member's kidneys balk at donating the liver. The reason, I believe, is that liver donation and transplantation are not yet as well known and accepted as kidney transplantation.

Most public education efforts in some way try to go beyond mere information giving and try to involve the audience in solving the problem by encouraging the completion and carrying of universal organ donor cards. Legislation has been enacted in all fifty states making such cards legal instruments for the post mortem donation of organs. As I have mentioned, however, all organ procurement programs with which I am familiar also require family consent, although legally it is not required if a donor card is available. The success of organ donor cards in increasing the number of donor organs in minimal; relatively few donors each year are identified as card carrying donors.

Our program has only one or two such donors each year out of 50 to 60 donors in our region. The primary problem, I believe, is that our death is a very fearful prospect for most of us. We defend ourselves against this fear by avoiding any activity which tends to confirm our mortality. Completing and signing a donor card affirms our appointment with death and, as a result, most of us never get around to getting or completing a card.

Like most other organ procurement programs, we distribute donor cards—as many as 10,000 a year. This is not a large number compared to our region's population of approximately 3.5 million people, however. In Pennsylvania we have also had donor cards distributed with drivers' licenses for several years, yet our program has not seen an increase in card-carrying donors as a result of this program. A recent survey in Maryland, where the donor card is on the drivers' license, found that only 1.5% of the people chose to complete and sign the card.[5]

Organ donor cards do have some utility. Their availability stimulates discussion and contribution to a positive climate of awareness regarding the need for organs. Many times I have been told by donor families that receipt of a donor card with a driver's license engendered a family conversation, during which

Appendix 2, 1983 National Organ Transplant Hearings, D. Denny Testimony

the deceased indicated his willingness to be a donor. These discussions are remembered at the time of death <u>if</u> organ donation is offered to the family, even though the deceased did not fill out the card. These families inevitably donate.

I have always believed that the public education should include the subject of brain death, as well as organ donation and transplantation. Many of my colleagues do not agree with me, believing that the subject is too complex for the lay public to comprehend or that there is a danger of brain death being misconstrued as so-called "transplant death." This latter possibility exists primarily because of the medical profession's hesitancy in educating the public about brain death, a syndrome which is undoubtedly clinically associated with many more nondonors than donors. If brain death is mentioned only in conjunction with organ donation, so the argument goes, the public will believe the syndrome is diagnostic of death only when the organs are sought, that brain death is not "real" death but a shortcut designed to make organ recovery possible.

On the contrary, I find the public intuitively sophisticated and ready to comprehend that death of the brain in diagnostic of death of the person if they are given accurate information and the discussion is in lay terms which can comprehend. Not being candid about brain death and its relationship to organ donation is potentially very dangerous. If the public does not understand and accept it, they are much more likely to experience suspicion and disbelief when they are faced with it. We are all more ready to reject what we have not heard of or do not understand.

Our emphasis on brain death education led us to seek enactment of legislation giving statutory recognition to brain death. Such legislation was not necessary to give legal standing to the syndrome as diagnostic of death, but was perceived as a means of educating the public. Public acceptance and passage of the brain death bill also, we hoped, would reassure a medical community fearful of putative public inability to understand and accept brain death. Our programs worked collaboratively with the other organ procurement program in the state, the Delaware Valley Transplant Program, Philadelphia, the Pennsylvania Department of Health, the Pennsylvania Catholic Conference, the Pennsylvania Medical Society and the Hospital Association of Pennsylvania in aggressively seeking passage of the Uniform Determination of Death Act during 1982. We conducted a vigorous letter writing campaign seeking medical professional and public support, sought and received press attention for the Bill and testified at legislative hearings in support of passage. This educational effort was very successful, surprisingly little opposition was encountered and the Bill was passed during December 1982. It is too early to tell whether or not the passage of this legislation will reassure the many physicians who hesitate to cooperate in organ procurement because of their fear that the public cannot accept brain death pronounced on the basis of destruction of brain function.

Perhaps one of the less well-recognized functions of public education is the impact it has on health professionals. Doctors and nurses are also media consumers and public education can help to persuade health professionals that organ procurement and brain death are acceptable to the general public. The health professions are generally conservative and frequently tend to follow rather than to lead public opinion. Yet, I am skeptical of the utility of costly advertising efforts, as I have seen them employed in this area in the past. Professionally produced public service announcements focusing on organ donation have almost always been directed toward the educated, white middleclass audience. Much more effective, I believe, would be programming and public service announcements directed toward segments of the population, i.e., working class ethnics, black Americans, Spanish-speaking Americans and other population subgroups. I feel that little is to be gained through educational efforts which do not employ the mass media; highly labor intensive public speaking campaigns directed toward schools and civic groups, for example, have little impact. The American Advertising Council does take on projects for non-profit organization and activities. Perhaps this group of professionals could be prevailed upon to contribute time and talent to the production of effective mass market public education.

Since, in my experience, approximately four out of five families offered the opportunity to donate will decide favorably, I believe that the most effective allocation of current funding available would be to invest in the education and motivation of health professionals to recognize and refer potential donors.

Appendix 2, 1983 National Organ Transplant Hearings, D. Denny Testimony

Despite very heavy favorable media attention to organ donation, transplantation and brain death in the greater Pittsburgh area, no more than one out of ten donor referrals to our program is at the request of the family. The death of a loved one is so painful, the families are generally so preoccupied with their loss, that they do not think of organ donation. <u>It must be offered to them</u>. The role of the physician and nurses who care for the patients and are in a position to recognize donors and to refer them to the local organ procurement programs therefore becomes critical. The education of health professionals and the establishment of institutional policies which will enhance organ donation should, I believe, be the primary areas for the investment of time, energy and money. I must recognize, however, that many of my colleagues do not agree with me. This is the philosophy which has been followed at both organ procurement programs with which I have been associated as Director.

I joined the newly formed Transplant Foundation at the University of Pittsburgh School of Medicine in January 1978, after nearly four years with the Delaware Valley Transplant Program. Both programs were established to the outset as independent not-for-profit corporations governed by Boards of Directors composed of physicians closely involved with transplantation at associated university medical centers. Financial and corporate independence allows for flexibility in establishing and implementing programs designed to achieve procurement goals. This Committee will hear evidence presented by other expert witnesses which strongly suggests that such independent organ procurement agencies are more economical and more successful than are programs which are functions of hospitals or universities.

In describing the philosophy and the programs which I have found successful of organ procurement, I will focus on the Transplant Foundation at the University of Pittsburgh and our efforts during the past five years. Although kidney transplantation had been initiated by the University's School of Medicine in 1964, the programs had remained relatively small until it was Reorganized in 1977 under the direction of Thomas R. Hakala, M.D. Growth of the transplant program had not been limited by the number of patients referred for renal transplantation, witness the fact that almost 100 ESRD patients were on our waiting list in late 1977. Instead, the major handicap had been the shortage of available kidneys. Until 1978, the University was entirely dependent upon kidneys which could be recovered at the University Health Center of Pittsburgh or could be imported from other centers in the nation. No organized effort existed to seek the collaboration of other area hospitals in recognizing and referring donors. In the fourteen-year history of the renal transplant program at Pitt prior to 1978, only one donor had provided organs at a hospital outside the University Health Center. Clearly the community hospitals offered an untapped source of organ donors.

Two major programs were planned and implemented during—1978 for developing organ procurement at approximately 90 hospitals in a geographic area including western Pennsylvania, eastern Ohio and northwestern West Virginia: (a) an educational program for health professionals and (b) a comprehensive organ retrieval Program, which would provide 24 hours-a-day services for the coordination of the donation process and for the surgical retrieval and preservation of donor kidneys in outlying hospitals.

The educational program emphasized dissemination of information concerning the need for kidneys, donor criteria, evaluation and management, the medicolegal aspects of donation and brain death, the psychology of grief and its effect on organ donation, the surgical techniques of organ retrieval and the services provided by the Transplant Foundation team. I was given responsibility for implementing this program.

We followed a five-step plan. First, the need for educational materials was recognized and appropriate brochures, posters, phone stickers and handbooks were developed. Secondly, a direct mail campaign utilizing personal letters and follow-up phone calls was initiated to establish contact with physicians in influential positions within area hospitals for the purpose of scheduled and carried out a meetings of medical staffs, critical care nurses and hospitals administrators. Fourth, in those hospitals in which contacts could not be made with supportive staff through mail and phone efforts, I sought cooperation and speaking opportunities through unscheduled individual contacts with key hospital personnel. Fifth, follow-up personal contacts were planned and carried out on a regular basis on strengthen and maintain the level of awareness and to facilitate to formation of strong purposeful relationships with important keystone professionals.

Appendix 2, 1983 National Organ Transplant Hearings, D. Denny Testimony

We have continued to follow this program throughout the past five years. Experience has proven the value of personal contacts through phone, mail and direct visits with physicians and nurses in critical care areas. Too frequent contact can be interpreted as unwarranted invasion of professional responsibility, whereas very infrequent contacts do not maintain the visibility for organ donation we strive to achieve. We find that contacts approximately four times a year are more effective. An effort is made to enhance identification of these health care professionals with our program through the distribution of inexpensive calendars, penlights, pens and other items with our logo, name and telephone number. Personnel changes in area hospitals frequently necessitate repeat educational programs.

Our efforts to acquaint physicians and nurses with our need for organs and to excite them about the possibility of cooperating with us were and are today met with a variety of responses. Many health professionals were warmly receptive, hungry for information and eager to assist for purely humanitarian reasons. Many others were indifferent and unresponsive or aloof and unwilling to help because of perceived medicolegal problems. A few were interested in helping because they anticipated that cooperation would possibly be used to their benefit politically. If their needs were not met, they quickly lost interest. And, finally, a very few were openly hostile; more than once I was summarily ejected from a hospital or told that I was presumptuous for seeking cooperation in establishing our donor program in a hospital. One became rather thick-skinned and if one approach does not work there are usually other approaches which can be taken. Almost always we can find someone in a given hospital who is interested, receptive and helpful. What I want to emphasize, however, is that the direct humanitarian appeal is sometime not effective in securing cooperation of health care professionals.

Health care is not unlike other areas of human endeavor in that it is affected by politics, power struggles, inertia, fear, vanity and money. Motivation is often, but not always, complex, and frequently includes factors other than a desire to help others. Development and the growth of a donor program must recognize and accept this reality and, if possible without compromising individual and program principles, work with it or, if necessary, work around it.

The most important inducements which are effective are the solace organ donation provides the health professional and the humanitarian appeal of helping others, both the donor family and the transplant recipients. Health professionals like all of us, dislike failure. The death of a patient is an assault on their feelings as caring people and an affront to their professional competence and identify. Their tendency in the face of patient death is often to attempt to distance themselves emotionally from the pain of failure. What we can offer doctors and nurses is a way of diminishing pain failure. We do not put it that way to them, of course. We talk instead of the lives of the recipients which can be saved and the solace the family can realize through transplantation of the donor's organs.

There is genuine satisfaction for a physician or nurse in helping both the family and the recipients through participating in organ donation, but what most get out of the experience, I believe, is a restoration of their own self-regard and emotional equilibrium. Participating in organ donation tends to diminish their sense of loss and failure. But, again, for some this is not enough. And for a very few, nothing appears to be enough to secure their active involvement.

The personal relationship developed between the representative of the organ procurement team and physicians, nurses and other hospital staff is also a major factor in developing an organ procurement program. In our program, the organ procurement coordinators (there are now four of us) are the most visible of the team members. We make initial contacts, provide the education programs for doctors and nurses, receive donor referrals, collaborate on-the-scene throughout the entire donor process (evaluation, management, discussions with family, surgical removal of the organs), call, write and return in person to provide feedback about the transplant outcome. In the process we strive to develop a relationship based on trust, collaboration, recognition, personal regard and shared experience. The strength of which may be operational.

Nothing succeeds like success, however, and a positive experience of being involved in recovering organs from a donor is very reinforcing for most physicians and nurses. Their sense of satisfaction almost always guarantees their future support. But, in order to provide this kind of positive experience, the entire

Appendix 2, 1983 National Organ Transplant Hearings, D. Denny Testimony

process must be handled efficiently, tactfully and knowingly from beginning to end. The second major component of our program, the system for coordinating the donor process and recovering the organs is based on our belief that only transplant professionals have the time, commitment and attention to detail which are necessary to ensure that the experience and the outcome are both positive. Some organ procurement programs appoint a nurse or physician on the staff of a community hospital to coordinate organ donation in that institution. Some programs also train local transplant center. We feel that reliance on indigenous health professionals is fraught with too many opportunities for error, misunderstanding and omission of important procedural steps. The organ donor process from beginning to end is a very complex one, involving critical clinical, medicolegal and psychological variables.

Problems, when they occur, need to be handled expeditiously and sensitively. If they are not the concept of organ procurement suffers and the enthusiasm for cooperating with our program is damaged. For these reasons, we believe it is necessary to have one of our coordinators present in the donor hospital whose sole purpose is to make the donation process work. Similarly, in the Operating Room our transplant surgeons are responsible for performing the donor surgery. The techniques are specialized and not understood by untrained surgeons. Additionally, the transplant surgeon's commitment to a positive experience for the donor hospital's staff and the recovery of viable organs is more focused because he knows that the success of his program and the well being of his recipients is directly at stake.

In summary, the establishment and success of an organ procurement program is not an enterprise which lends itself to a mechanistic or bureaucratic approach. As with any endeavor which requires collaboration of people from disparate professions with differing agendas and dissimilar institutional loyalties, organ procurement requires consent attention to the establishment, maintenance and repair of a delicate fabric of relationships, as well as dissemination of substantive information and technical competence.

Yet, no program is so successful that it can sustain itself solely with organs recovered in its immediate region. Organ sharing between 110 organ procurement programs has developed over the past dozen years in response to need and technical capabilities. Fully half the kidneys transplanted today have been surgically recovered by distant procurement programs and transported to the transplanting center. Kidney sharing is facilitated by our technical ability to preserve these organs for 48 hours and sometimes longer. Since kidney transplantation is seldom if ever life-saving therapy and since, until recently, demonstrably improved transplant survival occurred when attention was given to matching donor and recipient tissue types, the sharing of kidney on the basis of computer matching of immunologic factors has been enthusiastically supported by almost all centers.

The United Network for Organ Sharing (UNOS) is an informal network of approximately 130 transplant and organ procurement programs which register their patients waiting for renal transplants on a central computer owned and operated by the South-Eastern Organ Procurement Foundation (SEOPF) in Richmond, Virginia. SEOPF itself is a regional cooperative organization of 39 transplant programs, although its computer provides nationwide services for distribution of kidneys. The concept of computer matching for kidneys must not be misunderstood to mean that the computer directs the placement of that available kidney. Instead the computer merely sorts through the thousands of potential recipients to identify those which appear to be suitable matches. The sending center then selects the recipient center(s) to which it may wish to offer the available organ, contacts that center by phone and makes arrangements to transport the kidney if it is acceptable. Sharing of kidneys is not infrequently influenced by non-immunologic factors, such as the proximity and close relationship between sending and receiving centers.

The emergence of extrarenal organ transplantation as an acceptable therapy for end-stage heart and liver failure patients has in the past few years resulted in a modification of this informal organ sharing effort: the collaboration of two or three programs in surgically recovering organs from a single donor. In this form of sharing the donor is identified in a regional hospital of one program. The host program is almost always eager to recover the kidneys, but has no use for the extrarenal organs. Rather than see the organs wasted, the host program invites one or two other procurement programs in need of extrarenal

Appendix 2, 1983 National Organ Transplant Hearings, D. Denny Testimony

organs to fly to the donor hospital for the purpose of retrieving the heart and/or liver. In this model the on-scene coordination of all clinical, medicolegal and logistics aspects of the donation process is handled by the host program coordinator. Telephone communication between the host coordinator and his colleagues from the extrarenal center(s) facilitates the carrying out of specialized requirements for the extrarenal centers prior to the convergence of all the teams in the donor hospital Operating Room. All of the programs participating in organ recovery share in assuming the responsibility for the costs.

The Transplant Foundation at the University of Pittsburgh did not initiate intercenter collaborative organ retrieval (that distinction belongs to the University of Colorado and the Medical College of Virginia), but it unquestionably has the most experience in this form of organ (or, more properly, donor) sharing and has developed the system far beyond its early stages.

This form of intercenter collaboration was first attempted by Pitt in 1980 with the inauguration of our cardiac transplant program and has become a commonplace activity during the past two years with the relocation of the nation's largest liver transplantation program to Pittsburgh. Our program was unable to generate sufficient numbers of donors for heart and liver transplantation within our own region and necessarily turned to other program with a request for help. The need for help from other program is not just a function of the number of available donors locally. We have rather large donor program and annually recover kidneys from 50 to 60 donors in our region. For several reasons, an available donor may not be suitable for heart or liver donation. First, patients accepted for heart and liver transplantation are terminal and will die within days or weeks unless successfully transplanted. There is often no time to wait for a local donor. Secondly, unlike kidney, heart and livers must come from size compatible donors. Especially in the case of pediatric recipients, this presents a major problem since relatively few small children succumb to brain death.

Our liver transplant waiting list now includes over 30 potential pediatric recipients under the age of five years. Intercenter collaboration is imperative especially for these youngsters.

Our experience in seeking the cooperation of other procurement programs recapitulated our experience in asking for the help of hospitals in our own area. A few programs enthusiastically came to our aid immediately, most were suspicious and slow to respond and a very few were indifferent or hostile and totally uncooperative. The primary concern initially voiced by our colleagues to other programs was their fear that the surgical technique required for extrarenal procurement would jeopardize the quality of their donor's kidneys. This is not true but time, persistence and published data were required to convince many initially reluctant programs within the eastern half of the United States which are unwilling to collaborate with us in the recovery of extrarenal organs. Some of these programs are merely insular, some are unwilling to help because of the extra effort required and some are reluctant to work with us because they fear our involvement will somehow compromise their own procurement efforts.

Although intercenter collaboration was difficult for us to establish, the concept has become increasingly popular. The statistics reveal our success. During 1981, we received 175 referrals of extrarenal donors from other programs and were able to recover 20 livers and 9 hearts in cooperation with distant renal procurement teams. In 1982, we received over 520 referrals from other programs and recovered 63 livers and 18 hearts with outside help. Three-fourths of the livers and four-fifths of the hearts transplanted at the University Health Center were recovered through the generous collaboration of other regional procurement programs. We are proud, too, that Pittsburgh is also a major provider of extrarenal organs to other centers.

When we are unable to utilize an available extrarenal organ from a donor in our region, we always seek to work collaboratively in the recovery of these organs with other programs in need.

One of the major factors which aided us in developing intercenter cooperation was the opportunity for communication and the development of trust afforded by the professional association of organ procurement coordinators, the North American Transplant Organization (NATCO). Workshops on extrarenal organ procurement sponsored by NATCO provided an opportunity for concerns to be discussed and resolved. NATCO's annual training course for procurement coordinators provides intensive orientation through extrarenal procurement for new procurement personnel.

Appendix 2, 1983 National Organ Transplant Hearings, D. Denny Testimony

NATCO has also been a major force for the sharing of extrarenal organs. The major system used by procurement personnel to locate recipients for available extrarenal organs is sponsored by NATCO. At this time, approximately 17 transplant centers are involved in extrarenal organ transplantation in the United States and Canada. This number will become swollen during the next several months when at least five additional centers will inaugurate heart transplant programs and another six centers will begin transplanting livers.

Last year, NATCO recognized the problem faced by organ procurement personnel in locating suitable recipients for extrarenal organs which may become available in local community hospitals. The UNOS computer system has great utility in helping to distribute kidneys, but is much less effective in the area of extrarenal organ sharing. Because of very limited capability for preservation of extrarenal organs (hearts can be preserved for no more than 4 hours and liver for approximately 10 hours), these organs cannot be removed from the donor before a suitable recipient is identified. Transplantation must occur immediately after the donor surgery. Size, blood type compatibility, geographic distance and urgency of need are the primary factors considered to coordinating recipient selection of extrarenal organs.

Procurement coordinators who receive a donor referral during non-office hours or who are evaluating a donor at a community hospital and wish to discuss extrarenal donation with the donor family cannot access the UNOS computer to review current extrarenal needs across the country. NATCO recognized the problem and established a 24 hour-a-day telephone service for informing organ procurement programs of extrarenal needs. This free, volunteer service utilizes a recorded message system which can be accessed from any phone in the United States or Canada. Updated as needed (usually once or twice a day) the recording lists by center the type of organs needed, a priority status code indicating urgency of recipient need, the donor criteria (size, weight, blood type), geographic limitations to procurement, the name of the procurement coordinator to be contacted and the phone number of each participating extrarenal center. Fifteen extrarenal centers now use the system to acquaint organ procurement programs with their donor needs.

During the first six months of service, the NATCO 24-ALERT System (the name is taken from the System's mnemonic phone number) facilitated the recovery and transplantation of 30 hearts at 9 centers, 48 livers at 5 centers and 1 heart-lung bloc. Success of the 24-ALERT System and temporal limitations which prevent heart and liver procurement much beyond 1,000 miles from an extrarenal center have prompted NATCO to plan to divide the System into two complimentary geographic components. Within the next month a 24-ALERT WEST will establish to handle the western half of the country, while the original System will continue to convey information of relevance for the eastern half of the nation.

The System is not perfect but it works better than anything else available at this time. The UNOS computer, in fact, is used only infrequently for extrarenal organ sharing because of the greater effectiveness of the NATCO 24-ALERT System. As is the case with the UNOS computer program for kidney sharing, the current System provides information to the donor program staff and leaves up to them the decisions concerning which extrarenal program is to be contacted. Undoubtedly some extrarenal programs are often not contacted because of factors unrelated to the urgency of their need. Center-specific problems with the quality of their procurement services are a major impediment, for example, for some extrarenal programs. No distribution system will be effective which attempts to compel cooperation between programs which do not trust on another.

Inter-regional extrarenal procurement is expanding rapidly. The University of Pittsburgh alone worked cooperatively with over 40 other organ procurement programs during the past two years. On 12 occasions we have participated with two other programs in simultaneously recovering organs from a single donor. At this time the necessary trust in the technical competence of other transplant surgeons which would allow distant procurement and sharing of extrarenal organs (rather than donor opportunities) is not well developed; most extrarenal transplant surgeons still desire to have donor organs removed by members of their own team. With experience and time, however, this inhibition will be overcome and hearts and livers will be exchanged as kidneys are now.

Appendix 2, 1983 National Organ Transplant Hearings, D. Denny Testimony

One major problem will probably continue to exist for the foreseeable future. Because of the delicate nature of lung tissue, long distance procurement of heart-lungs and single isolated lungs now require the transportation of the donor from the donor hospital to the center where transplant surgery will be performed. Recent success with the transplant of heart-lung blocs warrants continued efforts in the transplantation of these organs. The willingness of most organ procurement programs to transport a local donor hundreds or thousands of miles to an extrarenal center for the recovery of heart-lungs or isolated lungs is strongly inhibited at this time by the fear of the procuring program that the quality of the kidneys will be jeopardized.

Another factor limiting the availability of these organs is that many families which are willing to donate are unwilling to subject their loved ones to transportation to the donor center for organ retrieval. The University of Pittsburgh and Stanford University have the only heart-lung transplantation programs in the United States and both are seriously compromised in their ability to offer heart-lung transplantation to the many candidates for this surgery because of the shortage of suitable donors. Montefiore Hospital, New York City has a similar problem in developing their lung transplantation program.

The current system for the procurement and sharing of kidneys and extrarenal organs is essentially sound, I believe. The existing system of regional procurement programs is in principle the most effective means of cultivating the growth of donor program at the community hospital level. Regionalization facilitates the personal contacts which are essential and regional idiosyncrasies are best recognized and respond to on a regional basis.

Inter-regional collaboration will continue to grow as need and familiarity with the benefits of donor and organ sharing increase. Yet the fact that no more than one-third of the potential donors in this nation now yield organs for transplantation indicates that the system for organ procurement at the regional level needs strengthening, especially at its weakest point: the interface between the organ procurement programs and the health professionals in the community hospitals who are in a position to recognize and refer donors. I have the following recommendations:

(1.) It is time that transplant and organ procurement professionals seek the help of others outside the transplant community. A national task force should be formed of representatives of organ procurement and transplant specialty groups and other significant health professional's organization to identify problems inhibiting referral of organ donors to regional programs and to recommend solutions on a national level. Such a task force should include leaders from organizations—which represent physicians and nurses likely to encounter donors, i.e., neurosurgeons, neurologists, critical care physicians, emergency physicians, pediatricians, critical care nurses, as well as leaders from organizations of hospital administrators and other relevant groups.

(2.) Rules and regulations should be enacted on the state and/or national level which would require that every hospital seeking certification (a) enact a policy and operational protocol for the determination of brain death; and (b) develop a policy and protocol for the recognition and referral of potential organ donors to the nearest regional procurement program. (In Pennsylvania, with the support of the Secretary for Health, efforts are now underway to have both of these regulations adopted by the State Department of Health as requirements for hospital certification.)

(3.) A financial incentive should be built into the federal Medicare reimbursement system, which would reward hospitals from which port mortem donor kidneys are recovered for transplantation. No new legislation should be required, since Medicare now funds renal transplantation and kidney procurement. This should be especially attractive to the taxpayers and the federal government since kidney transplantation is considerably less expensive than chronic dialysis. (Most post mortem kidney donors are also potential extrarenal donors and this incentive system would also enhance opportunities for extrarenal organ procurement.)

(4.) Areas of this country still exist which provide few if any organs for transplantation. The problem in part is the failure of the regional organ procurement programs effectively to educate

Appendix 2, 1983 National Organ Transplant Hearings, D. Denny Testimony

    physicians and nurses. Strengthening education for health professionals is essential. One step in this direction has recently been taken by NATCO, which has established a 24 hour-a-day organ donor information and referral hotline for doctors, nurses, and other hospital staff who have questions about donation or want to refer potential donors but do not know how to contact their local procurement program. Staffed by trained organ procurement coordinators, the hotline (dial 800/24-DONOR) needs wide exposure in the medical community to be effective. Support for this and other efforts to strengthen professional education is sorely needed.

(5.) Public education efforts should be stepped up, with emphasis given to developing mass media educational opportunities focused on subgroups of the population. The National Advertising Council should be asked to take on a national project for public education.

(6.) My final suggestion is one which should be self evident from my testimony. There is a real need for the accumulation of data on organ donation, organ distribution and transplantation. Some data is now collected on renal donation and transplantation by the Health Care Financing Administration, but no figures are available for the country as a whole concerning the number of potential donors, the number of potential donors referred to organ procurement programs but from whom organs are not recovered, the number of extrarenal organs needed, recovered and transplanted. Some very practical questions need to be answered. For instance, how many suitable pediatric donors between the ages of six months and five years are potentially available? The number of small children being referred for liver transplantation is growing geometrically; we may be faced with the fact that there will never be a sufficient number of younger donors to meet the need. We won't know unless we investigate.

BIBLIOGRAPHY

(1) Cooper, K.D., et al., "The Potential Supply of Cadaveric Kidneys for Transplantation." Transactions of the American Society of Artificial Organs, vol. 23, pp. 416-421 (1977)

(2) Project to Reduce Waiting Times for Cadaveric Kidney Transplants in Michigan: Phase I Final Report, Transplantation Society of Michigan (1982)

(3) Barb, K.J., et al, "Cadaveric Kidney for Transplantation: A Paradox of Shortage in the Face of Plenty", Transplantation, Vol. 35, no. 5, (1981)

(4) Statistical Abstracts of the United States, Department of Commerce, Bureau of the Census, 1982-1983 Council on Scientific Affairs of the American Medical Association, "Organ Donor Recruitment", Journal of AMA, Vol. 246, no. 19, (1981), p. 2157.

(5) Council on Scientific Affairs of the American Medical Association, "Organ Door Recruitment", Journal of AMA, vol 246, no. 19, (1981), p. 2157.

(6) Gallup Organization, Inc., Attitudes and Opinions of the American Public Toward Kidney Donation, (prepared for the National Kidney Foundation, Inc., New York), Princeton, N.J.

{AU: Where is reference 6, which is cited on p. 20?}

Questioning of Don Denny and Co-Panel Participants:

    Mr. GORE. Thank you very much, Mr. Denny. I commend your entire remarks to the attention of those reading this record and your recommendations will no doubt, many of them be included in the subcommittee's report.

    Dr. William Pfaff, past president of the South-East Organ Procurement Foundation at the University of Florida College of Medicine in Gainesville, and a noted kidney transplant specialist in his own right. We are delighted to have you here.

    Please proceed.

Appendix 2, 1983 National Organ Transplant Hearings, D. Denny Testimony

Dr. PFAFF. Thank you, I was asked to appear today to describe the South-East Organ Procurement Foundation [SEOPF]. SEOPF actually has been enlarged from its original membership of eight to some 40 members. Those of you who live north of here will be surprised to learn that New Jersey is also in the Southeast, as is Indiana. So the rough boundaries—

Mr. GORE. We are an ambitious region.

Dr. PFAFF. The rough boundaries are New Jersey to Indiana, Louisiana to Florida. Almost all of the programs that are transplanting and procuring organs in this area are members of our foundation.

SEOPF was established with the hope and expectation that tissue typing and tissue matching would result in improved graft survival. That was the first premise.

Second, there was a realization that an excess of supply at one site might coincide with a need at another site, that there was an advantage to mutual education and a discipline that was dramatically unfolding. Finally, there was a need for uniform tissue typing laboratory practices. As the organization has matured, it has continued to work at these goals, and then has established some others in a variety of activities.

The current means of exchange is heavily dependent upon our Computer network. We list, from the members alone, something in Excess of 2,200 patients. Approximately one-third of the patients who are being transplanted in the country receive their grafts among this membership of some 40 institutions. The means of distribution of kidneys is principally on the basis of tissue typing characteristics. We are trying to take advantage of the immunology that we have gradually uncovered over these years in order to provide a more successful graft, for there are some individuals who absolutely need a well-matched transplant in order to be successfully managed.

The computer network distribution system has been expanded to the rest of the country, and the organization that is an outgrowth of the SEOPF technology is called UNOS [the United Network for Organ Sharing.] Now some 138 transplant programs nationwide, thus, are using this single means of distributing kidneys. When I left Gainesville yesterday, on the plane with me there was a kidney that was destined for Minnesota. Another had left on the earliest plane from Gainesville to go to Mississippi. By the same token we expect that Minnesota is going to return the favor for the same purpose, Namely, to provide, again, a well-matched organ.

In practical terms if a kidney becomes available at the University of Florida or one of our nearby hospitals—we are in a semi rural area—that we tissue type the donor, look at the computer readout and first priority, and that is to distribute the well-matched organ, irrespective of local need. We run the computer program and identify the potential recipients who are listed in priority of their organ matching characteristics and then call the appropriate center. Each of the centers has 24-hour members and 24-hour personnel to advise them of this Opportunity.

The level of activity of SEOPF members, included 604 kidney transplants from July 1 through December 31, 1982. During the same time period, half again that number of organs were procured. In other words, the transplant rate is 1,200 per year, the procurement rate is 1,800 per year. Thus there is an excess that is generated within the region and that is distributed to non-members as the net of about 250 or 260 excess kidneys per year. The total incidence of sharing amongst the donating centers is some 59 percent. The majority of the kidneys that are procured in the Foundation are shared with other centers, both within and without the Foundation.

The other areas in which we have become interested in is scientific data. Somewhere along the line we needed to find out what we were doing. The points that Mel Williams made to you earlier today regarding the five factors that have import and the varied success of transplantation are factors that have been covered, uncovered, sustained and demonstrated individually in other programs.

All of that information was generated within one program and that was from the cooperative efforts of the SEOFP membership, so that we achieved some specific knowledge about transplantation, about organ preservation, sharing, and procurement as a consequence of sharing our informational.

In 1973, with the institution of the Medicare law that covered renal failure, the funding for the voluntary registry that transplant programs have maintained for a good number of years ceased.

Chapter 1: THE HISTORY OF THE TRANSPLANT COORDINATOR

Appendix 2, 1983 National Organ Transplant Hearings, D. Denny Testimony

We were promised a medical information system. That has never happened. The only sources I have for making decisions about patients are the SEOPF data that addresses only transplant patients and my local network, that is, the Florida End-Stage Renal Disease Network. We have excellent data on every dialysis and transplant patient in the State of Florida. I know the relative risks of dialysis and transplantation, of different modes of transplantation, as that is expressed in age, causative disease and also associated diseases.

I would urge those of you who are interested in having information available to make such decisions that you reconsider the efforts that have been suggested in some areas of our own Government to cease funding of the networks. To me, it would be crippling.

Transplantation of heart, liver and pancreas is varied in this country, rapidly growing. You heard a number of people describe a number of existing programs. Frankly, within our own foundation we have not kept up with it. We have not established a program for sharing these organs. We cannot address the costs of distribution of other organs, at least as an addition to the elements of exchange to the End-Stage Renal Disease Program. We would have to establish some other form of Funding to do that, because of the disallowance you have heard discussed earlier today.

Can the basic system be used for organ exchange? Yes. The means by which we exchange organs really is adaptable, I think, to almost any organ. There are differing needs in terms of the ability to maintain the organ outside the donor, even in using the preservation techniques we have today. The heart is very urgent, the pancreas, perhaps, the most urgent of all. It appears that the liver can be preserved for at least a number of hours. The kidney can be sustained for 1 to 3 days. Each of those developmental problems of organ preservation is going to put different kinds of restrictions on us in terms of both procurement and, most importantly, sharing of organs.

Yet we come to the subgroup of our patient populations who absolutely need a well-matched organ in order to be successfully transplanted, and we need to address that question as we proceed.

We are increasing our success at all forms of transplantation. Each one of us looks at our own program and questions. "Have we done better this year?" We are proud if we have; we are disappointed if we haven't—we are dashed if we haven't.

The economics of transplantation are a matter of continued conversation in your sphere and in ours. For these new areas we don't have a solution. We have come to you for a solution. We need to expand this dialog, from successful kidney transplantation to increasing success in other areas.

The problems, as I see them, are identification of additional appropriate transplant recipients. That is based on the delivery of sound, scientific information, both to patients and to other professionals.

I think that you have heard that often enough. I would not reiterate further. We are doing a good job of kidney procurement in our area of the country. I think we are doing a fairly good job I terms of extra organ procurement. I would ask whether that is the product of our cooperative work, of our group effort, of our mutual pride, because I think that that is something that might be exported to other areas of the country.

There are very few large regional organizations. They tend to be metropolitan or a small area. Yet, much of our ease of working with one another has been through sera exchange, through the histocompatibility laboratories and through our computer network. I would favor expansion of the regional concept with interregional cooperation. We have some patients who have uncommon blood type; uncommon tissue types and their opportunity for a matched graft even within our rather sizable program may be infrequent. Thus, expansion of the number of cooperating centers will expand the potential for cross-matching between donor and recipient, we will have a much better likelihood of getting these long waiting individuals a successful transplant.

Thank you.

Mr. GORE. Thank you very much.

Mr. GORE. Congresswoman Schneider, would you introduce our final witness?

Mrs. SCHNEIDER. I am more than happy to introduce Mr. Coleman, who is a constituent of mine, and I must say that I am very honored to introduce him to us today because he will tell us the true-life story

Appendix 2, 1983 National Organ Transplant Hearings, D. Denny Testimony

of what was involved in having his best friend experience—have his child experience the need for a liver transplant and how he with a very cool, calm head reacted in a time of crisis.

I think this probably comes from his training as a policeman; how he organized as a citizen activist the solution toward solving this problem.

As I mentioned a little earlier today, because of his efforts and the efforts of many others, Justine Pinheiro is currently being operated on in Pittsburgh, and that is who Dr. Starzl was operating on last night. So as we sit here we are hopeful that her condition will be on the upswing. I might also mention that Justine's mother was most anxious to appear here today, but fortunately she is with her daughter. Also, there is in the audience a member of the board of directors for the Donor Alert Program that Mr. Coleman founded. His name is Al Skorupa.

I am delighted to have Mr. Coleman here today to tell us his story of frustration and success. Thank you.

Mr. COLEMAN. It was really short notice for me, as you probably know, and then with Monday, Justine getting notified—you will have to excuse my written testimony. I would like to read this to you.

My name is Raymond Coleman. I am a welding supervisor for General Dynamics, Electric Boat Division, and founding president of Donor Alert, Inc., a nonprofit organization founded in December 1982.

I because involved in organ procurement out of a desire to help a friend, Jose Pinheiro, whose daughter, Justine, hopefully not anymore, suffers from biliary atresia. This friend had been led to believe that if he made the public aware of his problem, he might increase his daughter's chances of getting a liver.

When he and I became frustrated in our efforts, I went to Mr. William Bennett, my general manager, for assistance. I felt that being a large corporation and dealing with the media they would know better than I how to approach the problem. Not only did they lend their expertise to the problem of awareness, they agreed to pay for Justine's operation. Members of their staff worked tirelessly with me asking for no recognition and were happy with the thought that through their efforts they may help same lives.

This is the same reason that I am involved. All my efforts have been voluntary. I and the others involved receive no pay and have nothing to gain by my speaking here. Our thoughts in starting Donor Alert were that if we went on a national scale by public awareness and education and establishing an 800 telephone number, and by using Justine and a representative of all people in need of transplant surgery, it would be possible to locate enough organs to reduce the waiting list, thus insuring Justine's survival and continuing the donor process.

Being an ex-policeman and having been involved in situations that met the criteria of potential donors, we decided to start our campaign with police departments. The criteria of being brain dead and on life support was not a normal condition of dying and the fact that auto accidents, violent crimes, child abuse and drug abuse was a major cause of this condition, made us believe that the police could be a big help.

We sent out on a national teletype a message that if they were involved in these situations, to please notify the hotline and we would notify local donor coordinators. Simultaneously with this message, ABC World News Tonight televised our efforts on national TV.

Since the inception of Donor Alert's 800 hot line on January 13, 1983, we have received over a thousand calls, have established chapters in six States, have registered hundreds of donors and have come to realize that besides the basic complexities of the area of procurement, it is fraught with problems.

Some of the problems we as layman have encountered include:

First, on the whole, the general public knows nothing of what is involved in organ transplants, what is necessary to become an organ donor, or how to become one, or what to do if they want to donate organs.

Second, although the entire organ donor procurement recipient transplant system is run, directed and controlled by medical professionals, and for the most part it should be, I have been told I have no right or business to be involved in organ procurement because we are layman. Coordinators have advised

Chapter 1 — THE HISTORY OF THE TRANSPLANT COORDINATOR

Appendix 2, 1983 National Organ Transplant Hearings, D. Denny Testimony

me that there is such a delicate balance between them and the medical profession that a "bumbling, unprofessional might spoil" what they have achieved.

Our thoughts as bumbling unprofessionals is that if, instead of the almost secretive way they approached us, that they educate the people, that transplants affect most of the laymen. This way the medical aspects would not be a problem. If a doctor was told by his patients that they accepted it and wished to be a donor, then if the opportunity to be a donor arose, the doctor, as a normal part of handling the situation, would offer this life-saving option to the next of kin.

This is not entirely the coordinator's fault. I have been told of cases of coordinators being called vultures and chased out of hospital rooms for their efforts. They have been accused of preying on the dead. This exists probably because a doctor feels that his first duty is to his patient. With proper education of the public and the medical profession, it is hoped that once a person reaches a state of being legally brain death, then again, as a normal consideration, a doctor would suggest or discuss the options and possibilities of lifesaving organ donations.

As you are aware, it appears that every State, in some cases, counties, cities, and regional areas, have organizations, some public, some private, some sponsored, involved in some sort of organ procurement.

These people work so hard in setting up their areas in different parts of procurement, such as eyes, kidneys, hearts and livers, that they feel it is their domain and seem to protect it with a vengeance. This not only occurs because of territorial protection, but extreme examples have been related to me of organs that have not been routed to an area because of personal conflicts.

When our national hot line was set up, it was in the hopes of coordinating these efforts. Professional or unprofessional, without the layman there would be no organs. With the tremendous advance in the medical procedures used in organ transplants and with the fantastic success that has been attained in liver transplants, I think that the time has come for a national computer network to be established which lists all patients awaiting transplants. If this could be accomplished, then when a donor was located, the information could be fed into the computer and a match done making the selection impersonal and guaranteeing the most critical and best match would receive the organ.

This would make the information available to all medical personnel on a national basis. This should enhance the availability of organs and success rate even more. If this is not done in an impartial manner, it could take years for all separate factions in organ procurement to become cohesive. I have yet to talk to anyone involved in organ procurement who doesn't speak of his area in a protective way, and rightly so, because of the hard work necessary to develop it, but this attitude has to be shed now that organ transplants are growing at such a rapid rate. Among the first calls we received on the hot line were people from NATCO and SEOPF. They stated that this was something that should have been done years ago.

NATCO stated that they would like to work with us on the hot line and invited us to Richmond, Va., to meet with members of their board. The discussion we had further strengthened my belief that a neutral party is needed if a national computer network was to be set up.

There is no room for any conflict when a human life is involved. One subject that all parties agreed on was that national programs of public awareness and education were necessary and the time had passed when they should have been implemented. Following the establishment of our national hot line, several other organizations have established them. It was felt that a lot of money would be needed to accomplish this, so it would be something to work on in the future.

We felt that it could be accomplished now and we proved it. Granted, to be as effective as we should be, we still need funding, but if the Government never gave us a penny, we would still continue to grow because we are driven by a desire to help these beautiful children and will not be stopped by any obstacle.

If there is Federal money available, the Government should get behind an educational program that has already been established rather than putting money into duplicating the efforts of caring people who volunteer their time in an effort to help. It is my understanding in some areas of transplant there is still a shortage of organs, but in liver transplants there are more organs than doctors to perform the surgery. Statistics show that the success rate in liver transplants has passed the trial and error stage and should be classified as a therapeutic and lifesaving procedure.

A CLINICIAN'S GUIDE TO DONATION AND TRANSPLANTATION

Appendix 2, 1983 National Organ Transplant Hearings, D. Denny Testimony

Without Government approval of this operation, hospitals and surgeons will not become involved and everyone's efforts will be in vain. My final statement to you is our experience has shown that once people are made aware, they are willing to donate their organs in order that others may live. In our short existence we have acquired hundreds, approaching a thousand signed donor cards. This has come about through what little exposure we were able to get. The next and probably greatest problem that exists with all cards and donors is that upon death, rarely is anyone sure of who they should call and, further, rarely does anyone check for donor cards. A number of people who signed our donor cards were already carrying some sort of a local card, whether it was for kidneys, eyes, hearts, lungs or livers. These people stated that they felt our national education efforts would enhance the chance of the card being looked for and an 800 number to call would enhance the availability of organs.

At one of our functions, a story was related to me of a woman's mother who before she died expressed a desire to donate her eyes so that another might see. Because no one knew who to call, the eyes were never donated. Stories like this have been told to me time after time. It isn't just the man in the street who doesn't know what to do, this also extend to some doctors in hospitals. For example, on March 3, we received a call from a hospital in Colorado with a potential donor. Luckily, they were aware of our 800 number and contacted us. We notified a donor coordinator, the liver was matched with a child in California.

What is needed is not 800 different 800 numbers, but 1 central 800 number that everyone is aware of and able to call for educational information or to either register as a donor or donate. This would not infringe on the medical aspects of transplant or local and regional efforts, as a local coordinator would immediately be notified.

This concludes my remarks.

Mr. GORE. Now, let me get this straight. We have two different 800 numbers. Is that correct?

Mr. DENNY. The 800 number established by the North American Transplant Coordinators Organization, 800-24-DONOR, has been established for the specific purpose, Chairman Gore, of providing information and referral services to physicians and nurses within the country.

It is staffed 24 hours a day by trained organ procurement professionals who are totally familiar with the identity of donors, the management of donor organ function, the psychological aspect of organ donation, the surgical recovery of the organs, and the network of regional programs throughout this Nation. This 800 number, we hope, if made available to the physicians and nurses in the country, will enhance the opportunity for the recovery of organs. We don't seek to complete with any other organization. We seek, however, to exercise our competence in terms of providing the health care professionals with the information that they need.

Mrs. SCHNEIDER. Would the chairman yield a moment?

Mr. GORE. Yes; delighted.

Mrs. SCHNEIDER. Is there any particular criteria—you refer to organ transplant professionals, is there some specific type of training or criteria that is followed in order to be acknowledged as a transplant professional?

Mr. DENNY. When I say transplant professionals, that is a generic term meaning the physicians, the surgeons, the transplant, or organ procurement coordinators. I think you refer especially to the organ procurement coordinators.

Mrs. SCHNEIDER. Yes.

Mr. DENNY. Those of us like myself who operate organ procurement programs and are available to do all of the necessary work in evaluating the donors and making the process work.

Mrs. SCHNEIDER. What I am trying to get at is whether or not we can see a new area of professionalism.

Mr. DENNY. There is a new area of competence—

Mrs. SCHNEIDER. Is there a recognized curriculum that one would take in going to school or the university or postgraduate studies?

Mr. DENNY. No; most organ procurement coordinators are either nurses or physician's assistants. Some of us are neither. Some of us have no background in medicine.

Appendix 2, 1983 National Organ Transplant Hearings, D. Denny Testimony

Mrs. SCHNEIDER. But are you certified? Is there a certification program?

Mr. DENNY. There is not yet a certification program, though I am sure that we will be moving in that direction. The North American Transplant Coordinators Organization does provide an intensive, annual educational program for organ procurement coordinators at the 110 programs in this country.

Mrs. SCHNEIDER. Thank you Mr. Chairman.

Mr. GORE. Then, what differentiates you from Mr. Coleman is your experience at it?

Mr. DENNY. Knowledge, experience, and the fact that we are In the hospitals, that we are involved with the donors in the intensive care units, that we sit down and approach the grieving families to offer them the opportunity for life. His effort is, I think, primarily, and appropriately primarily designed to educate the public. I have no quarrel with that at all. I think that it can be a valuable service.

Mr. GORE. Well, Mr. Coleman, you see it a little bit differently, don't you?

Mr. COLEMAN. First of all, I am not here to compete with the medical aspects of it. I bow to his expertise, as far as that is concerned. My opinion is that my line can just as—we both—I think both lines are needed. OK? That he has done it this way, I don't think was very—how can I say it?—fair. If he would have let me know, I would have worked with him to make two different lines, one for general information and one for medical.

I would have referred all my calls. I have 35 calls on my desk of doctors, nurses, emergency room personnel that want to know what to do. If I knew that this was what they were doing, I would have just given them his 800 number and done it that way. I think that there is room for both in this field. The general public needs, I think, the general public to tell it because they don't understand sometimes.

If somebody came up to me and said, will you donate your kidneys, I would say, no, I probably wouldn't, Right? But if somebody showed me why it was necessary, and if somebody showed me why it was necessary to donate my liver, then I sure would. I carry a donor card, and I have been close to it, and I think if you put it to the people that way, people would understand and they would donate their organs, and there wouldn't be some of the problems that we have today.

Mr. DENNY. May I mention something with regard to the NATCO 24-DONOR number? Let me describe to you something in a hypothetical situation, something of how the process works. A patient—this will be brief—a patient involved in an automobile accident, strikes his head against the windshield. He is brought into the hospital. He is bleeding profusely. His blood pressure is dropping down to the danger level where his heart function is compromised.

His oxygenation is impaired because his breathing is slowing down. He needs to be put on a ventilator to support the oxygenation of his blood, to sustain the viability of the organs. A doctor recognizes this patient as a probable victim of brain death. He is moving in that direction rapidly. It is a question of should the family be asked, should the family be approached, Should they be offered the chance to think about donation? He needs to talk with somebody immediately. Not only about should he talk with the family at that point, he needs to talk with somebody rapidly about what to do to sustain the vital organ function.

In dealing with victims of brain death, there are a number of physiological problems that occur that are not common to those of us who are living. Maintaining the organ function in somebody who is a victim of brain death is always a race against the clock. It is always a competition between nature and those of us in transplantation whether or not the organs will be recovered in time. A physician who calls an 800 number needs to talk to a professional immediately who knows what to do to stabilize the blood pressure, to maintain the oxygenation, to assess when and how to talk with the family, to determine who is a suitable prospective donor. He needs it rapidly. The fact that our 800 number, 800-24-DONOR, is manned by trained procurement professionals, is a vital service to the physicians and nurses in this country.

Mr. GORE. Well, I think I see the two points of view represented here. You just think that Mr. Coleman's group is not qualified to perform the function that you wish to perform.

Mr. DENNY. Mr. Coleman and I have spoken over the phone about this on a number of occasions, and we had breakfast this morning together. We concur in having the same shared sense of urgency. We concur in the sad realization that few of the available organs are, in fact, recovered.

Appendix 2, 1983 National Organ Transplant Hearings, D. Denny Testimony

Our concern, the professional organ procurement coordinator's concern is that the professional be educated—I think Mr. Coleman's primary concern is that the Nation be educated, the public be educated.

Mr. GORE. And he faults the professionals for failing to do that.

Mr. DENNY. Perhaps not without some justification. I think that we can do a better job. It is a question of money. I have 95 hospitals in a 150-mile radius of Pittsburgh to cover; approximately 15,000 beds. I don't know how many physicians and nurses.

Mr. GORE. Now, wait a second. You cover 90 hospitals in—

Mr. DENNY. Ninety-five hospitals.

Mr. GORE. Ninety-five hospitals in a tri-state area around Pittsburgh.

Mr. DENNY. Right.

Mr. GORE. Now, is there a feeling on the part of somebody in Texas, say, that if they plug into your network that is based in Pittsburgh, then facilities in Texas are going to be disadvantaged and patients in Texas are going to be disadvantaged relative to patients in the Pittsburgh.

Mr. GORE. But you wear two hats, right?

Mr. DENNY. The rest of the country is broken up into similar geographic areas. We wear the second hat in the sense that we share organs with other programs similar to ours.

Mr. GORE. Aren't some of those people that are wearing two hats in the rest of the country skeptical of your national group because it is co-located with your regional group?

Mr. DENNY. No, sir, it is not collocated with our regional group. It is, in fact, at this time manned by the coordinators at the University of Pittsburgh.

Mr. GORE. They are both in Pittsburgh.

Mr. DENNY. This function will be taken over within the coming 6 months by another group. Let me explain, Congressman Gore. No; it is an information and referral service. If this hypothetical emergency room physician calls 800-24-DONOR, his burning, urgent questions will be answered, and then he will be immediately put in touch with the organ procurement professionals at his regional group. If he is in Amarillo, Tex., we will put him in touch with the procurement people in San Antonio.

Mr. GORE. Maybe I heard you wrong, didn't you say in your testimony that there are 110 procurement groups around the country?

Mr. DENNY. Yes, sir.

Mr. Gore. Didn't you say that only 50 of them will communicate—

Mr. DENNY. No, sir, I alluded to the fact that the University of Pittsburgh has worked collaboratively with approximately 50 of these organ-procurement programs in recovering livers and hearts for transplantations.

Mr. GORE. I see. So, that was the other half.

Mr. DENNY. We have worked with 50. There are another 60 that we have not worked with either because geography or time constraints prevent us from flying to the coast, for instance.

Mr. GORE. OK. So, you are wearing your local hat when you are talking about 50 other regions that you have cooperated with.

Mr. DENNY. Yes, sir.

Mr. GORE. I see. Now, how many of the 110 procurement systems communicate regularly with your national organization, the North American—

Mr. DENNY. Almost all of them. Almost all of them make use of the NATCO 24-Alert System. We have two systems. Don't get them confused. The 24-Alert System is the recorded phone message system so that a procurement coordinator in Amarillo, TX., can call and find out where a patient is who needs an organ from a donor similar to the one that is located in Amarillo. OK?

Mr. GORE. Yes.

Mr. DENNY. That is the 24-ALERT System. Almost everybody in the country uses that system to find suitable recipients for available, extra-renal organ donors. For instance, the University of Arizona

Appendix 2, 1983 National Organ Transplant Hearings, D. Denny Testimony

transplant team flew to El Paso, Tex., over this past weekend and recovered a heart because the procurement people in El Paso had called 24-Alert, learned that the University of Arizona was looking for a heart from a doctor similar to the one they had. They, in turn, called Arizona, and the two teams got together to recover the organs.

Mr. GORE. Dr. Pfaff, we have talked about these two 800 numbers, the two hotlines, and I understand the difference. Mr. Coleman, would you publicly recommend that a doctor call Mr. Denny's hotline and that public citizens interested in information call yours?

Mr. COLEMAN. Yes; if I had a call from a doctor, I would refer to a local coordinator in his area, anyway.

Mr. GORE. That number, again, it is really easy to remember, is 800-24-DONOR.

Mr. COLEMAN: Coleman, what is your 800 number?

Mr. COLEMAN. 800-325-7001.

Mr. GORE. 800-352-7001; right?

Mr. COLEMAN. Yes.

Mr. GORE. Dr. Pfaff, in addition to there being these two numbers, there are, I understand, two computer registries; is that correct? One, the UNOS system, and the registry operated by Dr. Terasaki's group at UCLA; is that correct?

Dr. PFAFF. That is correct.

Mr. GORE. To what extent do these two computer registries overlap?

Dr. PFAFF. They do overlap.

Mr. GORE. They do?

Dr. PFAFF. Yes. UNOS membership and utilization is voluntary. All you have to do us buy a display terminal, pay your phone bill and pay for computer costs. In effect, it is the extension of the SEOPF's approach.

Mr. GORE. Wait a minute. The SEOPF?

Dr. PFAFF. South-East Organ Procurement Foundation. We will call it southeastern region. The southeastern region's technology just expanded nationally. Dr. Terasaki has a very large tissue typing laboratory that serves almost all of the southern California programs. Much of their work is unified in his laboratory or by exchange with other laboratories that are generally located in the southwest. There is no competition between the two. It can be complementary. My principal interest is in seeing the overall activities of our region perhaps adopted by other regions locally and then with inter-regional cooperation. As you mentioned, we have our own 800 number, too.

Mr. GORE. You do?

Dr. PFAFF. I don't know what the number is. Basically it is for people to call in and sign donor cards. I don't think that there is any agreement about a whole bunch of people doing some things that may overlap. The biggest message we have heard today is that the public does not know, some professionals don't know or that they need to be reminded over and over again, and so that there is not—it shouldn't be thought of as competition. I hope that there is a heck of a lot of supplementation. It took me a long time to learn how to read.

Mr. GORE. Unfortunately, it has taken a lot longer than that to get the awareness of the importance of organ donation.

Dr. PFAFF. We are doing a good job. For example, in our region. I will tell you, we are outstripping our use. That isn't the total matter, though. We are looking forward—and I agree with Mel, again, as to what should happen with transplantation. I say it should double in terms of kidney transplants. You have heard that liver transplantation is going to increase in numbers. We are going from a number of roughly a hundred a year to more than that. Cardiac transplantation is going from a hundred a year to more than that, so that we need to be looking towards the future. We need to modify our practices that we are using now. That is all. We need some help in doing that. I think many of the things that we have talked about we can do, the one that I can't do is to make sure that we are getting accurate information. You can really help us there.

Appendix 2, 1983 National Organ Transplant Hearings, D. Denny Testimony

Mr. GORE. There are, Mr. Denny, 35 children awaiting a liver transplant at Pittsburgh right now; is that correct?

Mr. DENNY. Yes. Approximately.

Mr. GORE. How do you assign a priority as to which one of those children gets a liver that becomes available, assuming that several have tissue compatibility and the rest.

Mr. DENNY. Let me explain one thing. In terms of liver transplantation, we do not look at tissue compatibility as we do in renal transplantation. That is why Mr. Coleman's suggestion that a nationwide computer system be established so that we could sort out suitability for an available liver on the basis of tissue typing is not practical. Let me answer your question on two levels.

Mr. GORE. We have to sort it out on the basis of size, don't you?

Mr. DENNY. Size and compatibility of blood type between donor and recipient.

Mr. GORE. I see. Let's suppose that you have several that have the same blood type compatibility and size compatibility, how do you assign priority?

Mr. DENNY. If a donor is referred to the University of Pittsburgh and we have several people who are equally suitable for transplantation, the decision is left up to the physicians. Dr. Starzl and some of his colleagues make the decision based on the urgency of need.

All of these youngsters are going to die. Some, unhappily, will die before others, and they should be given the priority. That, in fact, is what is done. Occasionally, we have to compromise. Occasionally, we have only an hour or two advance notice that a donor is available, and we may have a recipient who has an urgent need on the west coast 2,000 miles away, a slightly less urgent need recipient in Pittsburgh.

If we have only an hour or two to get that liver, we will have to, sometimes, select the less ill child. Generally speaking, all things being equal, we will pick the child, Dr. Starzl will pick the child, who is most desperately in need. In the case of the 24-Alert System, again, the telephone service is available to organ procurement people to help them understand where there is a need for a liver or a heart that a donor in their area might provide.

On the 24-Alert System, if you call it, you will hear that the University of Pittsburgh, the University of Tennessee, Massachusetts General Hospital, Sacramento, Calif., Davis Medical Center are all looking for livers. We prioritize the recipients in terms of the urgency of need. In other words, at the University of Tennessee for the last several days there has been recognized a very urgent need, what we call a priority one recipient.

That was the youngster that we saw this morning. This youngster is identified as a priority one recipient on the 24-Alert System, so that a calling coordinator, such as the coordinator in Virginia who called last night, is alerted to the fact that this need is perhaps more urgent than other needs for liver transplantation among children of the same size and blood type elsewhere in the country.

Mr. GORE. Very good. Let's suppose we could get hospitals to put up notice about the 800-24-DONOR number and for public information, your number, Mr. Coleman, that might be helpful, would it not? If emergency room physicians and critical care nurses and hospital administrators knew about this number, then they would—well, maybe it would make them think more often. That is, I am sure, the intent of both of you, partly, in establishing such numbers.

Dr. PFAFF. Congressman Gore, actually I think that there is another solution. For example, if somebody from northern Florida were to call their number to find out that they should call us and get some help, we have done a bad job. So I think that you have got to pay heed to—literally hundreds of people are active in organ transplantation these days, and they are scouring those hospitals. If we aren't scouring them well, we haven't done a good job.

Have all of our programs done good jobs? No. Some are doing great and some aren't doing so great. We need to push ourselves a little more, too. I should have made that point earlier. I don't think everything flows from a single source. Just as I differ with Don regarding making a potential recipient list available to donor hospitals in hard copy because that list is going to get awful lengthy.

Mr. DENNY. We don't differ on that.

Appendix 2, 1983 National Organ Transplant Hearings, D. Denny Testimony

Mr. GORE. Now, Mr. Denny, financial considerations enter into this priority. I guess you don't even get considered for priority typically unless the financial threshold has been crossed.

Mr. DENNY. The child has to be accepted for liver transplantation at that center providing—

Mr. GORE. The center typically turns down patients that don't have the ability to pay unless the mother can do what Mrs. Hall did and get a radio station and a lot of friends to help her raise the money from volunteer donations, poor people don't have the same chance, do they?

Mr. DENNY. It depends on what State the poor people live in. In some States Medicaid has been helpful for those who are sufficiently indigent to allow them to qualify for Medicaid.

Mr. GORE. In States where Medicaid will not pay, then they are out of luck.

Mr. DENNY. Occasionally, families have been forced to turn to their communities for help. We have transplanted several patients in this group. Families having turned to their communities, having found the generosity of the neighbors, have recovered the funds through fundraising drives in their own areas and have been transplanted. It does require that on occasion, yes.

Mr. GORE. Mr. Coleman, do you believe that the organ procurement effort in the country has been impaired by competition between different organ procurement systems?

Mr. COLEMAN. Yes. I have heard of different situations where that has happened. But, basically, I have to say this, they are hard working, dedicated people. When they started in this, it was almost considered a macabre thing. But today people accept it and it is growing so fast that I do believe that these personal conflicts or if somebody is mad at somebody else or something this, should be removed somehow. If it has to be forced upon them, removed. There shouldn't be any type of personal conflict in something like this when it involves a human life.

Mr. GORE. Mr. Coleman, I as looking at the list of organ procurement programs provided to us, and I notice that many cities around the country have more than one organ procurement system in the city, and some have as many as five different organ procurement systems or networks in the same city. How does that work? Does that cause problems?

Mr. COLEMAN. Again, I just go by the personal talks. The medical people can tell you more on that.

Mr. GORE. Dr. Pfaff.

Dr. PFAFF. Really, no, it shouldn't cause problems. Are they competing for the same attention? Yes. How did this ever happen? Organ Procurement is an outgrowth of transplant programs, in the main. In some areas, people have seen advantage to coalescence. It is like anything else that a bunch of people do together. There has to be not only a mesh of purpose, but very important, a mesh of personalities and some personalities don't get along with others.

Mr. GORE. Doesn't it makes sense—I mean, if we have a situation where we have 110 different systems around the country, as many as 5 separate systems in the same city in some cases. We clearly see on the horizon a dramatic upsurge in the number of transplant procedures being performed and the demand for organs for transplant. It really makes sense to have a national strategy to, if not coalesce them all into a single system, at least devote a sufficient amount of attention to get rid of any competition that is impairing the procedures and make it a more sensible and rational system.

Dr. PFAFF. The competition doesn't impair the procedures. As a matter of fact, one of the major coalescences was just a dismal failure. That really isn't the matter. It is really the question of effort, and the attention of a number of decisions that each of us make individually in terms of sharing organs and increasing production, of transplantation as a whole are all really scientific decisions in the end. I think if all of us see the need for more organ procurement, we will do it. If, as people have heard today, there is a shortage of pediatric donors for a particular problem, biliary atresia, coordinators are going to pay attention to that. Physicians are going to pay attention to it. Nurses are going to pay attention to it. They are going to hear it on the night news, I suppose.

Mr. GORE. Well, there is clearly a need for more organ procurement. I mean, there is not any doubt about that, is there?

Appendix 2, 1983 National Organ Transplant Hearings, D. Denny Testimony

Dr. PFAFF. Oh, I think in some areas there is doubt. In some areas, in some organs, I mean we are talking about now three liver programs in the country, ten cardiac programs.

Mr. GORE. We have got 35 children at this one hospital alone that are going to die if they don't get a liver. They are waiting for one now.

Dr. PFAFF. Thirty-five are waiting?

Mr. DENNY. Yes.

Dr. PFAFF. Are on the list?

Mr. DENNY. Yes.

Dr. PFAFF. That represents a very high proportion of probably the number of individuals in the country. I think that you need to understand that. In other words, their need is for us nationally to provide organs to them.

Mr. GORE. Let me conclude 1 second. I am a little unclear about this. I am told that there can be expected to be as many as 4,000 people whose lives might be saved by a liver transplant in this country compared with 5,000 kidney transplants annually.

Mr. DENNY. That is a projection based on epidemiological data. There are at least two problems in realizing the promise of liver transplantation. Certainly the first and foremost in funding, which we have heard today, and the second we have also heard today is the shortage of available organs. Liver transplantation, you have to realize, until 2 years ago had results which did not recommend it as a therapy to be frequently applied. It has only been within the past 2 years that liver transplantation has achieved the status that it has achieved. So we are talking about the future.

We are talking about something that is building dramatically. A year ago there was only one liver transplant program in the country. Then there were two. Then there were three. Now there are six. By this time next year there will be another six. The number is growing rapidly.

Mr. GORE. Dr. Starzl said that as these regional centers develop and more patients are identified and we are able to treat more patients, that it would approach the level of 4,000 a year. I mean, that is a lot bigger than 35.

Dr. PFAFF. Yes.

Mr. GORE. So, clearly, there is a need for—

Dr. PFAFF. If it grows to that point and if that is the need and the number of individuals with hepatic failure, clear hepatic failure, and that is not just all the hepatic diseases and not all of the hepatic diseases that may result in death—I am getting overly technical, but if that were to happen, clearly we are going to need a good deal more donors, but the same is true for transplantation of each of the other organs that you have mentioned.

Mr. GORE. Thank you for your indulgence, Congresswoman Schneider.

Mrs. SCHNEIDER. Of course. You are the chairman, after all. I must admit that after listening to the testimony by this particular panel, I am not at all convinced that despite the very dedicated efforts of keeping the public informed and providing a public service that it is as effective as it ought to be. I guess to express that in more specific terms, I had asked my staff person here, Don Rheem, to go to the telephone and call the operator for 800 numbers and see what kind of information he could find. I would like to relate to you the conversation that transpired. He called the operator and he said that "I have an organ to donate, and I would like the toll-free number, please." She said "May I have the agency name?" He said, "I have no agency name." She then said, "Well, just a moment, I will give you the supervisor."

Well, essentially the supervisor went through the same thing and then putting on her thinking cap said, "Well, why don't you call your local hospital." I am under the impression that if I were to call my local hospital now and ask for information on donating a particular organ, I would probably get nowhere.

It seems to me that there is a definite need to pursue the network of professional communication with the doctors and the nurses, but also the need for the public citizen information that would very clearly answer general questions such as if I wanted to donate my organ, who do I go to, where do I begin?

Appendix 2, 1983 National Organ Transplant Hearings, D. Denny Testimony

One of the things that I am concerned about is the regional aspects of the problem. I would certainly hope that when it is recognized that we have the interest of some very powerful professional groups and organizations, such as the AMA, and the American Hospital Association, we can get a great deal of public service work accomplished by groups like the American Heart Association, the Lung Association, and other citizens' associations that we ought to be able to solve this problem.

Now, my great concern is that, yes, here we are in a congressional hearing and so we always look for solutions that are derived from our jurisdiction, but it seems pretty clear to me that there is little we can do on this. Now, I wonder is there agreement by this panel with me that there is nothing that we can specifically do?

Dr. PFAFF. My statement earlier was we had to do a hell of a lot of it. There are a few things you can do. You can foster good information getting back to us about current success in dialysis and transplantation. This is a responsibility the Federal Government assumed and has not fulfilled. So that is one thing that you can help us with.

Mrs. SCHNEIDER. Information generation.

Dr. PFAFF. Information. You must, I think, participate in the argument about funding for these other organs.

Mrs. SCHNEIDER. That is the next topic that I would like to discuss, is the funding.

Mr. DENNY. Let me mention, again, I think, Congresswoman Schneider, that I think the Federal Government can do something that you as a Representative and your colleagues can do something.

The fact that Medicare now funds 94 percent of the kidney transplants in this country and is ostensibly very eager to increase the number of patients transplanted, argues that Medicare administratively should be in a position to implement a financial incentive system for those hospitals which generate donors of kidneys. The Health Care Finance Administration is in a position to implement something like that without any legislative alteration in the Social Security Act. On the other hand, they are not going to do it unless they get the pressure put on them to do it.

Dr. PFAFF. Are you suggesting a bonus system?

Mr. DENNY. I am suggesting a financial incentive of some kind.

Mrs. SCHNEIDER. Such as a tax credit or a reduction in a medical bill?

Mr. DENNY. For instance. I leave it to wiser minds than mine. But hospitals, you know, are heavily dependent upon Medicare. Medicare is heavily dependent upon the hospitals for the recovery of kidneys for transplantation, which is funded by the Government. It only makes sense to me to move in a direction—the heartstrings of the hospital are closely tied to the purse strings of the hospitals.

Mr. GORE. Will my colleague yield?

Mrs. SCHNEIDER. Sure.

Mr. GORE. I would hope my colleague would wait until the end of the 3-day hearing to make the judgment that there is nothing we can do. I think already we have had a number of recommendations that could be included in a list of productive actions on the part of the Federal Government, not least among them, changing the procedures at CHAMPUS that deny approval of the transplant operations for children such as Captain Broderick's daughter.

In addition, I anticipate that we will have a list, a lengthy list of recommendations, many of them involving changes in Federal law, none of them as productive as or as important as the effort to increase the public's awareness of making organs available, but all of them helpful and all of them perhaps contributing to that larger effort.

Mrs. SCHNEIDER. Mr. Chairman, my question was specifically addressed to the 800 numbers, to the information exchange and the two separate networks, and I don't think that there is really anything that we can do on that score. I would like to address the costs of the 800 numbers and the information exchanges that you do have.

Mr. Denny, can you give us an idea? We know now the breadth of your communications network. Can you give us an idea of the cost of that network?

Appendix 2, 1983 National Organ Transplant Hearings, D. Denny Testimony

Mr. DENNY. Again, I have to differentiate between the two telephone systems that the North American Transplant Coordinators Organization has in place. The 24-Alert System, the recording system, which is updated two or three times a day to acquaint organ procurement professionals with the need for hearts and livers is a minimal cost.

It is not an 800 number. The caller, the organ procurement professional who is the donor hospital has the burden of paying for the cost. That is not a problem. We all have credit cards. We just do it.

The cost of setting that up was less than $200. The cost of the 800 number that NATCO has established, annually will be—it depends on the times and charges——but we expect that it will run between $6,000 and $7,000 a year. That is merely for three lines.

Mrs. SCHNEIDER. How about for the people who are operating those lines? I mean your overall information network, total cost, is about how much?

Mr. DENNY. The indirect cost for the time of the organ procurement professionals?

Mrs. SCHNEIDER. Yes.

Mr. DENNY. I have no handle on that. Again, our system has only been in place for 10 days.

Mrs. SCHNEIDER. That is true. Are volunteers right now manning those phones?

Mr. DENNY. No, ma'am.

Mrs. SCHNEIDER. Paid professionals?

Mr. DENNY. Professionals like myself, my colleagues, yes.

Mrs. SCHNEIDER. Mr. Coleman, can you give us an idea of some of the costs of your information network?

Mr. COLEMAN. The line costs us, again, depending on how much time is used, it averages $180 a month. We pay $30 a month for a 24-hour answering service. The line is manned 24 hours a day. We pay $40 a month for an emergency beeper which I carry at all times. That is the cost of our line, about $250 a month. We started this whole organization with a couple hundred dollars and a lot of effort.

Mrs. SCHNEIDER. All right. Terrific. I have no further questions, Mr. Chairman. Thank you.

Mr. GORE. Dr. Pfaff, what effect do you expect the new prospective payment reimbursement systems to have on the organization and function of organ procurement programs?

Dr. PFAFF. Gosh, I am not sure what diagnostic category they are going to use. There actually is quite a range in costs from institution to institution. I can't tell you why. In some it is very high indirect cost. In university hospitals, they are having hard times. I think the efficiencies of different organizations varies rather substantially. If everything would be to a unified cost, of course, it is going to cause so many more problems for us than if we lump transplant patients with people with bladder infections, there is going to be a substantial difference between those two if they hit the same diagnostic related group. I would urge, frankly, that there be some greater uniformity, and yet the risk of creating it is to probably eliminate those groups that are a little more costly but that are still making a major contribution.

Mr. GORE. Well, some have expressed concern about the potential effect of the prospective reimbursement system on transplant procedures and organ procurement, in particular.

Dr. PFAFF. I would say it could have a chilling effect on those who are economically marginal but productive.

Mr. GORE. Yes. What about the business that Dr. Starzl raised, that is responsible for the Federal kidney program and apparently it sent a letter out to institutions participating that implied that their insurance coverage might be lost if they harvested extrarenal organs in addition to kidneys. Are you familiar with that?

Mr. DENNY. Yes sir.

Mr. GORE. Did that have a chilling effect?

Mr. DENNY. I have no direct evidence that it did.

Mr. GORE. Dr. Pfaff?

Dr. PFAFF. Well, it creates an impediment. I guess, quite honestly, there is no way to measure because we don't have accurate data on the potential utilization of multiple donor organs and, you know,

Appendix 2, 1983 National Organ Transplant Hearings, D. Denny Testimony

what is being done today. In other words, our performance record isn't defined as yet. Further, there are a good number of programs that are just getting into multiple organ donations.

The bottom line is this. Actually, that Aetna did advise us that the cost that related to procurement of other than kidneys could not be attributed to the renal Medicare program. We have followed that, but have done it by a variety of means. We have participated in the harvesting of both livers and hearts and have a very active program in terms of joints that we are doing with the orthopedic groups up and down the east coast.

In many instances we have some sources of funds. Truthfully, in dealing with the University of Pittsburgh our costs that particularly related to liver removal for the purposes of transplantation were then passed back to Pittsburgh. Heart donor costs were segregated to the point that we could and then were sent to the recipient institution. I don't know what the payment rate has been, but I suspect after all the conversation that I have heard these last several days that, indeed, because dollars are such an impediment to individuals who require that kind of management, that one of the first things that the recipient institution has been paying attention to is, indeed, the donor institutions.

Mr. DENNY. I think that we have to be careful and not imply that Aetna is at fault for this. Aetna is merely operating under the guidelines established by the Health Care Finance Administration following the legislation which was enacted in 1973 and subsequently.

Aetna is responsible as the intermediary between HCFA and the independent organ procurement programs to see to it that the regulations governing the financial aspects of organ procurement are adhered to. Their statement to us that we would not be covered by Medicare in the event of malpractice, for instance, and a court case involving malpractice surrounding organ procurement came also with the recommendation that we take out insurance on malpractice liability for extra-renal organ procurement. That is, in fact, what we did do.

Mr. GORE. In other words, it emanated from the Health Care Financing Administration through Aetna?

Mr. DENNY. Yes. Aetna is merely the intermediary.

Mr. GORE. We are going to have the Health Care Financing Administration on the third day of these hearings along with the Surgeon General. We will be exploring a lot of these reimbursement questions at that time.

A couple of other real brief questions. It seems as if—and I know this is a delicate area—it seems often desirable to maintain a potential donor on life support after brain death has occurred; is that correct, Dr. Pfaff?

Dr. PFAFF. That it is desirable? It is for the purpose of multiple organ removal in that, let's say, if somebody is coming from a heart transplant hospital to our institution, it might have a delaying factor, usually in a matter of hours, not more than that.

Mr. GORE. But you don't get into a conflict on who pays for the cost of care under those circumstances?

Dr. PFAFF. No. No. Well, for the purpose of the kidney donor, from the time of diagnosis of death, the renal Medicare program assumes the cost of continued care. But that is not for long, because these are unstable individuals in many instances. We are anxious to proceed.

Mr. GORE. But if the extra care is principally needed for the multiple organ—

Dr. PFAFF. We are still talking about hours.

Mr. GORE. But is it charged to the kidney program?

Dr. PFAFF. Quite honestly, I am not sure. I could imagine that potentially being a point of confusion at the time and to the billing personnel. I would guess that the receiving institution would assume at least part of those costs or the fair share of costs.

Mr. DENNY. Yes, sir. That, in fact, is what happens. We regularly pay for a liver anywhere between $1,000 and $3,000, sometimes as high as $4,000 of the share of the donor-related charges, the balance being picked up by the renal programs.

Appendix 2, 1983 National Organ Transplant Hearings, D. Denny Testimony

Mr. GORE. Let me note that in tomorrow's hearing we are going to lead off with the prospective beneficiaries and voluntary agencies, including Charles and Marilyn Fiske, the parents of Jamie Fiske, who will also be with us tomorrow.

In the second panel we are going to explore in-depth the bioethical considerations with a number of bioethicists, including the Executive Director of the Presidential Commission on Bioethics. Then we are going to look in the third panel closely at the legal considerations, and you got into this a little bit in your testimony, Mr. Denny, and I would say for the record to my colleague from Illinois that the counsel for the National Conference of Commissioners on Uniform State Law will be among the witnesses on that third panel. Then the third day of the hearing will be a little later on, but I wanted to close by thanking members of this panel particularly for your contribution here today, and to all of the witnesses who have helped us in this first day of the hearings, I want to express our thanks and appreciation and with that, the hearing will stand adjourned.

Dr. PFAFF. Thank you.

[Whereupon, at 2:45 p.m. the hearing was adjourned, to be reconvened the following day, Thursday, April 14, 1983, at 9:30 a.m.]

Mr. GORE. We are really under a time constraint now. I am going to start your testimony, Winifred Mack. We have a close and important vote on the floor, and we are going to have to finish up the hearing by 2 o'clock. So what I am going to do is start your testimony and then interrupt it for the vote shortly, and then we will come back and have some brief questions.

So please proceed. We will put your prepared statement in the record. If you could summarize portions of it, that would be fine.

Ms MACK. I have cut it down in my verbal testimony.

Appendix 3, 1983 National Organ Transplant Hearings, W. Mack Testimony

STATEMENT OF WINIFRED B. MACK, PRESIDENT
NORTH AMERICAN TRANSPLANT COORDINATORS ORGANIZATION, SUNY AT STONY BROOK

Ms MACK. Mr. Chairman and members of the committee, as president of the North American Transplant Coordinators Organization, I welcome the privilege of testifying before this committee on behalf of the members of NATCO.

The North American Transplant Coordinators Organization is a national, nonprofit organization representing 365 professionals in the United States and several foreign countries. Our dedication is that there be a better quality of life for the thousands of patients with end-stage organ failure and a respect for those who shared.

NATCO members represent various aspects of the transplant community, including physicians, nurses, and allied health professionals working with the organ recipient as well as those whose main objective is to obtain and distribute the valuable human tissue so direly needed by the waiting victims of end-stage organ failure. To this end, our members provide information to medical personnel and the general public regarding all aspects of organ transplantation. In addition, NATCO works to disseminate information concerning new techniques in organ procurement, preservation, and transplant surgery to its members.

Kidney recovery and transplantation became a reality in 1972 when the Federal Government enacted H.R. 1, which provided, under Medicare, that persons with kidney failure would receive full medical treatment. To support these activities, a new breed of professional known as the transplant coordinator evolved. Most often, coordinators come from some other health background. Many of us are nurses or physicians' assistants; some are medical laboratory technologists; a few from related areas such as social work or psychology.

With the guidance of transplant surgeons and other physicians as well as input from the clergy, public relations and media persons, administrators, legal consultants, and other experts, the profile of the transplant coordinator was developed.

Today, although still young by comparison to other groups of health professionals, NATCO has established a training program for new coordinators as well as ongoing continuing education programs to assist in the sharing of information and techniques utilized by its members. Additionally, several transplant institutions have opened their doors to other centers wishing to train new personnel.

The term "coordinator" aptly describes the essence of our function, and the role may vary according to institutional needs. Specific details are in my written testimony. Some coordinators deal specifically with the transplant recipient. Other coordinators have responsibilities primarily to organ procurement, which includes development of local hospitals as donor referral sources. Each procurement center has a 24-hour hotline, and a coordinator is available day or night to assist the donor hospital with the legal issues, medical management of the donor, obtaining consent from the appropriate next of kin, and organizing the surgical team for the recovery of organs.

If the organ cannot be used by the local transplant organ, using a national computer system, the coordinator may arrange for sharing and transporting of the recovered organ to another center in a time period short enough to insure its viability.

Transplant centers have long recognized the need for public education. As individuals, or in concert with other organ recovery programs, their coordinators have developed materials such as brochures, donor cards, bumper stickers, poster campaigns, slide shows, et cetera, for presentation in schools, local community groups, civic organizations, churches, health fairs, and the like.

They keep channels of communication open with the media, being available to answer reporters' questions, perhaps speak on local and national television and radio programs, and encourage and/or assist in the development of public service announcements. Needless to say, one person cannot handle all the

A CLINICIAN'S GUIDE TO DONATION AND TRANSPLANTATION   Chapter 1

Appendix 3, 1983 National Organ Transplant Hearings, W. Mack Testimony

responsibilities described, and many programs have few persons hired under the general title of transplant coordinator.

It must be recognize, however, that these centers work under conditions of extreme austerity, and coordinators have learned to tap all available resources to insure the efficacy of their programs.

Collectively, transplant coordinators, under the aegis of NATCO, have addressed some of the problems existing on a national level.

On September 23, 1982, NATCO inaugurated a formal system to disseminate information concerning the need for extrarenal organ donors to procurement programs throughout the United States and Canada and to assist transplant coordinators and physicians in the placement of these organs for transplantation.

Mr. GORE. Ms Mack, if you could pause there, we will recess for approximately 7 minutes and come back and finish up your testimony.

Ms MACK. Fine.

[Short recess taken.]

Mr. GORE. The subcommittee will come back to order.

Ms MACK, you were proceeding with your statement. Please go ahead.

Ms MACK, Thank you, Mr. Chairman.

A recorded telephone message updated approximately twice a day provides a listing of urgently needed hearts, livers, lungs, heart/lungs, and pancreata for patients awaiting transplantation at participating centers.

The 24-ALERT system operates 24 hours a day and gives details of extrarenal donor requirements when needed, geographical recovery area, and 24-hour referral number. There are currently 15 transplant centers listing their extrarenal organ needs with 24-Alert.

To date, 24-Alert has facilitated the recovery and transplantation of 90 extrarenal organs, including the livers recovered for Jaime Fiske and Brandon Hall and Justine Pinheiro, cases which have received recent media attention.

NATCO 24-ALERT is a free, voluntary service easily accessible by telephone to coordinators in hospitals anywhere in the country by simply dialing 24-ALERT. I wish to stress, however, that informal referral of extrarenal organs has been in existence and common among our members since 1978.

On April 4, 1983, 800-24-DONOR was established by NATCO; 800-24-DONOR is an information and referral number for professionals, possibly to be expanded for public information in the near future. Staffed by NATCI members, it is designed to facilitate and enhance procurement programs throughout the country by referring the caller to the nearest organ recovery center in his area.

Steps are currently being taken to publicize this number through professional journals and mailings to the community it will best serve.

As previously mentioned, the NATCO training and development course is the only established professional training course provided for new coordinators at this time. In addition, a desk-side reference manual is now in the final stages of preparation for use both by procurement and recipient coordinators.

Annual educational meetings serve to update, improve, and share current knowledge pertaining to organ procurement, preservation, and transplantation. Recognized leaders from various areas of transplantation, as well as representatives from governmental and private agencies, are invited to speak to our membership on topics of common interest related to procurement, preservation, general education and clinical application.

All future meetings will be held in conjunction with other important meetings of the transplant community, enabling our members to glean information from these prestigious groups. In addition to the above major endeavors accomplished by NATCO, individual committees are working diligently on projects, short and long term, to attain specific goals and objectives of the organization.

With the general background of transplant coordinators and their representative organization, NATCO, presented herein, I feel qualified to present the following recommendations to this committee for your consideration.

Appendix 3, 1983 National Organ Transplant Hearings, W. Mack Testimony

Although over 30 States have thus far enacted some form of brain death legislation, for the remaining States, the physicians' and hospitals' fear of litigation looms ominous. Passage of a brain death law, and the media attention which generally accompanies it, also serves to educate the public about this difficult-to-understand phenomenon.

Imagine yourself, Mr. Gore, standing before the grieving family of an 18-year-old boy who, while on his way to a part-time job, was shot in the head by a couple of joy riders passing by. The respirator hisses every few seconds; the cardiac monitor beeps; and the boy lies motionless in his bed. The doctors have just informed his parents that he is dead, but they know there is a heartbeat, and heartbeat has always meant life to them.

Yesterday, they had a perfectly healthy, normal son. Today, they are told their son is brain dead, whatever that means. Imagine yourself trying to explain to this family that brain death is really death. And then imagine asking them to think of somebody else and to donate his organs for transplantation. They are frightened, they are confused, they are angry, and the question which comes to mind is, "Is our son really dead, or do they just want his organs?"

Brain death legislation will not answer all the questions all of the time, but if the issue is out in the open with legal support, it somehow becomes clearer, and the consideration of organ donation by individuals before their death becomes more likely.

We suggest that, using the definition recommended by the National Conference of Commissioners on Uniform State Laws, you strongly urge the 50 States to adopt brain death legislation.

Second, although our efforts at a local level in our own donor referral hospitals have gone a long way, we in this field are painfully aware of the lack of understanding by our colleagues in the health professions as to the legal, ethical, and medical issues surrounding organ donation and transplantation.

We hope that NATCO's 800-24-DONOR number will alleviate some of the problem. However, we recognize that a more broad based program is needed. An aggressive campaign of presentations such as seminars to groups of professionals via local and national associations and distribution of written materials would be helpful.

NATCO offers the following specific suggestions:

(A) Appropriation of funds, perhaps in the form of NIH grants, would assist in the development of professional educational programs and tools.

(B) Recommendations to State agencies entrusted with the responsibility of licensing of health professionals that information related to organ transplantation and donation be incorporated into curricula and questions pertaining to these issues be included in certifying examinations.

(C) A requirement that all hospitals receiving Medicare reimbursement be mandated to have written policies and procedures for brain death and organ donation.

We have, during these hearings, witnessed the testimony of desperate parents anxiously awaiting the availability of a cadaver donor organ for their children. Our hearts ache for these parents, and we truly appreciate their need to do all humanly possible to achieve their goal.

However, transplant coordinators are acutely aware that there are many Jaime Fiskes and Brandon Halls in this country in need of livers and thousands of patients awaiting the availability of renal as well as extrarenal cadaver donor organs.

It is easy to relate to one innocent baby's face as it comes across the TV screen into our homes. And we as coordinators acknowledge that the plea made for one child indeed increases, albeit only temporarily, organ donation in general. But what of the mother of two young children who fears that, for lack of a transplantation, she will not live long enough to see her babies reach adulthood; or the man in whom renal failure has caused sterility and who may never realize the joy of fathering a child?

It is imperative that the citizens of this Nation become aware that organ transplantation is a therapeutic modality past stages of experimentation and a viable alternative to life on a dialysis machine or blindness or, worst of all, death.

A CLINICIAN'S GUIDE TO DONATION AND TRANSPLANTATION

Appendix 3, 1983 National Organ Transplant Hearings, W. Mack Testimony

Great concern has been expressed during these hearings as to the equitability of organ distribution to the waiting recipients. Suggestions have been made in the form of a computerized matching system or a first-come, first-served basis.

National systems such as the computer available through the United Network for Organ Sharing, or NATCO's 24-Alert, already exist to facilitate the most effective utilization of recovered donor organs. It must be appreciated, however, that in the world of medical science, a computer is only a tool to assist but not to substitute for the trained clinical judgment which must be exercised in the care of the human patient.

In varying degrees, depending on the specific organ in question, recipient selection is made on the basis of tissue matching, medical urgency, length of time a patient may be waiting on the list, geographical location, donor-versus-recipient age, size and weight, or any combination of factors. What looks good in the computer printout is not necessarily good in clinical application.

The family that donate the organ with the expressed intention that it go to a particular recipient, or even a patient of the same race, ethnic background, or age of the donor should be told that such stipulations might result in the inability to find such a compatible recipient, or, more importantly, the inevitable rejection of the transplanted organ.

Education of the general public about specific advances in therapy have often resulted in pressure on the medical community to utilize new techniques or alter long-accepted practices. We believe that mass public education will raise the consciousness of American citizens, help them to more fully understand the complexity of these issues, and ultimately stop the senseless waste of valuable human tissue.

NATCO makes the following suggestion:

(a) A national coalition of organizations who have interest in the recovery of human organs—eyes, skin, kidneys, liver, heart, bone, et cetera—could poor their efforts and expertise to produce both public and professional educational materials on all aspects of organ donation and transplantation.

With the input from the fields of medicine, advertising, media, and public relations, fundraising, law, clergy, et cetera, a national campaign could be launched to provide this informational source. Once again, money in the form of grants could be used to seed this agency.

(b) NATCO's Education Subcommittee for Public Education has worked with both the National Kidney Foundation and the American Medical Association to increase organ donation. This year, the first session of the 98th Congress introduced Senate Joint Resolution 78, to authorize and request the President to issue a proclamation declaring this week, April 24-30, 1983, as National Organ Donation Awareness Week. We ask this committee to recommend that such a week be identified annually.

Finally, the Members of Congress, each represent leadership in their local constituencies. We urge this committee to request each of its colleagues to return to their home States, ask for time from their local television stations, and publicly sign an organ donor card such as the one you have before you.

This demonstration of moral leadership by political leaders will go a long way in establishing organ donation as a natural sequel to death.

I thank you very much.

Appendix 4, 1983 National Organ Transplant Hearings, A. Peele Testimony

STATEMENT OF AMY S. PEELE, PRESIDENT
NORTH AMERICAN TRANSPLANT COORDINATORS ORGANIZATION

Ms PEELE. Representative Waxman, members of the committee, my name is Amy S. Peele, president of the North American Transplant Coordinator's Organization and senior transplant coordinator at Rush-Presbyterian-St. Luke's Medical Center, Chicago, Ill. I welcome the invitation to testify before this committee on behalf of the members of NATCO.

The North American Transplant Coordinators Organization is a national, nonprofit organization representing 400 professionals in the United States, Canada, and several foreign countries.

Our dedication is "that there be a better quality of life for the thousands of patients with end-stage organ failure, and a respect for those who shares."

I want to elaborate on the members and what are the responsibilities of each coordinator. I will simply state there are various duties assigned to the coordinator, depending on the instituition's need for that coordinator.

That may entail procurement or it may entail the responsibility and care of the recipient after they have received that said organ. With the Medicare involvement for end-stage renal disease in 1972, a network of procurement agencies was established throughout the entire United States.

So, ladies and gentlemen, since that time, there has been a mechanism established across the country to obtain and distribute cadaver organs and tissues for transplantation.

The Government reimburses that system through Medicare but fails to recognize its existence and continues to mislead the public by claiming there is no system to facilitate the sharing of human organs. And that myth is perpetuated by reports from the news media.

It is only by chance that 30,000 patients in the United States received cadaver kidney transplants since 1972, nor is it by chance that last year over 90 patients underwent liver transplants and less than half that amount received heart and heart/lung transplants.

It is only through the efforts and dedication of the transplant community that these patients received new leases on life. The organ sharing system does work, but there is room for improvement and expansion.

The National Organ Transplant Act can improve and expand that organ sharing system, thereby allowing thousands more end stage organ disease patients another chance at life that only a healthy donor organ can bring.

Title I of the National Organ Transplant Act authorizes a program of grants for the development and expansion of local organ procurement organizations throughout the Nation. In theory, this is an excellent idea, however, the application of those funds to these organizations should not take place without a thorough review of the procurement systems already in place. That review would include:

One, an understanding of the Health Care Finance Administration's current level of involvement towards procurement efforts.

Two, the already established 32 regional end-stage renal disease networks currently funded by the Federal Government.

Three, the successful involvement at the Aetna Insurance Co.'s relationship with all independent organ procurement agencies.

Four, the United Network of Organ Sharing and its success in distributing cadaver kidneys via a computer system.

Five, NATCO's two 24-hour telephone hotlines to facilitate the retrieval and distribution of donor organs.

The NATCO 24-ALERT system began on September 23, 1982. This system, accessed by telephone, gives the caller a listing of urgently needed livers, hearts, and hear/lung combinations from the 15 transplant centers that perform these operations across the United States and Canada.

Appendix 4, 1983 National Organ Transplant Hearings, A. Peele Testimony

Since its inception 1 year ago, the 24-ALERT system has facilitated the transplantation of 122 livers at 9 centers, 73 hearts at 9 centers and 2 heart/lung combinations at 2 centers. The system's success is due to the fact it was designed by transplant coordinators to meet their specific needs. It is also successful because it is easily accessed by telephone. This telephone system can complement the Computerized system mentioned as part of the National Organ Transplant Act.

Title II of the bill revises title XVIII of the Social Security Act to permit the Secretary to pay for Organ transplants and other investigative procedures at a limited number of specialized centers. NATCO strongly supports this provision of the bill because it will increase the number of Medical centers performing extra-renal organ transplants across the country.

There has been much discussion over the past several months about the lack of donor livers for transplantation. The reality is that the University of Pittsburgh received 523 calls alerting them to the availability of donor livers in 1982.

Only 80 of those livers were recovered and transplanted by the Pittsburgh Program. 102 of the donor livers offered were declined by the Pittsburgh group because the transplant team was exhausted or the hospital could not accommodate another liver transplant patient.

However, I must note that all those potential referrals were then passed on, if not immediately, to all the other liver transplant programs in the country.

So, the shortage of donor livers is not as dramatic as portrayed by the news media. It is the lack of adequate liver transplant programs that precludes a larger number of patients from receiving therapeutic liver transplants.

Exempting organ procurement activities from the Medicare prospective payment plan shows a great deal of foresight on the part of Representative Gore. This action will continue to support the present system and allow for its growth.

NATCO supports the revision of title XIX of the Social Security Act to require States to develop written policies for the payment of transplant procedure under Medicaid, to require the State Medicaid programs participate in any transplant program established under Medicare, and that designated transplant centers serve Medicaid patients.

NATCO strongly agrees with title III of the bill prohibiting the sale of human organs and the penalties for violating this act. Our final recommendation to this committee is to suggest that the Federal Government, through the Joint Commission on the Accreditation of Hospitals, mandate the establishment of policy and procedures in every hospital for the declaration of brain death and for the referral or organ and tissue donors for transplantation.

JCAHO should require that upon every death in an accredited hospital, the deceased's next of kin be asked their position regarding organ and tissue donation.

In closing, I thank you for the opportunity to discuss NATCO's position regarding the National Organ Transplant Act.

We, as coordinators, are aware that although a successful organ procurement system exists, there is need for improvement and expansion. The National Organ Transplant Act with our recommendations can bring about this improvement and expansion, especially in the areas of public education and professional participation in the transplanting of human organs and tissues.

[The statement of Ms. Peele follows:]

Appendix 4, 1983 National Organ Transplant Hearings, A. Peele Testimony

TESTIMONY OF
AMY S. PEELE, PRESIDENT
NORTH AMERICAN TRANSPLANT COORDINATOR'S ORGANIZATION

Representative Waxman; Members of the Committee:

My name is Amy S. Peele, President of the North American Transplant Coordinator's Organization (NATCO) and Senior Transplant Coordinator at Rush-Presbyterian-St. Luke's Medical Center, Chicago, Illinois. I welcome the invitation to testify before this committee on behalf of the members of NATCO.

The North American Transplant Coordinators Organization (NATCO) is a national, non-profit organization representing over 400 professionals in the United States, Canada and several foreign countries. Our dedication is "THAT THERE BE A BETTER QUALITY OF LIFE FOR THE THOUSANDS OF PATIENTS WITH END-STAGE ORGAN FAILURE...AND A RESPECT FOR THOSE WHO SHARED."

The members of NATCO represent various aspects of the transplant community, including physicians, nurses and allied health professionals working with the organ recipients and those whose main objective is to obtain and distribute the valuable human organs and tissues so desperately needed by the waiting victims of end stage organ failure. NATCO members provide information to medical personnel and to the general public regarding all aspects of organ transplantation. In addition, NATCO disseminates information to its members concerning new techniques in organ procurement, preservation and transplant surgery.

The role of transplant coordinators varies greatly across the country according to the needs of the institution for which they work. Some coordinators only deal with the recipient, assisting physician with determining a patient's medical suitability for transplant, arranging for necessary laboratory and diagnostic testing, communicating with other health care providers (physicians, dialysis units, etc.) to keep current on the status of the patient, providing for the collection of frequent blood samples for tissue matching with specific donor organs, and educating and preparing the patient emotionally and otherwise for the future transplant procedure.

Procurement coordinators are specifically responsible for organ recovery. This includes developing a network of hospitals within a geographical area whose staffs will refer donors for organ and tissue recovery. The coordinator travels to these hospitals to meet with administrators, medical boards, nursing and other ancillary personnel to assist in formulating policies and procedures for the determination of brain death and organ donation. Frequent surveillance visits and continuing-education programs are offered as a means of keeping organ donation "alive: in the minds of the professionals in these hospitals. Procurement coordinators develop protocol manuals, posters, slide shows, telephone stickers, etc., for distribution in hospital emergency rooms and critical care units, the places where donor identification is likely to occur. A procurement center has a 24-hour "hot line" and a coordinator is available day and night to assist the donor hospital with the legal issues, medical management of the donor, obtaining consent from the appropriate next-of-kin, and organizing the surgical team for the recovery of organs and tissues.

When the organs or tissues are obtained, coordinators may be present in the operating room to help in the participation and preservation for transplantation. Within the transplant center they may arrange for the final cross-matching and then admission of the suitable recipient. If the organ cannot be used by the local transplant program, the coordinator, using a national computer system, may arrange for the sharing and transporting of the recovered organ to another center—all in a time period short enough to ensure its viability.

Needles to say, one person cannot handle all the responsibilities described and many programs have a few persons hired under the general title of Transplant Coordinator. It must be recognized , however, that these centers work under conditions of extreme austerity and coordinators have learned to tap all available resources to ensure the efficacy of their programs.

Appendix 4, 1983 National Organ Transplant Hearings, A. Peele Testimony

With the Medicare involvement for end-stage renal disease in 1972, a network of procurement agencies was established throughout the entire United States So ladies and Gentlemen, since that time, there has been a mechanism established across the country to obtain and distribute cadaver organs and tissues for transplantation. The government reimburses that system thru Medicare but fails to recognize its existence and continues to mislead the public by claiming there is no system to facilitate the sharing of human organs. And that myth is perpetuated by reports from the news media.

It is not by chance that 30,000 patients in the United States have received cadaver kidney transplants since 1972, nor is it by chance that last year over 90 patients underwent liver and less than half that amount received heart and heart/lung transplants.

It is only through the efforts and dedication of the transplant community that these patients received new leases on life. The organ sharing system does work but there is room for improvement and expansion.

The National Organ Transplant Act can improve and expand that organ sharing system thereby allowing thousands more end-stage organ disease patients another chance at life that only a healthy donor organ can bring.

Title one of the National Organ Transplant Act authorizes a program of grants for the development and expansion of local organ procurement organizations throughout the nation. In theory this is an excellent idea, however, the application of those funds to these organizations should not take place without a thorough review of the procurement systems already in place.

That review would include:
1. an understanding of the Health Care Finance Administration's current level of involvement towards procurement efforts.
2. the already established 32 regional end-stage renal disease networks currently funded by the federal government
3. the successful involvement of the Aetna Insurance company's relationship with all independent organ procurement agencies
4. the United Network of Organ Sharing and its success in distributing cadaver kidneys via a computer system
5. NATCO's two 24-hour telephone "hot lines" to facilitate the retrieval and distribution of donor organs.

The NATCO 24-ALERT system began on September 23, 1982. This system, accessed by telephone, gives the caller a listing of urgently needed livers, hearts and heart/lung combinations from the 15 transplant centers that perform these operations across the United States and Canada. This system is not in competition with the computerized United Network for Organ Sharing.

Since its inception one year ago, the 24-ALERT system has facilitated the transplantation of 122 livers at 9 centers, 73 hearts at 9 centers and 2 heart/lung combinations at 2 centers. The system's success is due to the fact it was designed by transplant coordinators to meet their specific needs. It is also successful because it's easily accessed by telephone. This telephone system can complement the computerized system mentioned as part of the National Organ Transplant Act.

Title two of the bill revises title XVIII of the Social Security Act to permit the Secretary to pay for organ transplants and other investigative procedures at a limited number of specialized centers. NATCO strongly supports this provision of the bill because it will increase the number of medical centers performing extra-renal organ transplants across the country.

There has been much discussion over the past several months the lack of donor livers for transplantation. The reality is that University of Pittsburgh received 523 calls alerting them to the availability of donor livers in 1982. Only 80 of those livers were recovered and transported by the Pittsburgh program. 102 of the donor livers offered were declined by the Pittsburgh group because the transplant team was exhausted or the hospital could not accommodate another liver transplant patient.

Appendix 4, 1983 National Organ Transplant Hearings, A. Peele Testimony

So the shortage of donor livers is not as dramatic as portrayed by the news media. It the lack of adequate liver transplants programs that precludes a larger number of patients from receiving therapeutic liver transplants.

Exempting organ procurement activities from the Medicare prospective payment plan shows a great deal of foresight on the part of Representative Gore. This action will continue to support the present system and allow for its growth.

NATCO supports revision of Title XIX of the Social Security Act to require states to develop written policies for the payment of transplant procedures under Medicaid, to require that state Medicaid programs participate in any transplant programs established under Medicare, and that designated transplant centers serve Medicaid patients.

NATCO strongly agrees with Title III of the billing prohibiting the sale of the human organs and the penalties for violating this act.

Our final recommendation to this committee is to suggest that the federal government, through the Joint Commission on Accreditation of Hospitals (JCAH), mandate the establishment of policy and procedures in every hospital for the declaration of brain death and for the referral of organ and tissue donors for transplantation.

JCAH should require that upon every death in an accredited hospital, the deceased's next-of-kin be asked their position regarding organ and tissue donation.

In closing, I think you are for the opportunity to discuss NATCO's position regarding the National Organ Transplant Act. We, as coordinators, are aware that although a successful organ procurement system exists, there is need for improvement and expansion. The National Organ Transplant Act with our recommendation can bring about this improvement and expansion especially in the area of public education and professional participation in the transplanting of human organs and tissues.

3. Because of conflicting views and programs developing under federal auspices, I support an office within the Public Health Service to coordinate federal organ and tissue transplantation policies. An example is the reimbursement policies for the care of dialysis patients that provide an incentive for physicians to eliminate a consideration of transplantation therapy for ESRD patients.

4. Because of the embarrassing discrepancy between the national records of the
United States related to patients receiving transplantation and dialysis therapy and the excellent reports of the European Dialysis and Transplantation Association, I support a scientific registry of patients with the basic facts concerning their therapy and results. This is essential information for the federal government to have in order to monitor programs almost exclusively financed by federal entitlement programs.

5. Because of the inevitable development of interests in communities across these United States for transplantation, I recommend development with collaboration and discussion with the medical profession and standards for centers conducting transplantation in regard to the selection of patients and in regard to the qualifications of the center for personnel, facilities, relation to community needs, and the like. The setting of national standards is desirable for maintaining high quality of care. The separate issue of cost control of medical care should not be addressed by federal programs limiting the number of institution authorized to carry out transplantation therapy, but by programs capping total costs. This leaves the choice of hospital and medical profession activities to the local medical care system without dictating specific solutions.

6. Because of the need for a national review on an annual basis of transplantation policies and therapies, I support a task force with the mandate to review the medical, legal, ethical, economic, and social issues presented by human organ and tissue procurement and transplantation.

7. Because of the artificial and irrational division of payment for medicines and drugs on the basis of hospitalization or otherwise, I recommend outpatients having their medicines and drugs fully covered by federal programs if they are eligible for transplantation therapy in the first instance.

Chairman JACOBS. I think we will proceed with Ms. Peele first, and then see if there are any questions that can be propounded.

Appendix 4, 1983 National Organ Transplant Hearings, A. Peele Testimony

STATEMENT OF AMY S. PEELE, PRESIDENT, NORTH AMERICAN TRANSPLANT COORDINATOR'S ORGANIZATION

Ms PEELE. You paint a very euphoric picture, and it is nice that you can do it in Boston, maybe some day in Chicago, in terms of regionalization. I am going to be brief in my comments because I don't want to be redundant, and I realize that I am clean up here, so I would like to finish up. You have my testimony for the record, and I wish you would accept that.

Chairman JACOBS. Without objection.

Ms PEELE. I just want to make a few comments. The group that I represent, North American Transplant Coordinator's Organization, is composed of over 400 coordinators throughout the United States, North America, and Canada. We are what you would probably refer to as the trench people.

We are the people who ask for organ donations. We approach the family. We orchestrate the events that culminate in organ donation, be it multiple or singular. We try to make it occur in a very professional manner, so that the grieving family is not feeling anymore taxed than they already are.

We also have in our membership professional clinical coordinators who care for those patients who receive those organs, who have new lease on life. That is the construction of our group. When looking at the Gore bill, and we have for some time, we have supported it in general and we continue to support it. Under title I, in terms of the grant programs. It is nice to know that you can set up an independent organ procurement program and it will be funded my Medicare, but that is after you receive or take a loan out for about $125,000, which is not something that a lot of people can do.

The types of funds that they are talking about in this bill would promote an independent organ procurement agency in the areas that maybe it is not functioning. It would offer them a startup with those funds, and then to expand. There are also programs that could probably expand, but financially can't. I understand that once a loan is taken out for the independent organ procurement agency, then each organ that is acquired through that has a certain amount of funds tacked on to it to pay for that loan on a long-term basis, so that you are not running in the red, so to speak.

The network that you, I think, Mr. Moore, referred to today, you asked about the United Network of Organ Sharing and the kidney sharing that occurs, and was there something similar in the case in terms of liver, heart, and lung. Yes, indeed, there is and it is called the NATCO 24-hour alert system. It is a telephone line, and you access it simply by calling on the phone. Currently, it is in the process of being updated to a talking computer. Pretty much, whenever we find that we have a donor anywhere in the United States—we, meaning procurement coordinators before we approach the family to obtain multiple consent, we call that number and we get a listing of every patient in the United States who is waiting for a heart, a liver, or a heart and lung. That way, when we go to the family to have them sign the consent, we can tell them that Minnesota is going to take the heart, or Pittsburgh is coming to take the liver. It is sort of the tally list or the given that we have walking into a procurement situation to obtain consent, and then bring in the teams.

Since its inception, which was about a year ago, we have recovered about 122 livers through the use of that, about 93 hearts, and 2 heart and lungs, and these were transplanted at multiple centers. We found it to be extremely successful. We have worked very long to get the funds to computerize it, so that it is much more efficient than it currently is. We are very pleased with the progress.

The network that is spoken about under the bill probably, if you want to look into the crystal ball, would include the UNOS system, the computer system in the NATCO 24-hour alert system, which is the phone system, both of which probably don't have the funding currently to own it, to continue to put it under a national framework, and make it available at a low cost to everybody.

In terms of the task force, it is really vague as to how it would function, but I think one thing that is very important here is that we need to get some bottom line numbers—how many kidneys, how many hearts, how many livers are we going to need, and how many potential recipients are there going to be, and what is the feasibility. This may be something that this task force could get their hands on and get back with numbers.

Chapter 1 — THE HISTORY OF THE TRANSPLANT COORDINATOR

Appendix 4, 1983 National Organ Transplant Hearings, A. Peele Testimony

It would be unfortunate if the Congress were accused again, as they were in 1972 after they passed the ESRD legislation, of medicareless in granting funds from Medicare to pay for the ESRD program, not really knowing well what the expenses were going to be that they incurred. I think that they far outweighed what they actually had though that they would.

In terms of allowing extra programs to do transplantation, liver specifically and heart, we see that there is definitely a need for other programs. In 1982, Pittsburgh did get enormous numbers of calls to the tune of 523 offers for livers. Eighty of those were only used, and the rest of the calls were passed on to the other 14 programs that perform extra-renal transplants.

There is a problem because, as Dr. Starzl has already referred to and other people, when you call the program that is doing the extra-renal transplant, the team may be exhausted, they may be in the process of retrieving another organ, or they may not have a bed in their ICU to accommodate the recipient, all of which are things that could be solved if other programs started doing extrarenal transplantation.

Last, in terms of the buying and selling of organs, we suggest that that definitely be supported. It would be unfortunate to see that take place. The Blook Commission, I believe, or the American Red Cross, I forget where the origin was, did see a dramatic drop when blood was being bought and sold, and it took them a long time to recover in terms of voluntary donations.

One thing that probably could be done without any legislative effort is to encourage Joint Commission on Accreditation of Hospitals to include in all the hospitals that are accredited by them that when brain death occurs, or a death in the hospital, that the family be approached about organ donation to continue receiving Medicare funds.

These are pretty much all the comments I have. If you have any questions, I will be glad to answer them.

[The prepared statement follows:]

STATEMENT OF AMY S. PEELE, PRESIDENT, NORTH AMERICAN TRANSPLANTCOORDINATOR'S ORGANIZATION

Representative Jacobs; Members of the Committee: My name is Amy S. Peele, President of the North American Transplant Coordinator's Organization (NATCO) and Senior Transplant Coordinator at Rush-Presbyterian-St. Luke's Medical Center, Chicago, Illinois. I welcome the invitation to testify before this committee on behalf of the members of NATCO.

The North American Transplant Coordinators Organization (NATCO) is a national, non-profit organization representing over 400 professionals in the United States, Canada and several foreign countries. Our dedication is "That there be a better quality of life for the thousands of patients with end-stage organ failure.... and a respect for those who shared."

The members of NATCO represent various aspects of the transplant community, including physicians, nurses and allied health professionals working with the organ recipients and those whose main objective is to obtain and distribute the valuable human organs and tissues so desperately needed by the waiting victims of end stage organ failure. NATCO members provide information to medical personnel and to the general public regarding all aspects of organ transplantation. In addition, NATCO disseminates information to its members concerning new techniques in organ procurement, preservation and transplant surgery.

The role of transplant coordinators varies greatly across the country according to the needs of the institution for which they work. Some coordinators only deal with the recipient, assisting physicians with determining a patient's medical suitability for transplant, arranging for necessary laboratory and diagnostic testing, communicating with other health care providers (physicians, dialysis units, etc.) to keep current on the status of the patient, providing for the collection of frequent blood samples for tissue matching with specific donor organs, and educating and preparing the patient emotionally and otherwise for the future transplant procedure.

A CLINICIAN'S GUIDE TO DONATION AND TRANSPLANTATION

Appendix 4, 1983 National Organ Transplant Hearings, A. Peele Testimony

Procurement coordinators are specifically responsible for organ recovery. This includes developing a network of hospitals within a geographical area whose staffs will refer donors for organ and tissue recovery. The coordinators travel to these hospitals to meet with administrators, medical boards, nursing and other ancillary personnel to assist in formulating policies and procedures for the determination of brain death and organ donation. Frequent surveillance visits and continuing-education programs are offered as a means of keeping organ donation "alive" in the minds of the professional in these hospitals. Procurement coordinators develop protocol manuals, posters, slide shows, telephone stickers, etc., for distribution in hospital emergency rooms and critical care units, the places where donor identification is likely to occur. A procurement center has a 24-hour "hot line" and a coordinator is available day and night to assist the donor hospital with the legal issues, medical management of the donor, obtaining consent from the appropriate next-of-kin, and organizing the surgical team for the recovery of organs and tissues.

When the organs or tissues are obtained, coordinators may be present in the operating room to help in the preparation and preservation for transplantation. Within the transplant center they may arrange for the final cross-matching and then admission of the suitable recipient. If the organ cannot be used by the local transplant program, the coordinator, using a national computer system, may arrange for the sharing and transporting of the recovered organ to another center—all in a time period short enough to ensure its viability.

Needless to say, one person cannot handle all the responsibilities described and many programs have a few persons hired under the general title of Transplant Coordinator. It must be recognized, however, that these centers work under conditions of extreme austerity and coordinators have learned to tap all available resources to ensure the efficacy of their programs.

With the Medicare involvement for end-stage renal disease in 1972, a network of procurement agencies were established throughout the entire United States. Since that time, there has been a mechanism established across the country to obtain and distribute cadaver organs and tissues for transplantation.

The National organ Transplant Act can improve and expand that organ sharing systems thereby allowing thousands more end-stage organ disease patients another chance at life that only a healthy donor organ can bring.

Title I of the National Organ Transplant Act authorizes a program of grants for the development and expansion of local organ procurement organizations throughout the nation and the establishment of U.S. Transplantation Network. In theory, this is an excellent idea, however, the application of those funds to these organizations should be appropriated with careful consideration to the potential recipient organizations. The establishment of U.S. Transplant Network would possibly include two national systems currently existing: The United Network of Organ Sharing—a computer that prints out most recipients awaiting a kidney and the NATCO 24-ALERT system.

The NATCO 24-ALERT system began on September 23, 1982. This system, accessed by telephone, gives the caller a listing of urgently needed livers, hearts and heart/lung combinations from the 15 transplant centers that perform these operations across the United States and Canada. This system is not in competition with the computerized United Network for Organ Sharing.

Since its inception one year ago, the 24-ALERT system has facilitated the transplantation of 122 livers at 9 centers, 73 hearts at 9 centers and 2 heart/lung combinations at 2 centers. The system's success is due to the fact it was designed by transplant coordinators to meet their specific needs. It is also successful because it's easily accessed by telephone. This telephone system can complement the computerized system mentioned as part of the National Organ Transplant Act.

NATCO supports the establishment of a Task Force to study carefully the various issues surrounding the field of transplantation. It is important that a clearer picture be obtained regarding the number of possible patients needing extra-renal transplants and the potential of available donors to meet those projected needs.

Title II of the bill revises title XVIII of the Social Security Act to permit the Secretary to pay for organ transplants and other investigative procedure at a limited umber of specialized centers. NATCO

Appendix 4, 1983 National Organ Transplant Hearings, A. Peele Testimony

strongly supports this provision of the bill because it will increase the number of medical centers performing extra-renal organ transplants across the country.

There has been much discussion over the past several months about the lack of donor livers for transplantation. The reality is that the University of Pittsburgh received 523 calls alerting them to the availability of donor livers in 1982. Only 80 of those livers were recovered and transplanted by the Pittsburgh program. 102 of the donor livers offered were declined by the Pittsburgh group because the transplant team was exhausted or the hospital could not accommodate another liver transplant patient.

So the shortage of donor livers is not as dramatic as portrayed by the news media. It is the lack of adequate liver transplant programs that precludes a larger number of patients from receiving therapeutic liver transplants.

Exempting organ procurement activities from the Medicare prospective payment plan shows a great deal of foresight on the part of Representative Gore. This action will continue to support the present system and allow for its growth. NATCO strongly agrees with title III of the bill prohibiting the sale of human organs and the penalties for violating this act.

The voluntary system of organ donation does work, buying and selling kidneys will only complicate the system not to mention the unethical aspects associated with this issue.

Our final recommendation to this committee is to suggest that the federal government, through the Joint Commission on The Accreditation of Hospitals (JCAH), mandate the establishment of policy and procedures in every hospital for the declaration of brain-death and for the referral of organ and tissue donors for transplantation. JCAH should require that upon every death in an accredited hospital, the deceased's next-of-kin be asked their position regarding organ and tissue donation.

In closing, I thank you for the opportunity to discuss NATCO's position regarding the National Organ Transplant Act. We, as coordinators, are aware that although a successful organ procurement system exists, there is need for improvement and expansion. The National Organ Transplant Act with our recommendations can bring about this improvement and expansion especially in the area of public education and professional participation in the transplanting of human organs and tissues.

Chairman JACOBS. Thank you.

Mr. MOORE. Thank you, Mr. Chairman.

Ms PEELE, the bill does call for the establishment of a task force on organ transplantation to conduct a comprehensive study, or study the very question you have raised. Would it appear to be more prudent for us to legislate perhaps a bill that would prohibit the sale of organs, and to set up a task force like this to find out what we are getting into, rather than pass a bill that regulates everything before we know what we are getting into?

Ms PEELE. In logic, that sounds very good, but I think there are a lot of patients right now who are suffering because they can't afford cyclosporine or transplantation. Some kind of effort needs to be extended, possibly legislatively, to at least start initiating or embarking on that journey, probably at the same time working with the task force.

Ms. MOORE. I see those questions as separate. There is no question that this Congress can address what it is going to pay for at any time, and we can do that. That to me is not so serious a question as having a better understanding of what we are getting into. Dr. Barnes stated he is strongly in agreement with moving ahead. I can understand his logic, even if I disagree with his conclusion. I wish my colleague, Mr. Rangel, had been here to hear how you very clearly say what the bill says, and that is my reading of the bill, too.

I just hate to tell Ms. Karsten that her 16 years worth of work is going out the window, because when I look at Houston, I see that there are two organizations there doing the same work. We have to choose one of the two. I don't want to be the one, and I don't think that HHS either wants to be the one to tell her that she is out of business.

There are too many people doing the soliciting, and there are too many people doing the collecting, I think that this was Dr. Barnes' statement. He suggested that we have to get down to a regionalized process in which one agency is doing that. To me this means that the Government, through its certification

Appendix 4, 1983 National Organ Transplant Hearings, A. Peele Testimony

program, has got to tell others to get out of the business. I am not really sure that we ought to do that without at least having the task force look into this deeper.

This way my question, doesn't the task force seem to be more logical to approach before we start getting into all of this certification business? We have the administration saying it doesn't want to do it, and many of us have grave questions about the necessity of doing it.

Ms PEELE. I follow your logic, but I think that it is a stalling tactic. I think that they need to get into it, but I think they have to come across with, either we are not going to do it, or we want to study it, and that is what we are going to do again. We are not making too much headway in terms of coming up with answers.

Mr. MOORE. I think the progress you all have made has been astounding, and it is very promising, it is very helpful. We are not living in a perfect world where every patient has got a donor. Don't think that the Government is going to create that perfect world, just look at some of the other programs that we have looked at, and draw that conclusion. Dr. Barnes, did you want to say something about my using your name in vain?

Dr. BARNES. I think the map here locating the organ procurement agencies really illustrates the problem. If you were trying to devise a distribution of organ procurement agencies on some rational basis, it wouldn't have the chaotic scatter that you see. Something has to be done to get them working together. It is really a multiregional operation. You can't have five in one or two counties, and it really doesn't make sense because of the elaborate nature of the operation of a tissue-typing laboratory and the costs of redundant preservation laboratories.

We think the existing interests in organ procurement that we have heard today about are just that: they are very strong, parochial interests. Someone with authority, and we see none except the Federal Government, has to bring these groups together and provide incentives to work together. The fragmentation will continue indefinitely as at present unless there is some incentive provided, and I only see it coming from Washington.

Mr. MOORE. You may be right, but I sure would like to see a task force stating that before we pass a bill saying what we have to do. The simple reason is my concern over undermining the motivation that could Mrs. Karsten, and the other individuals and organizations here, to do their work. We are then telling them, thanks, but no thanks, we don't need you anymore. We are going to have another group carry out these activities.

I see the same problem with raising money for universities. We can claim that there is too much diffusion in raising money for private universities, so we are going to have the Government determine that there is going to be one organization in a region that going to raise money for all the colleges around the country. It is not a lifesaving thing, but how we educate our children is very important. We raise money, and all kinds of people do it differently.

I am just yet unconvinced that the Federal Government has to come in and solve what I consider to be certainly growing pain problems, but not problems that require the heavy hand of the Federal Government. I am just not convinced of that yet, although I am totally in sympathy, and I don't think you are going to find anybody on this committee who doesn't agree 100 percent with what you are trying to get at. Where we part company, at least I do, is over the necessity of the Federal Government doing it for us.

I will go along with the study, this task force to look into it. If the study comes back and says, Congressman, you are all wet, we would think about it. She is a nice lady, and she is doing a great job. I hesitate to have the heavy hand of the Federal Government get involved in that. I have seen the Federal Government operate, and I am not fully impressed, to say the least, with what it has done so far in terms of helping people.

Chairman JACOBS. I would have to say this, Henson, in the U.S. Government versus Mrs. Karsten, I think she would win. [Laughter.]

Thank you for your testimony.

Appendix 4, 1983 National Organ Transplant Hearings, A. Peele Testimony

[Whereupon, at 2:20 p.m., the hearing was adjourned.]

[Submissions for the record follow:]

All of the NOTA testimony was taken from:

Bernard D. Reams. A Legislative History of Pub.L.No. 98-507. Volumes 1-3. ISBN 0-89941-691-8. William s. Hein and Company, Inc. 1990.

Reams is a Professor of Law and Director, Law Library for the Washington University in Saint Louis.

Tables

Table	Title of Table
1	Evolution of "Titles" for the Transplant Coordinator
2	Philosophy of Transplant Coordination–Early Statement
3	Syllabus from Second Meeting (First "Organized" Meeting) of US Transplant Coordinators, August 19-20, 1976
4	Syllabus from Third US Transplant Coordinators Meeting, April 6-7, 1978
5	Syllabus from Fourth Meeting of US Transplant Coordinators Meeting: May 30-31, 1979 (NATCO Founded at This Meeting)
6	American Board of Transplant Coordinators Chairmen, 1987
7	Purposes and Accomplishments and Activities of the American Board of Transplant Coordinators
8	Transplant Coordinator Societies
9	First International Transplant Coordinators Meeting, August 29, 1994

Chapter 1: THE HISTORY OF THE TRANSPLANT COORDINATOR

Table 1. EVOLUTION OF "TITLES" FOR THE TRANSPLANT COORDINATOR

Procurement of Organs *and* Care of Recipients–Dual Role
Transplant coordinator
Procurement Roles
Donor management—primary duty
Organ procurement officer
Transplant coordinator
Organ retrieval coordinator
Organ procurement coordinator
Organ recovery coordinator
Organ donation coordinator
Donation coordinator
Donation clinical specialist
Family requesting (consent)—primary duty
Requestor
Minority requestor
Family liaison
Donor family services coordinator
Family support coordinator, family support specialist
Operative recovery of organs—primary duty
Perfusion technician
Operating room technician
Assistant organ procurement coordinator
Donation support specialist
Development of hospital donation systems—primary role
Hospital development coordinator
Hospital development specialist
Hospital liaison
Donation system specialist
Clinical Roles
Clinical care of the transplant recipient—primary duty
Nurse coordinator
Transplant coordinator
Clinical transplant coordinator
Recipient coordinator
Transplant recipient coordinator
Pretransplant coordinator
Posttransplant coordinator
Transplant evaluation coordinator
Living donor workup coordinator

A CLINICIAN'S GUIDE TO DONATION AND TRANSPLANTATION

Table 2. PHILOSOPHY OF TRANSPLANT COORDINATION—EARLY STATEMENT

Philosophy of Transplant Coordination

Human life is sacred and valued; however, in instances in which life is certain to end but organs and tissues of the dying person would enable another to live or live more fully, donation to the living may result. To donate an organ or tissue is to give the gift of life itself. Organ and tissue donation represents a degree of sacrifice and the donor's next of kin must decide whether to donate. Human beings have the capability to make rational decisions, and deserve support and respect both during and following that decision-making process. They have the right to awareness of all alternatives before a decision can be exacted. All associated healthcare providers must be considered part of those affected when organ and/or tissue donation is being considered or has been decided by those legally responsible.

Transplant/Organ Procurement Coordinators are individuals with advanced skills and knowledge who work with affected persons, groups, agencies, and fellow healthcare team members in activities related to organ and tissue procurement and transplantation. These activities include, but are not limited to, explaining alternatives, obtaining consent, supporting grieving family members and significant others in their decisions (regardless of the direction of choice), managing details related to the procurement, preservation, transportation, and receiving of organs and tissues, and education of healthcare professionals and the general public as to the concept of organ and tissue donation.

Transplant/Organ Procurement Coordinators value human life and promote renewed quality of life. We value the psychological health of the grieving family and significant others as well as the physiological health of transplant recipients. We value the philosophies of life and death held by those who speak for the donors, and support whatever religious and/or ethical precepts **are** inherent in their decision process.

Our goal is to increase the number of organs and tissues available for transplantation, improve support to the family of the donor, facilitate the preservation and utilization of donated organs and tissues, and to increase public and professional awareness of the value of and need for organ and tissue donation and transplantation.

We serve a variety of clients. These include the dying patient (the donor), the donor's family, the affected healthcare providers, the support personnel who work with the family, the affected staff in the receiving center, and the general public.

Continued .....

Table 2. PHILOSOPHY OF TRANSPLANT COORDINATION–EARLY STATEMENT, continued

We provide the following professional services: 1) assessment of potential donors, 2) consultation with relevant persons, organizations, and groups, 3) management of details related to obtaining, preserving, and transporting of organs, 4) counseling with donor's families and obtaining consent. The Transplant/Organ Procurement Coordinator also develops systems of procurement for hospitals, collects follow-up data on recipients, receives imported organs and tissues and conducts surveillance of the patient population. In summary, our responsibilities include assessment, teaching consulting, counseling, management, data collection, and evaluation.

The settings for practice for the Transplant/Organ Procurement Coordinator may be defined as any setting in which a potential donor can be found. Typically, these settings include critical care areas for major vital organ donors, but may occur anywhere in the healthcare facility for tissue donors. The coordinator also practices when addressing community groups.

We, as coordinators, are responsible to the transplant physician(s), institutional policies, and to the attending and procuring physicians for the donor; however, in many respects, the coordinator is an independent practitioner, particularly in relation to the teaching, collaborative, counseling, and consultative roles.

Theories and principles used in practice by the Transplant/Procurement Coordinator may vary according to the function being performed and the coordinator's individual preferences; however, the theories and principles common to the practice of most of all coordinators include problem-solving, communication, management, and teaching-learning.

In order to educate individuals to assume or refine their role as Transplant/Organ Procurement Coordinators, certain approaches to education are preferable. These include active learning, role-play, simulations, and case studies. Learners are responsible for their own learning; instructors are responsible to identify needed content, help learners assess their own learning needs, and facilitate the learner's progress during the educational process.

These are the duties, goals, and philosophy to which we, as health care professionals, adhere, aspire toward and ever seek to attain. In summary, *primum non nocere*. The NATCO dedication displays our goal for the individuals we serve: "That there be a better quality of life for the thousands of patients with end-stage organ failure…and a respect for those who shared."

(source: *NATCO Procurement Training Course Manual*, 1985)[26]

Table 3. SYLLABUS FROM SECOND MEETING (FIRST "ORGANIZED" MEETING) OF US TRANSPLANT COORDINATORS, AUGUST 19-20, 1976

TRANSPLANT COORDINATORS WORKSHOP
August 19 and 20, 1976

New York Blood Center
310 East 67th Street
New York, NY 10021

This first Transplant Coordinators Workshop brings together the members of a newly evolving professional group dealing with organ procurement and clinical transplantation.

THURSDAY, AUGUST 19TH
- 8:00 Registration
- 9:00 Announcements - JUSTINE WILLMERT, R.N.
  Welcome - LOUIS BAKER, Ph.D.

I. Present and Future Roles of Organ Retrieval Coordinators
JOHN BLEIFUSS - Moderator
- 9:15 JOHN BLEIFUSS   MARY ANN FARNSWORTH, R.N.
       SHAWNEY FINE, R.N.   ROBERT HOFFMAN
       PAUL TAYLOR   KEITH JOHNSON, M.D.
- 10:45 Coffee Break

II. Clinical Transplant Coordinators
GLORIA HORNS, R.N. - Moderator
- 11:00 Job Description of Nurse Coordinator
  BARBARA SCHANBACHER, R.N.
- 11:15 Telephone Follow-up Care of the Transplanted Patient
  LOIS BARTELL, R.N.
- 11:30 Role of the Nurse Coordinator in the Selection of Cadaver Recipients
  RAIJA K. PONKANEN, R.N.
  (CAROLYN GYERDE was written in over the above name, which had been crossed through, in NATCO copy of brochure)
- 11:45 Discussion
- 12:00 Lunch

III. Discussion of Cadaver Kidney Sharing
WESLEY L. DIXON - Moderator
- 1:30 WESLEY L. DIXON   SHAWNEY FINE, R.N.
       GERDA H. LIPCAMAN   MILDRED YOUNG, R.N.
       GLORIA HORNS, R.N.   GENE A PIERCE
       GERALDINE RASMUSSEN   BERNARD COHEN, DRS.
- 3:30 Adjournment

Table 3. SYLLABUS FROM SECOND MEETING (FIRST "ORGANIZED" MEETING) OF US TRANSPLANT COORDINATORS, AUGUST 19-20, 1976, continued

FRIDAY, AUGUST 20TH

IV. **Transplant Patient Education**
   CYNTHIA FORSMAN, RN - MODERATOR
   (BARB *was written in over the above name, which had been crossed through, in NATCO copy of brochure*)

9:00	Transplant Patient's Viewpoint ELEANOR SHUGART, REPRESENTING NAPHT
9:15	Patient Teaching LINDA JONES, R.N.
9:45	Discussion
10:00	Coffee Break

V. **Public and Professional Education**
   GERALDINE RASMUSSEN - MODERATOR

10:15	Public Education - Prevention of Kidney Disease IRA GREIFER, M.D.
10:35	Comprehensive Approach to a National Education Program LAWRENCE CHILNICK
10:55	Approaching Potential Cadaver Families SAMUEL KOUNTZ, M.D.
11:15	Inclusion of Education Expenses in the Standard Kidney Acquisition Fee PHILIP JOS
11:35	Discussion
12:00	Lunch
1:30	**VI. Business Meeting** **BARBARA SCHULMAN, R.N. - MODERATOR**
3:30	Adjournment

Acknowledgements: Upjohn Drug Company

→ **Cocktail** ←
Party
at the New York Blood Center
Thursday, August, 19, 1976
5:00 P.M.
Hostess and Host:
Geraldine Rasmussen
And
Dr. Louis Baker

Table 4. SYLLABUS FROM THIRD US TRANSPLANT COORDINATORS MEETING, APRIL 6-7, 1978

TRANSPLANT COORDINATORS WORKSHOP
April 6-7, 1978
Fawcett Center for Tomorrow
2400 Olentangy River Road
Columbus, Ohio

8:00 a.m.	Registration
9:00 a.m.	Welcome
	James Cerilli, MD
9:05 a.m.	The Clinical Criteria of Brain Death
	George Poulson, MD
10:00 a.m.	Tissue Typing and its Relationship to the Nursing Care of the Renal Transplant Patient
	Paul Terasaki, PhD
11:00 a.m.	The role of the ESRD Coordinator/Advocate
	Pat King
11:30 a.m.	LUNCH – CENTER FOR TOMORROW
1:30 p.m.	11:30 a.m. Lunch - Center for Tomorrow
1:30 p.m.	The ALG Controversy and its Effects on Patient Care
	Dick Condie, M.D.
	Oscar Salvatierra, M.D.
	Pat Carr, R.N.
	Cindy Forsman, R.N., B.A.
3:00	2nd Transplant Coordinator's Business Meeting
4:30	Social Hour - Open Bar
Evening - Free	

Friday, April 7, 1978
CONCURRENT NURSING SESSIONS

Selections can be made from either group. Please select 2 sessions in the morning and 2 sessions in the afternoon. Indicate your selections I the space provided on the registration form. Do not select more than 4 sessions.

Morning

SESSION #1 9:00 a.m. Acute Renal Failure and Its Effects on Other Body Systems
Charold Baer, R.N., Ph.D.

SESSION #2 1:30 p.m. The Nursing Care of the Renal Transplant Diabetic Patient
Lois Bartell, R.N., B.S.
Milton Boisvin, R.N.

SESSION #3 10:30 a.m. Related Donors—Cost and Gains
Roberta Simmons, Ph.D.

**Table 4. SYLLABUS FROM THIRD US TRANSPLANT
COORDINATORS MEETING, APRIL 6-7, 1978, continued**

SESSION #4 10:30 a.m. Pathogenesis of Rejection
        James Cerilli, M.D.

11:30 a.m. LUNCH - Center for Tomorrow

Afternoon

(Sessions above repeated exactly as they are above, renamed Sessions 5, 6, 7 and 8; the times being 1:30 and 3:00 respectively. – Authors Note)

CONCURRENT ORGAN PROCUREMENT AND PRESERVATION SESSIONS

Selections can be made from either group. Please select 2 sessions in the morning and 2 sessions in the afternoon. Indicate your selections in the space provided on the registration form. Do not select more than 4 sessions.

Morning
SESSION A   9:00 a.m. The Cadaveric Donor Dilemma—Are We Educating or
        Alienating Our Supportive Resources?
                Pat Garrison, Transplant Coordinator
                Paul Taylor, B.S., Transplant Coordinator
                David Yashon, M.D.
                Richard Weil, lll, M.D.
                Don Wilson
                Dana Lee
SESSION B   9:00 a.m. The Role of Tissue Typing with Cadaver Donors
                Norman C. Kramer, M.D.
                Janis Ball, Chief Technologist
SESSION C 10:30 a.m. Physicians Assistant & Their Role in Cadaver Kidney
        Nephrectomy
                Ewing von Schmittow, P.A.
                Bruce Wilsom, P.A.
                Mark Reiner, P.A.
SESSION D 10:30 a.m. Emotional Factors of the Potential Cadaveric Recipient
                Joanne Bonish, R.N.

11:30 a.m. LUNCH – CENTER FOR TOMORROW

Afternoon

(Sessions above repeated exactly as they are above, renamed Sessions E, F, G and H; the times being 1:30 and 3:00 respectively—Authors Note)

Table 4. SYLLABUS FROM THIRD US TRANSPLANT COORDINATORS MEETING, APRIL 6-7, 1978, continued

OHIO STATE UNIVERSITY PROGRAM SPEAKERS		
Pat Carr, R.N. Head Nurse, Transplant Unit 9 West 410 W. Tenth Avenue Columbus, Ohio 43210	Pat King Administrative Associate 4950 University Hospitals Clinic Ohio State University Hospital Columbus, Ohio 43210	George Paulson, M.D. Clinical Professor of Neurology The Ohio State University 931 Chatam Lane Columbus, Ohio 43221
James Cerilli, M.D. Professor, Department of Surgery Transplant Program N-723 University Hospital 410 W. Tenth Avenue Columbus, Ohio 43210	Mr. Dana Lee Student Body President The Ohio State University Columbus, Ohio 43210	David Yashon, M.D. Professor of Surgery Department of Neurosurgery University Hospital Columbus, Ohio 43210
GUEST PROGRAM SPEAKERS		
Charold Baer, R.N., Ph.D. Project Director, ONA 4000 E. Main Street Columbus, Ohio	Oscar Salvatierra, M.D. Associate Professor of Surgery and Urology Chief, Transplant Service Univ. of California Medical Ctr. 3rd and Parnassus San Francisco, California 94943	Pat Garrison Transplant Coordinator Phoenix Transplant Coordination Service Good Samaritan Hospital 1033 East McDowell Road Phoenix, Arizona 85006
Milton Boisvin, R.N. Inservice Nurse Station 22 University of Minnesota Minneapolis, Minnesota 55455	Ewing von Schmittow, P.A. Director of Organ Procurement Nashville Transplant Program 2416 Hillsboro Road Nashville, Tennessee 37203	Paul Taylor, B.S. Transplant Coordinator University of Colorado 4200 East 9th Avenue, c-305 Denver, Colorado 80262
Lois Bartell, R.N., B.S. Transplant Patient Instructor Box 116 - Mayo Station 22 University of Minnesota Hospital Minneapolis, Minnesota 555455	Roberta Simmons, Ph.D. Professor of Sociology and Psychiatry 1067 Social Service Building University of Minnesota Minneapolis, Minnesota 55455	Paul Terasaki, Ph.D. Professor of Surgery UCLA 1000 Veterans Avenue Los Angeles, California 90024
Norman C. Kramer, M.D. Director, Tissue Typing Lab George Washington University MC Room 411 Ross Hall 2300 Eye Street, N.W. Washington, D.C. 20037	Janis Ball Chief Technologist George Washington University Medical Center Room 411 Ross Hall 2300 Eye Street, N.W. Washington, D.C. 20037	Richard Weil, III, M.D. Associate Professor of Surgery Director, Renal Transplant Program University of Colorado Medical Center Denver, Colorado 82602
Joanne Bonish, R.N. Akron City Hospital 525 E. Market Street Akron, Ohio 44309	Dick Condie, M.D. Instructor, Dept. of Surgery Director of ALG Program P.O. Box 383 University of Minnesota Hospital Minnesota, Minnesota 55455	Bruce Wilson, P.A. Nashville Transplant Program 2416 Hillsboro Road Nashville, Tennessee 37203
Mark Reiner, P.A. Nashville Transplant Program 2416 Hillsboro Road Nashville, Tennessee 37203	Cindy Forsman, R.N., B.A. Head Nurse Renal Transplant- Station 22 Univ. of Minnesota Hospital Minneapolis, Minnesota 55455	Don Wilson Associate Minister First Christian Church 6750 N. 7th Avenue Phoenix, Arizona 85006

Chapter 1 — THE HISTORY OF THE TRANSPLANT COORDINATOR

Table 5. FOURTH MEETING OF US TRANSPLANT COORDINATORS MEETING: MAY 30-31, 1979 SYLLABUS (NATCO FOUNDED AT THIS MEETING)

NORTH AMERICAN TRANSPLANT COORDINATORS ORGANIZATION
ANNUAL MEETING
MAY 30-31, 1979
HOLIDAY INN, CHICAGO CITY CENTRE
300 EAST CHICAGO STREET
312-787-6100

PROVIDING A SERVICE.....
FULFILLING A PURPOSE

GENERAL INFORMATION

This two day session will touch many aspects of the broad field of Organ Transplantation. The program is directed at persons who actively participate in transplant programs in an effort to disseminate relevant information, promote greater utilization of transplantable tissues and to apprise ourselves of current advances in the field.

A variety of group sessions are also included. Convention attendees are encouraged to participate so as to expand the scope of the topics.

* *

GUEST SPEAKERS

Jessie E. Hano, M.D. Chief, Section of Renal Disease Loyola University Medical Center Stritch School of Medicine Maywood, Illinois	James Wolf, M.D. Professor of Surgery Director, Organ Transplant Unit Northwestern University Medical Center Chicago, Illinois
Mary Ann Gideon, R.N., Ph.D. Albert Einstein Medical Center Philadelphia, Pennsylvania	Peter McConnachie, Ph.D. Memorial Medical Center Springfield, Illinois
Robert J. Corry, M.D. Professor of Surgery Director, Organ Transplant Unit University of Iowa Iowa City, Iowa	Israel Penn, M.D. Professor of Surgery Chief, Surgical Service Veterans Administration Hospital Denver, Colorado
Paul Balter, M.D. Nephrologist West Suburban Kidney Center Oak Park, Illinois	Thomas E. Starzl, M.D. Professor and Chairman Department of Surgery University of Colorado Medical Center Denver, Colorado

Table 5. FOURTH MEETING OF US TRANSPLANT COORDINATORS MEETING: MAY 30-31, 1979 SYLLABUS (NATCO FOUNDED AT THIS MEETING), continued

PROGRAM – WEDNESDAY, MAY 30, 1979

9:00 - 9:15   Welcome
Paul D. Taylor
Chairman
Steering Committee

9:15 - 9:35   Cost Effectiveness of Treatment of Chronic Renal Failure
Jessie E. Hano, M.D.
9:45 - 10:05   Quality of Life on Dialysis
Paul Balter, M.D.
10:05 - 10:25   Quality of Life With Transplantation
James Wolf, M.D.
10:45 - 11:45   Coffee Break
11:15 - 11:45   The Transplant Coordinator Thru The Eyes of a Transplant Surgeon
Robert J. Corry, M.D.
12:15 - 1:30   Lunch

PROGRAM – WEDNESDAY AFTERNOON, MAY 30, 1979

2:00 p.m.   BUSINESS MEETING (Badges Required for Admission)

         A.   Final Report, Minutes, Financial Report, Columbus Meeting
                 Justine Wilmert, R.N.
         B.   Approval of Agenda - This Meeting
         C.   Discussion of Proposed By-Laws. The Revisions, Amendments, Deletions, Vote to Adopt.

3:30 p.m.   Coffee Break

3:45 p.m.   A.   Affiliation Proposals
               B.   Long-Term Capitalization
                     (1)   Transplant Agency
                             Paul D. Taylor
                     (2)   Memberships - Each Person
                             Kate Hume
               C.   Unfinished Business
               D.   New Business
               E.   Election of Officers

5:00 - 6:30 p.m.

Cocktails

Table 5. FOURTH MEETING OF US TRANSPLANT COORDINATORS MEETING: MAY 30-31, 1979 SYLLABUS (NATCO FOUNDED AT THIS MEETING), continued

PROGRAM – THURSDAY, MAY 31, 1979
WORKSHOPS

9:00 - 10:00 a.m.

Session A. Modalities of perfusion
 (1) In-vivo
 (2) Ex-vivo
 Leaders: *Bob Hoffman and Sandy Seim*

Session B. Patient rights and liability of transplant personnel
 Leader:

Session C. Pre and post of patients care plan, instructions, tools & standards
 Leader: *Amy S. Peele*

10:15 - 11:15 a.m.
Session A. Concept of body image and nursing implications for the transplant nurse
 Leader: *Kate Hume*

Session B. Stress & acceptance of chronic renal failure
 Leaders: *Patricia Collins and Della Herzog*

Session C. Education of donor referral sources
 Leader: *Mary Ann Farnsworth*

11:30 - 12:30 p.m.

Session A. Procurement cost containment
 (1) Cadaver
 (2) Living Related
 Leader: *Bruce Crowthers*

Session B. Basic tissue typing & immunology
 Leader: *Peter McConnachie*

Session C. Psychological aspects of living related donor and his family
 Leader: *Trisha Barber*

12:30 - 2:00 p.m. Lunch (Do your own thing!)

Table 5. FOURTH MEETING OF US TRANSPLANT COORDINATORS MEETING: MAY 30-31, 1979 SYLLABUS (NATCO FOUNDED AT THIS MEETING), continued

PROGRAM – THURSDAY AFTERNOON, MAY 31, 1979
WORKSHOPS

2:00 - 3:00 p.m.

Session A. Cadaver Donor Criteria
            Leader: *Ewing von Schmittow*

Session B. How to Handle Public Relations Commercialism of Product
            Leader: *Paul D. Taylor*

Session C. Stress of Nursing Staff - The Burn Out Phenomenon
            Leader: *Peggy Snodgrass*

3:15 - 4:15 p.m.

Session A. The Concept of Sexuality and Nursing Complications in the Transplanted Patient
            Leader: *Israel Penn, M.D.*

Session B. Dealing with the Grieving Family (Death and Dying)
            Leader: *Mary Ann Gideon*

Session C. (1) Multiple Tissue Recovery
            (2) Cannulation of Multiple Arteries
            Leaders: *Bob Gosnell and Dave Mainous*

<u>Main Meeting Room</u>

4:30 - 5:00 p.m.   Past, Present and Future of Organ Transplantation
                   Thomas E. Starzl, M.D.

5:00 - 5:30 p.m.   General membership

                   (1) Passing out documents
                   (2) Program evaluation
                   (3) Etcetera!

Adjournment

Table 5. FOURTH MEETING OF US TRANSPLANT COORDINATORS MEETING:
MAY 30-31, 1979 SYLLABUS (NATCO FOUNDED AT THIS MEETING), continued

WORKSHOP PARTICIPANTS	
Sandra Seim Preservation Technologist Rush-Presbyterian St. Lukes Medical Center Chicago, Illinois	Peter McConnicy, Ph.D. Tissue Typist Memorial Medical Center Springfield, Illinois
Bob Hoffman Transplant Coordinator University of Wisconsin Madison, Wisconsin	Trisha Barber Nurse Practitioner University of Illinois Medical Center Chicago, Illinois
Dave Mainous Transplant Coordinator Indiana University Medical Center Indianapolis, Indiana	Robert Gosnell Director of Administration and Organ Recovery South Texas Organ Bank Inc. San Antonio, TX
Amy S. Peele, R.N. Transplant Coordinator Northwestern University Medical Center Chicago, Illinois	Paul D. Taylor Transplant Coordinator Department of Surgery University of Colorado Medical Center Denver, Colorado
Patricia Collins, R.N. Dialysis Nurse Veterans Administration Medical Center Hines, Illinois	Peggy D. Taylor Transplant Coordinator Department of Surgery University of Colorado Medical Center Denver, Colorado
Della Herzog, R.N. Dialysis Nurse Veterans Administration Medical Center Hines, Illinois	Peggy Snodgrass, M.S.N. Psychiatric Clinical Specialist Veterans Administration Medical Center Hines, Illinois
Mary Ann Farnsworth, R.N. Transplant Coordinator University of Oregon Medical Center Portland, Oregon	Howell Warner Transplant Coordinator Vanderbilt University Medical Center Nashville, Tennessee
Bruce Crowthers, B.A. Assistant to Executive Vice-President Northwestern Memorial Hospital Chicago, Illinois	Ewing S. von Schmittou Physician Assistant Nashville Transplant Program Nashville, Tennessee

A CLINICIAN'S GUIDE TO DONATION AND TRANSPLANTATION

Table 6. AMERICAN BOARD OF TRANSPLANT COORDINATORS, 1987

AMERICAN BOARD OF TRANSPLANT COORDINATORS

Board of Governors

CHAIRMAN
Louise M. Jacobbi
Louisiana Organ Sharing Program
P.O. Box 33932
1501 Kings Highway
Shreveport, LA 71130-33932

VICE CHAIRMAN *Anita Principe* Montefiore Hospital 111 E. 210th Street Bronx, NY 10467 (212) 920-5184	**CREDENTIALS – CLINICAL** *Sue Dutton* Post Transplant Coordinator UTMB B-23 Room IJ10.33 Galveston, TX 77550 (409) 761-1451 Committee Members: • Eileen DeMayo (CA), Elaine Vuyosevich (TN)
TREASURER/SECRETARY Michael L. Baker 800 South Wells, Suite 190 Chicago, IL 60607 (312)431-3600 or 3605	**JUDICIARY** Barbara Schulman ROPA of Southern California 1000 Veteran Avenue Los Angeles, CA 90024 (213) 825-7651
EXAMINATION – PROCUREMENT Robert Duckworth Nebraska Organ Retrieval 4060 Vinton Street, #102 Omaha, NE 68105 (402)553-7952 Committee Members: • Amy Peele (CA), Louise Jacobbi (LA), Barbara Schulman (CA), Jim Springer (MO), Jane Warmbrodt (KS), Michael Baker (IL)	**CREDENTIALS – PROCUREMENT** Amy S. Peele Transplant Resource Services 438 Chestnut Street San Francisco, CA 94133 (415) 391-9949 Committee Members: • Roger Smith (CA), Phyllis Weber (CA)
EXAMINATION – CLINICAL Barbara A. Schanbacher University of Iowa Hospital Department of Surgery Iowa City, IA 52242 (319) 356-3585 Committee Members: • Anita Principe (NY), Patricia Hansen (NY), Laurel Williams (NE), Sue Dutton m(TX), Louise Jacobbi (LA), Barbara Elick (MN)	**CONTINUING CERTIFICATION** Jane M. Warmbrodt Midwest Organ Bank 4006 Central Kansas City, MO 64111 (816) 361-8744 Committee Members: • Bonnie Sammons (FL), Howard Adams (CA), Linda Johnson (TX), Sue Ellen Marfriott (NE), Cheryl Westlake (CA)

Table 7. PURPOSES AND ACCOMPLISHMENTS AND ACTIVITIES OF THE AMERICAN BOARD OF TRANSPLANT COORDINATORS

- Established a national certification system for entry level procurement and clinical transplant coordinators,
- Maintains a registry of health care professionals who meet the standards for certification in transplant coordination,
- Conducts examination of eligible candidates who seek certification and recertification,
- Issues credentialing certificates to candidates who meet the certification and recertification requirements,
- Developed a recertification process for qualified candidates, and
- Promotes and acknowledges the profession and professionals practicing transplant coordination.

Table 8. TRANSPLANT COORDINATOR SOCIETIES

American Board of Transplant Coordinators	ABTC
Australasian Transplant Coordinators Association	ATCA
Canadian Association of Transplantation	CAT
European Transplant Coordinators Organization	ETCO
International Transplant Coordinators Society	ITCS
Japanese Transplant Coordinators Organization	JATCO
North American Transplant Coordinators Organization	NATCO
United Kingdom Transplant Coordinators Association	UKTCA

Table 9. FIRST INTERNATIONAL TRANSPLANT COORDINATORS MEETING, AUGUST 29, 1994

International Transplant Coordinators Meeting (ITCM)
(first meeting, held just prior to the ITCS formation)
Kyoto International Conference Hall

Kyoto, Japan
August 29, 1994

PROGRAM

15:05-15:15 Presidential Address
  Takagi, H. (Nagoya/Japan), ITCM Honorary President
  Hiraga, Seigo (Isehara/Japan), ITCM President

15:15-16:40 Workshop: International report of activity of transplant coordinators and transplant coordination

  Chairs: Taylor, Paul D. (Pittsburgh/USA)
    Tamaki Isao (Hachioji/Japan)

  1. Report on transplant coordination in the United States: background, profile. Shafer, Teresa (Fort Worth/USA)
  2. Coordinating organ donation and transplantation in Europe and the role of legislative, organizational and educational incentives. Roels, Leo (Leuven/Belgium)
  3. Transplant activities in Singapore. Tan, Sally (Singapore)
  4. Transplant co-ordination and co-ordination in Australia. Armstrong, Greg T. (Brisbane/Australia)
  5. Current state of transplant coordinators in Japan. Kato, Osamu (Nagoya/Japan)

16:45-17:35 Free Papers-Session 1

  Chairs: Shafer, Teresa (Fort Worth/USA)
    Hattori, C. (Osaka/Japan)

  1. Proposal concerning a standardized European professional education program for transplant coordinators. Karbe, Thomas (Hamburg, Germany)
  2. A review of donation and utilization of donated organs in Australia. Armstrong, Greg T. (Brisbane/Australia)
  3. Lessons learned from and lessons for Scandinavian cadaveric organ procurement programs. Gabel, Haken; Ahonen, J; Sodal, G; Lamm, L (Stockholm, Sweden)
  4. Current state and future challenges of a coordinator for organ transplantation. Nakahara, Noriko; Yuasa, Mitsutoshi; Yasui, Yutaka; Fujiwara, Masae; Konaka, Setsuko; Nojiri, Masahiro (Osaka, Japan)
  5. International training course on transplant coordination. Manyalich, Marti; Cabrer, C.A.; Valere, R.; Matesanz, R. (Barcelona/Spain)

Table 9. FIRST INTERNATIONAL TRANSPLANT COORDINATORS MEETING, AUGUST 29, 1994, continued

17:35-18:25 Free Papers-Session 2

    Chairs: Roels, Leo (Leuven/Belgium)
                     Ichiki, Junko (Saitama/Japan)

1. Transplant co-ordination in the U.K.
   Falvey, Susan J. (Cambridge/UK)
2. The role of the recipient transplant coordinator.
   Gleeson, Alice P; Jones, R.M. (Melbourne/Australia)
3. Legal basis, principles and unsolved problems in organization of organ donation in Russia. Konstaninov, Boris A; Dzemeshkevich, S.L.; Solovyvov, A.N. (Moscow/Russia)
4. Multi-organ procurement in Japan.
   Nishigaki, F., Hirano, T., Chikaraoka, T. (Sapporo/Japan)
5. The problems of domestic long distant kidney graft transportation in Japan. Nishigaki, Fumitaka; Hirano, Tetsuo; Chikaraoka, Tatsuya (Sapporo, Japan)

18:25-19:25 Free Papers-Session 3

    Chairs: Tan, S. (Singapore)
                     Nakata, A. (Ehime/Japan)

1. Heart transplant experience in University of Sao Paulo Medical School Hospital. Tominaga, Motomu E.; Stolf, N.A.G.; Nakira, K., Tsuzuki, S.; Jatene, A.D. (Sao Paulo/Brazil)
2. The role of kidney transplant coordinator in Okinawa and its nationwide distribution. Takaesu, Asao; Arakaki, Yoshitaka; Nakamura, Nobuyuki; Yogi, Takashi; Genka, Osamu; Iwasaki, Misuoki; Yakena, Tetsu (Okinawa/Japan)
2. Experience from a new transplant centre in Denmark
   Tram, Elise Marie (Aarhus/Denmark)
4. Tissue bank network in the Kinki region of Japan
   Niwaya, Kazuo; Motomura, Noburo; Yuasa, Mitsutoshi; Kitamura, Soichiro (Nara/Japan)
5. Transplant Procurement Management (TPM)
   Manyalich, Marti; Cabrer, C.A., Garcia-Fages, L.C., Valero, R., Salvador, L., Matesanz, R. (Barcelona/Spain)
6. Huge discrepancy between declared support of organ donation and actual rate of consent for organ retrieval. Schutt, Gabriele; Smit, Heiner; Dancker, Gernot (Kiel/Germany)

19:25-19:30 Closing Remarks: Mitsutoshi Yuasa (Osaka/Japan)
              ITCM Vice President, Director of Scientific Program Committee

19:40-21:45 Party in the room "SWAN " (B1F)

A CLINICIAN'S GUIDE TO DONATION AND TRANSPLANTATION

Chapter 1

Figures

Figure	Title of Figure
1	Second Transplant Coordinators Meeting, New York City, NY *(Technically, the first meeting was in Los Angeles—this was the first formal meeting with an organized agenda and brochure)*
2	First NATCO Committee Roster, 1979-1980
3	Second NATCO Committee Roster, 1980-1981
4	Third NATCO Committee Roster, 1981-1982
5	First National Proclamation of National Organ Donation Awareness Week
6	Notice of Organ Transplant Hearings, April 6, 1983
7	Brandon Hall Received a Liver During National Organ Transplant Hearings but Died Following Transplantation
8	Certificate of Merit Given to Faye Davis, Creator of NATCO Procurement Training Course, Shows Many Signatures of Pioneer Transplant Coordinators, 1982
9	NATCO Newsletter Article on 24-ALERT
10	UNOS Resolution Recognizing NATCO Upon Receiving 24-ALERT Computer Donor Organ Matching System From NATCO
11	Press Release: UNOS Receiving 24-ALERT from NATCO, pages 1 and 2
12	Story on Transplant Coordinators Features Amy Peele
13	The Typical Transplant Coordinator
14	First Publication of Transplant Coordinator Job Duties, 1980
15	Invitation to First International Transplant Coordinators Society Meeting Party, Kyoto, Japan, 1994
16	NATCO Procurement Training Course Brochure cover, October 21-27, 1985

Figure 1. Second Transplant Coordinators Meeting, New York City, NY
(Technically, the first meeting was in Los Angeles—this was the first formal meeting with an organized agenda and brochure)

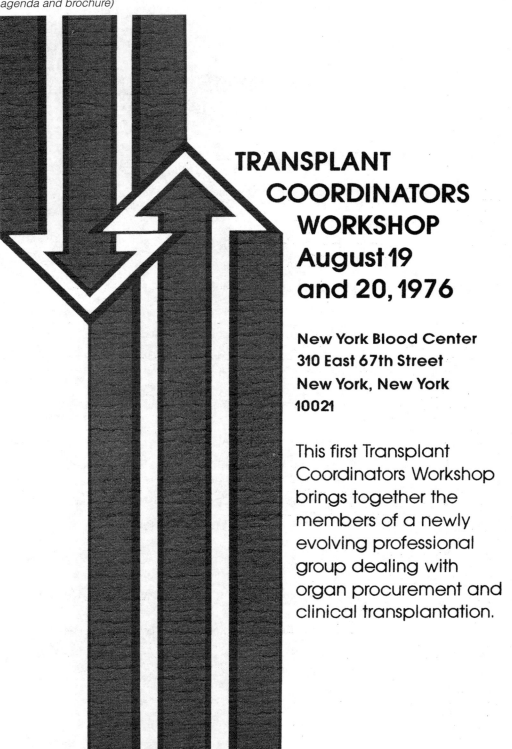

Figure 2. First NATCO Committee Roster, 1979-1980

NATCO Committee Roster

Membership Committee
Transplant Nursing Professionals
Linda Jones, R.N. — *Chairman*
Elizabeth Cameron, R.N.
Jane Waskerwitz, R.N.
Chris De Voe, R.N.
Professional Procurement Personnel
Roger Smith — *Chairman*
Geraldine Rasmussen
Jim Springer

Legal Committee
Michael Merriman, P.A. — *Chairman*
Sylvia Rogers, R.N.

Ethics Committee
Cecil Gunter — *Chairman*
Faye Davis, R.N.
Sylvia Rodgers, R.N.
Daniel Ferree

Newsletter Committee
Julie Hall, M.T.
— *Co-Chairman*
Mikki Masteller, R.N.
— *Co-Chairman*
Emi Yoshihara

Scientific Committee
Steve Raid — *Chairman*
Christine Gladden, R.N.
John Dennis
D. Bruce Schreiman
Howard Nathan
Laurie Sophie, R.N.
Bruce Sutphin
Barbara Elich, R.N.

Heart And Liver Procurement Committee
Louise Loring — *Chairman*
Herb Teachey
Paul Taylor

Cost And Regulations Committee
Paul Deutsch — *Chairman*
Charles Foxworth
Richard Metz
Roger Smith
Debora Nelson, R.N.
Patricia Prekup

Position Referral Service
Paul Taylor — *Chairman*
Eileen De Mayo, R.N.

1980 Boston Conference Committee
Kate Hume, R.N. — *Chairman*

Program Committee
Barbara Schanbacher, R.N. — *Chairman*
Steve Sammut
Mel Cohen
Tom Hagen
Gail Tyndall, R.N.
Phyllis Weber, R.N.
Barbara Self, R.N.

Publicity Committee
Winnifred Mack, R.N. — *Chairman*
Lea Emmett, R.N.
Rosemary Dressler
Douglas Miller

Registration And Budget Committee
Robert Gosnell — *Chairman*
Kathy Rudd

Hospitality Committee
Justine Willmert, R.N. — *Chairman*
Faye Davis, R.N.
Patricia Conway, R.N.
Cheryl Shimek, R.N.
Rita Menard, R.N.
Eileen De Mayo, R.N.
Mary Anne House, R.N.

Education Committee
Barbara Schanbacher, R.N.
— *Chairman*
Jacqueline Elkin, R.N.
Patricia Barber, F.N.P.
Lois Bartell, R.N.
Donna Tomky, R.N.
Claire Day, R.N.
Amy Peele, R.N.
Sylvia Rodgers, R.N.
Marge Maeser, R.N.
Cheryl Shimek, R.N.

By-Laws Committee
Kate Hume, R.N. — *Chairman*
Daniel Williams
Mary Jane Nevin, R.N.

Nominating Committee
Paul Taylor — *Chairman*
Mary Ann Farnsworth, R.N.
Mikki Masteller, R.N.

Figure 3. Second NATCO Committee Roster, 1980-1981

1980-81 NATCO Committee Roster

By-Laws Committee
Chairman
  Mark Reiner, P.A. — Gainesville, Florida
Secretary
  Cy Gilman — Gainesville, Florida
Members
  John Collins — Washington, D.C.
  Faye Davis, R.N. — Boston, Massachusetts
  Mary Ann Farnsworth, R.N. — Portland, Oregon
  Bruce Sutphin — Hartford, Connecticut
  M. Gail Tyndall, R. N. — Albuquerque, New Mexico
  Curtis Yaeger — Washington, D.C.

Communications Committee
Chairman
  Roger Smith — Los Angeles, California
Secretary
  Emi Yoshihara — Los Angeles, California
Members
  Carolyn Atkins — Dallas, Texas

Education Committee
Chairman
  Amy S. Peele, R.N. — Chicago, Illinois
Members
  Patricia Barber, R.N. — Chicago, Illinois
  Lois Bartell, R.N. — Minneapolis, Minnesota
  Claire Day, R.N. — Gainesville, Florida
  Cecil Gunter — Seattle, Washington
  Louise M. Jacobbi — Shreveport, Louisiana
  Ellie Nelson, R.N. — Minneapolis, Minnesota
  Eileen O'Toole, R.N. — Pittsburgh, Pennsylvania

Glenda Payne, R.N. — Dallas, Texas
Diana Prindle — Cleveland, Ohio
Sylvia Rodgers, R.N. — Atlanta, Georgia
Steve Sammut — Philadelphia, Pennsylvania
Barbara Schulman, R.N. — Los Angeles, California
Luke Skelly, R.N. — Knoxville, Tennessee
Laura Ruse Sophie, R.N. — Chicago, Illinois

Legal-Ethical Issues Committee
Chairman — Legal
  Michael Merriman, P.A. — Winston-Salem, North Carolina
Chairman — Ethical
  Cecil Gunter — Seattle, Washington
Members
  Faye Davis, R.N. — Boston, Massachusetts
  Sylvia Rodgers, R.N. — Atlanta, Georgia
  Jim Springer — Kansas City, Missouri
  Herb Teachey — Richmond, Virginia

Membership Committee
Chairman
  Patricia Prekup — Phoenix, Arizona
Secretary
  Mary Ann House, R.N. — Augusta, Georgia
Members
  Don Beavers — Tucson, Arizona
  Robert Hoffman — Madison, Wisconsin
  Linda Jones, R.N. — Columbus, Ohio
  Tony Samulari, M.D. — Rome, Italy
  Roger Smith — Los Angeles, California

Nominating Committee
Chairman
  Lea Emmett, R.N. — Brooklyn, New York
Secretary
  Claire Day, R.N. — Gainesville, Florida
Members
  John Collins — Washington, D.C.
  Rosemary Dressler, R.N. — Grand Rapids, Michigan
  Mary Ann Farnsworth, R.N. — Portland, Oregon
  Mikki Masteller, R.N. — San Diego, California
  O'Neil Matthews, R.N. — Chattanooga, Tennessee
  Barbara Schulman, R.N. — Los Angeles, California

Program & Publications Committee
Chairman
  Steve Sammut — Philadelphia, Pennsylvania
Secretary
  Phyllis Weber, R.N. — San Francisco, California
Members
  Sheila Alongi, R.N. — Baltimore, Maryland
  Carolyn Atkins, R.N. — Dallas, Texas
  Mel Cohen — Toronto, Canada
  Cecil Gunter — Seattle, Washington
  Julie Hall — San Diego, California
  Winifred Mack, R.N. — Long Island, New York
  Jane Reid — Kansas City, Missouri
  Mark Reiner, P.A. — Gainesville, Florida
  Ann Schafelette, R.N. — Hartford, Connecticut

M. Gail Tyndall, R.N. — Albuquerque, New Mexico
Jane Van Hook, R.N. — Minneapolis, Minnesota

Scientific Studies Committee
Chairman
  Laura Ruse Sophie, R.N. — Chicago, Illinois
Members
  Patricia Barber, F.N.P. — Chicago, Illinois
  Mel Cohen — Toronto, Canada
  John Dennis — Camden, New Jersey
  Barbara Elich, R.N. — Dallas, Texas
  Barbara Giordano, R.N. — Boston, Massachusetts
  Christine Gladden, R.N. — Camden, New Jersey
  Frank Lansden — Atlanta, Georgia
  Howard Nathan — Philadelphia, Pennsylvania
  D. Bruce Schreiman — Lansing, Michigan
  Bruce Sutphin — Hartford, Connecticut

Local Arrangements Committee
Co-chairman
  Peggy O'Connor — Chicago, Illinois
  Mary Jane Nevin, R.N. — Chicago, Illinois
Secretary
  Eileen DeMayo, R.N. — Chicago, Illinois
Members
  Lea Emmett, R.N. — Brooklyn, New York
  Kathleen Espee — Chicago, Illinois
  Justine Willmert, R.N. — Minneapolis, Minnesota

A CLINICIAN'S GUIDE TO DONATION AND TRANSPLANTATION

Figure 4. Third NATCO Committee Roster, 1981-1982

1981-82 NATCO Committee Roster

By-Laws Committee
Chairman
 Mark Reiner, P.A.
Members
 John Collins
 Dan Ferree
 Roger Smith

Communications Committee
Chairman
 Roger Smith
Members
 Carol Christiansen
 Lea Emmett, R.N.
 Lisa Watson
 Emi Yoshihara

Education Committee
Patient Subcommittee
Co-chairmen
 Lois Bartell, R.N.
 Laura Sophie, R.N.
Members
 Barbara Self, R.N.
 Marge Severeid

Public Subcommittee
Chairman
 Patty Prekup
Members
 Cathy Rudd, R.N.
 Sylvia Rodgers, R.N.

Professional Subcommittee
Chairman
 Kate Hume, R.N.
Members
 Tracy Fleeter, R.N.
 Glenda Payne, R.N.

Continuing Ed. Subcommittee
Members
 Carlos Castaneda
 Judith Lutton

Audio-Visual Subcommittee
Chairman
 Diana Prindle
Members
 Alice Curtis, R.N.
 Diane Kaschak

Bibliography Booklet Subcommittee
Chairman
 Patricia Barber, R.N.
Members
 Jackie Elkins
 Jane Reed

Federal Registry Subcommittee
Chairman
 Claire Day, R.N.
Members
 Lea Emmett, R.N.
 Julia Hall
NATCO-AANNT Liaison
 Cyrena Gilman, R.N.

Legal-Ethical Issues Committee
Chairman
 Jo Leslie, P.A.
Members
 Alice Curtis, R.N.
 Faye Davis, R.N.
 Judith Lucier, R.N.
 Michael Merriman, P.A.
 Mark Reiner, P.A.
 Luke Skelly

Membership Committee
Co-chairmen
 Burton Mattice
 Barbara Schulman, R.N.
Members
 Vicky Aslanian
 Caroline Buszta, R.N.
 Carol Christiansen
 Barbara Self, R.N.
 Julie Wade, R.N.

Multi-Organ Procurement Committee
Chairman
 Herb Teachey
Members
 Vicky Aslanian
 Faye Davis, R.N.
 Michael Merriman, P.A.

Nominating Committee
Chairman
 Lea Emmett, R.N.
Members
 Carol Christiansen
 John Collins
 Claire Day, R.N.
 Rosemary Dresser, R.N.
 Carol Lieberman, R.N.
 Burton Mattice
 Mikki Masteller, R.N.

Program & Publications Committee
Chairman
 Louise Jacobbi
Members
 Patricia Barber, R.N.
 Lois Bartell, R.N.
 Ronald Dreffer
 Julia Hall
 Diane Kaschak
 Carol Lieberman, R.N.
 Ann Martin, R.N.
 Gwen McNalt, R.N.
 Howard Nathan
 Amy Peele, R.N.
 Jane Reed
 Roger Smith
 Laura Sophie, R.N.

Scientific Studies Committee
Co-chairmen
 Anne Schefiliti, R.N.
 Bruce Sutphin
Members
 Patricia Barber, R.N.
 Mel Cohen
 Barbara Giordano, R.N.
 Christine Gladden, R.N.
 Steve Haid
 Howard Nathan
 Glenda Payne, R.N.
 Laura Sophie, R.N.
 Maxine Uniewski
 Jane Waskerwitz

Chapter 1

261

Figure 5. First National Proclamation of National Organ Donation Awareness Week

98TH CONGRESS
1ST SESSION
S. J. RES. 78

To authorize and request the President to issue a proclamation designating April 24 through April 30, 1983, as "National Organ Donation Awareness Week".

IN THE SENATE OF THE UNITED STATES

APRIL 7 (legislative day, APRIL 5), 1983

Mr. GORTON (for himself, Mr. DURENBERGER, Mr. LUGAR, Mr. BURDICK, Mr. STEVENS, Mr. HEFLIN, Mr. BUMPERS, Mr. D'AMATO, Mr. GLENN, Mrs. KASSEBAUM, and Mr. RANDOLPH) introduced the following joint resolution; which was read twice and referred to the Committee on the Judiciary

---

JOINT RESOLUTION

To authorize and request the President to issue a proclamation designating April 24 through April 30, 1983, as "National Organ Donation Awareness Week".

1   *Resolved by the Senate and House of Representatives*
2   *of the United States of America in Congress assembled,*
3   That the President is authorized and requested to issue a
4   proclamation designating April 24 through April 30, 1983,
5   as "National Organ Donation Awareness Week".

O

Figure 6. Notice of Organ Transplant Hearings, April 6, 1983

NEWS from:
Committee on Science and Technology
U.S. House of Representatives

DON FUQUA
Chairman

LARRY WINN, Jr.
Ranking Minority Member

FOR IMMEDIATE RELEASE
April 6, 1983
#97-42

GORE TO EXAMINE PROCESS OF OBTAINING HUMAN ORGANS FOR TRANSPLANTATION

Congressman Albert Gore, Jr. (D-Tenn.) announced today that the Subcommittee on Investigations and Oversight will hold hearings on April 13, 14, and 27 on the procurement and distribution of human organs for transplant surgery. The hearings will begin each day at 9:30 a.m. in Room 2325 of the Rayburn House Office Building, Washington, D.C.

Major strides in the transplantation of human organs have been made in the past few years. One year survival of liver, heart, and combined heart and lung transplants are now 70-85 percent. Recently, highly publicized cases of small children awaiting liver transplantation have highlighted the lack of sufficient organs to meet the increasing demands because of these improvements in transplant surgery.

The hearings were scheduled after Gore was contacted in January during a nationwide search to secure a liver for a 20-month old child then hospitalized in Memphis. "After learning of the difficulty in locating a suitable donor for this child, I realized there needed to be a better way to find transplantable organs than relying on bursts of publicity during what is an emotionally difficult time for the patient's family," said Gore.

"Through these hearings I hope that we in Congress can better understand the problems and determine if there is anything we can do to assist families and their physicians in solving this dilemma," Gore stated.

Rep. Joe Skeen (R-N. Mex.), the Ranking Minority Member of the Subcommittee, commented, "This is one of many areas where the introduction of information technology can make an enormous difference. The use of computers in managing an 'organ bank' information system could go a long way in solving the problem of matching organ donors with those in desperate need. This and other aspects or organ transplant placement practices will be examined in these important three days of hearings."

Among scheduled witnesses are some of the most eminent transplant surgeons in the world, including Drs. Norman Shumway of Stanford University, Thomas Starzl of the University of Pittsburgh and G. Melville Williams of Johns Hopkins University. The Fiske family, of Bridgewater, Massachusetts, who captured national attention after making a public plea in November for a liver donor for their daughter, Jaime, will also testify.

On April 27, the final day of the hearings, Dr. C. Everett Koop, Surgeon General, U.S. Public Health Service and Dr. Carolyn K. Davis, Administrator of the Health Care Financing Administration, Department of Health and Human Services, will testify.

The Subcommittee on Investigations and Oversight is part of the full Committee on Science and Technology chaired by Rep. Don Fuqua (D-Fla.).

A complete witness list appears on the reverse.

STAFF CONTACTS: Robert B. Nicholas, Staff Director, or Dr. Myron Genel of the Subcommittee at (202) 226-3636.

Chapter 1 — THE HISTORY OF THE TRANSPLANT COORDINATOR

Figure 7. Brandon Hall Received a Liver During National Organ Transplant Hearings but Died Following Transplantation

Thursday, May 12, 1983 — THE WASHINGTON POST

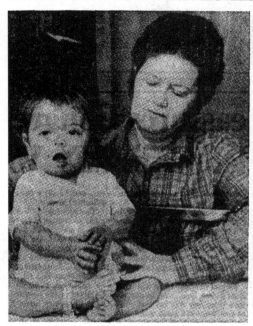 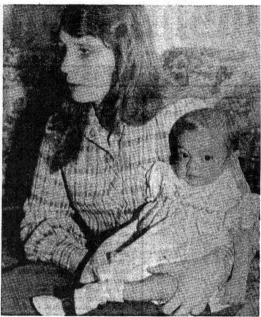

...don Hall, 13 months old, the recipient of two liver transplants, died of heart failure yesterday; Amy Hardin, 11 months old, received a transplant on Tuesday.

Brandon Hall Dies; Transplants Go On

By Victor Cohn
Washington Post Staff Writer

...ndon Hall, who at 13 months became the ...est human to get two liver transplants, ...f heart failure yesterday in Memphis.

...another city, the effort to make liver ...lants a regular and life-saving procedure ...n. Minneapolis surgeons reported that on ...ay they transplanted a liver into 11-...-old Amy Hardin, pairing her with Jamie ...of Massachusetts as the youngest recip-...f liver transplants.

...h Amy and Jamie, who received her new ...purifying organ last Nov. 5, were 344 ...ld at the time of their operations at the ...rsity of Minnesota.

...ndon Hall, the subject of two appeals for ...ably tiny liver, weighed 22 pounds when ...d at 4:30 a.m. EDT at Le Bonheur Chil-...Medical Center. That was four pounds ...than he weighed when he got his first ...ransplant a month ago, but the gain was ...l by an unhealthy buildup of fluids.

blood pressure, lowered kidney output and a faltering heart.

"The [latest] liver functioned very well throughout the whole ordeal, but it began to fail slightly toward the end," a hospital spokesman said. The cause of death was cardiac arrest.

John Donica, a spokesman for the medical center, described Brandon's death as a "slow and sure total system failure."

The child, who was born without bile ducts, got his first liver transplant on April 13 just after his mother, Billie Hall, had testified before a House subcommittee with her son in her arms. The liver came from a 9-month-old Virginia girl who had died in a traffic accident.

Twice during the first operation, Brandon's heart went into arrest; interrupted blood flow caused the lung damage. A week later, a blood clot formed in an artery and blocked blood flow to the new liver.

A nationwide alert went out, and on April 22 Brandon got another liver from a 5-month-old Kentucky girl who was an alleged victim of...

without media help "Brandon probably would not have gotten his liver transplants."

She donated Brandon's corneas to an eye bank, and said she hoped his death would help someone else.

"I loved those eyes," she said, "but I gave them to somebody else ...."

"If there's any good that's come out of Brandon's death, maybe it is worth it, I don't know," she said after returning to her home in Walnut, Miss.

On Capitol Hill, a House Science and Technology subcommittee headed by Rep. Albert Gore Jr. (D-Tenn.) has been seeking ways to find donors for all persons in need of transplants, ending the need for emotional appeals.

The University of Pittsburgh has established a toll-free national coordinating number—800-243-6667, or 800-24-DONOR—for use in lining up organs from injured and brain-dead but still breathing patients.

The liver transplanted in Amy Hardin, of Cahokia, Ill., came from 7½-month-old Daniel Sakellarios of Monticello, Fla., who died Friday

Figure 8. Certificate of Merit Given to Faye Davis, Creator of NATCO Procurement Training Course, Shows Many Signatures of pioneer transplant coordinators, 1982

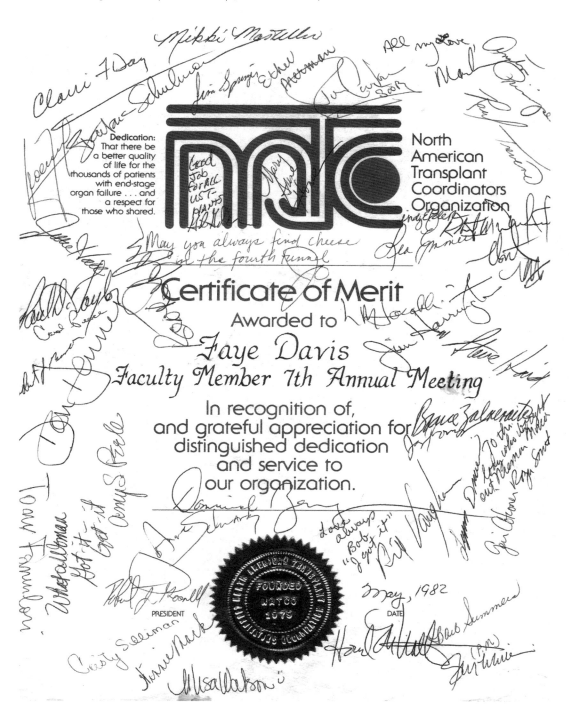

Figure 9. NATCO Newsletter Article on 24-ALERT

Some Thoughts on 24-ALERT

A recent meeting in Pittsburgh, with some of the people who have made 800-24 ALERT a possibility (and a reality) prompted me to write this article.

This system has come a long way since the early 1980's when it was first conceived at a coordinator's meeting. Today, NATCO owns computer hardware worth just a little less than one hundred thousand dollars and a software package developed for the 800-24 ALERT system that has attracted world-wide attention. Now I know that many of you are thinking that this system can't be so hot if you can't get on to run a donor in the middle of the night or, your updates don't make it into the system within a reasonable period of time or the telephone numbers aren't understandable. Just remember, this system is operated by volunteers. People who are among the very busiest, if not *the* very busiest, coordinators in the United States. And there are more of you out there than them. Cut them a little slack whenever you can. They are doing their very best. (Yes, Virginia, this is the voice of experience speaking. I remember it only too well.) Something to think about next time you get back after a donor run and want to delete a patient at 3:00 am. You may not have been the only one up all night!

A brief spiel about prioritization of our recipients.

Way back when, we (meaning collectively the Multi-Organ Committee) developed a system of prioritization for the listing of extra-renal recipients. We didn't have any special knowledge that endowed us with the wisdom necessary to develop such a ranking system. We did have a need for such a system and set out to satisfy that need. It seemed that no one else had the time or desire to undertake this project. (Today, everybody has a better idea.) The result is the current system that we all "use" (or abuse as the case may be) today.

To refresh your memory, STATUS THREE for those patients well enough to await transplantation at home, STATUS TWO for those patients that require hospitalization but not intensive care, STATUS ONE for those patients in very poor condition that not only require hospitalization, but continuous intensive care on a round the clock basis and finally, STATUS NINE for those patients that are extremely critical or those that have been transplanted and require regrafting on an urgent basis.

We envisioned this as a reasonable system for the ranking of recipients and so did most of the physicians that we approached about the feasibility of such a system. The initial belief behind such a system was that we could all trust one another and our colleagues, the transplant surgeons. We had no misconceptions about being able to "police" such a ranking scheme and/or "punish" those who repeatedly violated our collective trust and abused the system. We knew that, as voluntary organization, we had no such capabilities. In the days since this system was implemented, we've taken a lot of flak about what a poor system this is and how it lends itself to flagrant abuse and so on and so forth. The truth is that this is not a perfect way of going about ranking patients who need lifesaving transplants. BUT, it is the only system that we have and neither my boss nor yours has come up with anything better. At least anything that all the other "bosses" of the transplant world will agree upon and use. Since we have to use this system, lets *ALL* vow to decrease our abuses and try to make this system work in the manner and spirit intended. (To those of you who never abuse the system, my apologies for the blanket accusation.)

On to happier things, the VMS Multi-Tasking System is now up and operational. Hopefully this will end many of the irritations which the smaller, single channel systems provided to many of you. You can expect more clear speech synthesis and very, very short turnaround time once you've entered your donor data. Again, the system is not perfect but, that *IS* our goal.

A small reminder about your bitches and gripes as they relate to the 800-24 ALERT system.

If you are having problems with the system, please call and let someone know what is happening. We can't fix what we don't know about. It's your system and only you can make it work. Contact the P.T.F. or Herb or me if you have problems or maybe just feel like chewing on someone because of something we did or didn't do. (NOTE — The management reserves the right to chew back.) We do want this system to operate as efficiently and appropriately as humanly possible. We can't accomplish this without your input.

Finally, a long overdue and much deserved thanks to the people of NATCO for their tremendous efforts in developing, funding and maintaining this system. A special thanks is owed to the people of the Pittsburgh Transplant Foundation. They are the ones who, on a daily basis, have been down in the trenches slugging it out with this project. We owe more than we can repay for their efforts and continued support.

Let me not forget Rick Sheppeck (now M.D.) who, through many long nights, wrote the software that runs on this system. In terms of financial value, there is no way this organization could ever have afforded to pay for this software development. As we have so often done, we turned to our greatest resource, our members, and again, we got the job done. THANKS RICK!!

P.S. Multi-Organ Sub-Committee Chairpersons: Hope that your broken arms all heal soon. Write when you can. We would like to know how things are coming along. □

Figure 10. UNOS Resolution Recognizing NATCO Upon Receiving 24-ALERT Computer Donor Organ Matching System From NATCO

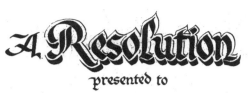

A Resolution presented to North American Transplant Coordinators Association

Whereas, The formation of the National Organ Procurement and Transplantation Network signifies the beginning of a strong allegiance among transplant surgeons, physicians, transplant coordinators, histocompatibility personnel, directors of transplant-related organizations across the nation, and the general public; and

Whereas, The United Network for Organ Sharing (UNOS) sees this the perfect opportunity to meld ideas, beliefs, and technologies for the ultimate good of the transplant community and the society it serves; now, therefore be it

Resolved, that UNOS would like to express gratitude to the North American Transplant Coordinators Association (NATCO), for donating their 24-ALERT voice-activated computer system to the newly recognized national organization.

UNOS looks forward to a fruitful association with NATCO and all other transplant organizations and facilities in the future, in hopes of further expanding the capabilities of the NATIONAL ORGAN PROCUREMENT AND TRANSPLANTATION NETWORK

Signed this 5th day of December, 1986.
Richmond, Virginia

John C McDonald
President, UNOS

Figure 11. Press Release: UNOS Receiving 24-ALERT from NATCO, page 1

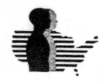

UNOS
United Network for Organ Sharing
3001 Hungary Spring Road P.O. Box 28010 Richmond, Virginia 23228 Telephone (804) 289 5380

December 5, 1986

President
John C. McDonald, M.D.
Louisiana State University, Shreveport

Vice-President
H. Keith Johnson, M.D.
Nashville VA Hospital

Secretary
Robert J. Corry, M.D.
University of Iowa Hospitals & Clinics

Treasurer
James S. Wolf, M.D.
Northwestern Memorial Hospital, Chicago

Past President
Oscar Salvatierra, Jr., M.D.
University of California, SF

Councillors

Region 1
Donald A. Leeber, M.D.
Maine Medical Center

Region 2
J. Wesley Alexander, M.D.
University of Cincinnati

Region 3
William W. Pfaff, M.D.
University of Florida

Region 4
Martin G. White, M.D.
Southwest Organ Bank

Region 5
Ben A. VanderWerf, M.D.
Phoenix Transplant Center

Region 6
John A. Hansen, M.D.
Puget Sound Blood Center, Seattle

Region 7
Howard S. Shapiro, M.D.
William Beaumont Hospital, Michigan

Region 8
Richard Weil III, M.D.
University of Colorado, Denver

Region 9
Felix T. Rapaport, M.D.
State University at Stony Brook, NY

Executive Director
Gene A. Pierce
Richmond, Virginia

FOR IMMEDIATE RELEASE

CONTACT: Barbara Ettne
UNOS
(804) 289-060

24-ALERT SYSTEM TRANSFERRED TO RICHMOND

24-ALERT, the voice-activated organ matching computer system of the North American Transplant Coordinators Organization (NATCO), has been transferred to Richmond, Virginia, to consolidate computer procurement and transplantation facilities nationwide. The 24-ALERT system will be housed at the United Network for Organ Sharing (UNOS), along with UNOS' Organ Center, a computerized organ matching system staffed 24-hours-a-day. Official announcement of the transfer was made Friday, December 5, 1986, in Richmond, Virginia.

"NATCO is transferring its 24-ALERT system for extrarenal matching in an effort to contribute to a unified computerized donor matching program for the organ procurement and transplantation network," Stephen D. Haid, President of NATCO, said. Extrarenal organs include the heart, lungs, liver, pancreas, and tissues; and exclude the renal organs, kidneys.

UNOS was named recipient of a federal contract to establish the national network on September 30, 1986.

The National Network For Tissue And Organ Registration, Procurement And Sharing

Figure 11. Press Release: UNOS Receiving 24-ALERT from NATCO, page 2

```
24-ALERT Transfer
Page Two
```

The 24-ALERT system, founded in 1983, was funded through a grant from the Mellon Foundation. Amy Peele, President of NATCO in 1983, said the organization saw the need for an organized system to place extrarenal organs, but did not anticipate that 24-ALERT would be as widely used as it has been. The computerized system serves the United States and Canada, and has been housed at the University of Pittsburgh Medical Center, Pennsylvania, since its inception.

As of September 1, 1986, 24-ALERT has facilitated the matching and transplantation of 2,568 organs, including 1,209 livers, 1,168 hearts, 65 heart-lungs, 4 lungs, and 122 tissue donations. 88 centers were listed as part of the 24-ALERT system as of that date. Currently, UNOS has 176 transplant centers, 27 independent organ procurement agencies, and nine tissue-typing laboratories throughout the nation as its members.

"We hope that the 24-ALERT system will continue to offer an easily accessible approach to extrarenal matching by transplant coordinators across the country," Haid said.

# # #

Figure 12. Story on Transplant Coordinators Features Amy Peele

Living

PAGE 43

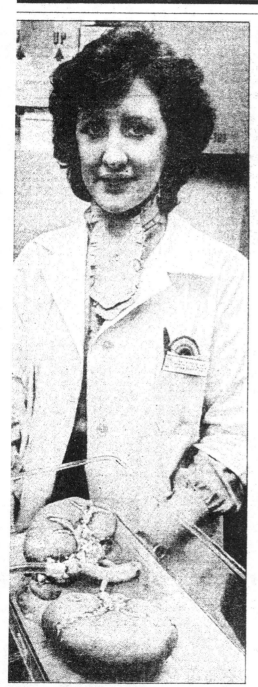

ordinator of an organ recovery program, helps send organs such as these tients needing transplants. (Sun-Times Photo by Barry Jarvinen)

The gift that keeps on living

Barbara Varro

Amy Peele good-naturedly tolerates comments about her work. "I've been called Dr. Frankenstein," she says. "And people often ask, 'Got any spare parts?'"

Peele is a registered nurse and senior coordinator of the organ and tissue recovery program at Rush-Presbyterian-St. Luke's Medical Center. Her job is to find functioning organs that will become gifts from the dead to the living.

Peele's bailiwick is a laboratory that looks like any other at the medical center, except for a huge freezer filled with human bones. There also are several machines that feed oxygen to keep kidneys viable until they can be transplanted.

It is in this laboratory where organs and tissues—kidneys, corneas, livers, hearts and bones—are collected for use by surgeons in 40 hospitals in Illinois and cities throughout the United States and some international destinations.

BEFORE THE DRAMA of the medical transplant takes place, organs and tissues must be found. There are dire shortages of organs throughout the country. More than 11,000 potential transplant patients in the United States are awaiting kidneys; 600 kidney patients in Illinois are on a waiting list, reports the Illinois Transplant Society. A spokeswoman for the Illinois Eye Bank says that 300 people in Illinois and 20,000 nationally are waiting for corneal transplants.

Peele maintains close contact with many hospitals in Illinois, where organs may become available from donors. She also keeps in touch, via computer, with hospitals throughout the country where patients need organs. She also coordinates the efforts of a team of surgeons, nurses and technicians involved in procurement. As part of this job, she is on call 24 hours a day, seven days a week and must be ready on short notice to put the procurement program into action.

QUICK WORK IS essential in retrieving viable organs. Once a donor is pronounced brain dead, that person must be kept on life-support systems until organs are removed. The heart must be kept beating because organs and tissue need blood flow to be in good condition for transplantation. Although bones can be kept viable for as long as two years by freezing them, a kidney can be properly maintained outside of the body for only three days. Hearts and livers must be transplanted within hours.

The part of her job Peele characterizes as the most difficult is talking to the family of a hospital patient who is a potential donor. "You can imagine how difficult it is to talk to a dead patient's loved ones about organ removal procedures," she said. "But I have to be there to answer whatever questions they have about the procedure. I recently talked to the parents of a 19-year-old boy who committed suicide. They told me that by permitting their son's organs to be donated, 'perhaps someone else's life will be saved.'"

It is gratifying to Peele to know how much good a single donor can do. "We acquired a heart, kidneys, corneas and a parathyroid from a 15-year-old boy who was involved in a fatal car accident. That one boy benefitted six people who received transplants with his organs."

The process of acquiring organs usually begins with a phone call from a hospital about a potential donor—often someone who has been in an accident and is brain dead. Peele rushes to the hospital and consults with doctors and nurses to review the potential donor's medical history.

Not everyone is a candidate for organ donation, she explained. The person's organs must be in excellent condition. Donors must be under 65 and those with heart disease, cancer, hypertension or diabetes are ruled out.

IF THE DONOR IS accepted, he or she is given fluids and chemicals necessary to keep blood and oxygen pumping through the body's organs and tissues. Then, the organs are surgically removed and placed in storage cases designed to keep them viable until transplantation.

Peele deals primarily with kidneys, which are stored in a profusion machine that maintains oxygen flow and infuses organs with a solution that approximates human albumen. Another method of storage is packing kidneys in a plastic bag containing "slush," a cold solution similar to a human's intercellular fluids.

To transport organs such as kidneys from one city to another rapidly, they are placed in a portable renal system that is like a mock heart to sustain oxygen flow. The metal module containing the kidneys is rushed to an airport, where it is put on a flight to its destination. "The farthest we've sent kidneys so far is to a hospital in Kuwait," Peele said.

Peele's work has its share of rewards. "It is gratifying to see patients who have had successful transplants," she said. "The quality of their lives is vastly improved."

She longs for the day when there will no longer be shortages of organs for transplantation. "I feel that the public is becoming more aware of the crucial need for organ donation because transplantation is becoming more acceptable," she said. "If would be great if rejection [of organs] could be conquered to raise the rate of successful transplants."

CONSIDERABLE INCREASES in the rate of successful transplants soon may be realized because of a new drug—Cyclosporin—that has proved effective in clinical tests. The drug, which is isolated from fungi, suppresses the production of T-lymphocyte cells involved in the body's natural defense against foreign tissue. The American Medical Association points out that the drug has spurred a resurgence in transplantation surgery.

Peele's job as a kind of go-between for the medical center and other hospitals is a crucial one involving hundreds of thousands of dollars. She said that a kidney transplant—from procurement through transplantation—costs about $45,000.

"That is a lot of money," she conceded, "but it is less than the $25,000 to $30,000 it costs per year to maintain a patient on dialysis. The government, which budgeted $1.8 billion for dialysis in the last year, is coming around to realizing that transplants are more cost-effective."

A CLINICIAN'S GUIDE TO DONATION AND TRANSPLANTATION

Figure 13. The Typical Transplant Coordinator

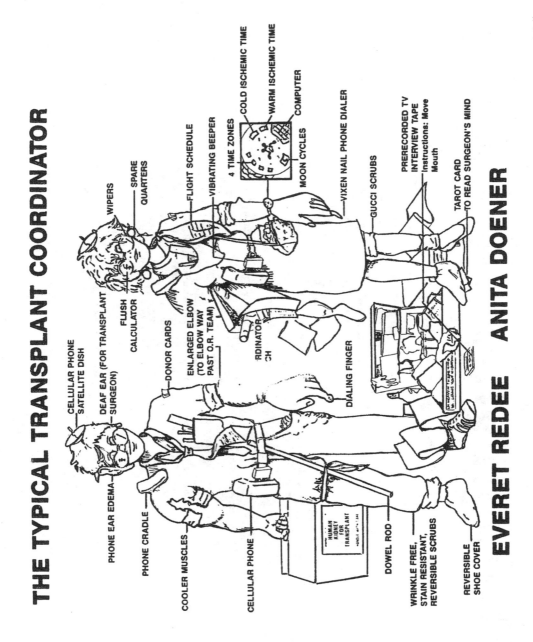

Chapter 1 — THE HISTORY OF THE TRANSPLANT COORDINATOR

Figure 14. First Publication of Transplant Coordinator Job Duties, 1980

ESRD Regulation Follow-Up

After a study of the Transplant Coordinators' job description from 7 different centers, there are some generalizations that can be made. Although this is by no means a comprehensive list of everything a transplant coordinator has ever been known to do, it is a general listing of the areas of responsibility covered by most coordinators. The areas of responsibility can be broken down into 5 general groups. Some centers have a separate individual to handle each group; some have two or three individuals covering primarily one area with overlap into one or two areas; and some centers have one unfortunate person to deal with all of the responsibilities.

1. Organ Procurement

a) Establish organ recovery programs at own local and referral hospitals (including ER, ICU, OR, Administration and Billing).
b) Establish policies and procedures about donor identification and maintenance and also organ recovery, preservation and sharing.
c) Arrange tissue typing of cadaver donors and send blood samples.
d) Obtain consent from next-of-kin of potential cadaver donors.
e) Assist families of cadaver donors with grief process.
f) Coordinate the sharing of organs with other centers when unable to use locally.
g) Assist with organ harvest (scrub and/or circulate in O.R.).
h) Maintain appropriate preservation of organs.
i) Keep information (ischemic times, flow rates, etc.) on cadaver organs.
j) Arrange shipment and/or transport of organs not used locally.
k) Work with coroner's offices.
l) Keep records and gather statistics about all functions performed for local, regional, network, and federal use.
m) Function as contact person for fiscal information.

2. Patient Services (Recipient)

a) Coordinate recipient identifications with local and referring nephrologists and dialysis units.
b) Coordinate blood work for ABO and tissue typing, MLC's, and preformed antibody screening.
c) Orient prospective recipient and family about renal program and treatment options.
d) Plan, schedule, and coordinate recipient workup.
e) Educate patient and family concerning all phases of transplantation.
f) Facilitate patient's progress through system.
g) Provide emotional support to patient and his family.
h) Schedule transplant date.
i) Instruct patient about post-transplant medications, diet, and clinic visits as well as monitor compliance.
j) Coordinate post-transplant outpatient follow-up and care.
k) Maintain records and statistics.
l) Function as contact person for financial information.
m) Attend Transplant Committee meetings.

3. Patient Services (Donor)

a) Coordinate bloodwork of all available family members for ABO, tissue typing, and MLC's.
b) Select best donor.
c) Plan, schedule, and coordinate donor workup.
d) Educate patient and family concerning all phases of transplantation.
e) Schedule transplant date.
f) Facilitate patient's progress through system.
g) Provide emotional support to both patient and family.
h) Function as contact person for financial information.

4. Education

a) Communicate frequently with physicians, nurses, and technicians in ERs and ICUs about cadaver donor identification.
b) Prepare and present lectures, demonstrations, and inservice training programs.
c) Prepare and present technician training programs.
d) Orient and establish working relationships with law enforcement personnel, EMT's fire rescue teams, etc.
e) Prepare written material and/or AV aids about transplant and organ donation for distribution.
f) General public education through presentations to schools, social groups, TV, radio, newspapers.
g) Help the local Kidney Foundation in their education efforts.
h) Distribute literature and Uniform Donor Cards.

5. General Duties (Application to each of the preceding 4 categories)

a) Provide 24 hour coverage.
b) Establish and update protocols.
c) Order supplies and equipment.
d) Maintain equipment.
e) Hire and fire subordinates.
f) Formulate and monitor budget.
g) Other administrative functions.
h) Assist in research projects.
i) Hold active membership in professional organizations.

Only two of the job descriptions specified education criteria for transplant coordinators. These were 1) P.A. or R.N. with B.A. or B.S. and 2) experienced preservation and acquisition professional. Certainly these are desireable qualifications for any of the four areas mentioned above. These would be most appropriate for entry into practice in the future, although all professionals currently active in any of these areas should remain eligible.

These criteria were forwarded to Thomas Morford, Director, Office of Standards and Certification, Health Standards and Quality Bureau, 1840 Gwynn Oak Ave., Baltimore, Md. 21207.

Claire F. Day, R.N.
Adult Transplant Coordinator
Gainesville, Florida

Figure 15. Invitation to First International Transplant Coordinators Society Meeting Party, Kyoto, Japan, 1994

Invitation to ITCM Party

Welcome Address

Kazuo Ota — Chairman, the 15th International Congress of the Transplantation Society

Tsuyoshi Ogata — Representative, the Japan Ministry of Health & Welfare

Toast

Seigo Hiraga — President, the International Transplant Coordinators Meeting

Congratulatory Address

Teresa Shafer — President, the North American Transplant Coordinators Organization

Leo Roels — President, the European Transplant Coordinators Organization

Entertainment

Keiko Iwai — Japanese Traditional Art "Gagaku"
the Traditional Court Music of Japan

Closing Remarks

Isao Tamaki — President, the Japan Transplant Coordinators Organization

Date : August 29, 1994 7:40 – 9:15 pm

Place : Kyoto International Conference Hall Room Swan (B1F)

Chapter 1 — THE HISTORY OF THE TRANSPLANT COORDINATOR

North American Transplant Coordinators Organization

presents

An Introductory Training Course on Procurement for Transplant Coordinators

October 21-27, 1985
Rolling Ridge Conference Center
North Andover, Massachusetts

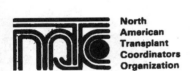

North American Transplant Coordinators Organization

Non-Profit Organization
U.S. Postage Paid
Augusta, GA
Permit No. 394

That there be a better quality of life for the thousands of patients with end-stage organ failure... and a respect for those who shared.

NATCO Sub-Committee for Training and Development

CHAIRPERSON
Faye Davis, B.A., M.S.N.
Washington Hospital Center, Washington DC

COURSE COORDINATORS
Mary Anne House, R.N., M.S.N.
Medical College of Georgia, Augusta, Georgia

Charles McCluskey, P.A.
University of Florida, Jacksonville, Florida

COMMITTEE MEMBERS
Gwen Mayes
Atlanta Regional Organ Procurement Agency, Atlanta, Georgia

Irv Koehler
Florida Hospital, Orlando, Florida

Del Steckler
American Red Cross, St. Paul, Minnesota

Mary Sloan
George Washington University, Washington, D.C.

Gary Hall
University of Tennessee, Memphis, Tennessee

Holly Franz
New England Organ Bank, Boston, Massachusetts

Richard Metz
Phoenix Transplant Center, Phoenix, Arizona

Bill Vaughn
Regional Transplant Labs, Nashville, Tennessee

Ken Trachy
University of Miami, Miami, Florida

Dave Mainous
Indiana University Hospitals, Indianapolis, Indiana

Bruce Zalneraitis
New England Organ Bank, Boston, Massachusetts

MEDICAL ADVISORY COMMITTEE

B.A. Barnes, M.D.
New England Organ Bank, Boston, Massachusetts

John M. Barry, M.D.
University of Oregon, Portland, Oregon

John D. Whelchel, M.D.
Alabama Regional Organ Bank, Birmingham, Alabama

Jimmy A. Light, M.D.
Washington Hospital Center, Washington, D.C.

G. Melville Williams, M.D.
Johns Hopkins University, Baltimore, Maryland

A CLINICIAN'S GUIDE TO DONATION AND TRANSPLANTATION Chapter 1

Historical Photos

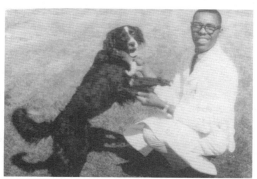

Paul Taylor. 1964. Denver Colorado at the University of Colorado. Dog 1 year post liver transplant – was taken off Imuran after four months. Survived 11 years. (Photo courtesy of Paul Taylor)

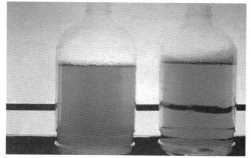

Folkert Belzer and Robert Hoffmann's scientific discovery: cryoprecipitate. 1964-1966. San Franciso General Hospital, UCSF. "This was a big breakthrough. At the time, plasma was the perfusate being used in dog kidney experiments on the pump. Most effective. The bottle on the left is plasma in its natural state. The bottle on right was passed through a .22 micron milipore filter removing unstabilized lipoprotein. With this purer perfusate, we could perfuse kidneys up to 3 days successfully. This is what made it possible to successfully perfuse kidneys. Prior to that, with our experiments and using the unfiltered plasma, after 20 minutes on the pump, the pressure in the kidney would increase dramatically to unacceptable levels. Notice that you can see through the line behind the bottle on the right."
Robert Hoffman

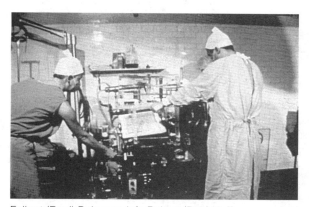

Folkert (Fred) Belzer on left, Robert (Bob) Hoffmann on right with Kidney Preservation machine. 1967. San Francisco General Hospital. Working on machine. They took the machine to the hospital where the donor was because these were non-heart-beating donors. As soon as the kidneys were removed, they were put on the machine and then the machine was put in the van for transport. This was the prototype of the Belzer machine.

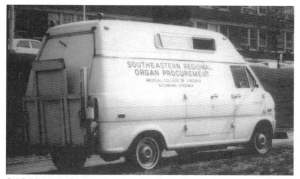

SEOPF Van. Circa 1973-74. Richmond, VA.

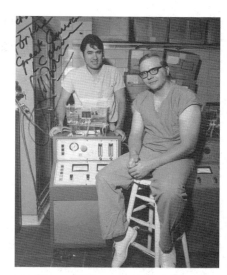

Les Olsen, sitting, on right. Dr. Louis Toledo behind MOX-100 Console Perfusion Machine. 1972. Minneapolis, MN. Taken in basement research lab at the University of Minnesota.
(Photo courtesy of Les Olsen)

Chapter 1 — THE HISTORY OF THE TRANSPLANT COORDINATOR

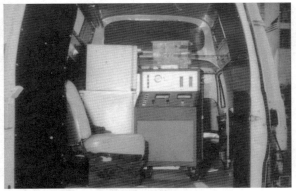

Inside SEOPF van. There was a refrigerator on left, a chair for the coordinator to sit in (left) and a generator, to avoid use of batteries as had been done in the beginning, for running the machine. With the generator, they could travel four to five hundred miles with the kidneys on the pump. Circa 1973. Duke University. MCV, Johns Hopkins, Maryland, and UNC all had vans. People started designing vans to load this machine and take to hospitals. The kidney preservation vans had a uniform design.

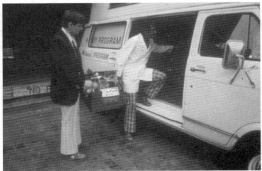

Bill Anderson and John Sampson. 1975. Duke University Medical Center emergency room. "I had a great time talking to both Mike Phillips and Bob Hoffmann about this photo. Bob's only remark about this photo was, 'Look at those pants. What a fashionable group.'" *Teresa Shafer*

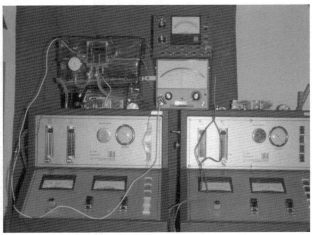

Two kidney preservation consoles at Duke University in 1976. Research: Testing core temperatures of kidneys (note temperature probes).

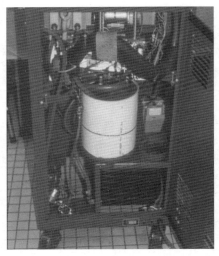

1976, Duke University. Inside the preservation machine. These machines were not portable early on. Antifreeze in white barrel. The lines contained CO2 and oxygen. Before the new synethetic perfusate was developed, oxygen and CO2 were used to change the pH of the perfusate. Use of the new synthetic perfusate removed the need for the use of the oxygen and CO2 canisters and the system was self-contained. Mike Phillips remembers setting the alarms, laying down on a guerny and getting some sleep. Bob Hoffmann on the other hand said his team never slept with the kidneys, but went home to conserve energy to be ready for the next day of surgery and work.

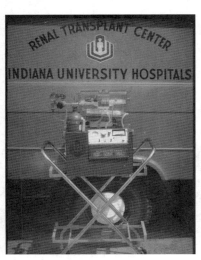

Kidney van – used to transport shared kidneys on the large preservation machine. Circa 1976. Bowman Gray, Duke, UNC, Charlotte and Indianapolis all had them – note the oxygen tanks.

A CLINICIAN'S GUIDE TO DONATION AND TRANSPLANTATION

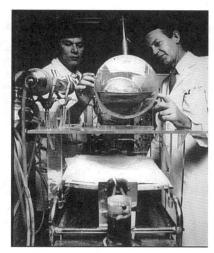

First working kidney preservation machine. Robert Hoffmann (left) and Fred Belzer. 1977, University of Wisconsin. "I had just finished an experiment and someone took our picture. I have this picture hanging today in my office. It was difficult to perfuse with plasma because of the risk of hepatitis and other such blood-borne diseases. The use of the synthetic perfusate allowed us to perfuse kidneys up to 5 days for the first time." *Robert Hoffmann*

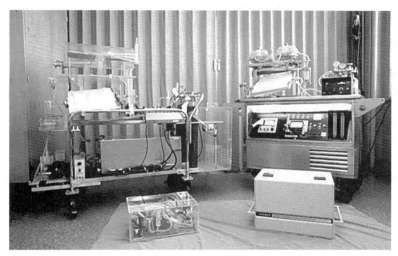

Belzer and Hoffmann's evolution of pumps photo: First machine on left, Belzers machine on right. On floor: Baby Belzer on left, portable Belzer on right. The Baby Belzer was designed to fit underneath an airplane seat.

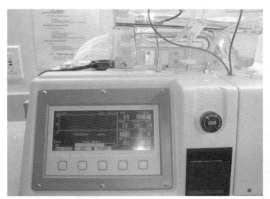

New Waters Preservation machine. Circa 2000. "This is an excellent machine. The computer system works great. It will tell you how much resistance your kidney has." *Bob Hoffmann*

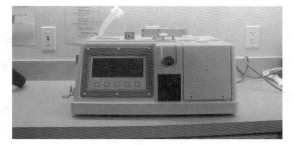

New Preservation machine. New waters machine.

*Photos on pages 1-3, unless otherwise noted, are courtesy of Michael Phillips and Robert Hoffman.

Chapter 1 — **THE HISTORY OF THE TRANSPLANT COORDINATOR**

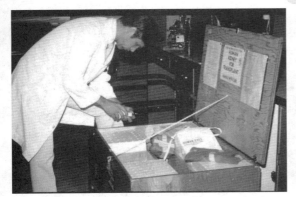

Mike Phillips. 1975. Duke University Medical Center. The big box contained everything Mike needed to recover kidneys and eyes by himself.
(Photo courtesy of Michael Phillips and Robert Hoffman)

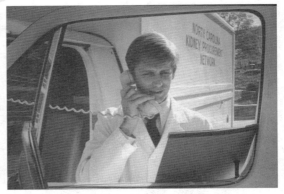

Mike Phillips. 1975. Duke University Medical Center. State purchased van for Duke and UNC.
(Photo courtesy of Michael Phillips and Robert Hoffman)

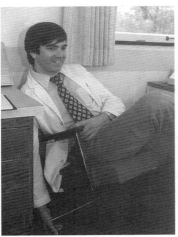

Stephen Kelley. 1975. University of Iowa.
(Photo courtesy of Stephen Kelley)

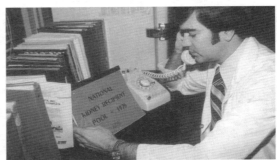

Stephen Kelley with Paul Terasaki's National Kidney Recipient Pool List of patients awaiting renal transplantation (predates SEOPF and UNOS organized sharing). 1976. University of Iowa. This was a national listing. Not everyone sent in the information on their patients, but about 4/5 of the centers did do so. After transplantation Steve would send in the list of patients who had been transplanted in order that they would be taken off.

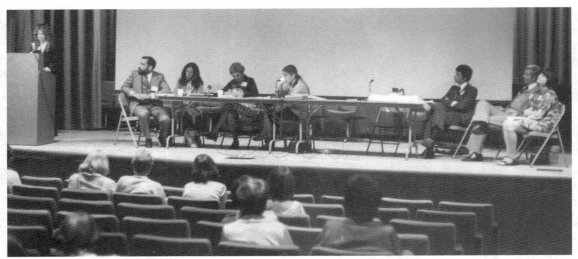

At podium: Mildred Young at lectern. Seated (l to r) Wesley Dixon, Shawney Fine, Gerda Lipcamann, Gloria Horns, Bernard Cohen, Gene Pierce, and Geraldine "Geri" Rasmussen. August 19 & 20, 1976. New York Blood Center on East 67th in NYC. First Official (and what became known as 2nd Annual) Transplant Coordinator Meeting.

*All photos in remainder of chapter are courtesy of the NATCO Archives, unless otherwise noted.

A CLINICIAN'S GUIDE TO DONATION AND TRANSPLANTATION

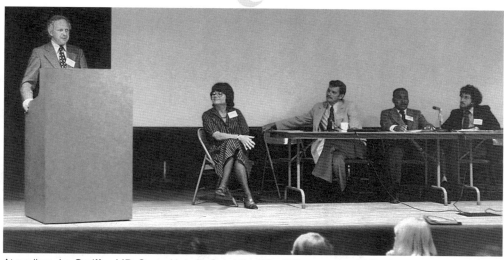

At podium: Ira Greiffer, MD, Seated L to R: Geraldine "Geri" Rasmussen., Philip Jos, Lawrence (Larry) Chilnick, Samuel Kountz, MD. August 19 & 20, 1976. New York Blood Center on East 67th in NYC. First Official (and what became known as 2nd Annual) Transplant Coordinator Meeting.

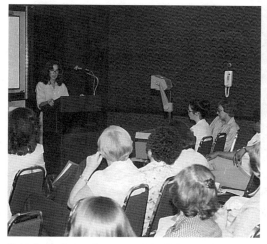

Patricia Barber at lectern. 1979. Chicago, IL. Third Annual Transplant Coordinator Meeting. This was the meeting where NATCO was formally created.

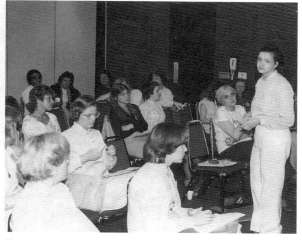

Kate Hume, standing. Justine Willmert is at her right hand, sitting. Linda Jones in front row, far left. 1979. Chicago, IL. Third Annual Transplant Coordinator Meeting. This was the meeting where NATCO was formally created.

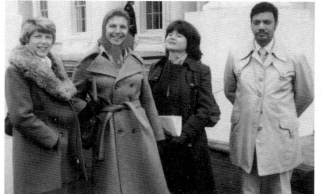

Gerda Lipcaman, Linda Jones, Geraldine (Geri) Rasmussen, and Curtis Yeager. 1977. Washington, D.C. Meeting to plan the April 6-7, 1978 Columbus transplant coordinator meeting – this was prior to the formation of NATCO.

THE HISTORY OF THE TRANSPLANT COORDINATOR

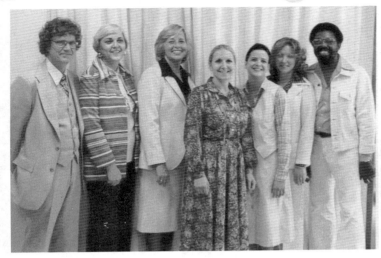

First NATCO Board.
(L-R): Robert Gosnell, Justine Willmert, Barbara Schanbacher, Barbara Shulman, Kate Hume, Winifred Mack, Paul Taylor. 1979. Chicago, IL.

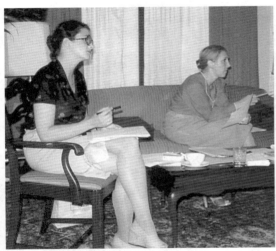

Kate Hume, Barbara Schulman. 1980. Boston.

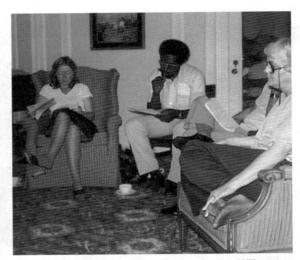

Winifred (Winnie) Mack, Paul Taylor, Justine Willmert. 1980. Boston.

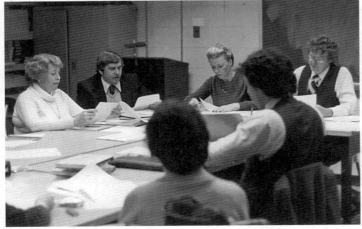

Barb Schanbacher, Burt Mattice, Winnie Mack, Bob Gosnell. November 19-20, 1981. Washington, DC. NATCO Administrative Council Meeting.

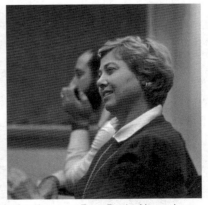

Herb Teachey, Faye Davis. November 19-20, 1981. Washington, DC. NATCO Administrative Council Meeting.

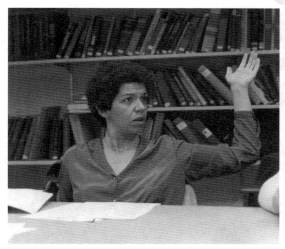

Louise Jacobbi. November 19-20, 1981. Washington, DC. NATCO Administrative Council Meeting.

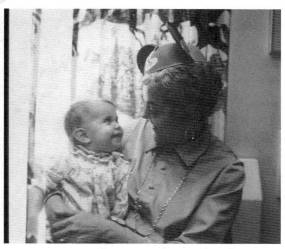

Justine Willmert with one of her kidney transplant patients. Circa 1975. In Justine's office at the University of Minnesota. "The hat really belonged to her, but she thought it was terribly funny when I wore it."

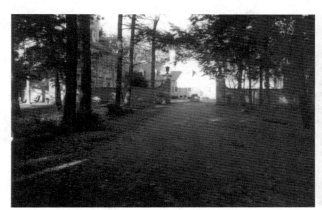

Road to Rollling Ridge. 1985. Rolling Ridge Retreat Conference Center, North Andover, MA. NATCO Procurement Training Course.

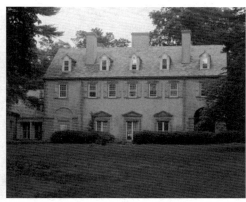

Main House at Rolling Ridge. 1985. Rolling Ridge Retreat Conference Center, North Andover, MA. NATCO Procurement Training Course.

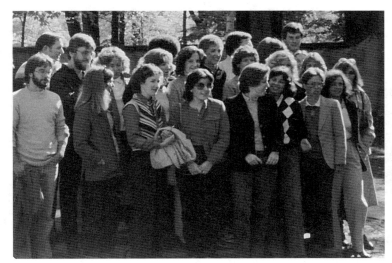

First Class of NATCO Procurement Training Course. 1982. Rolling Ridge Retreat Conference Center, North Andover, MA.

Chapter 1

THE HISTORY OF THE TRANSPLANT COORDINATOR

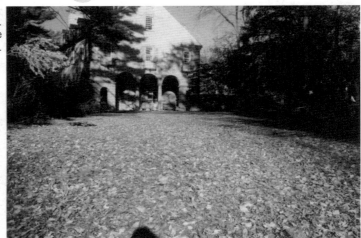

Rolling Ridge in October – beautiful. 1985. Rolling Ridge Retreat Conference Center, North Andover, MA.

Faculty at First NATCO Procurement Training Course.
Row 1: Faye Davis, Linda Jones, Howard Nathan
Row 2: Don Denny, Louise Jacobbi, Mary Anne House, Mark Reiner, John Welchel, MD
Row 3: Jim Springer, Bob Duckworth, Ron Dreffer, Marcia Blech, Bill Vaughn
1982
Rolling Ridge Retreat Conference Center, North Andover, MA.

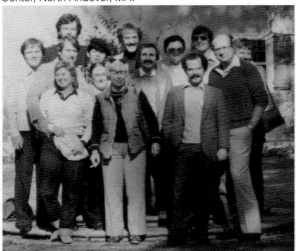

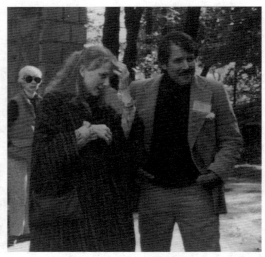

Jane Van Hook, Don Denny. 1982. Rolling Ridge Retreat Conference Center, North Andover, MA. NATCO Procurement Training Course

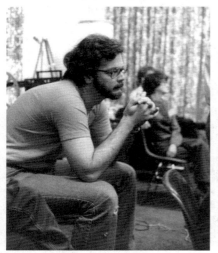

Bob Duckworth. 1982. Rolling Ridge Retreat Conference Center, North Andover, MA. NATCO Procurement Training Course.

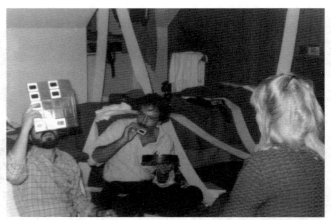

Howard Nathan and Ron Dreffer sorting through slides – everyone had roommates at Rolling Ridge. 1982. Rolling Ridge Retreat Conference Center, North Andover, MA. NATCO Procurement Training Course.

A CLINICIAN'S GUIDE TO DONATION AND TRANSPLANTATION

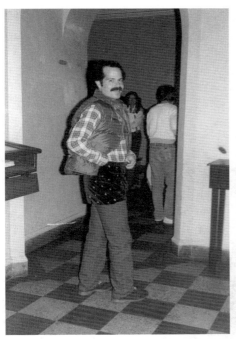

Howard Nathan. 1982. Rolling Ridge Retreat Conference Center, North Andover, MA. NATCO Procurement Training Course.

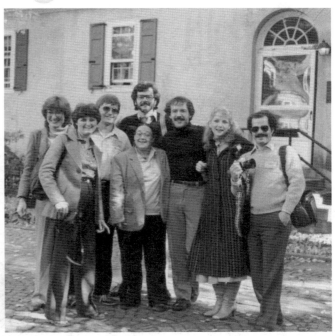

Jane Warmbrodt, Susan Hopper, Bill Vaughn, Mary Anne House, Bob Duckworth, Ron Dreffer, Jane Van Hook, Howard Nathan. 1982. Rolling Ridge Retreat Conference Center, North Andover, MA. NATCO Procurement Training Course.

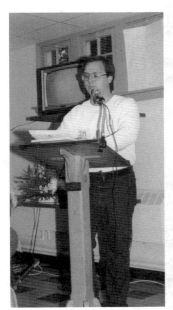

Jim Springer. 1983. Rolling Ridge Retreat Conference Center, North Andover, MA. NATCO Procurement Training Course.

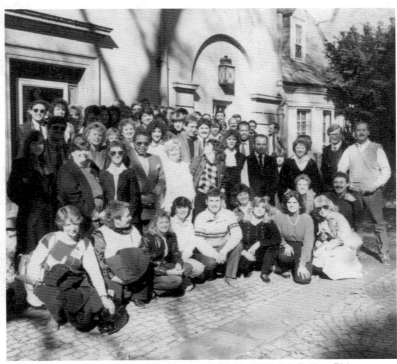

Another Rolling Ridge Procurement Course Class. 1983-84. Rolling Ridge Retreat Conference Center, North Andover, MA. NATCO Procurement Training Course.

Chapter 1 — **THE HISTORY OF THE TRANSPLANT COORDINATOR**

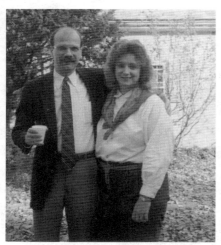

Tom Peters, MD and Teresa Shafer. 1985. Rolling Ridge Retreat Conference Center, North Andover, MA. NATCO Procurement Training Course.

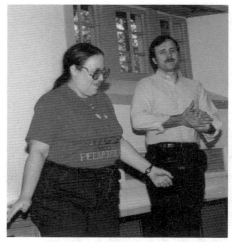

Mary Anne House and R. Patrick Wood, MD. 1984. Rolling Ridge Retreat Conference Center, North Andover, MA. NATCO Procurement Training Course.

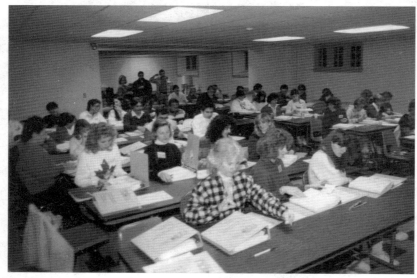

Classroom at Rolling Ridge for the Procurement Course. 1984. Rolling Ridge Retreat Conference Center, North Andover, MA. NATCO Procurement Training Course.

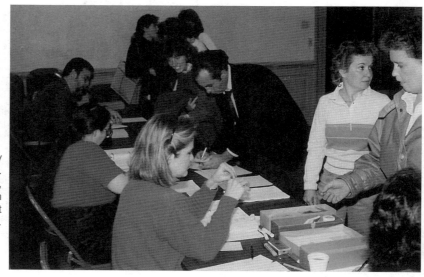

Robert Duckworth, Mary Anne House, Gwen Mayes. 1983-84. North Andover, Mass. Checking students in to the NATCO Procurement Training Course.

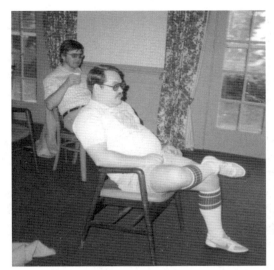

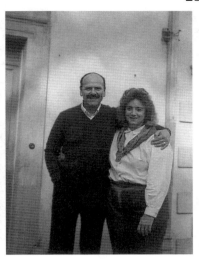

Gary Hall, Teresa Shafer. 1985. Rolling Ridge Retreat Conference Center, North Andover, MA. NATCO Procurement Training Course.

Bill Vaughn, Scott Woolley relaxing at night after class in main living area – pretty Spartan digs. 1985. Rolling Ridge Retreat Conference Center, North Andover, MA. NATCO Procurement Training Course.

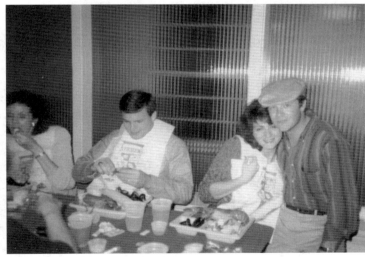

Jason Harrell, Allison (Ballew) Smith, Larry Cochran. 1985. Rolling Ridge Retreat Conference Center, North Andover, MA. NATCO Procurement Training Course.

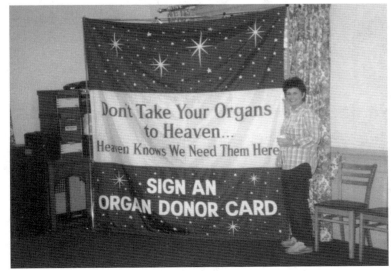

Don't Take Your Organs to Heaven – Heaven Knows we Need Them Here – banner set up in main living area. 1985. Rolling Ridge Retreat Conference Center, North Andover, MA. NATCO Procurement Training Course.

Chapter 1: THE HISTORY OF THE TRANSPLANT COORDINATOR

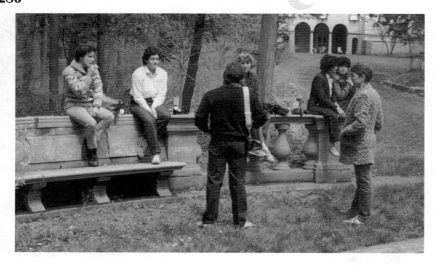

Hanging out at Rolling Ridge. 1985. Rolling Ridge Retreat Conference Center, North Andover, MA. NATCO Procurement Training Course.

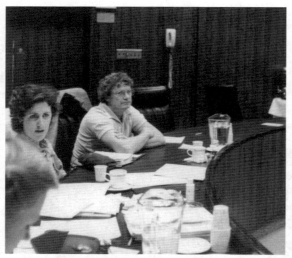

Amy Peele, Robert Gosnell. 1982. NATCO Board Meeting.

Claire Day. 1982. NATCO Board Meeting.

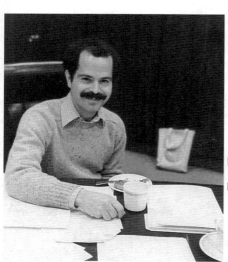

Howard Nathan. 1982. NATCO Board Meeting.

A CLINICIAN'S GUIDE TO DONATION AND TRANSPLANTATION

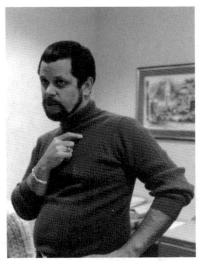

Roger Smith. 1989. San Francisco. NATCO Annual Meeting.

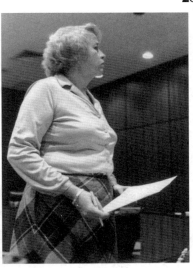

Barbara Schanbacher. 1982. NATCO Board Meeting.

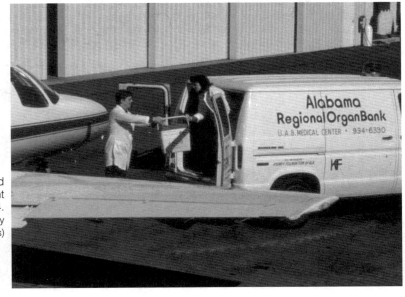

Laura Rudy and Paul Gaines, transplant coordinators. 1984.
(Photo courtesy Michael Phillips)

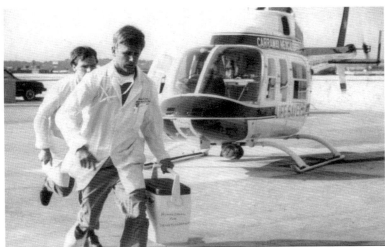

Early 1980's. David McGiffin, MD, University of Alabama heart surgeon and Michael Phillips, PA.
(Photo courtesy Michael Phillips)

Chapter 1 — **THE HISTORY OF THE TRANSPLANT COORDINATOR**

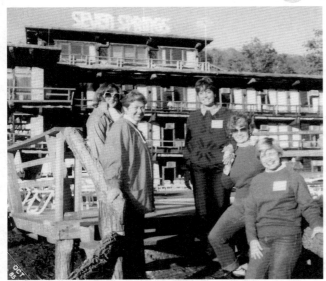

Instructors: (l to r) Patricia Barber, Faye Davis, Anita Principe, Claire Day, Barbara Elick. 1985. Seven Springs Mountain Resort, Champion, PA. NATCO Clinical Training Course.

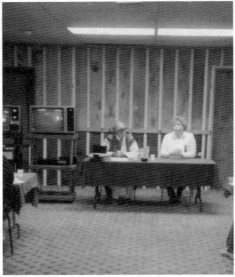

Barb Elick and Barb Schanbacher. 1983-84. Seven Springs Mountain Resort, Champion, PA. NATCO Clinical Training Course.

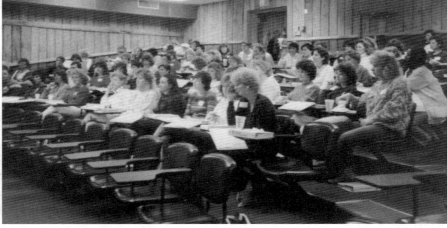

Participants at Clinical Training Course. 1983-84. Seven Springs Mountain Resort, Champion, PA. NATCO Clinical Training Course.

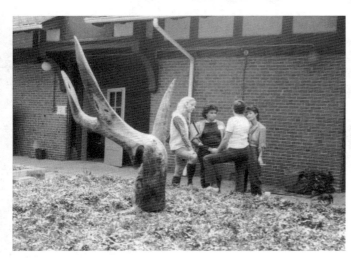

Hanging out at Seven Springs – Clinical Course. 1983-84. Seven Springs Mountain Resort, Champion, PA. NATCO Clinical Training Course.

A CLINICIAN'S GUIDE TO DONATION AND TRANSPLANTATION Chapter 1

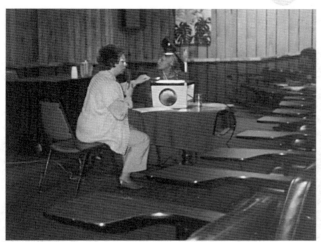

Sue Dutton, Barb Elick. 1983-84. Seven Springs Mountain Resort, Champion, PA. NATCO Clinical Training Course.

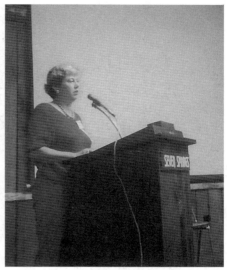

Faye Davis. Circa 1983-84. Seven Springs Mountain Resort, Champion, PA. NATCO Clinical Training Course.

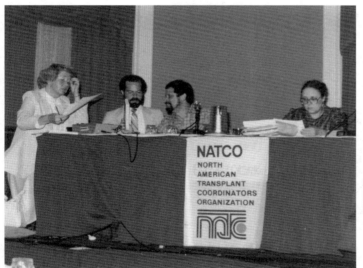

Barbara Schanbacher, Howard Nathan, Roger Smith, Mary Anne House, 1984-85.

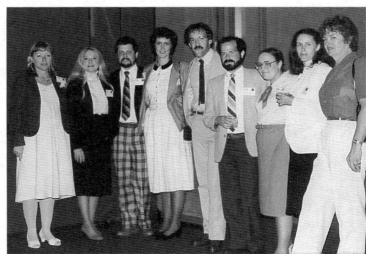

Winifred Mack, Lea Emmit, Roger Smith, Amy Peele, Ron Dreffer, Howard Nathan, Mary Anne House, unknown, Claire Day. 1983.

Chapter 1 — THE HISTORY OF THE TRANSPLANT COORDINATOR

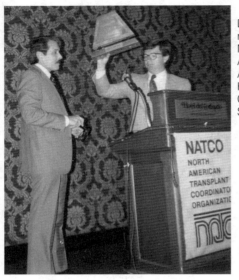

Don Denny receiving NATCO/Sandoz Achievement Award. 1985. Hotel Del Coronado, San Diego.

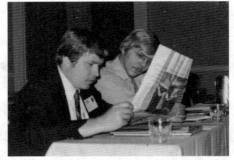

Burt Mattice, Ken Richardson. 1983.

Winifred Mack. 1983. New York City. Annual Meeting.

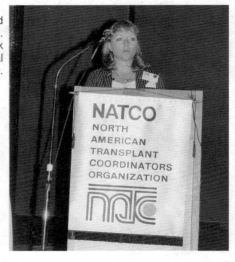

Anita Principe, Faye Davis, Claire Day. 1986. Seven Springs Mountain Resort, Champion, PA. NATCO Clinical Training Course.

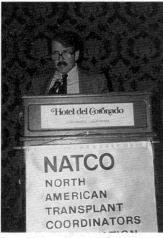

Donald Denny. 1985. San Diego Annual Meeting.

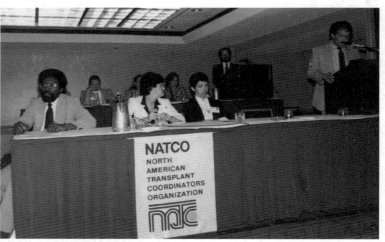

Paul Taylor, left. Louise Jacobbi, next to podium. Ron Dreffer at podium in front, Howard Nathan at podium in back. Barbara Schulman, far left, Patricia Barber next to Howard Nathan. 1985. One of the first "Ethics" section at a NATCO Annual Meeting.

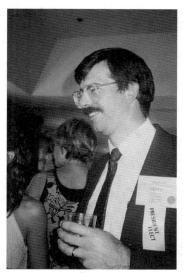

Stephen Haid. 1987.
Philadelphia, PA.

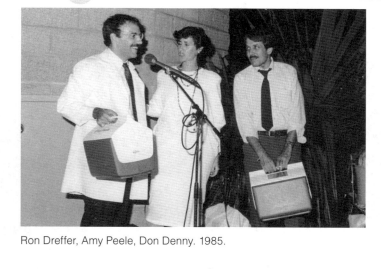

Ron Dreffer, Amy Peele, Don Denny. 1985.

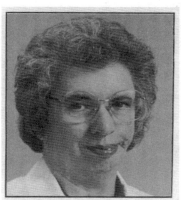

Suzanne B. Dutton

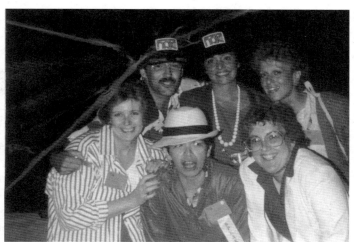

Eileen DeMayo, Louise Jacobbi, Mikki Mastellar, Back: Ron Dreffer, Anita Principe, Tina Kress. 1985. San Diego. Annual Meeting.

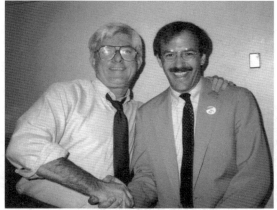

Phil Donahue, talk show host, and Ron Dreffer. 1985. Donahue show.

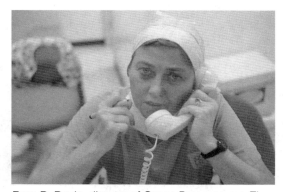

Faye D. Davis, director of Organ Procurement, The Methodist Hospital/Baylor College of Medicine Multi-Organ Transplant Center, Houston, TX. 1986. Reprinted with permission from The Methodist Hospital, Houston, TX.

THE HISTORY OF THE TRANSPLANT COORDINATOR

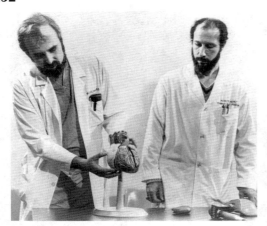

Mitch Goldman, MD, Herb Teachey.

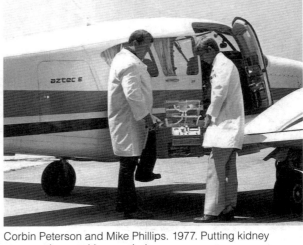

Corbin Peterson and Mike Phillips. 1977. Putting kidney preservation machine on airplane.
(Photo courtesy Michael Phillips)

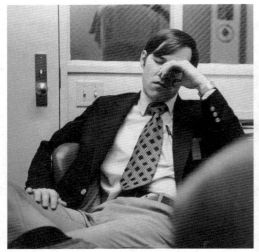

Brian Broznick.

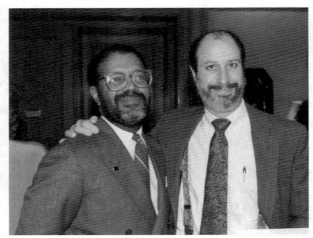

Rudy Morgan, Herb Teachey 1989. San Francisco. Annual Meeting NATCO.

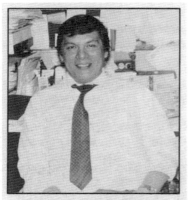

Robert M. Hoffman

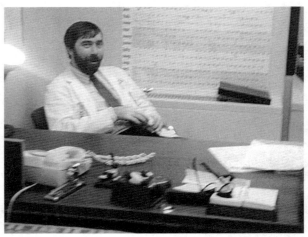

Lynne Driver. 1985. Methodist Hospital in Indianapolis.

A CLINICIAN'S GUIDE TO DONATION AND TRANSPLANTATION

Chapter 1

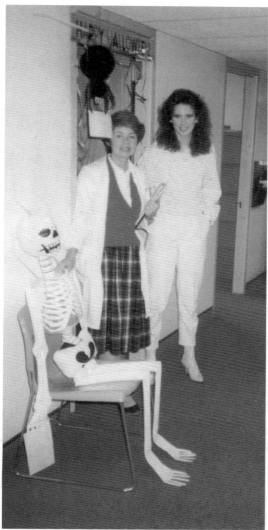

Christine Gilmore, far left. 1985. Methodist Hospital in Indianapolis. Someone left Chris an October 31 surprise.

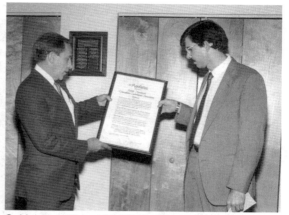

G. Melville Williams, UNOS President, and Steve Haid, NATCO President. December, 1986. Turning 24 Alert over to UNOS.

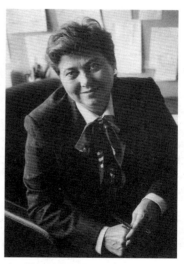

Faye D. Davis, RN, MSN, director of Organ Procurement, The Methodist Hospital/Baylor College of Medicine Multi-Organ Transplant Center, Houston, TX. 1986. Reprinted with permission from The Methodist Hospital, Houston, TX

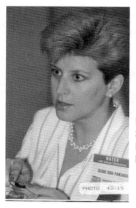

Dede Panjeda. 1989. San Francisco, CA. NATCO Annual Meeting.

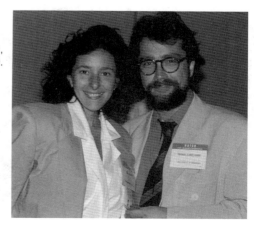

Jolie (Savas) Slaton, Thomas (Lang) Karbe. 1989.

Chapter 1 — **THE HISTORY OF THE TRANSPLANT COORDINATOR**

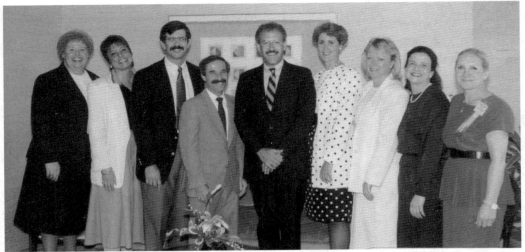

Barbara Schanbacher, Anita Principe, Steve Haid, Mark Reiner, Ron Dreffer, Amy Peele, Winifred Mack, Kate Hume, Barbara Schulman. 1989. San Francisco, CA. NATCO Annual Meeting.

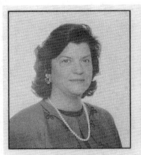
Carolyn Atkins

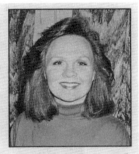
Alesha Hammond

1989.

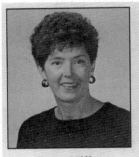
Joan Miller

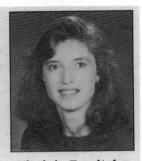
Virginia Travitzky

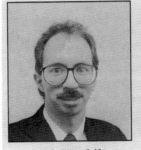
Rob Kochik

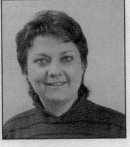
Jayne Meyer

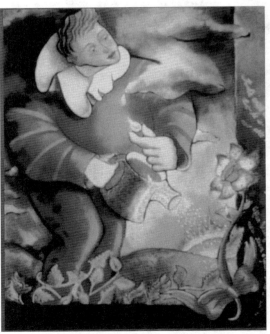

NATCO Art Poster. 1990. NATCO commissioned this painting. It was to be a fund raising effort for the organization.

A CLINICIAN'S GUIDE TO DONATION AND TRANSPLANTATION *Chapter 1*

Sandra Staschak-Chicko, CCTC, Senior Transplant Coordinator, University of Pittsburgh, Past Co-Chair NATCO Introductory Course for Transplant Coordinators; Barbara Elick, CCTC/CPTC, Chief Transplant Coordinator, University of Minnesota, NATCO President. At the White House, Wahington, D.C. 1991.

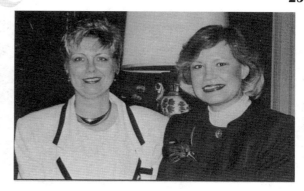

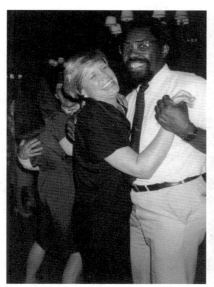

Barb Elick, Paul Taylor. 1991.

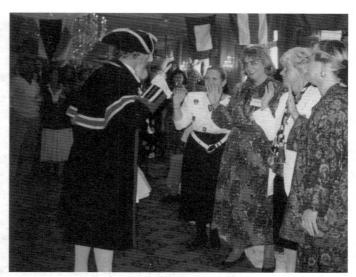

Barbara Schulman, Teresa Shafer, Linda Jones, Barbara Elick. 1991. Halifax, Nova Scotia. First (and only) NATCO Annual Meeting held out of the country.

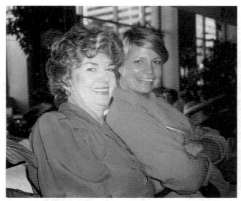

Claire Day, Barbara Elick.

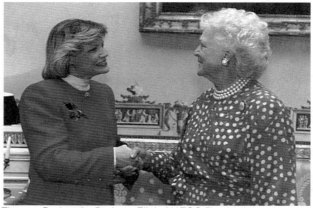

The two Barbara's: Barbara Elick, NATCO President, and Barbara Bush, first lady. 1991. White House Washington, D.C.

Chapter 1

THE HISTORY OF THE TRANSPLANT COORDINATOR

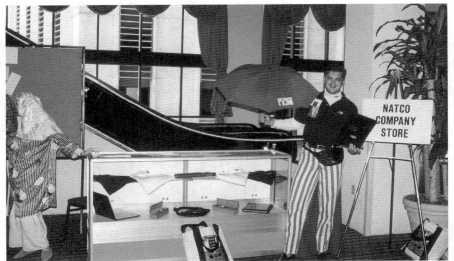

Bruce Nicely. 1994. New Orleans. NATCO opened the company store to sell NATCO items – a fund raising effort for the organization. This was the first time we rolled it out – in New Orleans. Bruce dressed the part and walked into the Annual meeting wearing many of the items for sale.

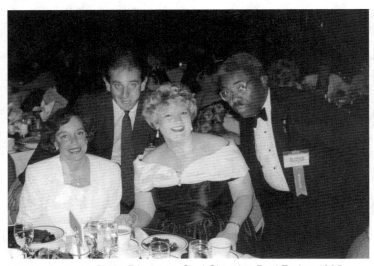

Marilyn Bartucci, Barry Friedman, Gayl Chrysler, Paul Taylor. 1995. Kansas City.

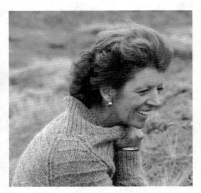

Celia Wight. Circa 2000. United Kingdom. First President, UKTCA. (Photo courtesy of Celia Wight)

Walter Graham, Executive Director, UNOS. August, 1994. Kyoto, Japan. 15th International Congress of the Transplantation Society.

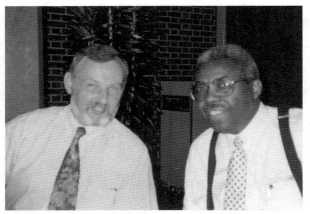

Leo Roels, Paul Taylor. August, 1994. Kyoto, Japan. 15th International Congress of the Transplantation Society.

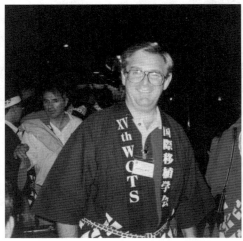

A CLINICIAN'S GUIDE TO DONATION AND TRANSPLANTATION

Chapter 1

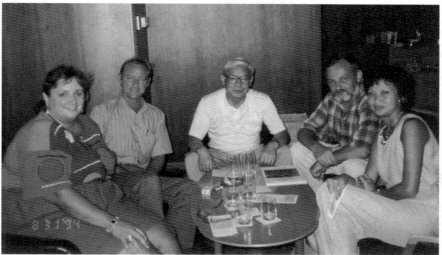

Formation of the International Transplant Coordinators Society: Founding Members: Teresa Shafer (US), Greg Armstrong (Australia), Seigo Hiraga, MD (Japan), Leo Roels (Belgium), Sally (Tan) Kong (Singapore). August, 1994. Kyoto, Japan. Kyoto Takaragaike Prince Hotel, in the bar. 15th International Congress of the Transplantation Society.

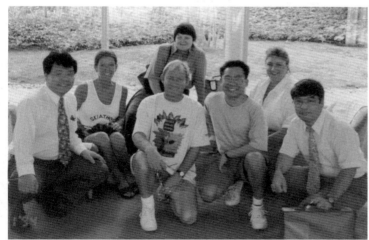

Isao Tamaki, President, JATCO
Celia Wight, Past President, UKTCA
Sue Falvey, President, UKTCA
Greg Armstrong, Australia
Teresa Shafer, President, NATCO
Don Akagi (Teresa Shafer's husband)
Osamu Kato, Japan. August, 1994. Kyoto, Japan
Kyoto Takaragaike Prince Hotel. 15th International Congress of the Transplantation Society.

Leo Roels, President, ETCO
Osamu Kato, Teresa Shafer, President, NATCO
Seigo Hiraga, President ITCM
Sally (Tan) Kong, Greg Armstrong, Paul Taylor . August 29, 1994. Kyoto International Conference Hall, Kyoto, Japan. 1st International Transplant Coordinators Meeting (ITCM) Party.

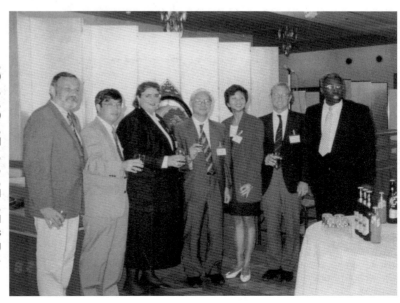

Chapter 1 — **THE HISTORY OF THE TRANSPLANT COORDINATOR**

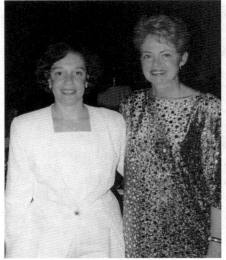
Marilyn Bartucci, Christine Gilmore. 1995.

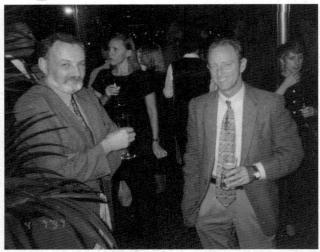
Leo Roels, Greg Armstrong. 1997. Canberra, Australia. Australasian Transplant Coordinators Association (ATCA) meeting.

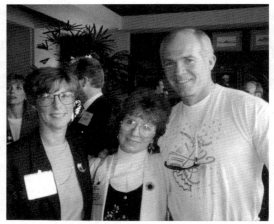
Ellen French, Linda Ohler, Jim McCabe. Linda Ohler is editor of Progress in Transplantation (PT) and Ellen French is with Innovision, the publisher for PT.

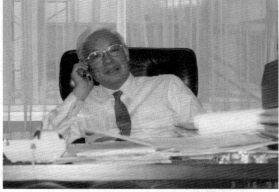
Siego Hiraga, MD. 1998. Mishima, Japan. Seigo Hiraga was key in forming the Japanese Transplant Coordinators Organization. He was also first President of the International Transplant Coordinators Organization.

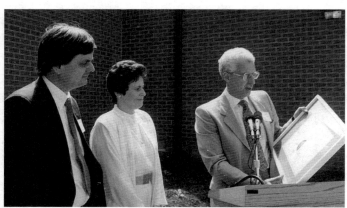
Bill Anderson, Helen Leslie Bottenfield, Richard Hurwitz, MD. 1998. Dr. Richard Hurwitz, one of the three co-founders of LifeNet. (Photo courtesy of LifeNet)

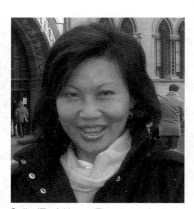
Sally (Tan) Kong, First transplant coordinator in Singapore.

A CLINICIAN'S GUIDE TO DONATION AND TRANSPLANTATION

Chapter 1

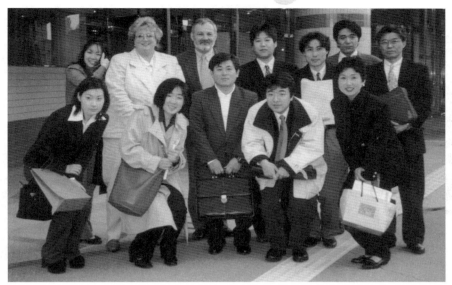

Teresa Shafer and Leo Roels with Japanese transplant coordinators. 1998. Shizuoka, Japan. Travel to Japan on a Human Science Foundation grant to review Japanese transplant system.

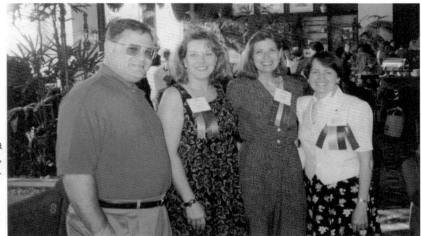

Richard Metz, Laura Stephens, Nancy Senst, Jamie Blazek. 1996.

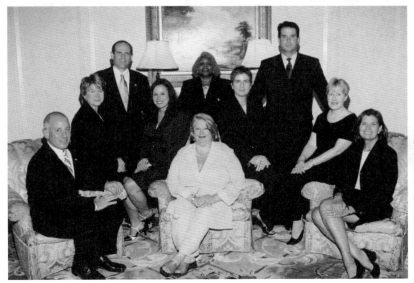

Barry Friedman, Holly Warren, Keith Stevens, Dianne LaPointe Rudow, Cozzie Watkins, Marian O'Rourke, Charlie Alexander, Mary Beth Drangstveit, Nancy Senst, President Judy Graham in front. 2002. Washington, D.C.

Chapter 1: THE HISTORY OF THE TRANSPLANT COORDINATOR

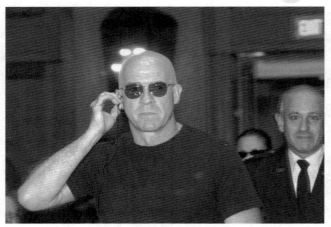

Jim McCabe, Barry Friedman. 2003. New Orleans, LA.

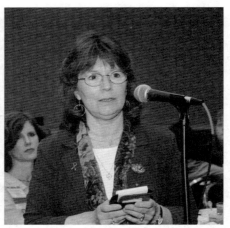

Linda Ohler. 2003. New Orleans, LA.

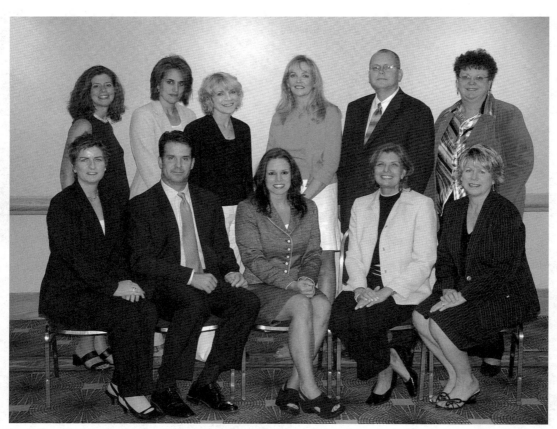

Back Row (l to r): Gina Dunne-Smith, Carrie Comellas, Barbara Nuesse, Jan Finn, David Zimmerman, Nancy Boyle Front Row (l to r): Marian O'Rourke, Charlie Alexander, Dianne LaPointe Rudow, Nancy Senst, Holly Warren. 2004. San Francisco, CA.

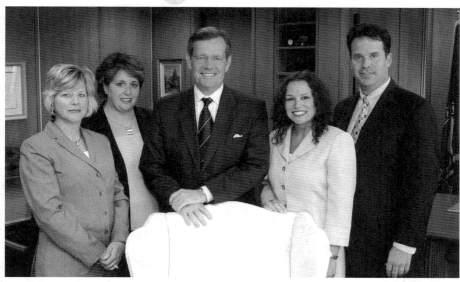

Dede Gish Panjeda, Amy Demske, DHHS Secretary Michael Leavitt, Dianne LaPointe Rudow, Charlie Alexander. 2005. Washington, D.C.

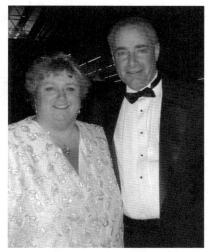

Teresa Shafer, John Chessare, MD. Co-Chairs, Organ Donation Breakthrough Collaborative. May, 2005. Pittsburgh, PA. First National Learning Congress – following completion of Organ Donation Breakthrough Collaboratives 1 & 2.

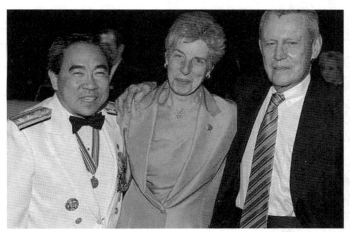

U.S. Deputy Surgeon General Kenneth Moritsugu, MD, Lisa Kory, RN, and Thomas Starzl, MD. National Learning Congress, Pittsburgh, PA, May, 2005. Lisa, a former transplant coordinator and NATCO President, and Dr. Moritsugu were married in 2000.

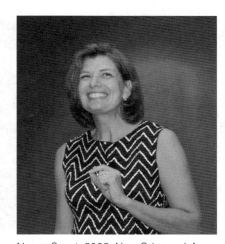

Nancy Senst. 2003. New Orleans, LA.

THE HISTORY OF THE TRANSPLANT COORDINATOR

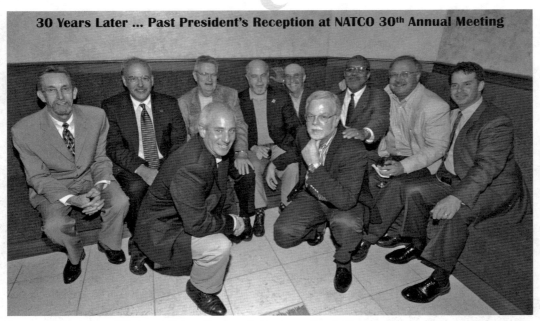

30 Years Later ... Past President's Reception at NATCO 30th Annual Meeting

Front row (l to r): Barry Friedman, Robert Duckworth. Back row (l to r): Charles Bearden, Ron Dreffer, Robert Gosnell, Howard Nathan, Mark Reiner, Rudy Morgan, James Springer, Charlie Alexander. August, 2005. Atlanta, GA. Past President's Reception at 30th NATCO Anniversary, Annual Meeting.

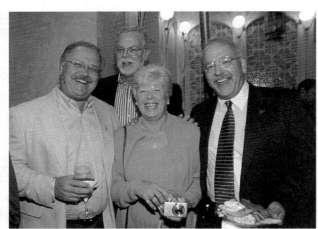

James Springer, Robert Duckworth, Linda Jones, Ronald Dreffer. August, 2005. Atlanta, GA. Past President's Reception at 30th NATCO Anniversary, Annual Meeting.

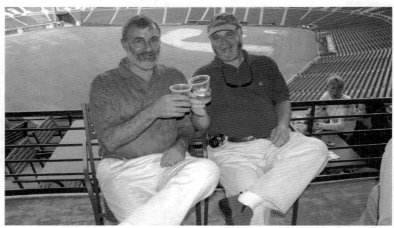

Jim Warren, Editor, *Transplant News*, Howard Nathan. August, 2005. Atlanta, GA. NATCO Annual Meeting.

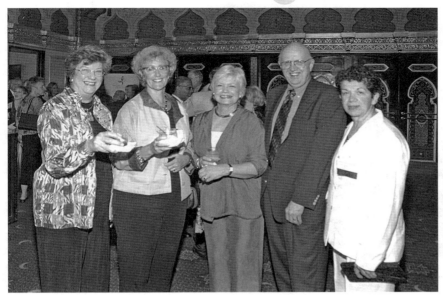

Carolyn Atkins, Amy Peele, Barbara Elick, Jim Atkins (Carolyn's husband), Louise Jacobbi. August, 2005. Atlanta, GA. Past President's Reception at 30th NATCO Anniversary, Annual Meeting.

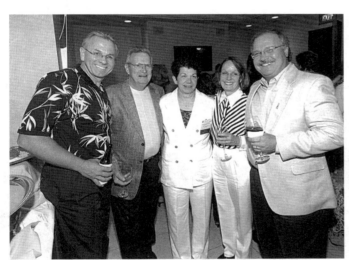

Laurie's husband, Duane, Bob Gosnell, Louise Jacobbi, Laurie Williams, Jim Springer. August, 2005. Atlanta, GA. Past President's Reception at 30th NATCO Anniversary, Annual Meeting.

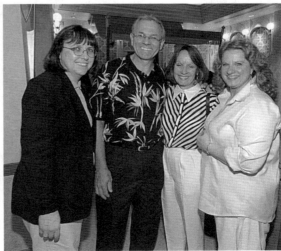

Frances Hoffman, Laurie's husband, Duane, Laurie Williams, Mary Ann Palumbi. 2005. Atlanta, GS. Past President's Reception at 30th NATCO Anniversary, Annual Meeting.

Chapter 1 — THE HISTORY OF THE TRANSPLANT COORDINATOR

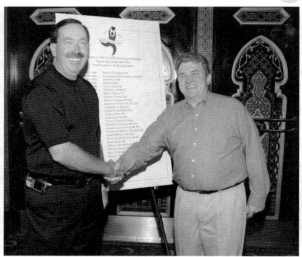

Lynne Driver, Burt Mattice. August, 2005. Atlanta, GA. Past President's Reception at 30th NATCO Anniversary, Annual Meeting.

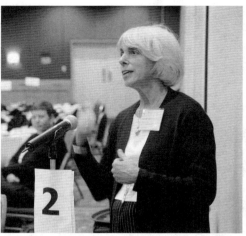

Elaine Vuyosevich. August, 2005. Atlanta, GA. NATCO Annual Meeting.

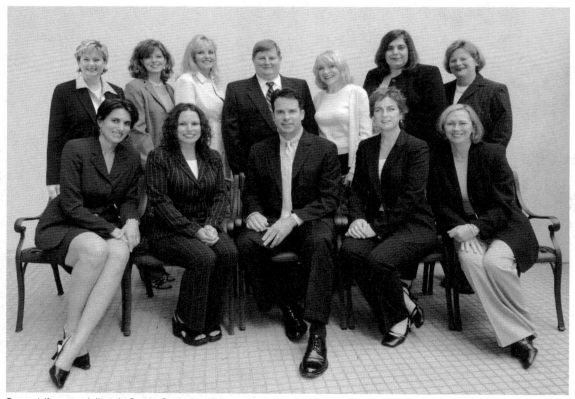

Seated (front row) (l to r): Carrie Comellas, Dianne LaPointe Rudow, Charles Alexander, Marian O'Rourke, and Lori Coleman. Standing (back row) (l to r): Nancy Harrington, Gina Dunne-Smith, Jan Finn, Bill Hasskamp, Barb Nuesse, Lindsay Arnott, and Cathy Garvey. 2005. 2005 Board of Directors.

References

1. Rife M. NATCO – a display of determination. *Dial Transplant* 1981;10(9):769.
2. Vincent MC, Repper SM, Peters TG. Education, pay, and job status: a national survey of transplant coordinators. *Prog Transplant.* 2002;12:212-216.
3. Kalson S. A link to life: coordinators of organ procurement programs are transplantation's "unsung heroes." *New York Times Magazine.* June 19, 1983;20.
4. Kootstra G. History of organ donation and sharing. In: Hakim NS, Papalois VE, eds. *History of Organ and Cell Transplantation.* London: Imperial College Press; 2003:55-75.
5. Day C. Transplant coordinator as part of ESRD regulation. *NATCO Newsletter.* 1981;2(1):1.
6. Denny D. How organs are distributed. *Hastings Center Rep.* December 1983;13:26-27.
7. NATCO: an organization dedicated to serve those with end stage organ failure. *Nephrol Nurse.* Sept-Oct 1982;4:31-33.
8. Mandefield H, Wellington F, Morgan V. Introduction of the certificate in transplant coordination in the United Kingdom. *Prog Transplant.* 2001;11:14-16.
9. Teixeira JF, Fiuza C, Cruz J, Araujo R, Fonseca J, Teixeira A. Key tasks for the transplant coordinator. *Organs Tissues.* 2003;3:175-181.
10. Dutton SB. Certification of transplant coordinators by the American Board of Transplant Coordinators. *J Transplant Coord.* 1996;6:210-214.
11. Falvey S. The role of the transplant coordinator. *J R Soc Med.* 1996;89(S29):18.
12. Soh P, Lim SM, Tan ED. Organ procurement in Singapore. *Ann Acad Med Singapore.* 1991;20:439-442.
13. Matesanz R, Lopez Navidad A. The transplant coordinator in Spain. In: Matesanz R, Miranda B, eds. *Organ Donation for Transplantation: The Spanish Model.* Madrid: Aula Medica Madrid; 1996:57-66.
14. Wight C. The role of the transplant coordinator. In: Collins GM, Dubernard JM, Land W, Persijn GG, eds. *Procurement, Preservation and Allocation of Vascularized Organs.* Kluwer Academic Publishers; 1997:241-247.
15. Wight C. Transplant coordinators and organ procurement in Western Europe. *J Transplant Coord.* 1991;1:39-41.
16. Bergstrom C, Gabel H. Organ donation and organ retrieval programs in Sweden, 1990. *J Transplant Coord.* 1991;1:47-51.
17. Colpart JJ, Noury D, Cochat P, Kormann P, Moskovtchenko JF. Organization of organ transplantation in France. *Pediatrie.* 1991;46:313-322.
18. Karbe T. Standardized education program in organ procurement for transplant coordinators. *Transplant Proc.* 1991;23:2539-2540.
19. Soeda E. A role of recipient coordinators in Japan. *Nippon Rinsho.* 2005;63:1928-1934.
20. Filipponi F, De Simone P, Mosca F. Appraisal of the coordinator-based transplant organizational model. *Transplant Proc.* 2005;37:2421-2422.
21. Matesanz R. Factors that influence the development of an organ donation program. *Transplant Proc.* 2004;36:739-741.
22. Tolboe NO. The role of the transplant coordinator: a newly emerging professional. In: Chatterjee SN, ed. *Renal Transplantation: A Multidisciplinary Approach.* New York, NY: Raven Press Books; 1980:43-57.
23. Schulman, B. Founders share a bit of history. *NATCO Newsletter.* 1984;5(2):6.
24. Elick B. Transplant coordinators. In: Chapman JR, Deirhoi M, Wight C, eds. *Organ and Tissue Donation for Transplantation.* New York, NY: Oxford University Press; 1997:325-343.
25. Donaldson TA. The role of the transplant coordinator. In: Cupples SA, Ohler L, eds. *Transplantation Nursing Secrets.* Philadelphia, Pa: Hanley & Belfus, Inc;2003:17-26.
26. Gutkind L. *Many Sleepless Nights.* New York, NY: W.W. Norton and Company, Inc.; 1988.
27. Tilney NL. *Transplant: From Myth to Reality.* New Haven, Conn: Yale University Press; 2003.
28. Starzl TE. *The Puzzle People: Memoirs of a Transplant Surgeon.* Pittsburgh, Pa: University of Pittsburgh Press;1992.
29. Mackinney L. *Medical Illustrations in Medieval Manuscripts.* Berkeley, Calif: University of California Press; 1965.
30. Dewhurst J. Cosmos and Damian, patron saints of doctors. *Lancet.* 1988;2:1479.

31. Smith SL. Historical perspective of transplantation. In: Smith SL, ed. *Organ Transplantation: Concepts, Issues, Practice, and Outcomes*. Electronic Publication, Medscape, June 2002. Available at: http://www.medscape.com/viewarticle/436532. Accessed January 25, 2006.
32. History of transplantation. In: *The Gift of a Lifetime: Organ and Tissue Transplantation in America*. Available at: http://www.organtransplants.org/understanding/history/. Accessed October 4, 2005.
33. Churchill WLS. *My Early Life, a Roving Commission*. London: T Butterworth Ltd;1930:211.
34. Sharma S, Unruh H. Heart and heart-lung transplantation. In: Shapiro R, Talvera F, Sudan DL, Zevitz ME, Mancini MC, eds. *History of Adult Transplantation*. August 15, 2004. Available at: http://www.emedicine.com/med/topic3497.htm. Accessed February 19, 2006.
35. Reitz, BA. History of heart and heart-lung transplantation. In: Baumgartner WA, Reitz B, Kasper E, Theodore J, eds. *Heart and Lung Transplantation*. Philadelphia, Pa: W B Saunders Co; 1995:3-14.
36. Papalois VE, Hakim NS, Najarian JS. The history of kidney transplantation. In: Hakim NS, Papalois VE, eds. *The History of Organ and Cell Transplantation*. London: Imperial College Press; 2003:79.
37. Edwards WS, Edwards PD. *Alexis Carrel: Visionary Surgeon*. Springfield, Ill: Charles C Thomas; 1974.
38. Malinin TI. *Surgery and Life: The Extraordinary Career and Alexis Carrel*. New York, NY: Harcourt Brace Jovanovich; 1979.
39. Quinton W, Dillard D, Scribner BH. Cannulation of blood vessels for prolonged hemodialysis. *Trans Am Soc Artificial Organs*. 1960;6:104.
40. Scribner BH, cited in Fox RC Swazey JP. *The Courage to Fail*. Chicago: University of Chicago Press; 1974:240-279.
41. Mollaret P, Goulon M. Le coma dépassé (mémoire préliminaire). *Rev Neurol*. 1959;101:3-15.
42. Wijdicks EFM. The Landmark "Le Coma Dépasse". In: Wijdicks EFM, ed. Brain Death. Lippincott Williams and Wilkins, 2001:1-4.
43. Williams GM. History of transplantation. In: Phillips MG, ed. *Organ Procurement, Preservation and Distribution in Transplantation*. 2nd ed. Richmond, Va: William Byrd Press, Inc;1991:7-12.
44. Machado C. Historical neurology: the first organ transplant from a brain-dead donor. *Neurology*. 2005;64:1938-1942.
45. Murray JE. Organ transplantation: the practical possibilities. In: Wolstenholme GEW, O'Connor M, eds. *Ethics in medical progress: with special reference to transplantation*. Boston, Mass: Little Brown, 1966.
46. Lock M. *Twice Dead: Organ Transplants and the Reinvention of Death*. Berkeley, Calif: University of California Press;2002.
47. The Heart: Miracle in Cape Town. *Newsweek*, December 18, 1967:87.
48. Sharma S, Unruh H. Evolution of organ donation and procurement. In: Shapiro R, Talvera F, Sudan DL, Zevitz ME, Mancini MC, eds. *History of Adult Transplantation*. August 15, 2004. Available at: http://www.emedicine.com/med/topic3497.htm. Accessed: February 19, 2006.
49. American Medical Association House of Delegates. Definition of death. *JAMA*. 1974;227:728.
50. A definition of irreversible coma: report of the Ad Hoc Committee of the Harvard Medical School to Examine the Definition of Brain Death. *JAMA*. 1968;205:337-340.
51. Chabalewski F, Taylor GJ, Johnson K, Evers KA, McGaw LJ, Sampson D, Newman MB. Policy and practice in organ transplantation. In: Organ Transplant, 2002 Medscape. Available at: http://medscape.com/viewarticle/436539_print. Accessed: January 25, 2006.
52. Hoffmann RM, Miller DT. Cadaver kidney preservation and procurement. In: Schoengrund L, Balzer P, eds. *Renal Problems in Critical Care*. New York, NY: John Wiley & Sons:1985:269-274.
53. Cranford RE. Brain death. In: Phillips MG, ed. *Organ Procurement, Preservation and Distribution in Transplantation*. Richmond, Va: William Byrd Press, Inc; 1991:23-38.
54. Culpepper MI Jr. Legal aspects of organ and tissue procurement in transplantation. In: Phillips MG, ed. *Organ Procurement, Preservation and Distribution in Transplantation*. Richmond, Va: William Byrd Press, Inc; 1996:23-38.
55. Guidelines for the determination of death: report of the medical consultants on the diagnosis of death to the President's Commission for the Study of Ethical Problems in Medical and Biomedical and Behavior Research. *JAMA*. 1981;246:2184-2186.
56. Altman LK. Norman E. Shumway, 83, Who Made the Heart Transplant a Standard Operation, Dies. *The New York Times*. February 11, 2006. Available at: http://www.nytimes.com/2006/02/11/health/11shumway.html?pagewanted=2&_r=1. Accessed February 12, 2006.
57. Norman E. Shumway, MD, PhD (1923-2006). *Am J Transplant*. 2006;6:1091-1092.
58. Shafer TJ, Schkade LL, Warner HE, et al. The impact of medical examiner/coroner practices on organ recovery in the United States. *JAMA*. 1994;272:1607-1613.
59. Strama BT, Burling-Hatcher S, Shafer TJ. Criminal investigations and prosecutions not adversely affected by organ donation: a case law review. *Newsletter of Medicine and Law Committee*. Tort and Insurance Practice Section, American Bar Association; Summer 1994:15-21.
60. Goldstein B, Shafer TJ, Greer D, Stephens BG. Medical examiner/coroner denial for organ donation in brain-dead victims of child abuse: controversies and solutions. *Clin Intensive Care*. 1997;8:136-141.

61. Shafer TJ, Schkade LL, Siminoff LA, Mahoney TA. Ethical analysis of organ recovery denials by medical examiners, coroners and justices of the peace. *J Transplant Coord.* 1999;9:232-249.
62. Shafer TJ, Schkade LL, Evans RW, O'Connor KJ, Reitsma W. The vital role of medical examiners and coroners in organ transplantation. *Am J Transplant.* February 2004;4:160-168.
63. Shafer TJ. The forensic nurse examiner and organ donation: a partnership for life. In: Lynch V, ed. *Forensic Nursing.* St. Louis, Mo: Elsevier/Mosby;1995:217-234.
64. Voelker R. Can forensic medicine and organ donation coexist for the public good? JAMA. 1994;271:891-892.
65. Medical examiners limiting organ use. *Pittsburgh Post Gazette.* November 23, 1994.
66. Organ releases needlessly delayed. *San Francisco Examiner.* November 23, 1994.
67. Study finds examiners sometimes delay organ release for no reason. *Northwest Herald* (Woodstock, Ill). November 23, 1994.
68. Chinnock RE, Bailey LL. Letter to the Editor. JAMA. 1995;273:1578.
69. Toledo LH, Toledo AH. 1954. *J Invest Surg.* 2005;18:285-290.
70. Murray JM. *Surgery of the Soul: Reflections of a Curious Mind.* Canton, Mass: Science History Publications; 2001.
71. Murray JE, Merrill JP, Harrison JH. Renal homotransplantations in identical twins. *Surg Forum.* 1955;6:432.
72. Merrill JP, Murray JE, Harrison JH, Guild WR. Successful homotransplantations of the human kidney between identical twins. JAMA. 1956;160:277.
73. Murray JE, Merrill JP, Harrison JH. Kidney transplantations between seven pairs of identical twins. *Ann Surg.* 1958;148:343.
74. Joseph E. Murray—Nobel Lecture. Available at: http://nobelprize.org/medicine/laureates/1990/murray-lecture.html. Accessed April 16, 2006.
75. Starzl TE. The mystique of organ transplantation. *J Am Coll Surg.* 2005;201:160-170.
76. Hume DM, Merrill JP, Miller BF, Thorn GW. Experiences with renal homotransplantations in the human: report of nine cases. *J Clin Invest.* 1955;34:327-382.
77. Goodwin WE, Mims MM, Kaufman JJ. Human renal transplantation III: technical problems encountered in six cases of kidney homotransplantations. *Trans Am Assoc Genitourin Surg.* 1962;54:116.
78. Goodwin WE, Kaufmann JJ, Mims MM, et al. Human renal transplantation I: clinical experiences with six cases of renal transplantation. *J Urol.* 1963;89:13.
79. Hamilton D. Kidney transplantation: a history. In: Morris PJ, ed. *Transplantation Principles and Practice.* Philadelphia, Pa: W B Saunders Co;1994:1-7.
80. Ullman E. Tissue and organ transplantation. *Ann Surg.* 1914;60:195.
81. Nagy J. A Note on the early history of renal transplantation: Emerich (Imre) Ullmann. History of dialysis and transplantation. *Am J Nephrol.* 1999;19:346-349.
82. Kuss R, Bourget P. *An Illustrated History of Organ Transplantation.* Rueil-Malmaison, France: Laboratoires Sandoz; 1992.
83. Sharma S, Unruh H. Kidney transplantation. In: Shapiro R, Talvera F, Sudan DL, Zevitz ME, Mancini MC, eds. *History of Adult Transplantation.* August 15, 2004. Available at: http://www.emedicine.com/med/topic3497.htm. Accessed February 19, 2006.
84. Stefoni S, Campieri C, Donati G, Orlandi V. The history of clinical transplant. *J Nephrol.* Available at: http://www.sin-italy.org/jnonline/Vol17n3/475.html. Accessed April 21, 2006.
85. Wardener H. Interview of Dr. Gabriel Richet, Charing Cross Hospital, 1997. In: *International Society of Nephrology.* Available at: http://cybernephrology.ualberta.ca/ISN/VLP/Trans/Richet.htm. Accessed April 22, 2006.
86. Murray JW, Merrill JP, Harrison, Wilston RE, Dammin GJ. Prolonged survival of human kidney allografts by immunosuppressive drug therapy. *N Engl J Med.* 1963;268:1315.
87. Starzl TE. *Experience in Renal Transplantation.* Philadelphia, Pa: W B Saunders Co;1964.
88. Welch CS. A note on transplantation of the whole liver in dogs. *Transplant Bull.* 1955;2:54-55.
89. Starzl TE. History of Liver and Other Sphlanchic Organ Transplantation. In: Busuttil R, Klintmalm G, eds. *Transplantation of the Liver.* Philadelphia, Pa: W B Saunders Co;1996:3-22.
90. Cannon JA. Brief Report. *Transplant Bull.* 1956;3(7).
91. Calne RY. History of liver transplantation. In: Hakim NS, Papalois VE, eds. *History of Organ and Cell Transplantation.* London: Imperial College Press; 2003:100-119.
92. Sharma S, Unruh H. Liver and pancreas transplantation. In: Shapiro R, Talvera F, Sudan DL, Zevitz ME, Mancini MC, eds. *History of Adult Transplantation.* August 15, 2004. Available at: http://www.emedicine.com/med/topic3497.htm. Accessed February 19, 2006.
93. Calne RY, White DJG, Thiru S, et al. Cyclosporin A in patients receiving renal allografts from cadaver donors. *Lancet.* 1978;2:1323-1327.
94. Starzl TE, Weill R III, Iwatsuki S, et al. The use of cyclosporin A and prednisone in cadaver kidney transplantation. *Surg Gynecol Obstet.* 1980;151:17-26.

Chapter 1 — **THE HISTORY OF THE TRANSPLANT COORDINATOR**

95. Starzl TE, Klintmalm GBG, Porter KA, et al. Liver transplantation with the use of cyclosporin A and prednisone. *N Engl J Med*. 1981;305:266-269.
96. Starzl TE, Todo S, Fung J, et al. FK506 for human liver, kidney and pancreas transplantation. *Lancet*. 1989;2:1000-1004.
97. Todo S, Fung JJ, Starzl TE, et al. Liver, kidney and thoracic organ transplantation under FK506. *Ann Surg*. 1990;212:295-305.
98. Starzl TE, Iwatsuki S, Van Thiel DH, et al. Evolution of liver transplantation. *Hepatology*. 1982;2:614-636.
99. Starzl TE, Marchioro TL, Von Kaulla KN, et al. Homotransplantation of the liver in humans. *Surg Gynecol Obstet*. 1963;117:659-676.
100. Kang YG, Martin DJ, Marquez J, et al. Intraoperative changes in blood coagulation and thrombelastographic monitoring in liver transplantation. *Anesth Analg*. 1985;64:888-896.
101. Carrel A, Guthrie CC: The transplantation of vein and organs. *Am Med*. 1905;10:1101-1102.
102. Shumaker HB Jr. *The Evolution of Cardiac Surgery*. Indianapolis, Ind: Indiana University Press; 1992:317.
103. Heart, Heart-Lung, and Lung Transplantation. The Cardiothoracic Surgery Network. Available at: http://www.ctsnet.org/edmunds/Chapter1section15.html. Accessed April 28, 2006.
104. Demikhov VP: Experimental transplantation of an additional heart in the dog. *Bull Exp Biol Med* (Russia). 1950;1:241.
105. Lower RR, Shumway NE: Studies on orthotopic homotransplantation of the canine heart. *Surg Forum*. 1960;11:18.
106. Brock R: Heart excision and replacement. *Guys Hosp Rep*. 1959;108:285.
107. Demikhov VP. *Experimental Transplantation of Vital Organs* [authorized translation from the Russian by Basil Haigh]. New York, NY: Consultants Bureau; 1962.
108. Spencer F. Intellectual creativity in thoracic surgeons. *J Thorac Cardiovasc Surg*. 1983;86:172.
109. Hardy JD, Chavez CM, Kurrus FD, et al: Heart transplantation in man: developmental studies and report of a case. JAMA. 118:1132:964.
110. The James D. Hardy Archives: A Pioneer in Surgery. The University of Mississippi Medical Center. Available at: http://www.umc.edu/hardy/. Accessed: April 28, 2006.
111. Barnard CN: A human cardiac transplant: an interim report of a successful operation performed at Groote Schurr Hospital, Capetown. *S Afr Med J*. 1967;41:1271.
112. Gift of a heart. *Life Magazine*. December 15, 1967;63(24):24-31.
113. Denise Darvall. 1943–1967. Available at: http://www.sahistory.org.za/pages/people/Denise-d.htm. Accessed February 12, 2006.
114. Kroshus TJ, Kshettry VR. The history of heart transplantation and heart valve transplantation. In: Hakim NS, Papalois VE, eds. *History of Organ and Cell Transplantation*. London: Imperial College Press; 2003:197-208.
115. Michler RE. Xenotransplantation: risks, clinical potential, and future prospects. *Emerg Infect Dis*. January-March 1966;2(1). Centers for Disease Control. Available at: http://www.cdc.gov/ncidod/eid/vol2no1/michler.htm. Accessed June 12, 2006.
116. Surgeon kept heart transplant field alive. *Los Angeles Times*. February 11, 2006. Available at: http://www.latimes.com/news/science/la-me-shumway11feb11,1,1049847.story?page=2&coll=la-news-science. Accessed February 12, 2006.
117. Wikipedia. Norman Shumway. Available at: http://en.wikipedia.org/wiki/Norman_Shumway. Accessed February 12, 2006.
118. Sharma S, Unruh H. Lung transplantation. In: Shapiro R, Talvera F, Sudan DL, Zevitz ME, Mancini MC, eds. *History of Adult Transplantation*. August 15, 2004. Available at: http://www.emedicine.com/med/topic3497.htm. Accessed February 19, 2006.
119. Kroshus TJ, Kshettry VR. The history of lung transplantation. In: Hakim NS, Papalois VE, eds. *History of Organ and Cell Transplantation*. London: Imperial College Press; 2003:209.
120. Cooley DA, Bloodwsell RD, Hallman GI, et al. Organ transplantation for advanced cardiopulmonary disease. *Ann Thorac Surg*. 1969;8:300.
121. Lillehei CW. Discussion of Wildevour CRH, Benfield JR. A review of 23 human lung transplantations by 20 surgeons. *Ann Thorac Surg*. 1970;9:489.
122. Losman JG, Campbell CD, Replogle RL, et al. Joint transplantation of the heart and lungs: past experience and present potentials. *J Cardiovasc Surg*. 1982;23:440.
123. Gray DWR. A short history of the development of islet transplantation. In: Hakim NS, Papalois VE, eds. *History of Organ and Cell Transplantation*. London: Imperial College Press; 2003:152-170.
124. Sutherland DER, Groth CG. History of pancreas transplantation. In: Hakim NS, Papalois VE, eds. *History of Organ and Cell Transplantation*. London: Imperial College Press; 2003:120-151.
125. Kelly WD, Lillehei RC, Merkel FK. Allotransplantation of the pancreas and duodenum along with the kidney in diabetic nephropathy. *Surgery*. 1967;61:827-835.
126. Sutherland DER. International human pancreas and islet transplantation registry. *Transplant Proc*. 1980;12:229.

127. Najarian JS, Sutherland DER, et al. Kidney transplantation for the uremic diabetic patient. *Surg Gynecol Obstet.* 1977;144:682.
128. Piccolo, CM. Transplant Timeline—Kidney Transplantation. Available at: http://www.medhunters.com/articles/transplantTimelineKidney.html. Accessed April 9, 2006.
129. Johnson HK, Broznick BA, Shires DL. Organ procurement organizations. In: Phillips MG, ed. *Organ Procurement, Preservation and Distribution in Transplantation.* 2nd ed. Richmond, Va: William Byrd Press, Inc; 1991:47-58.
130. Fitzgerald LM, Bartyn BN. The evolution of the transplant coordinators in Australia. *Transplant Proc.* 1992;24:2051.
131. Smit H, Sasse R. Organization of transplantation and organ donation DSO. *Organs Tissues.* 1998;2:79-80.
132. Second European Congress for Transplant Coordinators. *NATCO Newsletter.*1983;4(2):4.
133. Hall G. Organ procurement system. *NATCO Newsletter.* 1985;6(2):6.
134. Schaeffer MJ, Alexander DC. System for organ procurement and transplantation. *Am J Hosp Pharm.* 1992;49:1733-1740.
135. Davis FD. Coordination of cardiac transplantation: patient processing and donor organ procurement. *Circulation.* 1987;75(1):29-39.
136. Heyl AE, Staschak S, Folk P, Fioravanti V. The patient coordinator in a liver transplant program. *Gastroenterol Clin North Am.* 1988;17:195-206.
137. Colorado University Organ Transplant Coordinator. *Odyssey West.* September/October 1983;2(8).
138. Schanbacher B. A Tribute to Justine. *NATCO Newsletter.* 1981;2(3):1.
139 Meet your officers. *NATCO Newsletter.* 1980;1(1):1.
140. A look at your officers. *NATCO Newsletter.* 1982;4(2):1.
141. Joan Miller. Heart Transplant – Our Team. Stanford Hospital and Clinics. Stanford University Medical Center. Available at: http://www.stanfordhospital.com/clinicsmedservices/coe/heart/hearttransplant/ourTeam.html. Accessed August 23, 2006.
142. *On The Beat.* New York Organ Donor Network newsletter. Volume 6, Issue 1. Winter-Spring 2003. Available at: http://www.nyodn.org/pdf/onthebeat_w03.pdf Accessed March 8, 2006.
143. Donald W. Denny Testimony. Procurement and Allocation of Human Organs for Transplantation. Hearings before the Subcommittee on Investigations and Oversight of the Committee on Science and Technology, U.S. House of Representatives. 98th Congress, first Session. In: April 13,1983.
144. Slate of Candidates for NATCO Board Positions. *NATCO Newsletter.* March 1989;9:12.
145. Press Release. The American Society of Transplantation Announces Dr. Richard N. Fine as President-Elect. American Society of Transplantation. Mt. Laurel, NJ, July 7, 2004.Available at: http://www.a-s-t.org/news/June_2004/04FinePresElectRls.pdf. Accessed February 20, 2006.
146. Daye C. Spotlight on Gloria Horns. *NATCO Newsletter.* 1984;5(2):3.
147. Faye Davis curriculum vitae, circa 1985. In: *Care of the Recipient.* NATCO Training Course Binder. Lenexa, Kan: NATCO; 1985.
148. Betty Irwin curriculum vitae, circa 1985. In: *Care of the Recipient.* NATCO Training Course Binder. Lenexa, Kan: NATCO; 1985.
149. Schulman, B. President's Message. *NATCO Newsletter.* 1980;1(2):1.
150. Dreffer R. Presidential address. *NATCO Newsletter.* 1985;7(1):9.
151. Carroll N. An interview with past presidents—Barbara Schulman, Mark Reiner and Barry Friedman. *NATCO Newsletter, In Touch.* 30(4):1.
152. Call for Leadership. *NATCO Newsletter.* 1983;4(2):7.
153. Schulman B. Choose Life. History of NATCO. Presented at: the 30th annual meeting North American Transplant Coordinators Organization, Atlanta, Ga, July 31, 2005.
154. Organ Transplants. Hearings before the Subcommittee on Investigations and Oversight of the Committee on Science and Technology, US House of Representatives. 98th Congress, first Session. April 13, 14, 27; November 7, 9, 1983.
155. National Organ Transplant Act. Hearings before the Subcommittee on Health and the Environment of the Committee of Energy and Commerce. House of Representatives. 98th Congress. First Session. July 29, October 17, 31, 1983.
156. National Organ Transplant Act. Hearing before the Subcommittee on Health of the Committee on Ways and Means. House of Representatives. 98th Congress, Second Session. February 9, 1984.
157. Procurement and Allocation of Human Organs for Transplantation. Hearings before the Subcommittee on Investigations and Oversight of the Committee on Science and Technology, U.S. House of Representatives. 98th Congress, first Session. November 7, 9, 1983.
158. Reams BD. Jr, ed. *The National Organ Transplant Act of 1984: A Legislative History of Pub. L. No. 98-507.* Buffalo, NY: William S. Hein & Co, Inc; 1990.
159. Peele A. Amy Peele testimony in National Organ Transplant Hearings. April 13, 1983. Hearings before the Subcommittee on Investigations and Oversights of the Committee on Science and Technology, U.S. House of Representatives, 98th Congress, First Session. In: Reams BD. Jr, ed. *The National Organ Transplant Act of 1984: A Legislative History of Pub. L. No. 98-507.* Buffalo, NY: William S. Hein & Co, Inc; 1990.

160. North American Transplant Coordinators Organization. 1980 Conference. June 1980. Copley Plaza Hotel, Boston Massachusetts. *NATCO Newsletter*. 1980;1(2):4.
161. Davis F. Five-day course on procurement. *NATCO Newsletter*. 1983;4(1):4.
162. A training course on procurement for transplant coordinators. *NATCO Newsletter*. March/April 1984;5:6.
163. A training course on clinical care of the transplant patient. *NATCO Newsletter*. March/April 1984;5:3.
164. A first for organ procurement. *NATCO Newsletter*. March/April 1983;4:6.
165. Roels L. Transplant coordination in Europe or the charms and challenges of a hodge-podge. *NATCO Newsletter*. March/April 1994;15:8.
166. Karbe T. Standardized education program in procurement for transplant coordinators. *Transplant Proc*. 1991;23:2539-2540.
167. Paez G, Valero R, Paredes D, et al. Evaluation of transplant procurement management courses: an educational project as a tool for the optimization of transplant coordination. *Transplant Proc*. 2003;35:1638-1639.
168. Paredes D, Manyalich M, Cabrer C, et al. [The TPM Project (Transplant Procurement Management): international advanced training of transplant coordination] *Nefrologia*. 2001;21(suppl 4):151-158.
169. Paredes D, Valero R, Navarro A, et al. Transplant procurement management: a training tool to increase donation. *Transplant Proc*. 1999;31:2610-2611.
170. Manyalich M. Transplant procurement management training: concentration of responsibilities.*Transplant Proc*. 1997;29:1633-1634.
171. Cabrer C, Manyalich M, Valero R, Garcia-Fages LC. Timing used in the different phases of the organ-procurement process. *Transplant Proc*. 1992;24:22-23.
172. Belzer FO, Ashby BS, Gulyassy PF, et al. Successful 17-hour preservation and transplantation of human-cadaver kidney. *N Engl J Med*. 1968;278:608.
173. Belzer FO. Stanford University Medical Center. Kidney Transplantation: Past, Present and Future. History. Available at: http://www.stanford.edu/dept/HPS/transplant/html/belzer.html. Accessed April 15, 2006.
174. Van J. Transplants now a phone call away. *The Chicago Tribune*. May 10, 1983.
175. Correspondence, John M. Tew, Jr MD, President, Congress of Neurological Surgeons, to Carl Watts, MD and Hal Hankinson, MD, instructing them to print 24-Donor Alert notification in Congress newsletter and *Neurosurgery*. Copied to Donald Denny. May 4, 1983. NATCO Archives. Lenexa, Kan: NATCO; 1983.
176. NATCO 24-ALERT system and its role in extrarenal organ sharing. *N Engl J Med*. 1984;310:1465.
177. Correspondence, Frank R. Wren MD, President, American Association of Neurological Surgeons, to Donald Denny with commitment to print 24-Donor Alert notification in AANS in-house publication. June 2, 1983. NATCO Archives. Lenexa, Kan: NATCO; 1983.
178. Correspondence, Ulys H. Yates, Editor, *Practical Cardiology*, to Donald Denny, committing to print 24-Donor Alert notification in *Internal Medicine for the Specialist*. May 26, 1983. NATCO Archives. Lenexa, Kan: NATCO; 1983.
179. Correspondence, Herbert Sloan, MD, President, Congress of Neurological Surgeons, to Henry T. Bahnson, MD notifying him that a 24-Donor Alert notification will appear in The *Annals of Thoracic Surgery*. Bahnson copied Donald Denny with a note that it would also appear in *Journal of Thoracic and Cardiovascular Surgery*. May 4, 1983. NATCO Archives. Lenexa, Kan: NATCO; 1983.
180. If you want to donate a body organ. *U.S. News and World Report*. May 23, 1983:58.
181. 24-ALERT, Abstract. *NATCO Newsletter*, July/August 1983;4:3.
182. Larsen G. Lifeguard. *Raytheon Magazine*. Spring 1985:28-29.
183. Duckworth R. *NATCO Newsletter*. July/August 2005;30:2.
184. Nathan H. 24-ALERT: How it works for me and all of us! *NATCO Newsletter*. 1984;5:5.
185. Dreffer R. Presidential message: Closing remarks of the ninth NATCO meeting. Minneapolis, Minn. *NATCO Newsletter*. January/February1985;6(1):1.
186. Extra Renal Transplant Centers. *NATCO Newsletter*. March/April 1984;5:3.
187. Scanlon T. Captain's Announcement. *NATCO Newsletter*. July/August 1983;4:1.
188. *NATCO Newsletter*. January/February 1980;1:1-6.
189. *NATCO Newsletter*. 1980;1(2):1-6.
190. Committee Reports. *NATCO Newsletter*. 1980;1(1):3.
191. McAtee R. The perils of organ transportation. *NATCO Newsletter*. January/February 1980; (1):5.
192. Diliberto G, Neuhaus C. The desperate hunt for life. *People*. May 2, 1983;19:42-45.
193. Clark J, Witherspoon D, Gosnell M, et al. The new era of transplants. *Newsweek*, August 29, 1982:38-44.
194. Pick G. The gift of life. *American Way*. October 1984:65-69.
195. Proctor P. Midnight lifeguard. *Professional Pilot*. September 1984:122-132.
196. Saving lives through transplantation. *Ebony*. April 1984:58-62.
197. Uniform donor information one more time. *NATCO Newsletter*. March/April 1983;4:4.
198. Second European Congress for Transplant Coordinators. *NATCO Newsletter*. January/February 1983;4(2):4.

199. Van der Vliet JA, Vroeman JPAM. Attention: Transplant Coordinators. International Congress on Organ Procurement. *NATCO Newsletter*. May/June 1983;4(3):7.
200. About ITCS. International Transplant Coordinators Society. Available at: http://med.kuleuven.be/itcs/about/about ITCS.html. Accessed April 1, 2006.
201. First International Transplant Coordinators Meeting. Meeting Syllabus. August 29, 1994. International Transplant Coordinators Society; 1994. Available from: NATCO Archives, Lenexa, KS.
202. Merriman M. Who is a Transplant Coordinator? *NATCO Newsletter*. January/February 1981;2:1.
203. Warren J. In memoriam—Bill Anderson, LifeNet CEO, passes away May 21. *Transplant News*. May 28, 2002;12:1-2.
204. Editorial: He made a difference / Brian Broznick was an apostle of organ transplantation. Monday, November 10, 2004. *Pittsburgh Post-Gazzette*. Available at: http://postgazette.com/pg/03314/238024.stm. Accessed March 16, 2006.
205. Aspiotes G. Man helped 300,000 get transplants. *Pittsburgh Tribune Review*. Tuesday, November 4, 2003. Available at: http://www.pittsburghlive.com/x/tribune-review/news/s_163322.html. Accessed March 16, 2006.
206. In Memoriam: Brian Broznick, CORE CEO, passes away November 2. *Transplant News*. November 15, 2003.
207. UNOS website. UNOS Statement regarding Brian Broznick of CORE. Available at: http://www.unos.org/news/newsDetail.asp?id=292. Accessed March 14, 2006.
208. Snowbeck C. Susan Stuart / New CORE director succeeds late husband. Monday, May 10, 2004. Newsmaker: Health Science and the Environment. *Pittsburgh Post-Gazette*. Available at: http://www.post-gazette.com/pg/04131/313955.stm. Accessed March 16, 2006.
209. Rapaport FT. The Life and Times of a Transplant Immunosurgeon. In: Terasaki, PI, ed. *History of Transplantation: 35 Recollections*. Los Angeles, CA: The Regents of the University of California; 1990:351-377.
210. New circulatory model. William Harvey. In: Wikipedia, the free encyclopedia. Available at: http://en.wikipedia.org/wiki/William_Harvey. Accessed June 2, 2006.
211. Transplantation Timeline. History of Transplantation. Available at: http://biomed.brown.edu/Courses/BI108/BI108_2005_Groups/06/timeline.htm Accessed April 28, 2006.
212. Leacock JH. On transfusion of blood in extreme cases of haemorrhage. *Med Chir J Rev*. 1817;3:276-284.
213. John Henry Leacock: The Critical Animal Experiments. British Medical Journal online. Available at: http://bmj.bmjjournals.com/cgi/content/full/325/7378/1485#B3. Accessed April 28, 2006.
214. Blundell J. Experiments on the transfusion of blood by the syringe. *Med Chir Transact*. 1818;9:56-92.
215. Blundell J. Some remarks on the operation of transfusion. In: *Researches, Physiological and Pathological*. London: E Cox and Son, 1825:63-146.
216. The Early Development of Dialysis and Transplantation. In: Royal Infirmary of Edinbrugh Renal Unit. Available at: http://renux.dmed.ed.ac.uk/edren/Unitbits/historyweb/HDWorld.html. Accessed June 2, 2006.
217. McCann SR. History of bone marrow transplantation. In: Hakim NS, Papalois VE, eds. *History of Organ and Cell Transplantation*. London: Imperial College Press; 2003:293-308.
218. Hamblin T. Historical review: historical aspects of chronic lymphocytic leukaemia. *Brit Jour Haem*. 2000;111:1023-1034.
219. Ernst Neumann. In: Available at: http://www.ernst-neumann-koenigsberg.de/Ernst_Neumann/ernst_neumann.html. Date accessed: September 3, 2006.
220. Williams PW. Notes on diabetes treated with extract and by grafts of sheep's pancreas. *Br Med J*. 1894:2:1303-1304.
221. Landsteiner K. Ueber Agglutinationserscheinungen normalen menschlichen blutes. *Wien Klin Wchnschr*. 1901;14:1132.
222. Carrel A. La technique operatoire des anastomoses vasculaires et la transplantation des visceres. *Lyon Med*. 1902;98:859-864.
223. Ullmann E. Experimentelle Nierentransplantation. *Wien Klin. Wochenschr*. 1902;15:281.
224. Decastello A. Von. Experimentelle nierentransplantation. *Wien Klin. Wochenschr*. 1902;15:317.
225. Rostron CK. History of corneal transplantation. In: Hakim NS, Papalois VE, eds. *History of Organ and Cell Transplantation*. London: Imperial College Press; 2003:274-292.
226. First corneal transplant. Wikipedia. Available at: http://en.wikipedia.org/wiki/Eduard_Zirm. Accessed May 2, 2006.
227. Moffatt SL, Cartwright VA, Stumpf TH. Centennial review of corneal transplantation. *Clin Experiment Ophthalmol*. 2005;33:642-657.
228. Zirm ME. Eduard Konrad Zirm and the "wondrously beautiful little window." *Refract Corneal Surg*. 1989;5:256-257.
229. Fanta H. Eduard Zirm (1863–1944) *Klin Monatsbl Augenheilkd*. 1986;189:64-66.
230. Snyder C. Alois Glogar, Karl Brauer, and Eduard Konrad Zirm. *Arch Ophthalmol*. 1965;74:871-874.
231. Lesky E. Eduard Konrad Zirm (1863–1944). On the 100th anniversary of his birth (18 March 1963). *Wien Klin Wochenschr*. 1963;75:199-201.
232. Bock J. The jubilee of the first successful optic keratoplasty by Eduard Zirm. *Wien Klin Wochenschr*. 1958;70:381-383.
233. Jaboulay M. Greffe de reins au pli du coude par soudures arterielles et veineuses. *Lyon Med*. 1906;107:575-577.
234. Carrel A. Results of the transplantation of blood vessels, organs and limbs. *JAMA*. 1908;51:1662-1667.
235. Lexer E. Joint transplantations and arthroplasty. *Surg Gynecol Obstet*. 1925;40:782-809.

Chapter 1   THE HISTORY OF THE TRANSPLANT COORDINATOR

236. Hejazi SN. Gefäßchirurgie: ein historischer Rüblick. In: Medizin: Geschichte. Available at: http://www.laekh.de/upload/Hess._Aerzteblatt/2001/2001_08/2001_08_10.pdf. Accessed: June 16, 2006.
237. Unger E. Nierentransplantation. *Wien Klin Wochenschr.* 1910. 47:573-578.
238. Reemsta K, McCracken BH, Schlegel et al. Renal heterotransplantation in man. *Ann Surg.* 1964;160:384-410.
239. W. Drukker. Hemodialysis: a historical review. In: Maher JF, ed. *Replacement of Renal Function by Dialysis.* 4th ed. Dordrecht, Netherlands: Kluwer Academic Publishers, 1978:20-86.
240. Abel JJ, Rowntree LC, Turner BB. On the removal of diffusable substances from the circulating blood by means of dialysis. *Trans Assoc Am Physicians.* 1913;28:51.
241. Quinton W, Dillard D, Scribner BH. Cannulation of blood vessels for prolonged hemodialysis. *Trans Am Soc Artificial Organs.* 1960;6:104.
242. Gilleyboeugh T. The famous doctor who inserts monkey glands into millionaires. Available at: http://www.gvsu.edu/english/cummings/issue9/Gillybo9.htm. Accessed April 28, 2006.
243. Testicular transplantation (editorial). *Boston Medical and Surgical Journal.* 1924;191:1024.
244. Moore C. Physiologic effects of non-living testis grafts. JAMA. 1930;92:1912.
245. History: Islet Transplantation. Available at: http://biomed.brown.edu/Courses/BI108/BI108_2004_Groups/Group09/history.htm. Accessed April 22, 2006.
246. Banting FG, Best CH. The internal secretions of the pancreas. *Journal of Laboratory and Clinical Medicine.* 1922;7:251.
247. Banting FG. The history of insulin. *Edinburgh Medical Journal.* 1929;36:1.
248. Neuhof H. *Transplantation of Tissues.* New York, NY: Appleton and Co; 1923
249. Haas G. Ueber Versuche der Blutauswaschung am Lebenden mit Hilfe der Dialyse. *Naunyn Schmiedebergs Arch Pharmakol.* 1926;116:158.
250. Alexis Carrel biography. Available at: http://www.charleslindbergh.com/heart/carrel.asp. Accessed April 9, 2006.
251. Carrel A, Lindbergh CA. The culture of whole organs. *Science.* 1935;81:621.
252. Collins GM. History of Organ Preservation. In: *Organ Procurement, Preservation, and Distribution.* Editor: Michael G Phillips. The William Byrd Press, 1991:101-103.
253. Voronoy U. Sobre bloqueo del aparato reticuloendotelial del hombre en algunas formas de intoxicacion por el sublimado y sobre la transplantacion del rinon cadaverico como metodo de tratamiento de la anuria consecutiva a aquella intoxicacion. [Blocking the reticuloendothelial system in man in some forms of mercuric chloride intoxication and the transplantation of the cadaver kidney as a method of treatment for the anuria resulting from the intoxication.] *Siglo Medico.* 1936;97:296-297.
254. Hamilton DNH, Reid WA. Yu Yu Voronoy and the first human kidney allograft. *Surg, Gyn & Obstet.* 1984:159:289.
255. Mirskili MB. Soviet surgeon Yu Yu Voronoy, pioneer of allotransplantation of the cadaveric kidney in the clinic." *Klinches Kaya Zhurnalya.* 1973;5:76.
256. Voronoy YY. Transplantation of a conserved cadaveric kidney as a method of biostimulation in severe nephritides." *Vrachebnoe Dyel.* 1950;9:813.
257. Smith S. Progress in clinical organ transplantation. Available at: http://www.medscape.com/viewarticle/408767. Accessed April 22, 2006.
258. Gibson T, Medawar PB. The fate of skin homografts in man. *J Anat.* 1943;77:299-310.
259. Piccolo CM. Transplant timeline: other and unusual transplantation. Available at: http://www.medhunters.com/articles/transplantTimelineOtherUnusual.html. Accessed April 9, 2006.
260. Medawar PB. The behavior and fate of skin autografts and skin homografts in rabbits. *J Anat.* 1944;78:176-199.
261. Brown ME, Oyer PE. Donor Heart-Lung Retrieval. In: Phillips MG, ed. *Organ Procurement, Preservation, and Distribution.* The William Byrd Press, 1991:91-95.
262. The Eye Bank for Sight Restoration. Available at: http://www.eyedonation.org/. Accessed: September 2, 2006.
263. Moore FD. Give and Take: The Development of Tissue Transplantation. Philadelphia: W.B. Saunders; 1964:15
264. Gorer PA, Lyman S, Snell GD. Studies on the genetic and antigenic basis of tumour transplantation: linkage between a histocompatibility gent and "fused" in mice. *Proc R Soc Lond B.* 1948;135:499-505.
265. Kroshus TJ, Kshettry VR. The history of lung transplantation. In: Hakim NS, Papalois VE, eds. *History of Organ and Cell Transplantation.* London: Imperial College Press; 2003:209-224.
266. Metras H. Preliminary note on lung transplants in dogs. *Compte Rendue Acad Sci.* 1950;231:1176.
267. State of Illinois General Assembly. House Resolution Acknowledging Little Company of America as site of the first kidney transplant in the U.S. 91_HR0203. Available at: http://www.ilga.gov/legislation/legisnet91/hrgroups/hr/910HR0203LV.html. Accessed April 25, 2006.
268. R. H. Lawler, Pioneer Of Kidney Transplants. United Press International. *New York Times,* July 27, 1982. Archives. Available at: http://query.nytimes.com/gst/fullpage.html?res=9406E7DD1239F934A15754C0A964948260. Accessed: April 25, 2006.
269. Dubost C, Oeconomos N, Nenna A, Milliez P. Resultats d'une tentative greffe renale. *Bull Soc Med Hop Paris.* 1951;67:1372-1382.

270. Servelle M, Soulie P, Rougelle J. Greffe d'une rein de supplicie a une malade avec rein unique congenital, atteinte de nephrite chronoque hypertensive azatemique. *Bull Soc Med Hop Paris*. 1951;67:99-104.
271. Küss R, Teinturier J, Milliez P. Quelques essais de greffe rein chez l'homme. *Meme Acad Chir*. 1951;77:755-764.
272. Young JB. Organ transplantation in perspective: transition from an experiment. A publication of The Methodist Hospital, Houston, TX. The Journal. Special Issue 1986;25(1):1-7.
273. Michon L, Hamburger J, Oeconomos N, et al. Une tentative de transplantation renale chez l'homme: aspects medicaux et biologiques. *Presse Med*. 1953;61:1419-1423.
274. Hyatt GW, Turner TC Bassett CAL et al. New methods of preserving skin, bone, and blood vessels. *Postgrad Med J*. 1952;12:239.
275. Bogardus GM, Schlosser RJ. Influence of temperature on ischemic renal damage. *Surgery*. 1956;39:970.
276. Pegg DE, Calne RY, Pryse-Davies J, et al. Canine renal preservation using surface cooling and perfusion cooling techniques. *Ann NY Acad Sci*. 1964;120:506.
277. Brunius U, Fritjofsson A, Gelin LE. Microcirculatory aspects of the preservation of kidneys for transplantation. *Bibl Anat*. 1967;9:374.
278. Billingham RE, Brent L, Medawar PB. "Actively acquired tolerance" of foreign cells. *Nature*. 1953;172:603-606.
279. Piccolo CM. Transplant timeline: heart and heart-lung transplantation. Available at: http://www.medhunters.com/articles/transplantTimelineHeartLung.html. Accessed April 9, 2006.
280. Piccolo CM. Transplant timeline: bone marrow transplantation. Available at: http://www.medhunters.com/articles/transplantTimelineBMT.html. Accessed April 9, 2006.
281. Thomas ED, Lochte HL, Lu WC, Ferrebee JW. Intravenous infusion of bone marrow in patients receiving radiation and chemotherapy. *N Engl J Med*. 1957 Sep 12;257(11):491-496.
282. Jean Dausset. The Nobel Prize in Physiology or Medicine 1980. In: Nobelprize.org. Available at: http://nobelprize.org/nobel_prizes/medicine/laureates/1980/dausset-bio.html. Date accessed: September 2, 2006.
283. Murray JE, Merill JP, Dammin GJ, et al. Successful homotransplantation of the human kidney between non-identical twins. *N Engl J Med*. 1960;262:1251-1260.
284. Hamburger J, Vaysse J, Crosnier J, at al. Renal homotransplantation in man after radiation of the recipient: experience with six patients since 1959. *Am J Med*. 1962;32:854-871.
285. Wertheimer P, Jouvet M, Descotes J. [Diagnosis of death of the nervous system in comas with respiratory arrest treated by artificial respiration.] *Press Med*. 1959;67(3):87-88.
286. Descotes J, Jouvet M. [The limits of respiratory reanimation; the diagnosis of death of the central nervous system in comas with respiratory arrest.] *Anesth Anal*. 1959;16:344-352.
287. Murray JE, Merrill JP, Dammin GJ, et al. Study of transplantation immunity after total body irradiation: clinical and experimental investigation. *Surgery*. 1960;48:272-284.
288. Hamburger J, Vaysse J, Crosnier J, et al. Transplantation of a kidney between nonmonozygotic twins after irradiation of the receiver: good function at the fourth month. *Presse Med*. 1959;67:1771-1775.
289. Hamburger J, Vaysse J, Crosnier J, at al. Renal homotransplantation in man after radiation of the recipient: experience with six patients since 1959. *Am J Med*. 1962;32:854-871.
290. Schwartz R, Dameshek W. Drug-induced immunological tolerance. *Nature*. 1959;183:1682-1683.
291. Schwartz R, Dameshek W. The effects of 6-mercaptopurine on homograft reactions. *J Clin Invest*. 1960;39:952-958.
292. Meeker W, Condie R, Weiner D, et al. Prolongation of skin homograft survival in rabbits by 6-mercaptopurine. *Proc Soc Exp Biol Med*. 1959;102:459-461.
293. Calne RY. The inhibition of renal homograft rejection in dogs by 6 mercaptopurine. *Lancet*. 1960;1:417.
294. Zukoski C, Lee HM, Hume DM. The prolongation of functional survival of canine renal homografts by 6 mercaptopurine. *Surg Forum*. 1960;11:470.
295. Küss R, Legrain M, Mathé G, et al. Homologous human kidney transplantation: experience with six patients. *Postgrad Med J*. 1962;38:528-531.
296. Lower RR, Shumway NE: Studies on orthotopic homotransplantations of the canine heart. *Surg Forum*. 1960;11:18.
297. Calne RY, Alexandre GPJ, Murray JE. The development of immunosuppressive therapy. *Ann NY Acad Sci*. 1962;99:743
298. David Hume biography. Medical College of Virginia Hospitals. The Hume-Lee Transplant Center. Available at: http://www.vcuhealth.org/transplant/bio_hume.htm. Accessed September 21, 2005.
299. Hardy JD, Webb WR, Dalton ML, Walker GR. Lung homotransplantation in man. *JAMA*. 1963;186:1065-1074.
300. Reemtsma K, McCracken BH, Schlegel JU, et al. Renal heterotransplantation in man. *Ann Surg*. 1964:160:384-410.
301. Starzl TE, Marchioro TL, Peters GN, et al. Renal heterotransplantation from baboon to man: experience with 6 cases. *Transplantation*. 1964;2:752-776.
302. Starzl TE. Patterns of permissible donor-recipient tissue transfer in relation to ABO blood groups (37-47). In: Starzl TE, ed. *Experience in Renal Transplantation*. Philadelphia, Pa: W B Saunders; 1964.
303. Hardy JD, Chavez CM, Kurrus FD, et al. Heart transplantation in man. *JAMA* 1964;188:114-122.
304. Terasaki PI, McClelland JD. Microdroplet assay of human serum cytotoxins. *Nature*. 1964;204:998-1000.

Chapter 1 THE HISTORY OF THE TRANSPLANT COORDINATOR

305. Terasaki PI, Vredevoe DL, Mickey MR, et al. Serotyping for homotransplantation. VI. Selection of kidney donors for thirty-two recipients. *Ann NY Acad Sci.* 1966;129:500-520.
306. Pierce GA. UNOS history. In: Phillips MG, ed. Organ Procurement, Preservation and Distribution in Transplantation. Richmond, Va: William Byrd Press, Inc; 1991: 1-6.
307. Ferree DM. Cadaveric Organ Sharing: The Organ Center. In: Phillips MG, ed. *Organ Procurement, Preservation, and Distribution.* The William Byrd Press, 1991:129-144.
308. Lower RR, Dong E Jr, Shumway NE. Long-term survival of cardiac homografts. *Surgery.* 1965;58:110-119.
309. Lustinek K. Vasoconstrictor properties of blood in perfusion experiments. *Physiol Bohemoslov.* 1965;14:583.
310. Humphries AL, Russell R, Stoddard LD et al. Three-day kidney preservation: perfusion with hypothermic, diluted blood or plasma. *Surgery.* 1968;63:646.
311. Starzl TE, Marchioro TL, Porter KA, et al. Factors determining short- and long-term survival after orthotopic liver homotransplantation in the dog. *Surgery.* 1965;58:131-155.
312. Baumgartner WA, Traill TA, Cameron DE, et al. Unique aspects of heart and lung transplantation exhibited in the 'domino-donor' operation. JAMA. 1989 Jun 2;261(21):3121-5.
313. Perper RJ, Najarian JS. Experimental renal heterotransplantation. I. In widely divergent species. *Transplantation.* 1966;4:377-388.
314. Perper RJ, Najarian JS. Experimental renal heterotransplantion. II. Closely related species. *Transplantation.* 1966;4:700-712.
315. History of Eurotransplant. Available at: http://www.eurotransplant.nl/index.php/files/flash/files/statistics/rss/index.php?id=history. Accessed April 9, 2006.
316. Van Rood JJ. A proposal for international cooperation in organ transplantation: Eurotransplant. *Histocompatability Testing* 1967:451.
317. Starzl TE, Marchioro TL, Porter KA, et al. The use of heterologous antilymphoid agents in canine renal and liver homotransplantation and in human renal homotransplantation. *Surg Gynecol Obstet.* 1967;124:301-318.
318. Starzl TE, Groth CG, Brettschneider L, et al. Orthotopic homotransplantation of the human liver. *Ann Surg.* 1968;168:392-415.
319. Groote Schuure Hospital. The world's first heart transplant. Available at: http://www.gsh.co.za/ab/heart.html. Accessed February 12, 2006.
320. Kantrowitz A, Huller JD, Joos H, et al. Transplantation of the heart in an infant and an adult. *Am J Cardiol.* 1968;22:782-790.
321. Belzer FO, Ashby BS, Dunphy JE. 24- and 72-hour preservation of canine kidneys. *Lancet.* 1967;2:536.
322. Hoffmann RM, Belzer FO. Organ Preservation: Kidney, Liver, Pancreas. In: Phillips MG, etc. *Organ Procurement, Preservation, and Distribution.* The William Byrd Press, 1991:105-119.
323. Gatti RA, Meuwissen HJ, Allen HD, et al. Immunological reconstitution of sex-linked lymphopenic immunological deficiency. *Lancet.* 1968;2:1366-1369.
324. Piccolo CM. Transplant timeline: other and unusual transplantation. Available at: http://www.medhunters.com/articles/transplantTimelineOtherUnusual.html. Accessed April 9, 2006.
325. The Uniform Anatomical Gift Act of 1968, amended 1987. National Conference Of Commissioners On Uniform State Laws. Available at: http://www.law.upenn.edu/bll/ulc/fnact99/uaga87.htm. Accessed June 12, 2006.
326. SoRelle, R Transplants spur Houston's growth as a medical center. Houston Chronicle. April 2, 2001. Available at: http://www.chron.com/disp/story.mpl/first100/866560.html . Date accesssed: September 9, 2006.
327. Derom F, Barbier F, Ringoir S, et al. Ten-month survival after lung homotransplantation in man. *J Thorac Surg.* 1970;9:489.
328. Kluyskens P, Ringoir S. Follow-up of a human larynx transplantation. *Laryngoscope.* 1970 Aug;80(8):1244-50.
329. Lillehei RC, Simmons RL, Najarian JS, et al. Pancreaticoduodenal allotransplantation: experimental and clinical observations. *Ann Surg.* 1970;172:405-436.
330. Southeastern Organ Procurement Foundation. Brief History. Available at: http://www.seopf.org/intro.htm. Accessed April 15, 2006.
331. Pierce GA, McDonald JC. UNOS History. In: Phillips MG, ed. Organ Procurement, Preservation and Distribution in Transplantation. 2nd ed. Richmond, Va: William Byrd Press, Inc; 1996:1-5.
332. Collins GM, Bravo-Shugarman M, Terasaki Pl. Kidney preservation for transportation: initial perfusion and 30 hours' ice storage. *Lancet* 1969;2:1219.
333. Dausset J. The HLA adventure. In: Terasaki PI, ed. History of HLA: 10 Recollections. Los Angeles, Calif: The Regents of the University of California; 1990:1-20.
334. Upton H. Origin of drugs in current use: the cyclosporine story. The Discovery of Cyclosporine. 2001. Available at: http://www.world-of-fungi.org/Mostly_Medical/Harriet_Upton/Harriet_Upton.htm. Accessed June 12, 2006.
335. Kemp CB, Knight MJ, Scharp DW, Ballinger WF, Lacy PE. Effect of transplantation site on the results of pancreatic islet isografts in diabetic rats. *Diabetologia.* 1973;9:486-491.

336. Starzl TE, Porter KA, Andres G, et al. Long-term survival after renal transplantation in humans: with special reference to histocompatibility matching, thymectomy, homograft glomerulonephritis, heterologous ALG, and recipient malignancy. *Ann Surg*. 1970;172:437-472.
337. Mickey MR, Kreisier M, Albers ED, et al. Analysis of HLA incompatibility in human renal transplants. *Tissue Antigens*. 1971;2:57-67.
338. Morris PJ. Cyclosporine. In: Morris PJ, ed. *Kidney Transplantation: Principles and Practice*. Philadelphia, Pa: W B Saunders Co;1994179-201.
339. Dreyfuss M, Harri E, Hoftmann H, et al. Cyclosporin A and C. New metabolites from *Trichoderma polysporu* (Lind ex Pers.) Rifai. *Eur J Appl Microbiol* 1976;3:125.
340. Nitschke P. Shirley Nolan. Available at: http://www.exitinternational.net/shirley_nolan.htm. Accessed: September 4, 2006.
341. A fact sheet. Unrelated bone marrow and cord blood stem cells transplants. Available at: http://www.worldmarrow.org/fileadmin/Press_Releases/FACT_sheet.pdf#search=%22bone%20marrow%20%22Shirley%20Nolan%22%22. Accessed: September 4, 2006.
342. First unrelated bone marrow transplant. National Marrow Donor Program. Available at: http://www.marrow.org/NMDP/history_of_transplants.html. Accessed April 28, 2006.
343. About the Diabetes Institute. Second Chance: Newsletter of the Diabetes Institute for Immunology and Transplantation. Fall 2002;10. Available at: http://www.diabetesinstitute.org/img/assets/9507/Fall%202002%20second%20chance.pdf. Accessed June 12, 2006.
344. First Transplant Coordinators Workshop Brochure. New York, NY: August 1976.
345. Borel JF, Feurer C, Gubler HU, et al. Biological effects of cyclosporin A, a new antilymphocytic agent. *Agents Actions*. 1976;6:468-475.
346. Borel JF, Kis ZL. The discovery and development of cyclosporine (Sandimmune). *Transplan Proc*. 1991;23:1867-1874.
347. Borel JF, Feurer C, Gubler HU, Stähelin H. Biological effects of cyclosporin A: a new antilymphocytic agent. *Agents Actions*. 1976:6:468-475.
348. Colpitts DB, Freitag CL. Organ donation and transplantation in the Canadian healthcare system. *J Transplant Coord*. 1977;7:59-66.
349. Gevers S, Janssen A, Friele R. Consent systems for post mortem organ donation in Europe. *Eur J Health Law*. 2004;11:175-186.
350. World Health Organization. *Legislative Responses to Organ Transplantation*. The Netherlands: Martinus Nojhoff Publishers. 1994.
351. United Network for Organ Sharing. Who we are: history. Available at: http://www.unos.org/whoWeAre/history.asp. Accessed April 15, 2006.
352. Pudlo P. European transplant programs: what can the U.S. learn? *J Transplant Coord*. 1993;3:138-140.
353. Ting A, Morris PJ. Powerful effect of HLA-DR matching on survival of cadaveric renal allografts. *Lancet*. 1980;2:282-285.
354. Calne RY, Rolles K, White DJG, et al. Cyclosporin A initially as the only immunosuppressant in 34 recipients of cadaveric organs; 32 kidneys, 2 pancreases, and 2 livers. *Lancet*. 1979;2:1033-1036.
355. NATCO celebrates 30 years! The history of NATCO. In Touch, NATCO Newsletter July/August 2005;30:8-10.
356. Reis CE. Brain death. In: Neurology. Available at: http://www.medstudents.com.br/neuro/neuro5.htm. Accessed March 1, 2006.
357. Barber PL. Last Call – Research and Publications Survey. NATCO Newsletter. July/August 1981;2:4.
358. Gohke M. I'll take tomorrow. New York, M Evans, 1985.
359. Reitz BA, Wallwork J, Hunt SA, et al. Heart-lung transplantation: Successful therapy for patients with pulmonary vascular disease. *N Engl J Med* 1982;306;557.
360. Haid S. Articles of interest from the scientific community. *NATCO Newsletter*. May/June 1981;2:2.
361. Cosimi AB, Colvin RB, Burton RC,Rubin RH et al. Use of monoclonal antibodies to T-cell subsets for immunologic monitoring and treatment in recipients of renal allografts. N Eng J Med. 1981 Aug 6;305(6):308-314.
362. Cosimi AB, Colvin RB, Burton RC, Rubin RH et al. Immunologic monitoring with monocloncal antibodies to human T-cell subsets. *Transplant Proc*. 1981 Sep;13(3):1589-1593.
363. Haid S. Articles of interest from the scientific community. *NATCO Newsletter*. May/June 1982;3:2.
364. Joyce LD, DeVries WC, Hastings WL, Olsen DB, Jarvik RK, Kolff WJ. Response of the human body to the first permanent implant of the Jarvik-7 total artificial heart. *Trans Am Soc Artif Intern Organs*. 1983;29:81-87.
365. *NATCO Newsletter*. January/February 1983;4:2.
366. Bundesgesetzblatt fuer die Republik Oesterreich. 1983;273:1161-1162.
367. Smit H, Sasse R. Organisation of transplantation and organ donation Deutsche Stiftung Organtransplantation. *Organs Tissues*. 1998;2:79-80.
368. Surgeon General's Workshop on Solid Organ Procurement for Transplantation. Program Brochure, June 7,8,9, 1983. Project HOPE Health Sciences Education Center, Millwood, Va. Located in NATCO Archives, Book 2.

369. Winifred B. Mack, RN, BSN. "Who Procures Organs, How They Do It and How Well They Do It." Testimony for Surgeon General's Workshop on Solid Organ Procurement for Transplantation. June 7,8,9, 1983. Project HOPE Health Sciences Education Center, Millwood, Va. Located in NATCO Archives, Book 2.
370. Toronto Lung Transplant Group. Unilateral lung transplantation for pulmonary fibrosis. *N Engl J Med.* 1986;314:1140-1145.
371. UPMC News Bureau. Milestones at the University of Pittsburgh. Available at: http://newsbureau.upmc.com/MediaKits/LiverTransplant/Milestones.htm. Accessed: September 6, 2006.
372. Dreffer R. Presidential message. *NATCO Newsletter.* March/April 1985;6(2):1.
373. S.B. 2048. Title: A bill to provide for the establishment of a Task Force in Organ Procurement and Transplantation and an Organ Procurement and Transplantation Registry, and for other purposes. 10/19/1984 Became Public Law No: 98-507. Available at: http://thomas.loc.gov/cgi-bin/bdquery/z?d098:SN02048:@@@L%7CTOM:/bss/d098query.html. Accessed June 12, 2006.
374. Broznick B, Johnson HK. History of Organ Procurement Organizations. In: Phillips MG, ed. *Organ Procurement, Preservation and Distribution in Transplantation.* Richmond, Va: William Byrd Press, Inc; 1991:21-22.
375. Starzl TE, Bilheimer DW, Bahnson HT et al. Heart-liver transplantation in a patient with familial hypercholesterolemia." *Lancet.* 1984;1(8391):1382-1383.
376. Bilheimer DW, Goldstein JL, Grundy SM et al. Liver transplantation to provide low-density-lipoprotein receptors and lower plasma cholesterol in a child with homozygous familial hypercholesterolemia. *N Engl J Med.* 1984;311:1658-1664.
377. Bailey LL, Nehlsen-Cannavella SL, Concepcion W, Jolley WB. Baboon to human cardiac xenotransplantation in a neonate. JAMA 1985;254:3321-3327.
378. Bollinger RR, Sugarman J. The history of ethical issues in transplantation. In: Hakim NS, Papalois VE, eds. *History of Organ and Cell Transplantation.* London: Imperial College Press; 2003:384-418.
379. United Network for Organ Sharing. *NATCO Newsletter.* July/August 1984;5:3.
380. Panel on Transplants Named. United Press International. January 27, 1985. Available at: http://query.nytimes.com/gst/fullpage.html?sec=health&res=9C0DE2DC123BF934A15752C0A963948260. Accessed: September 6, 2006.
381. *Belgisch Staatsblad*, 14 February 1987:2129-2140.
382. Cooper JD, Pearson FG, Patterson GA, et al. Technique of successful lung transplantation in humans. *J Thorac Cardiovasc Surg.* 1987;93:173-181.
383. Starzl TE, Hakala T, Tzakis A, et al. A multifactorial system for equitable selection of cadaveric kidney recipients. JAMA. 1987;257:3073-3075.
384. Abu-Elmagd K. History of intestinal transplantation. In: Hakim NS, Papalois VE, eds. *History of Organ and Cell Transplantation.* London: Imperial College Press; 2003:171-193.
385. Starzl TE, Rowe MI, Todo S, et al. Transplantation of multiple abdominal viscera. JAMA. 1989;261:1449-1457.
386. Starzl TE, Rowe MI, Todo S, et al. Transplantation of multiple abdominal viscera. JAMA. 1989;261:1449-1457.
387. History of transplantation timeline. Available at: http://www.transweb.org/reference/timeline/historytable.htm. Accessed April 25, 2006.
388. Belzer FO, Southard JH. Principles of solid-organ preservation by cold storage. *Transplantation.* 1988;45:673.
389. Kalayoglu M, Sollinger HW, D'Alessandro AM, et al. Successful extended preservation of the liver for clinical transplantation. *Lancet.* 1988;1:617.
390. Grant D, Wall W, Mimeault R, et al. Successful small bowel/liver transplantation. *Lancet.* 1990;335:181-184.
391. Pichlmayer R Ringe B, Gubernatis G, et al. Transplantation einer spender-leber auf zwei Empfanger (Splitting-Transplantation) – Eine neue Methode in der Weiterentwicklung der Lebersegmenttransplantation. *Langenbecks Arch Chir* 1988;73:127.
392. Strong RW, Lynch SV, Ong TN, et al. Successful liver transplantation from a living donor to her son. *N Engl J Med* 1990;322:1505-1507.
393. Adult living donor liver transplantation: another Pandora's box? *Med J Aust.* 2001;175:179-180. Available at: http://www.mja.com.au/public/issues/175_04_200801/mccaughan/mccaughan.html#refbody3. Accessed April 28, 2006.
394. Goulet O, Revillon Y, Brousse N, et al. Successful small bowel transplantation in an infant. *Transplantation.* 1992;53:940-943.
395. Starnes VA, Barr ML, Cohen RG. Lobar transplantation: indications, technique, and outcome. *J Thorac Cardiovasc Surg.* 1994;108:403-410; discussion 410-411.
396. Scharp DW, Lacy PE, Santiago JV, et al. Insulin independence after islet transplantation into type I diabetic patient. *Diabetes.* 1990;39:515-518.
397. Warnock GL, Kneteman NM, Ryan E, Seelis REA, Rabinovitch A, Rajotte RV. Normoglycemia after transplantation of freshly isolated and cryopreserved pancreatic islets in type I (insulin-dependent) diabetes mellitus. *Diabetologia.* 1991;34:55-58.
398. Starzl TE, Fung J, Tzakis A, et al. Baboon to human liver transplantation. *Lancet.* 1993;341:65-71.
399. Chari R, Collins BH, Magee JC, et al. Treatment of hepatic failure with ex vivo pig-liver perfusion followed by liver transplantation. *N Eng J Med.* July 28, 1994;331:234-237.

400. Starzl TE, Demetris AJ, Murase N, et al. Cell migration, chimerism, and graft acceptance. *Lancet.* 1992;339:1579-1582.
401. Cohen B, Persigjn G. European transplant programs: what can we learn? *J Transplant Coord.* 1993;3:128-133.
402. Upstate New York Transplant Services. History of transplantation. Available at: http://www.unyts.org/timeline.htm. Accessed April 22, 2006.
403. A simple act: the Nicholas effect. Available at: http://www.transweb.org/reference/articles/donation/a_simple_act.html. Accessed April 28, 2006.
404. Green R. The Nicholas effect: A boy's gift to the world. Sebastopol, Calif: O'Reilly & Associates, Inc.; 1999.
405. Todo S, Tzakis A, Abu-Elmagd K, Reyes J, Furukawa H, Nour B, Fung J, Demetris A, Starzl TE. Abdominal multivisceral transplantation. *Transplantation.* 1995 Jan 27;59(2):234-40.
406. Vito R. One year later, transplant patient has new lease on life. In: Health Story Page, CNN.com. December 20, 1996. Available at: http://www.cnn.com/HEALTH/9612/20/nfm/mega.transplant/index.html?eref=sitesearch. Date accessed: September 2, 2006.
407. Kootstra G. The asystolic or non-heart-beating donor. *Transplantation.* 1997;63:917-921.
408. Organ Transplant. Available at: http://en.wikipedia.org/wiki/Organ_transplant. Accessed April 22, 2006.
409. Ratner LE, Ciseck LJ, Moore RG, Cigarroa FG, Kaufman HS, Kavoussi LR. Laparoscopic live donor nephrectomy. *Transplantation.* 1995 Nov 15;60(9):1047-9.
410. Smithers F. The pattern and effect of on call work in transplant coordinators in the United Kingdom. *Int J Nurs Stud.* 1995;32:469-483.
411. Kita Y, Aranami Y, Aranami Y, et al. Japanese organ transplant law: a historical perspective. *Prog Transplant.* 2000;10:106-108.
412. Swinbacks D. Japan reaches a compromise on organ transplants. *Nature.* 1997;387:835.
413. Saegusa A. Japan's transplant law "is too stringent"…but the pill may be legalized at last. *Nature.* 1999;398:95.
414. Takagi H. Living and cadaveric donor issues in Japan. *Organs Tissues.* 1998;2:105-106.
415. Milanes CL, Hernandez E, Gonzalez L, et al. Organ and tissue procurement system: a novel intervention to increase organ donation rates in Venezuela. *Prog Transplant.* 2003;13:65-68.
416. Singh P. What ails cadaveric transplant programs in India: perspectives of a transplant coordinator. *Prog Transplant.* 2002;12:49-51.
417. Strome M. Human laryngeal transplantation: considerations and implications. *Microsurgery.* 2000;20(8):372-4.
418. Hakim JS. The history of arm transplantation. In: Hakim NS, Papalois VE, eds. *History of Organ and Cell Transplantation.* London: Imperial College Press; 2003: 309-319.
419. Hand transplantation: organ replacement. Available at: http://biomed.brown.edu/Courses/BI108/BI108_2003_Groups/Hand_Transplantation/history.html. Accessed April 22, 2006.
420. Dubernard JM, Owen E, Herzberg G, et al. Human hand allograft: report on first 6 months. *Lancet.* 1999 Apr 17;353(9161):1315-20.
421. Dubernard JM, Owen E, Lefrancois N, et al. First human hand transplantation. Case report. *Transpl Int.* 2000;13 Suppl 1:S521-4.
422. Shapiro JM, Lakey JR, Rya EA. Islet transplantation in seven patients with type 1 diabetes mellitus using a gluococorticoid-free immunosuppressive regimen. *N Engl J Med.* 2000;343:230-238.
423. Diabetes Breakthrough. Faculty of Medicine and Dentistry News. June 2000;2:1-5. Available at: http://www.med.ualberta.ca/documents/fn/fn-vol2-num4.pdf. Accessed June 17, 2006.
424. *Critical Care Nurse.* Organ Donation Issue. April 1999;19(2).
425. U.S. Surgeons Perform First U.S. Hand Transplant. CNN Interactive. Available at: http://www.cnn.com/HEALTH/9901/25/hand.transplant.02/. Accessed February 12, 2006.
426. Jones JW, Gruber SA, Barker JH, Breidenbach WC. Successful hand transplantation. One-year follow-up. Louisville Hand Transplant Team. *N Engl J Med.* 2000 Aug 17;343(7):468-73.
427. Dubernard JM, Henry P, Parmentier H, et al. [First transplantation of two hands: results after 18 months] *Ann Chir.* 2002 Jan;127(1):19-25.
428. Petruzzo P, Badet L, Gazarian A, et al. Bilateral hand transplantation: six years after the first case. *Am J Transplant.* 2006 Jul;6(7):1718-24.
429. Fageeh W, Raffa H, Jabbad H, Marzouki A. Transplantation of the human uterus. *Int J Gynaecol Obstet.* 2002 Mar;76(3):245-51.
430. Milanes CL, Gonzalez L, Hernandez E, Armenio A, Clesca P, Rivas-Vetencourt A. Transplant coordination program: a useful tool to improve organ donation in Venezuela. *Prog Transplant.* 2003;13:296-298.
431. US Department of Health and Human Services. Organ Donation Breakthrough Collaborative. From Best Practice to Common Practice. About the Collaborative. Available at: http://www.organdonationnow.org/index.cfm?fuseaction=Page.viewPage&pageId=471. Accessed April 22, 2006.
432. Shafer TJ, Wagner D, Chessare J, Zampiello, FA, McBride VA, Perdue J. Increasing organ donation through system redesign. *Crit Care Nurse.* February 2006;26:33-48.

Chapter 1 — **THE HISTORY OF THE TRANSPLANT COORDINATOR**

433. Kermer C, Oeckher M. [Tongue transplantation]*Wien Klin Wochenschr*. 2004 Oct 30;116(19-20):643-4.
434. Sheehy E, Conrad SL, Brigham LE, et al. Estimating the number of potential organ donors in the United States. *N Engl J Med*. 2003;349:667-674.
435. Tokalak I, Karakayali H, Moray G, Bilgin N, Haberal M. Coordinating organ transplantation in Turkey: effects of the National Coordination Center. *Prog Transplant*. 2005;15:283-285.
436. Kyoto University Hospital Islet Program. Achievements. Available at: http://islet.eriko.com/index_en.html. Accessed April 22, 2006.
437. Woman has first face transplant. BBC News, November 30, 2005. Available at: http://news.bbc.co.uk/1/hi/health/4484728.stm. Accessed February 12, 2006.
438. Devauchelle B, Badet L, Lengele B, et al. First human face allograft: early report. *Lancet*. 2006 Jul 15;368(9531):203-9.
439. Johns Hopkins Medicine. News and information services. Available at: http://www.hopkinsmedicine.org/Press_releases/2005/index.html. Accessed April 25, 2006.
440. Montgomery RA, Gentry SE, Marks WH, et al. Domino paired kidney donation: a strategy to make best use of live non-directed donation. *Lancet*. 2006 Jul 29;368(9533):419-21.
441. Jordan M, Brown D. Girls heart recovers; surgeons remove donor heart. *The Washington Post*. Friday, April 14, 2006. In: *Fort Worth Star Telegram*, 24A.
442. *Critical Care Nurse*. Transplantation issue. 2006;26(2).

Full Page photos following references:

Photo: page 319 – Herb Teachey, transplant coordinator. Photograph by Russell Munson. Published in *Raytheon* magazine, 1985. **Photo © Russell Munson** (*Duplicated as originally published – in full page layout.*)
From: Larsen G. Lifeguard. *Raytheon Magazine*. Spring 1985:28-29.

Photo: page 320 – Amy Peele, transplant coordinator. 1984. (*Duplicated as originally published – in full page layout.*) Photo: David Kogan/The 11th Hour Pictures Ltd.
From: American Airlines *In Flight* magazine.

A CLINICIAN'S GUIDE TO DONATION AND TRANSPLANTATION — Chapter 1

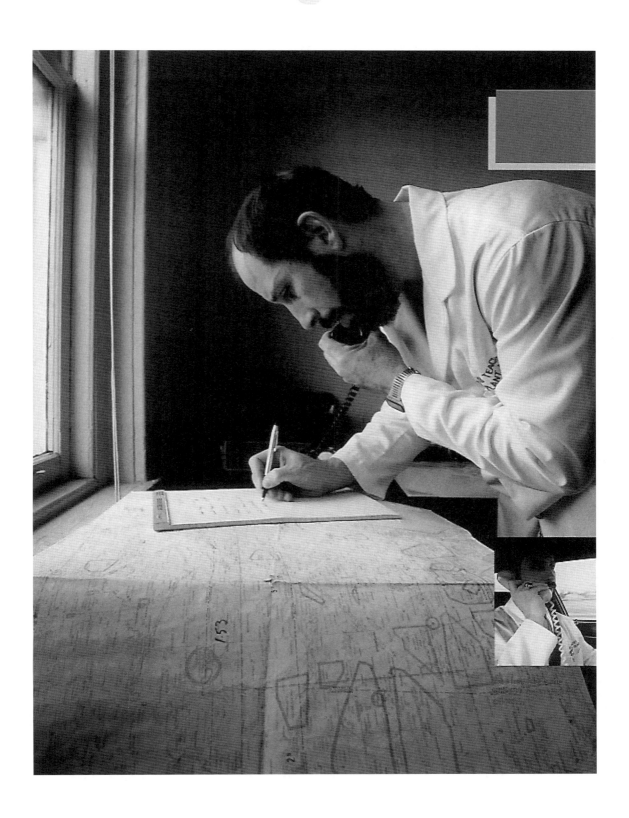

Chapter 1 — THE HISTORY OF THE TRANSPLANT COORDINATOR

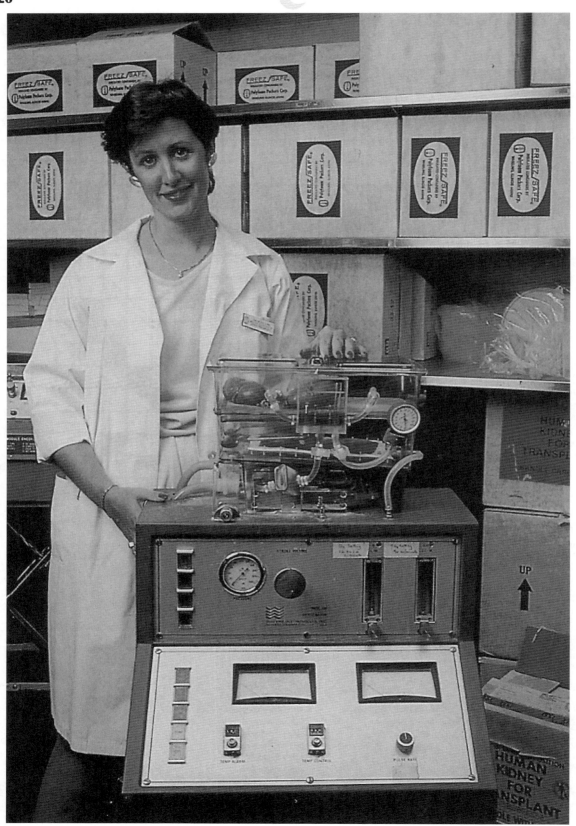

Organ Allocation

Walter Graham
Lin Johnson McGaw, RN, MEd
Kim Johnson, MS
Deanna C. Sampson, BS, JD
Cindy M. Sommers, Esq.
Roger Brown, BS, CPTC

Introduction

Organ allocation in the United States is governed by federal law and regulation under a program operated by the US Department of Health and Human Services (DHHS) by contract with a private entity comprising the nation's organ transplant community. The National Organ Transplant Act (NOTA) of 1984 authorized the establishment of the Organ Procurement and Transplantation Network (OPTN) and empowered the OPTN to maintain "a national list of individuals who need organs, and a national system, through the use of computers and in accordance with established medical criteria, to match organs and individuals included in the list."[1]

NOTA also established the modern system of organ procurement organizations (OPOs), with exclusive, defined service areas in which the OPOs have responsibility for promoting organ donation as well as procuring organs from deceased organ donors. According to NOTA, OPOs are required to have a system that will allow donated organs to be allocated equitably among transplant patients according to established medical criteria[2] and that the OPTN assists OPOs in the nationwide distribution of these organs.[1] Central to these requirements is the law's stipulation that allocation is to be based on *medical criteria*, as opposed to social criteria such as social worth or economic criteria such as wealth and *equity*, (i.e., fairness) with distribution of organs *among patients* rather than distribution among transplant centers or physicians who then choose the patient to receive the organ (although physicians may exercise medical judgment and are not required to accept an organ for a particular patient).

In 2000, DHHS issued regulations governing the operation of the OPTN authorized by NOTA. The OPTN Final Rule[3] provides the legal basis for organ allocation policies to be developed by the OPTN and requires that allocation policies:

- Be based on sound medical judgment;
- Seek to achieve the best use of donated organs;
- Preserve the ability of a transplant program to decline an offer of an organ or not to use the organ for the potential recipient;
- Be specific for each organ type or combination of organ types to be transplanted into a transplant candidate;
- Be designed to avoid wasting organs, to avoid futile transplants, to promote patient access to transplantation, and to promote the efficient management of organ placement;
- Be reviewed periodically and revised as appropriate;
- Include appropriate procedures to promote and review compliance including, to the extent appropriate, prospective and retrospective reviews of each transplant program's application of the policies to patients listed or proposed to be listed at the program; and
- Not be based on the candidate's place of residence or place of listing, except to the extent required by the foregoing considerations.

Equitable Allocation

A primary goal of the OPTN is the maximization of the benefit of transplantation to patients with end-stage organ failure while also minimizing the burden of that organ failure. At the same time, the policies for equitable organ allocation must also minimize organ wastage and maximize transplant benefit and patient safety along with system efficiencies that increase the number of viable organs for transplantation. Equity is frequently understood as being synonymous with the concept of distributive justice, and the classic definition of justice espoused by Aristotle is that "equals must be treated equally, and unequals must be treated unequally."[4(p227)] In other words, the allocation system must be perceived as being fair and unnecessarily impartial, all things being considered equally.

Medical Benefit

In keeping with Kant's ethical imperative to do the most good for the most people, the OPTN's organ allocation policies seek to maximize the number of people who receive a transplant and thereafter benefit from an enhanced quality of life. In developing organ allocation policies, the OPTN takes into account the "burden of disease" for patients before and after transplantation, so that an allocation policy will select candidates and time the transplantations in an attempt to minimize the net burden of disease and to maximize the number of life years gained.

The elements of "burden of disease" include factors such as the patient's potential for early mortality, morbidity or the relative incidence of disease, potential for disability/impairment, psychological and emotional distress, quality of life, and functional status. It includes, of course, patient survival, both before and after transplantation, which, as the lung allocation policy incorporates the concept, translates into the risk of death while waiting and the probability of survival after transplantation. In examining the benefit of particular policy for organ allocation, the OPTN also takes into account other important factors including cost, resource utilization, and the availability of alternative treatments.

Another important consideration is the possibility of prioritizing patients on the basis of consequences of their underlying disease. Should the policy give preference to a patient with kidney failure who may not be well suited for dialysis or a patient who has lost kidney function because of diabetes and is in the process of losing other functions because of his or her diabetes, such as sight? How does the allocation system evaluate the benefit for each patient? If the patient who is not well-suited for dialysis does not receive a kidney transplant, he or she may die. If the patient who needs a kidney together with a pancreas from the same donor does not receive such a transplant, he or she may become blind, lose a leg, or even die. Is one more compelling than the other? What is the "net benefit" in each instance? These are but a few of the tough issues OPTN organ allocation policies must consider.

Balancing Equity and Benefit

This balancing is a major challenge in organ allocation. The DHHS Office of the Inspector General has issued several reports that are critical of organ allocation policies because minorities wait on average much longer than others for a kidney transplant. The reasons for this difference can be explained on the basis of biological and other medical factors, but it has been well established that an allocation policy that seeks to maximize benefit may result in disadvantage for minorities because of those biological factors. On the other hand, it has long been established that more medical benefit in kidney transplantation ensues from better histocompatibility matches between donor and recipient. Thus, were the allocation system to be focused solely on net benefit measured by the post-transplant survival of recipients (e.g., post-transplant life-years gained), it is possible that the system could result in inequity, which would be contrary to the OPTN's mission as defined by NOTA and the OPTN Final Rule. Likewise, it has long been understood that as a group, women have a poorer rate of posttransplant survival in kidney transplantation than men.

The Impact of Geography

The organ allocation system in the United States has always been based primarily on a "local first" philosophy. The "local" area for initial distribution is typically the designated service area of the OPO procuring the organ, unless an alternative local area has been approved by the OPTN. The traditional rationale for a local first policy was the rapid deterioration of organs after recovery. Thoracic organs show significant deterioration after 4 to 6 hours. However, kidneys are now routinely transplanted successfully after 24 to 36 hours following recovery. This causes questions to arise regarding the appropriateness of a local first priority policy for kidneys. Will there be a negative impact on local efforts to maximize organ recovery if organs are not allocated locally first? Is the national system considered "equitable" when one part of the country has a much longer average wait for a transplant than another part of the country? The OPTN final rule established that the candidate's place of residence or listing may not be a factor in allocation except to the extent the final rule's other policy objectives determine otherwise. The final rule also establishes an allocation performance objective that organs are to be distributed over as broad a geographic area as feasible in keeping with those policy objectives. It also includes a performance objective of reducing the intertransplant program variance to as small as can be reasonably achieved.

Objectives of Equitable Organ Allocation

The goal of the OPTN's organ allocation system must be to achieve the following fundamental objectives:

- Maximize the number of organs available for transplantation;
- Maximize patient and graft survival, including maximizing the number of life-years gained;
- Minimize the number of deaths while waiting for a transplant;
- Minimize disparities in the opportunity to receive a transplant among similarly situated transplant candidates; and
- Enhance the public's trust in the fairness and effectiveness of the allocation system.

OPTN Operations

In 1986, the Health Resources & Services Administration of DHHS awarded a contract to the United Network for Organ Sharing (UNOS) to establish and operate the OPTN. UNOS, a not-for-profit membership corporation, maintains the OPTN's board of directors and committee structure for the development of policies and standards, including organ allocation policies. UNOS also facilitates the process of organ allocation via a centralized computer network, UNet^{SM}, which links organ donor, transplant, recipient, and potential transplant patient information in all OPOs and transplant centers in a secure, real-time environment. UNet^{SM} is accessible 24 hours a day, 7 days a week, and is used by UNOS members as well as organ placement specialists in the Organ Center to assist OPOs and transplant centers allocate organs.

When a deceased organ donor is identified, a transplant coordinator accesses the UNet^{SM} system. Each patient on the National Transplant Waiting List is matched by the system against the organ donor characteristics. The system then generates a list of patients, called a "match run," for each donated organ procured in a ranked order according to organ allocation policies.

Factors affecting the rank order may include medical urgency, tissue match, blood type, length of time on the National Transplant Waiting List, immune status, and the geographic distance between the patient and organ donor. Therefore, the UNet^{SM} system generates a differently ranked list of patients for each donor organ.

The organ is offered to the transplant team of the first person on the list. Often, the top patient will not get the organ for 1 of several reasons. When a patient is selected, he or she must be available, healthy enough to undergo major surgery, and willing to receive a transplant immediately. Also, a laboratory test to measure compatibility between the organ donor and patient may be necessary. If the organ is refused for any reason, the transplant hospital of the next patient on the National Transplant Waiting List is contacted. The process continues until a match is made. Once a patient is selected and contacted and all testing is complete, surgery is scheduled and the transplantation takes place.[1]

Those Involved

- **The Organ Center.** Staffed with organ placement specialists, the Organ Center, located in Richmond, VA, coordinates the efforts of many transplant professionals in OPOs and transplant centers with the needs of the patient.

- **The Organ Donor.** A person who has died, is compatible with the recipient, and meets certain criteria.
- **The Transplant Patient.** A person who needs a new organ because he or she has suffered from end-stage organ disease. A transplant center has evaluated this patient, determined that he or she is a patient for an organ transplant, and has added him or her to the national Transplant Candidate List.
- **The Transplant Recipient.** A person who has received an organ transplant.
- **The Procurement Team.** A group of professionals who work at an OPO or transplant center and coordinate the recovery of the organ. They remove the organs from the donor's body for transplantation.
- **The Transplant Team.** Healthcare personnel who perform the transplant operation. They also take care of the patient before, during, and after the transplant operation.
- **UNet[SM].** A secure Internet-based transplant information database, created by UNOS for the nation's organ transplant centers and OPOs to register patients for transplants, match donated organs to transplant patients, and manage the critical data of all patients. This computer network is accessible 24 hours a day, 7 days a week.[5]

Heart Allocation

Heart allocation policies use the following factors for prioritization: time accumulated on the National Transplant Waiting List, ABO compatibility, and geography. Waiting time is accumulated by transplant patients and will affect their rank on the National Transplant Waiting List within the status they are listed. To ensure donor organ quality and reduce ischemic time, donor hearts are allocated first to patients within local areas before being distributed to increasingly larger allocation zones.

Adult patients awaiting heart transplantation are assigned a status code, which corresponds to how medically urgent it is that the patient receive a transplant. More specifically, status 1A heart patients have the most urgent status, and are listed having (1) mechanical circulatory support for acute hemodynamic decompensation that includes at least 1 of the following: left and/or right ventricular assist device implanted, total artificial heart, intra-aortic balloon pump, or extracorporeal membrane oxygenator; (2) mechanical circulatory support with objective medical evidence of significant device-related complications such as thromboembolism, device infection, mechanical failure, and/or life-threatening ventricular arrhythmias; (3) continuous mechanical ventilation; or (4) continuous infusion of a single high-dose intravenous inotrope or multiple intravenous inotropes, in addition to continuous hemodynamic monitoring of left ventricular filling pressures. Status 1B heart patients have at least 1 of the following devices or therapies in place: left and/or right ventricular assist device implanted or continuous infusion of intravenous inotropes. Status 2 heart patients are all other patients awaiting a heart who do not meet the criteria for status 1A or 1B. Status 7 is available for heart patients who are considered temporarily unsuitable to receive a thoracic organ transplant.

A patient who does not meet the criteria for status 1A or 1B may nevertheless be assigned to such status upon application by his or her transplant physician(s) and justification to the applicable Regional Review Board that the patient is considered, using acceptable medical criteria, to have an urgency and potential for benefit comparable to that of other patients in the status applied for as defined above. A patient's listing for status 1A under this exceptional provision is valid for 14 days.

Pediatric patients awaiting heart transplantation are assigned a status code that corresponds to how medically urgent it is that the patient receive a transplant. Medical urgency is assigned to a heart transplant patient who is younger than 18 years of age at the time of listing, as follows: pediatric heart patients who remain on the National Transplant Waiting List at the time of their 18th birthday without receiving a transplant qualify for pediatric standing. A status 1A pediatric heart patient requires assistance with a ventilator, requires assistance with a mechanical assist device (e.g., extracorporeal membrane oxygenator), requires assistance with a balloon pump, is younger than 6 months old with congenital or acquired heart disease exhibiting reactive pulmonary hypertension at greater than 50% of systemic level, requires infusion of high-dose or multiple inotropes, or does not meet the criteria specified above and has a life expectancy

A CLINICIAN'S GUIDE TO DONATION AND TRANSPLANTATION

without a heart transplant of fewer than 14 days. A status 1B pediatric heart patient requires an infusion of low-dose single inotropes, is younger than 6 months old, and does not meet the criteria for status 1A or has growth failure on the basis of the National Center for Health Statistics for pediatric growth curves. Status 2 pediatric heart patients do not meet the criteria for status 1A or 1B. Status 7 is available for pediatric heart patients who are considered temporarily unsuitable to receive a thoracic organ transplant.

A pediatric patient who does not meet the criteria for status 1A may nevertheless be assigned to such status if the patient has a life expectancy without a transplant of fewer than 14 days. In addition, a pediatric patient who does not meet the criteria for status 1B may nevertheless be assigned to such status upon application by his or her transplant physician(s) and justification to the applicable Regional Review Board that the patient is considered, using acceptable medical criteria, to have an urgency and potential for benefit comparable to that of other patients in this status as defined above.

Within each heart status, a heart retrieved from an adolescent organ donor shall be allocated to a pediatric heart patient before the heart is allocated to an adult patient. In addition, as mentioned earlier, thoracic organs are allocated locally first, and then in a specific sequence of 4 zones. Zone A will extend to all transplant centers that are within 500 miles from the donor hospital but not in the local area of the donor hospital. Zone B will extend to all transplant centers that are at least 500 miles from the donor hospital but not more than 1000 miles from the donor hospital. Zone C will extend to all transplant centers that are at least 1000 miles from the donor hospital but not more than 1500 miles from the donor hospital. Zone D will extend to all transplant centers that are located beyond 1500 miles from the donor hospital. A heart is allocated to the local area first, to status 1A then status 1B then status 2 patients; then the heart is allocated to zone A, to status 1A then 1B patients; then to zone B, to status 1A and 1B patients; then to zone A, to status 2 patients; then to zone B, to status 2 patients; then to zone C, to status 1A, status1B and then status 2 patients; and lastly to zone D, to status 1A, 1B, and then status 2 patients.

ABO typing is important when matching a donor heart with a recipient. The following criteria apply within heart status categories. An O donor heart must go to an O or B recipient. An A donor heart must go to an A or AB recipient. A B donor heart must go to a B or AB recipient and an AB donor heart must go to an AB recipient. If a patient meeting these match requirements is not available, then the heart is offered to a compatible patient.

Sensitized Patient Allocation

The transplant surgeon or physician for a patient awaiting thoracic organ transplantation may determine that the patient is "sensitized," that is, the patient's antibodies would react adversely to certain donor cell antigens. It is permissible to forgo thoracic organ allocation policies of a particular thoracic organ when all thoracic organ transplant centers within an OPO and the OPO agree to allocate the thoracic organ to a sensitized patient because results of a cross-match between the blood serum of that patient and cells of the thoracic organ donor are negative.

Blood Type "Z"

For pediatric patients younger than 1 year of age who will accept a heart from a donor of any blood type, the blood type Z designation may be added as a suffix to the actual blood type (e.g., AZ) or used alone if actual blood type is not known for *in utero* patients.[6,7]

Lung Allocation

Patients awaiting a lung transplant, whether it is a single or a double lung transplant, will be grouped together for allocation purposes. If one lung is allocated to a patient needing a single lung transplant, the other lung will be then allocated to another patient waiting for a single lung transplant. Lungs from adult donors will first be offered to patients age 12 and older, and then to patients 0 to 11 years old. Lungs from donors 0 to 11 years old are first offered to patients age 0 to 11, and then to those between 12 and 17 years of age, then to adults.[7] Lungs from donors 12 to 17 years old are first offered to patients age 12 to 17, then to those between 0 and 11, then to adults. Lung patients who are 0 to 11 years old are ranked by waiting time and patients age 12 and above are ranked by Lung Allocation Score.

ORGAN ALLOCATION

The Lung Allocation Score is generated by an algorithm that considers predictions of waiting list survival and post-transplant survival. These predictions are based on clinical data such as forced vital capacity, age, and ventilator use. The higher the resulting score, the higher priority a patient will receive on the waiting list. If the NYHA Classification or Assisted Ventilation questions are unanswered, the patient is automatically assigned a Lung Allocation Score of 0. The Lung Allocation Score is calculated using the following measures: (1) waiting list urgency measure (expected number of days lived without a transplant during an additional year on the waitlist), (2) post-transplant survival measure (expected number of days lived during the first year after transplantation), and (3) transplant benefit measure (post-transplant survival measure minus waiting list urgency measure). The calculations define the difference between transplant benefit and waitlist urgency, where the raw allocation score equals Transplant Benefit Measure minus Waitlist Urgency Measure.

Similar to heart allocation, lung allocation is influenced by location, ABO typing, and medical urgency. Lungs are allocated to their local area first, then to zone A, B, C, and D, in that order. Within each zone and patient age group, the organs are allocated to ABO-identical patients before ABO-compatible patients.

Sequence of Adult Donor Lung Allocation

Patients age 12 and older awaiting a lung transplant, whether it is a single or a double lung transplant, will be grouped together for adult (18 years old and older) donor lung allocation. Lungs from adult donors will be allocated locally first, then to patients in zone A, B, C, and D, in that order. In each of those 5 geographic areas, patients will be grouped so those who have an ABO blood type that is identical to that of the donor are ranked according to applicable allocation priority; the lungs will be allocated in descending order to patients in that ABO-identical type. If the lungs are not allocated to patients in that ABO-identical type, they will be allocated in descending order according to applicable allocation priority to the remaining patients in that geographic area who have a blood type that is compatible (but not identical) with that of the donor.

Patients age 0 to 11 years old awaiting a single or double lung transplant will be grouped together for allocation purposes. If one lung is allocated to a patient waiting for a single lung transplant, the other lung will be allocated to another patient waiting for a single lung transplant.

Patients 12 to 17 years old awaiting a single or double lung transplant will be grouped together for pediatric (0-17 years old) donor lung allocation. If one lung is allocated to a patient waiting for a single lung transplant, the other lung will be allocated to another patient waiting for a single lung transplant.

Lungs from donors who are 0 to 11 years old will first be offered to patients age 0 to 11; then to patients age 12 to 17; then to patients 18 years and older. Lungs will be allocated locally first, then to patients in zone A, B, C, and D, in that order. In each of those 5 geographic areas, patients will be grouped so those who have an ABO blood type that is identical to that of the donor are ranked according to applicable allocation priority; the lungs will be allocated in descending order to patients in that ABO-identical type. If the lungs are not allocated to patients in that ABO-identical type, they will be allocated in descending order according to applicable allocation priority to the remaining patients in that geographic area who have a blood type that is compatible (but not identical) with that of the donor.[6,7]

Lungs from donors age 12 to 17 years old will first be offered to patients age 12 to 17; then to patients age 0 to 11; then to patients 18 years and older. Lungs will be allocated locally first, then to patients in zone A, B, C, and D, in that order. In each of those 5 geographic areas, patients will be grouped so that patients who have an ABO blood type that is identical to that of the donor are ranked according to applicable allocation priority; the lungs will be allocated in descending order to patients in that ABO-identical type. If the lungs are not allocated to patients in that ABO-identical type, they will be allocated in descending order according to applicable allocation priority to the remaining patients in that geographic area who have a blood type that is compatible (but not identical) with that of the donor.[6,7]

Heart-Lung Allocation

Patients for a heart-lung transplant are registered on the individual National Transplant Waiting List for each organ. When the transplant patient is eligible to receive a heart, the lung will be allocated to the heart-lung patient from the same donor. When the patient is eligible to receive a lung, the heart is allocated to the heart-lung patient from the same donor if no suitable status 1A isolated heart patients are eligible to receive the heart. In addition, ABO-matching requirements are applied for heart-lung patients, per the individual organ policy, when these patients are included in the respective heart or lung match run results.[6,7]

Liver Allocation

Livers are allocated on the basis of 3 tiers of geographical sharing units: local, regional, and national. In addition, patients awaiting a liver transplant are assigned a status code of 1A or 1B on the basis of their medical condition or a mortality risk score corresponding to the degree of medical urgency, referred to as the Model for End-Stage Liver Disease (MELD) and the Pediatric End-Stage Liver Disease (PELD). Following status 1, livers will be offered to patients with the highest medical urgency on the basis of these scores, with the patient having the highest probability ranking receiving the highest priority and being offered the liver before it is offered to patients having lower probability rankings. The most urgent need category is status 1 for both adults and pediatric patients. Adults will have fulminant failure, primary nonfunction, hepatic artery thrombosis of a transplanted liver, or acute decompensated Wilson disease and be assigned to status 1A. Pediatric patients will be in the intensive care unit, have fulminant failure, primary nonfunction, hepatic artery thrombosis of a transplanted liver, or acute decompensated Wilson disease and be assigned to status 1A. Pediatric patients in the intensive care unit with chronic liver disease can be assigned to status 1B if certain specified criteria are met. The next highest rank is based on MELD score for adults and MELD or PELD scores for pediatric patients.

The allocation ranking is as follows within the geographical sharing units: status 1 is based on points, ABO, and time waiting; MELD/PELD score (morality risk system) with the highest score having the highest ranking and ABO and time waiting within each MELD/PELD score. More specifically, adult liver allocation follows this order: local status 1A patients, regional status 1A patients, local status 1B patients, regional status 1B candidates, local MELD/PELD score of 15 or greater in descending order, regional MELD/PELD score of 15 or greater in descending order, local MELD/PELD score of less than 15 in descending order, regional MELD/PELD score of less than 15 in descending order, then national status 1A followed by status 1B, then MELD/PELD scores in descending order.

Pediatric liver allocation follows the similar adult local, regional, and national order, with a few exceptions; pediatric patients take priority over adult patients within each allocation group and pediatric PELD patients age 0 to 11 years old take priority over pediatric MELD patients age 12 to 17 years old.

ABO typing for liver allocation is such that O donor livers must first be offered to O patients or B patients with a MELD/PELD score of greater than or equal to 30. The exception is a status 1 patient. Patients with a MELD/PELD score of greater than or equal to 25 and status 1A or 1B patients may be listed to accept incompatible ABO. In addition, within each MELD/PELD score, the ABO is allocated to an identical match, then to an ABO-compatible match, and lastly to an ABO-incompatible patient.

Sequence of Allocation for Patients with PELD or MELD Scores Less Than or Equal to 6

Adult patients and pediatric adolescent patients with a MELD score of 6 are considered together with pediatric patients younger than 12 years, with a PELD score less than or equal to 6. These patients will be initially ranked on the basis of waiting time. National Transplant Waiting List positions assigned to pediatric patients on the basis of this initial ranking (e.g., if the 3rd and 5th positions on the ranked list are held by pediatric patients) will then be redistributed among the pediatric group on the basis of PELD or MELD score, with the patient with the highest PELD or MELD core receiving the highest available pediatric ranking position. The next available pediatric ranking position will be assigned to the pediatric patient with the next highest PELD or MELD score. Redistribution of pediatric patients continues until the pediatric patient with the lowest PELD or MELD score is assigned the last pediatric ranking position.

Allocation of Livers for Segmental Transplantation

A transplant center that accepts a liver for segmental transplantation shall offer the remaining segment:

(i) in sequence, as determined by the deceased donor liver allocation algorithm set forth in liver allocation policy and defining "local" on the basis of the host OPO's local area, to the highest-ranking patient on the transplant candidate list of patients; provided, however, that the host OPO places the liver segment(s) by the time the donor organ procurement procedure has started, or

(ii) into patients listed with the recipient program or any medically appropriate patient on the transplant candidate list, if, after reasonable attempts by the host OPO to place the remaining portion(s) of the donor liver, the liver segment(s) is not placed by the time the donor organ procurement procedure has started.

Additional Consideration

A liver shall not be used for other methods of hepatic support before being offered for transplantation. The liver shall first be offered by the UNOS organ center in descending point order to all status 1A and 1B patients, followed by all patients in order of their MELD/PELD scores (probability of patient death) in the host OPO's region, followed by status 1A and 1B patients, and then by all patients in order of the MELD/PELD scores (probability of patient death) in all other regions. If the liver is not accepted for transplantation within 6 hours of attempted placement by the organ center, the organ center shall offer the liver to status 1A and 1B patients, followed by all patients in order of their MELD/PELD scores (probability of patient death) for whom the liver will be considered for other methods of hepatic support. Livers allocated for other methods of hepatic support shall be offered first locally, then regionally, and then nationally in descending point order to transplant patients designated for other methods of hepatic support.[6,8]

Intestinal Allocation

Intestinal organs include the stomach, small and/or large intestine, and any portion of the gastrointestinal tract. Intestinal organs are allocated first to size-compatible and ABO-identical patients, followed by patients who have a blood type that is compatible to the organ donor. Allocation is based on length of waiting time and in accordance with the following sequence: local status 1 then local status 2; regional (host OPO's region) status 1 then regional (host OPO's region) status 2; then status 1 patients in all other regions and lastly status 2 patients in all other regions. Status 1 patients have liver function test abnormalities and/or no longer have vascular access through the subclavian, jugular, or femoral veins for intravenous feeding, or have other medical indications that warrant intestinal organ transplantation on an urgent basis. Status 2 patients do not meet the criteria for status 1 and status 7 patients are temporarily inactive; however, the patient continues accruing waiting time up to a maximum of 30 days.[6,9]

Intestinal-Liver Allocation

For patients awaiting a combined intestine-liver transplant, the liver may be allocated by the local OPO to a local or regional intestine recipient on the basis of priority for receipt of the intestine using the intestine transplant waiting list, unless there is a status 1 liver patient locally or regionally. If the liver is voluntarily offered with the intestine regionally, a liver of identical blood type shall be referred back to the host OPO from the next acceptable donor procured by the recipient OPO.[6,9]

Kidney Allocation

The objectives for allocating and distributing deceased donor kidneys are to provide patients with a donor kidney best suited to them as quickly as possible while balancing other medical considerations that contribute to organ transplantation and overall system utility, as well as medical factors unique to particular patient populations; increasing the availability of organs; and preserving the public's trust in the national allocation system. A combination of factors determines who receives which organ. These factors include human leukocyte antigen (HLA) matching between donor and patient, blood type, blood antibody levels, length of time spent on the transplant candidate list, whether the potential organ recipient is a child, body size of both donor and recipient, and geographic factors. Points will not be assigned to recipients on the basis of medical urgency for regional or national allocation of kidneys. HLA matching has been a factor in kidney allocation since its inception. Differences in HLA or tissue type between kidney donor and recipient stimulate the recipient's immune system to reject the donor kidney. Pharmacologic immunosuppression is required to impede the immune responses and, hopefully, prevent rejection and enable long-term acceptance of the donor kidney transplantations between HLA-matched recipients and donors generally function longer and with less immunosuppression, thereby maximizing utility of the donor's organs. Significant improvement in transplantation outcomes because of HLA matching is currently demonstrated only with a zero antigen mismatch (the highest level of match based on the degree of HLA identity between donor and recipient), and matches at the DR locus. HLA match also provides the greatest opportunity for transplant candidates who have developed anti-HLA antibodies directed against a relatively substantial proportion of the donor pool, as discussed below. Therefore, for both standard and expanded criteria donor kidneys, priority is given nationally to zero antigen mismatched patients, because of the documented graft survival benefit experienced by recipients of such kidneys and enhanced access to transplantation for sensitized patients. These zero antigen mismatched patients are stratified on the basis of a number of factors, including blood type, panel reactive antibody (PRA), payback status, age, and location.

Blood Group Compatibility

The systems for allocating standard and expanded criteria donor kidneys are similar also in ensuring compatibility between donor and patient ABO blood group, which is necessary for success of the transplant procedure, allocating organs on the basis of blood group identity or to particular compatible blood groups to avoid disadvantaging these patients because of blood type.

Wait Time

Wait time is an additional factor used in the allocation of standard as well as expanded criteria donor kidneys. Patients with end-stage kidney failure can be sustained on dialysis over a period with good results, with exceptions noted below for children. However, dialysis therapy has adverse quality of life implications. In addition, studies show improved long-term patient survival for recipients of kidney transplantation versus individuals waiting for kidney transplantation while receiving dialysis. Differences in survival may be affected by patient medical condition such as diabetes, glomerulonephritis, or other causes of end-stage renal disease. The potential patient survival advantage attributable to kidney transplantation and its role in the allocation system is being explored. At present, however, relative patient waiting time plays a unique role in kidney allocation in defining system fairness. In general, kidneys are allocated locally first, then regionally, then nationally.

Standard Kidney Allocation

Within the standard donor allocation system, additional allocation priority is awarded as follows: points are awarded for less than the optimal (zero antigen mismatch) degree of HLA identity between donor and patient on the basis of significantly improved transplant outcomes with matching at the DR locus. Kidney transplant recipients who have been exposed to the HLA antigens of another individual as a consequence of pregnancy, blood transfusions, or previous transplantation are at risk for developing antibodies against foreign HLA antigens. Anti-HLA antibodies prevent patients from receiving transplants from donors with HLA antigens to which the antibodies are directed. Recipients who have developed high levels of these antibodies generally need donor organs with a very good HLA match to avoid rejection. Because of the documented difficulty such patients experience in obtaining a donor kidney with a negative cross-match, they are assigned extra points.

Previous Living Donors

Patients who need a kidney and have previously donated a living donor organ for transplantation are awarded additional points when listed, with the intent of encouraging organ availability through living donation and acknowledging these patients' sacrifice and exposure to medical risk.

Age for Pediatric Patients

Young children and adolescents experience unique problems associated with dialysis, including disruption of expected growth and development processes because of renal failure. Early reversal of uremia through transplantation can avoid the complications of dialysis and ameliorate many of the adverse effects of end-stage renal disease that confront these patients. Rapid treatment provides the best opportunity for reversing the growth and development deficits and preventing lifelong adverse consequences. Additional priority is, therefore, assigned to children in allocating kidneys from donors younger than 35 years. The intent is to expedite access for these patients to donor kidneys considered medically suitable for use in pediatric transplant patients.

Expanded Criteria Donor Kidney Allocation

The allocation algorithm for expanded criteria donor kidneys allocates kidneys to patients who have agreed to accept them only on the basis of accrued waiting time and blood type considerations after the zero antigen mismatched level of priority. The intent is to maximize procurement and use of these kidneys, providing a mechanism for more rapid placement of the organs while minimizing cold ischemic time. An expanded criteria donor is 60 years or older, or 50 to 59 years old with 2 or more of the following conditions present: a creatinine level greater than 1.5 mg/dL, cause of death due to a cerebral vascular accident, and a history of hypertension.

The policy recognizes the additional risk expected with expanded criteria donor kidney transplantation and establishes a protocol for offering them under conditions intended to improve acceptance and enhance outcomes. Pediatric patients waiting for a kidney transplant generally are not considered good patients for expanded criteria donor kidneys because of long-term graft survival concerns and possibility of sensitization. It is anticipated that ongoing review of outcome data will help in better defining the most appropriate patients for such kidneys.[6,10]

Double Kidney Allocation

For a recipient to be able to accept 2 kidneys from the same adult donor, 2 of the following criteria must be met by the donor: older than 60 years, an estimated creatinine clearance of less than 65 mL/min on the basis of the serum creatinine level upon admission, rising creatinine level of greater than 2.5 mg/dL at time of retrieval, long-standing hypertension or diabetes mellitus, and between 16% and 50% glomerulosclerosis.[6,10]

Allocation of Kidneys With Discrepant HLA Typing

Allocation of deceased donor kidneys is based on the HLA typing identified by the donor histocompatibility laboratory. If the recipient HLA laboratory identifies a different HLA type for the donor, the kidney may be allocated in accordance with the original HLA typing, or the recipient center may reallocate the kidney locally, according to UNOS policy.[6,10]

Pancreas Allocation

In general, pancreas allocation is first done locally, then regionally, and then nationally on the basis of certain geographic zones. For local pancreas allocation, recipients may be selected from patients awaiting an isolated pancreas, kidney-pancreas combination, or a combined solid organ islet transplant from the same donor, unless there is a patient on the transplant candidate list who meets the requirements of a zero antigen mismatch offer. Patients accrue waiting time while registered on the transplant candidate list, and are considered for the selection of organ recipients. Patients continue to accrue waiting time while registered on the transplant candidate list as inactive. For combined kidney-pancreas patients, blood type O kidneys must be transplanted into blood type O recipients, unless there is a zero antigen mismatch between the patient and donor and the patient is highly sensitized. If the pancreas is not placed locally for an isolated or combined whole organ transplant, a combined solid organ islet transplant, or to a zero antigen mismatch patient, and if procured from a donor 50 years old or younger and with a body mass index of less than or equal to 30 kg/m^2, the pancreas shall be allocated for whole organ or combined kidney whole organ transplantation regionally and then nationally, or for whole pancreas to patients listed for facilitated pancreas placement. Regional whole pancreas allocation is based on the transplant patient's length of time waiting in the following categories: isolated pancreas and combined kidney-pancreas. Blood type O kidneys must be transplanted into blood type O recipients. If the pancreas is not allocated within the region, it will be allocated nationally in the same manner as within the region.

Mandatory Sharing of Zero Antigen Mismatch Pancreas

Differences can exist in the HLA or tissue type between the pancreas donor and patient that will stimulate the patient's immune system to reject the donor pancreas. Pharmacologic immunosuppression is required to impede the immune responses and, hopefully, prevent rejection and enable long-term acceptance of the donor pancreas. Data no longer indicate improved transplant outcomes on the basis of HLA match between recipients of kidney-pancreas combinations and donors, even at the highest level of match on the basis of degree of HLA identity between donor and patient. For isolated pancreas transplantation there is a trend toward improved outcomes, although the results do not demonstrate statistical significance. HLA match does, however, provide the best candidates opportunity for transplant who are sensitized against a relatively substantial proportion of the donor pool. Optimally (zero antigen mismatched) matched organs provide the best chance for avoiding rejection for these patients and a large donor pool provides greater options for locating such matches.

If there is a patient on the transplant candidate list for whom there is a zero antigen mismatch with the donor, the pancreas from that donor shall first be offered to the appropriate OPTN member for any highly sensitized patient waiting for a combined kidney-pancreas transplant with a zero antigen mismatch; first locally, then regionally, and then nationally, on the basis of length of time waiting. The pancreas shall then be offered to the appropriate OPTN member for any highly sensitized (i.e., PRA level $\geq$ 80%) patient waiting for an isolated pancreas transplant with a zero antigen mismatch, first locally, then regionally, and then nationally, on the basis of length of time waiting, unless there is a patient listed on the host OPO's local patient transplant candidate list for combined kidney-pancreas or isolated pancreas transplantation who is mismatched with the donor and also has a PRA level of 80% or greater on the basis of historical or current serum samples, as used for cross-match to determine suitability for transplant, and there is a negative preliminary cross-match between the donor and that patient. In this event, for local allocation, the pancreas shall be offered for the mismatched patient(s) with a PRA level greater than or equal to 80% and a negative preliminary cross-match (on the basis of length of time waiting if more than 1 patient meets these criteria) before being offered for highly sensitized zero antigen mismatched isolated pancreas transplant patients regionally and nationally.

After zero antigen mismatched patients, allocation of pancreata is dependent on characteristics of the donor. The distinction is based on analyses of organ discard rates and pancreas islet cell yields. The intent is to balance transplant opportunities for whole organ patients with opportunities to test the efficacy of islet transplantation by providing first priority for local use of pancreata to patients in need of whole organ transplantation, and then allocating those pancreata most suitable for islet transplantation for patients in need of islets, first locally, then regionally, and then nationally. Pancreata procured from donors 50 years or younger and with a body mass index less than or equal to 30 kg/m^2 are allocated locally for isolated pancreas patients, combined kidney-pancreas patients, or combined solid organ islet patients on the basis of waiting time. The rationale for local donor service area emphasis is to minimize cold ischemic time and maximize graft survival. Such pancreata would then be allocated regionally and nationally for whole organ transplantation or combined kidney-pancreas transplantation on the basis of waiting time and then for islet cell transplantation.

Pancreata procured from donors 50 years and older or with a body mass index greater than 30 kg/m^2 are allocated locally to isolated pancreas patients, combined kidney-pancreas patients, or combined solid organ islet patients, and then to clinical islet patients on the basis of medical need and length of waiting time. The intent is to determine whether islet cell transplantation is a viable alternative for diabetics taking insulin, ensure the application of medical judgment, and minimize the wastage of pancreata and islet cells.[6,11]

Facilitated Pancreas Allocation

The pancreas allocation system provides a further mechanism to minimize organ wastage and maximize organ utilization. The facilitated pancreas allocation system is available after 5 hours of placement effort or if organ retrieval is anticipated within 1 hour. Transplant centers must notify the organ center of their intent to participate in the facilitated pancreas system and an expedited placement is managed on the basis of patient waiting time. The pancreas shall be offered, on the basis of the transplant patient's length of waiting time within each of the following categories: isolated pancreas patients and combined kidney-pancreas patients. Again, blood type O kidneys must be transplanted into blood type O recipients.[6,11]

Islet Transplantation

If the donor is 50 years old or younger and has a body mass index less than or equal to 30 kg/m^2 and a suitable recipient is not identified by the allocation criteria specified in the pancreas allocation policies, the host OPO shall offer the pancreas locally for clinical islet transplantation. If the organ is not used locally, the host OPO shall offer the pancreas regionally and then nationally for clinical islet transplantation. If the organ is not used for transplantation, the host OPO should offer the pancreas for research. If the donor is older than 50 years or has a body mass index greater than 30 kg/m^2 and a suitable recipient is not identified at the local level of organ allocation by the criteria specified in the pancreas allocation policy, the host OPO shall offer the pancreas locally for clinical islet transplantation. If the organ is not used locally, the OPO shall offer the pancreas regionally and then nationally for clinical islet transplantation, and then regionally followed by nationally for whole organ transplantation. If the organ is not used for transplantation, the OPO should offer the pancreas for research.[6,11]

Islet Allocation

Allocation of pancreata for islet transplantation shall be to the most medically suitable patient on the basis of need and the transplant candidate's length of waiting time. If the islet preparation is medically unsuitable for the patient after islet processing is completed, the islets from that pancreas will be reallocated to the next most suitable patient within the OPO that the Investigational New Drug application allows. The purpose of this policy is to allow for the application of medical judgment and to avoid islet wastage.[6,11]

Allocation for Organs Not Specifically Addressed

For organs not specifically addressed, points are assigned for medical urgency as follows: A status 1 patient is assigned 4 points and is at home functioning normally; a status 2 patient is assigned 8 points and is at home, requiring continuous medical care that can be self-administered; a status 3 patient is assigned 12 points and is at home, requiring continuous medical care with the assistance of an attendant; a status 4 patient is assigned 16 points and is continuously hospitalized; a status 5 patient is assigned 20 points and requires continuous hospitalization as well as intravenous inotropic drug therapy; and a status 6 patient is assigned 24 points and requires continuous hospitalization and a mechanical assist device for survival.

The following points are also assigned for the distance between the transplant center and the donor as well as for the distance between the recipient and the transplant center, respectively: between 0 and 50 miles 12 points and 6 points; between 50 and 500 miles, 10 points and 5 points; between 500 and 1000 miles, 8 points and 4 points; between 1000 and 1500 miles, 6 points and 3 points; between 1500 and 2000 miles, 4 points and 2 points; between 2000 and 2500 miles, 2 points and 1 point; and for greater distances, no points are assigned.[12]

Allocation to Multiple Organ Transplant Patients

Patients who are transplant candidates for multiple organs, of which one of the required organs is a heart, lung, or liver shall be registered on the individual transplant candidate list for each organ. When the patient is eligible to receive a heart, lung, or liver, the second required organ shall be allocated to the multiple organ patient from the same donor if the donor is located with the same local organ distribution unit where the multiple organ patient is registered. If the patient is listed outside the local organ distribution unit where the donor is located, voluntary sharing of the second organ is recommended. When the second organ is shared, the same organ of an identical blood type shall be referred back to the host OPO from the next acceptable donor procured by the recipient OPO, unless the second organ is a kidney, in which case the organ shall be referred back according to standard kidney allocation policy. This policy shall not apply to the allocation of heart-lung combinations. Heart-lung combinations shall be allocated in accordance with thoracic allocation policies or an approved variance to these policies. For patients awaiting a combined liver-intestine transplant, the liver may be allocated using the intestine list unless there is a status 1 liver patient listed in the region.[12]

Alternative Allocation/Distribution System

Alternative allocation/distribution (AAD) systems have different organ allocation from the standard organ allocation. These systems are designed to increase organ availability and/or quality while addressing possible distribution inequities that are unique to that geographical area. The AAD systems exist in the forms of (1) alternative local units, (2) sharing arrangements and agreements, (3) alternative point assignment protocols, and (4) protocols that may include components of more than 1 of these AAD systems.[13]

Organ Allocation Policies

OPTN member organizations, transplant patients, transplant recipients, and donor family members work together to develop organ allocation policies that will provide transplant patients with an opportunity to receive the organ they need. Organ allocation policies are always reviewed and revised as part of an ongoing effort to improve the transplantation process. Organ allocation policies are designed as equitable as possible, while making the best use of the limited number of donor organs. Ethnicity, gender, religion, socioeconomic status, and personal and behavioral history are not taken into account in organ allocation policy.[14]

How Policies Are Made That Influence Allocation

Transplantation is the only field in medicine in the United States in which patients have a formal role in making policies. There are 6 basic steps to developing organ distribution policies (see Figure):

1. An individual, such as a member of the public, brings an issue to the attention of OPTN/UNOS.

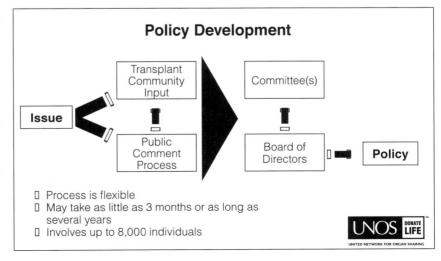

2. OPTN/UNOS committees discuss the issue and consider recommending a new policy or policy change.
3. Patients, OPTN/UNOS members, and the public comment on any proposed policy change or new policy.
4. The OPTN/UNOS committee considers all public comments before recommending a policy change to the OPTN/UNOS Board of Directors.
5. The OPTN/UNOS Board of Directors votes on whether to adopt the policy change or new policy.
6. OPTN/UNOS submits the policy to the DHHS for review and approval. Organ allocation policy is voluntary until approved by the DHHS.

Through its various committees, anyone, at anytime, can bring an issue to the attention of the OPTN/UNOS.[13]

References

1. National Organ Transplant Act of 1984 (NOTA). 42 USC § 274
2. National Organ Transplant Act of 1984 (NOTA). 42 USC § 273
3. Allocation of Organs. 42 CFR §121.8 (1999).
4. Beauchamp TL, Childress JF. Principles of Biomedical Ethics. 5th ed. Oxford, England: Oxford University Press; 2001:227.
5. Transplant Living. Available at: http://www.transplantliving.org/beforethetransplant/allocation/matchingOrgans.aspx. Accessed June 17, 2005.
6. OPTN Evaluation Plan. Available at: http://www.unos.org/SharedContentDocuments/050520_Evaluation_Plan_FINAL.pdf. Accessed June 17, 2005.
7. United Network for Organ Sharing. Organ Distribution: Allocation of Thoracic Organs. Available at: http://www.unos.org/PoliciesandBylaws/policies/docs/policy_9.doc. Accessed June 17, 2005.
8. United Network for Organ Sharing. Organ Distribution: Allocation of Livers. Available at: http://www.unos.org/PoliciesandBylaws/policies/docs/policy_8.doc. Accessed June 17, 2005.
9. United Network for Organ Sharing. Organ Distribution: Intestinal Organ Allocation. Available at: http://www.unos.org/PoliciesandBylaws/policies/doc/policy_13.doc. Accessed June 17, 2005.
10. United Network for Organ Sharing. Organ Distribution: Allocation of Deceased Kidneys. Available at: http://www.unos.org/PoliciesandBylaws/policies/docs/policy_7.doc. Accessed June 17, 2005.
11. United Network for Organ Sharing. Organ Distribution: Pancreas Allocation. Available at: http://www.unos.org/PoliciesandBylaws/policies/docs/policy_10.doc. Accessed June 17, 2005.
12. United Network for Organ Sharing. Organ Distribution: Allocation System for Organs Not Specifically Addressed. Available at: http://www.unos.org/PoliciesandBylaws/policies/docs/policy_11.doc. Accessed June 17, 2005.
13. United Network for Organ Sharing. Organ Distribution: Definitions. Available at: http://www.unos.org/PoliciesandBylaws/policies/docs/policy_3.doc. Accessed June 17, 2005.
14. Transplant Living. Available at: http://www.transplantliving.org/beforethetransplant/allocation/allocationPolicies.aspx. Accessed June 17, 2005.

General Medical Ethics – Organ Donation and Transplantation Snapshots

Gloria J. Taylor, RN, MA, CPTC

Science cannot stop while ethics catches up–and nobody should expect scientists to do all the thinking for the country. – Elvin Stackman

General Medical Ethics

Historically, medical ethics had maintained a certain level of consistency from the time of Hippocrates until the mid-1990s. The advances in the health, biological, and technological sciences of the later 20th century required a critical review of the traditional notions regarding moral obligations of all healthcare professionals to the sick and injured. Unraveling the relationship between patient and healthcare provider, as well as clarifying the rights, responsibilities, and requirements of such a relationship, remains a daunting task. As health, biological and technological sciences continue to merge at alarming rates and produce more modern medical innovations; the accompanying moral and ethical challenges can only escalate.

As healthcare professionals, procurement and transplant coordinators have moral, ethical, and professional obligations to an expanding number of donation-and transplantation-related stakeholders. The ethical knowledge and skills needed to practice competently in the transplantation arena intensify with each new practice, procedure, or challenge. This chapter aims to support coordinators and address some of the contemporary ethical issues in the field of donation and transplantation.

Morality Versus Ethics

The terms "morality" or "morals" and "ethics" are often interchanged without any distinction offered. In ancient times, the Greek and Latin words both meant *character* and had similar connotations. As humankind has evolved, distinct differences and variations in these 2 terms have arisen. Morality is now understood to indicate the norms of right or wrong conduct. Therefore, morality can be considered as the "rightness" or "wrongness" of an act or thought. In addition, morality is thought to be a commonly held belief in a particular culture or subculture.[1]

The term ethics has several meanings in today's society. It can refer to a person's character or behavior. However, for the purposes of this discussion, ethics will be defined in a more systematic nature and offered as the perspective from which individuals view, examine, or understand an issue. Ethics can be termed as the "why" or actual underpinning for a thought or action.[1]

Some historic examples of general moral beliefs might include the notions of not killing, not stealing, or not lying. Although individuals may agree with 1 or more of these widely held beliefs, each person may support a single belief for a different reason depending upon his or her perspectives. An individual's perspective(s) can be influenced by his or her culture or ethnicity, religion or spirituality, upbringing, education, socioeconomic status, or a number of other factors.

As shown in Figure 1, the relationship between ethics and morality can be viewed as table-like in nature. An individual's ethics (perspectives and personal values) provides support for whatever moral belief or issue being considered.

Ethical Theories and Principles

In the existing body of ethics literature, numerous authors refer to various ethical reflections, arguments, or systems of thought as well as principles, styles, theories, or rules. In this chapter, distinctions will be made and addressed by referencing ethical theories per se and ethical principles. (Note that the ethical theories mentioned are by no means an all-inclusive list and are offered as examples.)

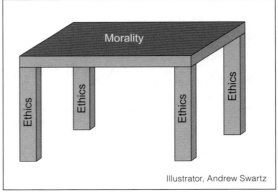

Figure 1. The Relationship of Ethics to Morality

Utilitarianism

Often associated with the phrases, "the greatest good for the greatest number" and "the end justifies the means," utilitarianism promotes maximizing the good consequences while minimizing the bad consequences. The right act is the one that generates the best overall results. Utilitarianism is the most well-known consequence-based ethical theory.[2]

Kantianism

The ethical thoughts formulated by Immanuel Kant (1724-1804) are the foundation for Kantianism. This ethical theory is based on the *categorical imperative* that any choices made must be such that the person would be willing for everyone else to make the same choices. Categorized as deontological, Kantian ethical theory proposed a method often referred to as *formalism*. Kantianism and deontological ethical models are duty- or obligation-based in concept and purport that actions are intrinsically or inherently right or wrong. Many consider these as "Golden Rule" type theories.[2-5]

Virtue

Virtue theory is based on the tradition of Plato and Aristotle, and gives paramount status to *virtuous character*. Virtue is frequently understood as character traits of moral value (ie, compassion, courage, truthfulness, and wisdom). Through virtue ethics, the focus falls upon the person performing the act and his or her character or intent. If the person's intention is to do good, then it is considered ethical even if the outcome is less than desired or bad.[4-6]

Liberal Individualism

Considered a rights-based theory, liberal individualism promotes a doctrine of basic human rights. Preservation of certain basic liberties and interests of individuals is the essence of this theory. Liberal individualists use a language of rights to strengthen ethical and political debate. The expression of rights is the foundation of the Anglo-American legal language and system.[2]

Communitarianism

The common good, community ideals, societal goals, and traditional values are fundamental to communitarianism. In communitarianism, the social nature of life and institutions and organizations, loyalties, traditions, and customs figure more prominently. This ethical theory would require that individuals adhere to codes, respect traditions, and conform to societal laws. Community acceptance forms the basis of requisite moral rules or social practice whether in a professional, family, or town setting.[2]

Ethics of Care

Although having no chief moral principle, the ethics of care focuses on relationships and a willingness to act on another's behalf. Having an emotional commitment to an individual or individuals and striving to maintain or restore relationships is essential to this form of ethics. Those who ascribe to the ethics of care would respond to the needs of others in a responsible and sensitive way without taking into account what they might consider abstract standards.[2,7]

Casuistry

Rather than rely totally on theories, some practitioners concentrate on resolving a specific case or even types of cases. This case-based approach to ethics is referred to as casuistry and addresses the complexities of real life decision making. Casuistry supporters highlight the need for *practical wisdom*, as coined by Aristotle, by which appropriate decisions are made on the basis of the particular circumstances of the case. Casuistry practitioners are skeptics when it comes to rules, theories, and rights that are disassociated from cases, precedents, circumstances, or history. Frequently called a bottom-up style of thinking, casuistry is a methodology that can be useful when ethical theory or principle practitioners find themselves at an impasse.[2,7]

Principles

There are various sets of principles in medical and biomedical ethics today. However, the principles of bioethics initially proposed by Tom L. Beauchamp and James F. Childress in 1979 in *Principles of Biomedical Ethics*[2] are thought to be the most widely applied.[5] The 4 principles enumerated by Beauchamp and Childress[2] are the following:

- Respect for autonomy
- Nonmaleficence
- Beneficence
- Justice

Respect for autonomy highlights the need to defer to the choices and wishes of competent persons. It also requires protecting those who have lost their autonomy or those who have never had any autonomy.[2,5,8] The concept of autonomy, generally defined as self-determination or self-governance, and the respect for such an ideal are often in direct opposition to paternalism. Paternalism in medicine often involves overriding a person's known preferences with the intent to do good or avoid harm.[2]

The principle of nonmaleficence emphasizes the obligation of not inflicting harm on others or preventing or avoiding harm to persons; whereas the principle of beneficence requires contributing to the welfare of persons. Beneficence entails helping or benefiting persons. These 2 principles most often work in tandem. There is a continuum of sorts from not inflicting harm to providing benefit, and there is usually a balancing act that takes place. When a balancing of benefits and risks or burdens occurs, utility is the product resulting in the best overall result obtainable.[2,8] Conflicts occur between the principles of beneficence and respect for autonomy when paternalistic governments and healthcare providers seek to do "what is best for the patient" while disregarding the patient's autonomous choice to forego treatment.

The principle of justice has elements of fairness and equality. This principle seeks to give persons their "due," or what they are entitled to, and to treat similar cases the same. In the language of Aristotle, equals must be treated equally, and unequals must be treated unequally. Often, the terms fair, equitable, and appropriate are used in defining what is due or owed to persons when referencing the principle of justice.[2,8] Some authors purport that patients have a right to receive equal care and be treated fairly in light of the principle of justice.[4]

The ethical principles of Beauchamp and Childress are most prevalently used in attempting to resolve organ and tissue donation- and transplantation-related ethical conflicts and therefore will be employed throughout this chapter.

GENERAL MEDICAL ETHICS – ORGAN DONATION AND TRANSPLANTATION SNAPSHOTS

Working Toward Ethical Solutions

Ethically Acceptable Options

When striving to identify possible ethical solutions in particular situations, polar opposites are generally easy to identify. However, it is much more difficult to realize that there are 180 degrees of ethically acceptable options that exist between those distinct, black and white, polar opposites (Figure 2). In the realm of organ and tissue donation, people authorize or refuse the option of donation every day (polar opposites); or they select some variation of an ethically acceptable option (ie, kidneys only, liver and kidneys, corneas and lungs). In the transplantation arena, candidates exercise their options when deciding to be listed or not, as well as during the informed consent process when they decide whether to accept various types of organs (e.g., hepatitis-positive organs, extended criteria donor organs) or not. It is the individual's prerogative to decide which organs they would want to accept if offered.

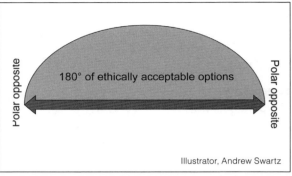

Figure 2. Degrees of Ethically Acceptable Options

Identifying Stakeholders

When trying to identify a course of action in certain circumstances, it is extremely important to identify all persons having standing in the situation. Stakeholders are persons who will be affected in some fashion by the outcome of the circumstance (ie, patients, family members, significant others, physicians, nurses, and the hospital).

Ethically Relevant Considerations

When dealing with the complexities of ethically charged cases, it is important to contemplate the following ethically relevant considerations (these ethically relevant considerations were adapted for organ donation and transplantation)[1]:

- identification of stakeholders;
- balancing benefits and harms;
- disclosure, informed consent, and shared decision making;
- patient and family values;
- responsibilities of all healthcare providers in relationship contexts;
- professional integrity;
- societal norms of cost-effectiveness and allocation of resources (also known as resource stewardship);
- cultural and religious/spiritual distinctions;
- considerations of power; and
- psychosocial issues, including compliance.

The balancing of benefits and harms is innate to the practice of medicine, and donation- and transplantation-related cases are no exception. The principles of beneficence and nonmaleficence demand no less. There is a delicate balance necessary in maximizing benefits to patients, donor families, and recipients, while minimizing or avoiding harm and pursuing the goals of donation and transplantation.

Disclosure, informed consent, and shared decision making considerations have changed the landscape of donation and transplantation dramatically in recent years. No longer does a single healthcare provider have unilateral authority to determine what medical treatment is best for a patient or family. The principle of respect for autonomy has paved the way for donor, donor family, surrogate decision makers, and patients to have a true voice. It is no longer acceptable for healthcare providers to make paternalistic decisions–

donors, donor families, and transplant candidates are consulted; information is disclosed in a truthful and transparent fashion; and shared decision making takes place. Whether an organ procurement coordinator or family services professional is interacting with a donor family or a transplant surgeon or clinical coordinator is interacting with a transplant candidate, disclosure, informed consent, and shared decision making considerations must be evident.

The values of the patient and family are relevant with regard to both donation and transplantation. Rarely does a donor or patient present without loved ones. Depending on the donor's or transplant candidate's age, rights and responsibilities of the family differ. In the totality of donation and transplantation cases, family members provide assistance, support, or resistance and are vital to the outcome. Therefore, it is essential to consider all familial factors in donation or transplantation cases.

The responsibilities of donation- and transplantation-related healthcare providers in relationship contexts are the focal point of numerous ethics cases. As healthcare providers, there is a fiduciary responsibility to care for the sick and injured. However, not communicating truthfully and respectfully with the donor, family, or candidate would be disrespectful; even though they are often considered vulnerable groups, they are owed respect and must participate as fully as possible in the decision-making processes.

Professional integrity has a role in determining whether a request made by a donor or donor family or candidate or candidate family is ethical and appropriate. Although the principle of autonomy protects a patient from having treatment forced on them, they are not entitled to receive *any* treatment desired. In donation and transplantation circumstances, transplant professionals are not required to provide treatment that is not medically indicated, and organ procurement organizations (OPOs) are not responsible to provide services not indicated or appropriate. If a family requests money to consent to donation or demands that all funeral expenses be paid by the OPO, there is no obligation on the OPO's part to comply. If a patient demands to be listed at a transplant center and does not meet the center's evaluation criteria, the transplant center is under no obligation to list that patient.

The societal norms of cost-effectiveness and allocation of resources are reflected in the ethical principle of justice. With a focus on treating similar cases similarly, the allocation of organs is governed by policies that have been developed with the principle of justice in mind. However, every organ donated is not equal (e.g., deceased donor pediatric organs, expanded criteria organs, and donation after cardiac death organs); therefore, distribution of some types of organs is augmented and they are distributed to transplant centers that will accept particular types of organs. In addition, more OPOs are negotiating hospital rates for organ recovery in an effort to make this process as cost-effective as possible. Transplant centers now have financial coordinators in place to help make transplantation financially possible for candidates who may or may not have adequate insurance and to provide indigent or charity care in some instances. These issues directly affect cost-effectiveness questions in ethically charged cases.

Cultural and religious and/or spiritual distinctions are often faced by OPO and transplant center staff. A family's culture may place the decision making capacity with a member of the family other than the patient or the legal next of kin. This presents challenges to the healthcare providers who interact with the patient and/or family. The respect for autonomy of a particular patient may be nonexistent in a family's culture. These types of cultural considerations create highly divergent situations for families and healthcare providers alike. In some instances, religious or spiritual values, although rare, may be in conflict with donation or transplantation. Each of these considerations will need to be addressed individually with the utmost respect.

Considerations of power are often the foundation of ethically problematic circumstances. Healthcare providers are constantly in a position of power with respect to patients, donors, and their families, because they have knowledge and information. In order for patients, donors, and families to make informed decisions, they need information and respect for their autonomy, which culminates in a sharing of power. Power considerations are also present in professional relationships. There can be struggles that occur among OPO staff and hospital staff regarding the presentation of the option of donation to the potential donor family or the management of the donor in the intensive care unit. Other interprofessional power considerations can manifest when OPOs deal with anesthesia providers, various transplant recovery teams, or ancillary healthcare service providers in the hospital.

Psychosocial issues, including patient compliance, are relevant to successful transplantation. Although it is difficult to measure compliance empirically, medical professionals often approach this issue subjectively. Potential transplant candidate psychosocial evaluations need to be conducted as a means of evaluating nonmedical criteria. Transplantation should be cautiously considered for patients who have historically or currently demonstrated the inability to comply with previous or existing treatment.[9] Responsible stewardship requires that such evaluations be performed to reduce the risk of organ wastage through noncompliance. Without such evaluations, the utility of the system would be jeopardized.

Setting the Stage

The Donation and Transplantation Continuum

Each year in the United States, thousands of people donate organs and tissues for transplantation and thousands of people receive transplants. These are morally commendable acts supported by sound ethical principles that promote good. However, the reality is that thousands more people continue to wait, the supply does not meet the demand, thousands of people die annually awaiting organ transplants, and potential harms exist because of varying interests. This continuous challenge is reflected in Figure 3.

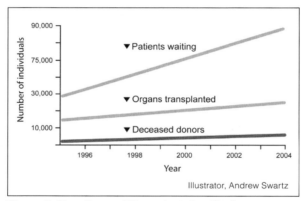

Figure 3. Donation and Transplantation Challenge

Donation and Transplantation Stakeholders

Identification of organ donation and transplantation stakeholders varies depending on the circumstances (e.g., living donation, an individual case, and the community at large). The following are some of the proposed stakeholders involved in organ donation and transplantation:
- potential organ donors, their families and significant others;
- transplant candidates, their families and significant others;
- transplant recipients, their families and significant others;
- transplant physicians, surgeons, and coordinators;
- donor hospitals, physicians, nurses, and allied healthcare providers;
- OPOs and their staff;
- histocompatability laboratories and their staff;
- payors (government and private insurers);
- pharmaceutical companies;
- researchers;
- donation- and transplantation-related organizations;
- news media; and
- general public.

Potential Conflicts

There are at least 2 types of conflicts inherent in medical ethics situations, conflicts of interest and conflicts of ethical principles. A conflict of interest consists of a set of conditions in which professional judgment concerning a primary interest (e.g., patient welfare and research validity) is liable to be unduly influenced by a secondary interest (e.g., recognition and financial gain). The primary interest is dictated by the person's professional duties whether a physician, nurse, scholar, or researcher. A secondary interest is generally not illegitimate in itself, and may even be desirable or necessary. The impact of the secondary interest on professional decisions is the problematic circumstance.[10] A conflict of ethical principles arises when 1 or more ethical principles exist on both sides of a choice or issue.[8] When conflicts of ethical principles occur, decision makers are usually left to determine which of the principles should be given the most weight or how the principles can be balanced. Some procurement coordinators may think they have a direct responsibility to transplant candidates, others may think their responsibility is to donor families, and some procurement coordinators believe they can do both without any conflict of interest. Yet, what is the procurement coordinator's primary interest, and where do their obligations to the OPO and the hospitals in their service area reside? Other procurement and transplant professionals consider transplant surgeons and physicians serving on OPO boards of directors as a conflict of interest because they directly benefit from the work of the OPO.

Ethical Challenges in Donation and Transplantation Environments
Prehospital Environment

The 3 common mechanisms to express voluntary donation wishes are donor cards, advance directives, and donor registries. The parameters of the donor card are delineated by the Uniform Anatomical Gift Act (UAGA).[11] Although donor cards may take many forms (e.g., 1-part, 2-part, and driver's license), they all must contain the basic components outlined in the UAGA.[12]

Advance directives were created by the Patient Self-Determination Act of 1990.[13] Living wills, durable power of attorney for healthcare, or healthcare proxies are forms of advance directives.[14] The type of advance directive and the information necessary in these documents vary by state; some states may require 2 signatures, whereas others may require 3 signatures.

Donor registries are generally formed through state legislation or by state agencies. Three types of donor registries exist: those that are associated with driver's licenses through state motor vehicle departments, those that are independent stand-alone registries, and those that are a combination of the first two. For combination registries, the motor vehicle department generally records the person's voluntary donation wish in a database and, on a scheduled basis, transfers the registrations to the registry database.[15] More important than the design of the registry, the type of donor card or advance directive is the purpose of the communication. All these mechanisms for communicating voluntary donation wishes express the person's intent. There are important questions to be asked regarding a person's intent to donate, not the least of which, *Is a person's intent to donate sufficient?* Other significant questions that *need* to be addressed are, *Do these individuals have enough information to make donation decisions? Does it matter if they do or do not?* and, *Would you be comfortable acting on someone's expressed intent?* Additional questions that need to be asked are, *Do people need to know what organs and tissues can be donated? Do they need to know the size of the surgical incision? Do they need to know how the body will look after donation?* and, *Do they need to know anything about the donor suitability testing?*

Models of Informed Consent

The highly specific process of informed consent used to secure consent for organ donation is based on the medical model of informed consent. The elements of the informed consent process that have evolved within the field of bioethics are capacity, voluntariness, disclosure of information, recommendation, understanding, decision, and authorization.[2,16]

One essential element of informed consent is capacity, which is the functional ability to make a decision.[16] Do not confuse capacity with competence, as competency is determined by legal standards.

Voluntariness entails exercising a choice that is free of coercion or any other form of controlling influence exerted by another person. Rarely, if ever, is anyone totally free of known or unknown pressures that can affect his or her choices.[2,16] Disclosure is the obligation to supply the necessary information in a such format that a person can make an informed decision. The disclosed information should include the nature of the therapy, as well as purpose, risks, consequences, benefits, probability of success, feasible alternatives, and a prognosis if the therapy is not given.[2,16] A recommendation is a routine part of the disclosure portion of the informed consent process. If asked directly by a patient what should be done, a physician is expected to respond. However, the recommendation is normally outlined in the treatment plan. Understanding or comprehension on the part of the patient is a vital requirement of informed consent. A patient best demonstrates understanding by describing the information imparted by healthcare professionals in his or her own words.[2,16] Subsequently, a decision needs to be made and recorded. The patient's decision is communicated in some fashion and noted, generally on some type of form that can be signed. The patient's decision can be to accept or decline the proposed therapy, and either decision is of equal value and standing. Even "irrational" decisions made by patients with the functional capacity for decision making must be respected by the medial team. A signed consent or authorization form does not constitute a "valid consent"–legally or ethically.[16] The described bioethical informed consent process is thought to be impractical for the organ donation consent process because it cannot be fully implemented.

The American Association of Tissue Banks, Association of Organ Procurement Organizations, and Eye Bank Association of America worked collaboratively to formulate the "Model Elements of Informed Consent for Organ and Tissue Donation" (Appendix A). This model was implemented in November 2000 and contains basic elements of informed consent, as well as additional elements of informed consent for indicated situations. This collaborative effort is an attempt to address the unique circumstances and challenges that surround the organ and tissue donation consent process.

The North American Transplant Coordinators Organization (NATCO) position statement on donor registries supports the autonomy of Americans to make personal choices, including those regarding organ donation. In addition, the NATCO statement supports and encourages thorough study of registries and commends those who are honoring the wishes of a donor.[17]

Potential conflicts of ethical principles regarding voluntary donor intent mechanisms loom large. Although donor cards, advance directives, and registries track the person's autonomous choice, is this document of a person's intent enough? How can the benefits and risks of such donation intentions be balanced? If a "yes" on a donor card or driver's license is honored, must a "no" be honored also? Can a person's autonomous choice be disregarded? What if registries or state motor vehicle departments record only "yes" or "unknown" and not "no?"

Potential Donation Hospital Environments

Before a potential donation consent process begins, the patient has presented at the hospital with a terminal illness or a critical, life-threatening injury. In these instances, healthcare providers are rendering end-of-life care, and are faced with potential conflicts, including the fiduciary obligations to the patient, shared end-of-life decision making, and the obligation to refer potential donors, according to the Medicare conditions of participation. In addition, procurement coordinators may face conflicts such as dealing with early referrals, evaluation of donation potential, and existing hospital processes. Coupled with these conflicting scenarios are the challenges of competing ethical principles. Is the potential donor's autonomy to be respected in these cases? Are there harms that need to be prevented? What good can be done now? What might justice look like in these instances?

If a patient meets the criteria set forth in the Medicare conditions of participation and the hospital refers the potential donor, conflicts of interest may materialize. In order for the option of donation to be presented, the healthcare team must admit the inability to sustain life, step aside, and either support or obstruct the process. At the same time, the OPO staff is sometimes conflicted regarding the control of the process, taking care of the family while trying to gain consent, and attempting to give full disclosure to fulfill the requirements of informed consent. How can benefits be realized in this situation? How can harms be minimized? Will autonomous choices be supported? Can there be just treatment for all? The answers to these ethical questions can be drastically different depending on the presenting circumstances.

What if the patient had not expressed any donation wishes and the family is in disagreement regarding the option of donation? If the patient had expressed a desire not to donate, could the family override that wish, demanding that donation of organs or tissues take place? Some states are not allowing the patient's donation wishes to be overruled by family members and have amended the state UAGA to make a person's donation intent irrevocable. Donor authorization, as some states refer to this UAGA amendment, is not universally accepted in every state.[18] However, the number of states with donor authorization continues to increase each year. Although states are considering this issue, some donor hospitals do not want to complicate matters and allow families to override donor consent. Hospitals fear the threat of negative publicity or legal action by family members.

Often, the question arises, who should speak with families to offer the option of donation? If a poll was taken, the answers would range from trained OPO staff to the nurse providing care to the potential donor, with many options in between. Every person presenting the option of donation can have conflicts of interest; whether it is the overworked, sleep-deprived OPO staff person who would rather be home in bed, the staff nurse who really does not believe in donation, or the OPO family services staff. Whoever interacts with the family needs to be well versed regarding the relevant laws, myths, and misconceptions regarding donation, allocation policies, and possible familial fears.

Postconsent Environment

There are plenty of postconsent circumstances that have ethical importance as well as potential conflicts, not the least of which are prompted by donor suitability issues that are manifested through the performance of a medical and social history and serology testing. The need for a true and complete medical and social history for the sake of the transplant candidates is a very important aspect of donor suitability. When this necessary practice is coupled with the desire to care for the donor family and show respect and sensitivity, it may be difficult to balance benefits and burdens. If a serology test result eliminates any donation possibility, the potential transplant candidate's harms have been avoided, but what about the potential harm to the donor's family with the revelation of such news?

Ethical challenges and conflicts are prevalent in the organ allocation, placement, and distribution processes. The 1999 Organ Procurement and Transplantation Network (OPTN) Final Rule[19] and the ethical principles of justice and medical utility, along with input from the OPTN committees, membership, and the public at large, affected the formulation of the current allocation policies. The mere existence of policies does by no means imply that they are followed by all OPTN members. OPOs struggle to place donated organs via a computerized match list of potential candidates that is dependent on all transplant programs listing patients properly, with ranges and fields completed accurately. Transplant programs participate in good faith, hoping that no other program is "gaming the system." If patient ranges are inaccurate, this practice results in increased placement time, increased ischemic time, possible decreased organ function, or, worst case scenario, wastage of an organ. Do transplant centers have an obligation only to their candidates or to all transplant candidates as a whole?

Expanded criteria donor organs present yet another allocation and placement challenge. What does it mean to exhaust "the list"? Is it permissible to expedite the placement of organs to transplant centers an OPO knows will take the organ?

Transplant Candidate and Recipient Issues

Behavior or Status as Factors

Historically, the behavior of potential liver transplant candidates has been scrutinized. People questioned why an alcoholic should be allowed to be listed for a possible liver transplant. If transplant candidate behavior is the issue, then why not include smokers who need lungs, drug abusers who need hearts because of cardiomyopathy, and those who are overweight and/or hypertensive who do nothing to care for themselves and end up needing kidneys? People who are against letting alcoholic cirrhotic patients receive transplants generally maintain that these individuals are to blame for their condition because of their "misconduct." If so, however, then should all the other examples listed above be treated the same? Or should medical decisions simply be based on medical criteria?

Prisoners and nonresident aliens, by virtue of their status, often become media targets regarding their need for a transplant. Prisoner-related transplant candidacy dialogue falls along a broad continuum from a person serving a limited term who will return to be a productive member of society to the death row inmate whose debt to society is to be paid with his or her life. The rationale for some of the prisoner debate goes back to the conduct or behavior issue. In addition, there is widespread concern that prisoners who receive transplants will not obtain good posttransplant medical care in the prison system.

The OPTN/United Network for Organ Sharing (UNOS) Ethics Committee's statement regarding convicted criminals and transplant evaluation is as follows:

…absent any societal imperative, one's status as a prisoner should not preclude them from consideration for a transplant; such consideration does not guarantee transplantation. Acknowledged are medical and non-medical factors that may influence one's candidacy for transplant however prisoner status is not an absolute contraindication. Although one's status as a prisoner may evoke legitimate medical concerns (i.e., infectious diseases), as well as psychosocial issues (i.e., character disorders and substance abuse problems that may compromise compliance), judgments regarding these medical and non-medical factors are the purview of individual transplant teams. Consideration of prisoners as well as others for transplantation includes evaluation of medical and non-medical factors relative to their impact on transplant outcome. Screening for all potential recipients should be done at the candidacy stage and once listed; all candidates should be eligible for equitable allocation of organs."[20]

The Committee did not directly address the death row inmate as a potential transplant candidate. However, in their General Considerations in Assessment for Transplant Candidacy, the Committee did address the issue of life expectancy by stating: "While the Committee would not recommend arbitrary age or co-morbidity limits for transplantation, members generally concur that transplantation should be carefully considered if the candidate's reasonable life expectancy with a functioning graft, based on factors such as age or co-morbid conditions, is significantly shorter than the reasonably expected 'life span' of the transplanted organ."[9] Life expectancy of a death row inmate would be limited and transplantation could be questionable.

Nonresident aliens may be viewed as competing for healthcare resources in the United States, and transplants make no exception. OPTN/UNOS policy allows no more than 5% of a transplant program's organ recipients to be nonresident aliens. In addition, the same policy outlines nondiscrimination in allocation of organs regarding factors such as political influence and national origin.[21] The OPTN/UNOS Ethics Committee explored the topic of nonresident aliens and transplantation in April 1999 and March 2003 (OPTN/UNOS, unpublished data, 1999 and 2003). The Committee's consensus on both occasions was that a person's status as a nonresident alien should not preclude him or her from consideration for a transplant, and that consideration (in the form of evaluation) does not guarantee a nonresident alien or anyone a transplant.

What if a person has already received an organ transplant? Should his or her status as a recipient keep him or her from receiving or reduce his or her priority for an additional transplant? Some utilitarians would argue that it would be unfair or unjust to give a person a second organ while others are awaiting their first transplant.[6] Others would argue that retransplantation is the only option for patients with extrarenal graft failure.

Some ethical issues in transplantation have to do with an individual's religious beliefs. For example, should Jehovah's Witnesses be transplant candidates and receive a transplant? These individuals could refuse a needed posttransplant blood transfusion, die and waste the organ. Or will they even accept an organ to begin with, knowing that someone else's blood was circulating through the particular organ?

Should an individual's infectious disease status affect his or her ability to be evaluated or listed for transplantation? Few transplant programs accept human immunodeficiency virus (HIV)-positive patients as possible transplant candidates. Yet, the initial data regarding HIV-positive transplant recipients' outcomes are comparable to other categories of recipients.

A CLINICIAN'S GUIDE TO DONATION AND TRANSPLANTATION

Organ Acceptability and Other Risks

In the era of expanded donors, donation after cardiac death, and limitations of some preprocurement screening, the variation in the quality of organs available for transplantation and the other potential risks to transplant candidates need to be acknowledged. A transplant candidate can, in the shared decision making process with his or her transplant team, opt to accept or reject certain types of organs, whereas other candidates might defer to their transplant surgeon's clinical expertise in selecting appropriate organs. No matter which decision the candidate makes, should the candidate be told the quality and characteristics of the organ during the organ acceptance process? Would this be respecting the candidate's autonomy? Would proceeding without any candidate input be expressed paternalism?

How does a transplant program mitigate the risks of transmissible disease and malignancies for the transplant recipient? How can risks be minimized in the organ offer process? What does a transplant program's organ offer protocol entail? Does it include serology results as well as any other potential disease-related information during the offer? Balancing the benefits and risks of transplantation for candidates is a complex task. Do all transplant coordinators take offers in the same manner for every candidate? To ensure that the principle of justice is applied equally (ie, treating similar cases similarly), this seems to be necessary.

What about transplant candidates who choose to travel to another country for an organ transplant? In addition to the apparent risks of being in another country, with an entirely unfamiliar transplant team, working within another healthcare system, trusting additional unfamiliar allied healthcare professionals, and the uncertainty of the origin of the organ, what other repercussions might exist for the transplant recipient? Upon returning to the United States, the transplant recipient may find it difficult to secure healthcare follow-up. How do transplant programs in the United States deal with this form of medical tourism? The American Medical Association's Code of Ethics[22] explains that although physicians are free to choose their patients, they should respond to emergent cases and not neglect patients. This code also addresses the ability of physicians to terminate relationships with patients, but they cannot do so without giving advance notice so that another physician can be secured.[22] In March 2004, the OPTN/UNOS Ethics Committee opined that first and foremost, medical professionals should "do no harm," and that in nonemergent situations, the physician has the right to offer a list of alternative care providers and can dissolve the contractual relationship in 30 days and is no longer legally obligated to care for the patient.[22]

Access Issues

In the United States, access to organ transplantation is a function of a person's general medical care or lack thereof and insurance coverage or lack thereof, which both relate directly to socioeconomic status. Once listed for a transplant, another access issue tied to candidates' socioeconomics status is multiple listing, which means that a candidate is actually placed on more than 1 local transplant list. In order to multiply list, a candidate must have the resources to undergo additional evaluation at a cost unlikely to be covered by insurance; time, and ability to travel to another geographic area. Multiple listing increases a candidate's chances to receive an organ,[6] and OPTN/UNOS policy allows multiple listing.[23] Some transplant programs do not allow their candidates to multiply list, and in New York candidates are only allowed to list at single state transplant center. How does multiple listing address the principle of justice? How can the transplantation system balance the risks and benefits for all candidates when socioeconomic advantages exist?

Another way of limiting transplant candidates' access to organs is through directed donation. Some families have asked that their loved one's organs not go to alcoholics, because a drunk driver was responsible for the death of their family member. Other families may want to direct their donation to a particular religious group, ethnicity, or even gender. The UAGA currently allows directed donation to a specified list of donees. Is it ethical to discriminate for or against a class of people regarding donated organs? Some individuals think that a person should only be allowed to receive an organ transplant if he or she has signed a donor card. However, what about people who cannot donate because of existing medical conditions?

Potential Living Donor Issues

Organ transplantation began in the mid-1950s with kidney transplantation between living twins.[12] Simultaneously, living donor ethical issues were immediately recognized. As the field of donation and transplantation advanced in achievement and complexity, so did the ethical issues. With the expansion of various types of living donation, the ethical issues have grown exponentially.

The NATCO position statement regarding living donor transplantation endorses the use of living donors and defines guidelines for donor evaluation and informed consent. This position statement also addresses living donor follow-up, financial considerations, and sources of living donors.[24]

Relationship Issues

Although the historic paradigm for living donation has been from one living relative to another, the last decade has seen a huge shift in who can and now wishes to be a living donor. It is no longer necessary to be related to the transplant candidate by blood to donate. Living donor "relationships" have changed, and a spouse, a coworker, or an individual who has an emotional link or tie with the candidate can donate an organ or organ segment. Perfect strangers off the street have become anonymous donors to particular transplant centers and the transplantation system itself. Should there be some type of relationship between the organ donor and transplant candidate? If not, how can coercion, payments, or "deals" be monitored or prevented? Is there a way to ascertain the motivation of the potential donor?

Technology has made it possible for nearly everyone to be electronically connected via the Internet. Are relationships established via the Internet any less legitimate than others? After all, people have even married after meeting on the Internet and developing relationships. Is it any different when a person publicizes or announces his or her need for an organ on the Internet? Let's say a person reads the Internet posting of a candidate in need of an organ and autonomously decides to help this person—is that permissible? What if another person reads the same posting, has a loved one who died, and directs a donation of an organ to the candidate in need? Is there a difference? One helps to decrease the transplant candidate list by a living donation, the other changes the queue in the list by directing a deceased donor organ to a particular individual. If taken a step further, what about the transplant candidate who uses billboards or ads in newspapers to publicize his or her need for an organ? There are many opinions on these issues, from allowing living autonomous adults to donate to whomever they wish, to those who are against any deceased donor scheme that undermines the existing allocation system.

Consent Issues

The informed consent process highlighted earlier in this chapter has implications in this section as welll. The need for attention to capacity, voluntariness, disclosure, recommendation, understanding, decision, and authorization is present in dealing with living donors—even more so because these donors are typically otherwise healthy individuals who are placing themselves at risk for the good of another. Living donors do not generally benefit medically from donation and would not routinely be considered "patients."[25] If the potential living donor is a child, additional ethically related concerns arise. If the child is donating to a parent, is this a coercion-free environment? What child would not want to help a parent? What child would not be afraid of a parent dying? In addition, who is the surrogate decision maker for the child? Would it be the parent needing the transplant or the other parent? Or should it be neither? Does the age of the child matter? Generally, children under the age of 18 who can and do agree with their surrogate decision maker's decision to donate, assent rather than consent. This is a term reserved specifically for this situation.[16]

Living lobular liver donors unearth an entirely new set of informed consent issues. This type of donation is such a recent phenomenon that there are insufficient data available to let these potential donors know what their lives will be like 5 or 10 years after donation surgery. The lack of outcome data for these living liver donors presents a problem when attempting to disclose their potential risks, benefits, or expectations for what their future health issues may be. In this instance, the routine medical model for informed consent may fall short. The OPTN/UNOS Ethics Committee recommends a stricter standard of informed consent likened to a research standard for these cases.[25] The NATCO Living Donor Transplantation position statement's informed consent guidelines are also more stringent.

Should someone who had previously donated a kidney be allowed to donate a segment of his or her liver? Should someone who had previously donated a kidney be allowed to donate his or her other kidney? Who will set limits on the autonomous choices of living donors?

Conclusion

Organ donation and transplantation give rise to medical ethics questions that are not easily answered. From its inception as a potential therapeutic modality for end-stage kidney failure, by transplanting 1 twin's kidney into another, to today's multiple combinations of needed organs and people willing to donate, the ethical issues have continued to increase in a limitless fashion. As medicine, technology, and people continue to collide at warp speed, the challenges faced by clinical and procurement transplant coordinators will only escalate. All transplant coordinators should prepare by identifying and using every ethically related resource possible, including the NATCO Code of Ethics for the Transplant Practitioner (Appendix B), other applicable professional codes of ethics (e.g., nursing, social workers, physician assistants, and physicians), organizational position statements, protocols and policies, OPTN policy, ethics committees opinions, historic ethical and legal cases, classes, or workshops. Furthermore, coordinators should be intimately familiar with all state and federal laws associated with their professional practice.

APPENDIX A

Model Elements of Informed Consent for Organ and Tissue Donation
American Association of Tissue Banks
Association of Organ Procurement Organizations
Eye Bank Association of America

Adopted November 30, 2000

Human organ and tissue transplantation has become an important and growing part of modern medical practice. Advances in medical science have made it possible for millions of Americans to receive these life-saving and life-enhancing gifts. None of this would be possible, however, were it not for the tens of thousands of donors and donor families who give their organs and tissues to help their fellow men and women.

The decision to donate must, therefore, be an informed consent, and it must be conducted under circumstances that are sensitive to the consenting person's situation. Information concerning the donation should be presented in language and in terms that are easily understood by the consenting person. The consent should be obtained under circumstances that provide an opportunity to ask questions and receive informative responses. An offer should be made regarding the availability of a copy of the signed consent form, and information should be provided regarding ways to reach the recovery organization following donation. Consent should be obtained in accordance with federal, state and/or local laws and/or regulations. The person seeking the consent should be trained to appropriately answer any questions that the consenting person may have. In addition, coercion should not be exerted in any manner, nor monetary inducement offered to obtain consent for donation. The identification of who may be the appropriate person to consent to donation, and whether the consent of any person in addition to the donor needs be obtained, should be evaluated in accordance with the applicable laws and organizational policy and is not addressed in this statement.

The following list of "Basic Elements of Informed Consent" is intended to highlight the information that may be considered critical to informed decision making by a family member or other legally authorized person, who is being approached for consent to organ and/or tissue donation. This listing, whether communicated verbally or included on consent forms, is not intended to preempt any applicable federal, state, or local laws or regulations that may require more or less information to be disclosed for informed consent to be legally effective.

Basic Elements of Informed Consent

In seeking informed consent, the following information should be provided to the person(s) being approached for consent:

1. A confirmation/validation of the donor's identity and his or her clinical terminal condition.
2. A general description of the purposes (benefits) of donation.
3. Identification of specific organs and/or tissues (including cells) that are being requested for donation (with subsequent information provided on specific gifts recovered).
4. An explanation that the retrieved organs/tissues may be used for transplantation, therapy, medical research, or educational purposes.
5. A general description of the recovery process (including timing, relocation of donor if applicable, contact information, etc.).
6. An explanation that laboratory tests and a medical/social history will be completed to determine the medical suitability of the donor, including an explanation that blood samples from the donor will be tested for certain transmissible diseases.
7. An explanation that the spleen, lymph nodes, and blood may be removed, and cultures may be performed, for the purpose of determining donor suitability and/or used to determine compatibility of donor and recipient.
8. A statement granting access to the donor's medical records, and that the medical records may be released to other appropriate parties.
9. An explanation that costs directly related to the evaluation, recovery, preservation, and placement of the organs and tissues will not be charged to the family.
10. An explanation regarding the impact the donation process may have on burial arrangements and on appearance of the body.
11. Any additional information required by federal, state and/or local laws and/or regulations.

Additional Elements of Informed Consent

1. In some situations, there may be additional information that should be known by the consenting person(s), or that might be helpful for family decision making. At a minimum, if the donor family inquires about any of these or additional matters, explanations should be provided.
2. The guiding principle for the use of these "Additional Elements of Informed Consent" is to advance simplicity and reasonableness in seeking informed consent, i.e. include these elements or additional comments if they are appropriate and might clarify any exigencies. For example, if there is the likelihood that the patient will become a Medical Examiner's case, then it should be appropriate to so inform the family. If it is unlikely that donated tissue is going to be used for aesthetic surgery, then it would not be reasonable to address this issue in the family approach.
3. One or more of the following elements of information may also be appropriate for communication to the person(s) being approached for consent, depending upon the circumstances surrounding the donation and the potential gift(s):
4. A description of any involvement by the Medical Examiner and/or Coroner, including an explanation that an autopsy may be performed.
5. An explanation that transplantation may include reconstructive and aesthetic surgery.
6. A reference to the possibility that the final gift may take a different form than originally recovered.
7. An explanation that multiple organizations (nonprofit and /or for profit) may be involved in facilitating the gift(s).
8. Reference to the possibility that tissue and/or organs may be transplanted abroad.

APPENDIX B

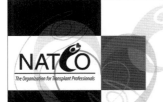

Code of Ethics
for the
Transplant Practitioner

The Transplant Practitioner...

...maintains the highest standards of professional conduct

...assumes responsibility and accountability for individual judgments and actions

...gains and maintains proficiency of practice

...participates in efforts to establish, implement and improve standards of practice

...contributes to the growth of professional knowledge

...respects individual privacy and holds confidential all information obtained in the course of practice

...maintains a cooperative, respectful relationship with other transplant practitioners and other health care professionals

...serves the public regardless of race, ethnicity, culture, social or economic status, personal ideology or religious belief

...educates the public on donation and transplantation issues

...acts to protect the public when health care and safety are endangered

References

1. Fletcher JC, Miller FG, Spencer EM. Clinical ethics: history, content, and resources. In: Fletcher JC, Hite CA, Lombardo PA, Marshall MF, eds. *Introduction to Clinical Ethics*. Frederick, Md: University Publishing Group, Inc; 1995:3-17.
2. Beauchamp TL, Childress JF. *Principles of Biomedical Ethics*. 5th ed. New York, NY: Oxford University Press; 2001.
3. Ashley BM, O'Rourke KD. *Ethics of Health Care: An Introductory Textbook*. 2nd ed. Washington, DC: Georgetown University Press; 1994.
4. Schroeter K, Derse A, Junkerman C, Schiedermayer D. *Practical Ethics for Nurses and Nursing Students*. Hagerstown, Md: University Publishing Group, Inc; 2002.
5. Mappes TA, DeGrazia D. *Biomedical Ethics*. 5th ed. New York, NY: McGraw-Hill; 2001.
6. Veatch RM. *Transplantation Ethics*. Washington, DC: Georgetown University Press; 2000.
7. Lo B. *Resolving Ethical Dilemmas: A Guide for Clinicians*. 2nd ed. Philadelphia, Pa: Lippincott Williams & Wilkins; 2000.
8. Wicks AC, Spielman BJ, Fletcher JC. Survey of ethical orientations and theories. In: Fletcher JC, Hite CA, Lombardo PA, Marshall MF, eds. *Introduction to Clinical Ethics*. Frederick, Md: University Publishing Group, Inc; 1995:239-247.
9. Organ Procurement and Transplantation Network/United Network for Organ Sharing Ethics Committee. General Considerations in Assessment for Transplant Candidacy. Available at: http://unos.org/resources/bioethics.asp?index=4. Accessed June 15, 2005.
10. Thompson DF. Understanding financial conflicts of interest. *N Engl J Med*. 1993;329:573-576.
11. Uniform Anatomical Gift Act. 23 Bus L 919. 1968.
12. Task Force on Organ Transplantation. *Organ Transplantation: Issues and Recommendations*. Washington, DC: US Department of Health and Human Services; 1986.
13. Patient Self Determination Act. 42U.S.C. 1395 cc (a). 1990.
14. King NMP. *Making Sense of Advance Directives*. Revised edition. Washington, DC: Georgetown University Press; 1996.
15. Office of Inspector General. *Organ Donor Registries: A Useful, but Limited, Tool*. Washington, DC: Department of Health and Human Services; 2002.
16. Boyle RJ. *The Process of Informed Consent*. In: Fletcher JC, Hite CA, Lombardo PA, Marshall MF, eds. *Introduction to Clinical Ethics*. Frederick, Md: University Publishing Group, Inc; 1995:81-95.
17. North American Transplant Coordinators Organization. Position Statement: Donor Registries. Available at: http://www.natco1.org/documents/DonorRegistries_000.pdf. Accessed June 15, 2005.
18. Metzger RA, Taylor GJ, McGaw LJ, Weber PG, Delmonico FL, Prottas JM, for the UNOS Research to Practice Steering Committee. Research to practice: a national consensus conference. *Prog Transplant*. 2005;15:379-384.
19. Organ Procurement and Transplantation Network, Final Rule, 42 CFR part 121 (1999). OPTN Final Rule
20. Organ Procurement and Transplantation Network/United Network for Organ Sharing Ethics Committee. Convicted Criminals and Transplant Evaluation. Available at: http://unos.org/resources/bioethics.asp?index=2. Accessed June 15, 2005.
21. United Network for Organ Sharing. Policy 6.0 Transplantation of Non-resident Aliens. Available at: http://www.unos.org/PoliciesandBylaws/policies/pdfs/policy_18.pdf. Accessed June 15. 2005.
22. American Medical Association Council on Ethical and Judicial Affairs. *Code of Medical Ethics: Current Opinions With Annotations*. 2004-2005 edition. Chicago, Ill; 2004.
23. United Network for Organ Sharing. Policy 3.2.2 Multiple Listing Permitted. Available at: http://www.unos.org/PoliciesandBylaws/policies/pdfs/policy_4.pdf. Accessed June 15, 2005.
24. North American Transplant Coordinators Organization. Position Statement: Living Donor Transplantation. Available at: http://www.natco1.org/documents/LivingDonorTransplantation_000.pdf. Accessed June 15, 2005.
25. Taylor GJ, Allee MR, Fox MD, Barrett W, McGee Jones C, Mozes MF. Informed consent for living anonymous adult donors: truth or dare. In: Gutmann T, Daar AS, Sells RA, eds. *Ethical, Legal, and Social Issues in Organ Transplantation*. Lengerich, Germany: Pabst Science Publishers; 2004.

Multi-Cultural Considerations in Organ Donation and Transplantation

Karen Garcia, MS
Clifton McClenney, MSM
Victoria Dent, BSW
Melissa Zinnerman, RN

Introduction

As the transplant community drives into the era of the collaborative, process improvement models and other ways to increase organ donation and transplantation, there are four important issues on the road to increased organ donation and transplantation.

First, it is important that cultural competency remains part of the transplant community. The nation's demographic makeup has and will be changing during the next 10 years. It is vital that educational efforts regarding organ donation and transplantation are consistent with this change. Second, as the demographics of the nation change, it will be important to enhance the public's knowledge of the transplant system. One way to do this is to find ways to increase input from the general public especially underserved populations when organ transplant policies are developed. Third, the transplant community must continue to address the challenges faced when attempting to increase organ donation in multicultural communities. Finally, some of the obstacles that the transplant community must overcome during the organ donation process parallel the issues potential organ recipients face.

Cultural Competency

The demographic composition of the US population will change dramatically in the next few decades. Within the next 10 years, the population will become significantly more diverse, making it paramount that potential donor families receive culturally competent and linguistically appropriate care. For example, by 2010, Latinos/Hispanics will be the largest minority group in the United States, comprising nearly 20% of the population.[1] This demographic shift will have important implications for donor hospitals, organ procurement organizations, tissue and eye banks, and transplant centers, as a greater number of minorities will constitute a growing proportion of the potential donor pool, thereby having a significant impact on donation rates. To assure that opportunities for donation among multicultural groups are not lost, it is critical for organizations dedicated to saving lives through organ and tissue donation to be able to provide families with culturally competent and linguistically appropriate care during the consent process.

Cross et al[2] describe cultural and linguistic competence as "…a set of congruent behaviors, attitudes, and policies that come together in a system, agency, or among professionals that enables effective work in cross-cultural situations. 'Culture' refers to integrated patterns of human behavior that include the language, thoughts, communications, actions, customs, beliefs, values, and institutions of racial, ethnic, religious, or social groups. "Competence' implies having the capacity to function effectively as an individual and an organization within the context of the cultural beliefs, behaviors, and needs presented by consumers and their communities.[2]

The requisite for cultural and linguistic competence can be validated by the need to respond to demographic changes; improve the quality of care provided to potential donor families; create a culturally sensitive environment for families; improve communications with families; increase consent rates among minority populations; support workforce diversity initiatives; and, perhaps in the future, meet accreditation mandates. The Joint Commission on Accreditation of Healthcare Organizations (JCAHO) currently views the provision of services in a culturally and linguistically appropriate manner as a significant healthcare quality issue and encourages organizations to offer equitable services across diverse communities.

Across the nation, healthcare organizations are having a difficult time effectively meeting the needs of racially, ethnically, culturally, and linguistically diverse populations, including organizations involved in requesting consent for organ donation. A potential contributing factor to this difficulty is the need for a more culturally competent and culturally diverse health professional workforce. Two leading national donation-related organizations are acutely aware of the need for a culturally diverse workforce and organizational competence within the industry.

Established in 1992, the American Society of Multicultural Health and Transplant Professionals (ASMHTP) is a multicultural organization that serves health and transplant professionals by providing leadership in a national capacity on matters of ethnic diversity in the transplant industry. The ASMHTP seeks to advance cultural competency among organ procurement organizations, transplant centers, and individual members, via the introduction of ethnic minority groups to health and transplant professions.

In 2002, the Association of Organ Procurement Organizations (AOPO) established the Task Force on Multicultural Issues to address the needs of diverse population groups. The task force, comprising multicultural professionals, developed a national minority recruitment video for OPOs experiencing difficulty in finding diverse staff and has served to integrate multicultural issues and objectives into the scope of work of AOPO committees, councils, task forces, and ongoing activities. Additionally, in 2003, the task force spearheaded the inclusion of Multicultural Needs Standards in the AOPO Standards and Accreditation Program, which state the following: the OPO shall review the linguistic, ethnic, and cultural composition of its service area; the OPO shall identify the unique needs for donation in distinct populations; the OPO shall assess the availability of staff, services, and volunteers and seek to ensure effective primary language communication and educational support to substantially sized and distinct linguistic, ethnic, and cultural communities, as determined by the OPO; the OPO shall identify and encourage the distribution of communication tools to expand the awareness of donation and the benefit of transplantation among targeted linguistic, ethnic, and cultural groups throughout the OPO donor service area; and the OPO shall monitor the consent and conversion rates of distinct linguistic, ethnic, and cultural groups it has previously identified and sought to serve through specific programming.[3]

All AOPO-accredited organ procurement organizations are held to these standards, which serve as the impetus for each OPO to seek cultural competency. Both AOPO and ASMHTP have strategically made efforts to recruit under-represented minorities in donation and transplant professions and bring cultural competency to the forefront of donation processes.

Several organ and tissue recovery agencies have employed ethnically "like requestors" to increase cultural sensitivity when approaching diverse families. It is important to note that requestors, whether or not they are members of a minority group, should receive cultural competency training. Cultural competency extends beyond cultural awareness or sensitivity. Requestors must possess knowledge of and respect for different cultural perspectives and use their skills effectively when handling cross-cultural situations. Cultural competency among professionals who are in direct contact with potential donor families may serve to enhance trust between the requestor and family, result in the diffusion of more appropriate care and services, and improve consent outcomes and the families' overall experience with organ donation. Evidence of a requestor's cultural competence may include knowing not to rely on other family members to translate but rather using an interpreter who is trained in medical terminology and the donation process; knowing not to rely on the first available administrative staff member who speaks the families' language; having insight regarding the families' religious beliefs, which so many times impedes the donation process; being able to eliminate stereotypical beliefs when approaching families for consent; and being familiar with cultural beliefs and attitudes toward death and dying.

A universally accepted approach to building cultural competency or creating a culturally competent workplace does not exist. Approaches to the realization of competency tend to differ between organizations and the needs of the communities they serve. A guideline to help healthcare organizations move toward higher levels of cultural competence was developed by the Office of Minority Health. The guideline, known as the Culturally and Linguistically Appropriate Services in Health Care (CLAS) Standards, are 14 recommendations that can provide a blueprint for health care organizations that want to create culturally competent organizations. These 14 standards are organized by themes: Culturally Competent Care (Standards 1-3), Language Access Services (Standards 4-7), and Organizational Supports for Cultural Competence (Standards 8-14).[4]

As outcome measures, some programs have focused on structural changes, such as training bilingual staff, instituting translation services, and developing culturally and linguistically specific materials.[5]

An increase in consent rates is the outcome measure that will indicate whether implementing training programs, policies, and culturally or linguistically appropriate standards makes a difference when requesting an organ for donation. Cultural competency, implemented in a strategic manner, also can be supportive of the quality improvement process. For example, an organization can analyze patterns of refusals for consent, examining variables such as age, gender, or race/ethnicity. If the analysis reveals that blacks have the highest rate of refusals, the organization can use specific strategies for this group. Does the requestor understand the culture's bereavement process? Would working with a community pastor or hospital chaplain increase the likelihood of consent?

The changing demographics and growing awareness of cultural issues and their relationship to consent outcomes among diverse populations is likely to motivate organizations to acquire new tools to assess their level of cultural competency as well as that of their staff, especially those who interact with potential donor families. Improved cultural competency on the part of donation/transplant organizations is important and, perhaps, a decisive component of any approach to addressing refusals to donate and improving outcomes among minorities and diverse populations.

Input From Minorities During the Organ Procurement Transplant Network (OPTN)/United Network for Organ Sharing (UNOS) Public Comment Period

In 2004, the OPTN/UNOS Minority Affairs Committee initiated discussion regarding the public comment process. Review and response to public comments is one of the steps in the OPTN/UNOS Policy Development Process. One issue addressed by the Minority Affairs Committee was how to increase specific ethnic minority groups' access to proposals that are currently available for public comment. The OPTN/UNOS Minority Affairs Committee reviewed the Federal Public Comment Process. The Federal Register Act, enacted July 26, 1935, establishes the basic legal structure of the federal regulatory system. The Federal Register is a single uniform publication for Executive agency rules and notices and Presidential documents. The Code of Federal Regulations (added in 1937) codifies the rules once finalized. Federal Register publications are produced by the Office of the Federal Register and the Government Printing Office and are available online at no charge to the public. In addition, a free federal Web site provides access to any item issued for public comment from any federal agency without the need to visit each individual agency Web site. As required by the National Organ Transplant Ace (NOTA), the OPTN process closely replicates the federal process, with some distinctions noted. Both are available in electronic and hard copy format for public response. Hard copies of the OPTN public comment document are available upon request; however, copies of the Federal Register are available only by subscription. Both provide notice of proposed policy/rule and an opportunity to comment, and both provide notice of final policy/rule prior to implementation.

The OPTN/UNOS Minority Affairs Committee continued its discussion by developing ways to enhance the level of participation in and understanding of the OPTN/UNOS Public Comment Process. Suggestions included the following:

- Presentations at dialysis facilities and hospital waiting rooms. These could include presentations prepared in advance in video format and played using equipment already available in these sites. An advantage of using this type of medium rather than written documentation is the opportunity

for better understanding and translation into multiple languages. These also could include training candidate advocates to assist with such presentations.
- Funding to provide computers and Internet access for dialysis facilities and hospital waiting rooms. Individuals to provide training on using the computers and responding to proposals distributed for public comment also would be needed.
- Enlistment of the services of the National Association for Transplant Coordinators (NATCO) to garner transplant center support for these initiatives.
- Appeals to each potential transplant recipient to determine the means of communication/outreach that best suits their needs.

The OPTN/UNOS Minority Affairs Committee has also discussed the need for a National Survey on organ donation and transplantation.

As a result of these discussions and a subsequent report that included 3 resolutions for deliberation, the OPTN/UNOS Board of Directors approved a proposal to promote participation in the public comment process, including the simplification of public comment summary information so that interested parties from all constituencies are provided opportunities to participate in the process.[6]

The Board also approved a proposal to initiate a national survey to determine baseline information on the views of the general public regarding transplantation. The third resolution approved by the Board directed that simplified language used in the public comment and the national survey to determine the views of the general public regarding transplantation shall be undertaken in a culturally competent method and subject to the availability of personnel and financial resources.

The OPTN/UNOS Minority Affairs Committee will continue working on the issue of how to create a public comment process that captures the full breadth of interested opinion regarding organ procurement and transplantation issues.

After examining the process in depth, a Subcommittee on Public Education and Outreach Initiatives was formed to assist with efforts to foster constituency and stakeholder participation in and understanding of the public comment process, additional opportunities for public education about and awareness of transplantation as an option for minorities, and greater inclusiveness in the development of allocation policy.[7]

The Challenges Transplant Professionals Face Related to Donation Rates in Multicultural Communities

In the field of transplantation, many challenges exist when attempting to educate multicultural communities. An organization should view education in multicultural communities as an opportunity and not a challenge. By employing culturally competent staff, as mentioned previously in this chapter, opportunities to educate multicultural communities can flourish. A challenge is a stimulating task or problem, and an opportunity is defined as a good chance for advancement or progress. The word opportunity gives the transplant field a fresh approach to an issue that continues to remain a topic of discussion during staff meetings across the country.

The transplant field has the opportunity to include multicultural education and outreach programs as an integral part of any transplant agency's mission. As professionals, do we over prepare ourselves for the challenge and under prepare for the opportunity? Can professionals in the transplant field work more diligently to address the needs of multicultural communities and achieve higher donation rates? These questions should be addressed by the upper management of organizations throughout the field. Once we embrace the value of diversity at the management level, opportunities that were once cloudy will become clear. "Diversity is an environment where differences are valued and comprehensively integrated into an organization's daily business functions. Diversity is synonymous with people and the inherent differences they bring to everything they do. These differences include the ways people are (human diversity); the ways people think (cultural diversity); and the ways people naturally do things (systems diversity)."[1] The way we conduct our internal affairs affects the manner in which we interact with our external affairs. An organization like this has the opportunity to garner relationships through education and outreach efforts of a properly trained staff, and develop a highly visible relationship with the community. An organization like this will see the benefits of their efforts, potentially an increase in donation rates. When community members see that an organization is visible and supportive of community events, they may begin to take an interest in the organization and its mission, particularly if they see staff and volunteers who are representative of their culture. Once an organization has "buy-in" from the community, their support can be invaluable and immeasurable. "Collaborating with religious, social, and civic community groups who support and share the mission of increasing donation and transplant awareness is vital."[8]

Transplant organizations should take the opportunity to educate multicultural communities on organ and tissue donation. This education will provide people with a better understanding of how organ and tissue donation may affect their families. When promoting awareness of the diseases that multicultural communities face on a daily basis, it is important to educate these communities about the prevalence of diabetes and heart disease, which can lead to organ failure, and the importance of healthy eating habits. This information offers people a sense of empowerment by giving them the tools they need to do something to decrease their risk of needing a transplant.

The biggest opportunity to influence multicultural communities is the chance to promote discussion among family members. When multicultural families talk about organ donation prior to the sudden death of a loved one, the decision to donate becomes less burdensome. As a donor daughter, the initial shock was enough to say no to donation. I wanted my father back; I did not want to make a decision regarding donation. Of course, my family knew what my father wanted, but now I know firsthand how difficult the decision would have been if we had never discussed it. Knowing my father's decision made ours an easier one to make. Because of my father's gift, two people can see.

Pre-transplant Issues Affecting Post-transplant Potential

Before discussing the post- transplant experience of ethnic minority patients, we must address the issues that arise in the pre-transplant phase. Transplant professionals can attest to the experience that pre-transplantation for some ethnic minority patients does not exist because of access problems and disparities in healthcare. Access to healthcare has created disparities in caring for ethnic minority patients and individuals with low levels of education, inadequate and unsafe living conditions, and low socioeconomic status.[2] Notwithstanding the fact that transplantation is an option in some cases, ethnic minority patients are usually not informed about the transplant process and are less likely to be identified as transplant candidates by nephrologists.}show that ethnic minority patients receive fewer cardiac diagnostic tests, less pain medication in the emergency room, and less treatments that involve surgery for operable lung cancer. With advancements in therapies, patients are often treated medically, while many of these patients are placed on suboptimal treatment in cases where a transplant workup is clearly warranted but the disparities in healthcare provide must be overcome for transplantation to considered an option. Until issues related to access to health care are resolved, disparities surrounding healthcare in the ethnic minority and low socioeconomic status populations of our society will always exist.

How many healthcare professionals have heard statements from patients indicated that the patients were told it was too early for them to be considered as transplant candidates by physicians who were not a part of the transplant community. Disparities in the level of healthcare represent a real issue that has been well documented.[8] According to an article by Betancourt et al,[2] the Institute of Medicine (IOM) report on organ transplantation states that several factors, such as stereotyping, prejudice, and healthcare worker misperceptions, contribute to disparities in healthcare. A diverse healthcare team, education, and awareness will help improve the quality of healthcare that ethnic minority groups receive.[9]

It's important that healthcare workers recognize these factors because they will have an effect on how healthcare practitioners educate patients before and after transplantation. According to Foster, the education process will have an effect on compliance and patient survival after transplantation.[10]

Multicultural Sensitivity in Education

Issues that will affect transplantation include religion, mistrust of the medical community, communication, and educational differences. In addition, misperceptions among healthcare professionals may hinder the amount of educational information provided to post-transplant candidates.

In *Webster's New College Dictionary*,[17] religion is defined as belief in and reverence for a supernatural power accepted as the creator and governor of the universe. Religion and spirituality definitely play a role in a patient's perception and willingness to participate in his or her well-being. Westlake et al[1] made mention of how religion and spirituality can affect how patients view their overall quality of life. In our society, a myriad of religious beliefs and practices exist, and sometimes a person's religious beliefs are in conflict with those of a healthcare worker. When approaching families about organ donation, it is important that their religious beliefs are respected; therefore, transplant professionals must understand religious attitudes about organ donation and transplantation (Table 1). Knowledge is power, and understanding someone's religious beliefs can help open a door. Families will feel respected if they see that a healthcare worker has taken the time to understand their religious and cultural views, which, in turn, can encourage communication.[9] Another way to open the door is to make sure patients' dietary requirements and accommodations for prayer and religious practice are available. It is also important to take time to teach a medication regimen that accommodates time for prayer.

Table 1. RELIGIOUS BELIEF ON ORGAN DONATION AND TRANSPLANTATION

Religion	Organ Donation	Transplantation
Anglican	Acceptable	Acceptable
Baha'I	Acceptable	No Official Position
Baptist	Acceptable	Acceptable
Buddhist	Individual Decision	Individual Decision
Catholicism	Acceptable	Acceptable
Christian Scientists	Individual Decision	Individual Decision
Church of Jesus Christ of Latter Day Saints (Mormons)	Individual Decision	Individual Decision
Greek Orthodox Church	Acceptable	Acceptable
Gypsies	Generally Oppose	Generally Oppose
Hinduism	Individual Decision	Individual Decision
Islam	Acceptable	Acceptable
Jehovah's Witnesses	Individual Decision	Individual Decision
Judaism	Acceptable	Acceptable
Lutheran	Acceptable	Individual Decision
Seventh-Day Adventist	Acceptable	Acceptable
Society of Friends (Quakers)	Individual Decision	Individual Decision
United Church of Christ	Acceptable	Acceptable
United Methodist	Acceptable	Acceptable

Mistrust of the medical community is a real factor for ethnic minority groups. While conducting a study on diabetes in the ethnic minority community, Robert Anderson[6] became aware of the mistrust patients have for the medical community. This mistrust dates back to the exportation of patients associated with the Tuskegee Experiment when patients with syphilis went years without treatment even though treatment was available. The Tuskegee Experiment lasted from 1932 to 1972, when 399 black men with syphilis were not treated so that the medical community could study the effects of untreated syphilis.[7] The history of this travesty lives on in the minds of blacks; it was a critical event that created mistrust of public health institutions and biochemical studies. The Tuskegee Experiment was so devastating to the community in Macon County, Alabama, and to countless lives that President Clinton gave a public apology for the racism in medicine, misconduct by physicians, and governmental abuse.[7]

Many factors have an effect on learning when educating patients; therefore, it is important that healthcare practitioners avoid any barriers that may affect the learning process. Healthcare workers must remember that there are verbal and nonverbal forms of communication. Most families are willing participants and want to learn; however, sometimes a minor intrusion, strange look, or misunderstanding of a cultural practice can cause families and/or patients to withdraw. During the education process, it is essential that patients don't feel hurried to learn their post-transplant responsibilities. A straightforward approach is the best policy, and taking a moment to learn what the family knows about transplantation may help open the door for the healthcare provider.

There are no educational differences between ethnic minority and non-minority patients. An important fact to remember when teaching families about organ donation and transplantation is that different people have different learning styles. The first step to being a good educator is to be familiar with the three different types of learning styles: visual, auditory, and tactile/kinesthetic. Visual learners learn by what they see; therefore, illustrations and actually being able to see post-transplant drugs will improve retention of information. Auditory learners learn by what they hear; they need to talk things through and hear discussions about the topics. Tactile/kinesthetic learners benefit from a hands-on approach; they must move, do, and touch in order to learn. Tactile learners cannot sit still; they need to move around or they will become distracted. When educating post-transplant candidates, each learning style should be incorporated. According to Foster et al,[3] when educating patients within the dialysis unit, support groups, and local community hospital, written materials and videos helped reach patients who were not auditory learners.

When using written materials, they should be in a language with which patients feel comfortable. If your patient population doesn't speak English, provide patients with materials in their native language. Don't be afraid to ask if family members and transplant candidates need further instructions or if they understand the instructions that were provided. Use verbal or written tests to assess a patient's level of comprehension regarding the educational materials covered. Utilize real-life stories to make the process of transplantation more real for transplant patients. Teaching materials should not contain too much information so that patients will not feel overwhelmed. Providing education on transplantation to patients a few hours before they are discharged is an unacceptable practice and shows a lack of interest for patients' overall outcome.

Transplant professionals should follow up with families and patients regarding their opinions of the educational efforts provided on transplantation. Healthcare practitioners must allow themselves to be evaluated by the individuals they are teaching and should not assume patients will speak up when confused. As transplant professionals, we must be willing to receive constructive criticism so that we can improve our educational techniques. After transplantation, patients especially those in underserved areas who do not have the resources to choose other areas to receive care face many risks: organ rejection, infection, graft failure, and even death. Too often after transplantation these patients must deal with issues related to health insurance, medication coverage, and immunological challenges.[5] With all of this in mind, education pitfalls should not hinder patients during their new lease on life. Included in Table 2 on the following page are graft survival rates that show minorities do well with transplantation when given the opportunity. The Scientific Registry of Transplant Recipients documented graft survival by ethnicity and many other factors related to pre- and post-transplant statistics. The Web site of the Scientific Registry of Transplant Recipients (http://www.ustransplant.org/)[18] is very informative and provides statistics based on several factors. The information on this Web site is based on data that the United Network of Sharing collects from OPO and transplant centers across the nation.

It is vital that the transplant community maintain cultural competency, utilize input from ethnic minority groups as organ transplant policies are developed, and understand the challenges regarding organ donation rates in multicultural communities as well as pre-transplant issues that affect post-transplant potential on its agenda as the transplant community works toward increasing organ donation and transplantation.

Table 2. ADJUSTED GRAFT SURVIVAL, DECEASED DONOR NON-ECD KIDNEY TRANSPLANTS SURVIVAL RATE AT 3 MONTHS, 1 YEAR, 3 YEARS, AND 5 YEARS AFTER TRANSPLANTATION

		3 Months			1 Year			3 Years			5 Years		
		N	%	Std. Err.	N	%	Std. Err.	N	%	Std. Err.	N	%	Std. Err.
Total	All	13,924	94.9%	0.2%	13,924	90.6%	0.3%	13,480	79.4%	0.4%	13,177	68.8%	0.4%
Recipient Race	White	8905	95.1%	0.2%	8905	91.4%	0.3%	8832	81.8%	0.4%	8711	72.2%	0.5%
	Asian	622	95.5%	0.8%	622	92.6%	1.1%	596	84.1%	1.5%	609	75.9%	1.8%
	Black	4145	94.1%	0.4%	4145	88.4%	0.5%	3809	72.2%	0.7%	3638	58.9%	0.8%
	Other/ Multi-race	250	94.5%	1.4%	250	90.9%	1.8%	243	81.6%	2.5%	217	77.0%	3.0%
	Unknown	2	*	*	2	*	*	0	-	-	2	*	*

Data from OPTN/SRTR Data as of May 3, 2004.

*Values not determined because of insufficient follow-up.;

-Values not determined because there were no transplants in the category. Cohorts are transplants performed during 2001-2002 for survival at 3 months and 1 year; { 1999-2000 for rate of survival at 3 years; and 1997-1998 for rate of survival at 5 years.

Graft survival follows individual transplants until graft failure.Counts for patient and graft survival are different because a patient may have had more than one transplant for a type of organ. Center volume = Center's yearly transplants performed during the base period, based on kidney and kidney-pancreas transplants. Multiorgan transplants are excluded.

Survival rates are adjusted to the characteristics of the 3-month and 1-year cohort. See Technical Notes for details.

References

1. US Bureau of the Census. *Population Projections for States, by Age, Sex, Race, and Hispanic Origin: 1993 to 2020. Current Population Reports.* Washington, DC: US Bureau of the Census. 1994.
2. Cross TL, Bazron BJ, Dennis KW, Issacs MR. *Towards a Culturally Competent System of Care.* Washington, DC: CASSP Technical Assistance Center. 1992.
3. Association of Organ Procurement Organizations. *AOPO Task Force on Multicultural Issues: Multicultural Needs Standards.* McLean, Va: Association of Organ Procurement Organizations. 2003.
4. Office of Minority Health. *National Standards for Culturally and Linguistically Appropriate Services in Health Care* [Executive summary]. Washington, DC: US Department of Health and Human Services. 2001.
5. US Department of Health and Human Services. *Proceedings of the National Conference on Cultural Competence and Women's Health Curricula in Medical Education, October 1995.* Washington, DC: US. Department of Health and Human Services. 1998.
6. Williams W, Young C Parker D, Sommers C. OPTN/UNOS Minority Affairs November 2004 Board Report.
7. Williams W, Young C Parker D, Sommers C. OPTN/UNOS Minority Affairs June 2005 Board Report.
8. Westlake C, Dracup, K. Role of spirituality in adjustment of patients with advanced heart failure. *Prog Cardiovasc Nurs.* 2001;16:119-125.
9. Bentancourt JR, Ananeh-Firempong II O. Not me! Doctors, decisions, and disparities in health care. *Cardiovasc Rev Rep.* 2004;25:105-109.
10. Foster CE 3rd, Philosophe B, Schweitzer EJ.A decade of experience with renal transplantation in African-Americans. *Ann Surg.* 2002;236:794-805.
11. {Need author info here.} What are learning styles? Available at: http://www.ldpride.net/lerningstyles.MI.htm. Accessed June 10, 2005.
12. Young C, Kew C. Health disparities in transplantation: focus on the complexity and challenge of renal transplantation in African Americans. *Med Clin North Am.* 2005;89:1003-1031.
13. Anderson, Robert M, EDD, (2005), Is It Ethical to Assign Medically Underserved African Americans to a Usual-Care Control Group in Community-Based Interventions in Research? *Diabetes Care.* 2005;28:1817-1820.
14. Gamble VN. Under the shadow of Tuskegee: African Americans and health care. *Am J Public Health.* 1997;87:1773-1778.
15. Press R, Carrasquillo O, Nickolas T, Radhakrishnan J, Shea S, Barr, RG. Race/ethnicity, poverty status, and renal transplant outcomes. *Transplantation.* 2005;80:917-924.
16. Ott B B, Al-Khadhuri J, Al-Junaibi S. Preventing ethical dilemmas: understanding Islamic health care practices. *Pediatr Nurs.* 2003;29:227-230.
17. *Webster's New College dictionary* {incomplete reference. Need to add edition number, editors, city and state of publisher, etc., to this reference.}
18. Scientific Registry of Transplant Recipients (http://www.ustransplant.org/

The Economics of Organ Donation and Transplantation

G. Kent Holloway, MSF
Helen M. Hauff, RN, MBA, CCTC, CPTC

Background

Transplantation is an effective therapy and, in most cases, the only therapy available to patients with end-stage organ failure. Financial analysis of the cost of ongoing renal dialysis compared with the cost of transplantation indicates that transplantation could be a clinically effective mode of treatment as well as cost effective.[1] One report published by the Office of the Inspector General in 1987 concluded that "Each transplant of a Medicare beneficiary generates a 5-year cost savings of $75,000."[1] This finding generated great hope and enthusiasm for successful, cost-effective, and lifesaving transplants.

Support grew for a national program that would guarantee each individual entitled to Medicare benefits the opportunity for a kidney transplant regardless of his or her ability to pay. Ultimately, a 1972 Social Security Amendment guaranteeing access to renal transplantation became law. According to this amendment, nearly all citizens requiring renal dialysis and/or transplantation were guaranteed treatment. Under Medicare Part A, qualified dialysis and transplantation programs were guaranteed cost reimbursement for these services.[2] In 1987, Congress passed legislation that extended payment for kidney transplantation coverage from 12 months to 36 months and added a provision that authorized full reimbursement for reasonable costs associated with the acquisition of deceased donor kidneys. This legislation established the fundamentals for accumulating costs and for reimbursing applicable services related to the acquisition of all transplantable organs.

Medicare has approved reimbursement for all transplants for Medicare beneficiaries. Medicare reimbursement for transplantation of these organs was approved in the following years: heart, 1987; liver, 1991; lung, 1995; simultaneous kidney and pancreas, 1999; and pancreas after kidney, 1999. In 1981, Medicare introduced language defining Medicare as a secondary payor (MSP) for patients with end-stage renal disease for the first 12 months of entitlement. Subsequent rules have extended the MSP provision to its present limit of 30 months from entitlement.

The economics of donation and transplantation in the 21st century are grounded in these early programs. In addition to clinical advancements in the specialty of transplantation, there are now patient reimbursement programs and patterns that mirror those of other highly specialized modes of treatment.

THE ECONOMICS OF ORGAN DONATION
Organ Procurement Organization Overview

In the early years and in general, organ donation occurred only in centers that had both a transplant program and a trauma center. In some cases, these transplant programs established potential donor notification agreements with trauma centers in institutions without a transplant program. Organ sharing and allocation were born from these independent transplant programs and their partner hospitals and were managed according to local priority, expertise, and preference–this is not today's model!

Chapter 5 THE ECONOMICS OF ORGAN DONATION AND TRANSPLANTATION

Currently, 58 organ procurement organizations (OPOs) are certified by the Centers for Medicare and Medicaid Services (CMS). These OPOs service the entire country, including Puerto Rico. Of these 58 programs, only 8 are hospital-based OPOs (HOPOs); the other 50 organizations are independent OPOs (IOPOs), as defined by the National Transplant Act of 1984.[3] This act also made provisions for an organ procurement transplant network (OPTN). The OPTN would be a nonprofit, contracted agency that would, among other responsibilities, establish one national list of potential candidates to receive a deceased donor organ. All OPOs, whether IOPO or HOPO, must be members in good standing of the OPTN and must abide by its sharing algorithms.

All OPOs must be accredited by the CMS and are assigned a donation service area (DSA). DSAs do not overlap; however, OPOs may share a common metropolitan area but must contract specifically with hospitals in the area to create distinct service affiliations. OPOs were recertified every 2 years until President Clinton signed the Public Health Improvement Act in 2000. This act specifically cites limitations in the recertification process for OPOs, mandates a recertification cycle of 4 years, requires the recertification process to incorporate an evaluation of process improvement measures as well as outcome performance measures, and provides for the development of an equitable process for appeals. Interestingly, this law includes language prohibiting the creation of any new OPO.

In response to the Public Health Improvement Act, revised CMS conditions for coverage for OPOs were released in the Federal Register for public comment in January 2005 in concert with revised conditions for coverage for transplant centers and end-stage renal disease facilities. All OPOs were recertified by CMS by December 31, 2005, and from that point forward began the 4-year recertification cycles for all OPOs.

Reimbursement

In July 1974, the Department of Health, Education, and Welfare, Social Security Administration[4] released Part A Intermediary Letter No. 74-23. The title of this letter is Determining Costs Associated With the Renal Disease Provisions of Public Law 92-603. The purpose of this document was to add definition and detail to this law's provision for "reimbursement for the variety of medical services that are required to support a quality transplant program where it is appropriate to have such a program."[4] This intermediary letter established the concept of an "organ acquisition cost center" for the purposes of setting a standard acquisition charge (SAC) for a transplantable organ, specifically for a transplantable kidney.

The following is a quote from Section I: General of the letter:

"...there were two principal areas of concern. First, it was necessary to ensure that Medicare would pay its share of the costs of organ procurement recognizing that in live donor organ procurement there would be a considerable amount of medical costs incurred in evaluating potential donors prior to the possible selection of a donor and that in the cadaver organ procurement program not all organs excised would eventually be transplanted. Second, an equitable means had to be developed for covering and reimbursing necessary medical services provided to potential donors and recipients, recognizing that in some situations these services would be provided prior to the effective date of the potential transplant recipients Medicare entitlement. For example, patients (recipients) or potential donors may be blood or tissue typed shortly after end-stage renal disease is diagnosed and transplantation is being planned. However, the specific patient's date of entitlement to Medicare may not occur until much later when the dialysis waiting period is satisfied or the patient is transplanted. Where no dialysis treatments are given, entitlement would not occur until the month of transplant (or the month before the month of transplant if the patient was admitted to the hospital in that month in preparation for and in anticipation of a transplant).

Therefore, in order to determine costs of Medicare covered services which are normally provided in preparation for a transplant and for kidneys acquired for the purpose of providing Medicare beneficiaries with renal transplant and to encourage the consideration of this treatment modality; i.e., allowing beneficiaries who are acceptable candidates for transplantation the opportunity to be transplanted irrespective of economic factors, the concept of the kidney acquisition cost center was developed. In addition to supporting the above objections, the use of the kidney acquisition cost center (formerly referred to as a kidney excision cost center) also provides the mechanism for reviewing the cost of services provided between hospitals under arrangements. It also provides the mechanism to make more current reimbursement for some costs which, using preexisting reimbursement policy could not be reimbursed by the program until they could be added to the billable service which is generated by a participating hospital.[4]

Included in this letter were definitions for acceptable costs for acquiring a deceased donor kidney. Typical costs were determined to include intensive care costs; surgeon's services; anesthetist's services; operating room fees; preservation materials and equipment; preservation technician's services; donor evaluation and support; pathology, transportation, and packaging; administration costs, and overhead costs. Specific instructions were given to "non-transplant center" donor hospitals to establish a kidney acquisition cost center to ensure accurate cost reimbursement for kidney acquisition. This document established that all kidney acquisition costs from deceased donors were cost reimbursed by the Medicare program.

General guidelines from this 1974 intermediary letter still apply to the 8 remaining HOPO programs. Costs are accumulated in cost centers specific to acquisition type; for example, kidney, heart, and tissue should all have distinct cost centers to account for direct acquisition costs. HOPO program expenses are reported on the appropriate hospital cost report, and appropriate SACs are established and billed for each recovery service provided by these entities.

Cost Account for Independent Organ Procurement Organizations

The majority of deceased donation in the United States is facilitated by IOPOs. All 50 IOPOs report to one Medicare Intermediary, Riverbend Government Benefits Administration (Riverbend GBA). Each IOPO is considered a Medicare provider under Part A and must complete a statement of reimbursable costs, form 216-94, by the last day of the fifth month following the end of the IOPO's fiscal year.

Cost accounting for IOPOs is similar to that established years ago for HOPOs. Renal acquisition is cost reimbursed by Medicare. Riverbend GBA must approve all renal SACs for IOPOs but cannot mandate SACs; however, SACs are *strongly* recommended based on current and/or projected renal program costs, as reported in the most recently filed cost report or estimated report of reimbursable costs. It is the responsibility of each IOPO to manage reimbursable costs under this program to avoid risk of lost revenue.

Medicare does not guarantee reimbursement for extra renal procurement services or, for that matter, any other service provided by the IOPO. The IOPO is responsible for establishing appropriate charges for services provided that sufficient revenue is produced to fund operations. All IOPOs must be classified by the Internal Revenue Service (IRS) as nonprofit corporations. All IOPOs should responsibly manage their business to keep revenue margins within acceptable standards for businesses of similar purpose and IRS status.

In general, IOPO costs can be categorized in the follow groups: renal acquisition, extra renal acquisition, tissue acquisition, and other program service lines. Each service line will have direct costs, acquisition overhead costs, and administrative and general costs.

Direct costs are costs directly attributed to a service or function. For example, a heart catheterization is a direct cost of a heart acquisition. Some direct costs are allocated. For example, operating room costs will be allocated to the cost centers associated with the organs and/or tissue procured in each specific donation. As simple as this concept may seem, the lines are sometimes gray regarding how to best allocate direct expense and to which categories an expense applies.

Acquisition overhead costs, as defined by the CMS cost report 216-94, include procurement staff salary and benefits, professional education expenses, community education expenses, and other acquisition expenses. Other acquisition expenses would include costs associated with a donor referral triage service.

Administrative and general costs, as with most businesses, include, for example, the costs for administrative personnel, office space, and general operating equipment. Some general business costs may not be eligible for Medicare reimbursement to the renal acquisition program; if such costs occur, they will be offset for reimbursement purposes, and the non-renal programs will assume responsibility for generating the necessary revenue for these operations.

Overhead costs and administrative and general costs must be allocated to each recovery program to determine Medicare reimbursement and to determine the approximate cost of doing business in each service line. The method for allocation of these expenses is defined by Medicare. Overhead costs, for example, are allocated based on a ratio established by the number of actual organs procured with the intent of transplantation plus the number of tissue donors recovered multiplied by an approved ratio to allow for variance of effort required between an organ donation and a tissue donation.

Direct costs are added to allocated overhead costs to arrive at a subtotal for each service line. Administrative and general costs are allocated to each service line based on a rate determined by dividing the service line's subtotal of accumulated costs by the total of all direct costs and overhead costs for the accounting period.

This complicated system of allocation and cost accumulation has well defined rules and an elaborate structure. Still, some areas are gray. In recent years, as service lines and the practice of organ and tissue acquisition have evolved, the rules have changed. In some cases, these changes have caused reduced Medicare funding for kidney acquisition. In nearly all cases in which funding has been reduced, it has been done retrospectively. IOPOs are not classified as standard Medicare providers. The options for appeal for IOPOs are limited, and the opportunities for negotiation and standardization as an industry are not guaranteed to this group. The Association for Organ Procurement Organizations continues to address this issue for its membership.

"How Much Is That Organ in the Window?"

Although much is written in this chapter about the structure of reimbursement and cost accounting for organ and tissue recovery, the truth is that there is tremendous variability between OPOs in every imaginable aspect from size of DSA to basic service provided to the transplant centers in their DSA. In addition, much of this profession is regulated. Often with increased regulation comes increased overhead. Details within these 2 primary categories help to explain the wide variation of donor organ SACs charged by OPOs across this country.

The Association of Organ Procurement Organizations surveys its membership on an annual basis to better understand these variances. There has yet to be 100% membership participation, and therefore a definitive list of organ SACs has never been fully reported. However, Riverbend GBA is under obligation to report all renal SACs for IOPOs; this information is available on their Web site at www.riverbendgba.com.

Because these SACs, by definition, approximate costs and standardization per transplantable organ, one could argue that they are a good general indicator of shifts in organ recovery costs over time. Examining the shift in renal SACs from December 1, 2002 to December 1, 2004 indicates a growth in average SAC from 2002 to 2004 of about 6% per year. The gap between minimum and maximum SAC on a national basis widened from a $12,000 gap in 2002 to a $14,500 gap in 2004.

Another notable statistical change from 2002 to 2004 was in the modal rate. The modal charge for a kidney increased to $23,000 in 2004 after remaining at $19,000 in 2002 and 2003; this is a 21% increase in the most frequently occurring renal SAC for IOPOs nationally.

The SAC detail provided in Table 1 is too limited to analyze to any great extent, but it confirms what any transplant program knows to be true: The cost of a transplantable organ from one OPO to another is highly variable. This fact begs the question: How can such variances exist when the fundamental service–delivery of a viable organ for transplant–is the same? The answer to this question is not simple or straightforward, but there are some overarching facts that lend themselves to explaining the inconsistencies.

Although the procurement industry is highly regulated from a service and reimbursement standpoint, huge variances exist in practice between IOPOs with regard to the detail of service provided. Some organizations coordinate long distance travel and some do not. Some organizations coordinate the sharing (importing) of organs from one DSR to another, thus assuming responsibility for the import SAC, and some do not. Some IOPOs provide services such as pulsatile perfusion for their transplant programs and build this cost into their SAC, and some do not.

Diversifying service lines can help reduce allocated overhead and administrative cost burdens to organ acquisition costs centers. Many IOPOs also recover donated tissue. Efficiently blending this service

A CLINICIAN'S GUIDE TO TRANSPLANTATION AND DONATION

Table 1. SHIFT IN RENAL STANDARD ACQUISITION CHARGES, 12/02 TO 12/04

	Renal SAC*, $ Effective 12/1/02	Renal SAC*, $ Effective 12/1/03	Renal SAC*, $ Effective 12/1/04
Minimum	12 500	14 000	13 500
Maximum	24 000	28 000	28 000
Mean	19 483	20 633	21 850
Median	19 100	20 500	22 150
Mode	19 000	19 000	23 000

*SAC indicates standard acquisition charge.

into an IOPOs day-to-day operations can help reduce allocated costs. These types of services that serve the mission of the organization are ideal opportunities for improving efficiency.

DSAs vary in size and character across the country. Depending on the demographics in each DSA, success in facilitating organ and tissue donation will vary. Some DSAs require extensive travel to sparsely populated regions, whereas other DSAs rarely facilitate long-distance travel to service their populations.

Changes in Medicare rules for participation can affect costs. In 1997, Medicare required all deaths to be reported to the OPO assigned to a hospital's service area. The additional expense needed to establish call centers equipped to handle the thousands of calls that resulted have added overhead expense to each OPO. This is a good example of well-intended regulation having an inflationary effect on the cost of transplantable organs.

One of the biggest indicators for cost variance in an OPO has to do with the number of organ donors per service area coupled with the average number of viable and billable organs per donor. Even for OPO's with larger service areas, the fact is that the number of potential and actual donors per DSA is small. The key to efficient and effective OPO operation within any DSA, regardless of demographics, lies in the ability to increase and maintain a donation conversion rate approximating that of the most effective OPOs, 75% or greater. Coupling a quality conversion rate with average viable organs per donor greater than 3.0 provides the option to keep inflation of SACs in check and in line with national healthcare pricing.

Transplant Center Economics: An Overview

Transplant center economics was largely driven by Congress and the U.S. Department of Health and Human Services, with Medicare now being the primary payor for 55.4% of all kidney transplants.[5] The regulations and cost accounting requirements for kidney transplants were later expanded to include heart, lung, liver, and intestinal programs, with limited inclusion for islet cell transplant in 2004. The cost reporting mechanism related to kidney transplantation was much broader than that for other organs until January 1, 2004, when the word "kidney" was replaced by "organ" in the regulatory wording. All transplant programs now use the cost reporting mechanism; for this reason, transplant center economics needs to be taken into consideration with Medicare certification, organ acquisition cost centers, managed care contracting, and reimbursement revenue streams when determining budgeting and business planning for organ transplantation. The financial intricacies of transplant administration make it one of the most complex administrative specialties in healthcare today.

Medicare and Transplantation

The primary responsibility of transplant services involves Medicare-certified transplant hospitals. To bill Medicare and participate in the cost reporting mechanism, the transplant center must first be Medicare approved. This approval process is based on sound clinical outcomes and demonstration that all aspects of transplant care and staffing are in place (Table 2). The 2-year requirement to meet and achieve Medicare certification was adjusted in 2000 to a volume per year requirement.[6]

The proposed 2005 CMS regulations seek to change this approval process.[7] Currently, Medicare certification for transplant centers is held by the hospital that is accountable for the program's outcomes;

Chapter 5 THE ECONOMICS OF ORGAN DONATION AND TRANSPLANTATION

Table 2. VOLUME CRITERIA

Organ	Volume/Year	1-Year Actuarial Survival, %	2-Year Actuarial Survival, %
Heart	12	73	65
Liver	12	77	60
Kidney	N/A	N/A	N/A
Lung	10	69	62
Small bowel	10	65	N/A

Facility requirements for transplant centers.[6]
*N/A indicates not applicable.
Not taken from a soucre but collected from Medicare manuals

however, the entire transplant team, particularly the surgeon, bears most of the accountability. To set up a new program requires an experienced surgical and medical director whose previous experience is not taken into consideration during the application process until the mandatory clinical outcomes have been met at the new center during a 2-year period, as stated previously, even if the program director has achieved superior outcomes at a previous institution. The proposed new certification process will allow experienced surgeons and teams with high volume of transplants {high volume of *what*?} to use center volume and clinical outcomes in lieu of the 2-year minimum experience period when there is a high probability that the clinical outcomes will be met. This process will allow hospitals to become Medicare certified sooner and will encourage hospitals to provide transplant services. The implementation of these new regulations is still pending.

In addition to the Medicare process for certification, some states require that hospitals obtain a certificate of need to provide transplant services and State Department of Health Approval that all conditions of participation have been met. Applications must demonstrate a clinical need for transplant services that is not adequately provided for within the local or state region.

Medicare certification becomes important in determining the overall cost-benefit analysis for the transplant center. During the 2 years that the institution is performing transplantations to meet the volume and outcome criteria, there is no revenue for Medicare beneficiaries who receive transplants at the center. Medicare will not cover a Medicare beneficiary if an organ transplantation is performed at a non-certified center. Likewise, managed care organizations, especially those that certify transplant centers as centers of excellence, will likely not approve their members for transplantation at a non-Medicare–certified transplant center, giving the institution no choice but to formulate a business plan that will pay for the transplants until Medicare certification is obtained. This cost is burdensome, and many centers find themselves paying for pre-transplant costs, the transplant procedure, transplant-related admissions, and follow-up care for as many as 10 years in some cases. Therefore, it is imperative for any new transplant center to become Medicare certified as soon as possible, especially because Medicare is the primary payor in more than 50% of transplant cases nationwide.[5]

Organ Acquisition Cost Centers (OACC)

Kidney transplant was the first organ to be covered by the Medicare program when Medicare was extended to include end-stage renal disease (ESRD) services under the entitlement program. This created the kidney organ acquisition cost center in which services and costs associated with the determination of suitability of a candidate for transplantation were allowable costs on the Medicare cost report. Costs are not the same as charges. Charges are the fees charged for the service, and costs are the cost of producing the service. Allowable costs do not include costs associated with ongoing or concurrent care or the diagnosis of disease. Patients referred to transplant centers for evaluation have already been diagnosed and are receiving treatment; therefore, the costs associated with the transplant center pertain to the evaluation of the candidate and/or living donor (e.g., tests and medical/surgical consultations to determine if the candidate is a potential transplant recipient) but not to treatment of the disease before transplantation.{Please check to make sure that I did not alter the intended meaning of the sentence.} These direct costs incurred by the transplant program are described in 4 categories and pertain to pre-transplant activities only.[8]

1. Program operating costs
   - Space-related costs, telephone, supplies, computers, utilities, insurance, photocopiers, and office equipment
   - All pre-transplant personnel, including transplant coordinators, patient financial coordinators, and data coordinators
   - United Network for Organ sharing registration costs
   - Program administration, medical director services
   - Standard institution fees such as continuing education meetings, seminars, travel to transplant-related meetings, and membership dues and subscriptions
   - Patient education materials
2. Services associated with the determination of suitability of the recipient and donor for transplant
   - Tissue typing
   - Laboratory and non-laboratory clinical tests
   - Physician fees for consultation services for recipients and living donors
   - Social services
   - Nutrition
   - Dental evaluation
   - Psychiatric evaluation services
   - Inpatient and outpatient testing services
3. Maintenance of the evaluated patient on the wait list for transplant, including ongoing re-evaluation of potential recipients
   - Repeat antibody screening
   - Re-evaluation services to determine ongoing suitability for transplantation
4. Costs associated with organ acquisition, deceased and living donor.
   - OPO charges for organ acquisition, including surgeon organ procurement fees, preservation and perfusion costs, and transportation
   - Costs related to in-house procured and transplant kidneys
   - Hospital costs associated with the living donors at the time of transplant, operating room, and other ancillary services
   - Laboratory costs associated with final cross matching and kidney acquisition
   - Costs associated with an intended transplant that is subsequently aborted

At the actual time of transplantation, costs associated with the surgery for the recipient are considered treatment costs. For this reason, the professional fees are no longer allowable organ acquisition costs. The professional fees are billed to the primary payor as usual, as is true of all post-transplant care. These direct costs associated with the program and the indirect costs (i.e., the proportionate share of the hospital's overall operating expense allocated to the transplant program [hospital overhead]) are also included. All of the costs are calculated separately for each organ and become the organ acquisition charge.

The evaluation costs associated with a potential kidney or pancreas recipient are easier to identify. However, with heart, liver, small bowel, and lung transplantation, evaluation testing is co-mingled with concurrent medical care making it difficult to distinguish between treatment costs versus costs associated with medical care. The recent wording change by CMS in 2005 has had a significant impact on transplant administration. Transplant centers now need to differentiate between an evaluation cost and ongoing, concurrent care, which is not a part of organ acquisition. Therefore, transplant centers need finance department staff members who are very familiar with the pre-transplant evaluation process for each organ type and a systematic billing process that can review individual charges received for each patient.

Chapter 5 THE ECONOMICS OF ORGAN DONATION AND TRANSPLANTATION

Implications for Administrators

Oversight of the cost reporting issues described previously falls to the hospital finance department in conjunction with the transplant administrator. All pre-transplant costs are required to be identified if the true costs for pre-transplant services are to be determined accurately, ensuring that Medicare reimburses for its proportionate share of pre-transplant costs. The OACC is not a profit center; it is a means of revenue to reimburse for the costs incurred in providing services to Medicare beneficiaries. Understanding the "reasonable and customary" allowable costs is important. However, ensuring that all costs are captured requires a multidisciplinary approach from all hospital departments, making transplant centers the gatekeepers for organ acquisition costs. All services provided to the recipient and donor are typically reviewed by the transplant program to verify that the service was a pre-transplant service and then sent to OACC for payment or to the primary payor, thereby ensuring that all pre-transplant costs are captured and documented for cost-reporting purposes. The transplant administrator will need to:

- Ensure all salary expenses are accounted for and allocated to pre-transplant services.[9]
  - Require all staff members to complete timesheets for 1 week each month to ensure that salary expenses are allocated correctly to pre-transplant services.
  - Include medical director salary for administrative services.
- Account for all expenses other than salary expenses associated with pre-transplant expenses,.
  - Set up separate cost centers for each organ for pre-and post-transplant expenses so that expenses can be allocated correctly.[9] Pre- and post-transplant expenses should not be on one cost center.
- Assess space for pre-transplant services.
- Account for all professional fees for pre-transplant evaluation services.
- Establish organ acquisition charges for all organs and living donors.
- Monitor all OPO organ acquisition charges, transportation, tissue typing, UNOS registration. and organ procurement fees.
- Report all in-house deceased donors for inclusion on the cost report.
- Monitor all laboratory and non-laboratory clinical testing expenses.
- Establish policies and procedures to maintain compliance with organ acquisition reporting regulations.
- Account for all Medicare primary and Medicare secondary recipients for cost- reporting purposes.
- Track all aborted transplants to capture costs on the cost report.
- Establish a relationship with the hospital's CMS intermediary.

The transplant administrator's role is not only to monitor these expenses and ensure that appropriate pre-transplant costs are allocated on the cost report, but also to understand the importance of the budgetary impact of the cost report on transplant services. Medicare pays its portion of total costs incurred by the transplant center for providing pre-transplant evaluation services; therefore, total costs need to be reported. The Medicare portion is calculated as the total number of Medicare beneficiaries who have received transplants, including any deceased donor kidneys that are excised at the transplant center, divided by the total number of patients who have received transplants at the center, thus providing a ratio of Medicare usable organs to total usable organs. This ratio is applied to the total costs for pre-transplant evaluation services and then the transplant center is reimbursed for Medicare's portion for services provided to Medicare beneficiaries. Knowing the Medicare ratio for each organ is important. If kidney recipients represent greater than 50% of the total number of patients who have received transplants, the transplant administrator can predict that more than 50% of the pre-transplant costs will be reimbursed and use this information when deciding whether to expand pre-transplant services for the purposes of business planning or preparing annual budgets.

Medicare Beneficiaries: Financial Implications

The Medicare cost report is vital to the success of a transplant program, hence the need for hospitals to become Medicare certified. Understanding Medicare benefits, pre-entitlement, entitlement, and Medicare beneficiaries is another key component. A patient is entitled to hospital insurance benefits if:

1. He or she is medically determined to have ESRD
2. He or she is fully or currently insured under the social security program or would be fully or currently insured if his or her employment (after 1936), as defined under the Railroad Retirement Act, is entitled to monthly social security or Railroad Retirement benefits, or if he or she is the spouse or a dependent child who meets the requirements stated previously
3. He or she has filed an application for Medicare Part A and
4. He or she has met the required waiting period.

The waiting period for coverage for ESRD patients begins on the first day of the third month after the month in which the individual initiates a regular course of dialysis maintained throughout the waiting period. Coverage can begin sooner if there is a pre-emptive kidney transplant or self-dialysis training. For a pre-emptive transplant, coverage begins on the first day of the month in which the kidney transplant was performed. For a patient admitted to a Medicare-certified transplant center or renal dialysis center for procedures prior to the transplant, coverage begins on either 1) the first day of the month in which he or she enters the hospital if the transplant is performed in that month or in the next 2 months or on 2) the first day of the second month before the month of the kidney transplant if the transplant is delayed more than 2 months after the initial hospital stay.

Pre-entitlement is defined as the "period during which services are furnished in anticipation of a transplant after the patient has been diagnosed to have end-stage renal disease, but prior to the patient's actual Medicare entitlement."[4] {A beneficiary is a person entitled to Medicare benefits; the importance of this is not only to ensure patients have adequate coverage for transplantation but also to calculate the Medicare ratio because entitled patients are considered Medicare beneficiaries.

The rules do vary when a potential patient has primary insurance through a commercial payor and is entitled to Medicare benefits and may have Medicare as a secondary payor. However, Medicare will become the primary payor for a transplant after a 30-month coordination of benefits period even if the recipient has alternative medical coverage. Under this coordination of benefits period, it is quite possible for the commercial payor to pay for an evaluation and for Medicare to be the primary payor at the time of transplant. In these cases, the commercial payor would need to be reimbursed for the services paid if the transplant is outside of the coordination of benefits period and Medicare is deemed the primary payor at the time of transplant.

Global Contracts

Global contracting plays a significant role in transplant finances. When transplantation costs soared in the early 1990's, commercial payors began to enter into global contracts. A fixed rate was negotiated for services, including re-transplantation if required due to graft failure, with a predetermined length of stay. Global contracting is widely associated with transplantation and other costly procedures; it is used as a means to control costs for the payor, spread financial risk, and it ensures business for the transplant center, as large payors can promote centers as "Centers of Excellence" and guarantee business. Transplantation is divided into 4 distinct phases for the purpose of contracting:

- Phase I: Evaluation to listing for transplant
- Phase II: Maintenance phase, waiting for a transplant
- Phase III: The transplant event Yes you did change the meaning.
- Phase IV: Post-transplantation.

Typical global contracts originally included phase I (evaluation) and phase III (transplantation) including defined periods of care post-transplant. The rate included hospital charges and professional fees for testing and procedures. Today, this type of contract has been replaced by what is termed a "hybrid" global contract. Typically, a case rate is set only for the procedure itself, i.e., phase III. All other services are provided as fee for service, with or without a discounted rate or set in accordance with pre-existing contracts. Organ acquisition, immunosuppressive medication, home care, rehabilitation, and dental care are usual exclusions as are any mechanical devices. It is not uncommon for a negotiated rate to be either a percentage of charges, a discounted rate, or set at a percentage of the prevailing Medicare rate for services.

The hybrid global contract evolved as the traditional global contract became increasingly difficult to manage by both payor and hospital. In all contracts. it is essential that financial billing staff be extremely knowledgeable about the clinical transplant process and the actual contract itself. Evaluations can be performed years before the transplantation actually occurs, creating issues regarding when the contract should be paid if the evaluation period is included. Today, most contracts require a fee-for-service for phases I, II, and IV and a case rate for phase III. When possible, post-transplantation care is limited to 3 months. The longer the contracted post-transplantation phase, the greater the financial exposure to the institution, as readmission costs will be included in the original transplant case rate. Contract language and management of length of stay (LOS) is vital in reducing the financial risk for the hospital. Essentially, hospitals are receiving a fixed payment for a set number of days for the procedure. If discharge occurs before the contracted LOS, the same amount is paid. If the LOS is extended, the hospital incurs an increased cost with no additional payments until the outlier provision is met. Once the contracted outlier day criteria have been met, additional payments will be made at a reduced rate; hospitals are offered some compensation for highly complicated cases. Re-transplantation within the contracted period is usually at a discounted rate and is highly costly to the program.

Global contracting has increased as payors try to contain costs in return for volume. It is not uncommon for global contracts to comprise more than 40% of a transplant center's business. Pricing strategies, understanding the total costs involved in providing transplantation services, and aligning hospital and provider services is required if the case rate is to be profitable for both transplant center and physicians, and if the financial exposure of the transplant program is to be minimized. Typically, despite global contracts, Medicare still remains the best payor for transplantation. If the global rate of the contract is less than the cost of providing the service, no amount of volume will ever make the center financially viable.

Medicaid

Most states provide Medicaid reimbursement for transplantation services; however, emergency Medicaid does not cover transplantation. The reimbursement rates under Medicaid, while acceptable for hospital reimbursement, create a huge financial burden on physician reimbursement s, as the rates are substantially lower than Medicare rates. {This info is given again later in this same paragraph.} It is not uncommon for Medicaid to reimburse surgeons less than $1000 for a liver transplant, making it impossible for these surgeons to generate enough revenue to cover their expenses. Hospitals do make a profit from the hospital admission of these patients and therefore many hospitals provide salary support to transplant physicians to compensate for a high Medicaid patient population and to encourage the provision of services to patients with Medicaid. . Reimbursement issues are especially common in reimbursement for pediatric transplantation. Medicaid HMO and capitation are adversely affecting reimbursement by placing a dollar limit per patient per year on medical care. This capitation also applies to transplantation services, creating a financial risk for transplant centers.

Diagnostic Related Groups

Diagnostic related groups (DRGs) define the payments for each organ transplantation based on a prospective payment system. Hospitals are paid a set amount that is based on a DRG relative weight used to assess complexity, labor and wage, {indices} graduate education costs if applicable, and non-labor–related costs. The result is a fixed payment per admission based on the assigned DRG. Only one DRG is assigned per admission. Outlier payments can be applied for if a particular case has unusually high expenses. Transplantations are complex and resource intensive; however, complex cases in which complications occur are paid at the usual DRG rate, regardless of costs. Because the complexity of a case does not affect reimbursement, transplant centers where complex cases are routinely undertaken are adversely affected,, particularly when a case involves the insertion of a left ventricular assist device

A CLINICIAN'S GUIDE TO TRANSPLANTATION AND DONATION

(LVAD) and transplantation occurs in the same admission. The prevailing {Is this word necessary here?} heart transplant DRG is paid because only one DRG is payable; therefore heart transplant programs must discharge pre-transplantation patients before transplantation to receive reimbursement for both the LVAD and the transplantation.

The current DRG payments for transplant are in Table 3.

Table 3. FEE SCHEDULE FOR DIAGNOSTIC RELATED GROUPS

Organ	DRG	Payment, $
Heart	103	126 341
Liver	480	63 771
Kidney	302	20 365
Lung	495	57 150

*DRG indicates diagnostic related group.

Medicare Physician Fee Schedule

The physician "?can be either and referred to as either} is based on relative value calculations for the effort and work involved in performing certain services and is known as the resource-based relative value system. Similar to hospital reimbursements, predetermined reimbursements g yes it is the meaning. .} are made for services. Procedures are given CPT codes, and modifiers apply that can alter the reimbursement for the CPT, especially when more than one physician is required for a procedure. Other factors included in the resource-based reimbursement schedule are geographic area and a national conversion factor for the procedure. CPT codes are re-evaluated every 5 years and are required to remain budget neutral. In 2002, reimbursement to kidney transplant surgeons { decreased by reduced 15% {, and reimbursement for liver transplantations decreased9% {[11] {

Summary

During the last 10 years, the transplantation market has changed dramatically. Once a rare procedure, transplantation is now much more commonplace. Living related and non-related donation, as well as extended criteria donors, have increased the supply of available organs while advances in technology have increased demand. Patients have more choices in terms of selecting from a variety of transplant center, which has changed pricing strategies for global contracts and increased competition between patients for organs, as more patients become eligible for transplantation. High-risk transplant cases, extended donor programs, and extended criteria donors all affect transplant economics. In addition, physician and nursing shortages have increased salary expenses. Increased transplant center competition has caused global contract reimbursement to decrease, while transplant center costs increase, as centers compete for scarce resources and manage the overall escalation in healthcare costs with new technologies and therapies. The overall impact is a decline in profitability for transplantation. As contribution margins decrease, profitability reduces. Transplant centers are pressured to offer services more efficiently and effectively to remain viable financially. The business of transplantation should be continuously evaluated as follows:

- Hospital revenues, direct and indirect costs per transplantation
- Physician revenues and costs per transplantation
- Contribution margin to hospital profitability
- Medicare cost report ratio
- Ancillary service revenues.
- Revenue generated through research
- Potential philanthropy to support academic ventures
- Payor mix (percent of commercial versus Medicare versus Medicaid payors) to monitor for changes in reimbursement
- Uninsured losses in which no payments were received, or charity care
- Revenue cycle management, ensuring all charges are captured and paid at the expected rate
- Accurate cost reporting of all transplantation costs
- Monitoring of transplantation-related costs and assessment of all organ acquisition charges.

It is only by considering all of these components that the financial health of a transplant program can be assessed and strategic decisions can be made as to whether to increase transplant services in a given area.

Chapter 5 THE ECONOMICS OF ORGAN DONATION AND TRANSPLANTATION

As reimbursement decreases, transplant centers will be under increasing pressure to reduce costs and streamline services. Innovation and advances in technology and novel therapies are certain to add increased burdens to an already costly enterprise. In addition, the proposed CMS regulations are likely to place additional financial burdens on transplant centers, as centers strive to meet the mandated reporting requirements, process requirements, and re-certification of transplant centers every 3 years. The business of transplantation is one of the most complicated and highly regulated areas of medicine.

References

1. Organ Procurement & Transplantation Manual. Laws, Regulations & Guidelines. National Health Publishing, May 1989 No.4. Reports & Studies. *The Access of Dialysis Patients to Kidney Transplantation.* Health and Human Services Office of the Inspector General, March, 1987. Pages 1392-1394.
2. United States Statutes at Large. *Social Security Amendments of 1972, October, 30, 1972.* Section 2991, e, 3.
3. Organ Procurement & Transplantation Manual. Laws, Regulations & Guidelines. National Health Publishing, May 1989 No.4. Federal Law. *National Organ Transplant Act Public Law 98-507, October 19, 1984.* Pages 2003-2013.
4. Department of Health, Education, and Welfare, Social Security Administration. *Determining Costs Associated With the Renal Disease Provision of Public Law 92-603.* 200 Independence Avenue, S.W., Washington, D.C. 20201 (Renamed U.S. Department of Health and Human Services in 1979): Department of Health, Education, and Welfare, Social Security Administration; 1974. Part A Intermediary letter No. 74-23.
5. United Network for Organ Sharing. Primary source of payment for U.S. transplants: January 1, 1994 to September 30, 1998. United Network for Organ Sharing; Richmond, 1998.
6. Coding Solutions for the Healthcare Industry. Program Memorandum Intermediaries/Carriers. Facility requirements for transplantation centers, transmittal AB-00-95. Available at: http://www.irp.com/refinfo/hcfapm/AB-01-28.htm. Accessed April 9, 2006.
7. Centers for Medicare & Medicaid Services. (2005). Medicare program: hospital conditions of participation: requirements for approval and re-approval of transplant centers to perform organ transplants. Proposed rule CMS-3835-P. 42 CFR Parts 405, 482, and 488. {Federal Register, 70, 23.
8. Centers for Medicare & Medicaid Services. CMS Intermediary Manual. Accessed May 7, 2006 at http://www.cms.hhs.gov/CFCsAndCoPs/11_transplantcenter.asp#TopOfPage.
9. Burke RL. HHS OIG targeting organ transplant services in 2004. *Medicare Report.* Washington, DC: Bureau of National Affairs; 2004.
10. Centers for Medicare & Medicaid Services. Physician fee schedule. Available at: http://www.cms.hhs.gov/physicianfeesched/. Accessed April 9, 2006.
11. Workforce Safety and Insurance. DRG fee schedule. Available at: http://www.workforcesafety.com/medical-providers/managedcare.asp. Accessed May 7, 2006.

The Gift of Tissue and Eye Donation

Scott A. Brubaker, CTBS
Nancy Senst, RN, BSN, CPTC

Family Perspective and Public Understanding

If you turn on the local news, you may hear a story about a family who donated the organs of a loved one and hear about the recipients whose lives had been saved. In contrast, a story on tissue donation is rare, even though it's estimated there are more than 40,000 tissue donors per year compared with 8,000 organ donors. Tissue donation does not seem to provide the high impact that newscasters are looking for to grab listeners' attention. Even when providing public education, donation agencies tend to focus on life-saving organ transplantation, even though some tissue donations (i.e., skin for burn patients, heart valves for pediatric recipients) are life-saving and not restricted to only improving the quality of life. For donor families, their loved ones' gifts of tissue donation are just as important and significant as organ donations are to the families of those donors. The legacy of their mother, father, aunt, uncle, sister, or brother, for example, which may have enhanced the lives of numerous tissue allograft recipients, remains a proud and everlasting testament of good will.

Generally, the public is unaware of where tissue grafts come from or that tissue donation is an option. Ironically, tissue donation is a more common possibility upon death than is organ donation. Of the estimated 1.2 million people who die in hospitals each year, 11,000 to 14,000 of them die in circumstances that allow them to be organ donors, and in contrast, at least 100,000 meet the general criteria for tissue donation.[1] Many times, families are not aware that this option exists until it is presented to them soon after the death of their loved one. This lack of understanding and awareness of tissue donation emphasizes the need for the health care team, which includes you as a transplant professional, to provide an informative dialogue when obtaining authorization or a donor history during the family discussion for tissue donation. This chapter will help prepare you to gain the wealth of knowledge required to be able to share information adequately and answer intuitive questions you may receive during this process.

Historical Overview: Growth and Development

During 2004, organ transplantation celebrated its 50th anniversary. In 1954, the first kidney transplantation was performed in Massachusetts. However, the history of *tissue* donation extends to the third century. Historical records from Catholicism show that the idea for tissue transplantation started around AD 287, when Saints Cosmas and Damian reportedly attempted to transplant the leg of a recently deceased Moor to take the place of the diseased/ulcerated leg of a nobleman (a Roman, Christian verger).[2] In the 1600s, van Meekeren reported good results after a Russian surgeon transplanted bone from a dog's skull to repair a defect in the cranium of a soldier.[3] Possibly, this was the first xenograft; however, it's also reported that the Church ordered removal of the graft (the first explant?). In 1869, Swiss surgeon Jacques Louis Reverdin reportedly began transplanting fresh allograft skin.[4]

The first known official publication of successful human-to-human bone transplantation was authored by Sir William MacEwen in the *Proceedings of the Royal Society of London* in 1881, and it was titled, "Observations Concerning the Transplantation of Bone."[5] The patient was reportedly a 4-year-old boy who had an osteosarcoma removed from his humerus and had the amputated tibia from a donor diagnosed with rickets used as the diaphyseal bone graft replacement. In the early 1900s, Dr. Alexis Carrel became known as the "father of vascular surgery" and, among other transplant discoveries, developed procedures to anastomose vessels, which led to further clinical experimentation.[6] History surrounding the use of allograft heart valves and vascular tissues from deceased persons closely resembles that of organ donation's beginnings in that the first known use of "homograft" tissues for vascular reconstructions was reported in 1948 by Gross.[7] The first successful implants using the human aortic valve were reportedly done in London by Sir Donald Ross and in New Zealand by Sir Brian Barratt-Boyes in 1962.[8]

In 1949, the US Navy established the first true "modern" bone bank.[9] This bank remained the primary tissue bank in the United States for almost 30 years and was under the direction of a physician to whom tissue banking owes much gratitude, George W. Hyatt, MD. Although the primary focus of the Navy was the development of treatments for traumatic blast/burn injuries to personnel injured on the battlefield, their research made significant advances in tissue banking–including the procedures for obtaining consent from families of deceased servicemen and explaining the potential uses of the donated tissues. They were also instrumental in developing the first support services for donor families. The US Navy Tissue Bank pioneered the processing, freeze-drying (lyophilization), and storage methods for allografts that have led to widespread application and further development of these processes today.

Navy researchers began to communicate with those who were creating the early independent tissue banks and exchanged ideas, organized and shared research activities, and improved processes. This interaction resulted in the formation of an association of tissue banks that eventually created ethical guidelines, developed a book of standards, and formalized a tissue bank accreditation program. This voluntary organization was founded in 1976 and was named the American Association of Tissue Banks (AATB). Its set of *Standards for Tissue Banking*[10] preceded federal regulatory oversight and development of tissue banking guidelines worldwide by well over a decade and these guidelines have been used as a basis for rule making, guidance documents, and eventual development of international standards for cell and tissue transplantation.

As allograft use grew, many hospitals established their own bone bank (termed "surgical bone banking"). Bone grafts were stored that originated from patients who had hip replacement/repair procedures–with or without their knowledge/consent or any donor screening or testing being performed. A piece of the excised femoral head or ilium would be placed in the hospital's "living bone bank" and used in future cases as needed. As regional tissue banks formed throughout the United States in the 1970s and 1980s, hospitals/surgeons became aware of the availability of higher quality bone grafts (generally from younger donors or donors without compromised bone quality) supplied through the tissue bank, and surgical bone banking operations began to dwindle throughout the United States. Also, to further the decline of this practice, a transmission of human immunodeficiency virus (HIV) occurred in the mid-1980s that involved the use of "surgical bone," and the cause was determined to be improper screening of the living donor.[11] Through the latter part of the 1980s and into the early 1990s, it was realized that new types and forms of allografts were being made available that could be used for multiple clinical applications and could be stored easily at ambient temperatures. The high maintenance required to house a freezer and the realization of the inherent risks associated with untested/unscreened donors led to a fairly rapid decline in surgical bone banking, which had been estimated to exist at approximately 300 US hospitals.[12] Then, in 1993, with the publication of interim federal regulations that required screening and testing of donors of tissues for transplantation,[13] hospital surgical bone banks that recovered/stored allogeneic bone became nonexistent. Independent, university, and hospital-based tissue banks that screen, recover, process, package, label, store, and distribute a variety of allograft types (eg, bone, soft tissues, skin, veins, and heart valves) emerged.

Of note, the Food and Drug Administration's (FDA's) first concerted efforts in 1993 to broadly regulate human tissues for transplantation (musculoskeletal, skin) began because they intercepted tissues being brokered and offered for export and distribution to the United States from Russia, Eastern Europe, and Central America and South America. Their investigations uncovered a threat to public health because these donors and tissues were not properly screened or tested to prevent transmission of infectious diseases. These federal regulations were never originally intended to provide the comprehensive regulatory oversight like that which has developed during the past 12 years.[1]

The year 2005 marked the 100th anniversary of the first corneal transplant.[14] It took place in Austria (an area that's now the Czech Republic) and was performed by Dr. Eduard Zirm, who restored sight to one eye of a patient who had suffered burns to the eyes a year earlier. Although it was many years later that the first eye bank in the United States opened in New York in 1944, the United States has evolved as the leader of the global eye-banking community. The Eye Bank Association of America (EBAA) was established in 1961 by the American Academy of Ophthalmology's Committee on Eye Banks, which makes the EBAA the oldest national association of transplantation organizations in the country. The EBAA has developed and maintains Medical Standards that are endorsed by the American Academy of Ophthalmology and member eye banks that operate not only in the United States, but also in Canada, England, Italy, Saudi Arabia, Japan, and Taiwan. The EBAA reports that there are more than 40,000 cornea/eye donors annually that result in approximately 46,000 transplants yearly. In addition to the donated cornea, the sclera can also be used for ocular graft surgery in the treatment of cancer and other diseases, so whole-eye donation can help up to 10 patients. More than 10,000 corneal grafts have been exported from the United States to help those in need in foreign countries throughout the world. The EBAA website[14] provides details on all the above information and up-to-date statistics.

Although organ donation has been slow to increase, tissue donation has increased significantly. In 1994, there were less than 10,000 tissue donors (Figure 1). By 2002, this number had grown to approximately 30,000 eye and tissue donors. Organ procurement organizations (OPOs) are also involved in retrieval of tissues, but their recovery activity is not specifically tracked and reported. The AATB requires that AATB-accredited tissue banks participate in an annual survey, which includes tissue donor recovery activities. However, as of 2005, only 25% of the federally designated OPOs had attained accreditation by the AATB, so OPO-specific data on tissue referral, screening, and recovery are not currently being collected or reported. Routine referral legislation in 1998 had a significant effect on the number of potential tissue donors. Through this steady increase, tissue transplants now improve over a million lives annually. Unlike organ transplants, tissue transplants can be performed at most community hospitals, outpatient surgical suites, and medical and dental offices.

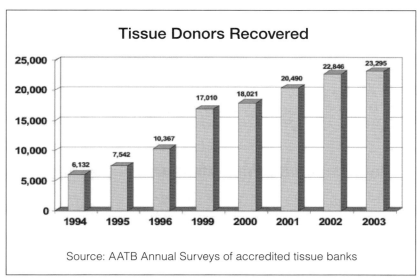

Figure 1. Tissue Banks Accredited by the American Association of Tissue Banks: Tissue Donation in the United States (1994-2003)

Profit and Not-for-Profit Agencies

Federal law prohibits the sale of human organs and tissues; however, organ and tissue banks are allowed to request reasonable payment for expenses associated with the donation of the organ or tissue. There is widespread misunderstanding of the designations of for-profit and not-for-profit companies, especially how this relates to tissue banks and OPOs. These are legal terms that classify and describe an organization's corporate structure, governance, and administration. These terms do not confirm whether or not an organization actually makes a monetary profit. This fact should be realized by transplant clinicians when discussing these issues with donor families. All businesses–for-profit and not-for-profit alike–need to break even financially, or make a profit, to stay in business. A perception, or message often sent to prospective donors and donor families, is that for-profit companies will make a profit from their donation, but not-for-profit firms will not. In the US experience, the term for-profit does not mean that the tissue bank firm actually clears substantial revenue above operating costs[15] that results in dividends paid to shareholders, and the term, not-for-profit does not mean the firm operates with no financial gain at all.[16] Profit experienced by a not-for-profit agency is returned to, or used by, the organization. It would not be distributed to shareholders, which can happen when a for-profit agency makes a profit. The community should benefit from the financial gain experienced by a nonprofit organization, whereas individual stakeholders could gain financially from profits made by a for-profit company.

It's well known that to remain viable, a medical, technology-based organization must make funds available for research and development to explore new possibilities for advanced care. Research and development has been the basis for countless advances in transplantation that continue to improve outcomes of all kinds for both organ and tissue recipients. For-profit pharmaceutical and medical device companies may fund up to 14% of their overall sales for research and development operations.[17] Corporate spending on research and development remains the driving force behind innovation. Not-for-profit tissue banks have strategic alliances and partnerships with for-profit companies to obtain expertise in research and development, to use their marketing capabilities and sales force to increase representation to the end user (i.e., hospital, physician), and/or to offer some financial stability for the near future over the term of such a contractual relationship.

The US health-care system relies largely on private enterprise. It should be understood that some monetary profit is made by all businesses, in this case OPOs and tissue banks, recognizing that those profits are necessary to keep these organizations operating to help the patients who need transplants. It is suggested that consent (authorization) documents additionally include an explanation that multiple organizations may be involved in facilitating the gift, some of which could be nonprofit and/or for profit.[18] To obtain a thorough understanding of what these terms mean in our particular field of practice, transplant clinicians are encouraged to investigate financial statements of the agencies in partnership with the OPO/tissue bank.

International Distribution and Importation

As previously described, thousands of corneas are exported from the United States to many countries to offer the gift of sight. Any tissues for transplantation that are exported have been appropriately screened, tested, and processed like any tissues for transplantation distributed within our national borders. Specific export data for conventional tissue banks in the United States is not tracked because of the multitude of allograft types. It is known that tissue grafts are distributed to more than 30 countries worldwide.[19] This overseas distribution normally involves tissue graft types whose demand in our nation is met, so export to other nations in need is logical. In order to fully meet the expectations of the donation, the gift should be used (maximized) to its fullest extent to help mankind, no matter where the recipients may reside. The potential that the tissue donation could result in transplantation abroad is listed as a suggested additional element of informed consent as described in the "Model Elements of Informed Consent for Organ and Tissue Donation."[18]

Importation of conventional tissue grafts is not tracked and is not likely to occur. Some US tissue banks import unprocessed tissues, process them under contractual arrangements, then return the processed allografts to the country of origin for distribution to countries other than the United States. However, some tissues can be recovered from foreign donors who are screened and tested following appropriate FDA regulations and accreditation standards, sent to the United States to be processed, and distributed.

Increasing Role of the FDA

As mentioned earlier, the FDA interjection into regulating tissue banking in 1993 occurred as a focused response to a specific public health threat.[13] Tissue brokers were identified who were attempting to sell cadavers originating from other countries to tissue banks in the United States.[1] These donors had inadequate medical records, suspicious test results, and were accompanied by questionable blood specimens. This event caused the FDA to respond by publishing an immediate ruling, without public comment, that required certain screening and testing for tissue donation. The authority to do so was referenced to Section 361 of the Public Health Services Act, which authorizes the Secretary of the Department of Health and Human Services to make and enforce such regulations as judged necessary to prevent the introduction, transmission, or spread of communicable diseases from foreign countries into the states or from state to state.[1]

As they began to review past allograft-associated infections and experienced investigations of new infections, FDA oversight grew. Some of the infections reviewed included multiple incidents of transmission of Creutzfeldt-Jakob disease (CJD) recognized during the late 1980s[20] (caused by pooling/commingling of dura mater during processing at a facility based in Germany that exported to the United States) and HIV transmissions originating from a single organ/tissue donor that occurred in 1985 but were identified and reported only years later in 1992.[21] The latter case brought to light 3 shortcomings: (1) the limitations of testing because the donor tested negative for the HIV antibody (identified as anti-HTLV-III at that time), (2) the lack of organized reporting mechanisms to identify infections in organ and tissue recipients, and (3) the difficulty tracing tissues from the hospital (end user) to the recipients.

During the 1990s, the FDA began to notice new allograft problem cases: probable transmission of CJD through cornea/ implantation[22] and the removal and replacement of an allograft heart valve that was contaminated with *Candida albicans*.[23] At the beginning of this decade, more cases involving transplantation were reported, most notably the death of a 23-year-old recipient of an allograft resulting from an elective knee surgery (the allograft was later proven to be contaminated with *Clostridium*)[24]; a West Nile virus infection was thought to have been transmitted via blood and organ donation (no tissue was transplanted from this case)[25]; and HCV transmissions occurred from a single organ/tissue donor to 3 organ recipients and more tissue recipients.[26] Again, in this last case, results of conventional antibody testing were negative, but nucleic acid testing (NAT) performed on an archived donor blood sample revealed a viremic hepatitis C donor.

These and other sentinel events coupled with the knowledge of the rapidly expanding clinical uses for tissue grafts in the United States raised concern. Also, because of advances in tissue processing, it is now possible that there could be 100 tissue recipients from 1 infected donor and public expectation for safety is high.[1] A proposed regulatory approach was announced in 1997 that was described as comprehensive and tiered according to risk.[26] The FDA determined that their authority would include regulations for human cells, tissues, and cellular and tissue-based products (HCT/Ps), defined to encompass these various allograft types: conventional musculoskeletal tissue and skin; ocular tissue such as corneas and sclera; reproductive tissues such as semen and ova; cellular therapies (including therapies derived from adult and embryonic stem cells), hematopoietic stem cells derived from umbilical cord blood or peripheral blood; human heart valves; dura mater; and combination products such as cells combined with a matrix for wound healing.

A final rule and accompanying guidance document was published by the FDA in 1997 that described specific requirements for tissue donor screening and testing for infectious diseases.[27,28] Then, registration and listing became a reality via rules published that described what constitutes a tissue establishment.[29] An entity is considered a "manufacturer" of HCT/Ps if it performs any of the following functions: donor screening, recovery, donor testing, processing, packaging, labeling, storage, or distribution. Subsequent rule making such as the Donor Eligibility Rule[30] and Guidance Document[31] as well as the Current Good Tissue Practices Final Rule[32] and its future Guidance, are all applicable to tissue establishments. Organ procurement agencies can qualify as tissue establishments under the rule, and their personnel are expected to comply with all of the applicable tissue regulations for the functions they perform. These regulations are detailed and require thorough review and implementation as the FDA has the authority to inspect a registered tissue establishment at any time. Tissue associations actively communicate with FDA personnel to clarify interpretations of these comprehensive regulations that became effective on May 25, 2005.

Gift-Specific Donation to Transplantation Details

It is estimated that, as an average, more than 50 people benefit from 1 generous tissue donation. There are many phases of tissue donation that lead to transplantation: consent/authorization, screening, testing (See Table 1), recovery, processing, packaging, labeling, storage, distribution, and ultimately transplantation. Most tissue recovery agencies complete only 1 or some of the early phases; the processing partner generally handles the rest of the process. In turn, tissue processors may either partner with a distributor or have their own marketing team supply the tissue allografts to the end user (eg, hospitals, physicians' offices).

Table 1. INFECTIOUS DISEASE TESTING FOR TISSUE DONATION

Tests required by the Food and Drug Administration
1. anti-HIV-1 and anti-HIV-2
2. HBsAg;
3. anti-HBc–total, meaning IgG plus IgM
4. anti-HCV
5. syphilis test
Additional tests required by the American Association of Tissue Banks
1. HIV-1 NAT
2. HCV NAT
3. anti-HTLV-I and anti-HTLV-II

Abbreviations: HBc, hepatitis B core; HbsAg, hepatitis B surface antigen; HCV, hepatitis C virus; HIV, human immunodeficiency virus; HTLV, human T-lymphotrophic virus; IgG, immunoglobulin G; IgM, immunoglobulin M; NAT, nucleic acid testing.

Sources: References 31 and 10

The overall goals of tissue donation are to:
- maximize the gift of donation to sufficiently meet the clinical need,
- ensure the safety of the allograft,
- support the donor's family throughout the process, as needed, and
- afford respect to the donor.

Musculoskeletal Donation

Other than cornea donation, the most common tissue donated is musculoskeletal tissue, which includes bone and soft tissue (eg, tendons, ligaments, fascia, pericardium). Although some tissue processing is time-sensitive like organ transplantation (ie, allografts offered as fresh, such as fresh skin for burns, wet-stored and refrigerated osteochondrals [bone plus cartilage], and tissues that will be cryopreserved, such as heart valves and vessels), most musculoskeletal tissue processing takes place months after recovery. It can sometimes be a year or more after donation before musculoskeletal allografts are distributed. Usually, preservation methods (ie, cryopreservation, freezing, lyophilization) can extend the expiry of allografts up to 5 years after completion of processing. The tissues recovered and subsequent grafts processed from the donation are dependent on many tissue bank-specific factors: donor age, medical history, tissue quality, the variety of tissue forms that can be produced, and clinical need.

Bone and soft tissues can be recovered from the upper and lower extremities and the pelvis. Individual bones may include the radius, ulna, humerus, femur, tibia, fibula, and ilium or hemipelvis. Some recovery agencies may also recover the scapula, ribs, intercostal cartilage, the mandible, and specific vertebra. Whole joints (knee, ankle) may be recovered intact when there is a specific need. When discussing donation with the family, the donation coordinator may ask if the family has decided what kind of funeral service they anticipate and if the deceased might wear long or short sleeves, or a dress. If the family is having an open casket funeral, upper and lower arm bones may be deferred from recovery depending on the donor's expected funeral attire. Generally, short sleeves worn by the deceased at their open casket funeral would rule out arm recovery options and a planned heart-for-valves donation may not be appropriate if the female donor will wear a dress style that would show this incision. The goal is to ensure that the family can have whatever funeral they desire without the chance that incision lines may show. Alternatively, if the consenting person wishes to donate all possible tissues and the donor's attire can be flexible, necessary pathways of the incisions can be explained and the clothing styles needed to cover them could be discussed. Whatever discussions take place, the decisions that are made must be communicated to the personnel who will perform the recovery of the tissues. Regardless of the type of funeral planned, the body is reconstructed after the recovery.

Soft/connective tissue is usually recovered only if consent/authorization is also given for bone. Generally, the same incision that is made for bone recovery is used for soft-tissue recovery. Except for fascia lata (the tissue that covers the thigh muscle) and specific tendons, connective tissue grafts typically are recovered with bone on one or each end, which can be fashioned for use to anchor the graft into place when implanted. Advances in sports medicine surgery have steadily increased the need for connective tissue grafts. In general, people are now more active in fitness activities than ever before and want their injuries repaired so they may return to the same active lifestyle to which they were accustomed before the injury. Soft tissues that are routinely recovered include tendons (eg, posterior and anterior tibialis, gracilis, semitendinosus, and Achilles), patellar ligaments, fascia lata, pericardium, and rotator cuffs (of the shoulder socket).

As each musculoskeletal tissue is recovered, the gifts are cultured and individually dry-wrapped by using sterile bags and moisture barriers. After each tissue is properly labeled, it is then placed on wet ice in a qualified, insulated box, labeled as quarantined, and transported to the tissue processor via priority shipping (same-day or next-day). Upon receiving the tissue, the processor either processes time-sensitive tissues (osteochondrals, fresh tissues, tissue to be cryopreserved) or places the tissue in quarantine freezers until all records, including autopsy reports, and blood and tissue culture results are reviewed for suitability by technical personnel and the medical director. In this latter scenario, it may take from 3 to 6 months before the tissue is released to a plan for processing.

To prevent cross contamination, each donor is processed separately. Pooling of tissues from different donors is not allowed.[10,32] The tissue is usually cleansed/treated with various solutions to remove adventitious agents (microorganisms, viruses) as well as lipids and bone marrow elements (such as red blood cells and leukocytes). The processing rooms offer a controlled, monitored environment to reduce the potential for contamination and cross-contamination. Specially trained technicians must wear appropriate attire in these rooms, and the air is circulated through high-efficiency particulate air (HEPA) filters to maintain a controlled environment. The bone and soft tissues are processed into specific forms and freeze-dried or processed as frozen, all of which is dependent on the quality of the donor's individual tissues and the clinical need for specific graft types. Advancements in tissue-processing methods and how allografts are shaped and constructed allow a variety of possibilities for uses of the donated tissues. Current requests of the end users are constantly monitored so that processing plans coincide with clinical need.

Preprocessing cultures for each tissue being recovered are mandatory per AATB's standards.[10] However, some culture techniques (ie, swab cultures) are not highly specific or sensitive, so it can be difficult to assess bioburden.[33] Also, irradiation treatments of various dosages may be used to pretreat musculoskeletal tissues to reduce or eliminate the level of bioburden at processing. Irradiation is also being used in low doses after processing to ensure the safety of the graft. Tissue processors have developed in-process and end-process culturing methods that are sensitive and verified not to be prone to interfering substances that could cause a false-negative culture result. Validated processes that ensure a sterile allograft have also been developed and are in use today. Using input from a variety of tissue banking experts, the AATB developed and published guidance that offers methods to control contamination and cross-contamination at recovery,[33] which can obviate taking more drastic measures at processing (ie, irradiation treatments).

When tissues (ie, any tissue type) have reached the end of the many stages of processing and testing, records are thoroughly reviewed by responsible experts to ensure that established technical parameters have been met. The detailed donor suitability review, which contains all relevant medical records, is performed by quality assurance personnel and ultimately completed by the tissue bank's medical director.[10] Only then are tissues labeled and sent from quarantined inventory to released inventory for distribution.

The final phase of the tissue process is distribution. In this final step, the tissue is returned to the community for the recipient. Allografts may be distributed by a recovering tissue bank, the processor, or a third party. The distributor could also be an intermediary who hospitals call with a specific need. The intermediary places calls to various processors until the hospital's order is filled. Some tissues are distributed through a partnership between the processor and a medical device company.

Hospitals and surgery centers may maintain a preferred vendor status with a tissue processor that offers them priority access to specific allografts. If the hospital partners with a tissue recovery agency that supplies tissue to the processor from whom they receive the grafts, the hospital may receive additional priority. Through this donor-user loop, special grafts that are frequently scarce (eg, those used in sports medicine or neurosurgery) can be more readily available for the hospitals where tissue donations and recoveries also occur.

In the past, distributors worked with surgeons to provide them with grafts that best met their patients' needs. It is now becoming more common that tissue provider agreements are placed out for bid through a hospital's materials management department. Regardless of tissue provider agreements, if hospitals need grafts, they will work with the processor/distributor who can provide them with what they need. Table 2 lists the types of specialties that use allografts. More hospitals are requiring that vendors who supply tissues meet specific qualifications, such as providing evidence of their registration with FDA, state tissue banking licenses held, as well as their certificates proving AATB or EBAA accreditation.

Table 2. SURGICAL SPECIALTIES THAT USE ALLOGRAFTS

Spine:	**Hand Surgery:**
Cervical Fusion (anterior and posterior)	Fusions
Multi-level Cervical Fusion	Carpal Fractures
Lumbar Fusion (anterior and posterior)	Distal Radius/ulna Fractures
	Metacarpal Fractures
General Orthopedics :	
Osteo Defects	**Foot/Ankle Surgery:**
Acetabular Repair	Metatarsal Osteotomy
Total Joint Revisions	Fusions
	Metatarsal Fractures
Sports Medicine:	Talus/Malleolar Fractures
Osteochondral Defects	
Anterior Cruciate Ligament Repair	**Dental :**
Soft Tissue Reattachment	Periodontal Surgery
Meniscal Transplantation	
Ostoechondral Transplantation	**Urology**:
	Bladder Neck Suspension
Oncology:	
Tumor Resection	**Specialty:**
Large Graft Matching	Bone grafts, eg, femurs or whole joint
Joint Transplant	- grafts matched patient specific

(Source: www.mtf.org. Reprinted with permission from MTF)

Tissue establishments are required to maintain records for 10 years after the last date of expiration, distribution, or utilization, whichever is latest.[10,32] All association standards and federal regulations require that there be a unique or distinct donor identification system in place so that tissues can be traced from the donor to the end-user and vice versa. The end user is responsible for tracing the allografts to the recipients who benefit from them. Those entities that maintain accreditation by the Joint Council on Accreditation of Healthcare Organizations (JCAHO) are required to keep records that permit the traceability of all tissues from the donor or source facility to all recipients or other final disposition.[34] AATB-accredited tissue banks who distribute cells and/or tissues must also establish protocols for collection of follow-up data on recipients.[10]

Skin Donation

Donated skin is recovered as either split thickness or full thickness grafts. Split thickness grafts are generally regarded as one of the life-saving tissues because it can be used to cover severe burns to decrease the chance of infection and to assist with fluid retention. Although the overall criteria for skin donation are the same as for musculoskeletal donation, the recovery team assesses each donor's skin integrity for abrasions/trauma, moles, or tattoos; then a final decision is made to recover skin, or not. Skin is usually recovered before other tissues that have been consented/authorized for donation.

After the team assesses the skin, the area is prepped and shaved. Skin can be recovered from the donor's back, abdomen, and the posterior and anterior surfaces of the legs. Mineral oil is usually used to lubricate the dermatome blade and skin surface area to glide the dermatome across the skin. After the skin is carefully removed, it's placed in a container for culturing and rinsing, then placed in media containing antibiotics, properly labeled, and shipped to the processor on wet ice under quarantine status.

Skin can be conventionally processed as fresh or cryopreserved. Surgeons determine the applications for which they will use the various skin allografts that are made available to them. Preferences are based on their experiences and patients' needs. For instance, some surgeons believe that fresh skin adheres to the wound better and hastens revascularization of the area; however, fresh skin has a relatively short refrigerated shelf life (about 7-14 days),[10] which makes it difficult to maintain a supply at the burn center. Fresh skin presents a higher level of risk management for its use because it must be released before final cultures and autopsy results are available. For many reasons, shortages of cryopreserved skin for burn use in the United States can occur. Fresh skin is much more difficult to provide continuously.

When the skin arrives at the tissue bank processor for conventional processing, it is maintained refrigerated and typically processed within 1 or 2 days. Initially, the skin is rinsed and agitated in isotonic solutions to remove any residual fluid, dirt, or shaved hair. It is examined for uniformity of thickness (standard thickness is 12-18/1000th of an inch) and width. It is also assessed for excessive hair, moles, scars, and tattoos. Measurements can differ from processor to processor, but as an example, the skin can be spread on a fine mesh gauze (sterile) and trimmed into segments of 3 in. x 8 in. (7.62 cm x 20.32 cm) and 2 inches x 8 inches (5.08 cm x 20.32 cm, or approximately 1/6 square foot). It is covered again with the same type of mesh, then allowed to equilibrate with isotonic sodium chloride solution amended to include 10% glycerol, which helps protect the skin during cryopreservation. After this, each measured piece can be arranged, folded in half, and placed in a foil package. The package is then sealed and control-rate frozen by using the heat-sink method or a computer-controlled process. The cryopreserved skin usually has a shelf life of 5 years and is shipped to the end user at dry ice temperatures.

Most burn centers have an agreement with a skin processor outlining annual usage by the square foot and maintenance of an inventory achieved. Generally, fresh skin is less expensive for the burn center than cryopreserved skin because there is less processing involved. Skin allografts can be prioritized for the regions where recovery of skin takes place; however, the method in which skin is recovered by the recovery agency determines what skin allograft types (eg, for burn use or otherwise) the processor can provide.

According to the American Burn Association,[35] skin grafts are used for burn victims and those in need of reconstructive surgery. Unfortunately, 1 million people are burned annually. There are approximately 700,000 emergency room visits resulting in around 45,000 hospitalizations, with 6% of these patients dying while in burn units. In addition, 5,000 people will require reconstructive procedures. These recipients have suffered second- and third-degree (partial and full thickness) burns over much of their body. These life-saving grafts protect these victims from infection and fluid loss. Allograft skin used for burns is a temporary covering that will reject and slough after 10 to 20 days. The grafts stimulate blood supply to the area and allow the patient to heal until autografts can be recovered and applied in their place.

Full thickness skin grafts can be used for reconstructive surgery. Some processing methods remove the cellular components and remnants of the skin to produce an acellular matrix that can be packaged as layers or cryofractured and supplied as injectable allografts. For skin allografts used for reconstructive surgery, the processing steps remove the epidermis and the cells that can lead to rejection and graft failure without decreasing the overall integrity of the skin. When used in various applications, the biological components that remain in some decellularized skin allografts allow the body to heal itself. These types of grafts can be used for surgeries such as abdominal wall reconstruction, breast reconstruction after mastectomy, surgeries on the bladder, and plastic reconstructions of the head and neck.[36]

Veins and Arteries

Vein and artery grafts can provide hope to recipients to salvage their limb or provide relief from angina. Donor vessel criteria are similar to criteria for other tissue types except that some processors accept only male donors, may have more defined donor age limitations, and may have restrictions that allow only certain donor blood types. Vessels are matched with recipients by blood type, although such matching is not proven to affect outcome. Females are not optimal vessel donors because the lumen size of the veins and arteries of the legs are smaller than in men. Small lumen size can adversely affect patency rates in recipients.

The same incision is used for recovery of the greater saphenous vein as is used for the recovery of bone and connective tissue. The vessels are usually recovered first after this incision is made. After prepping the leg, anatomic landmarks are used to identify the greater saphenous vein to cannulate it distally. The vein is then gently flushed with a room-temperature tissue culture medium or an isotonic solution that is amended with a smooth muscle relaxant (ie, papaverine). Some processors additionally prefer that the perfusion solution include an anticoagulant such as sodium heparin. In any case, it is of extreme importance to use these solutions only after they have reached room temperature. Use of chilled perfusion solution or transport solution can damage the endothelial lining of the vessels and lead to early occlusion or aneurysm after implantation into a future recipient. Time limitations for perfusion of vessels is currently 12 hours from asystole but some variances have been approved that allow perfusion up to 24 hours past asystole as long as established body cooling parameters were also met.

After the vessel is gently perfused, it is surgically removed using a no-touch technique, which leaves approximately 1 cm of adipose and connective tissue surrounding the length of the vessel. This practice decreases the potential to inadvertently nick the vessel during recovery and avoids pulls on the vessel and its tributaries that can damage the vascular wall. After recovery, the vessel is again gently rinsed with room-temperature perfusion or transport solution. It is then placed in a sterile plastic jar with room-temperature media amended with papaverine, the lid is screwed on, and this bundle is doubled bagged to maintain a sterile packaging system. It is labeled appropriately, then placed on wet ice in a qualified, insulated box to gradually chill the grafts. This box is priority shipped (same day or overnight) under quarantine status to the processor.

When the vessels arrive at the processor, the box and contents are examined for acceptable temperature and package integrity. Processing begins soon after receipt, as time limitations apply to vessels. Preprocessing cultures are obtained before the vessels are submitted to antibiotic-containing fluids. A filter-culturing technique is widely used for this tissue type. This technique has an increased sensitivity over swabbing methods because it allows both qualitative and quantitative identification of microorganisms that may be present. Sized, representative tissue samples are also used for cultures.

During processing, the vessels are carefully examined and some adventitial layer is surgically removed. Any noted nicks or clots will shorten the graft. Long vessel grafts are desired because they can be used in more clinical application scenarios and can avoid use of 2 segments to complete the clinically needed length. Vessels are processed in a Class 100 clean room environment as required by AATB standards,[10] and processing must be completed within 48 hours of asystole. After a validated disinfection period, the processed vessels are rinsed and final cultures are obtained. The grafts are then individually packaged with a cryoprotectant media, placed in a freezing chamber, and subjected to a cooling rate of approximately 1°C/min using bursts of liquid nitrogen. This cooling is controlled by a specific computer program that has been established by the processor. Programs are designed to compensate for the latent heat of fusion that occurs just below the freezing point of the vessel tissue. At this point, heat is released from the tissue when it freezes. Rapid cooling of the chamber is required to maintain a steady cooling/freezing rate of the tissue. The end point for the cryopreservation program is at approximately −40°C or below, after which placement and storage is at liquid nitrogen vapor temperatures (colder than −100°C but warmer than −196°C). Package expiration dates have historically been set at 5 years unless validations prove otherwise. Surgery departments may contact the processor when they have a patient with a need, or this type of graft may frequently be ordered as needed to replenish an inventory that is maintained in an ultracold, liquid nitrogen freezer at the hospital. These cryopreserved tissues must be shipped and stored at temperatures colder than −100°C.[10]

Cryopreserved vessel allografts are used when the patient has no suitable autologous veins or arteries and when a graft is needed for placement into an infected field (eg, synthetic bypass graft has become infected). The allografts are carefully removed from ultracold storage, allowed to warm briefly for a few minutes at room temperature, and then quickly thawed for use. Quick thawing is desirable, followed by serial dilution of the cryoprotectant. Surgeons typically use these grafts for peripheral artery bypass applications and less often for coronary bypass. In the heart, the grafts replace coronary arteries that provide blood to the heart muscle. In the leg, when the patient's own arteries are blocked because of atherosclerotic disease or blood clots, or if a synthetic bypass graft has failed or become infected, allograft may be selected to attempt to save the patient from limb amputation. Vessels such as femoral veins and arteries may also be used as shunts for dialysis access. Long-term allograft vessel patency is not expected; however, allografts can successfully be used with other therapies that result in limb salvage.

Heart Valves/Conduits

The recovery of the heart specifically for valves may occur during the recovery of other tissues or immediately after procedures for recovery of solid organs. In organ donation cases, there are times when the heart may not be medically suitable for whole-heart transplantation but it may still be used for valve donation. In both instances, the entire heart is aseptically recovered to prevent contamination. Cardiectomy procedures are also designed to avoid damage to the valves during retrieval. It is important to remember that recovery of sufficient outflow tract lengths (of the ascending aorta and pulmonary arteries) is critical to a successful cardiectomy performed for valve donation. A heart that has been recovered with little or no outflow tracts, like that which is usually done for orthotopic heart transplantation, renders the valves unusable to a cardiac surgeon. Implantation of the allograft valve with its outflow tract is crucial to successful outcomes for recipients.

When the heart-for-valves donor is not also a solid organ donor, the incision that is made is similar to one performed for an autopsy that includes the thoracic cavity. This takes the shape of a "V" and decreases the chance that the incision might be seen during a funeral viewing. It also provides good exposure of the heart during the recovery. Otherwise, a median sternotomy is made and chest retractors are used to expose the pericardium, the heart, and its outflow tracts. The pericardium is carefully incised and reflected to establish a working field for the cardiectomy. After careful blunt and sharp dissection to expose and recover adequate lengths of the aorta and right and left pulmonary arteries, the heart is carefully rinsed several times with isotonic, sterile solutions in an effort to remove blood from all 4 chambers. The heart is then placed in a sterile bag, totally immersed in a fresh, sterile isotonic solution, excess air is expressed out, and the bag is knot-tied closed. This bundle is then labeled and placed in a sterile plastic jar, the lid is closed securely, and the jar is then bagged, closed, and labeled. The bagged jar is placed in a qualified, insulated box with sufficient amounts of wet ice, labeled as quarantined, and expedited by same-day or overnight shipment to the processor.

As with vessels described earlier, when the heart arrives at the processor, the box and contents are examined for acceptable temperature and package integrity. Processing begins as soon as possible because time limitations apply. Cardiac tissues are also processed in a Class 100 clean room environment as required by AATB standards[10] and processing must be completed within 48 hours of asystole. Preprocessing cultures are obtained before the cardiac grafts are submitted to antibiotic-containing fluids. A filter-culturing technique is widely used for this tissue type. This method has an increased sensitivity over swabbing methods and allows qualitative and quantitative identification of microorganisms that may be present. Sized, representative tissue samples are also used for culturing. The aortic valve and the pulmonary valve, both with their outflow tracts, are dissected free from the heart. During processing, the valves are carefully examined and only superficial adventitia is removed, with care not to excise too much of this supportive tissue. Conduit-use-only cardiac tissue grafts can be produced from the pulmonary outflow tract (pieces cut from the main pulmonary artery trunk as well as from bilateral pulmonary artery branches) and the ascending, transverse, or thoracic aorta, if sufficient lengths are recovered.

The valves and/or conduit grafts are then sized, quality observations are documented, and then the valves or grafts are placed into a disinfection solution. After a validated disinfection period, the grafts are rinsed and final cultures are obtained. The grafts are then individually packaged with a cryoprotectant media, placed in a freezing chamber, and subjected to a cooling rate of approximately 1°C/min by using bursts of liquid nitrogen. This cooling is controlled by a specific computer program that has been established by the processor. Programs are designed to offer a steady rate of freezing, which includes compensating for the latent heat of fusion that occurs just below the freezing point of the tissue. At this point, heat is released from the tissue when it freezes. Rapid cooling of the chamber is required to maintain a steady cooling/freezing rate of the tissue. The end point for the cryopreservation program is at approximately −40°C, after which placement and storage is at liquid nitrogen vapor temperatures (colder than −100°C but warmer than −196°C). Package expiration dates have historically been set at 5 years unless validations prove otherwise.

If requested by the medical examiner/hospital pathologist who is performing the autopsy of the donor, the heart tissue remaining after dissection can be returned for further examination, or a gross and microscopic examination of the heart can be performed and reported to them. The processor can provide dissection observations, microscopic slides of the myocardium, and digital photographs of the gross heart, as well as providing return of the archived remnants of the heart if desired.

This cryopreservation process allows a surgical center to develop a "valve bank," where valves of different sizes can be stored, providing a choice for surgeons. Active cardiac surgery programs may have a liquid nitrogen freezer at their hospital that holds an inventory of cryopreserved allograft valves so they are readily available for cases. After the cardiac surgeon determines that an allograft valve is the best option for a patient, the surgeon will request a specific valve size, or a range of sizes (sized by internal annulus, measured in millimeters) to be available for the surgery. An idea of the size that will be needed is determined by echocardiography. The suitable valve size will be confirmed after the chest has been opened and the recipient's annulus is measured or the appropriate size needed for reconstruction is determined (ie, for a child). Surgeons will typically transplant the largest valve possible in a child so that function will adapt as the child grows. In adults, large valve sizes are most often requested due to of the cardiomegaly caused by their disease process.

The aortic and pulmonary valves are used for replacement of a diseased native valve or to construct a missing valve (ie, hypoplastic left heart) and/or outflow tract. The nonvalved pulmonary conduit from the pulmonary artery, or conduit tissue from the aorta, can also be used as a patch or tube for pediatric and adult reconstructions. Typically, recipients of cryopreserved allograft cardiac tissue may include women of child-bearing age, active adults, children born with heart defects, and patients with infective endocarditis. The benefits and disadvantages of allograft valves are shown in Table 3.

Depending on the recipient's age and specific cardiac anomalies, allograft heart valve/conduit applications may be part of a staged, palliative plan. The patient may require a second allograft replacement/reconstruction later in life.

Table 3. BENEFITS AND DISADVANTAGES OF ALLOGRAFT HEART VALVES

Benefits

Good Durability
- 10- to 20-year experience with allograft valves
- Freedom from catastrophic structural deterioration

Low Complications
- Low incidence of endocarditis
- Low risk of thromboembolic events
- No need for anticoagulation therapy

Excellent Hemodynamics
- Low pressure gradients across a large effective orifice area
- "Designed by God" (quote: Sir Donald Ross – homograft valve pioneer)

Disadvantages

Availability
- Dependence on the number of donated hearts
- Specific sizes are in high demand, especially pediatric sizes and very large adult sizes

Relatively difficult to implant (technically)
- No supportive stent or sewing ring
- Potential for long cross-clamp time
- Potential for less than perfect result

Reference: Hopkins RA. Cardiac Reconstructions with Allograft Valves. Secaucus, NJ: Springer-Verlag, 1989. Reprinted with permission.

The Referral Process

In 1998 the Center for Medicare/Medicaid Services changed the hospital "Conditions of Participation" to ensure that every deceased patient was assessed for organ and tissue donation and that donation is discussed with the family by a trained requestor (at 42 CFR 482.45(a)(3)). The goal of the Center for Medicare/Medicaid Services was to increase donation by 20% in the next 2 years. Although organ donation did not immediately experience substantial increases, tissue donation did. It is estimated by AATB-accredited tissue banks that tissue donation activity increased by 62% after the Conditions of Participation were instituted.[1]

Patients who die outside of a hospital setting still have the opportunity to donate eye, bone, cardiac, vascular, and soft tissues. Tissue recovery agencies routinely partner with medical examiners' offices and funeral homes as referral sources. This partnership provides more donors and families with the donation option and more tissue allografts provided to the community. This relationship also builds an understanding of each other's role in caring for a family after the death of a loved one, supporting the family's options and decisions. In areas where no referral process is made available for certain death situations, the funeral home may be the only avenue to offering the donation option to the family of a deceased person who may have expressed the wish to be a donor. These scenarios exist when death occurs outside of a hospital setting, when the death is not unexpected, or when it is due to natural causes (results in no medical examiner involvement).

As stated, hospitals are mandated by the Center for Medicare and Medicaid Services to refer every death to the OPO. If the OPO does not have an agreement with the hospital for tissue donation and organ donation is not an option, the OPO must refer the potential donor to the tissue agency or agencies with which the hospital has a signed agreement. Typically a triage service takes the initial death call from the hospital. Very basic information is requestd to complete the initial assessment. The triage service then has the option to:

1. Page the organ donation coordinator for a potential organ donor,

2. Determine that the donor may qualify as a tissue and /or eye donor,
3. Rule out donation of conventional tissue but forward the call to the Eye Bank for possible cornea/eye donation,
4. Determine that the donor is ineligible for all tissue donation because of established criteria, or
5. Continue with an advanced assessment and discuss donation with the family as appropriate.

In the secondary assessment, very specific questions about the patient's current and past medical history are addressed. The length of the secondary assessment screening depends on the complexity of the patient's medical history and the length of the hospital stay. Questions surrounding the patient's body temperature, findings on chest radiographs, white blood cell counts (WBCs), and diagnoses are all essential to evaluate whether an infectious process might be present. Colloid, blood, and crystalloid intake is assessed in an effort to calculate plasma dilution. If a diluted blood sample is collected for testing, the infectious disease test results may be false-negative. During this assessment phase, the tissue recovery team works closely with the hospital staff and must communicate well with the funeral home director to ensure a hold is placed on the body so it is not retrieved and embalmed before the discussion of donation with the family has occurred and/or the recovery is scheduled. Communication and coordination with the local medical examiner/coroner is also warranted, when applicable.

The Request

In many states, donor designation, the documented wish of a person to donate, is assessed before donation is discussed with the next of kin. Most conversations about tissue donation occur via telephone rather than in person. After it is determined that the decedent is a potential donor, the nurse is asked to connect the family with the tissue recovery agency for the donation discussion. The family's cooperation is critical. If the family leaves the hospital, a phone number where they can be reached must be obtained. Even if donor designation is present, the recovery should not proceed without obtaining the past medical history and behavioral risk assessment information from a knowledgeable source.

If donor designation is present, the nurse will be asked to tell the family:

Your loved one has documented wishes to be a donor; the donation coordinator can help you fulfill your loved one's final wish to be a donor. You can discuss this opportunity with the donation coordinator immediately or in a few hours.

If no donor designation exists, the nurse will be asked to tell the family:

Your loved one has the opportunity to help others through tissue and eye donation. You can discuss this opportunity with the donation coordinator immediately or after you get home.

The tissue recovery agency will speak with the family, usually using a recorded line, and complete the authorization or disclosure (if donor designation is in place) form. The elements of consent are discussed with the family, including benefits of donation, funeral decisions, and timing. After the form is completed, the tissue recovery agency will complete an extensive medical/social history assessment with the family or the most suitable historian. The entire family call may last approximately 45 minutes. (See AATB's *Model Elements of Informed Consent*[18] and the National Donor Family Council/National Kidney Foundation position statement on tissue donation[37]).

After the family discussion, the tissue recovery agency will contact a tissue processor for final assessment of donor eligibility. The patient's hospital course, past medical history, and behavioral risk assessment will be reviewed. The processor will then determine whether or not the case will be accepted. If there are questions surrounding the history, more information may be requested from the hospital staff, or the processor's medical director may be requested to review the available information. If questions cannot be resolved, the donor may be deemed ineligible. If donation is ruled out, the tissue recovery agency will notify the family, the medical examiner, and the funeral home, as needed.

Medical History and Behavioral Risk Assessment

History of the Process

During the early years of organ transplantation, the review of the past history of the donor focused more on the donor's medical history and the clinical effect this might have on kidney function. Later, the focus was on how this history could affect performance of other organs as they began to be successfully transplanted. However, the donor history perspective evolved in a different direction with the emergence of HIV in the 1980s and transmission of this infection[21,38,39] and other infectious diseases from organ and/or tissue donors to recipients.[40-47] During the latter half of that decade and into the early 1990s, behavioral risk assessment for organ/tissue donors began to mimic the medical and social history screening required for blood donation in the United States.[48-55]

Today, a donor's medical history and its effect on the functional quality of organs for transplantation is still a consideration, but social risk behavior can now designate a donor as high risk for transmitting a communicable disease and results in a determination that the donor as ineligible for tissue donation. Infectious disease testing has improved in the past decade, but various window periods continue to exist for each disease screened by testing (ie, donor is infectious during this time frame but the screening test for the disease agent is negative). Testing methods (enzyme-linked immunosorbent assay, enzyme immunoassay, NAT, flocculation/precipitation) used in the available screening test kits that are approved, cleared, or licensed by FDA vary regarding their expected specificity and sensitivity that measures their ability to detect the disease marker for which they were developed. For these reasons, a potential tissue donor is determined ineligible if, after review of relevant medical records, the history suggests that the donor's behavior or treatments qualify as high risk. For cell and/or tissue donation, a positive determination of high risk by history overrides negative screening test results because of the possibility of the presence of an infectious disease agent that is undetectable by testing.

Since 1993 with the publication of the *Interim Rule for Donors of Human Tissues for Transplantation*,[13] the FDA has mandated not only screening tissue donors by testing for specific infectious diseases, but also screening for behaviors associated with communicable disease risk. The FDA risk criteria for donors of cells and tissues have been updated in subsequent publications of rules[27,30] and guidance.[28,31] In contrast, the only recommendation (screening for HIV risk) published for *organ* donors dates back to 1994.[56] Although this was a landmark publication and is still referenced in part today, the behavioral risk criteria listing has evolved and has been updated. In consultation with the Centers for Disease Control and Prevention and other FDA offices within the Center for Biological Evaluation and Research, the FDA officially updates through regulatory publications aimed at cell and tissue donor screening. The AATB maintains *Standards for Tissue Banking*[10] that have been updated with these evolving regulations. Historically, questionnaires are individually formulated by OPOs and tissue banks to meet federal regulations as well as their own unique needs. Although there is some uniformity to the questions, there remain many individualized approaches to this process. To most effectively meet the needs of all parties involved with the questionnaire (the interviewer, historian(s), and the entity determining eligibility/suitability for tissue release for transplantation), future questionnaires will need to contain transplant-industry approved questions that have been validated/qualified so that the information recorded is understood, applicable, and as complete and accurate as possible when relying on a historian other than the donor.

The Interview

The need to place strong emphasis on the importance of obtaining accurate past and current medical history and behavioral risk information to aid in the determination of tissue donor eligibility has never been more evident. Completing the questionnaire, obtained by interview mostly by telephone and sometimes in person, serves as documentation of the donor risk assessment interview, and is but one part of the process that must be followed to help ensure the safety of tissues for transplantation.

This significant step normally occurs near the beginning of the donor screening process. The answers from the next of kin or others will make the difference between an eligible or ineligible determination, or will suggest the need to obtain further information. The relationship of the historian(s) selected for the donor risk assessment interview must be documented and the individual or individuals should be selected who are able to provide the information sought in the interview.[12] For example, this may be the donor (if living), the legal next of kin, the nearest available relative, a member of the donor's household, other individual with an affinity relationship (caretaker, friend, significant life partner), and/or the primary treating physician.[30] The relevant social history includes questions to elicit whether or not the donor met certain descriptions or engaged in certain activities or behaviors that are considered to place potential donors at increased risk for a relevant communicable disease agent or disease (RCDAD).

The interviewer must be familiar with the purpose of each question and when to expand the questioning to gather relevant, detailed information. For each question or disease process, the interviewer should be aware of conditions that might lead to automatic rule out (eg, risks associated with RCDADs), and the interviewer should be able to recognize when contact with the donor's primary care physician, or when a different donor historian, may be required. The questionnaire should be administered by someone skilled in interviewing techniques who can be empathetic, supportive and respectful under the difficult circumstances of these interviews.

It is the responsibility of each OPO or tissue banking organization to determine what procedures are necessary to help ensure the safety of transplantable tissues and to keep abreast of government regulations related to screening tissue donors for risk behaviors. RCDADs are potentially infectious microorganisms, viruses, or other disease agents that may pose a risk of transmission to recipients of, or persons who come in contact with, cells and/or tissues. To be qualified as such, these disease agents/diseases should be significantly prevalent in the potential donor population. These diseases can cause life-threatening conditions, result in permanent impairment, necessitate medical or surgical interventions, and can cause death. They can also result from accidental or intentional release into the population (ie, bioterrorism, biological laboratory accident). Currently, RCDADs applicable to all cell and/or tissue donors include (but are not limited to) HIV-1 and HIV-2, hepatitis B virus, hepatitis C virus (HCV), human transmissible spongiform encephalopathies, syphilis, communicable disease risks associated with xenotransplantation, severe acute respiratory syndrome, West Nile virus, vaccinia, and sepsis. Donors of viable, leukocyte-rich cells and/or tissues must additionally consider the infectious potential of HTLV I/II and cytomegalovirus, and donors of reproductive cells and/or tissues must be screened and tested for *Chlamydia trachomatis* and *Neisseria gonorrhea*.[31]

Recovery

Review of Relevant Medical Records

Prior to tissue recovery, a thorough review of available, relevant medical records is performed. Upon donor referral, some basic information is collected but if donation is pursued, this verbal referral information must be verified and expanded by review of medical records before recovery. After authorization or disclosure for donation is completed, the investigation to determine donor suitability continues. Information is collected using the medical history and behavioral risk assessment questionnaire by interviewing a knowledgeable historian as well as reviewing all current clinical course records, which could contain valuable information regarding suitability for donation. The information that is available before recovery can vary from none to an entire medical record from a lengthy hospital admission. These documents can be photocopied and forwarded for the donor record file or significant/relevant information can be transcribed onto a well-designed form that is ultimately used by a tissue bank medical director to review the donor's suitability.

Federal regulations, as well as AATB[10] and EBAA[57] standards, require that this information be sought, and pertinent records should be shared with all tissue establishments that are involved with receiving any of the tissues recovered from the donor.[32] Relevant medical information can be found in records produced by the: ambulance service, emergency department, surgery, clinical laboratory, x-ray, medical examiner, and so on. If performed, the transcription of the patient's admission history and physical should be located and reviewed. If indicated, contact with the donor's primary care physician may be necessary to better understand specific medical or behavioral history information or treatments.

A thorough physical assessment of potential tissue donors is required by federal regulations[30,31] and industry standards.[10,57] This assessment must be done by a responsible (authorized, qualified, and trained) person before recovery, and all findings must be documented. Physical assessment of tissue donors is a significant step in the donor eligibility process. Staff training and evaluation of competency is mandatory. A physical examination/assessment of the donor may yield findings that indicate infection with, or high-risk behavior for, HIV or hepatitis, or these observations may alert recovery personnel to signs related to other active communicable diseases (ie, sepsis, vaccinia, trauma/infection) that can affect donor eligibility. The list of required signs to look for includes the following: jaundice, genital lesions, enlarged lymph nodes, recent tattooing/body piercing, white spots in the mouth (thrush), nonmedical injection sites (injection drug use) with a focus on inspection within tattoos, enlarged liver (hepatomegaly), perianal lesions and/or insertion trauma (evidence of anal intercourse), generalized rash, scabs, skin lesions (nongenital), blue or purple spots or lesions (can appear gray or black postmortem) that may be signs of Kaposi's sarcoma, trauma, or infection of potential retrieval sites, and abnormal ocular findings (eg, icterus, corneal scarring from vaccinia infection–smallpox).[31] Any suspect findings must be investigated. The AATB offers a best practices procedure and format for documenting the physical assessment process,[58] and the Association of Organ Procurement Organizations (AOPO) suggests that members use this sample form and standard operating procedure as an example of a best practice and as a useful resource.

Technical Recovery Practices

The procedures employed and the specific equipment used by agencies to recover various donated tissues can differ, but common goals among them also exist. Proper recovery of tissues to minimize the potential for contamination and cross-contamination (which includes following sterile technique) as well as recovering tissues without making extraction errors that could damage the tissue are 2 such goals. Tissue processing banks monitor the performance of their contracted recovery agencies by tracking and trending these outcomes via use of established indicators. This quality systems approach uses benchmarking to set levels of performance expectation and help identify areas that would require focused training or retraining to raise proficiency. Performance monitoring can include positive recovery culture rates, technical recovery errors (related to cardiectomy, skin yield, ilia and soft-tissue recoveries), and operational error/adverse event reports that affect individual tissue or entire donor dispositions. To assist with the control of contamination and cross-contamination at recovery, the AATB has published a Guidance Document,[33] which offers proven technical methods (isolation draping in the presence of trauma, using zone recovery techniques, and sequencing tissue recovery), guidelines for handling preprocessing cultures (reporting and sharing of records, discard organisms), and important considerations regarding current culturing shortfalls and relevance to different processing methods.

Time restrictions for tissue recovery are based on the tissue type, but generally, cornea/whole eye recovery should take place as soon as possible after asystole, and musculoskeletal, skin, cardiac, and vascular tissue recovery must occur within 24 hours of asystole. This time limitation is based on induced body cooling (algor mortis) that also must occur within 12 hours of asystole. If the body cannot be cooled or refrigerated, then the time limitation is reduced to recovery within 15 hours of asystole. If some body cooling occurs but is followed by extended periods of no cooling, there can be no more than 15 consecutive hours of the absence of cooling. Sufficient body cooling and time limitations for commencement of recovery are in place to hopefully minimize the potential for organism proliferation postmortem. The AATB's Standards for Tissue Banking[10] describes these cooling/recovery time limit parameters and also offers this definition for asystole: "A reference time for cardiac death. A documented pronounced time of death is used as 'asystole' when life-saving procedures have been attempted and there were signs of, or documentation of, recent life (eg, agonal respirations, pulseless electrical activity). If a death was not witnessed, 'asystole' must be determined by the last time known alive. Asystole will be 'cross clamp time' if the tissue donor was also a solid organ donor."[59] This offers a uniform method of approach regarding this critical event and the various death scenarios that can be experienced when screening potential tissue donors. It should also be realized that the industry standard time limit of 1 day is also sensitive to the fact that the donor's family may have funeral arrangements to organize and the funeral home director/staff need sufficient time to properly prepare the body for viewing. Unexpected delays due to recovery operations can cause more stress to a family already experiencing duress.

Infectious Disease Testing

Another major screening parameter for tissue donation is evaluating the suitability of the blood sample for infectious disease testing. Some of these quality assurance methods are entirely applicable to organ donation as well, but are not required by the policies of the United Network for Organ Sharing/Organ Procurement and Transplantation Network or by AOPO standards. Plasma dilution of the donor blood sample being tested for infectious disease can cause a screening test result to be false-negative. Basically, when amounts of blood products and/or colloids transfused in the previous 2 days and amounts of crystalloids administered in the hour before blood specimen collection combine to add up to more than 50% of the patient's estimated plasma or blood volume, it's possible that infectious disease test results can be inaccurate. A qualifying plasma dilution algorithm, suggested by the FDA,[31] can be applied to calculate these factors to determine if this threshold has been eclipsed. This cutoff of 50% was, in part, derived from a study published in 1994.[60] In the 1994 sentinel document[56] regarding screening and testing of organ and tissue donors for HIV risk, a recommendation was made to consider possible hemodilution of the donor's blood sample when transfusions were received by an organ donor. These recommendations also cited an HIV transmission from a screened negative, but HIV-infected, organ donor to multiple recipients that occurred in 1987, partly as a result testing a diluted blood sample.[38]

The FDA requires that all laboratories that perform infectious disease testing for tissue donors be registered with their agency. The FDA also requires that the laboratories be certified to meet the requirements imposed by the Clinical Laboratory Improvement Act of 1988, or equivalent requirements as determined by the Center for Medicare and Medicaid Services.[30] This latter equivalency is to allow state accrediting bodies and Veterans Administration hospital laboratory certification to be acceptable for tissue donor testing sites. The FDA also mandates that tests kits used be those from manufacturers whose kits are FDA-licensed, approved, or cleared for donor screening.[30] These laboratory and test kit requirements are imposed to ensure that the laboratories being selected are following test kit manufacturers' instructions when performing the tests. The sensitivity and specificity of these test kits have been validated and are realized when properly used. Also, test kits labeled for patient diagnostic use, meaning those not intended for donor screening applications, cannot be used because of unknown (probably lower) sensitivity and specificity when screening donor populations for disease.

Test kit package inserts list specific blood sample types (serum, plasma collected in various tubes containing anticoagulants) that are acceptable for testing. Knowledge of these sample requirements and specific handling/storage instructions is required and should be written into procedures as references and made available to all tissue donor screening and recovery staff. The FDA also imposes a time frame limitation for collecting the tissue donor blood sample(s) that matches a well-established AATB standard. This states that, "a blood specimen shall be collected at the time of donation or within seven days prior to or after donation"[10] (D4.351 Specimens, page 37). This new rule also requires that when the donor is 1 month of age or less, the mother's blood must be collected and used for infectious disease testing instead of the baby's. Operational issues must be overcome to be able to offer the option of donation to these families as well as to continue to provide this life-saving allograft (heart valves) to surgeons because there is no man-made substitute that can be used instead. Porcine valves and mechanical valves cannot be manufactured that offer an orifice size this small without causing an unacceptable obstruction to blood flow. Current federal tissue donor testing requirements include: HIV-1/2 antibody, hepatitis B surface antigen, hepatitis B core antibody (total), HCV antibody, and an FDA-cleared serological test for syphilis.[31] The AATB additionally requires HTLV I/II antibody testing and HIV-1/HCV NAT assays.[61] See Table 1. Expectations are that the FDA will also eventually address the use of new test kits for various RCDADs that are, or will be, approved for cadaveric blood specimen testing by the NAT method.

Sites of Recovery

In recent times, more consideration has been given to qualifying the site of tissue recovery because the arena of recovery can affect the potential for microbial contamination of the tissue. By AATB annual survey, most tissue recoveries performed by accredited banks occur in a hospital operating room; however, other sites of recovery also exist. These include dedicated tissue recovery suites (at a tissue bank or medical examiner's office), medical examiner autopsy suite, hospital morgues, and funeral home embalming rooms. With the publication of the FDA's Final Rule for Current Good Tissue Practices (CGTPs),[32] consideration must be given to controlling contamination and cross-contamination during any stage of the tissue manufacturing process. Tissue recovery is considered a part of tissue manufacturing that must be controlled. Site parameters that are being established and documented by banks include adequate control of the room's location (eg, no direct access to the outside environment exists), ventilation and airflow not suspect as a source of contamination, adequate lighting to perform a physical assessment and recovery, and adequate space to perform an aseptic recovery and packaging of the tissues. The area should also have available working surfaces that can be disinfected, room construction that is in a good state of repair, control of human traffic, and cleanable floors and walls. If a site is deemed unsuitable, tissue recovery cannot take place at the site unless the deficiency can be rectified quickly. This control ensures that the site of recovery does not lend to contamination of the recovered tissues.

Donor Reconstruction

Immediately after tissue recovery, the donor is reconstructed and skin incisions closed so that the body is presentable for autopsy, embalming, funeral services, and/or cremation. Under certain circumstances, such as when a pathologist will perform a full or limited autopsy immediately after tissue recovery, or when a funeral home director will prepare the body for cremation or embalming immediately following the recovery, a request can be received by the recovery personnel that incision closures be made (farther apart, loose not tight) that allow access to underlying tissues for the requestor's individual reasons. The donor's body is reconstructed with care using prosthetic devices to replace recovered bones to maintain the respect and dignity of the person and the donation decision. The reconstruction process is also important for the closure to the donation process for the recovery team. The external body is cleansed and made presentable for transport. A waterproof body coverall is often supplied by the team to protect the body and those who handle it during transport.

Donor Family Support

The AATB's standards require that services to donor families or referral to a support system must be offered to the donor's family. Also, subsequent communications shall be documented, maintained, and readily available. The AOPO has similar policies for accreditation and allows organizations to develop and maintain their own systems.

The Future

The AATB and the EBAA have long-standing, respectable histories and are currently the only recognized accreditation organizations for tissue banks in the world. Almost all eye banks in the United States are accredited by the EBAA but by comparison, a slightly lesser percentage of conventional tissue banks are accredited by the AATB. Most of the tissue processors in our country with the highest distribution activity maintain accreditation by the AATB.

As of 2005, all tissue establishments must meet more stringent federal regulations that are similar to, but not as detailed as, AATB's standards. All recovery organizations (OPOs, tissue banks, eye banks) are now required by federal regulations[32] to have standard operating procedures that adequately cover steps they perform (includes any of the following: donor screening, recovery, donor testing, processing, packaging, labeling, storage, and distribution activities), and the forms being used to document these steps must accurately record the events that took place so they may be traced. For many years, AATB accreditation has required tissue banks to design and follow a quality assurance/quality control program but now there is federal mandate for the establishment and maintenance of the quality program concept, making it universal. As the new millennium has emerged, so has the realization that control of processes and the monitoring of their successes and failures must be a daily practice for organizations performing any aspect of the tissue banking process. Obtaining an informed consent for donation has evolved to be better termed as obtaining authorization for recovery, and now more disclosures are provided, all of which honor the decision the donor made prior to death as well as the authorization that can be granted by the donor's relatives.

When screening, we must realize that we live in a global community. International travel occurs regularly, quickly, and is available to millions daily. The potential for a novel disease to cross species barriers and eventually become a part of our lives is not unrealistic. It is now understood that, even in our modern times, disease agents and diseases could quickly evolve and spread uncontrollably and decimate populations on a global scale. In regard to the controls and regulations that also emerge, we, as transplant professionals, must maintain a positive attitude to ensure provision of safe tissues for transplantation to the public (recipients) whom we also serve. The screening of organ and tissue donors has never been more extensive or more interesting, and we must continue to be vigilant to keep abreast of worldwide emerging infectious diseases. Tissue processing methods will continue to evolve to offer even safer tissues for transplantation and provide more healing capabilities. We must always screen donors appropriately so what risk remains is minimal or nonexistent. Advancements will continue to be made in the provision of tissue in various forms, and the successful clinical application of these advancements will improve the quality of life for many of us. The potential for this success will only increase as the future unfolds for lifetimes to come. Tissue donation is truly a unique gift that offers an individual the ability to benefit dozens of lives with one selfless decision.

To successfully meet the expectations of tissue donors, donors' families, and recipients, it takes extensive coordination by many dedicated individuals who perform unique functions throughout the donation process.

References

1. Warner JH, Zoon KC. The view from the Food and Drug Administration. In: Younger S, Anderson M, Schapiro R, eds. *Transplanting Human Tissue: Ethics, Policy, and Practice*. New York, NY: Oxford University Press; 2004:5.
2. Kahan BD. Cosmas and Damian revisited. *Transplant Proc*. 1983;15:2211-2216.
3. Haeseker B. Van Meekeren and his account of the transplant of bone from a dog into the skull of a soldier. *Plast Reconstr Surg*. July 1991;88:173-174.
4. History of transplantation. Available at: http://www.transweb.org/reference/timeline/historytable.htm. Accessed July 6, 2006.
5. Macewan W. Observations concerning transplantation of bone. *Proc R Soc London*. 1881;32:232.
6. Sade RM. Transplantation at 100 years: Alexis Carrel, pioneer surgeon. *Ann Thorac Surg*. 2005;80:2415-2418.
7. Gross RE, Hurwitt ES, Bill AH Jr, Peirce EC 2nd. Preliminary observation on the use of the human arterial grafts in the treatment of certain cardiovascular defects. *N Engl J Med*. 1948;239:578-579.
8. The Ross procedure. Available at: http://ps4ross.com/ross/history.html. Accessed July 6, 2006.
9. Strong DM. The US Navy Tissue Bank: 50 years on the cutting edge. *Cell Tissue Banking*. 2000;1:9-16.
10. AATB. *AATB Standards for Tissue Banking*. 10th ed. McLean, Va: AATB; 2002.
11. Centers for Disease Control and Prevention. Epidemiologic Notes and Reports. Transmission of HIV through bone transplantation: case report and public health recommendations. *MMWR Morb Mortal Wkly Rep*. October 7, 1988;37:597-599.
12. Leslie H, Bottenfield S. Donation, banking, and transplantation of allograft tissues. *Nurs Clin North Am*. 1989;24:891-905.
13. U.S. Department of Health and Human Services, Food and Drug Administration. Human tissue intended for transplantation, Interim Final Rule. 58 *Federal Register* 65514-65521 (December 4, 1993) (codified at 21 CFR §1270).
14. The Eye Bank Association of America. Hall of History. Available at: http://www.restoresight.org. Accessed July 6, 2006.
15. NASDAQ. Available at: http://ticker.nasdaq.com [then query stock activity by using ticker for any for-profit tissue bank]. Accessed July 6, 2006.

16. Guidestar. Available at: http://www.guidestar.org/ [then enter query for any nonprofit tissue bank by name, city, and state then view previously filed IRS Form 990s]. Accessed March 6, 2006.
17. Technology Review, MIT. *Special Report, R&D '04*. Cambridge, Mass: Massachusetts Institute of Technology; December 2004.
18. American Association of Tissue Banks, Association of Organ Procurement Organizations, Eye Bank Association of America. Model Elements of Informed Consent for Organ and Tissue Donation, adopted November 30, 2000. Available at: http://www.aatb.org/model.htm. Accessed July 6, 2006.
19. AATB. *AATB Annual Survey of Accredited Tissue Banks, 2003*. McLean, Va: AATB; 2004.
20. Centers for Disease Control and Prevention. Epidemiologic Notes and Reports Update: Creutzfeldt-Jakob disease in a second patient who received a cadaveric dura mater graft. *MMWR Morb Mortal Wkly Rep*. January 27, 1989;38:37-38,43
21. Simonds RJ, Holmberg SD, Hurwitz RL, et al. Transmission of human immuno-deficiency virus type 1 from a seronegative organ and tissue donor. *N Engl J Med*. 1992;326:726-732.
22. Heckmann JG, Lang CJG, Petruch F, et al. Transmission of Creutzfeldt-Jakob disease via a corneal transplant. *J Neurol Neurosurg Psychiatry*. 1997;63:388-390.
23. Centers for Disease Control and Prevention. *Candida albicans* endocarditis associated with a contaminated aortic valve allograft: California, 1996. *MMWR Morb Mortal Wkly Rep*. March 28 1997;46:261-263.
24. Centers for Disease Control and Prevention. Public Health Dispatch–Update: unexplained deaths following knee surgery: Minnesota, 2001. *MMWR Morb Mortal Wkly Rep*. December 7, 2001;50:1080.
25. Centers for Disease Control and Prevention. Hepatitis C virus transmission from an antibody-negative organ and tissue donor: United States, 2001-2002. *MMWR Morb Mortal Wkly Rep*. 2003;5(2):273-276.
26. Proposed approach to the regulation of cellular and tissue-based products, February 1997. Available at http://www.fda.gov/cber/tissue/docs.htm. Accessed July 6, 2006.
27. U.S. Department of Health and Human Services, Food and Drug Administration. Human Tissue Intended for Transplantation, Final rule. July 29, 1997 (Volume 62, Number 145). Available at: http://www.fda.gov/cber/genadmin/frtissue.pdf. Accessed July 6, 2006.
28. U.S. Department of Health and Human Services, Food and Drug Administration. Guidance for industry, screening and testing of donors of human tissue, intended for transplantation, U.S. Department of Health and Human Services, Food and Drug Administration, Center for Biologics Evaluation and Research, July 1997. Available at: http://www.fda.gov/cber/gdlns/tissue2.pdf. Accessed July 6, 2006.
29. U.S. Department of Health and Human Services, Food and Drug Administration. Human cells, tissues, and cellular and tissue–based products; establishment registration and listing: final rule. 66 *Federal Register* 5447 (January 19, 2001). Available at: http://www.fda.gov/cber/rules/frtisreg011901.pdf. Accessed July 6, 2006.
30. U.S. Department of Health and Human Services, Food and Drug Administration. Eligibility Determination for Donors of Human Cells, Tissues, and Cellular and Tissue-Based Products; Final Rule. 69 *Federal Register* 29785 (May 25, 2004). Available at: http://www.fda.gov/cber/rules/suitdonor.pdf. Accessed July 6, 2006.
31. US Department of Health and Human Services, Food and Drug Administration. Draft guidance for industry: eligibility determination for donors of human cells, tissues, and cellular and tissue-based products (HCT/Ps), dated May 2004. Available at: http://www.fda.gov/cber/gdlns/tissdonor.pdf. Accessed July 6, 2006.
32. U.S. Department of Health and Human Services, Food and Drug Administration. Current good tissue practice for human cell, tissue, and cellular and tissue-based product establishments; inspection and enforcement; final rule, dated May 2004. Available at: http://www.fda.gov/cber/rules/gtp.pdf. Accessed July 6, 2006.
33. American Association of Tissue Banks. Guidance document no. 2, prevention of contamination and cross-contamination at recovery: practices and culture results, October 2004. Available at: http://aatb.org/. Accessed July 6, 2006.
34. Joint Council on Accreditation of Healthcare Organization (JCAHO) Standard PC.17.20. Available at: http://www.jcrinc.com/subscribers/perspectives.asp?durki=9159&site=10&return=6061. Accessed July 6, 2006.
35. American Burn Association. Burn incidence and treatment in the US: 2000. Available at: http://www.ameriburn.org/pub/BurnIncidenceFactSheet.htm. Accessed July 6, 2006.
36. Lifecell Web site. Applications and procedures. Available at: http://www.lifecell.com/products/6/. Accessed July 6, 2006.
37. Position statement on tissue donation. Available at: http://www.kidney.org/transplantation/donorFamilies/infoPolicyPosition.cfm. Accessed July 6, 2006.
38. Epidemiologic Notes and Reports: Human Immunodeficiency Virus Infection Transmitted From an Organ Donor Screened for HIV Antibody, North Carolina. *MMWR Morbid Mortal Wkly Rpt*. May 29, 1987;36(20):306-308.
39. Simonds RJ. HIV transmission by organ and tissue transplantation. *AIDS*. November 7, 1993(suppl 2):S35-S38.
40. Samuel D, Castaing D, Adam R, et al. Fatal acute HIV infection with aplastic anaemia, transmitted by liver graft. *Lancet*. 1988;1(8596):1221-1222.
41. Kumar P, Pearson JE, Martin DH, et al. Transmission of human immunodeficiency virus by transplantation of a renal allograft, with development of the acquired immunodeficiency syndrome. *Ann Intern Med*. 1987;106:244-245.

42. Prompt CA, Reis MM, Grillo FM, et al. Transmission of AIDS virus at renal transplantation [letter]. *Lancet.* 1985;2:67.
43. Penn I. Occurrence of cancers in immunosuppressed organ transplant recipients. In: Cecka JM, Terasaki PI, eds. *Clinical Transplants 1994.* Los Angeles, Calif: UCLA Tissue Typing Laboratory; 1994:99-109.
44. Lampros TD, Cobanoglu A, Parker F, Ratkovec R, Norman DJ, Hershberger R. Squamous and basal cell carcinoma in heart transplant recipients. *J Heart Lung Transplant.* 1998;17:586-591.
45. Penn I. Occurrence of cancers in immunosuppressed organ transplant recipients. In: Cecka JM, Terasaki PI, eds. *Clinical Transplants 1990.* Los Angeles, Calif: UCLA Tissue Typing Laboratory; 1990:53-62.
46. Brennan D C. Cytomegalovirus in renal transplantation. *J Am Soc Nephrol.* 2001;12:848-855.
47. Singh N, Carrigan DR. Human herpesvirus-6 in transplantation: an emerging pathogen. *Ann Intern Med.* 1999;124:1065-1071.
48. Title 21, Code of Federal Regulations, Parts 640.3, 640.12, 640.21, 640.31, and 640.51 Available at: http://a257.g.akamaitech.net/7/257/2422/01apr20051500/edocket.access.gpo.gov.cfr_aprqtr/21cfr64. Accessed April 15, 2006.
49. Deferral of donors who have received human pituitary-derived growth hormone: FDA memorandum to blood establishments, November 25, 1987. Available at: http://www.fda.gov/CBER/memo.htm. Accessed July 6, 2006.
50. Clarification of FDA recommendations for donor deferral and product distribution based on the results of syphilis testing: FDA memorandum to blood establishments, December 12, 1991. Available at: http://www.fda.gov/CBER/memo.htm. Accessed July 6, 2006.
51. Revised recommendations for the prevention of human immunodeficiency virus (HIV) transmission by blood and blood products: FDA memorandum to blood establishments, April 23, 1992. Available at: http://www.fda.gov/CBER/memo.htm. Accessed July 6, 2006.
52. Exemptions to permit persons with a history of viral hepatitis before the age of eleven years to serve as donors of whole blood and plasma: alternative procedures. 21 CFR §640.120 (April 23, 1992).
53. Donor suitability related to laboratory testing for viral hepatitis and a history of viral hepatitis: FDA memorandum to blood establishments, December 22, 1993. Available at: http://www.fda.gov/CBER/memo.htm. Accessed July 6, 2006.
54. Recommendations for deferral of donors for malaria risk: FDA memorandum to blood establishments, July 26, 1994. Available at: http://www.fda.gov/CBER/memo.htm. Accessed July 6, 2006.
55. Recommendations for the deferral of current and recent inmates of correctional institutions as donors of whole blood, blood components, source leukocytes and source plasma: FDA memorandum to blood establishments, June 8, 1995. Available at: http://www.fda.gov/CBER/memo.htm. Accessed July 6, 2006.
56. Centers for Disease Control and Prevention. Guidelines for preventing transmission of HIV through transplantation of human tissues and organs. *MMWR Recomm Rep.* May 20, 1994;43(RR8):1-17.
57. EBAA. *EBAA Medical Standards, June 2004.* Washington, DC: Eye Bank Association of America; 2004.
58. American Association of Tissue Banks. Guidance document no. 1, version 2, tissue donor physical assessment form. Available at: http://aatb.org/ Accessed July 6, 2006.
59. American Association of Tissue Banks. Memorandum to designated representatives of accredited tissue banks: changes in the standards for tissue banking, page 5, November 4, 2003. Available at: http://aatb.org/. Accessed July 6, 2006.
60. Heck E, Baxter C. Guidelines for preventing dilution false negatives in in-vitro laboratory testing of the donor population. *Cornea.* 1994;13:290-293.
61. American Association of Tissue Banks. Bulletin to designated representatives of accredited tissue banks: implementation of nucleic acid testing (NAT), no. 04-42, September 9, 2004. McLean, Va: AATB; 2004.

Section 2: Clinical Transplantation

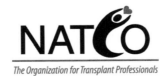

Kidney Transplantation

Marilyn Rossman Bartucci, MSN, APRN, BC, CCTC

Introduction

Despite ever-improving healthcare and new advances in medical technology, the number of Americans with end-stage renal disease (ESRD) continues to increase. Diabetes remains the leading cause of new cases (36%), followed by hypertension (27%) and glomerulonephritis (8%). In 2001, there were 392 023 patients with ESRD in the United States and 287 494 (73%) receiving dialysis therapy.[1]

Despite increased knowledge and skill in the management of ESRD, the most efficient dialysis techniques used today provide only 10% to 12% of the small solute removal of 2 normal kidneys and even less efficient removal of large solutes. Even in adequately dialyzed patients, progressive cardiovascular disease, peripheral and autonomic neuropathy, bone disease, and sexual dysfunction are common. Patients receiving dialysis often have impaired quality of life, fatigue, and malaise despite better management of anemia with erythropoietin; dependence on others for physical, emotional, and financial assistance; and poor rehabilitation.

The advances made in organ procurement and preservation, surgical technique, tissue typing and matching, understanding the immune mechanisms that lead to organ rejection, and the development of potent immunosuppressive drug regimens that effectively prevent and treat rejection have lead to excellent 1- and 5-year patient and graft survival rates (Table 1). Kidney transplantation is the renal replacement therapy of choice for patients with ESRD because it offers the greatest potential for a longer, healthier, productive life. A comparison of survival rates of patients receiving dialysis and those receiving a deceased or living donor kidney transplant revealed lower survival rates for patients receiving dialysis at 1, 2, 5, and 10 years compared to kidney transplant recipients, regardless of the donor source. The difference in the survival rate worsened between dialysis and transplantation at each subsequent time point. By 10 years, the dialysis survival rate was 9%, compared to survival rates of 58.9% and 77.8% for deceased and living donor kidney transplant recipients, respectively (Table 2).[1] Wolfe et al[3] used the United States Renal Data System database to compute and compare "projected years of life" for primary deceased donor kidney recipients and age-matched dialysis patients waiting for a kidney transplant. The results indicated

Table 1. UNADJUSTED 1- AND 5-YEAR PATIENT AND GRAFT SURVIVAL FOR KIDNEY TRANSPLANT RECIPIENTS[2]

Patient	1-year survival (%)		5-year survival (%)	
	2001-2002	*2002-2003*	*1997-2002*	*1998-2003*
Deceased donor	94.2	94.5	80.7	81.0
Living donor	97.5	97.6	90.1	89.8
Graft				
Deceased donor	88.7	89.0	65.7	66.2
Living donor	94.3	94.6	78.6	79.2

KIDNEY TRANSPLANTATION

Table 2. SURVIVAL RATES OF PATIENTS RECEIVING DIALYSIS, DECEASED DONOR KIDNEY TRANSPLANTS, AND LIVING DONOR KIDNEY TRANSPLANTS AT 1, 2, 5, AND 10 YEARS[1]

Years	Dialysis (%)	Deceased donor kidney transplantation (%)	Living donor kidney transplantation (%)
1 (2000-2001)	77.8	93.7	97.6
2 (1999-2001)	62.9	91.6	96.4
5 (1996-2001)	31.9	80.6	90.4
10 (1991-2001)	9.0	58.9	77.8

[[Used reference no. 1 instead of listing the source.]]

that transplantation offers a survival advantage over dialysis-based renal replacement therapies for all age groups. The survival advantage was most striking for younger patients and those with diabetes mellitus. For example, nondiabetic patients between 20 and 39 years old with a kidney transplant had 31 projected life years compared to 20 years for waiting list patients. Diabetics in the same age group with a kidney transplant had 25 versus 8 projected life years for waiting list patients.

The number of patients waiting for kidneys has continued to increase, while the number of kidney transplantations performed each year has remained fairly constant. At the end of 2004, there were more than 60 000 patients on the kidney waiting list, but only 16 000 kidney transplantations were performed.[2] The consequences of the imbalance between supply and demand are an exponential increase in the number of patients waiting for a kidney transplant, increased waiting times, and an increase in the number of patients who die while waiting for a transplant. The US kidney transplant waiting list has grown steadily from 24 704 in 1993 to 60 000 in 2004 (Figure 1). As a consequence, the median waiting time has increased by approximately 2 years from 747 to 1599 days, and the number of patients who die while

Figure 1. Number of Patients on the Kidney Waiting List Versus Transplantations[2]

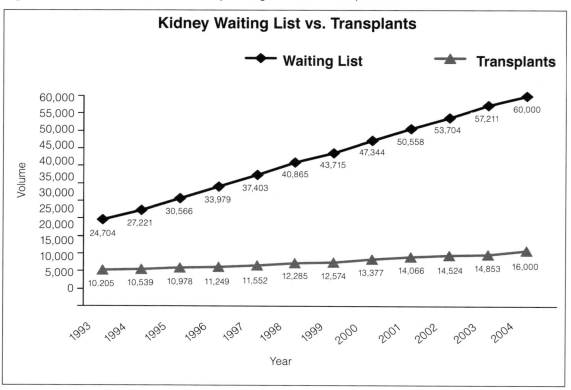

A CLINICIAN'S GUIDE TO TRANSPLANTATION AND DONATION Chapter 7

waiting for a transplant has more than doubled between 1993 and 2004; in 2004, 3201 patients died while waiting for a kidney transplant.[4]

Types of Donors

Kidneys for transplantation can be obtained from deceased donors, both heart-beating and non-heart-beating, and living donors.

Deceased Donors

Kidneys from deceased donors are removed en bloc (remaining attached to the aorta and vena cava), flushed with a sterile, cold preservation solution, and preserved in the cold solution via static or pulsatile perfusion for transport to the recipient's transplant center. Kidneys can be preserved for up to 72 hours, but most surgeons prefer to transplant kidneys before the cold ischemia time (the time between initiation of organ preservation in the donor and revascularization in the recipient) reaches 24 hours. Experience has shown that longer preservation time is associated with delayed graft function (DGF) from acute tubular necrosis, resulting in the need for dialysis until the acute tubular necrosis resolves.

Living Donors

With the shortage of deceased donors, longer waiting times, and evidence of a distinct survival advantage for transplant recipients over dialysis patients, there has been a rise in the number of living donors in the United States. In 2001, the number of living donors exceeded the number of deceased kidney donors for the first time, and this trend continues in 2005.[2] However, more deceased donor kidney transplantations are performed each year because 1 deceased donor can result in 2 transplants. As shown in Figure 2, the increase in living kidney donors has accounted for nearly all of the growth in kidney donation over the last decade.

The development of the laparoscopic donor nephrectomy, that is, the removal of a kidney through 4 small incisions using a laparoscope, has helped increase living donation. When the laparoscopic procedure

Figure 2. Number of Deceased Versus Living Kidney Donors[2]

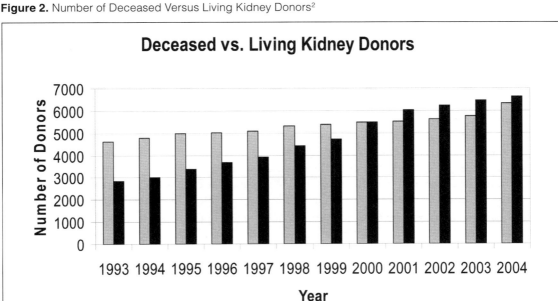

is compared to the standard open nephrectomy, there is a smaller incision with minimal scarring, a shorter stay in the hospital, less pain after surgery, and a more rapid return to normal activity, including work.[5]

Compared with deceased donors, living donors provide better patient and graft survival, permit transplantation to be performed electively when the recipient is in optimal condition, prevent the need for dialysis or shorten the time on dialysis, reduce the complications of organ procurement and preservation and thereby reduce the incidence of immediate and long-term kidney damage, permit immunologic conditioning and immunosuppression to begin before surgery, reduce the waiting period for transplantation, and perhaps improve rehabilitation.

Preemptive kidney transplantation is an alternative therapy for the initiation of dialysis when renal replacement therapy is medically necessary and there is a willing and medically suitable living donor. The morbidities associated with dialysis are avoided (e.g., vascular access-related problems, cardiac systolic dysfunction) and studies have demonstrated a distinct short- and long-term patient and graft survival advantage for preemptive transplant recipients compared with recipients who received their transplants after dialysis initiation.[6-9] These survival advantages have persisted despite substantial improvements in immunosuppression since 1994. Preemptive kidney transplantation is most successful when patients can be evaluated with sufficient lead time; that is, patients, as well as physicians, need to be educated about the detection of asymptomatic renal disease and the benefits of early referral to a nephrologist.

Expanded Criteria Donors

Attempts to expand the pool of kidneys from deceased donors have led to liberalizing criteria to include donors who would not have been considered previously. Such donors, called expanded criteria donors (ECD), include older individuals (up to 70 years) and those with medical conditions or other factors believed to be associated with decreased graft survival (e.g., diabetes, hypertension, certain infections, high-risk social behaviors but human immunodeficiency virus negative, some hemodynamic instability, some chemical imbalances, and increased organ preservation time). Sometimes transplantation of 2 kidneys into 1 recipient from such donors in order to maximize the mass of functioning nephrons has been employed to use organs that would previously have been discarded.

The United Network for Organ Sharing's registry database was used to compare the outcomes of 403 dual kidney transplantations and 11 033 single kidney transplantations performed between 1997 and 2000. The graft survival rate at 1 year was 7% lower in the dual kidney group; however, the graft survival rate was comparable to single kidney transplantations when donors in both groups were over 55 years of age.[10] These ECD donors have been estimated to add 25% to 39% to the organ donor supply.

A careful evaluation, including histologic assessment of the recovered kidneys, must be made before transplantation. If more than 20% of glomeruli are sclerosed on a wedge biopsy, the functional prognosis of the graft is poor, and these kidneys would be discarded.[11] In addition, careful long-term follow-up must be maintained to ensure that patient and graft survival rates are comparable to recipients of standard criteria deceased donor kidneys. The decision to transplant a kidney from an ECD donor requires not only a thorough anatomic and physiologic evaluation of the kidney, but a similar evaluation of the specific recipient that includes age, comorbid conditions, and immunologic compatibility. Much effort has gone into minimizing cold ischemia time, limiting the list of potential ECD kidney recipients to speed their allocation, and identifying patients who would most benefit from receiving an ECD kidney.

ECD kidneys are defined by the Organ Procurement and Transplantation Network as kidneys from donors over age 60 years or those aged 50 to 60 years who meet 2 of the following criteria: (1) a serum creatinine level greater than 1.5 mg/dL at the time of kidney recovery; (2) history of hypertension; or (3) death from a cerebrovascular accident. The use of ECD kidneys has increased from 11% in 1994 to 16% in 2003. ECD kidneys had lower graft survival rates than kidneys from standard criteria donors (SCD). The unadjusted 3-month, 1-year, 3-year, and 5-year graft survival rates were 90%, 81%, 67%, and 51%, respectively, for recipients of ECD kidneys, compared to 95%, 90%, 81%, and 68% for recipients of SCD kidneys.[12] The most appropriate use of ECD donor kidneys continues to be debated. Stratta et al[13] retrospectively studied 90 recipients of adult deceased donor kidneys transplanted between October 2001 and February 2003, and compared outcomes of ECD and SCD kidney transplantations. ECD kidneys were used by matching estimated renal function mass to recipient need and recipients were selected on the basis of older age, HLA-matching, low allosensitization, and low body mass index. Patient and kidney survival rates were similar between groups, as were the initial and mean serum creatinine levels up to 18 months after transplantation.

Recipient Selection Criteria

Because the supply of kidneys is limited, appropriate recipient selection is important for the best use of this scarce resource. The purpose of the pretransplant evaluation is to identify and treat all coexisting medical problems and psychosocial issues that may increase morbidity and mortality and adversely affect the posttransplant course. The physiologic and psychosocial parameters considered in the evaluation of the potential kidney transplant candidate are listed in Table 3. Contraindications to kidney transplantation are listed in Table 4.

Table 3. EVALUATION OF POTENTIAL KIDNEY TRANSPLANT RECIPIENTS: PHYSIOLOGICAL AND PSYCHOSOCIAL PARAMETERS

Rationale	Assessment

Cardiovascular
• Cardiovascular mortality rates 3 times higher than nonuremic patients, and diabetic dialysis patients 30 times higher
• Increased mortality related to atherosclerotic heart disease, myocardial infarction, congestive heart failure, and left ventricular hypertrophy mediated by systemic hypertension
• Increased frequency of coronary artery disease in long-term dialysis patients is related to hypertension, hyperlipidemia, and diabetes
• Increased prevalence of cardiovascular disease may be due to effects of increased oxidative stress, hyperhomocysteinemia, and accumulation of advanced glycation end products
	• Comprehensive history and physical examination
	• Cardiovascular tests
	   – 12-lead electrocardiogram
	   – 2D-Doppler echocardiogram*
	   – Noninvasive assessment of coronary arteries such as
	      – Conventional exercise stress test
	      – Thallium scintigraphy
	      – Dobutamine echocardiography
	   – Arteriogram to determine patency of iliac vasculature
	   – Coronary arteriogram*
	   – Carotid duplex*
	   – Cardiology consult* (for patients with diabetes, history of cardiac disease, and patients over 50 years of age)

Pulmonary
• Alteration in pulmonary capillary permeability resulting in pulmonary edema
• Pulmonary edema and pleural effusions due to increased total body fluid
• Cigarette smoking may add to pulmonary problems
	• Pulmonary tests
	   – Chest radiograph with posteroanterior (PA) and lateral views
	   – Pulmonary function studies* (for patients with asthma, chronic obstructive pulmonary disease, or smoking history)
	   – Tuberculin skin test

Hematologic
• Anemia due to decreased production of erythropoietin
• Dysfunction of coagulation cascade, platelet function, and vascular endothelium contribute to bleeding abnormalities
• Use of heparin during hemodialysis, antiplatelet agents, and warfarin therapy exacerbate bleeding abnormalities
• Some patients may demonstrate hypercoagulability
	• Hematologic tests
	   – Complete blood cell count with differential
	   – Prothrombin time
	   – Partial thromboplastin time
	   – International normalized ratio

Gastrointestinal (GI)
• Gastritis and hemorrhage in upper GI tract related to uremia
• Common lower GI tract abnormalities include diverticulosis, diverticulitis, spontaneous colonic perforation, and prolonged adynamic ileus (pseudo-obstruction)
	• GI tests
	   – Stool for occult blood
	   – Endoscopy*
	   – Colonoscopy*

Table 3. EVALUATION OF POTENTIAL KIDNEY TRANSPLANT RECIPIENTS: PHYSIOLOGICAL AND PSYCHOSOCIAL PARAMETERS (continued)

Rationale	Assessment

Hepatobiliary
• Hepatitis B and C common etiologic factors in long-term dialysis patients, especially if patient has received multiple blood transfusions
• Most with hepatitis B or C are asymptomatic
• Most with serologic evidence of hepatitis C have normal liver function tests
• Drug toxicity and alcohol abuse contribute to liver dysfunction especially if hepatitis present
• Hepatomegaly does not necessarily indicate primary liver disease, but may reflect chronic, passive liver congestion associated with fluid overload or cardiac disease
	• Hepatobiliary tests
	  – Liver function tests with coagulation profile
	  – Hepatitis B and C serologies
	  – Ultrasonography of gallbladder*
	  – Liver biopsy to look for cirrhosis*

Genitourinary
• The lower urinary tract should be sterile and continent without urinary retention before transplantation
• Pretransplant native nephrectomies are indicated for patients with ureteral reflux resulting in hydronephrosis or infection, polycystic kidney disease with grossly enlarged kidneys or frequently bleeding or infected cysts, or severe uncontrolled hypertension
	• Genitourinary tests
	  – Urinalysis, urine culture (if patient still making urine)
	  – Voiding cystourethrogram*
	  – Cystometrics*
	  – Gynecologic examination including Papanicolaou's smear for women who are sexually active or over 18 years of age
	  – Prostate examination and prostate specific antigen for men over 50 years of age
	  – Mammogram*

Neurological • Patients with seizure disorders on anticonvulsant agents have an increased rate of metabolism of calcineurin inhibitors (cyclosporine and tacrolimus) • Pretransplant neurology consult is useful in determining whether anticonvulsant therapy is mandatory	Neurology consultation*

Immunological
• All potential kidney transplant recipients are tissue typed to determine human leukocyte antigen (HLA) class I and class II; 6 HLAs are identified on A, B, and DR loci
• Kidney donors are also HLA typed; degree of compatibility between donor and recipient is defined by number of antigens mismatched at each HLA loci; there is mandatory sharing across the United States for all 6 antigen/0 mismatch kidneys
• Lymphocytotoxic antibodies obtained from multiparous women or from recipients of multiple blood transfusions used to determine presence of preformed antibodies to HLA antigens; results range from 0% to 100% and reflect percentage of antigens on test panel against which potential recipient has preformed antibodies; the higher the panel reactive antibody level, the more difficult it will be to find a donor with whom the potential recipient would have a negative t- and b-cell cross-match
	• Immunologic tests
	  – History of autoimmune disease, previous transplantations, blood transfusions, pregnancy (in women)
	  – Blood type
	  – Human leukocyte antigen testing
	  – Cytotoxic screening or panel reactive antibody testing
	  – T and B lymphocyte cross-match with potential donor

Immunizations • Because of their increased susceptibility to infection after transplantation, transplant candidates should have current immunization	• All immunizations current including pneumonia vaccine (Pneumovax), and Hepatitist B vaccine (Heptovax)

Table 3. EVALUATION OF POTENTIAL KIDNEY TRANSPLANT RECIPIENTS: PHYSIOLOGICAL AND PSYCHOSOCIAL PARAMETERS (continued)

Rationale	Assessment

Psychosocial
• Organic mental syndromes, psychosis, and severe mental retardation may seriously impair a patient's capacity to understand the entire transplant process and related complications
• Patients addicted to alcohol or any other drug should enter and successfully complete a rehabilitation program before being placed on waiting list
• Chemical dependency counselor must clear patient for placement on waiting list
• There is a relationship between pretransplant noncompliance and posttransplant outcomes; when compared with compliant recipients, noncompliant recipients have an increased mortality rate, more late acute rejection episodes, and lower graft survival rates
• Immunosuppressive agents and other medications can cost up to $20,000 per year. Although Medicare is often the primary payer for the kidney transplantation and related hospitalization, it only covers 80% of the cost of immunosuppression for 36 months from the day of hospital discharge, unless the recipient remains disabled. After 36 months, the recipient is personally responsible for the entire cost of medications, unless there is a supplemental insurance policy specifically covering prescriptions.
• Financial counselors and social workers help patients develop a plan to ensure medications can be obtained after transplantation
	• Psychosocial assessment (history and emotional stability)
	  – Patient's and family's ability to cope with illness
	  – Adjustment to and understanding of present illness
	  – Support system (family, friends, significant others)
	  – Preillness lifestyle
	  – Work history
	  – Education
	  – Previous transplant experience, if any
	  – Expectations of transplantation
	• Chemical dependency, if any
	  – Periodic random toxicology screening tests to ensure that patients with prior chemical dependency remain alcohol/drug free
	• Noncompliance
	  – Some programs require a period of acceptable compliance with specific, measurable criteria as a condition for placement on the waiting list
	• Financial/Insurance status

*As indicated.

Adapted from Bartucci MR, Hricik DE. Kidney transplantation. In: Cupples SA, Ohler L, eds. *Solid Organ Transplantation: A Handbook for Primary Health Care Providers*. New York, NY: Springer Publishing Company; 2002:193-198.

Table 4. CONTRAINDICATIONS TO KIDNEY TRANSPLANTATION

Malignancy

Chronic illness with short life expectancy

Chronic infection
- Human immunodeficiency virus – infected patients who are free of opportunistic infections, with a stable undetectable viral load, and CD4 lymphocyte count >300/mm3 may be considered
- Active hepatitis B
- Tuberculosis
- Peritonitis
- Chronic skin infection
- Chronic osteomyelitis

Untreated severe coronary artery disease

Cirrhosis of the liver

Chronic obstructive pulmonary disease

Noncompliance

Psychiatric illness

Active substance abuse

Lack of insurance or inability to pay for medication

After curative treatment of malignant disease, an interval of 2 to 5 years is recommended until transplantation is performed depending on the type of cancer. Patients with breast cancer and melanoma are at high risk for late recurrence warranting the longer interval between the treatment of the disease and transplantation. Patients with carcinoma in situ or low-grade cancers, such as basal cell carcinoma of the skin, can safely undergo transplantation earlier if treatment of the cancer was curative. Patients must be advised of the risk of recurrence and the risk of de novo carcinomas after transplantation.

Because the waiting list became so long, minimum listing criteria were established to ensure that only patients ready for transplantation were listed. A candidate for a kidney transplant from a deceased donor is any patient undergoing renal replacement therapy who is deemed medically suitable for transplantation by a transplant team. Those patients not requiring renal replacement therapy must have a creatinine clearance of ≤ 20 mL/min.

The United Network for Organ Sharing's policies for kidney allocation consider blood type, HLA tissue type, panel reactive antibody, and time on the waiting list. Additional points are given to children under age 18 because of the effect of uremia on skeletal growth, sexual maturation, cognitive performance, and psychosocial functioning and to candidates who have previously donated a kidney. Zero HLA-mismatched kidney candidates are given national priority regardless of their geographic location or points accrued. These allocation policies are continuously reviewed by the transplant community and the public, and updated on the basis of advances in medical science.

Waiting Period

With the increase in waiting time, the challenge is to ensure patient readiness for transplantation while minimizing the repetition of expensive testing. Many potential kidney transplant recipients develop new complications while waiting for a transplant. Cardiovascular disease often progresses rapidly in patients receiving maintenance hemodialysis, and approximately 5% die waiting each year.[4]

Although there are no studies specifically addressing patients on the waiting list, a strategy that uses guidelines targeting the general population but modified to meet the needs of patients with renal disease have been proposed by the American Society of Transplantation.[14] Candidates on the waiting list should undergo reevaluation every 1 to 2 years, including a history and physical examination, screening for infection and cancer, and cardiac testing as indicated. Cardiac testing is not necessary if the patient is asymptomatic and nondiabetic; however, it is recommended if a patient has at least 2 of the following risk factors: (1) receiving dialysis for more than 3 years; (2) primary disease with known arteriosclerotic risk (e.g., lupus); (3) male older than 45 years of age; (4) ischemic heart disease in a first-degree relative; (5) current cigarette smoking; (6) hypertension; (7) fasting total cholesterol higher than 200 mg/dL and/or high-density lipoprotein (HDL) cholesterol lower than 35 mg/dL; and (8) left ventricular hypertrophy and undergoes cardiac stress testing every 1 to 2 years. Patients with diabetes or documented asymptomatic cardiac disease should undergo annual stress echocardiography.[14] Ongoing communication is critical between dialysis units, patients, and the transplant center regarding health and psychosocial issues that are relevant to transplant candidacy.

Preoperative Management

A t- and b-cell cross-match is the final pretransplant immunologic screening step. A positive cross-match indicates that the potential recipient has preformed antibodies to the donor's HLA antigens and is a contraindication to transplantation. Because of the long waiting time, urgent reevaluation may be necessary to determine if the proposed recipient is an acceptable surgical candidate to decrease perioperative morbidity and mortality.

Care of the patient in the preoperative phase includes emotional and physical preparation for surgery. Because the patient and family may have been waiting 4 to 5 years for kidney transplantation, a review of the operative procedure and what can be expected in the immediate postoperative recovery period is warranted. For recipients of deceased donor kidneys, it is important to stress that there is a 10% to 30%

chance the kidney will not function immediately, and dialysis may be required for the first few weeks. In addition, the need for immunosuppressive medications and the importance of preventing infection after surgery must be stressed.

To ensure that the patient is in optimal physical condition for surgery, an electrocardiogram, chest radiograph, and laboratory studies are completed. The decision to dialyze a patient before transplantation depends on the timing of the previous dialysis, clinical assessment of volume status, and serum electrolytes, particularly potassium. Pretransplant dialysis is associated with an increased incidence of DGF. Because of the danger of intraoperative or postoperative hyperkalemia in oliguric patients, it is recommended that pretransplant dialysis be performed in patients with a serum potassium level of 5.5 mEq/L or greater. In well-dialyzed patients, preoperative dialysis for fluid removal is usually unnecessary. If fluid is removed, it should be done with care to maintain the patient at or slightly above their dry weight to facilitate postoperative diuresis. A patient supported by peritoneal dialysis must empty the peritoneal cavity of all dialysate solution before going to the operating room. Because dialysis may be required after transplantation, the patency of the vascular access must be maintained by avoiding blood pressure measurement, phlebotomy, or intravenous infusions in the affected extremity.

Operative Procedure

The kidney transplant procedure takes approximately 3 hours. A hockey stick shaped incision is made extending from the iliac crest to the symphysis pubis. The peritoneum is left intact and retracted upward while the common iliac, external iliac, hypogastric arteries, and common and external iliac veins are dissected. Any divided lymphatic vessels are ligated or cauterized to prevent future lymphocele formation. Intraperitoneal placement may be indicated in certain circumstances, such as in children in whom the transplanted kidney is too large to fit in the extraperitoneal space or in adults who have received previous transplants or have inadequate extraperitoneal vascular access.

Efficient revascularization is critical to prevent ischemic injury to the kidney. In a living donor kidney transplantation, an end-to-side anastamosis is made between the donor renal artery and the recipient hypogastric or internal iliac artery. In a deceased donor kidney transplantation, the donor renal artery with its aortic patch is anastamosed to the side of the recipient hypogastric or internal iliac artery.

The kidney is positioned in the iliac fossa, and the donor renal vein is clamped until the anastomosis to the recipient iliac vein is completed. When the clamp is released and blood flow to the kidney is reestablished, the kidney becomes firm and pink. Urine often begins to flow from the ureter immediately. Mannitol or furosemide may be administered intravenously to promote diuresis.

The donor ureter is tunneled through the bladder submucosa before entering the bladder cavity and is sutured in place in a procedure called ureteroneocystostomy. This allows the bladder to

Figure 3. Diagram of Diseased and Transplanted Kidney

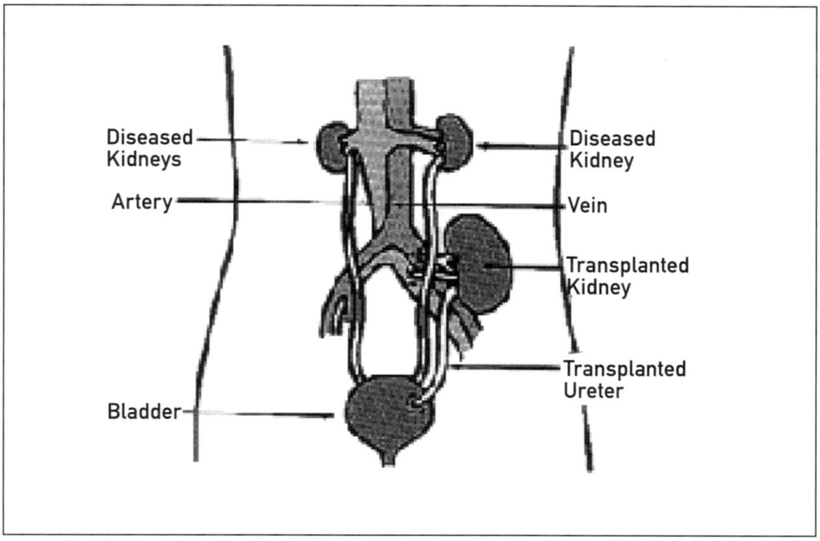

Reprinted with permission from the National Diabetes Information Clearing House. Available at: http://www.diabetic.com/education/pubs/esrd/esrd.htm. Accessed August 15, 2005.

clamp down on the ureter as it contracts for micturition, thereby preventing reflux of urine up the ureter into the transplanted kidney. Occasionally, a stent is placed in the ureter to prevent leaks and is removed via cystoscopy approximately 6 weeks after transplantation. After closing, a drain may be inserted adjacent to the incision to facilitate removal of excess blood and serum from the operative site. A closed drain, such as the Jackson-Pratt, is preferred because of a lower risk for wound infection. The recipient's native kidneys are not removed unless they are identified as a source of infection or uncontrolled hypertension (Figure 3).

Postoperative Management

The kidney transplant recipient has undergone major abdominal surgery and has care needs similar to the postoperative needs of any patient who undergoes abdominal surgery. These needs include hemodynamic monitoring, assessment of oxygenation and tissue perfusion, and fluid and electrolyte management.

Short-Term Complications

When successful, kidney transplantation eliminates the need for dialysis and the associated diet and fluid restrictions. Complications that contribute to increased length of stay or hospital readmission include: thrombosis, DGF, acute rejection, infection, obstruction, and urine leak (Table 5).

Immunosuppression

Immunosuppression in kidney transplant recipients is very similar to that used for recipients of other solid organs. The goal is adequate suppression of the immune response to prevent rejection, while maintaining sufficient immunity to prevent overwhelming infection. Many of the medications used to achieve immunosuppression have adverse effects of their own. By using a combination of medications that work in different phases of the immune response, lower doses of each drug produce effective immunosuppression while minimizing side effects. Immunosuppressive protocols vary among transplant centers. Immunosuppression for kidney transplant recipients includes induction, maintenance, and withdrawal and conversion regimens.

Induction. The benefits of using routine induction antibodies to reduce the risk of early acute rejection must be weighed against the cost of these agents and the potential for over-immunosuppression. There has been a progressive trend toward increasing use of induction agents in the United States. In 2003, 70% of kidney transplant recipients received induction therapy compared to 25% in 1994. The most commonly used induction antibody was rabbit antithymocyte globulin (34%) followed by basiliximab (22%), daclizumab (13%), horse antithymocyte globulin (1.1%), and muromonab-CD3 (0.4%).[2] Some centers reserve induction therapy for selected patients who are immunologically at high risk for acute allograft rejection (e.g., African Americans, second transplant recipients, and patients with high levels of preformed antibodies) or patients with DGF to postpone initiation of treatment with potentially nephrotoxic calcineurin inhibitors.

Maintenance. A small number of transplant recipients completely accommodate their allograft and allow cessation of immunosuppression. Because it is currently impossible to identify such individuals, lifelong immunosuppression is the current standard of practice. The challenge of maintenance immunosuppressive therapy is achieving the balance between enough immunosuppression to prevent rejection and avoiding excessive immunosuppression, which increases the risk of infection and malignancy. Most centers employ a triple therapy drug regimen, including corticosteroids, a calcineurin inhibitor (tacrolimus or cyclosporine), and a purine antagonist (azathioprine or mycophenolate mofetil) or mTOR (mammalian Target of Rapamycin) inhibitor (sirolimus) to minimize the toxicity of any single agent and to inhibit the immune response through separate, but additive or synergistic mechanisms. In 2003, at hospital discharge after kidney transplantation, 85% of patients received corticosteroids, 93% a calcineurin inhibitor (67% tacrolimus, 26% cyclosporine), 83% a purine antagonist (81% mycophenolate mofetil, 2% azathioprine), and 16% an mTOR inhibitor (sirolimus).[2]

Table 5. ETIOLOGY AND TREATMENT OF COMPLICATIONS IN THE IMMEDIATE POSTOPERATIVE PERIOD

Complication	Etiology	Assessment	Treatment options
Anuria (urine output < 50 mL/24 hours)	Most commonly due to acute tubular necrosis (ATN); may be due to urine leak, ureteral obstruction, or vascular thromboses	Serial measurements of urine output and serum creatinine concentration	Trial of intravenous (IV) diuretics to promote urine output
Oliguria (urine output < 400 mL/24 hours)	Most commonly observed after living donor transplantation, reflecting an osmotic diuresis in face of rapidly normalizing glomerular filtration rate (GFR)	Doppler ultrasonography or renal scans to determine structural abnormalities	Role of low-dose dopamine controversial
Polyuria	Some patients with ATN develop renal concentrating defect and may excrete large amounts of urine despite persistent azotemia	Serial measurements of urine output	Matching urine output with replacement IV fluids to avoid severe volume depletion in first 12-24 hours after transplantation
Hemodynamic instability	Ischemia due to organ procurement and/or denervation of allograft	Signs of volume depletion or volume overload Comparison of preoperative and postoperative weights Central venous pressure (CVP) monitoring Pulse oximetry or arterial blood gases	Maintenance of euvolemia by treating volume depletion with the administration of isotonic fluids to normalize blood pressure, heart rate, and CVP Treating volume overload with IV diuretics or dialysis, depending on urine output
Hypertension	Inability to take or reliably absorb antihypertensive medications	Blood pressure	IV medications such as nitroprusside, labetolol, hydralazine, enalapril
Electrolyte imbalance	Preexisting electrolyte or acid-base abnormalities	Serial assessment of serum electrolytes	
Hyperkalemia	Effects of surgical tissue destruction; impaired renal function		Dietary potassium restriction Cation exchange resins (e.g., sodium polystyrene sulfonate [Kayexalate]) Diuretics Dialysis
Hyponatremia	Excessive administration of hypotonic fluids in the presence of renal impairment		Water restriction Conversion of isotonic fluids
Hypomagnesemia	May be a manifestation of "high output" ATN; exacerbated by calcineurin inhibitors		IV magnesium sulfate for severe hypomagnesemia
Hypophosphatemia	Common when GFR suddenly normalizes in patients with preexisting hyperparathyroidism		Increased intake of dairy products

Table 5. ETIOLOGY AND TREATMENT OF COMPLICATIONS IN THE IMMEDIATE POSTOPERATIVE PERIOD (continued)

Complication	Etiology	Assessment	Treatment options
Metabolic acidosis	Impaired renal hydrogen ion excretion	Serial assessment of pH	Bicarbonate replacement when serum bicarbonate <15 mEq/L
DGF: need for dialysis during the first week after transplantation	Ischemic ATN (incidence varies from 10%-40%) Immunologic mechanisms (DGF is a risk factor for acute rejection; the combination of DGF and acute rejection portends a poor long-term prognosis for the allograft)	Serial measurements of urine output and serum creatinine concentration Percutaneous kidney biopsy to diagnose rejection	Dialysis Fluid restriction
Acute renal failure that develops after initial graft function has been established	Volume depletion Acute rejection (including delayed hyperacute rejection) Arterial of venous thrombosis (more common in patients with hypercoagulable states and recipients of pediatric kidneys) Urine leak Ureteral obstruction Anastomotic stricture Obstruction by perinephric fluid (e.g., hematoma, urinoma, lymphocele) Drug-induced nephrotoxicity Allergic interstitial nephritis Hemolytic uremic syndrome	Serial measurements of urine output and serum creatinine concentration Comparison of daily weights Percutaneous kidney biopsy to diagnose rejection Doppler ultrasonography to determine vascular or structural abnormalities	Fluid administration Treatment of rejection Correction of vascular abnormalities Drainage of hematoma, urinoma, or lymphocele Dose adjustment of nephrotoxic drugs Plasmapheresis

Adapted from Bartucci MR, Hricik DE. Kidney transplantation. In: Cupples SA, Ohler L, eds. *Solid Organ Transplantation: A Handbook for Primary Health Care Providers*. New York, NY: Springer Publishing Company. 2002; 205-208.

Withdrawal and Conversion. Because the use of newer immunosuppressants has been associated with lower rates of acute rejection, attention has focused increasingly on long-term minimization of immunosuppression to reduce drug toxicities in patients who are free of acute rejection during the early posttransplant period. Steroid- and calcineurin inhibitor-sparing protocols are examples of these types of regimens. With the availability of newer and more potent maintenance drugs, many centers convert recipients to a new maintenance regimen if acute rejection occurs while the patient is receiving another combination of drugs. An underlying concern that the calcineurin inhibitor may contribute to interstitial fibrosis and chronic graft dysfunction forms the basis for conversion protocols in which a new, nonnephrotoxic drug (most often either mycophenolate mofetil or sirolimus) is added to facilitate minimization or withdrawal of the calcineurin inhibitor in patients with chronic allograft nephropathy (CAN). Until long-term outcomes of clinical trials become available, withdrawal or dose reduction should be considered only after careful evaluation of risks and benefits for each individual patient.

Rejection

Hyperacute Rejection. Hyperacute rejection is mediated by preformed antibodies and may occur immediately following the vascular anastamosis or several days later (delayed hyperacute rejection or accelerated acute rejection). Necrosis of the renal parenchyma in this setting is often accompanied by a toxic state, including evidence of disseminated intravascular coagulation. Plasmapheresis and intravenous gamma globulin may be effective in removing and suppressing formation of the antibodies before irreversible damage occurs.

Acute Rejection. Although acute rejection is increasingly less common because of improvements in immunosuppression therapy, recognition, prompt diagnosis, and treatment remain an essential aspect of posttransplant care. Acute rejection can occur at any time following kidney transplantation, but the risk is highest in the first 6 months after transplantation. It is a t cell mediated immune response characterized by an abrupt deterioration in renal function, usually manifested by a rise in serum creatinine concentration. Fever, general malaise, graft tenderness, and decreased urine output are characteristic of severe acute rejection, but are rarely observed today because of the potent immunosuppressive agents in use.

Percutaneous biopsy remains the gold standard for diagnosis. Under ultrasound guidance, a needle is inserted through the skin and samples of kidney tissue are obtained for histological examination. The Banff classification was developed in an effort to provide a consistent approach for grading structural lesions in the transplanted kidney. Borderline rejection is characterized by patchy interstitial inflammation and mild tubulitis. Mild (grade 1) to moderate rejection (grade 2A) includes progressively worse interstitial inflammation, involving the renal parenchyma and tubulitis. Severe rejection includes interstitial inflammation, tubulitis, and mild (grade 2B) to severe intimal arteritis with necrosis and infarction (grade 3). In patients with acute rejection, the Banff grade can be predictive of recurrent rejection and subsequent graft failure. In addition, many centers choose treatment strategies based on the grade of rejection.

Timely administration of appropriate therapy can restore renal function to baseline, a response that confers significant statistical benefit in terms of long-term graft survival. Administration of high doses of corticosteroids for 3 to 5 days is the first-line therapy for acute rejection in most centers and can reverse approximately 60% of rejection episodes. Antilymphocyte antibodies are most often used in patients who fail to respond to pulse steroids, or as first-line therapy in patients with clinically or histologically severe episodes of rejection. The most commonly used agents are rabbit antithymocyte globulin and muromonab-CD3.

Chronic Rejection or Chronic Allograft Nephropathy. Chronic rejection or CAN generally occurs beyond the sixth posttransplant month. Thus, renal function must be monitored for the life of the allograft. It is characterized by a slow deterioration in the glomerular filtration rate manifested by a slow rise in serum creatinine concentration, often accompanied by proteinuria, and new or worsening hypertension. One third of patients develop heavy proteinuria and frank nephrotic syndrome (edema, hypoalbuminemia, and hyperlipidemia). On kidney biopsy, CAN is characterized by concentric intimal thickening of the small arterioles, interstitial fibrosis, tubular atrophy, and glomerulosclerosis. The histologic changes are a result of progressive ischemia from the obliteration of small blood vessels.[15]

Although the etiology of CAN is unknown, both immunologic and nonimmunologic factors are associated with its development. Immunologic factors include human leukocyte antigen mismatch, presence of preformed antibodies, retransplantation, and acute rejection following transplantation. Nonimmunologic factors include donor source (living or deceased), cold ischemia time of the transplanted kidney, donor age and cause of death (e.g., cerebrovascular accident vs motor vehicle accident), and length of dialysis before transplantation. To date, none of the available immunosuppressants has proven to be effective in treating established CAN. Aggressive treatment of hyperlipidemia and systemic hypertension, including the use of renal protective angiotensin inhibitors (angiotensin-converting enzyme inhibitors and angiotensin receptor blockers) is warranted, but the impact of these strategies on retarding the rate of renal functional deterioration remains to be proven. There is no convincing evidence that the addition of mycophenolate mofetil or sirolimus can alter the course of CAN. These drugs may allow discontinuation of calcineurin inhibitors, but this conversion strategy is associated with a 5% to 15% risk of inducing an acute rejection episode.

Long-Term Complications

The long-term care of kidney transplant recipients involves management of infection, cardiovascular disease (hypertension and hyperlipidemia), posttransplant diabetes mellitus, malignancy, skeletal disorders, hematopoietic abnormalities, and recurrent renal disease.[16]

Infectious Complications. Infections are frequent complications of systemic immunosuppression after transplantation. The principles of infectious disease management include: (1) identification of the organism, (2) identification of the organism's sensitivities to antimicrobials, and (3) localization of the site(s) of infections. Different types of infections occur at 3 periods after transplantation, first month, 2 to 6 months, and beyond 6 months (Table 6). Urinary tract infections are the most frequent bacterial infection in kidney transplant recipients. Predisposing factors include renal insufficiency, decreased urine flow through the urinary epithelium, prolonged bladder catheterization, and underlying diseases (e.g., diabetes and polycystic kidney disease). Causative organisms are the same as the general population, gram-negative enteric bacilli, enterococci, staphylococci, and *Pseudomonas aeruginosa*.

Cardiovascular Disease. The incidence of cardiovascular events is approximately 10 times higher in kidney transplant recipients than in the general population. Cardiovascular disease is the most common cause of death, responsible for about 40% of all deaths following successful kidney transplantation. This is no surprise because 50% of the transplant population has diabetes and hypertension. Reducing mortality from cardiovascular disease could improve long-term kidney allograft survival. Risk factors for ischemic heart disease events greater than 1 year after successful kidney transplantation include preexisting cardiovascular disease, advanced age, tobacco use, family history, diabetes, hypertension, hyperlipidemia, hyperhomocysteinemia, preexisting left ventricular hypertrophy, prior rejection episodes, and cumulative doses of corticosteroids. Cardiovascular monitoring including blood pressure, blood glucose, homocysteine, and lipid levels is highly recommended.[16]

Hypertension occurs in 80% of kidney transplant recipients and is associated with poorer long-term graft survival. The etiology is usually multifactorial and includes effects of retained native kidneys; renal insufficiency; parenchymal disease of the transplanted kidney (mediated by rejection or recurrent disease); hypertensive effects of immunosuppressants such as corticosteroids, cyclosporine, and tacrolimus; narrowing of the renal artery (renal artery stenosis); obesity; and essential hypertension. Hypertension may accelerate loss of allograft function, especially in African American patients.

Table 6. INFECTIOUS COMPLICATIONS AFTER KIDNEY TRANSPLANTATION

Period	Types of infections
First month	Wound – bacterial and fungal Urinary tract Nosocomial pneumonia Line-associated bacteremias and fungemias
2-6 months	Opportunistic – cytomegalovirus, *Pnemocystis carinii* pneumonia, invasive aspergillosis, disseminated toxoplasmosis, disseminated varicella zoster
After 6 months	Community acquired, tuberculosis, cryptococcus, reactivation of hepatits B and C, nocardiosis, and herpes zoster

Treatment with antihypertensive agents to achieve and maintain a blood pressure of 130/80 mm Hg or lower is recommended to preserve long-term renal function. There is no consensus about optimal therapy, but calcium channel blockers are used as first-line agents in many centers. In addition to controlling blood pressure, calcium channel blockers improve afferent arteriolar flow into the glomerulus and offset the effect of calcineurin inhibitors. Angiotensin-converting enzyme inhibitors and angiotensin-receptor blockers are effective as well. In addition to lowering blood pressure, they exert a renal protective effect. Because many kidney transplant recipients are at risk for or have ischemic heart disease, the use of beta blockers for adjunctive therapy is also effective.

The incidence of hyperlipidemia in long-term kidney transplant recipients is 60% to 80%, and is characterized by increased total cholesterol, increased or normal HDL, and increased low-density lipoprotein (LDL) with or without hypertriglyceridemia. The risk factors associated with the development of hyperlipidemia include poor kidney function, pretransplant hyperlipidemia, proteinuria, diabetes, obesity, diet, some antihypertensive agents (e.g., nonselective beta-blockers and diuretics), and immunosuppressants. Corticosteroids increase hepatic formation of lipoproteins and cyclosporine impairs bile acid synthesis and cholesterol excretion. The incidence and severity of hyperlipidemia are greater in patients receiving sirolimus. Although prednisone increases total cholesterol, it also increases HDL. Although corticosteroid withdrawal results in improvement in total cholesterol, this is offset by the reduction in HDL.

The treatment of hyperlipidemia to decrease cardiovascular risk is well established in the general population. Although there are no long-term, prospective, controlled studies in the transplant literature, it is fair to infer that transplant recipients will also benefit from similar treatment strategies. If adjustment of the immunosuppressive regimen, diet, and exercise are not successful in reducing lipid levels, drug treatment should be initiated. The most appropriate treatment for hyperlipidemia is the use of 3-hydroxy-3-methyl-glutaryl-CoA reductase inhibitors (statins), because the most common lipid abnormality is elevated total cholesterol and LDL. Fibric acid derivatives or nicotinic acid may be used adjunctively and are sometimes required for management of isolated hypertriglyceridemia.

Posttransplant Diabetes Mellitus(PTDM). PTDM occurs in 10% to 15% of patients and reflects the effects of corticosteroids and calcineurin inhibitors on insulin and glucose metabolism in genetically susceptible individuals. Risk factors for the development of PTDM include older age at transplantation; heavier body weight at transplantation; abnormal glucose tolerance before transplantation; African American, Hispanic, or Native American ethnicity; calcineurin inhibitors; corticosteroids; family history of type 2 diabetes; and posttransplant weight gain. Approximately two thirds of patients with PTDM require treatment with insulin, although the requirement for insulin may be eliminated with weight loss or minimization/withdrawal of steroids or calcineurin inhibitors.

Malignancy. Long-term transplant recipients have a 3- to 5-fold increase in the incidence of de novo malignancies compared to the general population. The mean incidence of malignancies of all types ranges between 1% and 18%, and there is substantial geographic variation in the incidence. Carcinomas of the lung, prostate, colon, and breast do not occur with increased frequency in transplant recipients. Neoplasms that occur with increased frequency are posttransplant lymphoproliferative disease (PTLD), skin cancer, Kaposi's sarcoma, and genital neoplasia.

The overall incidence of PTLD is 1% to 3% and commonly presents with unexplained fever or asymptomatic lymphadenopathy. Biopsy of affected lymph nodes or involved tissue is required for a definitive diagnosis. There are unusual features of PTLD compared to lymphomas in the general population. The majority (96%) are non-Hodgkin's lymphomas. Extranodal involvement (central nervous system, intestines, liver, transplanted organs) is common. There is a high rate of association with Epstein-Barr virus infection. Seronegative recipients of organs from seropositive donors are at highest risk (e.g., pediatric patients). The PTLD mortality rate is 50-fold higher than that of lymphoma in the general population. PTLD may respond to withdrawal or minimization of immunosuppression, antiviral therapy with ganciclovir or valganciclovir in patients with Epstein-Barr virus, and/or the anti-CD20 antibody, rituximab. In patients who do not respond to these therapies or who have progressive disease, chemotherapy and radiotherapy may be necessary.

Skin cancer is the most common posttransplant malignancy. The risk of developing skin cancer increases by 4- to 7-fold in areas with limited sun exposure and 20-fold in those with significant sun exposure compared with the general population. Unusual features compared to the general population include squamous cell carcinoma is more common than basal cell carcinoma; lesions develop at a younger age; multiple sites are often present at initial diagnosis; and squamous cell carcinomas are more aggressive, likely to recur after resection, and metastasize more frequently. Most skin cancers are easily treated with local excision. Recommendations to prevent skin cancer include avoiding sun exposure, wearing protective clothing, using sunscreen with SPF 30 or higher, conducting regular and thorough skin examinations, and referring suspicious lesions to a dermatologist.

In most series, up to 10% of all posttransplant malignancies are Kaposi's sarcoma. The most common sites of involvement are the skin, oropharyngeal membranes, and the conjunctiva. It presents as reddish blue macules and plaques. Treatment includes decreasing immunosuppression, chemotherapy, and radiotherapy.

Compared to the general population, female kidney transplant recipients have a 40-fold increase in vulvar and vaginal carcinoma and a 15-fold increase in cervical neoplasia. There is a higher incidence of human papilloma virus coinfection in transplant recipients than in nontransplant patients with cervical cancer. Because of the higher risk of cancer, aggressive gynecological screening is recommended for early detection and treatment.

Skeletal Disorders. Disorders of bone and mineral metabolism are significant problems in long-term kidney transplant recipients. Most transplant patients have 1 or more risk factors for bone disease at the time of transplantation, and many already have significant bone disease due to chronic kidney disease, including hyperparathyroidism, osteomalacia, and adynamic bone disease. Osteoporosis, a significantly decreased bone mineral density, may be present in up to 60% of kidney transplant recipients and frequently develops within the first 18 months after transplantation. Causes of osteoporosis include immunosuppressive medication (corticosteroids and calcineurin inhibitors), loop diuretics (e.g., furosemide), hypogonadism, hyperparathyroidism, cigarette smoking, and insufficient dietary calcium intake.

Monitoring of bone and mineral metabolism and institution of preventive measures is essential to minimize bone disease. Prevention of osteoporosis should begin before transplantation with measurement of bone density, thyroid function, serum calcium, vitamin D, and parathyroid hormone, and testosterone levels in men. Treatment of osteoporosis and low bone mass include calcium, vitamin D, and hormonal supplementation, if appropriate. Treatment with bisphosphonates should also be instituted.

Osteonecrosis occurs in up to 15% of patients in the first 3 years after transplantation. The femoral head is the most common site of involvement. The pathophysiology is uncertain, but corticosteroids are implicated as the major contributing factor. Treatment includes core decompression and total arthroplasty.

Hematopoietic Abnormalities. Posttransplant erythrocytosis occurs in 10% to 20% of kidney recipients. Pathophysiologic mechanisms are probably related to abnormal feedback regulation of erythropoietin metabolism. Treatment includes phlebotomy or angiotensin inhibitors. Pancytopenia is most often related to myelosuppressive immunosuppressants (azathioprine, mycophenolate mofetil, sirolimus). Anemia may be related to renal insufficiency.

Recurrent Renal Disease. The types of renal disease that may recur in transplant recipients are genetic and metabolic diseases, diabetic nephropathy, Fabry's disease, primary oxalosis, sickle-cell nephropathy, and amyloidosis. Patients with Alport's syndrome may develop antiglomerular basement membrane antibody-mediated glomerulonephritis. Table 7 lists renal diseases and rates of recurrence.

Table 7. RATES OF RECURRENT DISEASE AFTER KIDNEY TRANSPLANTATION

Disease	Frequency of recurrence (%)
Focal and segmental glomerulosclerosis	30-50
Membranoproliferative type 1	30-50
Membranoproliferative type 2	80-100
Diabetic nephropathy	80-100 (by histology)
Oxalosis	80-100
Immunoglobulin A nephropathy	40-60
Henoch-Schonlein purpura	75-85
Membranous nephropathy	10-30
Anti-GBM (glomerular basement membrane)	5-10
Hemolytic uremic syndrome	50-75
Lupus nephritis	3-10

Adapted from Siddqi N, Hariharan S, Danovitch G. Evaluation and preparation of renal transplant candidates. In: Danovitch GM, ed. Handbook of Kidney Transplantation. 4th ed. Philadelphia, Pa: Lippincott Williams & Wilkins; 2005:169-192.

Summary

Kidney transplantation is the treatment of choice for patients with ESRD because it offers the greatest potential for a longer, healthier life. Careful evaluation of the candidate and management of coexisting medical and psychosocial problems during the waiting period decrease the morbidity and mortality after transplantation. Management of infection, cardiovascular disease, diabetes mellitus, malignancy, skeletal disorders, hematopoietic abnormalities, and recurrent renal disease is key to long-term patient and graft survival. Successful outcomes depend on collaboration between the transplant team, patient, dialysis unit, and primary healthcare providers.

References

1. United States Renal Data System. USRDS 2003 Annual Data Report. Bethesda, Md: National Institute of Diabetes and Digestive and Kidney Diseases, National Institutes of Health (NIH), DHHS; 2003. Available at: http://www.usrds.org. Accessed May 11, 2005.
2. OPTN/SRTR. 2004 Annual Report. Available at: http://www.optn.org/AR2004. Accessed May 11, 2005.
3. Wolfe RA, Ashby VB, Milford EL, et al. Comparison of mortality in all patients on dialysis, patients on dialysis awaiting transplantation, and recipients of a first cadaveric transplant. *N Engl J Med.* 1999;341:1725-1730.
4. Davies DB, Harper A. The OPTN waiting list. 1998-2003. In: Cecka JM, Terasaki PI , eds. *Clinical Transplants 2004.* Los Angeles, Calif: UCLA Immunogenetics Center. 2005;27-40.
5. Jacobs S, Cho E, Dunkin B. Laparoscopic donor nephrectomy: current role in renal allograft procurement. *Urology.* 2000;55:807-811.
6. Meier-Kriesche HU, Port FK, Ojo AO, et al. Effect of waiting time on renal transplant outcome. *Kidney Int.* 2000;58:1311-1317.
7. Mange K, Joffe MM, Feldman HI. Effect of the use or nonuse of long-term dialysis on the subsequent survival of renal transplants from living donors. *N Engl J Med.* 2001;344:726-731.
8. Meier-Kriesche HU, Kaplan B. Waiting time on dialysis as the strongest modifiable risk factor for renal transplant outcomes. *Transplantation.* 2002;74:1377-1381.
9. Mange KC, Weir MR. Preemptive renal transplantation: why not? *Am J Transplant.* 2003;3:1336-1340.
10. Bunnapradist S, Gritsch HA, Peng A, Jordan SC, Cho YW. Dual kidneys from marginal adult donors as a source for cadaveric renal transplantation in the United States. *J Am Soc Nephrol.* 2003;14:1031-1036.

11. Kendrick E, Singer J, Gritsch HA, Rosenthal JT. Medical and surgical aspects of kidney donation. In: Danovitch GM, ed. *Handbook of Kidney Transplantation*. 4th ed. Philadelphia, Pa: Lippincott Williams & Wilkins. 2005;135-168.

12. OPTN/SRTR. 2003 Annual Report. Available at: http://www.optn.org/AR2003. Accessed February 26, 2004.

13. Stratta RJ, Rohr MS, Sundberg AK, et al. Increased kidney transplantation utilizing expanded criteria deceased organ donors with results comparable to standard criteria donor transplant. *Ann Surg.* 2004;239:688-695.

14. Matas AJ, Kasiske B, Miller L. Proposed guidelines for re-evaluation of patients on the waiting list for renal cadaver transplantation. *Transplantation*. 2002;73:811-812.

15. Joosten SA, VanKooten C, Paul LC. Pathogenesis of chronic allograft rejection. *Transpl Int.* 2003;16:137-145.

16. Cohen D, Galbraith C. General health management and long-term care of the renal transplant recipient. *Am J Kidney Dis.* 2001; 38(suppl 6):S10-S24.

Pancreas Transplantation

Daniel C. Steen, RN, BA
Mary Beth Drangstveit, RN, BAN, CCTC

The first pancreas transplantation was performed by Kelly and Lillihei at the University of Minnesota in 1966.[1] In 1 surgical procedure, both a kidney and pancreas from the same deceased donor were transplanted into an insulin-dependent diabetic with renal failure. This pioneering transplant surgery demonstrated that in addition to achieving freedom from dialysis, euglycemia independent of exogenous insulin and dietary restriction could be reestablished in individuals with type 1 diabetes mellitus and end-stage renal disease (ESRD). Since 1966, more than 23 000 pancreas transplants worldwide have been reported to the International Pancreas Transplant Registry.[2] Today, simultaneous transplantation of a pancreas and kidney from the same deceased donor into 1 recipient is the most frequently performed pancreas transplant surgery.

Pretransplant Considerations

Indications

More than 18 million people in the United States suffer from diabetes. Of these, 5% to 10% have type 1 diabetes; the remainder have type 2. Diabetes is now the leading cause of ESRD, accounting for more than 40% of new cases.[3,4] When these patients are referred for kidney transplant evaluation, they also should be screened to determine if they are candidates for a simultaneous pancreas-kidney transplant (SPK) or a sequential kidney transplant alone (KTA) followed by a pancreas after kidney transplant (PAK).

In addition to individuals with ESRD from type 1 diabetes, there are 2 cohorts of nonuremic insulin-dependent diabetics that are potential pancreas transplant candidates. First, for people who have potentially life-threatening complications of diabetes, such as hypoglycemic unawareness, severe insulin resistance, or extremely labile blood glucose levels, a pancreas transplant alone (PTA) restores euglycemia without the need for exogenous insulin. Second, for patients with surgical diabetes following native pancreatectomy, a functioning enteric-drained pancreas graft restores both pancreatic endocrine and exocrine function.

One of the most important benefits of pancreas transplantation is the protection the graft offers the transplanted kidney (in SPK and PAK) or native kidneys (in PTA) from diabetic glomerulopathy.[5] Proliferative retinopathy is stabilized so that, even though vision may not improve, injury to the retina usually does not progress as long as the pancreas graft continues to function.[6] Peripheral neuropathy and vascular disease, on the other hand, do improve as nerve conduction velocities increase and arterial intima-media thickness decreases after pancreas transplantation.[7,8] In quality-of-life studies, pancreas transplant recipients report that their lives are improved after transplantation.[9,10]

The numbers of patients to benefit from pancreas transplantation has increased as outcomes have improved. Currently, the 1-year recipient survival rate is greater than 95% in all categories, with 1-year graft survival between 76% and 85% (Figures 1 and 2).[2]

Transplant Evaluation

The goal of the evaluation is to determine for an individual patient whether the benefits of pancreas transplantation outweigh the potential risks associated with the surgical procedure and long-term immunosuppression. As part of the transplant evaluation, the patient's medical condition is assessed,

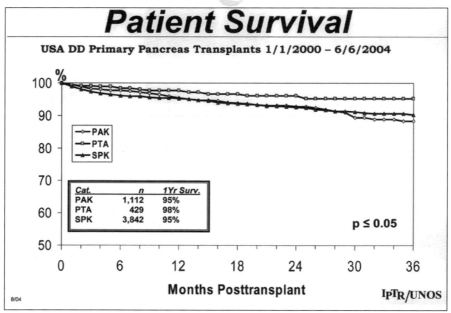

Figure 1. Patient Survival

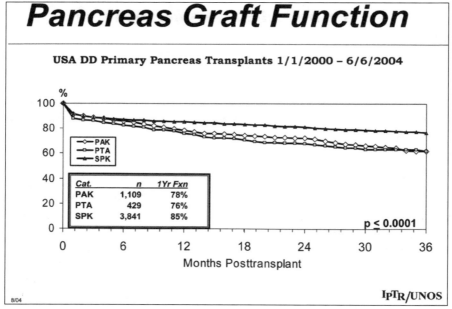

Figure 2. Pancreas Graft Function

Permission granted: Gruessner, A.C., Sutherland D.E.R. Pancreas Transplant Outcomes for United States (US) and Non-US Cases as Reported to the United Network of Organ Sharing (UNOS) and the International Pancreas Transplant Registry (IPTR) as of June, 2004. Clinical Transplantation: August 2005.

health status is optimized, and educational needs of the patient and family are addressed (Table 1).[11] The transplant process from referral through evaluation to transplantation is directed by the clinical transplant coordinator (CTC).

During the medical assessment, particular attention should be directed to coronary, cerebral, and peripheral vascular disease. Heart disease is the leading cause of death among diabetics. The death rate

Table 1. EVALUATION FOR PANCREAS TRANSPLANTATION

1. History and physical examination
2. Basic laboratory studies
   a. Blood typing (required to be checked twice)
   b. Chemistry, hematology panels
   c. Liver function tests, lipid profile
   d. Coagulopathy screening
   e. Virology screening
   f. Pregnancy test, if indicated
   g. Urinalysis, urine culture, stool guaiac
3. Immunology
   a. Tissue typing
   b. Panel reactive antibody
4. Diabetes laboratory studies
   a. Glycosylated hemoglobin
   b. C-peptide (if diabetes onset over age 30)
5. Kidney function
   a. Glomerular filtration rate
   b. Urinary protein
6. Cardiac evaluation
   a. Electrocardiogram, echocardiogram
   b. Stress test and/or coronary angiogram
7. Cancer screening
   a. Mammogram – all women over age 40
   b. Pap smear and pelvic examination – all women
   c. Colonoscopy – all individuals over age 50
   d. Prostate-specific antigen – all men over age 50
8. Radiology studies
   a. Chest radiograph
   b. Gallbladder ultrasound if history of gallstones
   c. Upper gastrointestinal endoscopy if history of bleeding or reflux
   d. Voiding cystogram if history of urinary tract infection or reflux
   e. Abdominal ultrasound to rule out aortic aneurysm if over age 55
9. Vascular evaluation – if claudication, diminished pulses, nonhealing wounds, ulcers, amputations, carotid bruit, stroke/transient ischemic attacks.
   a. Doppler ultrasound of iliac and femoral arteries and veins
   b. Magnetic resonance angiogram
   c. Dye angiogram – specific vessel(s)
   d. Carotid ultrasound
10. Respiratory evaluation – if history of smoking, sleep apnea
    a. Pulmonary function testing
    b. Sleep apnea study
11. Psychosocial evaluation
    a. Social worker assessment/counseling
    b. Psychiatric assessment if history of noncompliance, chemical dependency, cognitive disorder
12. Other consults as indicated
    a. Urology
    b. Neurology
    c. Gastrointestinal
    d. Hematology
    e. Dietician
13. Financial screening
    a. Assessment of adequate financial coverage for transplantation
    b. Financial counseling to maximize coverage
14. Transplant education
    a. Blood matching, cross-matching, antibodies
    b. United Network for Organ Sharing, organ allocation, waiting list
    c. Surgical procedures
    d. Benefits of transplantation
    e. Potential risks and complications
    f. Rejection
    g. Posttransplant routines and follow-up
15. Clinical transplant coordinator role
    a. Screens potential transplant candidates
    b. Coordinates evaluation process
    c. Assesses evaluation results and directs medical care as indicated
    d. Acts as liaison with community providers
    e. Collaborates with interdisciplinary team
    f. Documents actions and plans
    g. Assists with obtaining financial previous authorization for transplantation
    h. Completes UNOS waitlist process
    i. Educates patient and family throughout the pretransplant period

for adult diabetics with heart disease is 2 to 4 times higher than that of adults without diabetes. The risk for stroke is 2 to 4 times higher among people with diabetes.[3] Peripheral vascular disease with nonhealing wounds, claudication, or amputations further increases surgical and immunological risk.

Comorbidities identified during the evaluation phase should be addressed before transplantation to optimize the patient's medical condition before proceeding with major abdominal surgery. For example, if hemodynamically significant flow-limiting lesions are identified on coronary angiography, angioplasty or bypass grafting done before transplantation reduces the individual's cardiac risk at the time of transplant surgery.

Education of the patient and family regarding the risks and benefits of pancreas transplantation is crucial and should include information on rejection, infection, potential surgical complications, potential complications of immunosuppression, and posttransplant medical management. Education should be provided through a variety of media, including written materials, verbal presentations, one-on-one discussion, and visual aids.

Candidate Selection

The evaluation and candidate selection is done by a multidisciplinary team that may include the CTC, transplant surgeon, nephrologist, endocrinologist, social worker, dietician, financial counselor, and other consultants as indicated by the patient's medical condition.[12] On the basis of the evaluation, the team determines whether the individual meets the indication for pancreas transplantation and is medically suitable for the procedure. When the potential risks to the candidate outweigh the benefits, the individual is not a pancreas transplant candidate (Table 2). If the individual is an acceptable candidate, the team then discusses the transplant surgical options with the patient and family, and together determine the best approach for the individual.

Table 2. CONTRAINDICATIONS TO PANCREAS TRANSPLANTATION

Absolute contraindications
1. Active infection
2. Active or recent malignancy (noncutaneous)
3. Uncorrectable coronary artery disease
4. Severe peripheral vascular disease
5. ABO incompatibility
6. Positive T-cell cross-match
7. Morbid obesity
8. Age (per center standard)

Relative contraindications
1. Cardiovascular disease requiring revascularization (per center standard)
2. Obesity
3. Ongoing tobacco use
4. Active or recent substance abuse
5. History of noncompliance
6. Age less than 18 or greater than 45 (or per center standard)

Transplant candidates with type 1 diabetes and ESRD have 3 surgical options: (1) KTA as a definitive procedure, (2) SPK, or (3) KTA followed by PAK. Each transplant procedure or sequence of procedures has associated advantages and disadvantages (Table 3).

There are 2 distinct advantages of SPK over PAK. First, only 1 surgical procedure is needed to transplant both organs. Second, because both the kidney and pancreas come from the same organ donor, kidney graft function can be followed as a surrogate marker for rejection of the pancreas.[13] The main disadvantage of SPK is time on the transplant waiting list. Depending on the United Network for Organ Sharing region, the local organ procurement organization, and the recipient blood type, waiting time for SPK may be 3 to 5 years or longer because of the large waiting list for deceased donor kidneys. Preemptive kidney transplantation before starting dialysis becomes unlikely, and mortality and morbidity on dialysis while awaiting transplantation pose additional risks.

Table 3. TRANSPLANT OPTIONS FOR DIABETES

1. Simultaneous kidney-pancreas transplantation
   a. Insulin-dependent diabetes and end-stage renal disease.
2. Pancreas after kidney transplantation
   a. Previous kidney transplantation
   b. Prevent diabetic nephropathy in transplant kidney
3. Pancreas transplantation alone
   a. Hypoglycemic unawareness
   b. Failed standard insulin regimens
   c. Progressive secondary complications of diabetes
   d. Surgical diabetes secondary to native pancreatectomy
4. Kidney transplant alone
   a. Not a candidate for pancreas transplantation

There are 3 main advantages to PAK transplantations for patients with willing and medically suitable living donors.[14] First, a living donor KTA can be done before initiation of dialysis. Second, the quality of living donor kidneys is superior to grafts from deceased donors. Third, the transplant candidate can be added to the waiting list for a deceased donor pancreas and begin accumulating waiting time. As symptoms of uremia develop and need for dialysis approaches, KTA can be scheduled electively preemptive of dialysis while waiting time for PAK is minimized. Some transplant centers have placed both the living donor and recipient on call, so that if a deceased donor pancreas is allocated to the recipient, a simultaneous deceased donor pancreas and living donor kidney transplant can be done, obviating the need for 2 surgical procedures.[15]

There are 2 disadvantages to PAK over SPK. First, PAK requires 2 surgical procedures and 2 courses of induction immunosuppression. Second, because each organ originates from a different donor, kidney graft function cannot be followed for pancreas rejection, resulting in a slightly higher rate of immunological graft loss.[13] In bladder-drained PAK grafts, urinary amylase levels can be monitored as an independent parameter for early pancreas rejection.

For individuals with a constellation of serious comorbidities such as uncorrectable cardiovascular disease, extensive peripheral vascular disease, severe cerebral vascular disease, or obesity, the risk of major abdominal surgery may be too great to proceed with pancreas transplantation. Although high-risk candidates, they may be acceptable for KTA to improve quality of life and extend life expectancy.

For nonuremic insulin-dependent diabetics who are transplant candidates, PTA is the indicated procedure. However, if the patient has early diabetic nephropathy (eg, microalbuminuria, characteristic kidney biopsy findings, mild increase in serum creatinine, or hypertension), the options are not as clear.[5] Because calcineurin inhibitor nephrotoxicity is more severe in kidneys with chronic renal insufficiency, should the patient delay pancreas transplantation and wait for ESRD, then proceed with SPK or PAK? With glomerular filtration rates greater than 20 mL per minute, they are not eligible for the deceased donor kidney waiting list. However, if they have a willing and medically suitable living kidney donor available when needed, and they understand that progression to ESRD may be earlier with PTA, they may choose to accept the risks of PTA in exchange for the benefits.

Waiting List

The CTC is responsible for managing the waiting list and ensuring compliance with Organ Procurement and Transplantation Network procedures and regulations. While on the waiting list, there should be clear communication between the patient, their physician, and the CTC because changes in medical condition could affect the status of the candidate on the list. To screen for changes that might not be apparent, an annual medical evaluation including cardiac follow-up is required to remain active on the pancreas transplant waiting list.

Serum samples for the histocompatibility laboratory used for cross-matching with potential donors and serial monitoring of panel reactive antibody are needed every 1 to 3 months while waiting. If the patient has an immunizing event such as a blood transfusion, posttransfusion serum samples must be obtained to determine if the patient developed new anti-HLA antibody.

Pancreas Transplant Surgery

Organ Procurement and Bench Preparation

The spleen and duodenum are removed from the deceased donor *en bloc* with the pancreas as well as the pancreatic portion of the portal vein to provide venous outflow from the allograft.[16,17] The celiac access and common hepatic artery are sacrificed to procurement of the liver. Because the primary blood supply to the pancreas is from the splenic artery and superior mesenteric artery,, both of which originate from the celiac access, a segment of donor iliac artery, including the common iliac through the bifurcation to the internal and external branches, is removed to be used later to reconstruct arterial blood flow to the graft (Figure 3).

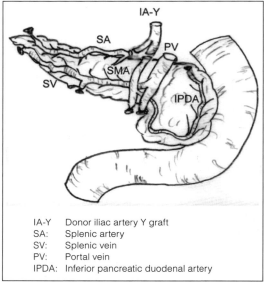

On a back table in the recipient operating room, the spleen is removed from the tail of pancreas. The duodenum is trimmed to capture exocrine secretions from the pancreatic and auxiliary ducts, creating a cuff to be used for the small bowel or urinary bladder anastomosis. Blood supply to the duodenal cuff comes from the pancreas via the inferior pancreaticoduodenal artery, a branch of the superior mesenteric artery. Next, the segment of donor iliac artery is brought onto the table to reconstruct arterial blood flow. The internal branch of the iliac artery is anastomosed end-to-end to the splenic artery. In a similar fashion the external branch of the iliac artery is anastomosed to the superior mesenteric artery, thus creating an interposition Y-graft to reestablish blood flow to the pancreas in the recipient.[18] The pancreas-duodenal allograft is then ready to be brought into the recipient surgical field for transplantation.

IA-Y   Donor iliac artery Y graft
SA: Splenic artery
SV: Splenic vein
PV: Portal vein
IPDA: Inferior pancreatic duodenal artery

Figure 3. Vascular Anatomy of the Pancreas

Transplant Surgical Procedure

In the recipient surgery, the peritoneum is entered via a midline abdominal incision. The right lower quadrant is dissected down to the iliac artery and vein. The portal vein of the donor pancreas is anastomosed end-to-side to the recipient's common iliac vein, resulting in systemic venous drainage of the allograft.[14] Alternatively, some transplant centers prefer portal venous drainage of the pancreas graft.[19] To accomplish this, an opening in the recipient's mesentery is created through which the distal end of the donor portal vein is passed and anastomosed end-to-side to the recipient portal vein.

Once venous outflow is established, the proximal end of the Y-graft (common iliac artery) is anastomosed to the recipient's right iliac artery to reestablish arterial blood flow. Vascular clamps are removed and the pancreas is reperfused. Attention is then focused on the exocrine pancreas.

Drainage of Exocrine Secretions

Enteric drainage is the most commonly used surgical technique for management of pancreatic exocrine secretions. Once blood flow to the allograft has been reestablished, the small bowel is followed from the ileum up the jejunum to the ligament of Treitz. The duodenal cuff of the pancreas is anastomosed to the jejunum as proximal as possible without creating tension via a side-to-side duodenojejunostomy (Figure 4).

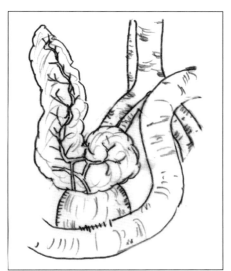

Figure 4. Pancreas Transplantation with Enteric Drainage

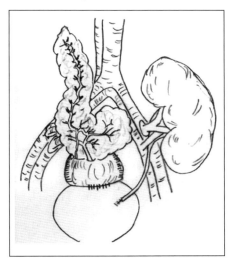

Figure 5. Pancreas Transplantation with Bladder Drainage

The pancreas also can be drained into a nonfunctional limb of jejunum via an end-to-side or side-to-side Roux-en-Y duodenojejunostomy.[20]

As an alternative to enteric drainage, pancreatic exocrine secretions can be diverted into the urinary tract via bladder drainage. In this technique, the bladder is exposed and a transverse incision is made through the bladder dome creating a cystostomy. The duodenal cuff of the pancreas is anastomosed to the dome via a side-to-side duodenocystostomy. Staples or sutures oversewn with bladder mucosa are used to reinforce the anastomosis (Figure 5).

There are 2 distinct advantages to bladder drainage over enteric drainage. First, bladder drained grafts have fewer and less severe early surgical complications. Because the urinary tract is sterile, the incidence of intra-abdominal infection is less. In addition, because there is less manipulation of the small intestine, bowel function returns earlier, the incidence of ileus is less, and hospital lengths of stay are usually shorter. Second, amylase levels in the urine can be monitored as an early indicator of rejection before onset of hyperglycemia (see Rejection). Bladder drained grafts, however, have more long-term complications; primarily metabolic and urological (see Urological Complications).

Enteric drainage, on the other hand, is the most physiological technique for management of the exocrine pancreas.[21,22] The metabolic and urological complications of bladder drainage are avoided. However, there is a higher incidence of early and more severe complications. For example, if an enteric anastomotic leak develops, spillage of bowel contents can lead to severe peritonitis, sepsis, and reoperation. With bladder drained grafts, a bladder leak causes painful chemical peritonitis from pancreatic enzymes, but the leak can be managed acutely with Foley catheter decompression of the bladder. Extended bladder decompression (4-6 weeks) gives the anastomosis a chance to heal without surgical intervention. If the leak persists, surgical repair of the bladder anastomosis or conversion of the graft to enteric drainage is indicated (see Enteric Conversion).

Simultaneous Kidney Transplant

In SPK transplantations, the kidney, like the pancreas, is placed within the peritoneum in 1 surgical procedure (Figure 5). The left lower quadrant is dissected to expose the iliac vein and artery, and urinary bladder. The renal vein and artery are anastomosed to the left iliac vessels and the ureter is implanted in the urinary bladder.

Postoperative Management

Early postoperative management of pancreas transplant recipients involves maintenance of hemodynamic stability and perfusion to the graft to prevent thrombosis, tight glycemic control, monitoring for excessive bleeding, and promoting return of bowel function.[23]

Thrombosis

Pancreas grafts are at increased risk for thrombosis compared with kidney grafts for 3 reasons.[24] First, reconstruction of blood flow with an interposition Y-graft and a deep portal vein anastomosis increases the risk of thrombosis as a technical complication. Second, unlike kidneys, which receive approximately 25% of cardiac output, the pancreas is a low-flow graft. Episodes of hypotension with systolic pressures less than 100 mm Hg decrease blood flow in an already low-flow graft, increasing the risk of thrombosis. Third, in response to surgical manipulation and cold ischemia, postoperative graft pancreatitis is common. Early pancreatitis is characterized by increased serum amylase and lipase levels and tenderness over the graft, and usually resolves within 1 to 3 days after surgery. Inflammation from pancreatitis creates pressure within the graft resulting in resistance to blood flow, further increasing the risk of thrombosis.

Clinical presentation of early pancreas graft thrombosis is characterized by a sudden spike in insulin requirements and a corresponding sudden drop in serum amylase and lipase levels to the low-normal range. If the graft is bladder drained, urine amylase levels also drop precipitously. If thrombosis is suspected, a STAT duplex Doppler ultrasound should be done to assess pancreas blood flow. If ultrasound results are in question or blood flow cannot be visualized, a magnetic resonance angiogram (MRA) of the graft should be obtained to demonstrate patency or confirm thrombosis.[25]

Early thrombosis always requires graft pancreatectomy. If not removed, hemorrhagic pancreatitis, tissue necrosis, peripancreatic inflammation, and intra-abdominal abscess and sepsis can develop. Late thrombosis, on the other hand, may not require graft pancreatectomy. The patient is observed for graft pain, fever and malaise, or other symptoms of dead tissue syndrome. If the patient remains asymptomatic, graft pancreatectomy can be avoided.

Venous thrombosis usually occurs within the first week and, in addition to the biochemical changes outlined above, is characterized by graft pain caused by outflow obstruction. Arterial thrombosis, however, may occur early from a technical complication or acute antibody-mediated rejection, or late as the end result of chronic rejection. Unlike venous thrombosis, arterial thrombosis can occur silently in the absence of pain (see Chronic Rejection).

To minimize graft loss from thrombosis, an intravenous bolus of heparin is given in the operating room before reperfusion of the pancreas. In addition, many transplant programs initiate low-dose heparin drip protocols later on the day of surgery.[26] Patients also start taking aspirin. Intravenous or subcutaneous octreotide may be used to decrease inflammation from early pancreatitis, thus reducing vascular resistance.[27] However, postoperative protocols to prevent thrombosis vary and tend to be center specific. Thrombosis accounts for less than 8% of pancreas graft loss.

Bleeding

When oozing is present in the operating room at the time of closing, surgical drains may be placed to monitor postoperative blood loss. Bleeding from the abdominal incision, if present, is reinforced with surgical dressings. Serial hemoglobins, drain output, physical examination of the abdomen, and hemodynamic values are monitored for signs of increased blood loss from continued oozing or vascular anastomotic bleeding. If there is evidence of excessive blood loss, heparin drips are decreased or discontinued and appropriate blood products are transfused. Hemodynamic compromise in the setting of active intra-abdominal bleeding is an indication for taking the patient to the operating room for exploratory laparotomy to surgically establish hemostasis.[28]

Postoperative bleeding into the intestinal tract from the enteric anastomosis in enteric drained grafts or hematuria in bladder drained grafts is common and usually self-limiting. Bladder drained grafts may require continuous bladder irrigation if clots obstruct the urinary catheter and patency cannot be maintained with intermittent manual irrigation. When hematuria is persistent and transfusions are required, cystoscopic fulguration of anastomotic bleeding may be necessary to control blood loss. In enteric drained grafts, it is uncommon that persistent bleeding necessitates surgical repair of the enteric anastomosis.

In rare cases, the source of bleeding is a vascular anastomosis, intrapancreatic arteriovenous fistula, or pseudoaneurysm. If bleeding presents as an acute abdomen with rapid distention, anemia, hypotension, and shock, emergent surgical intervention and vigorous blood and fluid resuscitation are required.

Early Glycemic Control

The 2 most common causes of early hyperglycemia are intravenous steroids given for induction immunosuppression and delayed pancreas graft function.[29] Most pancreas transplant recipients leave the hospital insulin free; however, some may need supplemental insulin for 2 to 4 weeks after surgery.

To maintain tight glycemic control in pancreas transplant recipients with early hyperglycemia, an insulin drip may be used for the first 2 to 3 days after surgery, if necessary, to keep blood glucose levels 80 to 120 mg/dL. When bowel function returns and the patient begins to eat, supplemental insulin, if necessary, is introduced to support basal glucose metabolism and the insulin drip is discontinued.

Infection

Intra-abdominal Infection

Intra-abdominal infection is a potentially serious postoperative complication.[30] Presenting symptoms usually include abdominal pain and fever. As part of the fever workup, computed tomography scans of the abdomen and pelvis should be obtained.[31] If a fluid collection or rim-enhancing abscess is identified, an interventional radiology consult is obtained for percutaneous drainage and fluid samples are sent for culture.[32] If the volume of the collection is large and the fluid appears purulent, a drain is left in place and broad-spectrum antibiotics are administered. When culture results become available, antibiotic therapy is focused on the basis of the organism and susceptibilities. When the patient improves clinically, drain output decreases, or follow-up computed tomography scan shows resolution of the fluid collection, the drain is removed.

When the abscess is the result of an enteric anastomotic leak or perforation of the duodenal cuff, the patient usually requires exploratory laparotomy for surgical repair of the defect and peritoneal lavage. If the resulting abscess involves the transplanted pancreas, graft pancreatectomy may be necessary.[33] Infected fluid collections in bladder-drained grafts usually respond to percutaneous drainage and antibiotics.[34] Management of bladder leaks is discussed in the section on Urological Complications.

Other Infections

Urinary catheters, central venous catheters, and surgical drains should be removed as early as practicable to reduce the risk of nosocomial infection. Similarly, aggressive pulmonary toilet and early ambulation are the standard of care to decrease postoperative complications. Antimicrobial prophylaxis protocols for abdominal surgery, cytomegalovirus, pneumocystis pneumonia, and oral and esophageal candidiasis are important preventative measures as well.[35]

Rejection

Acute Rejection

An acute cellular rejection episode can occur as early as 7 days after pancreas transplantation. The risk for acute rejection is highest in the first 3 months; however, it can occur anytime after transplantation. Acute rejection usually presents with signs and symptoms of graft pancreatitis characterized by increased serum amylase and lipase levels and graft tenderness. The patient may also complain of nausea and vomiting. Initially, blood glucose levels remain unchanged from baseline.[36,37]

In SPK recipients with enteric drainage, a corresponding increase in serum creatinine levels provides additional clinical evidence of acute rejection. The differential diagnosis for kidney and pancreas graft dysfunction includes acute rejection versus other etiologies such as urinary tract infection (UTI), dehydration, calcineurin-inhibitor nephrotoxicity, hydronephrosis, renal artery stenosis, graft pancreatitis, and peripancreatic abscess. The workup includes urine analysis and culture, calcineurin-inhibitor drug levels, oral hydration, sonogram for hydronephrosis, Doppler ultrasound of the kidney graft for renal artery stenosis (RAS), and repeat of laboratory studies. When the patient has fever and pancreas graft pain, blood cultures and computed tomography scan of the abdomen and pelvis should be obtained to evaluate for infection. If serum amylase, lipase, and creatinine remain elevated and other causes of graft dysfunction have been ruled out, then biopsy of the pancreas or kidney is indicated to make the diagnosis of rejection.[38,39]

Many SPK programs do not biopsy pancreas grafts. Because the donor source is the same, pancreas rejection is almost always concordant with the kidney, so the diagnosis of rejection can be made by kidney biopsy. If discordant rejection of the pancreas is suspected on the basis of clinical presentation, the patient may be treated for rejection empirically without a biopsy.

In bladder drained grafts with increased serum amylase and lipase levels and a corresponding 25% or greater decrease in urinary amylase levels from baseline, the differential diagnosis includes reflux graft pancreatitis or dehydration versus rejection or infection.[37] Orthostatic blood pressures and heart rates are obtained, and laboratory studies are reviewed for dehydration and acidosis, especially serum bicarbonate, potassium, and creatinine. Intravenous fluids and electrolytes are given, and the oral sodium bicarbonate dose and oral fluid intake are increased if indicated. A urine sample for analysis and culture is obtained and an indwelling urinary catheter is placed for bladder decompression to rule out reflux graft pancreatitis. If no cause for graft dysfunction is identified and repeat laboratory studies have worsened or not improved, then biopsy of the pancreas graft is indicated to make the histologic diagnosis of acute rejection.

Most acute rejection is graded mild when based on stains of pancreatic parenchymal tissue for inflammatory infiltrates.[40,41] Unlike heart, kidney, or liver grafts, rejection in pancreas grafts with a mild inflammatory grade usually is unresponsive to pulse steroids alone and requires a lympholytic polyclonal or monoclonal antilymphocyte antibody. In response to treatment, serum amylase and lipase levels should decrease to normal. In bladder drained grafts, urine amylase levels should increase to baseline. If pulse steroids are combined with or used as a premedication for antilymphocyte antibody, blood glucose levels may increase during treatment, but should return to normal once treatment has been completed.

Chronic Rejection

Chronic rejection is usually a late complication of pancreas transplantation. Although rare, it can occur within the first 3 months after transplantation. More commonly, however, chronic rejection occurs later than 6 months after transplantation. Patients who have had 1 or more acute rejection episodes are at increased risk for chronic rejection. Conversely, patients who have never had an acute rejection episode are at low risk for chronic rejection.

Chronic rejection usually presents with slowly increasing serum amylase and lipase levels. Over time, fasting blood glucose and glycated hemoglobin levels also may become elevated from baseline. In bladder drained grafts, urine amylase levels slowly decrease over time. A pancreas biopsy is necessary to make the diagnosis of chronic rejection versus acute rejection versus chronic graft pancreatitis.

On biopsy, histological changes such as fibrosis, scarring, and chronic inflammatory infiltrates are characteristic of chronic rejection.[42] As scar tissue replaces parenchymal acinar tissue, most patients with chronic rejection will eventually lose exocrine function and become hyperglycemic, once again requiring exogenous insulin for glucose management. In spite of severe chronic rejection with loss of exocrine function, selected patients will have preserved islets within a field of fibrosis and scarring. They continue to have islet endocrine function and remain euglycemic and insulin free.

Chronic rejection also may present as sudden onset hyperglycemia in the setting of low normal serum pancreatic enzyme levels. In the bladder drained graft, amylase secretion from the pancreas is no longer detectable in the urine. Doppler ultrasound and magnetic resonance angiography (MRA) of the pancreas should be done to evaluate for graft patency versus thrombosis.[25] If the graft is thrombosed, the patient is observed for fever and graft pain to determine the need for graft pancreatectomy, and insulin therapy is reintroduced.

Rejection Versus Graft Pancreatitis

Like rejection, graft pancreatitis presents with increased serum amylase and lipase, and graft pain. The patient may also have symptoms of anorexia, nausea, and vomiting. In bladder drained grafts, urine amylase levels are decreased.[37] On imaging studies, findings such as peripancreatic fluid collections or fat stranding are consistent with graft pancreatitis.[30] If the patient is febrile, the fluid is drained percutaneously and samples are sent for amylase and lipase in addition to gram stain, fungal, and bacterial cultures. In graft pancreatitis, the fluid is sterile but lipase levels are elevated in the 5000 to 10 000 units/L range.

When organisms are cultured from the fluid, the cause of graft pancreatitis is likely the intraperitoneal peripancreatic infection. With percutaneous drainage of the infected fluid and antibiotic therapy, the peritonitis and pancreatitis should resolve.[31]

In bladder drained grafts, a urinary catheter is placed for bladder decompression to rule out reflux graft pancreatitis. Peripancreatic fluid, in addition to the studies indicated above, should also be evaluated for creatinine and potassium levels to rule out an anastomotic urine leak (see Complications of Bladder Drainage). If a urine leak is present, creatinine and potassium levels in the fluid should be disproportionately higher than in serum. When the pancreatitis is caused by reflux, symptoms and laboratory findings should begin to improve within 24 hours. The catheter is left in place for 5 to 7 days and then removed.

Complications of Glucose Regulation

Transient episodes of hypoglycemia and hyperglycemia can occur in pancreas recipients. To better understand complications of glucose metabolism in the setting of pancreas transplantation, it is helpful to compare endocrine physiology in the native pancreas with a pancreas allograft.

Endocrine Function

There are approximately 1 million islets of Langerhans in the pancreas, which contain alpha and beta cells responsible for regulation of glucose metabolism.[43] In the native setting, beta cells secrete insulin into the portal vein in response to hyperglycemia. The insulin is delivered to the liver first to assist with storage of glucose for future use, before it enters systemic circulation to facilitate movement of glucose from the vascular space into the cell. As glucose levels normalize, insulin secretion ceases. Conversely, in response to hypoglycemia, alpha cells secrete glucagon. Portal circulation carries the glucagon directly to the liver, where is stimulates the release of glucose stores to raise glucose levels systemically. Glucagon secretion stops as serum glucose levels return to normal.

Hypoglycemia

In the transplant setting most pancreas grafts are revascularized to systemic venous drainage via the recipient iliac vein. In response to hyperglycemia, insulin secreted by the graft immediately enters systemic circulation, which can result in hyperinsulinemia and a rapid drop of serum glucose.[44] Although many pancreas transplant recipients have low normal glycosylated hemoglobin levels, 5% to 10% experience recurrent, symptomatic hypoglycemia. Clinically, these hypoglycemic episodes present as "reactive hypoglycemia" in response to systemic circulation of postprandial insulin, and nearly all patients respond to dietary changes.[45] By eating 6 small meals a day, insulin hypersecretion is spread over a longer period, leveling out high-peak insulin levels and corresponding low-glucose troughs.

Portal Venous Circulation

Chronic hyperinsulinemia and beta cell hypersecretion present potential risks for the patient. For example, long-term hyperinsulinemia has been shown to have detrimental effects on lipid and protein metabolism that could lead to accelerated atherosclerosis in a patient already at increased risk for vascular disease. Islet exhaustion from chronic insulin hypersecretion, on the other hand, may shorten the functional life of the graft. In response to these concerns, venous drainage of the pancreas into the recipient portal vein reestablishes portal venous circulation and normalizes islet cell regulation of glucose metabolism.[46] Proponents of portal venous drainage argue that, when combined with enteric drainage of exocrine secretions, the patient receives the most physiologically normal pancreas transplant.

Hyperglycemia

Although mild hyperglycemia is common and self-limiting in the first 1 to 2 weeks after pancreas transplantation, late hyperglycemia is more problematic. Hyperglycemia may be drug induced from steroids, tacrolimus, or other medications. Tapering or discontinuing steroids or converting from tacrolimus to cyclosporine should be considered; in addition, if other medications are implicated, alternatives should be considered. Hyperglycemia also may represent islet exhaustion or be the end result of chronic rejection for which there is no treatment.

When sudden onset hyperglycemia presents as a late complication, with serum glucoses levels from 300 to 600 mg/dL and with normal serum amylase and lipase levels, the likely cause is pancreas graft thrombosis related to chronic rejection.[47] Insulin therapy should be reintroduced; an insulin drip may be required initially. Unfortunately, there is no treatment to salvage graft function. Doppler ultrasound should be done to assess for graft thrombosis. A confirmatory MRA also may be ordered. If the graft has thrombosed and the patient develops fever and abdominal pain, graft pancreatectomy is indicated.

Complications of Bladder Drainage

Despite a less complicated early postoperative course, significant metabolic and urological morbidity is associated with the bladder drained technique in the long term.

Acidosis and Dehydration

In the heterotopic setting of a bladder drained pancreas graft, secretin and cholecystokinin, secreted from the duodenal mucosa in response to the delivery of a bolus of acidic chyme from the stomach to the intestine, are absorbed into the blood stream targeting the graft as well as the native pancreas. Unlike the setting of the native pancreas or enteric drained graft, bicarbonate ion and water secreted by the pancreatic ductules and duodenal cuff are not reabsorbed in the gut, but washed out of the bladder in the urine.[48] Without replacement of bicarbonate and water losses, bladder drained pancreas recipients develop severe acidosis and dehydration characterized by immobilizing orthostatic hypotension. Although most bladder drained graft recipients need 3 to 4 liters of fluid and 2.5 to 5 grams of sodium bicarbonate replacement daily, some may require in excess of 4 liters of fluid and 10 grams or more of bicarbonate to maintain hydration and acid-base balance.[49]

When bladder drained graft recipients are unable to replace fluid and electrolyte losses, serum bicarbonate levels less than 10 mmol/L and potassium levels greater than 6 mmol/L are not uncommon. The electrolyte changes place them at increased risk for electrocardiogram changes. The hypotension and intravascular volume contraction from dehydration increase the risk of pancreas thrombosis in a graft with baseline low-flow.

Hematuria

Blood in the urine is normal and almost always self-limiting in the first 1 to 2 weeks after bladder drained pancreas transplantation. New onset hematuria presenting later than 1 month after surgery occurs in 10% to 15% of bladder drained pancreas grafts. The source of blood loss most commonly is anastomotic at the duodenocystostomy from a small bleeder or an exposed staple or suture. Like postoperative hematuria, late bleeding is usually self-limiting. The patient is encouraged to hydrate to keep urine dilute to reduce the risk of clot formation and obstruction, and serial hemoglobins are checked to monitor blood loss. If clots obstruct the bladder outlet, a 3-way catheter is placed, clots are removed by mechanical irrigation to restore patency and continuous bladder irrigation by gravity drip is initiated. Anticoagulant agents should be withheld or discontinued if possible.[50,51]

When bleeding is persistent or recurrent and requires blood transfusions or patency of the urinary tract cannot be maintained by irrigation, a urology consultation is obtained for cystoscopy. Exposed staples or sutures are removed, bleeders are fulgurated and clots are evacuated. If it can be visualized by cystoscopy through the duodenocystostomy, the duodenal cuff is examined for ulcerations.[52] When hematuria continues or is recurrent in spite of cystoscopic interventions, enteric conversion should be considered.

Urinary Tract Infections

UTIs are a common long-term complication in recipients of bladder drained grafts. Risk factors for UTI include surgery of the urinary tract, maintenance immunosuppression therapy, and alkaline urine. If a staple or suture at the bladder anastomosis is exposed, it can become a nidus for recurrent infections from the same organism that can develop antibiotic resistance over time. Bladder stones can also form on exposed foreign bodies and become a nidus for infection. For recurrent UTI, in addition to treatment

Urethritis

Urethritis caused by inflammation from amylasuria occurs in 8% to 10% of men with bladder drained pancreas grafts. The inflammation causes severe pain with urination and increases the risk of developing urethral strictures or in rare cases urethral disruption. Both men and women are at risk for cystitis with inflammation and bleeding from the bladder mucosa. Women are at risk for developing excoriating lesions of the perineum. Often, the precipitating event is a vaginal yeast infection that compromises the integrity of perineal skin, leaving the exposed tissue vulnerable to excoriation from pancreatic enzymes in the urine. The first-line treatment for dysuria is placement of a Foley catheter to protect the injured tissue from the harsh pancreatic enzymes in order to reduce pain and allow for healing. If urethral or perineal complications recur after removal of the catheter, enteric conversion is indicated.[50,51]

Bladder Leaks

Urine leaks occur in 10% to 15% of patients with bladder drained pancreas grafts. The leaks develop from an anastomotic disruption at the duodenocystostomy. The clinical presentation is characterized by severe pain (10 on a Leichert scale of 1-10), which is relieved by placement of a urinary catheter. Serum amylase and lipase levels increase markedly from graft pancreatitis caused by exposure to pancreatic digestive enzymes. Serum creatinine levels increase because of reabsorption of creatinine from urine in the peritoneum. The extreme pain is caused by chemical peritonitis from exposure to pancreatic digestive enzymes. If the urine is sterile, the patient should not develop bacterial peritonitis.

A cystogram can be done to confirm a leak, but small leaks are often missed. Computed tomography cystograms may also miss small leaks; however, they also can be used to look for fluid collections.[53] Fluid collections should be drained percutaneously and fluid samples should be analyzed for amylase, lipase, creatinine, and potassium levels as well as gram stain and bacterial and fungal cultures. Lipase levels in peritoneal fluid in the 50 000 to 100 000 units/L range are consistent with a bladder leak. Creatinine and potassium levels, which are highly concentrated in urine, should be significantly higher in the peritoneal fluid compared to serum if a urine leak is present.

The urinary catheter is left in place while the diagnostic studies are being done. Once a leak is confirmed, a treatment plan is developed for the patient. For conservative treatment, the urinary catheter is left in place for 4 to 6 weeks to allow for healing of the anastomosis. If the leak is larger or the patient has other urological complications such as frequent UTIs and recurrent hematuria, enteric conversion is indicated.

Enteric Conversion

For patients with a bladder drained pancreas who have significant urological or metabolic complications, conversion of the graft from bladder to enteric drainage is indicated.[54] The abdomen is entered through the same midline incision used for the transplant surgery. The duodenal cuff is removed from the bladder. As described earlier, the pancreas graft is anastomosed side-to-side to the proximal jejunum via a pancreaticoduodenal jejunostomy. If there is increased risk for an enteric leak, the pancreas graft is anastomosed to a nonfunctional limb of jejunum via a Roux-en-Y pancreaticoduodenojejunostomy. The venous and arterial anastomoses are left undisturbed.

Long-Term Management

Pancreas transplant recipients must be committed to medical follow-up for the lifetime of their graft. Continued surveillance for complications of diabetes, side effects of immunosuppression, and pancreas graft dysfunction is critical to long-term success. Even after transplantation, the diabetic population remains at high risk for coronary artery disease and should have cardiology follow-up for life. Establishing primary care for routine health maintenance is especially important in this high-risk group.

Symptoms of pancreas graft dysfunction may be subtle and difficult to identify, making diagnosis and treatment of the underlying complications beyond the scope of practice for healthcare providers in the community who are not familiar with pancreas transplantation. Therefore, it is important that pancreas recipients and their physicians have easy access to the transplant center so that transplant-related complications, should they develop, can be addressed expediently.

Recipients who lose pancreas graft function may wish to pursue retransplantation. These patients need to be reevaluated for medical suitability in light of the surgical risks and outcomes of pancreas retransplantation.[55] Policies regarding pancreas retransplantation vary between transplant centers.

Summary

Until pancreatic islet transplantation is widely applied, transplantation of the pancreas remains the most effective method of restoring insulin independence. Despite steady progress in patient and graft survival, decreasing but significant complications are still associated with pancreas transplantation.[56,57] However, in patients for whom the benefits of the procedure outweigh the potential risks, a functioning pancreas graft can improve quality of life, stabilize complications of diabetes, and provide protection from diabetic nephropathy. Therefore, as immunosuppression therapies continue to improve and surgical morbidity decreases, continued growth of pancreas transplantation will be constrained only by the limitations of the deceased donor pool.

References

1. Kelly WD, Lillihei RC, Merkel FK, et al. Allotransplantation of the pancreas and duodenum along with the kidney in diabetic nephropathy. *Surgery.* 1967;61:827-837.
2. Gruessner AC, Sutherland DER. Pancreas transplant outcomes for United States (US) and non-US cases as reported to the United Network of Organ Sharing (UNOS) and the International Pancreas Transplant Registry (IPTR) as of June 2004. *Clin Transpl.* 2005;19:433-455.
3. National Center for Chronic Disease Prevention and Health Promotion. *National Diabetes Fact Sheet: General Information and National Estimates on Diabetes in the United States, 2002.* Atlanta, Ga: US Department of Health and Human Services, Centers for Disease Control and Prevention; 2003.
4. American Diabetes Association. Position statement: diagnosis and classification of diabetes mellitus. *Diabetes Care.* 2004;27(suppl 1):S5-S10.
5. Fioretto P, Steffes MW, Sutherland DE, et al. Reversal of diabetic nephropathy lesions by pancreatic transplantation. *N Eng J Med.* 1998;339:69-75.
6. Wang Q, Klein R, Moss SE, et al. The influence of combined kidney-pancreas transplantation on the progression of diabetic retinopathy, a case series. *Ophthalmology.* 1994;101:1071-1076.
7. Navarro X, Sutherland DE, Kennedy WR. Long-term effects of pancreatic transplantation on diabetic neuropathy. *Ann Neurology.* 1997;42:727.
8. Larsen LL, Colling BS, Ratanasuwan T, et al. Pancreas transplantation improves vascular disease in type 1 diabetes. *Diabetes Care.* 2004;27:1706-1711.
9. Hathaway DK, Hartwig MS, Milstead J. A prospective study of changes in quality of life reported by diabetic recipients of kidney-only and pancreas-kidney allografts. *J Transplant Coord.* 1994;4:12-17.
10. Suresh Kumar KK, Mubin T, Mikhael N, et al. Assessment of quality of life after simultaneous pancreas-kidney transplantation. *Am J Kidney Dis.* 2002;39:1300-1306.
11. Khwaja K, Humar A. Pretransplant evaluation and cardiac risk assessment. In: Gruessner RW, Sutherland DE, eds. *Transplantation of the Pancreas.* New York, NY: Springer-Verlag; 2004:103-109.
12. Freise CE, Narumi S, Stock PG, et al. Simultaneous pancreas-kidney transplantation: an overview of indications, complications and outcomes. *West J Med.* 1999;170:11-18.
13. Humar A, Kandaswamy R, Ramcharan T, et al. A multivariate analysis of risk factors for acute rejection in pancreas transplant recipients. *Am J Transplant.* 2001;1(suppl 1):212.
14. Gruessner RW. Recipient procedures. In: Gruessner RW, Sutherland DE, eds. *Transplantation of the Pancreas.* New York, NY: Springer-Verlag; 2004:150-178.
15. Farney AC, Cho E, Schweitzer EJ, et al. Simultaneous cadaver pancreas living donor kidney transplantation: a new approach for the type 1 diabetic uremic patient. *Ann Surg.* 2000;232:696-703.
16. Gill IS, Sindhi R, Jerius JT, et al. Bench reconstruction of the pancreas for transplantation: experience with 192 cases. *Clin Transpl.* 1997;11:104-109.

17. Bandlien KO, Mittal VK, Toledo-Pereyra LH. Procurement and benchwork procedures in preparation of pancreas allografts. *Am Surg.* 1988;54:578-581.
18. Mizrahi S, Boudreaux JP, Hayes DH, et al. Modified vascular reconstruction for pancreaticoduodenal allografts. *Surg Gynecol Obstet.* 1993;177:89-90.
19. Stratta RJ, Gaber AO, Shokouh-Amiri MH, et al. A prospective comparison of systemic-bladder versus portal-enteric drainage in vascularized pancreas transplantation. *Surgery.* 2000;127:217-226.
20. Prieto M, Sutherland DE, Goetz FC, et al. Pancreas transplant results according to technique of duct management: bladder versus enteric drainage. *Surgery.* 1987;102:680-691.
21. Stratta RJ, Gaber AO, Shokouh-Amiri MH, et al. Evolution in pancreas transplantation techniques: simultaneous kidney-pancreas transplantation using portal-enteric without antilymphocyte induction. *Ann Surg.* 1999;229:701-708.
22. Gruessner AC, Sutherland DE, Gruessner RW, et al. Enteric versus bladder drainage for solitary pancreas transplantation. *Transplant Proc.* 2001;33:1678-1680.
23. Leone JP, Christensen K. Postoperative management: uncomplicated course. In: Gruessner RW, Sutherland DE, eds. *Transplantation of the Pancreas.* New York, NY: Springer & Verlag; 2004:179-190.
24. Troppman C, Gruessner AC, Benedetti E, et al. Vascular graft thrombosis after pancreas transplantation: univariate and multivariate operative and nonoperative risk analysis. *J Am Coll Surg.* 1996;182:285-316.
25. Krebs TL, Daly B, Wong JJ, et al. Vascular complications of pancreatic transplantation: MR evaluation. *Radiology.* 1995;196:793-798.
26. Trollemar J, Tyden G, Brattstrom C, et al. Anticoagulation therapy for prevention of pancreatic graft thrombosis: benefits and risks. *Transplant Proc.* 1988;20:479-480.
27. Stratta RJ, Taylor RJ, Lowell JA, et al. Randomized trial of Sandostatin prophylaxis for prevention of injury after pancreas transplantation. *Transplant Proc.* 1993;25:3190-3192.
28. Troppman C, Gruessner AC, Dunn DL, et al. Surgical complications requiring early relaparotomy after pancreas transplantation. *Ann Surg.* 1998;227:255-268.
29. Tropmann C, Gruessner A, Papalois DB, et al. Delayed endocrine pancreas graft function after simultaneous pancreas-kidney transplantation: incidence, risk factors and impact on long-term outcome. *Transplantation.* 1996;61:1323-1330.
30. Benedetti E, Gruessner AC, Troppmann C, et al. Intra-abdominal fungal infections after pancreatic transplantation: incidence, treatment, and outcome. *J Am Coll Surg.* 1996;183:307-316.
31. Esterl RM, Stratt RJ, Taylor RJ, et al. Diagnosis and treatment of symptomatic peripancreatic fluid collections after pancreas transplantation. *Transplant Proc.* 1995;27:3057-3058.
32. Latourneau JG, Hunter DW, Crass JR, et al. Percutaneous aspiration and drainage of abdominal fluid collections after pancreas transplantation. *Am J Rad.* 1988;150:805-809.
33. Benedetti E, Troppman C, Gruessner AC, et al. Pancreas graft loss caused by intra-abdominal infection. *Arch Surg.* 1996;131:1054-1060.
34. Pirsch JD, Odorico JS, D'Alessandro AM, et al. Posttransplant infection in enteric versus bladder-drained simultaneous pancreas-kidney recipients. *Transplantation.* 1998;66:1746-1750.
35. Fishman JA, Rubin RH. Infection in the organ transplant recipient. *N Eng J Med.* 1998;388:1741-1751.
36. Gruessner RW, Sutherland DE. Clinical diagnosis in pancreas allograft rejection. In: Solez K, Racusen LC, Billingham ME, eds. *Solid Organ Transplant Rejection: Mechanisms, Pathology and Diagnosis.* New York, NY: Marcel Dekker; 1996:455-499.
37. Stratta RJ, Sollinger HW, Groshek M, et al. Differential diagnosis of hyperamylasemia in pancreas allograft recipients. *Transplant Proc.* 1990;22:675-677.
38. Lee BC, McGahan JP, Perez RV, et al. The role of percutaneous biopsy in detection of pancreas transplant rejection. *Clin Transpl.* 2000;14:493-498.
39. Aideyan OA, Schmidt AJ, Trenkner SW, et al. CT-guided percutaneous biopsy of pancreas transplants. *Radiology.* 1996;2001:825-828.
40. Papadimitriou JC, Drachenberg CB, Wiland A, et al. Histologic grading of acute allograft rejection in pancreas needle biopsy. *Transplantation.* 1998;66:1741-1745.
41. Kuo PC, Johnson LB, Schweitzer EJ, et al. Solitary pancreas allografts: the role of percutaneous biopsy and standardized histologic grading of rejection. *Arch Surg.* 1997;132:52-57.
42. Drachenberg CB, Papadimitriou JC, Klassen DK, et al. Chronic pancreas allograft rejection: morphologic evidence of progression in needle biopsies and proposed grading scheme. *Transplant Proc.* 1999;31:614.
43. Carola R, Harley JP, Noback CR. *Human Anatomy and Physiology.* New York, NY: McGraw-Hill; 1990.
44. Diem P, Abid M, Redmon JB, et al. Systemic venous drainage of pancreas allografts as an independent cause of hyperinsulinemia in type 1 diabetic recipients. *Diabetes.* 1990;39:534-540.
45. Katz H, Homan M, Robertson P, et al. Effects of pancreas transplantation on postprandial glucose metabolism. *N Eng J Med.* 1991;325:1278-1283.
46. Gaber AO, Shokouh-Amiri MH, Hathaway DK, et al. Results of pancreas transplantation with portal venous and enteric drainage. *Ann Surg.* 1995;221:613-622.

47. Kandaswamy R, Humar A, Gruessner AC, et al. Vascular graft thrombosis after pancreas transplantation: comparison of the FK506 and cyclosporine eras. *Transplant Proc.* 1999;31:602-603.
48. Nghiem DD, Gonwa TA, Corry RJ. Metabolic effects of urinary diversion of exocrine secretions in pancreatic transplantation. *Transplantation.* 1987;43:70-73.
49. Schang T, Timmerman W, Thedo A, et al. Detrimental effects of fluid and electrolyte loss from the duodenum in bladder-drained pancreas transplants. *Transplant Proc.* 1991;23:1617-1618.
50. Sollinger HW, Messing EM, Eckhoff DE, et al. Urological complications in 210 consecutive simultaneous pancreas-kidney transplants with bladder drainage. *Ann Surg.* 1993;218:561-568.
51. Elmahdi EE, Parminder SS, Mitchell LH, et al. Urologic complications following pancreas transplantation. *Transplantation Rev.* 1997;11:1-8.
52. Hakim NS, Gruessner AC, Papalois BE, et al. Duodenal complications in bladder-drained pancreas transplantation. *Surgery.* 1997;121:618-624.
53. Longley DG, Dunn DL, Gruessner RW, et al. Detection of pancreatic fluid and urine leaks after pancreas transplantation: value of CT and cystography. *Am J Rad.* 1990;155:997-1000.
54. Sollinger HW, Sasaki TM, D'Alessandro AM, et al. Indications for enteric conversion after pancreas transplantation with bladder drainage. *Surgery.* 1992;112:842-846.
55. Humar A, Kandaswamy R, Drangstveit, MB, et al. Surgical risks and outcome of pancreas retransplants. *Surgery.* 2000;127:634-640.
56. Steen DC. The current state of pancreas transplantation. *AACN Clin Issues.* 1999;10:164-175.
57. Humar A, Kandaswamy R, Granger D. Decreased surgical risks of pancreas transplantation in the modern era. *Ann Surg.* 2000;231:269-275.

Heart Transplantation

Debi Dumas-Hicks, RN, BS, CCTC

Historical Perspective

The development of the science of man, even more than that of other sciences, depends on immense intellectual effort. We must realize clearly that the science of man is the most difficult of all sciences.

Alexis Carrel, Nobel Laureate Medicine 1912.

The dream of human organ transplantation has existed for centuries and is referenced in both ancient mythology and the Bible. It would not be until the early twentieth century that the pioneering work of the French-American surgeon, Alexis Carrel, would serve as the catalyst that would lead to the first successful heart transplantation. Carrel's development of the surgical techniques for the anastomosis of blood vessels gave rise to a landmark paper in which Guthrie described a successful heterotopic transplantation of a heart of a small dog within that of a larger dog. His genius was rewarded with the Nobel Prize in physiology in 1912.[1]

Mann and Demikhov continued to pursue techniques for viable heterotopic heart transplantation in dogs. With the introduction of the cardiopulmonary bypass, heart surgeries became a clinical reality. Three physicians, Ross M. Brock (Guy's Hospital, London), Richard Lower (Medical College of Virginia), and Norman Shumway (Stanford), were responsible for the development of the technical aspects of orthotopic heart transplantation. This foundation made it possible for the first successful orthotopic heart transplant to be performed by Dr. Christian Barnard in South Africa in December 1967. In the year following Barnard's historic procedure, 102 heart transplants were performed in 17 centers throughout the world. Unfortunately, the results were less than optimal with less than a 15% survival rate. Considering the poor initial outcome, only a few medical centers continued to perform heart transplantation after 1969.[1]

The next breakthrough in transplantation would come in the 1980s with the introduction of cyclosporine A, an immunosuppressive medication, which dramatically improved patient survival by decreasing the threat of rejection.[1,2] This revolutionized the field of solid organ transplantation and increased the amount of transplant centers and transplant surgeries performed.[1,2] Although there are presently more than 140 heart transplant centers in the United States, fewer than 2300 heart transplantations are performed annually because the lack of donor availability. At present, approximately one third of patients on the waiting list for heart transplantation die before an appropriate donor organ can be procured.[1]

Expected Outcomes and Survival

According to the United Network for Organ Sharing (UNOS) and the International Society of Heart and Lung Transplant (ISHLT) 21st registry report (2004), the 1 year patient survival rate for heart transplant recipients has increased from 84% in 1994 to 87% in 2002 the 5-year survival rate is approximately 79% and the 10-year survival rate is approximately 65%.[2-4]

With improvements in surgical techniques, donor management, preservation solutions, immunosuppression and long-term management, the risk factors for prediction of mortality at 1 and 5 years have improved significantly (Tables 1 and 2).[3,4]

HEART TRANSPLANTATION

Table 1. RISK FACTORS FOR MORTALITY

First year
- Age of donor and / or recipient
- Transplant center volume and experience
- Recipient's bilirubin and creatinine levels
- Donor heart ischemic time.[2-5]

First 5 years
- Retransplantation
- Pretransplant coronary artery and/ or cerebrovascular disease
- Cytomegalovirus donor/recipient mismatch
- Treatment for infection before hospital discharge
- Presence of coronary artery vasculopathy and/or rejection in the first year.

First 10 years
- Diagnosis of pretransplant coronary artery disease
- Diagnosis of congenital heart disease
- Previous pregnancy
- Female recipient
- Retransplantation[2,3,5]

Table 2. CAUSES OF DEATH AFTER HEART TRANSPLANT

Within the first month
- Graft failure (41%)
- Multiorgan failure (13%)
- Non-CMV infection (14%)

Within the first year
- Non-CMV infection 35%)
- Graft failure (primary/nonspecific) (19%)
- Acute rejection (12%)

Within 5 years
- Cardiac allograft vasculopathy and subsequent graft failure (30%)
- Malignancies (24%)
- Non-CMV infection are the primary causes of death after five years.

Abbreviation: CMV, cytomegalovirus

Indications and Contraindications

Heart transplantation appears at the end of the treatment algorithm for patients with advanced refractory heart failure. The etiology of heart disease for potential transplant candidates has not changed through the years. The majority of patients have ischemic (44%) and dilated (43%) cardiomyopathies and a small percentage of patients (11%) have other diagnoses such as valvular, hypertrophic, peripartal and congenital cardiomyopathies.[2-4]

Standardized guidelines set by several organizations including the American College of Cardiology, American Heart Association, American Society of Transplant Physicians, UNOS, and the ISHLT have been created to assist physicians in the management of heart failure and to aid in the timing of appropriate referral of these patients for transplantation.[4]

Indications

The general consensus is that patients with end-stage heart disease refractory to optimal medical and pharmacotherapy and not amenable to any further percutaneous or surgical interventions are *potential* candidates for heart transplant surgery (Table 3).[1-7] Whether they meet the selection criteria for heart transplantation depends on the results of the evaluation process which is a thorough physical and psychosocial examination.

Table 3. INDICATIONS FOR ADULT HEART TRANSPLANT CANDIDATES

- New York Heart Association class III-IV with deterioration
- Ejection fraction < 0.20
- Max oxygen consumption per unit time <14 m/kg/minute
- Predicted life expectancy < 50 – 70% @ one year
- Refractory recurrent ventricular arrhythmias
- Refractory recurrent angina not amenable to medical, percutaneous, and/or surgical intervention
- Cardiogenic shock/low-output syndrome
- Mechanical assistance (e.g., ventilator, intra-aortic balloon counter pulsation, ventricular assist device)
- Continuous inotropic support and invasive monitoring

Contraindications

Absolute and relative contraindications for heart transplantation vary according to the philosophy of individual transplant centers, but there are some universally accepted tenets in deciding which patients would benefit from heart transplantation (Table 4).[2-5,7] The risk of multiple comorbidities of some patients and the sequelae of chronic damage to vital organs equates to inferior survival. With the scarcity of suitable donor hearts, this risk-benefit ratio must be considered.

Table 4. CONTRAINDICATIONS FOR HEART TRANSPLANTATION

- Fixed pulmonary hypertension (pulmonary vascular resistance > 6 wood units), pulmonary artery systolic pressure >70 mm Hg despite vasodilators, transpulmonary gradient (mean pulmonary artery pressure – pulmonary capillary wedge pressure) >15-20 mm Hg
- Irreversible hepatic, renal, and/or pulmonary disease
- Diabetes mellitus with end-organ damage
- Recent malignancy (< 5 years)
- Active untreated infection
- Chronic hepatitis
- Human immunodeficiency virus positive
- Active unresolved substance abuse
- Dementia, schizophrenia, severe mental retardation
- Severe cachexia
- Myocardial infiltrative and inflammatory disease
- Active peptic ulcer disease
- Morbid obesity

Evaluation of Potential Recipients

Patients referred for heart transplantation undergo a battery of diagnostic tests as well as consultations with specialty services to determine if they have contraindications for heart transplantation. (Table 5).[2-4] Tailoring the evaluation to save time and money can be done by performing tests in an orderly fashion to rule out absolute and relative contraindications first, before proceeding to more expensive tissue typing and other diagnostic tests. Emergent evaluation in the hospital setting can be performed for critical hemodynamically compensated patients.

Table 5. EVALUATION OF POTENTIAL HEART TRANSPLANT RECIPIENTS

Laboratory tests
- Complete metabolic profile), complete blood cell count, prothrombin time/international normalized ratio, partial thromboplastin time, lipid Profile, hemoglobin A1c
- Hepatitis Panel, human immunodeficiency virus, human T-lymphotropic virus 1, cytomegalovirus immunoglobulinG, Ebstein-Barr virus IgG, Varicella IgG, Toxoplasmosis IgG
- Screening prostate-specific antigen (men)
- ABO typing, HLA Tissue Typing (A, B, DR), panel reactive antibody

Noninvasive diagnostic tests
- Echocardiogram
- Chest radiograph, computed tomography of chest/ abdomen (if necessary)
- Cardiopulmonary Testing
- Pulmonary Function Studies with diffusing lung capacity for carbon monoxide
- Pap Smear and mammogram (women, age may vary)

Invasive diagnostic tests
- Left heart catheterization
- Right heart catheterization (if high pulmonary pressures, treat and repeat)
- Colonoscopy (if family history colon cancer or >50 years age)

Consultations
- Social Worker and/ or Psychiatrist
- Financial Coordinator
- Infectious disease physician (immunization record)
- Clearances by other services as warranted by comorbidities: (e.g., hematology/oncology for malignancy and endocrine for diabetes mellitus)

Selection and Listing of Potential Recipients

Selection of candidates for heart transplantation is performed by a committee composed of multidisciplinary team members, including heart transplant surgeons, cardiologists, transplant coordinators, social workers, dietician, and other professionals that may be involved with the care of particular patients to be presented. Candidates may be **permanently deferred, temporarily deferred** (i.e., infraction of substance abuse contract, new or active infection) or **listed** for heart transplantation. In the United States, the potential candidates for the solid organ transplantation are listed with United Network for Organ Sharing (UNOS) based in Richmond, Va. The criteria required for listing a potential heart transplant candidate are the following:[2-4,7]

1. ABO typing (needs to be verified twice by the blood bank and the two coordinators)
2. Weight range
   a. Based on height, weight, transpulmonary gradient (TPG)
   b. If the TPG is elevated, may need larger donor heart
3. Need for prospective donor-recipient crossmatch
4. Status of patient as defined by UNOS: 1A, 1B, 2

Reevaluation of listed patients is recommended at least every 6 months to determine if heart transplantation remains the best option for their heart disease. Patients can be deactivated to a status 7 if their heart function improves or they develop a serious infection and/or malignancy.[2-4,7]

The Waiting Period

After a potential transplant recipient is activated on the UNOS list for heart transplantation, the wait for an appropriate organ begins. During this period, the patient's general health may decline because of worsening pump failure (e.g., renal failure, refractory fluid overload, gastrointestinal distress, dyspnea, persistent hypotension, altered cognition).[4-6] Therefore, it is critical to aggressively intervene with frequent clinic visits and/or hospitalization. Treatment must include a combination of pharmacologic agents and devices such as implantable cardioverter defibrillators, intra-aortic balloon pumps and mechanical circulatory support devices to promote preservation of the potential recipient's vital organs.[4-6]

1. Pharmacological Bridging to Transplant

Strategies for treating patients with end-organ heart failure patient have evolved and improved through the years. Controversy still exists because of the broad and complicated nature of the heart failure milieu, but most clinicians would agree that it is of paramount importance to tailor medical therapy to the individual patient's needs.[4-7] Pharmacological approaches usually include all or combinations of angiotensin-converting enzyme inhibitors, vasodilators, diuretics, β-blockers and digoxin therapy. If congestion persists, placing a pulmonary artery catheter to objectively measure hemodynamic parameters aids in clarifying decisions on whether parenteral infusions of diuretics and/or renal dose dopamine (< 5mcg/kg/min) would be therapeutic. Hemofiltration, ultrafiltration and/or peritoneal dialysis may also be helpful in moving large quantities of volume, thus improving the patient's symptoms dramatically. In refractory advanced stages of heart failure, chronic parenteral infusion of dobutamine, dopamine, milrinone, nesiritide and/or combinations of these drugs may be used to improve the patient's symptoms and quality of life. These measures (apheresis therapy and inotropic/vasodilator chronic infusion) do not seem to increase survival, and are being evaluated in larger clinical trials to find out beneficial issues and clear recommendations in this specific population.[4] In the milieu of treating worsening heart failure, other comorbidities may go undetected (e.g., hypothyroid disease, diabetes mellitus, hypertension, chronic obstructive pulmonary disease, sleep apnea) and therefore untreated. Management of these conditions is essential for the success of a potential heart transplantation.[4] Antiarrhythmic drugs, except for low-dose amiodarone, should be avoided if possible, and alternative electrophysiologic intervention techniques (i.e., arrhythmia ablation, implantation of arrhythmia-terminating device, implantation of bi-ventricular pacing devices) might prove helpful. With the exception of the most severe end-stage heart failure, it is recommended that the patient still attempt to make prescribed lifestyle changes with dietary restriction of sodium and fluid; supplementation of vitamins, minerals and nutrients; along with tailored aerobic activity.

2. Mechanical Bridging to Transplant

The first circulatory support device was used in 1953 by Gibbon, a surgeon who used the cardiopulmonary bypass machine for open heart surgery.[8] Since that time, the quest for emergency, temporary, and permanent heart assist systems has persisted. Within the last decade, many advances have been made with mechanical circulatory support devices to "bridge" potential candidates for heart transplantation if pharmacological efforts fail. The ventricular assist device (VAD) is a surgically implanted device that is connected to the native heart to assist in decreasing myocardial workload by reducing preload and myocardial oxygen consumption and maintaining sufficient systemic circulation to perfuse vital organs. Depending on which side of the heart the VAD assists, it is referred to as right ventricular assist device RVAD), left ventricular assist device (LVAD), or bi-ventricular devices (BIVAD).[4,8-10] The VADS are categorized in 2 different groups:

1. Heart support
    a. Short-term support
    b. Long-term support
2. Pump-flow design
    a. Pulsatile or continuous
    b. Anatomic positioning of the VAD pump
        i. Paracorporeal (internal)
        ii. Extracorporeal (external).[1,3, 16,17]

The most commonly used assist devices approved by the Food and Drug Administration are the following:
1. Short term, pulsatile, paracorporeal VADS
    - Abiomed BVS: RVAD, LVAD, BIVAD (short-term)
    - Thoratec VAD: RVAD, LVAD, BIVAD (short- and long-term)

2. Long-term, pulsatile, extracorporeal VADS
   - Novacor LVAS: LVAD
   - Thoratec PVAD: LVAD
   - Thoratec IVAD: RVAD, LVAD, BIVAD (paracorporeal)
   - Heartmate XVE: LVAD

Survival in younger device recipients (< 30 years of age) is better than in those older than 50 years of age (the rate of death before transplantation is 13% vs. 37%, respectively). Complications include infection, bleeding, thrombosis and device failure. With the newly formed voluntary registry for circulatory support devices known as the Mechanical Circulatory Support Database, collecting patients' information related with device characteristics and complications, the hope is to be able to decrease the morbidity and mortality associated with these mechanical devices and to identify what patient populations would be better served with implantation of a mechanical device.[9-12]

Heart Transplant Surgery

1. Donor Management

Potential heart donors must meet the legally accepted criteria for brain death in the United States. These patients usually have suffered an irreversible catastrophic brain insult, with total cessation of brain function. At present, the only donors used for heart transplantation are non-heart-beating (deceased) donors.[1,4-6]

According to Organ Procurement and Transplant Network (OPTN) and UNOS policy, consent must be obtained from the next-of-kin. The deceased donor then undergoes a battery of tests to screen for malignancies, infectious diseases and pertinent pathology applicable to the use of a potential organ (in this case, the heart). The donor's family and friends are questioned regarding any psychosocial aspects of the potential donor's life (i.e., intravenous drug abuse) that may preclude the use of the donor's organs.[2,5,7]

The criteria for determining the suitability for heart transplantation may vary between transplant centers depending on the critical status of their patients and their experience in this arena (Table 6).[2-4,6,7] Determination of acceptability for heart transplantation depends on the donor's medical history (i.e., smoking, drug abuse, alcohol abuse, cardiac trauma) and the results of noninvasive diagnostic testing (i.e., echocardiogram, electrocardiogram) to check for hypokinesis, valvular abnormalities, and ejection fraction. In some cases, an angiogram is performed, if the donor is older than 45 to 50 years of age to determine if significant coronary artery disease is present.[2,4,6,7] (Some centers have an alternate list of older recipients who are willing to accept older as well as marginal donors.[3])

Matching the size of the donor heart to the recipient is critical to its functioning. The potential heart recipient is listed within a weight range based on height, weight, and TPG. Generally, the weight range is not more than 30% of the patient's actual weight and if the patient has pulmonary hypertension, the lower end of the weight range may be the actual weight of the patient. Oversizing the donor heart can produce a restrictive physiology and an inability to close the chest. If the donor's heart is too small for the potential recipient, hemodynamic instability may ensue (e.g., small donor heart into large male recipient).[2,4,7]

Table 6. DONOR CRITERIA FOR HEART TRANSPLANTATION

- Negative human immunosdeificiency virus serology
- Negative hepatitis B and C serology (some centers accept hepatitis C donor hearts for hepatitis C-positive recipients)
- Negative for systemic infections
- Negative for malignancies, except for primary brain tumor
- Cardiac criteria:
  – Negative for cardiac contusion
  – Negative for prolonged /repeated episodes of CPR
  – Negative for excessive inotropic support
  – Negative for abnormalities on echocardiogram (severe wall motion abnormalities)

The final decision to accept a potential donor rests with the cardiac surgeon because the transplant center's surgical team will perform a final inspection of the donor organ for potential contusions and general functioning of the organ before beginning the donor surgery. A very important maneuver for allograft survival during the donor surgery is the initial flushing of the heart with a cold cardioplegia solution to create a state of profound hypothermia to prevent cellular edema, to prevent acidosis and to maintain intracellular adenosine triphosphate for organ preservation. After removing the heart, the primary goal for transportation to the recipient's transplant center is to maintain hypothermia which is attained by placing the heart in a plastic bag submerged in a cold storage solution and ice.[1,4,5]

A key to successful heart transplantation is the minimization of the donor heart's ischemic time, which is measured from the time of aortic cross-clamping in the donor to the release of aortic cross-clamp in the recipient.[1,4,5,13] Four hours still remains the maximum acceptable cut-off time despite efforts to improve donor preservation solutions. As a result, great care in handling the donor heart must be taken during removal, transport and insertion into the recipient.

2. Transplantation Surgery

There are 2 procedures for placement of the cardiac allograft in the thoracic cavity: heterotopic and orthotopic. There are many inherent problems with the heterotopic procedure; therefore, it is rarely used except for patients with severe pulmonary hypertension. The orthotopic procedure, when recipient's heart is removed and the donor heart is inserted, is the most frequently used procedure for sewing in the cardiac allograft. The 2 surgical techniques for placement of the graft are the Biatrial and the Bicaval techniques (Table 7).[1-5,14] The period after the aortic cross-clamp is released is a critical for preservation of donor heart function. Reperfusion is initiated and a sinus rhythm is usually re-established within 1 to 3 minutes, sometimes with the aid of a coronary vasodilator such as intracoronary adenosine. Before and after discontinuation of cardiopulmonary bypass, transesophageal echocardiography is performed to assess each ventricle.

Surgical Problems

- Bleeding secondary to previous sternotomies (i.e., surgeries: cardiopulmonary arteries, valvular, and congenital surgery)
- Tricuspid Insufficiency (may relate to the newly constructed right atrium)
- Sinus node dysfunction (damage from procurement and implantation)
- Kinking of the main pulmonary artery
- Right ventricular dysfunction (during rewarming)
- Neurological events (implantation technique, mural thrombus, air embolism)

Table 7. SURGERY TECHNIQUES

Biatrial technique

- Original technique (Shumway-Lower)
- Removal of both the donor and recipient hearts at the mid-atrial level
- Preserves the pulmonary venous connections to the recipient's left atrium
- Great vessels are resected above the semi-lunar valves

Advantages: Simpler method and save approximately 1 hour ischemic time
Disadvantages: Atrial dysrhythmias, atrial dysfunction, thrombus formation, tricuspid valve dysfunction

Bicaval technique

- Introduction in 1991 by Drefous and colleagues
- Right atrium of recipient is excised leaving 2-3 cm cuff around each cava. (contrasts w/biatrial technique where atrial septum and large mass of recipient atrium are left behind)
- Donor heart is excised with right atrium and long segments of the superior vena cava

Advantages: Preserves integrity of right atrium (e.g., atrial contractility, sinus node function, tricuspid valve competence), lower diuretic dosing, less need for pacing, less mitral incompetence and possible shorter hospital stay
Disadvantages: Takes longer to complete, prolonging ischemic time

HEART TRANSPLANTATION

Post-Transplant Considerations

Upon hospital discharge, there is a period of adaptation as the heart transplant recipients adjust to independent roles in their care (e.g., taking vital signs; self-medication administration). Frequent surveillance for rejection, infection and other complications with laboratory tests, endomyocardial biopsies, echocardiogram and pertinent diagnostic tests become a routine part of their lives in the first year. The transplant team working in conjunction with the transplant recipients' local physicians monitors their progress tailoring the therapeutic regimen to the individual patient's needs.

A. Rejection

Rejection of the heart allograft is an immunologic process that can be devastating if the heart fails. Early detection is critical to preserving allograft function. The approach to determining rejection in a heart transplant recipient is three-pronged: clinical history and examination, non-invasive techniques, and invasive techniques.[2,4,13]

1. **Clinical History**
   - Donor cardiac history
   - Retrospective positive HLA donor-recipient crossmatch
   - History of donor surgery, organ transport and recipient surgery; reperfusion injury; prolonged ischemic time
   - Patient report of signs and symptoms such as dyspnea, fatigue, hypertension, low heart rate, papitations, increasing weight, swelling of the lower extremities and/or abdomen, nausea, vomiting, low-grade fever

2. **Physical Examination**
   - Head and neck: increased jugular venous pressure
   - Heart: Bradycardia, tachycardia, dysrhythmias, new S3 or S4, pericardial friction rub, hypotension
   - Lungs: presence of rales, increased respiratory rate
   - Abdomen: palpation of liver margins, increased abdominal girth
   - Extremities: pitting edema

3. **Non-Invasive Diagnostic Techniques for Rejection**
   - Color-flow Doppler echocardiography: Worsening indices of systolic and diastolic function, presence of a pericardial effusion, increasing thickness and decreasing motion of the walls of the heart, increasing left ventricular mass
   - Electrocardiogram: bradycardia, tacharrhythmias, atrial fibrillation, possibly low voltage (not as reliable for detection of rejection)
   - Bloodwork: immunosuppressive medication levels (cyclosporine, tacrolimus, sirolimus), inflammatory markers (brain natriuretic peptide assay, C-reactive proteins), panel reactive antibody level, immune cell function assay.

4. **Invasive Diagnostic Techniques: Endomyocardial Biopsy**

Techniques for diagnosing heart transplant rejection have continued to evolve since heart transplantation became a reality in 1967. With the introduction of the bioptome instrument for endomyocardial biopsy by Caves and Associates in the early 1970s, a standard for diagnosing rejection of the allograft was created.[2,3,8] Using the right/left internal jugular vein or the femoral vein, the bioptome is inserted into the right atrium across the tricuspid valve into the right ventricle to take samples of myocardial tissue for histological evaluation of allograft rejection. Though the endomyocardial biopsy is well-tolerated with few problems, complications can include carotid artery/myocardial perforation, pneumo- or hemothorax, transient dysrhythmias, and/or tricuspid regurgitation. Because it is invasive and interpretation of results lacks uniformity, the discussion whether the endomyocardial biopsy can be replaced by noninvasive testing is ongoing. Research in the field of molecular genomics holds promise for the future in the detection of rejection. The endomyocardial biopsy, however, has stood the test of time and it still continues to be the "gold standard" for detecting the presence of rejection. A histologic grading system for cellular rejection was created by Dr. Margaret Billingham, an eminent cardiac pathologist, and colleagues for the ISHLT in

1990.[1-4,15,16] This system underwent revision in 2004 by a multi-disciplinary team of immunopathologists, histopathologists and clinicians to clarify the diagnostic categories for rejection (Tables 8 and 9).[15-17]

Table 8. ENDOMYOCARDIAL BIOPSY GRADING SYSTEM FOR CELLULAR REJECTION

Cellular Rejection 1990

Grade 0	No evidence of celular rejection
Grade 1A	Focal perivascular or interstitial infiltrate without myocyte injury
Grade 1B	Multifocal or diffuse sparse infiltrates without myocyte injury
Grade 2	Single focus of dense infiltrates with myocyte injury
Grade 3A	Multifocal dense infiltrates with myocyte injury
Grade 3B	Diffuse, dense infiltrates with myocyte injury
Grade 4	Diffuse and extensive polymorphus infiltrate with myocyte injury May have hemorrage, edema, and microvascular injury

Cellular Rejection 2004

Grade 0 R	No rejection
Grade 1 R	Mild interstitial and/or perivascular infiltrate with up to one focus of myocyte damage
Grade 2 R	Moderate 2 or more foci of infiltrate with associated myocyte damage
Grade 3 R	Severe and Diffuse infiltrate with multifocal myocyte damage ±edema, ±hemorrhage ±vasculitis

Table 9. HUMORAL REJECTION

Humoral Rejection 1990

Humoral rejection (positive immunoflourescence, vasculitis or severe edema in absence of cellular infiltrate) recorded as additional required information

Humoral Rejection 2004

Light microscopic findings:
A. Intravascular polymorphonuclear leukocytes and macrophages with or without endothelial swelling
B. Vasculocentric, lymphocyte-poor inflammatory infiltrate
C. Myocyte injury including necrosis in areas adjacent to (affected?) vessels with infiltrates

Immunofluorescence microscopy findings:
Document the presence of immunoglobulins, complement, and, potentially, fibrin and HLA-DR positivity in the biopsy. At least 2 patterns exist:
A. The most common shows deposits in capillaries, arterioles, and small arteries.
B. The second pattern shows deposits around myocytes.

Immunohistochemistry findings:
It is common to distinguish between elongated macrophages and swollen endothelial cells by staining with CD68 and CD31 in adjacent sections.
Clinical pathology studies: Identification of donor specific antibody in serum

Classification

Antibody-mediated rejection 0
– Negative for acute antibody-mediated rejection (AMR)
– No histologic or immunopathologic features of AMR

Antibody-medicated rejection 1
– Positive for AMR
– Histologic features of AMR
– Positive immunofluorescence or immunoperoxidase staining for AMR
– Positive CD68, C4d

The frequency of endomyocardial biopsies after heart transplantation is specific to each transplant center, with the majority of these invasive procedures being performed in the first year after transplantation while aggressively tapering the immunosuppressive medications. The use of the endomyocardial biopsy diminishes after the first year, except as part of the patient's annual diagnostic tests and/or if the recipient exhibits signs and symptoms of rejection.

There are 3 categories of heart allograft rejection: Hyperacute, acute cellular and acute (vascular) humoral rejection. The use of the term "chronic rejection" can be confusing, therefore its use in the current literature is decreasing.

Hyperacute Rejection: If this type of lethal rejection occurs, it usually happens immediately after reperfusion of the allograft in surgery. This is secondary to an antigen-antibody reaction to preformed donor-specific antibodies that circulate through the coronary bloodstream. Because of pretransplant screening for reactive antibodies that signal a need for prospective crossmatching of the donor and recipient, hyperacute rejection is usually a rare event.

Cellular Rejection: This type of rejection may occur weeks and months, even years, after heart transplantation. The key histologic feature of these categories, ranging from "0" to "3R", is the amount of myocyte damage. Cellular rejection is an inflammatory predominantly lymphocytic response with extension into the myocardium along with myocyte degeneration and presence of eosinophils and plasma cells. Because the clinical symptoms can be vague and non-specific, diagnostic tests such as the endomyocardial biopsy, right heart catheterization and echocardiogram are necessary to support the diagnosis of cellular rejection. Determining the course of treatment depends on the severity of the grade of the biopsy, the time since transplantation, the patient's rejection profile and ventricular function as well as the presence of hemodynamic decompensation.

Treatment for Cellular Rejection:
- IV Solu-Medrol 500 mg – 1000 mg for 3 days and/or oral pulsed corticosteroids
  o Rebiopsy 2 to 4 weeks
- Augmentation of baseline immunosuppression
- IV cytolytic agents (antilymphocyte therapy)
- Other immunosuppressive agents (may be investigational)

Treatment for rejection with hemodynamic compromise is considered potentially life-threatening and usually requires hospitalization with more aggressive treatment with possible IV inotropic support, plasmapheresis and photopheresis.

Humoral Rejection: This type of rejection affects a significant number of heart transplant recipients (44-59%) who may present with unexplained graft dysfunction. It can be referred to as vascular humoral rejection, cardiac vascular (microvascular) rejection, allograft rejection or the newer nomenclature of antibody-mediated rejection.[4,15-17] It frequently occurs during the first month after heart transplantation but can affect the recipient many years later.

In the past, diagnosis of humoral rejection has been confusing because no standardized histologic criteria for humoral rejection have existed. A consensus for criteria for histologic evidence of humoral rejection was created by the same working group that rendered changes to the scoring of cellular rejection.[4,13] Within antibody-mediated rejection, the heart tissue usually has scant evidence of cellular rejection (ISHLT Grade 0 or 1A) with the presence of possible interstitial edema and/or hemorrhage, inflammatory infiltrates in the walls of microvessels (vasculitis) and endothelial cell necrosis. The heart tissue can be sent for frozen section analysis and evaluated with immunofluorescence to identify the deposition of fibrinogen, IgG, IgM or complement along with immunoperioxidate staining on paraffin blocks as confirmation. High right heart filling pressures and a lower systolic ejection fraction on echocardiogram and clinical examination may be used to support the diagnosis of humoral rejection.[4,15,16]

Treatment for Humoral Rejection:
- Hospitalization
- Plasmapheresis
- Cyclophosphamide (parenteral or oral) on the basis of its anti-B cell activity
- Rituximab (parenteral)

B. Infection

Because of the immunosuppressed state of the recipient, infections are a potentially life-threatening complication. Prevention, early diagnosis and aggressive treatment are the hallmarks of therapy.

Although infections can occur at any interval after heart transplantation, there are general guidelines in the type and the interval.

First month:
- Continuation of pretransplant infections
- Reactivation of latent viruses, bacterial nosocomial infections (e.g., mediastinitis)
- Donor-transmitted infections (e.g., toxoplasmosis in donor-recipient mismatch)

Two to six months:
- Opportunistic infections: cytomegalovirus (CMV), Epstein-Barr virus, varicella zoster, herpes simplex 1 and 2
    - CMV, mainly CMV pneumonia, carries the highest morbidity and mortality for transplant recipients and requires aggressive treatment

Six months and later:
- Community-acquired infections

C. Coronary Artery Vasculopathy

After the first year of transplantation, one of the major impediments to survival in heart transplant recipients' survival is coronary artery disease (CAD), commonly referred to as coronary artery vasculopathy (CAV) or allograft coronary artery disease (ACAD). Transplant CAV is an aggressive disease that differs from native CAD in that in CAV the lesions are concentric and diffuse, often affecting the entire length of the vessel. Immunologic and nonimmunologic donor/recipient risk factors increasing the likelihood of developing CAV, identified by the ISHLT 21st Registry are older donor age, CMV, humoral rejection, hypertriglyceridemia, and number of HLA DR mismatches.[3] In the early years of heart transplantation, CAV was thought to present as a "silent disease" because of the denervation of the heart allograft, however now there is evidence of focal and incomplete reinervation. As a result the heart transplant recipient may be able to feel angina pectoris.[4]

Invasive Diagnostic Tests

For heart transplant recipients, left heart catheterization is an integral part of their annual examinations, and the frequency of the procedure (e.g., yearly, every 5 years) is based on specific transplant center protocols. The angiogram is not completely sensitive to the diffuse concentric nature of CAV, but remains one of the best diagnostic tools. Using intravascular ultrasound during the catheterization has proved to be effective in the early diagnosis of intimal thickening leading to CAV.[2-4,15,16,18] Noninvasive diagnostic testing with dobutamine stress echocardiography, stress thallium scintigraphy, CAT Scan angiography and magnetic resonance imaging are used to aid in the determination of ischemia and myocardial injury.[2-4]

Management
- Aspirin 80 mg daily
- Folic acid supplementation (hyperhomocystinemia)
- 3-Hydroxy-3-methylgutaryl coenzyme A reductase inhibitors (hyperlipidemia)
- Percutaneous intervention: drug-eluting stents, balloon angioplasty
- Coronary bypass surgery

Treatment
Re-transplantation

D. Long-term Complications

1. Malignancy

One of the major contributing factors to heart transplant mortality is the development of neoplastic disorders. These disorders can be a recurrence of pre-existing malignancies, donor-related malignancy or *de novo* malignancy. All types of malignancies following transplantation can be found in heart transplant recipients, but cutaneous lesions (i.e., basal, squamous, melanoma), post-transplant lymphoproliferative disorders and lung malignancies account for the largest cohort of patients. The milieu that fosters the development of malignancies is a complex multifaceted interaction of immunosuppressive medications, potentially carcinogenic drugs, a disturbance in immune surveillance and regulation involving failure to recognize and destroy mutated cells.[2-4,5,15]

Management
- Reduction in immunosuppression
- Surgical resection if possible
- Chemotherapy and irradiation
- Annual surveillance for malignancy
  o Skin: dermatological screening
  o Lung: chest radiograph
  o Prostate: prostate-specific blood test; urology evaluation
  o Colon: occult blood test; digital rectal examination; colonoscopy in patients older than 50 years
  o Ovarian/Cervical: Pelvic examination; pap smear
  o Breast: Mammogram
- Patient surveillance for skin cancers, breast nodules

2. Gastrointestinal Complications

Gastrointestinal problems after transplantation can range from minor to major complications. Differential diagnosis is difficult to elucidate because many of the daily medications taken can cause gastrointestinal side effects (e.g., nausea, vomiting, constipation, and diarrhea). Major complications include diverticulitis, peptic ulcer disease, cholelithiasis, and pancreatitis. Chronic corticosteroid use can exacerbate pre-existing conditions creating serious life-threatening complications, such as intestinal bleeding and bowel perforation. Infections such as esophagitis candidiasis, invasive gastrointestinal CMV, and herpes simplex virus are often seen in the transplant recipients. These conditions are hard to elucidate because the symptoms are often vague and intermittent.[2-4]

Management
- Early and aggressive intervention
- Possible surgical intervention

3. Hypertension

Since the introduction of cyclosporine in the late 1980's, the incidence of hypertension in heart transplant recipients has been reported to range from 40% to 90%. Other risk factors, such as genetics, age, ethnicity, gender, diet, and obesity, may also contribute to hypertension. Secondary to denervation, the heart does not respond to sympathetic innervation, which normally maintains a balanced relationship between peripheral vascular resistance and the ventricular inotropic state. As a result, in a hypertensive state, the denervated heart responds poorly to increased afterload leading to systolic left ventricular dysfunction and left ventricular hypertrophy.[2-6,11]

Management
First Line Therapy:
- Calcium channel blocking agents (e.g., Diltiazem)
- Angiotensin-converting enzyme inhibitors (e.g., Ramipril)
- Aggressive sodium restriction
- Exercise
- Smoking cessation

Second Line Therapy:
- Diuretics: should be temporary adjunctive therapy; monitor for renal insufficiency
- α-Adrenergic blocking agents (i.e., catapres)
- β-Blockers: Not considered in the past because of relative chronotropic incompetence and inadequate heart rate response to exercise; currently, low doses have been used successfully.

4. Chronic Renal Disease

The major risk factors for renal dysfunction are the use of calcineurin inhibitors (cyclosporine and tacrolimus), but pretransplant co-morbidities contribute to the worsening of chronic renal disease.[2-5,11,14]

Management
- Reduction of calcineurin inhibitors (does not always guarantee progression of renal dysfunction)
- Aggressive treatment of hypertension, diabetes mellitus, obesity and hyperparathyroidism
- Early referral to nephrology

5. Hyperlipidemia

The causes of hyperlipidemia in transplant recipients are secondary to immunosuppressive agents (especially steroids) as well as the usual predisposing factors such as genetics, obesity, and diabetes.[2,3,6,18]

Management
- Aggressive dietary modifications
- Consistent and regular exercise program
- 2-Hydroxy-3-methylgutaryl coenzyme A reductase inhibitors (e.g., Pravastatin)
- Fibric acid derivatives (e.g., Gemfibrozil)
- Bile acid sequestrants
- Nicotinic acid
- Alterations in immunosuppression

6. Osteoporosis

Bone density loss after heart transplantation is progressive with the majority of bone loss occurring in the first 6 months. Risk factors that contribute to this bone loss are estrogen/testosterone deficiencies, excessive previous alcohol consumption, vitamin D and calcium deficiencies, renal insufficiency as well as posttransplant immunosuppressive medications (especially steroids and cyclosporine). The development of osteoporosis predisposes the patient to fractures and avascular necrosis (ischemic condition causing bone and cartilage death particularly in the femoral head). The quality of life of the heart transplant recipients is affected secondary to the acute and chronic pain from this condition along with limitations in mobility and activities of daily living.[2-4]

Management
- Daily exercise with strength and resistance training
- Weaning of steroids
- Calcium supplementation, vitamin D (not necessary with normal kidneys)
- Estrogen (women) and testosterone (men) supplementation
- Biphosphonates
- Posttransplant yearly dual energy x-ray absroptiometry scan

Final Thoughts

Since the 1980s, heart transplantation has been firmly established as a successful therapeutic modality in the treatment of end-stage heart failure. At present the number of potential candidates continues to exceed the availability of donor organs. This inadequate donor organ supply has placed extreme pressure on the transplant selection committee to critically examine the risk-benefit ratio for each candidate. Future strategies addressing donor-specific tolerance and more selective immunosuppressive therapies will aid in improving survival and quality of life for these patients. The promise of pharmacogenetics, myocardial regeneration, and stem cell therapy as potential treatments for the failing heart are being explored in clinical trials with the hope of offering viable alternatives to transplantation. In support of the proverbial contention, "an ounce of prevention is worth a pound of cure," the medical community must continue to strive toward changing lifestyles and decreasing the development of heart disease.

References

1. Myerowitz PD. The history of heart transplantation. In Myerowitz PD ed. *Heart Transplantation*. Mount Kisco, NY: Futura Publishing. 1987;1-15.
2. Cupples SA. Heart transplantation. In: Cupples SA, Ohler L. eds. *Transplantation Nursing Secrets*. Philadelphia, Pa: Hanley & Belfus. 2003;85-105.
3. Taylor DO, Edwards LB, Boucek MM, Trulock EP, Berkeley MK, Hertz MI. The Registry of the International Society for Heart and Lung Transplantation: 21st official Adult Heart Transplant Report 2004. *J Heart Lung Transplantation*. 2004;23:796-8.
4. Kirklin JK, Young JB, McGiffin DC. *Heart Transplantation*. Philadelphia Pa: Churchill Livingstone. 2002.
5. Baldwin JC, Wofgang TC, Shumway NE, Lower RR. Cardiac Transplantation. In: Flye MW, ed. *Principles of Organ Transplantation*. Philadelphia, Pa: W.B. Saunders Co. 1989;385-402.
6. Renlund DG. Cardiac Transplantation. In: Topol EJ, ed. *Textbook of Cardiovascular Medicine*. Philadelphia, Pa: Lippincott Williams & Wilkins. 1998;2327-2349.
7. Costanzo MR, Augustine S, Bourge R, et al. Selection and treatment of candidates for heart transplantation. *Circulation*. 1995;92:3593-3612.
8. Goldstein DJ, Oz MC. *Cardiac Assist Devices*. Armonk, NY: Futura Publishing. 2000.
9. Sweet LC, Coleman L. Ventricular assist devices as a bridge to cardiac transplantation: a comprehensive overview of device and patient management. In: Cupples SA, Ohler L, eds. *Transplantation Nursing Secrets*. Philadelphia, Pa: Hanely & Belfus. 2003;107-126.
10. Duke T, Perna J. The ventricular assist device as a bridge to cardiac transplantation. *AACN Clin Issues*. 1999;10:217-228.
11. Bowser D. Registry for Circulatory Support Devices Shows 50% Survival at 12 months. Medscape Medical News 2005. Available at: http://www.medscape.com/viewarticle/502719; Accessed at: August 1, 2005.
12. Deng MC, Edwards LB, Hertz MI, et al. Mechanical circulatory support device database of the International Society for Heart and Lung Transplantation: second annual report 2004. *J Heart Lung. Transplant*. 2004;23:1027-1034.
13. Dressler DK, Heart Transplantation, Organ Transplant 2002. Available at: http://www.medscape.com/viewarticle/436544. Accessed: June 21, 2005.
14. Miniati DN, Robbins RC, Reitz BA. *Braunwald: Heart Disease: A Textbook of Cardiovascular Medicine*. Philadelphia Pa: WB Saunders Co. 2001.
15. Kirklin, JK. Updates from the Annual Meeting of the International Society of Heart and Lung Transplantation. *J Heart Lung Transplant*. 2004;23:924.
16. Mehra MR, Kobashigawa JA. Advances in Heart and Lung Transplantation 2004: Report from the 24th International Society of Heart and Lung. Transplantation Annual Meeting, San Fancisco, Calif; April 21-24, 2004. *J Heart Lung Transplant*. 2004;23:925-930.
17. Muller FJ, vBaeyer H, Volk HD, et al. Treatment of humoral rejection after heart transplantation. *J Heart and Lung Transplantation*. 1998;17:1184-1194.
18. Luckraz H, Goddard M, Charman S, Wallwork J, Parameshwar J, Large S. Early mortality after cardiac transplantation: should we do better? *J Heart Lung Transplant*. 2005;24:401-405.

Lung Transplantation

Tracy Evans-Walker, RN, BSN, CCTC

Introduction

Lung transplantation became successful after the introduction of cyclosporine A in the 1980s, and has evolved from an experimental procedure into an accepted treatment option for patients with end-stage pulmonary diseases. According to the Organ Procurement and Transplantation Network (OPTN) database, more than 12,000 lung transplantations have been performed in the United States since 1988.[1] Before 2000, there were more single-lung transplantations performed than bilateral-lung transplantations. Since 2000, however, the number of bilateral-lung transplantations has surpassed that of single-lung transplantations.[2] Survival rates for all lung transplant recipients from January 1990 through June 2002 were 84% at 3 months, 74% at 1 year, 58% at 3 years, 47% at 5 years, and 24% at 10 years.[2] Survival rates for bilateral and single lung transplant recipients are similar in the first year after transplantation, but, overall, bilateral lung transplant recipients have a better survival rate long term.[2] The survival rates for lung transplantation are inferior to the corresponding rates for other solid organ transplantations, illustrating the difficulty of lung transplantation.

Indications for Transplantation

The common clinical indications for lung and heart-lung transplantation are listed in Table 1. The majority of adult patients who receive a lung transplant have the primary diagnosis of chronic obstructive pulmonary disease (COPD, 39%), followed by idiopathic pulmonary fibrosis (17%), cystic fibrosis (CF, 16%), α_1-antitrypsin deficiency emphysema (9%), and primary pulmonary hypertension (4.2%).[2] The common indications for pediatric patients are CF, idiopathic pulmonary fibrosis, pulmonary arterial hypertension (PAH), and congenital heart disease.[5] The type of transplant procedure performed is dependent on the age of the patient, the primary diagnosis, and the preference of the transplant center. Trends show that patients with COPD or idiopathic pulmonary fibrosis are more likely to receive a single lung transplant and those with PAH or Eisenmenger's syndrome are more likely to receive a bilateral lung transplant. Patients with α_1-antitrypsin deficiency receive a single or double lung transplant. Patients with a diagnosis of infectious lung disease, such as CF or bronchiectasis, receive a bilateral lung transplant.[2] Single-lung transplantation for infectious lung disease is not recommended because the transplanted lung would become contaminated from the bacterial colonization in the native lung and cause chronic infection.[6] The indications for heart-lung transplantation are few, but the procedure remains the only option for some patients with Eisenmenger's syndrome and irreparable heart disease.

Criteria for Transplant Recipient Selection

Lung transplantation is considered when medical and surgical therapies have failed and patients have a poor prognosis, usually an expected survival less than 12 to 24 months. Patients should be referred to the transplant center in a timely manner to ensure that they are evaluated and listed while they are healthy enough to survive the procedure. Delays in the referral or transplant evaluation can prevent patients from being considered for candidacy because they have become too debilitated and will have a poor outcome after transplantation.[7]

Table 1. COMMON CLINICAL INDICATIONS FOR LUNG TRANSPLANTATION[3,4]

Procedure	End-stage disease	Indications

Single lung	Obstructive lung disease
	    Emphysema
	    α_1-antitrypsin deficiency
	    Bronchiolitis obliterans
		After BD FEV_1 <25% predicted, and/or $PaCO_2$ ≥55 mm Hg, and/or increased pulmonary artery pressures with progressive deterioration

	Restrictive lung disease
	    Idiopathic pulmonary fibrosis
	    Drug/toxin-induced lung disease
	    Eosinophilic granuloma
	    Lymphangioleiomyomatosis
	    Sarcoidosis
		After BD FVC <60%-70% predicted, DLCO <50%-60%, PaO_2 <55 mm Hg, $PaCO_2$ ≥45 mm Hg, secondary pulmonary hypertension

	Pulmonary vascular lung disease
	    Pulmonary arterial hypertension
	    Eisenmenger's syndrome with correctable shunt
		Symptomatic progressive disease despite optimal medical/surgical intervention, NYHA III or IV

Bilateral Sequential	Infectious lung disease
	    Cystic fibrosis (CF)
	    Bronchiectasis
		After BD FEV_1, 30% predicted, FVC ≤40% predicted, PaO_2, 55 mm Hg, $PaCO_2$ ≥ 45 mm Hg, increasing bacterial resistance and clinical decline.

	Obstructive lung disease
	    Emphysema
	    α_1-antitrypsin deficiency
	    Bronchiolitis obliterans
		Same as single lung transplant

	Pulmonary vascular lung disease
	    Pulmonary arterial hypertension
	    Eisenmenger's syndrome with correctable shunt
		Same as for single lung transplantation

Heart-lung	Pulmonary vascular lung disease
	    Pulmonary arterial hypertension
	    Eisenmenger's syndrome with correctable shunt
	    End-stage lung disease with associated cardiomyopathy
	    End-stage lung disease with coronary artery disease
		Same as for single or bilateral sequential lung transplantation

Abbreviations: BD, bronchodilator; DLCO, diffusing lung capacity of carbon monoxide; FEV1, forced expiratory volume in 1 second; FVC, forced vital capacity.

The criteria for adult and pediatric lung transplantation can vary slightly from center to center; however, most centers follow the recommended guidelines developed by a joint committee of thoracic physicians and surgeons representing the American Society of Transplant Physicians, the American Thoracic Society, the European Respiratory Society, the International Society for Heart and Lung Transplantation, and the Thoracic Society of Australia and New Zealand.[3] The physiological age limit for single-lung transplantation is 65 years, and for bilateral lung transplantation and heart-lung transplantation it is 60 and 55 years, respectively. Patients must be nicotine free for at least 6 months to be considered for transplantation. Emotional stability, access to a good social support system, and a history of adherence to medical guidance are extremely important for a successful outcome after transplantation. Enrollment in a pulmonary rehabilitation program is mandatory at many transplant centers.

The Evaluation Process

The initial referral to the transplant center usually comes from the patient's local pulmonologist, primary care physician, or insurance company. The transplant coordinator conducts a brief telephone interview with the patient. During this interview, the coordinator gathers general information about the patient's medical history and assesses how much the patient knows about the transplant process. Patient education about the transplant process begins with the telephone interview and continues throughout the transplant process. The patient's demographic characteristics and current medical information are sent to the transplant center for review to determine if the patient has any contraindications to transplantation.

The identification of unsuitable candidates early in the evaluation process lowers costs and saves the patient from undergoing unnecessary testing.[8] Once a patient has been cleared as a possible candidate for transplantation the full evaluation workup begins. The evaluation consists of extensive diagnostic and laboratory testing, and a clinic visit with the transplant pulmonologist, surgeon, transplant coordinator, social worker, and financial counselor. Additional consults and testing are scheduled as needed. A list of diagnostic and laboratory tests and consults is presented in Table 2. During the evaluation, the transplant

Table 2. DIAGNOSTIC AND LABORATORY TESTS COMMONLY PERFORMED FOR EVALUATION OF THE LUNG TRANSPLANT CANDIDATE

Diagnostic tests
- Chest radiograph (pulmonary artery and lateral)
- High-resolution computed tomography of the chest
- Computed tomography of the sinuses (patients with chronic sinus infections and cystic fibrosis)
- Full pulmonary functions tests, including spirometry, lung volumes, diffusing lung capacity of carbon monoxide, and arterial blood gas values
- 6-minute walk distance (assess exercise tolerance)
- Quantitative perfusion scan
- 12-lead electrocardiogram
- Echocardiogram (transthoracic or transesophageal)
- Stress echocardiogram (dobutamine, dobutamine PET, or sestamibi)
- Left cardiac catheterization (patients 40 years of age and older)
- Right cardiac catheterization (assess pulmonary pressures)
- Papanicolaou smear (women of child-bearing age)
- Mammogram
- Prostate and testicular examinations
- Sigmoidoscopy or colonoscopy
- Computed tomography of the abdomen and pelvis (α_1-antitrypsin deficiency, cystic fibrosis, or history of possible cirrhosis)
- Esophageal function studies, including esophageal manometry, esophageal motility studies, pH probe (assess for gastric reflux disease, dysphagia, or other dysmotility problems)

Laboratory tests
- Histocompatibility
  - Tissue typing (human leukocyte antigens)
  - ABO blood type and cross-match
  - Panel reactive antibody
- Serology/Infectious disease
  - Cytomegalovirus
  - Epstein-Barr virus
  - Herpes simplex virus
  - Varicella zoster virus
  - Rapid plasma regain test
  - Human immunodeficiency antibody
  - Toxoplasmosis
  - Hepatitis B (antigen/antibody)
  - Hepatitis C antibody
  - Anergy panel skin testing for exposure to for mumps, Candida, *Histoplasma capsulatum*, and *Coccidiomycosis*
  - Purified protein derivative
  - Sputum for Gram stain, routine culture and sensitivity, fungal and Acid Fast Bacillus
- Chemistries
  - Complete blood cell count with differential
  - C-reactive protein
  - Antinuclear antibody
  - Rheumatoid factor
  - Erythrocyte sedimentation rate
  - Iron, Total Iron Binding Capacity, and transferrin
  - Liver function tests
  - Lipid panel
  - Partial thromboplastin time, prothrombin time/ international normalized ratio
  - Thyroid-stimulating hormone
  - Parathyroid hormone
  - 24-hour clearance for creatinine and protein
  - Urinalysis
  - Carcinoembryonic antigen
  - Prostate-specific antigen
  - Human chorionic gonadotropin, beta
  - Testosterone level
  - Nicotine/cotinine (urine or blood)
  - Immunoglobulin electrophoresis

Consults
- Social work
- Financial counselor
- Pulmonary rehabilitation/ physical therapy
- Psychiatry
- Chemical dependency evaluation
- Infectious disease (cystic fibrosis and bronchiectasis)
- Endocrine (osteoporosis or diabetes mellitus)
- Dietician
- Otolaryngology
- Hepatology
- Neurolgy

team can determine whether the patient has received proper management of his or her end-stage disease. Transplantation can be deferred in patients who are considered too well or have other medical or surgical options. Patients who are considered too debilitated for transplantation at the time of the evaluation may have to have optimization of medical therapy and be reevaluated by the transplant team if their health improves.

Contraindications to Transplantation

Relative and absolute contraindications to transplantation are listed in Table 3. Patients who have had previous thoracic surgery for lung volume reduction, congenital defect repair, or pleurodesis can be considered for transplantation. The surgical difficulty is increased in these patients because of scarring and adhesions from previous procedures, and they are at increased risk of bleeding during surgery. This is particularly true if the patient will require cardiopulmonary bypass. In addition, a severe case of musculoskeletal disease causing deformity of the thoracic cavity, such as scoliosis or kyphosis, would be considered a contraindication to transplantation.

Table 3. CONTRAINDICATIONS FOR LUNG TRANSPLANTATION[3]

Relative	Absolute
Collagen vascular disease without involvement of other organs	Significant cardiovascular disease
Previous thoracic surgery	Significant psychosocial problems, substance abuse or noncompliance
Chronic steroid use >3mg/kg/day	Current cigarette or nicotine use
Mechanical ventilation	End-stage hepatic or renal failure
Insulin dependent diabetes mellitus without end-stage organ disease	Active malignancy
Cachexia or obesity	Active, severe infection/pan-resistant organisms
Symptomatic osteoporosis	Progressive neuromuscular disease
Severe musculoskeletal disease	Human immunodeficiency virus
	Hepatitis C with biopsy-proven histologic evidence of disease
	Hepatitis B antigen positive

High-dose steroid use can cause increased incidence of infections, osteoporosis, hyperglycemia, poor surgical wound and anastomosis healing, and other serious complications; therefore, it is recommended that patients are weaned to a steroid dose of 20 mg per day or less.[3, 9] Patients who are dependent on invasive mechanical ventilation are considered too ill for transplantation. Cachexia and obesity can cause an increased risk for postoperative complications.[9-11] Patients who weigh more than 130% of predicted ideal body weight should be referred to a dietician or weight loss program. COPD and CF patients usually present with malnutrition issues.[12] Patients who weigh less than 70% of their ideal body weight should consider diet supplementation or placement of a percutaneous endoscopic gastrostomy tube for enteral nutrition to aid in weight gain.[9, 10,13]

Osteoporosis poses the risk of symptomatic fractures that can have a negative impact on long-term outcomes and quality of life after transplantation.[9, 14] Patients should be assessed for the presence of osteoporosis. Consultation with an endocrinologist for the treatment of severe osteoporosis is highly recommended.[9]

Cardiovascular disease is a relative contraindication if coronary artery disease is limited to 1 vessel or very mild left ventricular dysfunction.

An absolute contraindication for transplantation is current cigarette smoking. Patients should be nicotine free for at least 6 months before they can be evaluated for transplantation. This also applies to substance abuse such as alcohol, narcotics, or illicit drug use. Patients who have a current or recent history of substance abuse should be referred to a chemical dependency program for treatment and/or approval.

Patients with a current history of malignancy, except squamous cell or basal cell carcinoma of the skin, must be tumor free for at least 2 years before they can be considered for transplantation.[3] In cases of extracapsular renal cell tumors, breast cancer stage 2 or higher, melanoma level III of higher, and colon cancer stage higher than Dukes A, it is recommended that a 5-year waiting period is applied because of the high recurrence rate in these types of cancers.[3]

Active infection like sepsis is an absolute contraindication to transplantation. Patients with CF have problems with bacterial colonization of *Staphylococcus aureus* and *Pseudomonas aeruginosa* that can become resistant to antibiotic therapy. The *Pseudomonas* species *Burkholderia cepacia* is extremely difficult to manage because of its ability to become pan-resistant. Colonization with multiple or pan-resistant organisms is considered a relative contraindication; however, some transplant centers will consider the colonization with pan-resistant organisms or colonization with *B. cepacia* to be an absolute contraindication to transplantation. Consultation with a transplant infectious disease specialist should be made early in the evaluation period to develop a treatment plan for these patients.

Risks and Benefits of Lung Transplantation

Lung transplantation is considered the final treatment option for patients with end-stage lung disease. The goal of transplantation is to improve patients' quality of life and hopefully prolong their lifespan. The transplant team should reinforce the fact that lung or heart-lung transplantation is not a cure but a treatment for end-stage lung disease. Patients trade their current end-stage disease process for the consequences of transplantation, such as surgical complications, infection, rejection, malignancy, and the side effects from long-term use of immunosuppressive medication. The risks and benefits of transplantation are weighed against the patient's quality of life and life expectancy with end-stage disease.

The Waiting Period

Once the transplant team decides that the patient is an acceptable candidate for transplantation, he or she is placed on the United Network for Organ Sharing (UNOS) waiting list. The average waiting time for transplantation is 28 months for lung candidates and 36 months for heart-lung candidates.[15] Before May 2005, lung transplant candidates were listed by time only. As of May 4, 2005, OPTN and UNOS initiated a new lung allocation system for candidates 12 years and older.[15] The new system is based on waiting list urgency and transplant benefit. Each candidate receives a lung allocation score (LAS) of 0 to 100 on the basis of the variables listed in Table 4. A candidate with a higher score will have priority over candidates with lower scores. When a lung donor becomes available, allocation is determined by the LAS, blood type, age group, and distance between the candidates and the donor hospital.[15] OPTN and UNOS require transplant centers to update each candidate's clinical data every 6 months to keep data current. Transplant centers can update each candidate's data more frequently if the candidate has had a change in condition. The steps involved in the LAS calculation can be found under the Resources Section at www.UNOS.org.

Table 4. VARIABLES USED TO CALCULATE THE LUNG ALLOCATION SCORE[15]

New York Heart Association class
Assisted ventilation
Height
Weight
Diabetes
Supplemental oxygen
Actual forced vital capacity and percent predicted forced vital capacity
6-minute walk distance
Pulmonary artery systolic pressure
Mean pulmonary artery pressure
Pulmonary capillary wedge

Candidates who are younger than 12 years are listed by waiting time and blood type. Lungs from pediatric donors (those younger than 18 years of age) are offered to pediatric candidates (younger than 18 years of age) before they are offered to candidates 18 years and older. Lungs from donors younger than 12 years of age will be offered to candidates who are younger than 12 years of age first, then to candidates 12 to 17 years of age, and then to candidates 18 years and older. Lungs from donors who are 12 to 17 years of age are offered to adolescent candidates in the same age group first, then to candidates younger than 12 years of age, and then to candidates 18 years and older.

Patients who live more than 2 hours away from the transplant center will have to relocate or arrange for air transportation to bring them to the transplant center when an organ is available. Patients are provided with a pager so that the transplant team can contact them when a donor is available. Patients are encouraged to have a bag packed in advance, and to have enough medication and supplemental oxygen for at least 24 hours just in case the surgery is canceled.

Transplant education continues throughout the waiting period. Patients are encouraged to join support groups or be paired with a transplant mentor to help them cope with the stresses of "the waiting period."[16,17] Patients and families who have poor coping strategies may need a psychiatric consult for therapy.[18-20]

Pediatric patients should receive all of their childhood vaccinations before transplantation to ensure adequate protection against preventable diseases after transplantation. The use of live and live attenuated viruses is contraindicated after transplantation because of risk of infection.

Bridges To Transplant

Many transplant centers require their patients to be enrolled in a pulmonary rehabilitation program before being placed on the waiting list for transplantation. Pulmonary rehabilitation has helped patients improve their quality of life while waiting for transplantation, and maintenance of exercise tolerance improves postoperative outcomes.[21] Patients enrolled in pulmonary rehabilitation programs receive exercise training, education, optimization of medication therapy, breathing retraining, energy conservation techniques, nutrition assessment, and psychosocial support through support groups.[21]

Patients who have PAH can be managed with potent pulmonary arterial vasodilators. The prostacyclin analog epoprostenol (Flolan) has been used successfully for many years to improve the functional status of PAH patients.[22] Newer prostacyclin analogs include beraprost, iloprost, and treprostinil (Remodulin).[23] Endothelin-receptor antagonists such as bosentan (Tracleer) are also being used in these patients.[23] In some cases, transplantation can be delayed for patients who respond to vasodilator therapy. Atrial septostomy is another way to improve the systemic blood flow, organ function, and reduce right heart failure symptoms for PAH patients.

Lung volume reduction surgery may be used in patients with emphysema to remove part of the damaged lung, allow for lung expansion, and improve lung function.[24,25] Some patients who have had successful lung volume reduction surgery are able to delay transplantation.

Optimization of supplemental oxygen therapy and use of noninvasive positive-pressure ventilation such as bi-level positive airway devices have also been used as bridges to transplantation.

Reevaluation While Waiting

Patients should be reevaluated periodically for assessment of progression of disease during the waiting period. The frequency of clinic visits for reevaluation varies from center to center. The new OPTN/UNOS lung allocation policy for lung candidates 12 years and older requires laboratory data to be updated every 6 months.[15] The reevaluation testing should include routine blood tests, chest radiograph, spirometry, 6-minute walk test, and other tests, as indicated. Patients with CF or bronchiectasis should have sputum collected for cultures and sensitivity at every clinic visit to monitor for resistant organisms. Patients and their caregivers are instructed to call the transplant coordinator if they are sick or have been admitted to the hospital. Patients may have to be taken off the waiting list if their end-stage disease has progressed to the point where they are too ill or too well for transplantation.

The Surgery

Donor Criteria

The donor must be ABO compatible with the recipient. The donor-recipient size match is done by directly measuring the chest size, using chest radiology films, or predicting the total lung capacity and vital capacity on the basis of age, gender, and height. Donor lungs should be sized according to the recipient's underlying lung disease (COPD patients have huge lungs and chest cavities, whereas patients with pulmonary fibrosis have small lungs and chest cavities) to avoid significant oversizing or undersizing of the lungs.

The ideal donor for lung transplantation is younger than 55 years of age; has a smoking history of less than 20 pack/years; and has received mechanical ventilation for less than 72 hours, with a PaO_2 greater than 300 mmHg on 100% fraction of inspired oxygen and 5 cmH_2O of positive end-expiratory pressure (PEEP). In addition, the donor should have a clear chest radiograph, no significant chest trauma or any evidence of infection, a normal sputum Gram stain, and no evidence of aspiration noted during bronchoscopy. The potential donor should not have a previous history of cardiothoracic surgery, and the donor must be negative for hepatitis A, B, or C, and human immunodeficiency virus.

Few donors fulfill all these criteria and many transplant centers have extended the donor criteria to expand the pool of potential donors.[26] Lungs can come from deceased or non-heart-beating donors. Some centers have started living donor lobar programs to address the donor shortage for pediatric and small adult candidates who wait longer on the transplant list because of size issues.[27, 28] The ischemic time for lungs is 4 to 6 hours. The transplant team must work quickly to ensure that lungs are procured and transplanted within that short period.

The Surgical Procedure

Single-lung transplantation (see Figure 1) is performed using an anterolateral or a posterolateral thoracotomy through the fifth intercostal space. The recipient pulmonary artery, pulmonary veins, and bronchus are dissected free. The lung itself is freed and a pneumonectomy is performed. Care is taken to avoid damaging the phrenic nerve. Cardiopulmonary bypass (CPB) is used selectively depending on oxygen saturation and pulmonary and systemic hemodynamics. Patients who have high to moderate pulmonary artery pressures may require CPB; patients with normal to mildly elevated pulmonary artery pressures will likely not require CPB. Signs of hemodynamic instability, hypercarbia, hypoxemia, or right ventricular failure while the pulmonary artery is clamped indicates the need for CPB. Otherwise, CPB

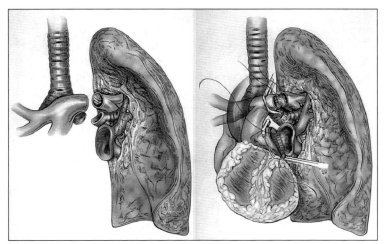

Figure 1. Single lung transplantation. The bronchial anastomosis is created first, followed by the pulmonary artery, and the left atrial cuff including the pulmonary veins.
Reprinted with permission of The Cleveland Clinic Foundation.

is placed on standby. Patients who are placed on CPB are at risk for postoperative bleeding because of systemic heparinization and postoperative coagulopathy. The donor lung is brought up to the surgical field after "back table" preparation. The bronchial anastomosis is created first, followed by the pulmonary artery and the left atrial cuff including the pulmonary veins. The pulmonary artery cross clamp is partially released and the lungs are slowly reperfused, inflated, and deaired through the left atrial suture line. If CPB is being used, the patient is quickly weaned off. Hemostasis is obtained, chest tubes are placed in the pleural space, and the chest is closed. A flexible bronchoscope is used to remove blood and secretions from the airway and to inspect the bronchial anastomosis.

The double lung en-bloc procedure has been replaced by bilateral sequential lung transplantation, which is 2 single-lung transplantations performed sequentially. Bilateral lung transplantation is performed through a bilateral transverse thoracosternotomy incision (also referred to as a "clamshell" incision) at the fourth intercostal space or through a median sternotomy dependent on surgeon preference. The lung with inferior lung function is generally transplanted first, using the same technique for single-lung transplantation. The newly transplanted lung supports the patient while the second lung is transplanted.

Heart-lung transplantation is performed through a median sternotomy incision. The heart and lungs are removed from the donor en bloc. During implantation, the heart-lung bloc is passed carefully behind the phrenic pedicles to avoid damage. The tracheal anastomosis is performed first. The right atrial anastomosis is created next, followed by the aortic anastomosis. The lungs are ventilated and the heart is deaired through the aortic vent. The aortic cross clamp is removed. Atrial and ventricular pacer wires are placed. The heart is defibrillated and the patient is weaned off CPB. Hemostasis is obtained. The chest tubes are inserted in the pleural cavities and mediastinum, and the chest is closed.

Surgical Complications

Surgical complications are usually seen in the early postoperative period. These complications include technical complications relating to bronchus, pulmonary artery, or veins; hemorrhage; reimplantation response; atrial arrhythmias; damage to the phrenic nerve; gastroparesis; ileus; and gastric or peptic ulcer.[4] Obstruction of the pulmonary artery is caused by stenosis of the anastomosis, thrombus, or a kink in the vessel.[4] Left atrial cuff anastomosis obstruction can occur because of poor surgical technique or thrombus that is obstructing the pulmonary veins.[4]

Postoperative bleeding can occur because of anticoagulation during the use of CPB. It can also occur because of trauma caused by cutting through pleural adhesions and scarring during the removal of the native lungs. Reexploration for evacuation of a hemothorax and hemostasis is indicated if excessive bleeding occurs.

Reimplantation response occurs to some degree in all transplant recipients. It is usually seen within hours up to the first few days after transplantation. Reimplantation response is caused by ischemia, surgical trauma, denervation, overhydration, and disruption of the thoracic lymphatic system. It is marked by hypoxemia and increased peak inspiratory airway pressures, and perihilar infiltrates are seen on chest radiograph. Patients are maintained on the ventilator, and fluid restriction is used to prevent worsening of the pulmonary edema. A small percentage of patients experience severe acute lung injury that presents similar to adult respiratory syndrome. Extracorporeal membrane oxygenation and nitric oxide have been used to support these patients.[29]

Atrial arrhythmias can occur after lung transplantation because of the irritation of the myocardium by clamps applied to the atria during surgery. Conversion to normal sinus rhythm can occur spontaneously, with medical therapy, or cardioversion. Heart-lung transplant recipients can also develop ventricular dysfunction due to ischemia or reperfusion injury.

Airway complications include anastomosis dehiscence, bronchial stenosis, or bronchomalacia.[30] Airway ischemia is the main reason for airway complications. A small dehiscence will be treated conservatively or with a stent placement across the anastomosis to allow healing. A large dehiscence can cause severe airway compromise, and in selected cases surgical correction may be necessary. Bronchial stenosis or bronchomalacia occur later in the postoperative period. Bronchial stenosis can be caused by granulation tissue or scar tissue from a healed dehiscence. Stenosis is treated by bronchoscopic balloon dilatation or stent placement.[31,32] Granulation tissue can be removed by surgical debridement or with bronchoscopic laser ablation. Bronchomalacia can be treated by stent placement in the affected airway.[31,32] In recent years, brachytherapy has also been used for this complication.

Unilateral or bilateral phrenic nerve damage can cause diaphragmatic paralysis. Evidence of elevation of one or both hemidiaphragms can be seen on chest radiograph. Observing diaphragmatic movement during a sniff test makes a definitive diagnosis of diaphragmatic paralysis. Patients with diaphragm dysfunction have dyspnea and difficulty clearing secretions, which puts them at risk for pneumonia and prolongs the need for mechanical ventilatory support.

Gastrointestinal complications are not uncommon among lung and heart-lung transplant recipients. Gastroparesis is a common complication that can be caused by analgesics and immunosuppression medications. Patients usually experience nausea and vomiting as a result from delayed gastric emptying, bloating, and constipation. Prokinetic agents are used to increase motility. Gastrointestinal reflux is treated with proton pump inhibitors. CF patients are susceptible to development of distal intestinal obstruction if they become dehydrated, use narcotics, or do not take the proper amount of pancreatic enzymes during meals.[33] Gastric ulcer, peptic ulcer, cholecystitis, and diverticulitis can develop and cause severe complications that prolong postoperative recovery.

Posttransplant Care

Immediate Postoperative Management

Lung and heart-lung transplant recipients are managed in the cardiothoracic intensive care unit until they are stable enough to be transferred to a surgical step-down unit or surgical nursing floor. Management of these patients is multidisciplinary and includes surgical and medical teams, nurses, respiratory therapy, nutritionist, physical therapy, social work, and other consultations, as needed during the postoperative period. Hemodynamic monitoring includes pulmonary and systemic arterial pressures, central venous pressures, and cardiac output and rhythm.

Respiratory Management

The standard protocol of ventilator management would apply to most lung transplant recipients. The fraction of inspired oxygen is adjusted to maintain PaO_2 80 to 120 torr. Standard ventilation is used with a tidal volume of 12 to 15 mL/kg and PEEP of 5 to 7.5. Special consideration must be made for the management of patients with pulmonary hypertension and COPD who receive a single lung transplant. Patients with pulmonary hypertension are at risk for right-heart failure if pulmonary artery pressures remain elevated in the postoperative period. Patients are sedated, paralyzed, and maintained on the ventilator for a longer period to prevent a pulmonary hypertensive crisis and pulmonary edema that can occur after reperfusion. In COPD patients, the tidal volume is reduced, the respiratory rate is increased, and lower levels of PEEP are used to prevent hyperinflation of the native lung, which would reduce cardiac filling and reduce ventilation of the transplanted lung. Single lung recipients should be positioned with the transplanted lung up to allow for better inflation and drainage of the transplanted lung. Patients should be extubated as soon as they are awake and alert, breathing spontaneously at a comfortable rate, have adequate pain control, and have good oxygenation and ventilation. Patients are usually extubated within 24 to 48 hours.

Denervation of the transplanted lung disrupts the communication of the autonomic nervous system, which causes changes in airway response, pulmonary vasculature, mucus production, and cilia movement. The deep cough reflex is lost distal to the anastomosis. The disruption of the thoracic lymphatics to the transplanted lung causes pulmonary edema in the initial postoperative period. Chest physiotherapy and suctioning are performed frequently to prevent mucus plugging and to promote drainage of secretions. Early ambulation and good pain control also help to encourage deep breathing and coughing. Patients are encouraged to use incentive spirometry to keep the alveolar sacs open to prevent pneumonia.

Surveillance bronchoscopy is performed periodically throughout the first year after transplantation. The bronchial anastomosis is inspected and bronchoalveolar lavage fluid is obtained. Bronchial washings are processed for culture and sensitivities. Transbronchial biopsies are obtained for determination of rejection. Surveillance bronchoscopy is usually performed 3 and 6 weeks after transplantation, then at 3 months, 6 months, and 12 months and for clinical indications of rejection or infection.

Cardiovascular Management

Hemodynamic stability must be maintained to avoid complications from systemic hypotension or hypertension. It is important to keep patients as hypovolemic as tolerated to protect the transplanted lung from pulmonary edema. If systemic hypotension occurs, vasoactive drugs should be used before fluid resuscitation to protect the lung graft from edema. Chest tubes should be monitored for evidence of excessive amounts of bloody pleural drainage that would indicate a hemorrhage.

Isoproterenol or atrial or atrial and ventricular pacing is used in the early postoperative period to augment the heart rate and improve ventricular function in heart-lung transplant recipients. The resting heart rate is usually increased because of the absence of parasympathetic influence. Heart-lung transplant recipients will need to have prolonged warm-up and cool-down periods when they exercise to allow circulating catecholamines to stimulate changes in the heart rate and contractility, otherwise orthostatic hypotension will occur.

Maintenance Immunosuppression

Most lung transplant programs use triple-drug immunosuppression protocols that consist of tacrolimus or cyclosporine, azathioprine or mycophenolate mofetil, and prednisone.[2,5] Induction with monoclonal or polyclonal antibodies is carried out routinely at several transplant centers.[2,5] Sirolimus can be used in recipients who have experienced calcineurin inhibitor neurotoxicity or nephrotoxicity.[34] Sirolimus should not be used in the early postoperative period because of reported complications with anastomotic healing.[35] Immunosuppression levels should be monitored frequently to ensure that therapeutic levels are maintained.

Nutrition

Patients must receive good nutritional support after transplantation to decrease the risk of complications from prolonged use of mechanical ventilation, infections, and poor wound healing.[11] Patients may require enteral or parenteral supplementation to achieve proper caloric intake that is needed for recovery.[11,12]

Infection

Infection is a significant cause of morbidity and mortality in lung transplant recipients.[2] Risk for infection is attributed to the lungs being exposed to the environment, changes in mucociliary movement, and the loss of the cough reflex distal to the anastomosis. Mediastinitis, sternal wound infections, catheter infections, and drainage catheter infections can also occur. Bacterial infections such as *P. aeruginosa*, *Stenotrophomonas maltiphilia*, *S. aureus*, *Haemophilus influenzae*, and *Streptococcus pneumoniae* are the most commonly seen in the first month after transplantation.[4,36,37] Patients are also at risk for *Clostridium difficile* diarrhea or infection because of the aggressive antibiotic therapy that is used in the postoperative period.[36] Other bacterial organisms that can cause infections after the first month after transplantation are *Nocardia asteroides*, *Listeria monocytogenes*, and *Legionella species*. Mycobacterial and parasitic infections may also occur at this time.

Fungal infections seen in the early postoperative period are caused by *Aspergillus* and *Candida* species. Both *Aspergillus* and *Candida* can colonize in the sinuses and respiratory tract, especially in patients with CF.[36,37] Aerosolized amphotericin B and itraconazole have been used by many centers for prophylaxis against fungal infection.[38] Invasive pulmonary infection by *Aspergillus* is difficult to treat. Patients who have invasive aspergillosis present with fever, dyspnea, cough with hemoptysis, and pleuritic chest pain. Fungal nodules, sometimes with cavitation, can be seen on chest radiograph and computed tomography scans. Amphotericin B, liposomal amphotericin, or voriconazole are be used for treatment. Caspofungin is used to treat refractory *Aspergillus* infection.[36]

On occasion, combination therapy is required. Disseminated aspergillosis can affect the brain, blood vessels, kidneys, liver, spleen, gastrointestinal tract, bone, and joints. The mortality rate for patients with *Aspergillus* infections is approximately 80%, but may be improving with the use of newer antifungal agents.[36] Fungal infections seen after the first month of transplantation include *Cryptococcus*, *Histoplasma capsulatum*, *Coccidioides*, Zygomycetes, and *Pneumocystis carinii*.[37] The occurrence of *P. carinii* infection has been reduced by the use of trimethoprim/sulfamethoxazole or dapsone (for sulfa allergic patients) for prophylaxis.

Viral infections are usually seen 2 to 3 months after transplantation. Cytomegalovirus (CMV) is the most common viral infection that occurs in lung transplant recipients.[4,36,37] Patients who are CMV seronegative are at high risk for primary CMV infection if they receive lungs from a CMV seropositive donor. CMV can cause viremia or pnuemonitis, and can also cause esophogitis, gastritis, colitis, retinitis, encephalitis, and polyradiculopathy.[36] Patients may be asymptomatic or have symptoms that may include fever, cough, shortness of breath, and leukopenia. CMV inclusions in lung tissue are seen histologically in patients with CMV pneumonitis. Prophylaxis with ganciclovir or valganciclovir, and CMV immunoglobulin is used to prevent infection.[37] Intravenous ganciclovir at 5 mg/kg twice a day for 14 to 28 days is used for treatment of CMV infection. Foscarnet can be used for resistant CMV infection.[36] Frequent monitoring of CMV DNA copies by quantitative polymerase chain reaction is useful for early detection of disease and for deciding the duration of therapy.[37,39]

Varicella zoster virus (VZV) can be a problem in pediatric and adult patients who have not been exposed to the virus before transplantation. Primary infection can cause pneumonia, skin lesions, pancreatitis, hepatitis, encephalitis, and disseminated intravascular coagulation.[36] Varicella zoster immunoglobulin can be given to VZV seronegative patients within 72 to 96 hours of exposure. Patients with primary VZV infection are treated with intravenous acyclovir. Patients who develop herpes zoster can be treated with oral acyclovir, famciclovir, or valacyclovir.[38]

Herpes simplex virus (HSV) infection usually manifests as oral lesions. Patients who are infected with HSV-2 may experience anogenital infection. Herpes esophagitis, bronchitis, and pneumonitis can develop early in the postoperative period. Acyclovir, valacyclovir, or famciclovir are used to treat infection. Low-dose oral acyclovir is used for prophylaxis against HSV infection.[36]

Epstein-Barr virus (EBV) can cause fever, malaise, headaches, swollen tonsils, and pharyngitis in EBV seronegative patients who receive lungs from EBV seropositive donors. EBV has been implicated in the development of posttransplant lymphoproliferative disorder (PTLD). The incidence of PTLD in lung and heart-lung transplant recipients is higher than in patients with other types of organ transplants because higher levels of immunosuppression are needed to maintain the lung graft. Pediatric patients are affected at higher rates than adults because of their lack of exposure to EBV before transplantation.[40] PTLD is caused by aggressive immunosuppression therapy that triggers uncontrolled proliferation and transformation of B-cells infected with EBV. PTLD can be found in the central nervous system, thorax, tonsils, cervical lymph nodes, and the gastrointestinal tract. Diagnosis of PTLD is made by histologic examination of biopsies taken from the affected area. PTLD is treated with antiviral agents, chemotherapy, and the reduction of immunosuppression medication therapy.[41] Anti-CD 20 monoclonal antibody (rituximab) has been used with positive results.[42] Antiviral prophylaxis has been shown to reduce the incidence of PTLD.[43]

Influenza and respiratory syncytial virus are common during the winter months. Patients and their families should be vaccinated against influenza every year. Stringent infection control and respiratory isolation are crucial for patients who are hospitalized with respiratory syncytial virus.

Discharge Planning

Discharge education should begin when patients are alert and rested, and pain is under control. Patients should learn how to recognize the symptoms of infection and rejection; monitor blood pressure, pulse, and temperature; and monitor their lung function by performing home spirometry using a microspirometer. The respiratory therapist is a valuable resource for patient teaching on the proper technique to use to obtain accurate forced vital capacity and forced expiratory volume in 1 second readings. Patients are also instructed on medication usage, diet restrictions, and exercise. Patients must avoid dust, chemical fumes, and second-hand smoke. Gardening is prohibited by many transplant centers because of the risk of exposure to fungal spores and other pathogens. Some centers permit patients to garden 1 year after transplantation, as long as they use a mask and gloves as protection. Once patients have demonstrated that they understand the discharge education, they can be discharged to home. Notification of the patient's discharge and all pertinent information about the patient's postoperative course and follow-up care should be shared with the patient's referring physician.

Signs and Symptoms of Rejection

Rejection in lung transplant recipients can present as acute (early) or chronic (late). The occurrence of acute rejection is common in the first few weeks to months after transplantation. Patients may be asymptomatic or experience mild to severe symptoms, including dyspnea, fatigue, a low-grade fever, a decrease in home spirometry readings or pulmonary function tests, and/or a decrease in oxygen saturation. Diffuse infiltrates, perihilar fluffiness, or pleural effusions may be seen on chest radiograph. A definitive diagnosis of acute rejection is made by using bronchoscopy to obtain transbronchial biopsies. The grading of rejection is summarized in Table 5.[44]

Table 5. GRADING SYSTEM FOR REJECTION

A. Acute rejection with/without
   A 0 – None
   A 1 – Minimal
   A 2 – Mild
   A 3 – Moderate
   A 4 – Severe
	B. Airway inflammation - Lymphocytic bronchitis and bronchiolitis
	   B 0 – None
	   B1 – Minimal
	   B2 – Mild
	   B3 – Moderate
	   B4 – Severe

C. Chronic airway rejection – bronchiolitis obliterans
   a. Active
   b. Inactive	

D. Chronic vascular rejection – accelerated graft vascular sclerosis	

Reprinted from Yousem SA, Berry GJ, Cagle PT, et al. Revision of the 1990 working formulation for the classification of pulmonary allograft rejection: lung rejection study group, part 2. J Heart Lung Transplant. 1996;15:1-15. ©1996. Used with permission from the International Society for Heart & Lung Transplantation.

Lung transplant recipients with acute rejection are treated with a bolus infusion of 500 mg to 1000 mg of methylprednisolone daily for 3 days, followed by an increase in the maintenance prednisone dose, then a taper over a few weeks back to the originally prescribed dose.[45] Transbronchial biopsy is repeated 3 weeks after the treatment for assess for the presence of rejection. Acute rejection is considered refractory after 3 consecutive episodes of failed treatment with steroids. When this occurs, treatment with polyclonal antibody (antilymphocyte globulin), monoclonal antibody (muromonab CD3), total lymphoid irradiation, extracorporeal photochemotherapy (photophoresis), or a change of immunosuppression therapy can be used.[45] Aggressive management of maintenance immunosuppression is recommended to prevent future episodes of rejection.

Chronic rejection in lung transplantation, called bronchiolitis obliterans or bronchiolitis obliterans syndrome (BOS), usually occurs after the first year of transplantation and is a major contributor to late mortality in lung transplant recipients.[2] Bronchiolitis obliterans is defined as the injury and inflammation of the small airways (bronchioles) that lead to fibrosis of the airways.[44] It can present suddenly with a rapid decline in lung function, or slowly with a persistent decline over a long period. Patients present with the symptoms of cough, dyspnea, and fatigue. Bronchiolitis obliterans is diagnosed by reviewing histological samples obtained from open lung biopsy.[46] A clinical diagnosis of BOS is defined by an irreversible drop

Table 6. GRADING SYSTEM FOR BRONCHIOLITIS OBLITERANS SYNDROME (BOS)

BOS 0: FEV_1 > 90% of baseline and FEF 25-75% > 75% of baseline
BOS 0p: FEV_1 81%-90% of baseline and/or FEF 25-75% ≤ 75% of baseline
BOS 1: 66%-80% of baseline
BOS 2: 51%-65% of baseline
BOS 3: 50% or less of baseline

Abbreviations: BOS, bronchiolitis obliterans syndrome; FEV1, forced expiratory volume in 1 second; FEF 25-75%, forced expiratory flow between 25% and 75% of FVC; FVC, forced vital capacity.

Reprinted from Estenne M, Maurer JR, Boehler A, et al. Bronchiolitis obliterans syndrome 2001: an update of the diagnostic criteria. J Heart Lung Transplant. 2002;21:299. Copyright 2002. Used with permission from the International Society of Heart & Lung Transplantation.

in forced expiratory volume in 1 second of 20% from a previously established baseline. The grading of severity of bronchiolitis obliterans and BOS is listed in Table 6.[47]

Bronchiolitis obliterans and BOS are difficult to treat. Early diagnosis and treatment are crucial to preserve existing lung function, because lung function that is lost is permanent. Treatment consists of modifying immunosuppression therapy or using methotrexate, photophoresis, or total lymphoid irradiation.[46] Retransplantation has been performed for BOS; however, it is considered controversial because of the small number of available donors and poor survival following the procedure.

Long-Term Management

Lung and heart-lung recipients usually remain under the care of the cardiothoracic surgeon or the transplant pulmonologist once they are discharged from the hospital. The frequency of posttransplant follow-up visits can vary from center to center. Patients are seen in transplant clinics for follow-up visits every week for the first month, then every 2 weeks for a month, then every 1 to 2 months thereafter for the first year. Patients who are clinically stable are seen less frequently after the first year. The clinic visit includes spirometry, chest radiograph, routine laboratory tests, and surveillance bronchoscopy (scheduled throughout the first year and as needed).

Long-term complications from immunosuppression medications include nephrotoxicity, neurotoxicity, hypertension, hyperlipidemia, diabetes, obesity, osteoporosis, and malignancy. Patients should have yearly health maintenance checkups for early detection of cancer and other problems. Health maintenance testing includes colonoscopy, digital rectal examination, and prostate-specific antigen (men older than 40 years of age), mammogram (women older than 40 years of age or earlier if high risk for breast cancer), and pelvic examination and Papanicolaou test (women of childbearing age and older). Bone mineral density should be checked annually for screening of bone loss. Patients should also have routine dental and eye examinations.

Most lung transplant recipients experience an improvement in functional status to the point of achieving independence with activities of daily living.[2] Lung transplant recipients who have participated in quality of life studies have reported improvement in overall health and function, as well as satisfaction with their quality of life after transplantation.[48-50] Recipients with BOS reported having a diminished quality of life.[48,49]

Recurrent Disease

End-stage lung diseases such as COPD and CF do not recur after transplantation. Recurrence has been reported in patients with sarcoidosis, lymphangioleiomyomatosis, and other interstitial lung diseases.[51,52]

Conclusion

Lung and heart-lung transplantation are viable treatment options for adult and pediatric patients with end-stage lung disease. The survival rates for lung transplant recipients are lower than for recipients of other organ transplants because of infection and chronic rejection; however, when successful, lung and heart-lung transplantation provides recipients with a better quality of life, and a longer life than they would have had without intervention.

Acknowledgment:
This work was supported in part by Health Resources and Services Administration contract 231-00-0115. The content is the responsibility of the author alone and does not necessarily reflect the views or policies of the Department of Health and Human Services, nor does mention of trade names, commercial products, or organizations imply endorsement by the US Government.

The author would like to thank Atul Mehta, MD, Marie Budev, DO, Gosta Pettersson, MD, David Mason, MD, and Robin Avery, MD, of the Cleveland Clinic Lung Transplant Program for their input.

References

1. 2003 Annual Report of the US Organ Procurement and Transplantation Network and the Scientific Registry of Transplant Recipients Transplant Data 1993-2002: Department of Health and Human Services, Health Resources and Services Administration, Healthcare Systems Bureau, Division of Transplantation, Rockville, Md; United Network for Organ Sharing, Richmond, Va; University Renal Research and Education Association, Ann Arbor, Mich.
2. Trulock EP, Edwards LB, Taylor DO, Boucek MM, Keck BM, Hertz MI. The Registry of the International Society for Heart and Lung Transplantation: twenty-first official adult lung and heart-lung transplant report-2004. *J Heart Lung Transplant.* 2004;23:804-815.
3. Maurer JR, Frost AE, Estenne M, Higenbottam T, Glanville AR. International guidelines for the selection of lung transplant candidates. *J Heart Lung Transplant.* 1998;17:703-709.
4. Ginns LC, Wain JC. Lung transplantation. In: Ginns LC, Cosimi AB, Morris PJ, eds. *Transplantation.* Malden, Mass: Blackwell Science; 1999:490-550.
5. Boucek MM, Edwards LB, Keck BM, Trulock EP, Taylor DO, Hertz MI. Registry for the International Society of Heart and Lung Transplantation: seventh official pediatric report-2004. *J Heart Lung Transplant.* 2004;23:933-947.
6. Mallory J, George B, Spray TL. Lung transplantation for cystic fibrosis in children. In: Franco KL, ed. *Pediatric Cardiopulmonary Transplantation.* Armonk, NY: Futura Publishing Company, Inc; 1997:277-301.
7. Nathan S. Lung transplantation: disease-specific considerations for referral. *Chest.* 2005;127:1006-1016.
8. Hauff H, Castro M. Reducing transplant evaluation costs by early identification of unsuitable patients. *Prog Transplant.* 2000;10:122-125.
9. Madison S, Ross DF, Kass RM. Management of patients awaiting lung transplantation. In: Baumgartner WA, Reitz B, Kasper E, Theodore J, eds. *Heart and Lung Transplantation.* 2nd ed. Philadelphia, Pa: WB Saunders; 2002:99-119.
10. Madill J, Gutierrez C, Grossman J, et al. Nutritional assessment of the lung transplant patient: body mass index as a predictor of 90-day mortality following transplantation. *J Heart Lung Transplant.* 2001;20:288-296.
11. Plochl W, Pezawas L, Artemiou O, Grimm M, Klepetko W, Hiesmayr M. Nutritional status, ICU duration and ICU mortality in lung transplant recipients. *Intensive Care Med.* 1996;22:1179-1185.
12. Schwebel C, Pin I, Barnoud D, et al. Prevalence and consequences of nutritional depletion in lung transplant candidates. *Eur Respir J.* 2000;16:1050-1055.
13. Teets JM, Borisuk MJ. Pediatric thoracic organ transplants: challenges in primary care. *Pediatr Nurs.* January-February 2004;30:23-30.
14. Spira A, Gutierrez C, Chaparro C, Hutcheon M, Chan C. Osteoporosis and lung transplantation: a prospective study. *Chest.* 2000;117:476-481.
15. United Network for Organ Sharing. Allocation of Thoracic Organs. http://www.unos.org/PolicesandBylaws/policies/docs/policy_9.doc. Accessed June 10, 2005.
16. Wright L. Mentorship programs for transplant patients. *Prog Transplant.* 2000;10:267-272.
17. Michalisko HO. Psychosocial evaluation. In: Baumgartner WA, Reitz B, Kasper E, Theodore J, eds. *Heart and Lung Transplantation.* 2nd ed. Philadelphia, Pa: WB Saunders;2002:74-77.
18. Burker EJ, Evon DM, Sedway JA, Egan TM. Appraisal and coping as predictors of psychological distress and self-reported physical disability before lung transplantation. *Prog Transplant.* 2004;14:222-232.
19. LoBiondo-Wood G, Williams L, Kouzekanani K, McGhee C. Family adaptation to a child's transplant: pretransplant phase. *Prog Transplant.* 2000;10:81-87.

20. Myaskovsky L, Dew MA, Switzer GE, et al. Avoidant coping with healthy problems is related to poorer quality of life among lung transplant candidates. *Prog Transplant.* 2003;13:183-192.
21. Kesten S. Pulmonary rehabilitation and surgery for end-stage lung disease. *Clin Chest Med.* 1997;18:173-181.
22. Cheever KH. An overview of pulmonary arterial hypertension. *J Cardiovasc Nurs.* 2005;20:108-116.
23. Badesch DB, Abman SH, Ahearn GS, et al. Medical therapy for pulmonary arterial hypertension: ACCP evidence-based clinical practice guidelines. *Chest.* 2004;126(suppl 1):S35-S62.
24. Glanville AR. Medical and surgical alternatives to pulmonary transplantation. In: Baumgartner WA, Reitz B, Kasper E, Theodore J, eds. *Heart and Lung Transplantation.* 2nd ed. Philadelphia, Pa: WB Saunders; 2002:83-89.
25. Bird GA, Macaluso S. Lung volume reduction surgery for emphysema. *Crit Care Nurs Clin N Am.* 1996;8:323-331.
26. de Perrot M, Snell GI, Babcock WD, et al. Strategies to optimize the use of currently available lung donors. *J Heart Lung Transplant.* 2004;23:1127-1134.
27. Horn MV, Schenkel FA, Woo MS, Starnes VA. Pediatric recipients of living donor lobar lung transplants: postoperative care. *Prog Transplant.* 2002;12:81-85.
28. Luciani GB, Barr ML, Starnes VA. Living-related pediatric lobar transplantation. In: Franco KL, ed. *Pediatric Cardiopulmonary Transplantation.* Armonk, NY: Futura Publishing; 1997:333-344.
29. Nguyen DQ, Kulick DM, Bolman R III, Dunitz JM, Hertz MI, Park S. Temporary ECMO support following lung and heart-lung transplantation. *J Heart Lung Transplant.* 2000;19:313-316.
30. Singer LG, Weinacker AB, Theodore J. Long-term management and outcome of heart-lung and lung transplant recipients. In: Baumgartner WA, Reitz B, Kasper E, Theodore J, eds. *Heart and Lung Transplantation.* 2nd ed. Philadelphia, Pa: WB Saunders; 2002:434-455.
31. Mughal MM, Gildea TR, Sudish M, Pettersson G, DeCamp M. Temporary self-expandable metallic stents in promoting healing of bronchial dehiscence. *Am J Respir Crit Care Med.* 2005;172:768-771.
32. Orons PD, Amesur N, Dauber JH, Zajko A, Keenan R, Iacono AT. Balloon dilation and endobronchial stent placement for bronchial strictures after lung transplantation. *J Vasc Interv Radiol.* January 2000;11:89-99.
33. Yankaskas JR, Aris R. Outpatient care of the cystic fibrosis patient after lung transplantation. *Curr Opin Pulm Med.* 2000;6:551-557.
34. Villanueva J, Boukhamseen A, Bhorade S. Successful use in lung transplantation of an immunosuppressive regimen aimed at reducing target blood levels of sirolimus and tacrolimus. *J Heart Lung Transplant.* 2005;24:421-425.
35. Groetzner J, Kur F, Spelsberg F, et al. Airway anastomosis complications in de novo lung transplantation with sirolimus-based immunosuppression. *J Heart Lung Transplant.* 2004;23:632-638.
36. Stosor V. Infections in transplant recipients. In: Stuart FP, Abecassis MM, Kaufman DB, eds. *Organ Transplantation.* Georgetown, Tex: Landes Bioscience; 2003:399-425.
37. Tucker PC. Infectious complications. In: Baumgartner WA, Reitz B, Kasper E, Theodore J, eds. *Heart and Lung Transplantation.* 2nd ed. Philadelphia, Pa: WB Saunders; 2002:355-371.
38. Dummer JS, Lazariashvilli N, Barnes J, Ninan M, Milestone AP. A survey of anti-fungal management in lung transplantation. *J Heart Lung Transplant.* 2004;23:1376-1381.
39. Zamora MR. Cytomegalovirus and lung transplantation. *Am J Transplant.* 2004;4:1219-1226.
40. Lim GY, Newman B, Kurland G, Webber SA. Posttransplantation lymphoproliferative disorder: manifestations in pediatric thoracic organ recipients. *Radiology.* 2002;222:699-708.
41. Muti G, Cantoni S, Oreste P, et al. Post-transplant lymphoproliferative disorders: improved outcome after clinico-pathologically tailored treatment. *Transplantation.* 2002;87:67-77.
42. Verschuuren EM, Stevens SJC, van Imhoff GW, et al. Treatment of posttransplant lymphoproliferative disease with rituximab: the remission, the relapse, and the complication. *Transplantation.* 2002;73:100-104.
43. Malouf MA, Chhajed PN, Hopkins P, Plit M, Turner J, Glanville AR. Anti-viral prophylaxis reduces the incidence of lymphoproliferative disease in lung transplant recipients. *J Heart Lung Transplant.* 2002;21:547-554.
44. Yousem SA, Berry GJ, Cagle PT, et al. Revision of the 1990 working formulation for the classification of pulmonary allograft rejection: lung rejection study group. *J Heart Lung Transplant.* 1996;15:1-15.
45. Ross DF, Kass RM. Treatment of acute lung allograft rejection. In: Baumgartner WA, Reitz B, Kasper E, Theodore J, eds. *Heart and Lung Transplantation.* 2nd ed. Philadelphia, Pa: WB Saunders; 2002:333-340.
46. Estenne M, Hertz MI. Bronchiolitis obliterans after human lung transplantation. *Am J Respir Crit Care Med.* 2002;166:440-444.
47. Estenne M, Maurer JR, Boehler A, et al. Bronchiolitis obliterans syndrome 2001: an update of the diagnostic criteria. *J Heart Lung Transplant.* 2002;21:297-310.
48. Chaparro C, Scavuzzo M, Winton T, Keshavjee S, Kesten S. Status of lung transplant recipients surviving beyond five years. *J Heart Lung Transplant.* 1997;16:511-516.
49. Rodrigue JR, Baz MA, Kanasky WF, MacNaughton KL. Does lung transplantation improve health-related quality life? The University of Florida experience. *J Heart Lung Transplant.* 2005;124:755-763.

50. Kugler C, Strueber M, Tegtbur U, Neidermeyer J, Haverich A. Quality of life 1 year after lung transplantation. *Prog Transplant*. 2004;14:331-336.
51. Bittman I, Rolf B, Amann G, Lohrs U. Recurrence of lymphangioleiomyomatosis after single lung transplantation: new insights into pathogenesis. *Hum Pathol*. January 2003;34:95-98.
52. Verleden G, Sels F, Van Raemdonck D, Verbeken E, Lerut T, Demedts M. Possible recurrence of disquamative interstitial pneumonitis in a single lung transplantation recipient. *Eur Respir J*. 1998;11:971-974.

Liver Transplantation

Marian O'Rourke, RN, CCTC

Introduction

Liver transplantation came of age in the 1980s with the introduction of cyclosporine-based immunosuppression after initial early efforts demonstrated the technical feasibility of liver transplantation.[1,2] It is now the treatment of choice for patients with end-stage chronic liver disease, various metabolic diseases, and fulminant hepatic failure (FHF).[3] The advances in pharmacology, preservation solutions, and surgical technique have led to significant improvements in both patient and graft survival in the past 15 years.[4-7] Current survival rates for patients at 1 year, 3 years, and 5 years are 87.6%, 79.9%, and 74.6%, respectively; graft survival rates at 1 year, 3 years, and 5 years are 82.4%, 73.5%, and 67.3%, respectively.[8] As outcomes have improved, the indications for liver transplantation have become broader, and is therefore now available to a greater number of patients. There has been a change in the distribution of liver diseases leading to liver transplantation, with increasing numbers of patients progressing to end-stage liver disease primarily due to hepatitis C virus (HCV) cirrhosis.[7] As of January 27, 2006, there were 17 667 liver transplant candidates on the Organ Procurement and Transplantation Network (OPTN) and United Network for Organ Sharing (UNOS) waiting list.[8]

This increased demand for liver transplants has not been met with an equivalent increase in the number of donor livers. Although the total number of liver transplantations performed in 2005 was 5438, as opposed to 3934 in 1995, the number of organs available limits the number of liver transplantations.[8] This has lead to increasing mortality for patients on the waiting list. In 2005, 8.1% of liver transplant candidates were removed from the OPTN/UNOS waiting list because of death, as opposed to 4.9% of candidates in 1995.[8] In addition, the significant range in mortality rates across UNOS regions, from 1.6% to 22.3% in 2005, is of concern.[8] As a result of the shortage of organs, novel techniques such as split liver transplantation, living donor liver transplantation (LDLT), and use of organs from donation after cardiac death donors and extended criteria donors have evolved to try to meet the increasing demand. Despite such advances, the number of patients in need of a liver transplant far outweigh the number of organs available. Expert medical management, expanding pharmacopoeia, surgical and radiological interventions, and careful selection criteria have been adapted to optimize the outcomes in liver transplantation. Advances in immunology, infectious disease management, and surgical technique have led to improved patient and graft outcomes in the setting of expanding the acceptable donor criteria.

Causes of Liver Disease

Chronic Liver Disease

The most common causes of liver disease leading to chronic liver failure in adults are outlined in Table 1. They can be broadly categorized into hepatocellular, cholestatic, malignant, metabolic, and vascular diseases. Currently, the leading indication for liver transplantation is HCV and it is one of the more controversial indications because of the rate and severity of recurrent disease after transplantation, leading to poorer survival relative to other diseases.[7] Liver transplantation for HCV now represents 31.8% of all liver transplantations in the United States versus 16.8% in 1996.[7] With the introduction of hepatitis B immunoglobulin and antiviral agents such as lamivudine, hepatitis B virus (HBV) infection is now considered an acceptable and even favorable indication for liver transplantation because of its relatively

LIVER TRANSPLANTATION

Table 1. CAUSES OF CHRONIC LIVER DISEASE IN ADULTS

Hepatocellular disease	Cholestatic liver disease
Hepatitis C	Primary biliary cirrhosis
Hepatitis B	Primary sclerosing cholangitis
Alcoholic liver disease	Secondary sclerosing cholangitis
Autoimmune hepatitis	Familial cholestatic disorders
Metabolic disorders	**Hepatic malignancy**
Primary hemochromatosis	Hepatocellular carcinoma
Wilson's disease (acute or chronic)	Epithelioid hemangio-endothelioma
α_1-antitrypsin deficiency	Neuroendocrine tumor – metastatic
Primary hereditary oxalosis	Cholangiocarcinoma
Hemophilia A and B	
Nonalcoholic fatty liver disease	
Nonalcoholic steatohepatitis	
Vascular	**Other**
Budd-Chiari syndrome	Cirrhosis secondary to total parental nutrition
Posttransplant complications	Caroli's disease
Portal vein thrombosis	Trauma
Hepatic artery thrombosis	Hematological disorders
Veno occlusive disease	

low rate of recurrence after transplantation.[9] Alcoholic liver disease is the second leading indication for liver transplantation, although it is declining.[7] Outcomes are excellent, but the impact of recidivism on patient and graft survival is not well defined.[10] Societal and ethical issues related to liver transplantation for alcoholic liver disease demand continued efforts at optimizing our ability to predict long-term sobriety. Autoimmune hepatitis, which is the third leading indication for liver transplantation in the United States, is an inflammatory liver disease of unknown etiology that can decompensate and cause life-threatening complications and is most commonly seen in young women.

Primary biliary cirrhosis (PBC) and primary sclerosing cholangitis (PSC) are chronic cholestatic liver diseases leading to destruction of the interlobular and septal bile ducts (PBC) and biliary ductal inflammation leading to strictures and obliteration of the biliary system (PSC).[11,12] Secondary sclerosing cholangitis and familial cholestatic syndrome are less common indications. Liver transplantation is indicated in a varied group of metabolic disorders of the liver in adults; hereditary or primary hemachromatosis, Wilson's disease, primary hereditary oxalosis, and α_1-antitrypsin deficiency are the most common. An emerging and concerning indication for liver transplantation in recent years has been nonalcoholic fatty liver disease and nonalcoholic steatohepatitis. These conditions are likely to account for a significant number of liver transplantations in the future because of the rate of increase in the incidence of insulin-resistant syndrome.[13]

Hepatocellular carcinoma (HCC) is the most common primary hepatic tumor and is seen in patients with cirrhosis related to HCV and HBV, although it has been diagnosed in other etiologies as well, such as hemachromatosis and PBC. There is a concerning increased incidence among patients with nonalcoholic fatty liver disease or nonalcoholic steatohepatitis. Advances in imaging techniques, more accurate diagnosis, and staging of HCC and better patient selections have lead to improved patient outcomes for this diagnosis. HCC as an indication for liver transplantation is discussed in more detail below. Cholangiocarcinoma has been excluded as an appropriate indication for liver transplantation except in selected patients because of aggressive recurrence rates and poor patient survival.[14] Hepatic epitheliod hemangioendothelioma is a rare indication for liver transplantation, but significant long-term survival has been reported even in the setting of extrahepatic tumor.[15] The outcome of liver transplantation for metastatic disease is extremely

Table 2. CAUSES OF LIVER DISEASE IN PEDIATRIC PATIENTS

Cholestatic disorders	Hepatocellular disorders
Biliary atresia	Autoimmune hepatitis
Alagille's syndrome	Cryptogenic cirrhosis
Familial cholestatic syndrome	Hepatitis B and C
Primary sclerosing cholangitis	Neonatal hepatitis
Malignancy	**Fulminant liver failure**
Hepatoblastoma	Wilson's disease
Hepatocellular carcinoma	Drug toxicity (acetaminophen, isoniazid)
Sarcomas	Viral etiology
Hemangioendoyhelioma	Toxins
Metabolic disorders	**Other**
α_1-antitrypsin deficiency	Caroli's disease
Wilson's disease	Budd-Chiari syndrome
Tytosinemia	Cystic fibrosis
Urea cycle defects	Cirrhosis due to total parental nutrition
Crigler-Najjar syndrome	
Primary hereditary oxalosis – familial	
Hypercholesterolemia	

poor with the exception of some neuroendocrine tumors. In carefully selected cases, there have been some good results reported.[16] Budd-Chiari syndrome is obstruction of the hepatic veins leading to progressive congestion, necrosis, and fibrosis of the liver and portal hypertension. Other vascular indications for liver transplantation occur as a result of complications of liver transplantation surgery, such as hepatic artery thrombosis (HAT) and portal vein thrombosis (PVT).

Biliary atresia is the leading indication for liver transplantation in children, with a wide range of metabolic disorders accounting for a large percentage of pediatric liver transplantation. Table 2 lists the common indications for pediatric liver transplantation.

Fulminant Hepatic Failure

FHF, as described by Bernuau et al,[17] is the onset of encepholopathy within 2 weeks of jaundice in combination with coagulopathy. However, the most commonly used definition as it relates to liver transplantation is the OPTN/UNOS liver allocation policy description, "the onset of hepatic encephalopathy within 8 weeks of the first symptoms of liver disease. The absence of pre-existing liver disease is critical to the diagnosis."[18] The etiology of FHF has a significant impact on the indication, timing, and outcome of liver transplantation.[19,20] Table 3 lists the most common causes of FHF in adults. Viral etiology accounts for most liver transplantations for FHF in the pediatric population (Table 2). Rapid

Table 3. CAUSES OF FULMINANT HEPATIC FAILURE IN ADULTS

Viral
Hepatitis A, B , D, and, rarely, C; Epstein-Barr virus, herpes simplex virus, coxsacki B virus, cytomegalovirus, unknown viral etiology
Drugs
Acetaminophen, isoniazid, rifampin, sodium valproate, halothane, sulfonamides
Toxins
Mushroom toxicity
Metabolic
Wilson's disease
Autoimmune hepatitis

and multidisciplinary evaluation, including neurological assessment and management of cerebral edema, is critical because the disease course is rapid and fatal if an organ is not identified within 24 to 48 hours. FHF has been associated with a high rate of mortality in the pediatric population.[21] Although FHF is associated with high initial posttransplant mortality, long-term (>1 year) survival parallels that of patients with cholestatic disease.[7]

Hepatocellular Carcinoma and Liver Transplantation

Transplantation for HCC has been a controversial subject since the first reports of dismal outcomes in patients with extensive tumors.[22] In 1985, a report from the Pittsburgh group[23] reopened the issue when they reported that a series of "incidental" tumors found on pathological examination of the explanted liver was associated with good patient survival. A pivotal study by Mazzaferro et al[24] in 1996 achieved 92% survival at 3 years by carefully selecting candidates with a single 5-cm lesion or candidates with 3 lesions or fewer, with each lesion less than 3 cm without evidence of metastases or vascular invasion. The Milan Tumor staging criteria were the basis for the OPTN/UNOS prioritized allocation policy adapted in recognition of sustained similar good outcomes in a number of other studies.

The current OPTN/UNOS policy has been criticized for being too restrictive, and proponents of a modest expansion in the criteria for prioritization have cited equally significant patient outcomes.[25] The less restrictive University of California, San Francisco, criteria may be better at predicting outcome than either the Milan or the UNOS criteria.[26] In an analysis conducted by Shetty et al,[27] the allocation system based on prioritization of T_1 (1 nodule $\leq$ 1.9 cm) and T_2 (1 nodule 2.0-5.0 cm; 2 or 3 nodules, all $\leq$3.0 cm) lesions did justice to the majority of patients in the absence of well-defined alternatives. The recent changes to the OPTN/UNOS prioritization for T_2 lesions have yet to be validated, but it is likely that the priority given to patients with HCC will continue to be reassessed.[18] The incidence of HCC in the United States is projected to increase for at least another 10 years, primarily because of the HCV epidemic. As a result, the number of patients who might need a liver transplant will also rise, requiring ongoing evaluation of this issue.

Evaluation for Liver Transplantation

Most patients present to the liver transplant center with advanced cirrhosis and a combination of complications of portal hypertension and decompensated synthetic function (Table 4). Patients may present with malnutrition, fatigue, muscle wasting, ascites, encepholopathy, spontaneous bacterial peritonitis, renal insufficiency, gastrointestinal bleeding, coaguloapathy, edema, jaundice, or a liver lesion. The evaluation should be a multidisciplinary process involving the hepatologist, transplant surgeon, transplant nurse coordinator, social worker, nutritionist, and financial counselor at a minimum. The goal of the evaluation is to (1) identify the cause of the liver disease as this may affect the rate of disease progression, and pretransplant and posttransplant management; (2) determine alternate therapeutic options that may prevent or delay progression to liver transplantation, (3) assess the severity of the disease and the risk/benefit of liver transplantation; and (4) identify if the patient is a suitable candidate from a medical, surgical, financial, emotional, psychosocial, and compliance perspective to undergo the procedure.[28]

Table 4. COMPLICATIONS OF CHRONIC LIVER DISEASE

Portal hypertension	Decreased hepatic mass/ synthetic dysfunction	Other
Ascites	Coagulopathy	Liver lesion
Hepato-hydrothorax	Fatigue	Hepatorenal syndrome
Peripheral edema	Malnutrition	Hepatopulmonary syndrome
Esophageal gastric varices	Hypoalbunemia	Spontaneous bacterial peritonitis
Portal gastropathy	Jaundice	
Hypersplenism	Pruritis	
Thrombocytopenia	Encepholopathy	

Initial Assessment

Patients referred for liver transplantation will typically undergo a detailed medical history review, including onset and severity of symptoms, family history, use of herbal substances, use of prescription and over-the-counter medications, alcohol and other illicit drug use, body piercing and tattoos, blood transfusions, and a dietary history. Information on functional status such as ability to work or attend school will help assess the impact of symptoms on quality of life. Assessment of growth, development, and nutritional parameters are important in pediatric candidates. Recent reports suggest that there is not a good correlation between the model for end-stage liver disease (MELD) score and quality of life, and that the Childs-Turcotte-Pugh (CPT) score may correlate better with quality of life probably because of the inclusion of ascites and encepholopathy.[29] A thorough review of all systems and current medication use and a detailed physical examination will complete the history and physical.

Laboratory Testing

Routine blood tests are outlined in Table 5, in addition to some disease-specific tests that are indicated. All patients should have a complete blood cell count (CBC) with differential and platelets, prothrombin time, international normalized ratio, serum urea nitrogen, creatinine, electrolytes and a fasting blood sugar, liver enzymes including alanine aminotransferase, aspartate aminotransferase, γ-glutamyl transpeptidase, alkaline phosphatase, total bilirubin and direct bilirubin, serum albumin, and total protein. A lipid profile and thyroid function tests should be considered. In addition, the blood tests should include basic serologies—antibody to HCV (anti-HCV), antibody to hepatitis A (anti-hepatitis A virus), HBV surface antibody, HBV surface antigen, HBV core antibody, human immunodeficiency virus (HIV), herpes simplex virus, cytomegalovirus (CMV), Epstein-Barr virus, and a blood type (ABO). Patients presenting with HCV cirrhosis should have a genotype drawn and a HCV RNA quantative assay, because this information will have an impact on the efficacy of both pretransplant treatment trials with interferon and ribavirin and posttransplant management strategies to prevent or treat recurrent HCV. The optimal treatment strategy for candidates with HBV will be determined on the basis of the degree of viral replication, so an HBV DNA and HBV e-antigen are indicated. In patients presenting with or suspected to have autoimmune hepatitis, antinuclear antibodies, antismooth muscle antibodies, and antibodies to liver/kidney microsome type 1 and antimitochondria antibodies should be drawn. These may also be useful in patients presenting with a diagnosis of PBC. Serum iron level and iron-binding capacity should be considered to exclude hemachromatosis. Some centers will screen for α_1-antitrypsin deficiency with α_1-antitrypsin phenotype, and serum ceruloplasmin to screen for Wilson's disease in patients younger than

Table 5. LABORATORY BLOOD TESTS

Routine	Liver disease specific
Complete blood cell count with differential and platelets	Primary biliary cirrhosis, primary sclerosing cholangitis, autoimmune hepatitis – ANA, AMA, ASMA, anti LKM1
Prothrombin time, international normalized ratio	HBV – HBV DNA, HBeAg, HBeAb, HBdAb
Serum urea nitrogen, creatinine, electrolytes, and fasting blood sugar	HIV – HIV DNA, CD4, T cell count
Liver enzymes, including AST, ALT, GGTP, alkaline phosphatase, total bilirubin, direct bilirubin, albumin, and total protein	HCV– HCV RNA quantative, HCV genotype
	Primary sclerosing cholangitis – CA 19-9, CEA
Lipid profile, thyroid function tests, alpha fetoprotein, iron studies, ABO	
Serologies; antibody to HCV antibody to hepatitis A virus, HBsAb, HBsAg, HBcAb, HIV, herpes simplex virus, cytomegalovirus, Epstein-Barr virus	

Abbreviations: ALT, alanine aminotransferase; AMA, antimitochondria antibodies ; ANA, antinuclear antibodies; ASMA, antismooth muscle antibodies; AST, aspartate aminotransferase; CEA, carcinoembryonic antigen; GGTP, γ-glutamyl transpeptidase; HBeAg, HBV e-antigen; HBeAb, HBV e antibody; HBdAb, HBV delta antibody; HBsAb, hepatitis B virus surface antibody; HBsAg, hepatitis B virus surface antigen; HBcAb, hepatitis B core antibody; HBV, hepatitis B virus; HCV, hepatitis C virus; HIV, human immunodeficiency virus; LKM1, liver/kidney microsome type 1.

50 years of age. All patients presenting with cirrhosis should have a serum alpha fetoprotein (AFP) level checked to screen for HCC.

Diagnostic Testing

Routine diagnostic testing for evaluation for liver transplantation is shown in Table 6. All liver transplant candidates should have a chest radiograph performed, in addition to an electrocardiogram. Pulmonary function tests may be indicated in patients with an abnormal chest radiograph, history of smoking, or intrinsic lung disease such as chronic obstructive pulmonary disease. Cardiac evaluation may include an echocardiogram and an exercise or pharmacological stress test to identify candidates at risk for cardiac complications perioperatively and postoperatively, which increase with age.[30] Of particular significance are preexisting cardiac diseases due to coronary artery disease (CAD), alcohol cardiomyopathy, and hereditary hemachromatosis.[31] Mortality in liver transplant recipients with a history of CAD has been reported as high as 50%.[32] Carey et al[33] reported that the incidence of moderate to severe CAD was 27% in candidates older than age 50 years, with diabetes being a significant predictive risk factor.[33] The most common cardiac condition in patients with cirrhosis is cirrhotic cardiomyopathy, which has been recognized only relatively recently and remains poorly described. It presents as impaired cardiac contractility in episodes of stress in these patients.[34] Patients with impaired left ventricular function should have cardiac angiography. Two other well-documented, although relatively rare, conditions are portopulmonary hypertension (PPH), defined as a mean pulmonary artery pressure (PAP) greater than 25 mm Hg, pulmonary vascular resistance greater than 120 dyne/cm^{-5}, and a pulmonary capillary wedge pressure less than 15 mm Hg, and hepatopulmonary syndrome, defined as hypoxemia (PaO$_2$ <70 mm Hg) or alveolar-arterial oxygen gradient greater than 20 mm Hg and pulmonary vascular dilatation, in the setting of advanced liver disease.[35] Hepatopulmonary syndrome was once considered an absolute contraindication to liver transplantation, but now, with treatment, patients may receive a transplant with successful outcomes.[36] The severity of PPH determines if it is a contraindication to liver transplantation. PAP greater than 50 mm Hg is associated with up to 100% mortality, with no mortality reported with a PAP less than 35 mm Hg in one study.[37] Right heart caterization with pressure measurements is the gold standard in patients with PPH, and should be performed preoperatively in any patient with evidence of PPH on echocardiogram.

Abdominal imaging, either computed tomography (CT) or magnetic resonance imaging (MRI), is performed to evaluate the anatomy of the bile ducts and the hepatic vasculature. In cases of PVT, the

Table 6. ROUTINE DIAGNOSTIC TESTING

- Chest radiograph
- Computed tomography/magnetic resonance imaging of abdomen
  Liver volume measurement
  Presence of and staging of hepatocellular carcinoma
  Assess status of portal vein, hepatic artery, and hepatic veins
- Electrocardiogram
- Echocardiogram, cardiac stress test
- *Hepatocellular carcinoma diagnosis*
  Bone scan – rule out bone metastases
  Chest computed tomography – rule out lung metastases
- Endoscopy – treatment strategies for varices
- Bone densitometry – age, gender, and disease specific
- Colonoscopy >50 years
- Mammogram – per American Cancer Society Guidelines
- Gynecologic examination including Pap smear
- Prostate cancer screening – men >40 years
- Dental evaluation

extent of the thrombus into the splanchnic venous circulation will determine if liver transplantation is technically possible. In patients with PVT it is essential to evaluate the patency of the superior mesenteric vein. CT or MRI is also used for screening for HCC and extrahepatic malignancies.[38] However, limitation in accurate staging of tumors and detection of small satellite tumors has been reported with both modalities.[27] A chest CT and possibly a bone scan may be indicated to rule out metastases in candidates with HCC. Angiography or tumor biopsy is rarely indicated to diagnose or stage HCC.

Consultations

The etiology of the liver disease, age, and the presence of comorbid conditions will for the most part determine the type of specialty consultation used to evaluate the liver transplant candidate. Table 7 outlines standard consultations for liver transplantation. Cardiology consultation may be indicated in the setting of abnormal findings on cardiac testing or the presence of multiple risk factors as identified by the American Heart Association. Compromised renal function is a complex and difficult finding to manage in liver transplant candidates. A nephrology consult may be indicated to identify the cause of abnormal renal function. Hepatorenal syndrome is a relatively common occurrence, particularly with longer waiting time to liver transplantation, and is in general reversible with liver transplantation.[39-41] Progressive, chronic intrinsic kidney disease is likely to be further compromised by the addition of calcinurine inhibitors and acute tubular necrosis after surgery and is therefore an indication to evaluate the efficacy of a combined liver-kidney transplantation. Acute decompensation of renal function in a cirrhotic patient demands a full evaluation to prevent further deterioration and to optimize existing renal function.

Table 7. CONSULTATIONS

Routine	As indicated
• Hepatologist • Surgeon • Clinical transplant coordinator • Social worker • Financial counselor • Nutritionist/Dietitian	• Psychiatry – history of recent substance abuse (6-24 months) or psychiatric disorder • Cardiology – abnormal electrocardiography or echocardiogram, presence of 2 or more risk factors for coronary artery disease, history of excessive alcohol use/abuse, hemachromatosis • Pulmonary – abnormal pulmonary function tests or chest radiography, clinical indications of intrinsic lung disease • Nephrology – hepatorenal syndrome, abnormal kidney function, cryoglobunemia in hepatitis C virus cirrhosis

Psychosocial evaluation is an essential component of the transplant evaluation. In most programs, potential candidates will be evaluated by a clinical social worker. Assessment of educational level, support structure, and compliance with previous treatments can give important insight into a patient's ability to cope with the stressors of chronic disease and the complexities of liver transplantation. In addition, a clinical psychologist or psychiatrist should evaluate for depression, anxiety disorder, and other psychiatric illness that may need to be treated or may be a contraindication to liver transplantation. In candidates with a history of substance abuse, the assessment will focus on issues related to compliance, period of abstinence, attendance in a substance abuse treatment program, risk of relapse, and insight into the disease. Rates of recidivism in liver transplantation for alcoholic liver disease range from 11.5% to 49%.[42] This report and others rarely cite graft failure as a result of recidivism. However, graft dysfunction rates have been reported ranging from 0% to 17% and mortality ranging from 0% to 5%.[43,44] Alcoholic liver disease remains a controversial indication for liver transplantation in respect to the allocation of a scarce resource to a population with a risk of recidivism and related posttransplant morbidity and mortality. A significant decline in 10-year survival rates has been reported in patients who relapse into alcohol use after liver transplantation for alcoholic liver disease compared with those who did not relapse.[45] Many programs require a minimum period of 6 months of abstinence as a predictor of sobriety after transplantation. It has been suggested that a good support network and insight into the disease process may be more predictive of sobriety after transplantation than 6 months of abstinence.[46] Programs may individualize their evaluation to include these factors to assist in predicting sobriety after transplantation, particularly if disease severity will not allow time to obtain 6 months of sobriety, particularly in cases with HCC.

The financial impact of liver transplantation on the patient, the family, the transplant center, and society as a whole is significant. The majority of medical insurance carriers and state and federal programs cover liver transplantation at approved centers. However, the extent of the coverage and the presence of coverage for medications vary significantly. A financial counselor is now an integral member of the multidisciplinary team at most programs and will provide a detailed financial and insurance assessment in addition to counseling to the patient and the family with limited resources.

In addition, referrals may be indicated to facilitate routine cancer screening such as colonoscopy, mammogram, Pap smear, and prostate cancer screening. A comprehensive screening for oral and pharahgeal cancer should be considered in patients with alcoholic liver disease who also use tobacco. Bone denisitometry should be considered in at risk patients. Vaccination protocols may be instituted for both HBV and hepatitis A where appropriate in adults, and every effort to complete the age-appropriate pediatric vaccination schedule before liver transplantation should be attempted (Table 8). Patients with chronic liver disease may be anergic and, despite accelerated double dosing schedules, may not seroconvert before transplantation.[47] Patients should also receive the pneumococcal vaccine every 5 years and the influenza vaccine annually. Some centers will do tuberculin skin testing on initial presentation or annually, but because of the significant prevalence of anergy in this population, skin testing is not a definitive screening tool for tuberculosis.

Table 8. VACCINATIONS FOR PEDIATRIC PATIENTS

Pretransplant vaccinations	Posttransplant vaccines
Inactive vaccines	Inactive vaccines
Diphtheria, pertussis, tetanus	Influenza
Polio	Pneumovax (>2 years old, give every 5 years)
Influenza	Live vaccines
Hepatitis A and B	Contraindicated in general
Pneumovax (>2 years)	
Rotavirus	
Live vaccines (do not give within 4-6 weeks of liver transplantation)	
Oral polio	
Varicella	
Measles mumps rubella	

Contraindications to Liver Transplantation

Absolute contraindications to liver transplantation have evolved over the years and are relatively few. Table 9 outlines the absolute and relative contraindications. The significance of comorbid conditions and their potential impact on a patient's quality of life and life expectancy can be the most difficult to assess and predict. However, severe cardiac and pulmonary diseases remain absolute contraindications to liver transplantation. Active sepsis should be treated before transplantation, although when the source is the liver itself (cholangitis), this may not be possible without removal of the diseased organ. Active use of alcohol in the setting of alcohol-related liver injury or illicit drug use and noncompliance is considered a contraindication to liver transplantation. Liver transplantation is not indicated in FHF cases with advanced coma and irreversible brain injury. HIV was once considered an absolute contraindication to liver transplantation; however, in the era of highly active antiretroviral therapy and subsequent significant increase in life expectancy, coupled with the evidence that end-stage liver disease related to coinfection with HBV or HCV is one of the leading causes of death among HIV-infected individuals, the transplant community has begun to address the efficacy of liver transplantation in highly selective HIV-positive individuals.[48,49] Early results are encouraging but longer follow-up in controlled studies needs to be evaluated to understand the long-term impact.[50,51] HCV coinfected recipients may not have a similar good outcome as recipients with other causes of liver disease.[52] Acquired immunodeficiency syndrome (AIDS) remains an absolute contraindication to liver transplantation.

Liver transplantation has been performed by some centers for patients with advanced HCC (>T_2) with promising results.[53,54] The presence of extrahepatic malignancy is generally a contraindication, except in cases of neuroendochrine tumors, hemangioendothelioma, and skin cancers. Candidates with a remote history of malignancy and who have had appropriate treatment and follow-up should not be excluded from consideration for liver transplantation. Advanced age is no longer a contraindication, with emphasis shifting from chronological to physiological age in determining candidacy. Keswani et al,[55] in a review of the impact of older age on patient survival after liver transplantation, found that CAD and de novo malignancy were the 2 main risk factors associated with survival after liver transplantation in this age group. Lower survival rates have been reported in recipients older than 60 years.[56] Candidates older than 60 years warrant thorough and comprehensive evaluation of comorbid disease severity and careful risk-benefit estimation in light of these findings. Seniors older than 65 years may have even worse outcomes than seniors aged 60 to 65 years.[55]

Liver transplantation in obese patients (body mass index >30), in addition to the risk of cardiac complications, is a technically difficult surgery and complications include impaired wound healing and higher risk of posttransplant infection. PVT was once a technical contraindication to liver transplantation, but embolectomy or a graft to the superior mesenteric vein can be performed. Diffuse mesenteric thrombosis may not be an absolute contraindication either, but would necessitate multivisceral transplantation.

Table 9. CONTRAINDICATIONS TO LIVER TRANSPLANTATION

Absolute contraindications to liver transplantation
Active substance abuse/noncompliance
Active sepsis
Severe pulmonary hypertension
Severe cardiac disease
Coma with irreversible brain injury
AIDS
Relative contraindications
Human immunodeficiency virus infection
Age
Extrahepatic malignancy

Minimal Listing Criteria

Standardized listing criteria were developed in the late 1990s primarily in response to the inequities associated with access to liver transplant evaluation and the inflated impact of time on the waiting list on liver allocation policies. Minimal listing criteria were identified to level the playing field.[57] The original criteria used the CPT scoring system (Table 10).[58] In order to be placed on the waiting list, a candidate should have a minimal CPT score of 7. Certain complications such as ascites, refractory variceal bleeding,

Table 10. CHILDS-TURCOTTE-PUGH SCORE[58]

	Points	Points	Points
	1	2	3
Encepholopathy	None	Moderate	Severe
Ascites	None	Slight	Moderate
International normalized ratio	< 1.7	1.7-2.3	>2.3
Albumin	>3.5	2.8-3.5	<2.8
Bilirubin *Primary biliary cirrhosis, primary sclerosing cholangitis*	1-4	4-10	>10
Bilirubin *All other diseases*	<2	2-3	>3

spontaneous bacterial peritonitis, and encepholopathy were given additional weight. Although still OPTN/UNOS policy, the impact of these minimal listing criteria is limited in the MELD/ pediatric end-stage liver disease (PELD) era. Placement on the OPTN/UNOS liver candidate waiting list is based on a candidates MELD/PELD score. The MELD/PELD scoring system for liver allocation allows transplant centers to approximate timing to transplantation for a specific candidate. There is variability across UNOS/OPTN regions in the MELD/PELD score that will potentially initiate an organ offer, which is in turn, may lead to variability in the minimal listing scores used by transplant centers.

Timing of Liver Transplantation

As the indications for liver transplantation have expanded over the past 15 years, and as the waiting time has lengthened, the optimal timing to liver transplantation has been the subject of much discussion and debate. Decompensated liver disease in the setting of life-threatening complications remains the leading indication for liver transplantation. Many investigators have reported on the impact of disease severity at the time of liver transplantation on posttransplant outcomes, demonstrating a better patient survival when transplantation is performed in less chronically ill candidates. However, the shortage of available organs in an allocation system, which triages the sickest patients first, has resulted in candidates with severely decompensated liver disease undergoing complex surgery with, sometimes, marginal organs. In a setting of unlimited organ availability, it is likely that the current indications and timing of liver transplantation would be based on very different criteria. Timing to liver transplantation has essentially become a function of the liver allocation policy, except where LDLT is an option. A triage methodology of organs has evolved out of this disparity between supply and demand, with the sickest patient (in greatest need) receiving the first available organ, replacing the earlier system, which emphasized time on the waiting list. The MELD/PELD (explored in detail in chapter 3) score is an evidence-based, dynamic allocation system that prioritizes candidates on the basis of disease severity measured on objective data elements. The MELD/PELD score is predictive of mortality within 3 months without liver transplantation. The MELD/PELD score has been shown to better predict short-term waiting list survival than the CPT score. Death on the waiting list has decreased by 3.5% since the adoption of MELD/PELD.[59] Studies have also shown a decreased benefit of liver transplantation in patients with a MELD score less than 10, with the risk of early postoperative mortality being greater than the risk of death on the waiting list.[60] Liver transplantation is generally not indicated in this group of patients except in select circumstances where the MELD score does not adequately assess disease severity and therefore accurately predict mortality. The MELD score will fall short in predicting mortality in 15% to 18% of patients with chronic liver disease.[61] Patients with hyperbilirubinemia secondary to Gilbert's disease, patients receiving anticoagulant therapy, and patients with impaired kidney function are unfairly advantaged by the MELD system. There is also growing data to suggest that patients with refractory ascites and hyponatremia have a higher mortality risk than predicted by their MELD score alone.[62] Prioritization for candidates with HCC has also evolved on the basis of evidence that too much weight was initially assigned to T_1 and T_2 candidates. As a result, adjustments have been made to give T_1 and T_2 HCC candidates appropriately weighted MELD scores. In summary, although the MELD/PELD system essentially determines the timing to liver transplantation, it continues to be in evolution in response to evidence-based research.[63]

Roberts et al[7] in a recent analysis of the UNOS database demonstrated the impact of disease-specific factors on posttransplant outcomes. This analysis also suggests that the characteristics that are predictive of survival on the waiting list are not identical to those that predict posttransplant survival. PELD does not seem to be as accurate a predictor of pretransplant mortality as MELD, and further analysis may be indicated.[63]

Management on the Waiting List and Bridges to Liver Transplantation

Management of liver transplant candidates includes, whenever possible, the treatment of the underlying liver disease. This may ameliorate aspects of decompensated disease either temporarily and postpone liver transplantation, or in some circumstances perhaps prevent the need for a liver transplant. The treatment of suspicious liver lesions has evolved into a significant field of expertise, with options including chemoembolization, percutaneous radiofrequency ablation, percutaneous ethanol injection, and, in carefully selected cases, liver resection.[64] The treatment of large lesions remains somewhat controversial, as downsizing tumors by size alone does not change their underlying biological behavior.

In compensated HCV-related cirrhosis, combination therapy with pegylated alpha interferon and ribavirin is indicated.[65] The response rate varies; however, the response rate for genotype 1 is significantly lower than genotype 2 and 3. The efficacy of treatment in decompensated liver disease remains controversial primarily because of the difficult dosing considerations and the potential for fatal complications.

In contrast, even in decompensated HBV-related cirrhosis, treatment with antiviral therapy is efficacious and well documented and can lead to inhibition of viral replication and clinical improvement and stabilization.[66] Long-term use is limited, however, by the high rate of drug-resistant mutant strains. Adefovir dipivoxil has been proven to be effective in suppressing lamivudine-resistant HBV[67]; however, the long-term outcomes for patients on the waiting list and posttransplant recurrence are not yet clear. As Lok[67] concludes in her analysis, the role of combination therapy with lamivudine and adefovir or monotherapy with newer agents such as entecavir or tenofovir remains to be determined.

There may be a role for immunosuppressive treatment of active autoimmune hepatitis, although the risk-benefit must be weighed against the higher incidence of drug-related complications in patients with cirrhosis. In quiescent or end-stage autoimmune hepatitis, drug therapy is not indicated.

Standard therapy for PBC is ursodeoxycholic acid, which slows the progression of the disease but does not lead to resolution. Because of the risk of osteoporosis in PBC patients, screening and early management are recommended and should follow current practice guidelines.[68] Ursodeoxycholic acid may have a role in PSC, although improvement in liver tests has not been proven to be associated with improvement in disease severity. Patients with PSC have an 8% to 12% risk of developing cholangiocarcinoma.[69] All transplant candidates with PSC should be tested with serum tumor markers carcinoembryonic antigen (CEA) and CA-19-9 and have an abdominal imaging study. Any acute increase in serum bilirubin, sudden weight loss or abdominal pain should be investigated aggressively. In patients with associated ulcerative colitis, screening for colon cancer should be performed because of the increased risk.[70] Management of complications of end-stage liver disease is a challenge for the clinician, particularly in areas where the waiting time for a liver transplant is significant and where the MELD/PELD score at which patients are receiving transplants is high. Complications of portal hypertension such as hepatic encephalopathy require identification and treatment of precipitating factors such as infection, gastrointestinal bleeding, dehydration, or electrolyte imbalance. Treatment of encephalopathy is generally supportive, with use of lactulose to produce 2 to 3 soft bowel movements a day. Antibiotics such as neomycin and flagyl can be efficacious because of the effect on ammonia production in the intestine, but should be used with careful monitoring of renal function. Renal insufficiency in patients with end-stage liver disease can be prerenal, intrarenal, or hepatorenal. The development of hepatorenal syndrome is associated with a poor prognosis, and transplant recipients with this condition have an increased mortality rate and longer hospital stay.[71] Hepatorenal syndrome is generally reversible with liver transplantation, although prolonged dialysis before transplantation may necessitate a combined liver-kidney transplant.

First time esophageal and gastric variceal bleeding has a mortality risk of 30% to 50%.[72] Prophylaxis includes beta blockers, endoscopic surveillance and therapy, and in some cases transjugular intrahepatic portosystemic shunt (TIPS). Encepholopathy, PVT, and HCC are contraindications to TIPS, and periodic assessment of patency of TIPS is required. Rebleeding is common. Hepato-hydrothorax, lower extremity edema, and ascites are a common occurrence and are generally managed by dietary restriction of sodium and diuretic therapy. TIPS has been effective in managing refractory ascites and hepato-hydrothorax. Refractory ascites is a challenging complication often requiring frequent large volume paracentesis and can be complicated by hyponatremia, hypotension, and renal insufficiency. Spontaneous bacterial peritonitis (SBP) must be treated aggressively to prevent overwhelming sepsis. SBP is associated with poor prognosis and active transplant candidates should be inactivated until the infection has been cleared.

Reevaluation on the Waiting List

With the introduction and maturation of the MELD/PELD allocation system, an added benefit is the ability to "predict" when a candidate's score is likely to generate an organ offer. This allows the transplant team to optimize their resources by reevaluating candidates who are likely to receive an offer. The MELD/PELD score itself determines the frequency of laboratory test (MELD: INR, creatinine, and bilirubin; PELD: INR, creatinine, bilirubin, and albumin) updates to maintain OPTN/UNOS waiting list status (discussed in detail in chapter 3). It is common practice to complete a full CBC with differential and platelets, electrolytes, including serum urea nitrogen and creatinine, and liver function tests on this frequency. AFP should be added every 3 months for surveillance and more frequently in patients with a rising AFP level. There may be efficacy to repeating previously negative serologies such as CMV, particularly if posttransplant prophylaxis regimens are based on recipient CMV status. For patients with HCV and HBV, as timing to recurrence and severity may be affected by rate of viral replication at the time of liver transplantation, it may be prudent to check HCV RNA quantative by polymerase chain reaction and HBV DNA as specific protocols determine. For HIV-positive candidates, frequent HIV DNA, CD4, and T-cell counts are indicated and may affect a candidate's suitability for liver transplantation. Abdominal imaging for surveillance of HCC should be considered every 6 months in candidates with cirrhosis. However, imaging studies for patients with rising AFP levels or known HCC should be at 2-3 month intervals. HCC prioritization on the OPTN/UNOS waiting list currently requires updated abdominal imaging every 3 months to maintain priority status. CT or MRI may be indicated as early as 1 month after HCC treatment. Status of the portal vein should be updated every 3 to 6 months. Other diagnostic tests may be repeated as indicated by the initial results and the predicted risk factors for disease progression.

Cardiac reevaluation will be indicated for patients with known cardiopulmonary disease, abnormal findings on initial evaluation, or prevalence of risk factors as identified by the American Heart Association. Similarly, repeat psychosocial and financial evaluation in candidates identified on initial evaluation to have less than optimal supports, questionable financial circumstances, limited coping mechanisms, and relatively recent abstinence from substance abuse or use, is prudent. Routine cancer screening following the American Cancer Society guidelines should be maintained.

Organ Source

The most common source of donor livers for transplantation has been from deceased brain-dead donors. In the majority of cases, the whole liver will be implanted. Split liver transplantation evolved out of the shortage of donor livers and the experience gained with reduced-sized livers from adult donors to accommodate the small size of the pediatric recipient. In a reduced-size procedure, part of the donor liver is removed and discarded. Split liver transplantation allows the liver to be split anatomically between 2 candidates, most commonly an adult and a pediatric patient or another small adult patient.[73,74] Only young, hemodynamically stable donors who have not had any significant compromise such as prolonged hypotension, aggressive use of pressure support, acidosis, or prolonged cardiac resuscitation are suitable candidates for splitting.[75,76]

Even with this innovative expansion of the donor pool, the supply has not kept pace with the demand, and alternate sources of organs have been explored. LDLT initially evolved in the early 1990s out of the need to identify a more available source of donor livers for the pediatric population.[77] In the late 1990s, LDLT was successfully applied to adult recipients.[78,79] Before the establishment of brain-death criteria, the use of organs from deceased after cardiac death donors or non-heart-beating-donors was explored. With the organ shortage of the late 1990s, interest was again focused on expanding this source of donor livers for transplantation and has continued to date with some caution, as the long-term outcomes still have to be determined.[80]

Donor Characteristics

Despite the number of liver transplantations almost doubling in the past 10 years, there has been a growing imbalance between supply and demand. This imbalance, coupled with an alarming and unacceptable mortality rate on the waiting list, has lead to the expansion of acceptable donor criteria. "Marginal" or extended criteria donor livers, such as livers from older donors (>60 years), obese donors, HCV-positive donors, HBV core antibody-positive donors, donors on vasopressors, and donors with a history of high-risk behaviors, are now routinely used.[81,82] HCV-positive livers are now routinely used in HCV-positive recipients.[83] Reports of transmission of the donor genotype has led transplant programs to limit this practice to genotype 1 recipients because of the risk of transmitting the more resistant genotype 1 from an untested donor into a recipient with genotype 2 or 3.[84,85] HBV core antibody-positive donor livers can be safely used in HBV surface antigen-positive recipients without added risk. Antiviral therapy and/or HBV immunoglobulin may prevent infection in the HBV naive recipient of a HBV core antibody liver, but some risk and the commitment to possible lifelong prophylaxis remain.[86-88] As a result of the more aggressive use of extended criteria donor livers, the quality of the average donor liver being used for transplantation has deteriorated over time,[89] which has led to reports of higher rates of primary graft nonfunction and lower patient survival.[90] Despite using extended criteria donor livers, up to 29% of all donor livers are discarded.[91] The dilemma facing the clinician and the patient in the middle of the night is the risk-benefit of accepting a marginal offer now, or waiting for a more ideal offer later, which may be too late. There has also been an accepted theory that a marginal liver in a sick patient will be poorly tolerated and therefore the "marginal" or extended criteria donor offer has traditionally been used in the less sick candidate.[89] A recent report by Amin et al[92] proposes a paradigm shift on the basis of their risk-benefit analysis, and suggests extended criteria donor livers be used in candidates with a MELD score greater than 20. It is clear that not every donor liver offer can or should be used in every recipient. Each offer must be judged with the specific recipient in mind and a risk-benefit analysis for each donor-recipient match. Recipient informed consent is critical before proceeding.

Living Donor Liver Transplantation

As the deceased donor shortage has continued, LDLT has become an option for many recipients. A comprehensive review of LDLT and care of the living donor is provided in chapter 11. There are many benefits to the recipient of a LDLT, including the benefits of elective scheduling of liver transplantation, ability to optimize the recipient's condition before surgery, shorter waiting time, shorter ischemic times, and generally younger donor age.[79,93,94] Careful selection of recipients, however, is warranted as not all recipients may be suitable candidates for LDLT. Severity of illness, degree of portal hypertension, previous abdominal surgery, obesity, and PVT are factors that may affect recipient outcomes and therefore selection criteria.[95,96] It is also important to match adequate liver volume to the degree of decompensated liver disease when selecting candidates for LDLT.[97] The greatest lifelong benefit and lowest posttransplant mortality risk may be in candidates with a MELD score of 14 to 25.[98] A report by Roberts et al[7] suggests that because of the impact of different variables on future outcomes, the optimal timing to LDLT may be different in different diseases. A recent analysis of the OPTN and the Scientific Registry of Transplant Recipients showed graft survival to be only slightly lower at 1 year and 3 years with LDLT.[99] Similar outcomes for rate and severity of recurrent HCV were reported in a comparison of LDLT to deceased donor liver transplantation.[100]

Liver Transplant Surgery

A bilateral subcostal incision with a midline extension to the xiphoid process, commonly termed a "Mercedes," is used to expose the entire liver and suprahepatic vena cava. The native liver is dearterialized by ligating the right and left hepatic arteries. The cystic and common hepatic ducts are ligated and divided. The portal vein is exposed from the level of gastroduodenal artery to its bifurcation. The inferior and superior vena cava are exposed and then clamped, and the liver is removed. Backtable, preparation of the donor graft is completed and may include arterial and/or venous reconstruction.

LIVER TRANSPLANTATION

The complexity of the implantation is dependent upon the type of graft being implanted. Implantation begins with the anastomosis of the suprahepatic and infrahepatic vena cava. An end-to-end portal vein anastomosis is done. The liver is flushed free of preservation solution before the circulation is reopened. The caval clamps are removed and normal portal flow is restored. Next the hepatic artery is reconstructed. The donor gallbladder is then removed. The final step is the biliary reconstruction using a choledocholedochostomy, with or without a T-tube, or a Roux-en-Y hepaticojejunostomy. The abdomen is closed, leaving 1 to 3 suction drains in place.

Complexities of Liver Transplant Surgery

The strategic location of the liver under the right costal margin; its intimate relationship to the portal vein and inferior vena cava; adhesions due to previous right upper quadrant surgery; PVT and other anatomical anomalies, make this a very complex and challenging surgery. There is an increase risk of bleeding because of portal hypertension, tissue fragility, and coagulation deficiencies commonly seen in the decompensated cirrhotic patient. Selection of the appropriate recipient of a split liver or a living donor liver is essential to optimize success.

Intensive Care Management of the Liver Transplant Recipient

After liver transplantation, patients are taken directly to the intensive care unit (ICU). ICU mortality following liver transplantation has been reported as high as 11.5%.[101] Complications related to mortality are acute renal failure, acute respiratory distress syndrome, low cardiac output, hemorrhage, pneumonia, and graft failure.[101] The length of time receiving mechanical ventilation will depend on the preoperative condition of the patient and initial graft function. Poor nutritional status, severe muscle wasting, refractory ascites or pleural effusions, and severe encepholopathy can prolong the period of ventilator support. Patients with chronic liver disease usually have a hyperdynamic circulation, which is more pronounced in patients with refractory ascites, hyponatremia, hypoalbunemia, and renal insufficiency. These patients present a unique challenge and often require the use of pulmonary arterial pressure monitoring, aggressive fluid resuscitation, and meticulous attention to metabolic and electrolyte imbalances. Common electrolyte imbalances after liver transplantation are outlined in Table 11. Adequate control of hypertension and appropriate pain management should be instituted. The use of an H_2 blocker, or proton pump inhibitors, is recommended to prevent gastric ulceration. Early enteral feeding is recommended once graft function is confirmed, because most patients with advanced liver disease are malnourished and in a hypermetabolic state after transplantation.[102] Renal dysfunction has been reported to occur in 64% of patients, but resolves in 69% of patients[103]; however, renal dysfunction will lead to prolonged or even permanent renal failure in a small number of cases.[104] Patients may require renal support therapy such as continuous venous-venous hemofiltration

Table 11. COMMON ELECTROLYTE IMBALANCES AFTER LIVER TRANSPLANTATION

Hyponatremia	Hypophosphoremia
Hypokalemia	Hypoglycemia
Hyperkalemia	Hyperglycemia
Hypocalcemia	Hypomagnesium

Table 12. INDICATORS OF LIVER FUNCTION AFTER LIVER TRANSPLANTATION

Hemodynamically stable
Normalizing renal function
Normal acid-base balance
Recovery of consciousness
Resolution of hypothermia
Euglycemia
Normal prothrombin time/international normalized ratio
Resolving aminotransferase
Decreasing bilirubin

or hemodialysis. Renal dose dopamine is commonly used for its vasodilatory effect. Antibiotics in the perioperative period is standard practice in combination with antiviral and antifungal prophylaxis. Protocol immunosuppressive therapy will be instituted perioperatively. (See chapter 16 for a comprehensive review of transplant pharmacology.) Graft function is of primary concern in the immediate postoperative period. Recovery of mental status, return to normalization of renal function, normalization of hemodynamic status, decreasing serum bilirubin, normalization of INR, and resolution of reperfusion injury as evidence by resolving alanine aminotransferase and aspartate aminotransferase levels are all indicators of a functioning liver (Table 12). Any indication of graft dysfunction warrants evaluation and appropriate, timely intervention.

Evaluation of Liver Dysfunction

A systematic approach to the assessment of liver allograft dysfunction should be defined to facilitate a clinical differentiation of cause (Table 13). It is not uncommon for overlapping in cause of injury to occur, and treatment for one cause can aggravate another. A meticulous review of the history, including original liver disease; donor characteristics; type of graft; review of surgical details such as size matching of donor-recipient vasculature; type of biliary reconstruction; donor and recipient serologies; ABO matching; previous complications and treatments; should be performed. Thorough review of symptoms, onset, severity, precipitating factors such as known side effects of the current medication regime, and adherence with medications will be helpful. Detailed review of trends in liver chemistries, bilirubin, renal function, and CBC should be included. Additional disease-specific markers such as HCV RNA quantative in HCV cases, HBV DNA and HBV surface antigen in HBV cases, autoimmune markers, AFP in HCC cases, and CMV antigenemia and Epstein-Barr virus polymerase chain reaction may be indicated. Doppler ultrasound of the liver is indicated to evaluate the vasculature and the biliary system, which can help rule out HAT and biliary dilatation secondary to bile duct stricture. A liver biopsy is indicated if no evidence of a biliary etiology is present on biochemical analysis and ultrasound. Examination of the biliary system with an endoscopic retrograde cholangiogram or percutaneous transhepatic cholangiogram depending on the type of biliary reconstruction is indicated if there is evidence of biliary dilatation.

Table 13. EVALUATION OF LIVER ALLOGRAFT DYSFUNCTION

1. Indication for liver transplantation – original liver disease, comorbid conditions
2. Donor characteristics – living or deceased donor, donation after cardiac death donor, deceased brain-death donor, standard donor criteria, extended donor criteria, donor serologies
3. Surgical details – reduced sizes graft, split liver graft, left lateral segment or right lobe graft from living donor, biliary reconstructions, vascular reconstruction, piggy-back or standard placement.
4. Histology – preperfusion and postperfusion liver biopsies
5. Donor/Recipient serology review
6. ABO matching
7. Previous posttransplant complications review
8. Medication review including side effects profile, toxicities, and drug interactions
9. Review of biochemical profile with trending
10. Disease-specific markers for recurrence of original disease, donor transmission of disease, common posttransplant infectious complications such as cytomegalovirus, Epstein-Barr virus
11. Complete review of systems and physical examination
12. Ultrasound and Doppler, computed tomography or magnetic resonance imaging
13. Liver biopsy
14. Evaluation of the biliary system – cholangiography
15. Angiography

Table 14. COMPLICATIONS AFTER LIVER TRANSPLANTATION

Immediately after transplantation (0-7 days)	Primary graft nonfunction
	Poor early graft function
	Hepatic artery thrombosis
	Portal vein thrombosis
	Bile leak
Early posttransplant period (<3 months)	Acute cellular rejection
	Biliary stricture/leak
	Opportunistic infections
	Complications of immunosuppression
Late posttransplant period (>3 months)	• Chronic rejection
	• Recurrence of original liver disease
	• Complication of long term immunosuppression
	◻ Chronic renal insufficiency
	◻ De novo malignancy
	◻ Hypertension
	◻ Hyperlipidemia
	◻ Diabetes mellitus
	◻ Metabolic bone disease
	◻ Obesity

Complications After Liver Transplantation

There are many causes of graft dysfunction and they can occur at any time. For the purpose of this discussion and to provide a framework to assist in a differential diagnosis, complications of liver transplantation are categorized on the basis of the most common timing of their occurrence. "Immediately after" transplantation refers to fewer than 7 days after liver transplantation, "early" refers to fewer than 3 months after transplantation, and "late" refers to more than 3 months after transplantation. Table 14 reviews the common complications after liver transplantation defined by these periods. Table 15 provides a synopsis of posttransplant complications, presentation, diagnosis, and treatment.

Long-term complications of immunosuppression are covered in chapter 13 and infectious disease is covered in chapter 14 and will not be discussed here. Pediatric issues in liver transplantation are covered in chapter 19.

Primary Graft Dysfunction

All transplanted livers have some degree of preservation injury characterized by elevated aminotransferases, which usually normalize within the first 7 days. Approximately 40% of patients with aspartate aminotransferase levels greater than 5000 IU/L within the first 72 hours after transplantation will develop primary graft nonfunction (PNF). Possible causes or contributing factors to developing severe preservation injury are outlined in Table 16. It may be difficult to differentiate between PNF and poor early graft function, the latter often being reversible. The treatment of PNF is retransplantation. The incidence of PNF is 2% to 5% in the United States. Risk factors include long ischemic times, severe donor hypernatremia, advanced donor age, and severe donor macrosteatosis.

Vascular Complications

HAT is the most common vascular complication in the early postoperative period.[105]

It is more common in pediatric recipients because their arterial reconstructions are much smaller, and often require the use of operative microscope. Doppler ultrasound is a good noninvasive screening study that is used in most programs. Thrombectomy may be corrective in cases of early diagnosis. Retransplantation

Table 15. PRESENTATION, DIAGNOSIS, CAUSE, AND TREATMENT OF LIVER TRANSPLANT COMPLICATIONS

Primary graft nonfunction

Presentation: coma, severe coagulopathy, oliguria, jaundice, and hypoglycemia

Diagnosis: clinical presentation, liver biopsy

Cause: unknown. Associated with >50% macrovesicular fat, prolonged ischemic time

Treatment: retransplantation

Poor early graft function

Presentation: prothromin time >20 seconds, decrease glucose production, slow lactate clearance

Aspartate aminotransferase (AST) >2000 IU/L, severe injury; AST >5000 IU/L, very severe injury

Diagnosis: clinical presentation, liver biopsy

Causes: ischemic, anoxic, or reperfusion injury

Treatment: supportive care; prostaglandin-E, prostacyclin

Hepatic artery thrombosis

Presentation: routine Doppler screening, rapid onset hepatic dysfunction

Diagnosis: angiography

Causes: unclear; pediatric patients are at higher risk; technical; rejection – decreased vascular compliance and edema

Treatment: attempt rearterialization, retransplantation

Portal vein thrombosis

Presentation: early;fulminant hepatic failure, ascites, renal failure, and hemodynamic collapse. late; ascites, pedal edema

Diagnosis: Doppler, venogram

Causes: technical, decreased portal flow

Treatment: early; retransplantation, late; dilatation, placement of stents, retransplantation

Bile leak

Presentation: fever, jaundice, high white blood cell count, sepsis, bilious drainage from incision/drains

Diagnosis: sonogram/computed tomography scan, cholangiography; exploratory laporotomy

Causes: technical, hepatic artery thrombosis (HAT), prolonged ischemia

Treatment: surgical repair, retransplantation

Acute cellular rejection

Presentation: increase in liver function tests, right upper quadrant pain, fever, asymptomatic.

Diagnosis: Doppler to rule out HAT and bile leak/stricture; liver biopsy

Treatment: steroid bolus +/- recycle, monoclonal antibody, +/- augmentation of maintenance immunosuppression

Chronic rejection

Presentation: increase in liver function tests

Diagnosis: rule out HAT and biliary stricture/leak; liver biopsy

Treatment: switch to tacrolimus; add mycophenolate mofetil and/or rapamycin; retransplantation

Associated with previous cytomegalovirus infection and nonadherence

Biliary stricture

Presentation: jaundice, pruritis, increase in bilirubin and alkaline phosphatase, fever, chills

Diagnosis: sonogram and Doppler, cholangiography

Treatment: dilatation and stent placement; surgical reconstruction of biliary anastomosis; rarely, retransplantation is required; usually ischemic in origin

Associated with late HAT

Table 16. POSSIBLE CAUSES OF PRESERVATION INJURY

Donor-related factors
- Older age
- Severe steatosis
- Hospital stay >3 days
- Acidosis before procurement
- Complication of procurement

Cold ischemic time
Warm ischemic time
Reperfusion injury
Recipient factors

---

may be necessary to salvage a patient with uncorrectable HAT or biliary ischemia. Late HAT should be suspected in patients who develop late (>3 months) biliary complications.

Early PVT usually necessitates retransplantation if early thrombectomy is not successful. Late PVT should be suspected in patients presenting with ascites or variceal bleeding. It can usually be managed with balloon dilatation and stenting, although retransplantation may be necessary.

Complications of the Biliary Tract

The overall biliary complication rate after liver transplantation has been reported to be 20.7%, including bile leakage 7.1% and anastomotic stricture 16.2%.[106] The bile duct is dependent on blood supply from the hepatic artery, so any disruption or decrease in blood flow through the hepatic artery will likely manifest in biliary tract complications such as bile leaks, biliary strictures, and bilomas. Bile leaks typically occur early and are from the anastomotic site or from the cut surface of the liver in a partial graft. Depending on the volume of bile leakage, in the absence of any evidence of sepsis, a trial of local drainage may lead to resolution without further intervention. In cases of more severe leaks, or when there is evidence of sepsis, surgical intervention is generally required. Biliary strictures occur later and may result from ischemic or technical issues. Nonanastomotic strictures are more likely ischemic in nature or related to recurrence of PSC, and have a lower success rate with treatment, either from interventional radiology or surgically.[107] Patients usually present with a cholestatic biochemical profile (increased bilirubin and alkaline phosphatase levels) and may have jaundice, pruritus, fever, or abdominal pain. Diagnosis is made on ultrasound if biliary dilatation is present. Endoscopic retrograde cholangiography or percutaneous transhepatic cholangiogram can identify the level of obstruction and treatment by dilatation or stenting may be possible. Surgery may be required in some cases. Ultrasound or computed tomography can be used to diagnose bilomas, and antibiotics and drainage is the optimal initial treatment. Obstruction due to biliary stones or sludge formation are also common. Patients with these obstructions should be treated with antifungal therapy, because there is a high incidence of fungal infections with biliary obstruction.

Allograft Rejection

Approximately 40% of patients may have at least 1 episode of acute cellular rejection, and the most common period is in the first 30 days after transplantation.[108] Definitive diagnosis is made on liver biopsy. The histology and the degree of biochemical abnormality and the original liver disease will usually be considered in defining the treatment. Mild acute rejection does not always warrant treatment with steroids, particularly in patients who received a transplant because of HCV. Often, increasing these patients' tacrolimus or cyclosporine levels will be sufficient. However, moderate to severe rejection is treated usually with a bolus of methylprednisolone followed by administration of antilymphocyte globulin or muronab-CD3 for steroid-resistant rejection. Maintenance immunosuppression may be augmented with the addition of mycophenolate mofetil or rapamycin and switching from a cyclosporine-based regimen to tacrolimus. Retransplantation for acute rejection is rarely necessary.

Chronic rejection, also referred to as vanishing bile duct syndrome or ductopenia, is a rare early occurrence in liver transplantation. Patients usually present many months to years after their liver transplantation with abnormal biochemistries, specifically abnormal bilirubin, γ-glutamyl transpeptidase, and alkaline phosphatase. Diagnosis is made on biopsy, and tacrolimus, rapamycin, or mycophenolate mofetil may stabilize and even reverse chronic rejection in many cases.[109]

Recurrent Disease

One of the most challenging issues in liver transplantation today is recurrence of the native liver disease. The impact of immunosuppression on the rate, severity, and timing of recurrence is not well understood. Graft failure due to recurrent disease is significant and survival rates after retransplantation are often much lower than primary graft survival rates. A complete review of disease-specific prophylaxis, diagnosis, and treatment is provided in Table 17.

Most liver diseases have been reported to recur, but the most common and currently the most challenging is HCV. Serologic HCV recurrence is essentially universal after liver transplantation but the effects on the allograft histology are varied and difficult to predict.[110,111] Approximately 10% of HCV-infected recipients

Table 17. RECURRENT DISEASE AFTER LIVER TRANSPLANTATION

Hepatitis B virus (HBV)
Prophylaxis: hepatitis B immunoglobulin, antiviral – lamivudine/famciclovir
Diagnosis: serological conversion to hepatitis B surface antigen positive, liver biopsy staining for HBV
Treatment: add or change antiviral therapy
Retransplantation considered (center specific)

Hepatitis C virus (HCV)
Prophylaxis: possible role for pegylated interferon/ribavirin, minimize immunosuppression
Diagnosis: liver biopsy for increased liver function tests, HCV RNA quantitative levels
Treatment: pegylated interferon/ribavirin, decrease immunosuppression
Retransplantation (center specific); associated with poorer outcomes

Autoimmune hepatitis
Prophylaxis: steroid maintenance considered
Diagnosis: liver biopsy for increased liver function tests, rule out other etiology
Treatment: steroids, cyclophosphamide, retransplantation (uncommon)

Primary biliary cirrhosis
Diagnosis: liver biopsy, rule out other etiologies
Treatment: ursodiol, retransplantation (rare)

Sclerosing cholangitis
Diagnosis: liver biopsy for increase in liver function tests; cholangiography to evaluate biliary tree; rule out other etiologies, difficult to distinguish from chronic rejection
Treatment: biliary stents, ursodiol, retransplantation

Relapse to alcohol abuse
Prevention: abstinence before transplantation, family support, insight into disease, continued alcohol rehabilitation or AA, return to work, develop hobbies, or goal in life
Diagnosis: liver biopsy for increase in liver function tests, clinical suspicion
Treatment: alcohol rehabilitation, supportive care, retransplantation not usually considered

Recurrent hepatocellular carcinoma
Prophylaxis: posttransplant adjunctive chemotherapy – efficacy unclear; size and number of lesions and presence of vascular invasion are predictive of recurrence risk
Screening and diagnosis: imaging studies, alpha fetoprotein
Treatment: local resection of lesion, chemotherapy, radiotherapy, supportive care

may die or lose their graft within 10 years after transplantation.[112] Fibrosis with progression to cirrhosis within 5 years of transplantation has been reported in 20% to 30% of patients.[113] Recurrent disease tends to have a more aggressive and rapid course after liver transplantation.[114] Risk factors for recurrent HCV after transplantation include older donor age,[115] immunosuppression,[116] and CMV infection.[117] Initial early reports of a higher incidence and more rapid progression of recurrent HCV in recipients of LDLT have not been supported uniformly and more data will be needed.[118] Retransplantation for HCV recurrence has had relatively poor overall results.[119] Risk factors predictive of a poor outcome after retransplantation for recurrent HCV are bilirubin levels greater than 5 mg/dL, renal insufficiency, and thrombocytopenia.[120,121] Early results with pegylated interferon and ribavirin have shown promise.[122]

Transplantation for HBV is now universally performed in the setting of prophylaxis with either antiviral therapy and/or HBV immunoglobulin.[123] HBV recurrence has decreased significantly as a result, but is higher in patients with active viral replication evidenced by the presence of HBV e-antigen or HBV DNA at the time of transplantation.[124] Pretransplant HBV viremia should be considered in optimizing posttransplant prophylaxis to prevent recurrence of HBV after liver transplantation.[125] Diagnosis of recurrent HBV is made by HBV surface antigen or HBV DNA in the serum or by presence of HBV surface antigen or HBV core antibody in the liver tissue. Treatment consists of adding an antiviral agent such as lamivudine, adefovir, or entecavir.[126] Drug-resistant mutant strains remain a challenge. Retransplantation for recurrent HBV has been reported but may be center specific.

Autoimmune hepatitis has been reported to recur after liver transplantation in addition to PBC and PSC. However, the impact of recurrent disease on patient and graft survival is not reported as significant.

HCC recurrence is well documented and in general treatment is supportive and retransplantation is not indicated.[127] Surveillance for recurrent disease should be part of the routine posttransplant treatment protocols.

Summary

Liver transplantation is a viable therapeutic option for patients with end-stage liver disease. Although graft and patient outcomes have improved considerably over the past 15 years, challenges continue to require our focus and ongoing research. As long as we have a shortage or donor livers, we will continue to struggle with identifying a fair and equitable way of allocating this scarce resource. Advances in outcomes related to the use of donor livers from extended criteria donors, donation after cardiac death donors, and living donors has helped, but the waiting list mortality remains a significant challenge. The liver allocation and distribution system in the United States will likely continue to evolve to try to meet the challenge of more patients needing a liver transplant.

As patient and graft survival has improved, our focus is shifting to address the challenges of the long-term survivor of liver transplantation. Management of renal insufficiency, recurrent liver disease, bone disease, coronary artery disease, malignancy, and infection continue to challenge us. Expansion in the pharmacopoeia available to clinicians managing liver transplant recipients allows for tailored, patient-specific drug cocktails, which will enhance our patient outcomes. Issues of quality of life after liver transplantation, functional status, and employment, school, financial, and emotional issues warrant continued and more focused attention.

Acknowledgment:
The author gratefully acknowledges the expert review of Sander Florman, MD.

References

1. Starzel TE, Demetris AJ, Van Thiel D. Liver Transplantation. N Engl J Med. 1989;329:1014–1092.
2. Ascher NL, Lake JR, Emond JC, et al. Liver transplantation for fulminant hepatic failure. *Arch Surg.* 1993;128:677-682.
3. Carithers RL Jr. Liver transplantation. American Association for the Study of Liver Diseases. *Liver Transpl.* 2000;6:122-135.
4. Starzl TE, Todo S, Fung J, et al. FK506 for human liver, kidney and pancreas transplantation. *Lancet.* 1989;2:1000-1004.
5. Starzel TE, Iwatsuki S, Van Thiel D, et al. Evolution of liver transplantation. *Hepatology.* 1982;2:614-636.
6. Starzl TE, Klintmalm GBG, Porter KA, et al. Liver transplantation with the use of cyclosporine A and prednisone. *N Engl J Med.* 1981;305:266-269.
7. Roberts MS, Angus DC, Bryce CL, Valenta Z, Weissfeld L. Survival after liver transplantation in the United States: a disease specific analysis of the UNOS database. *Liver Transpl.* 2004;7:886-897.
8. United Network for Organ Sharing. Available at: http://www.optn.org/latestData. Accessed February 5, 2006.
9. Markowitz JS, Martin P, Conrad AJ, et al. Prophylaxis against hepatitis B recurrence after liver transplantation using combination lamivudine and hepatitis B immune globulin. *Hepatology.* 1998;28:585-589.
10. Lim JK, Keefe EB. Liver transplantation for alcoholic liver disease: current concepts and length of sobriety. *Liver Transpl.* 2004;10(suppl 2):S31-S38.
11. Locke GR, Dickson ER. Transplantation for primary biliary cirrhosis. In: Busuttil RW, Klintmalm GB, eds. *Transplantation of the Liver.* Philadelphia, Pa: WB Saunders Company. 1996;101-107.
12. Crippin JS. Transplantation for scherosing cholangitis. In:, Busuttil RW, Klintmalm GB, eds. *Transplantation of the Liver.* Philadelphia, Pa: WB Saunders Company. 1996;108-112.
13. Burke A, Lucey MR. Non-alcoholic fatty liver disease, non-alcoholic steatohepatitis and orthotopic liver transplantation. *Am J Transplant.* 2004;4:686-693.
14. Heimbach JK, Haddock MG, Alberts SR, et al. Transplantation for hilar cholangiocarcinoma. *Liver Transpl.* 2004;10(10 suppl 2):S65-68.
15. Lerut JP, Orlando G, Sempoux C, et al. Hepatic haemangioendothelioma in adults: excellent outcome following liver transplantation. *Transpl Int.* 2004;17:202-207.
16. Florman S, Toure B, Kim L, et al. Liver transplantation for neuroendocrine tumors. *J Gastrointest Surg.* 2004;8:208-212.
17. Bernuau J, Rueff B, Benhamou J. Fulminant and sub-fulminant liver failure: definitions and causes. *Semin Liver Dis.* 1986;6:97-106.
18. United Network for Organ Sharing. Policy 3.6. Available at: http://www.unos.org. Accessed June 3, 2005.
19. Ostapowicz GA, Fontana RJ, Schiodt FV, et al. Results of prospective study of acute liver failure at 17 tertiary care centers in the United States. *Ann Intern Med.* 2002;137:947-954.
20. Wlliams R. Classification, etiology, and considerations of outcome in acute liver failure. *Semin Liver Dis.* 1996;16:343-348.
21. Bhaduri BR, Mieli-Vergani G. Fulminant hepatic failure: pediatric aspects. *Semin Liver Dis.* 1996;16:349-355.
22. Penn I. Hepatic transplantation for primary and metastatic cancers of the liver. *Surgery.* 1991;110:726-735.
23. Iwatsuki S, Gordon RD, Shaw BW Jr, Starzl TE. Role of liver transplantation in cancer therapy. *Ann Surg.* 1985;202:401-407.
24. Mazzaferro V, Rehalia E, Doci R, et al. Liver transplantation for the treatment of small hepatocellular carcinoma in patients with cirrhosis. *N Engl J Med.* 1996;334:693-699.
25. Yao FY, Ferrell L, Bass NM, et al. Liver transplantation for hepatocellular carcinoma: expansion of the tumor size limits does not adversely impact survival. *Hepatology.* 2001;33:1394-1403.
26. Leung JY, Zhu AX, Gordon FD, et al. Liver transplantation outcomes for early-stage hepatocellular carcinoma: results of a multicenter study. *Liver Transpl.* 2004;10:1343-1354.
27. Shetty K, Timmins K, Brensinger C, et al. Liver transplantation for hepatocellular carcinoma validation of present selection criteria in predicting outcome. *Liver Transpl.* 2004;10:911-918.
28. Wiesner RH. Current indications, contraindications, and timing for liver transplantation. In: Busuttil RW, Klintmalm GB, eds. *Transplantation of the Liver.* Philadelphia, Pa: WB Saunders Company. 1996;71-84.
29. Saab S, Ibrahim AB, Shapaner A, et al. MELD fails to measure quality of life in liver transplant candidates. *Liver Transpl.* 2005;2:218-223.
30. Kannel WB, McGee D, Gordon T. A general cardiovascular risk profile: the Framingham Study. *Am J Cardiol.* 1976;38:46-51.
31. Sharma P, Rakela J. Management of pre-liver transplantation patients – part 1. *Liver Transpl.* 2005;11:124-133.
32. Plotkin JS, Scott VL, Pinna A, Dobsch BP, De Wolf AM, Kang Y. Morbidity and mortality in patients with coronary artery disease undergoing orthotopic liver transplantation. *Liver Transpl Surg.* 1996;2:426-430.
33. Carey WD, Dumot JA, Pimentel RR, et al. The prevalence of coronary artery disease in liver transplant candidates over age 50. *Transplantation.* 1995;59:859-864.

34. Therapondos G, Flapan AD, Plevris JN, Hayes PC. Cardiac morbidity and mortality related to orthotopic liver transplantation. *Liver Transpl.* 2004;10:1441-1453.
35. Krowka MJ, Mandell MS, Ramsay MA, et al. Hepatopulmonary syndrome and portopulmonary hypertension: a report of the multicenter liver transplant database. *Liver Transpl.* 2004;10:174-182.
36. Carey EJ, Douglas DD, Balan V, et al. Hepatopulmonary syndrome after living donor liver transplantation and deceased donor liver transplantation: a single-center experience. *Liver Transpl.* 2004;10:529-533.
37. Krowka MJ, Plevak DJ, Rosen CB, Wiesner RH, Krom RA. Pulmonary hemodynamics and perrioperative cardiopulmonary-related mortality in patients with portopulmonary hypertension undergoing liver transplantation. *Liver Transpl.* 2000;6:443-450.
38. Rode A, Bancel B, Douek P, et al. Small nodule detection in cirrhotic livers: evaluation with US, spiral CT, and MRI and correlation with pathologic examination of explanted livers. *J Comput Assist Tomogr.* 2001;25:327-336.
39. Davis CL, Gonwa TA, Wilkinson AH. Identification of patients best suited for combined liver-kidney transplantation: part II. *Liver Transpl.* 2002;3:193-211.
40. Guevara M, Gines P. Hepatorenal syndrome. *Dig Dis.* 2005;23:47-55.
41. Cardenas A. Hepatorenal syndrome: a dreaded complication of end-stage liver disease. *Am J Gastroenterol.* 2005;100:460-467.
42. Pageaux GP, Bismuth M, Perney P. Alcohol relapse after liver transplantation for alcoholic liver disease: does it matter? *J Hepatol.* 2003;39:629-634.
43. Lucy MR, Carr K, Beresford TP, et al. Alcohol use after liver transplantation in alcoholics: a clinical cohort follow-up study. *Hepatology.* 1997;25:1223-1227.
44. Pageaux GP, Michel J, Costes V, et al. Alcohol cirrhosis is a good indication for liver transplantation, even for cases of recidivism. *Gut.* 1999;45:421-426.
45. Cuadrado A, Fabrega E, Casafont F, Pons-Romero F. Alcohol recidivism impairs long-term patient survival after orthotopic liver transplantation for alcoholic liver disease. *Liver Transpl.* 2005;4:420-426.
46. Summary of National Institute of Health Workshop on Liver Transplantation for Alcoholic Liver Disease. *Liver Transpl Surg.* 1997;3:197-347.
47. Arslan M, Wisner RH, Sievers C, Egan K, Zein NN. Double-dose accelerated hepatitis B vaccine in patients with end-stage liver disease. *Liver Transpl.* 2001;7:314-320.
48. Bica I, McGovern B, Dhar R, et al. Increasing mortality due to end stage liver disease in patients with human immunodeficiency virus infection. *Clin Infect Dis.* 2001;32:492-497.
49. Fung J, Eghtesad B, Patel-Tom K, DeVera M, Chapman H, Ragni M. Liver transplantation in patients with HIV infection. *Liver Transpl.* 2004;10(suppl 2):S39-53.
50. Moreno S, Fortun J, Quereda C, et al. Liver transplantation in HIV-infected recipients. *Liver Transpl.* 2005;11:76-81.
51. Roland ME, Stock PG. Review of solid-organ transplantation in HIV-infected patients. *Transplantation.* 2003;75:425-429.
52. Norris S, Taylor C, Muiesan P, et al. Outcomes of liver transplantation in HIV-infected individuals: the impact of HCV and HBV infection. *Liver Transpl.* 2004;10:1271-1278.
53. Gondolesi GE, Roayaie S, Munoz L, et al. Adult living donor liver transplantation for patients with hepatocellular carcinoma: extending UNOS priority criteria. *Ann Surg.* 2004;239:142-149.
54. Roayaie S, Llovet JM. Liver transplantation for hepatocellular carcinoma: is expansion of the criteria justified? *Clin Liver Dis.* 2005;9:315-328.
55. Keswani RN, Ahmed A, Keefe EB. Older age and liver transplantation: a review. *Liver Transpl.* 2004;10:957-967.
56. Collins BH, Pirsch JD, Beckker YT, et al. Long-term results of liver transplantation in older patients 60 years of age and older. *Transplantation.* 2000;70:780-783.
57. Lucey MR, Brown KA, Everson GT, et al. Minimal criteria for placement of adults on the liver transplant waiting list: a report of a national conference organized by the American Society of Transplant Physicians and the American Association for the Study of Liver Diseases. *Transplantation.* 1998;66:956-962.
58. United Network for Organ Sharing. Available at: http://www.unos.org. Policy 3.6 implemented January 19, 1998. Accessed February 6, 2006.
59. Wiesner RH. Evidenced- based evolution of the MELD/PELD liver allocation policy. *Liver Transpl.* 2005;3:261-263.
60. Merion RM, Schaubel DE, Dykstra DM, Freeman RB, Port FK, Wolfe RA. The survival benefit of liver transplantation. *Am J Transplan.t* 2005;5:203-204.
61. Wiesner RH, Edwards E, Freeman R, et al. The model for end-stage liver disease (MELD) and allocation of donor livers. *Gastroenterology.* 2003;124:91-96.
62. Heuman DM, Abou-Assi SG, Habib A, et al. Persistent ascites and low serum sodium identify patients with cirrhosis and low MELD scores who are at high risk for early death. *Hepatology.* 2004;40:802-810.
63. Olthoff KM, Brown RS Jr, Delmonico FL, et al. Summary report of a national conference: evolving concepts in liver allocation in the MELD and PELD era. *Liver Transpl.* 2004;10(10 suppl 2):A6-22.
64. Lu DS, Yu NC, Raman SS, et al. Percutaneous radiofrequency ablation of hepatocellular carcinoma as a bridge to liver transplantation. *Hepatology.* 2005;41:1130-1137.

65. Strader DB, Wright T, Thomas DL, Seeff LB. Diagnosis, management, and treatment of hepatitis C. *Hepatology*. 2004;39:1147-1171.
66. Villeneuve JP, Condreay LD, Williams B, et al. Lamivudine treatment for decompensated cirrhosis resulting from chronic hepatitis B. Hepatology. 2003;31:207-210.
67. Lok AS. Liver transplantation for patients with lamivudine-resistant HBV: what is the optimal prophylactic strategy? *Liver Transpl*. 2005;11:490-493.
68. Heathcote EJ,. Management of primary biliary cirrhosis. The American Association for the Study of Liver Disease practice guidelines. *Hepatology*. 2000;31:1005-1013.
69. Heimbach JK, Haddock MG, Alberts SR, et al. Transplantation for hilar cholangiocarcinoma. *Liver Transpl*. 2004;10(10 suppl 2):S65-68.
70. Stiehl A. Urosodeoxycholic acid therapy in treatment of primary sclerosing cholangitis. *Scand J Gastroenterol Suppl*. 1994;204:59-61.
71. Bataller R, Gines P, Guevara M, Arroyo V. Hepatorenal syndrome. *Semin Liver Dis*. 1997;17:233-247.
72. McCormick PA, O'Keefe C. Improving prognosis following a first variceal hemorrhage over four decades. *Gut*. 2001;49:682-685.
73. Broelsch CE, Emond JC, Thistlewaite JR, et al. Liver transplantation with reduced-size donor organs. *Transplantation*. 1988;45:519-524.
74. Kim JS, Broering DC, Tustas RY, et al. Split liver transplantation: past, present and future. *Pediatr Transplant*. 2004;8:644-648.
75. Busuttil RW, Goss JA. Split liver transplantation. *Ann Surg*. 1999;229:313-321.
76. Yersiz H, Renz JF, Farmer DC, Histake GM, McDiarmid SV, Busuttil RW. One hundred in situ split-liver transplantations: a single-center experience. *Ann Surg*. 2003;238:496-505.
77. Broelsch CE, Whitington PF, Emond JC, et al. Liver transplantation in children from living related donors. *Ann Surg*. 1992;214:428-439.
78. Marcos A, Ham JM, Fisher RA, et al. Single-center analysis of the first 40 adult-to-adult living donor liver transplants using the right lobe. *Liver Transpl*. 2000;6:296-301.
79. Miller CM, Gondolesi GE, Florman S, et al. One hundred nine living donor liver transplants in adults and children: a single center experience. *Ann Surg*. 2001;234:301-312.
80. Reddy S, Zilvetti M, Brockman J, McLaren A, Friend P. Liver transplantation from non-heart-beating donors: current status and future prospects. *Liver Transpl*. 2004;10:1223-1232.
81. Zhao Y, Lo CM, Liu CL, Fan ST. Use of elderly donors (>60 years) for liver transplantation. *Asian J Surg*. 2004;27:114-119.
82. Karatzas T, Olson L, Ciancio G, et al. Expanded liver donor age over 60 years for hepatic transplantation. *Transplant Proc*. 1997;29:2830-2831.
83. Vargas HE, Laskus T, Wand LF, et al. Outcome of liver transplantation in hepatitis C virus-infected patients who received hepatitis C virus-infected grafts. *Gastroenterology*. 1999;117:149-153.
84. Fan X, Lang DM, Xu Y, et al. Liver transplantation with hepatitis C virus-infected graft: interaction between donor and recipient viral strains. *Hepatology*. 2003;38:25-33.
85. Arenas JI, Vargas HE, Rakela J. The use of hepatitis C-infected grafts in liver transplantation. *Liver Transpl*. November 2003;9(suppl):S48-S51.
86. Saab S, Chang AJ, Comulada S, et al. Outcomes of hepatitis C- and hepatitis B core antibody-positive grafts in orthotopic liver transplantation. *Liver Transpl*. 2003;9:1053-1061.
87. Fabrega E, Garcia-Suarez C, Guerra A, et al. Liver transplantation with allografts from hepatitis B core antibody-positive donors: a new approach. *Liver Transpl*. 2003;9:916-920.
88. Burton JR Jr, Shaw-Stiffel TA. Use of hepatitis B core antibody-positive donors in recipients without evidence of hepatitis B infection: a survey of current practice in the United States. *Liver Transpl*. 2003;9:837-842.
89. Merion RM. Doc, Should I accept this offer or not? *Liver Transpl*. 2004;12:1476-1477.
90. Agnes S, Avolio AW, Magalini SC, Grieco G, Castagnero M. Marginal donors for patients on the regular waiting lists for liver transplantation. *Transpl Int*. 1996;9(suppl 1):S469-471.
91. Feng S, Bragg-Gresham JL, Dykstra DM, Punch JD, Greenstein SM, Merion RM. Definitions and outcomes of transplant using expanded criteria donor livers. *Hepatology*. 2004;38(suppl 1):S6.
92. Amin MG, Wolf MP, TenBrook JA Jr, et al. Expanded criteria donor grafts for deceased donor liver transplantation under the MELD system: a decision analysis. *Liver Transpl*. 2004;12:1468-1475.
93. O'Rourke M. Care of living liver donors. In: Couples SA, Ohler L, eds. *Transplantation Nursing Secrets*. Philadelphia, Pa: Hanley & Belfus. 2003;213-234.
94. Brown RS, Russo MW, Lai M, et al. A survey of liver transplantation from living donors in the United States. *N Engl J Med*. 2003;348:818-825.
95. Tojimbara T, Fuchinoue S, Nakajima I, et al. Factors affecting survival after living-related liver transplantation. *Transplant Int*. 2000;13:S136-S139.
96. Trotter JF. Selection of donors and recipients for living donor liver transplantation. *Liver Transpl*. 2000;6(suppl):S52-S58.

97. Schwartz ME, Miller CM. Critical graft size in adult-to-adult living donor liver transplantation: impact of the recipients disease. *Liver Transpl.* 2001;7:948-953.
98. Freeman RB. The impact of the model for end-stage liver disease on recipient selection for adult living liver donation. *Liver Transpl.* 2003;9:554-559.
99. Brown RS, Rush SH, Rosen HR, et al. Liver and intestinal transplantation. *Am J Transplant.* 2004;4(suppl 9):81-92.
100. Malus DG, Cotterell AH, Posner MP, et al. Adult living donor verses deceased donor liver transplantation: a six year single center experience [abstract]. *Am J Transplant.* 2004;4(suppl 8):532.
101. Seller-Perez G, Herrera-Gutierrez ME, Aragones-Manzanares R, Munoz-Lopez A, Lebron-Gallardo M, Gonzalez-Correa JA. Postoperative complications of liver transplantation: relationship with mortality. *Med Clin (Barc).* 2004;18:340-341.
102. Hasse J. Recovery after organ transplant in adults: the role of postoperative nutritional therapy. *Top Clin Nutr.* 1998;13:15-26.
103. Gallardo LM, Gutierrez ME, Perez SG, Curiel BE, Ortega F, Garcia QG. Risk factors for renal dysfunction in the postoperative course of liver transplant. *Liver Transpl.* 2004;11:1379-1385.
104. Jain A, McCauley J, Kshyap R, et al. Incidence of end stage renal failure amongst long-term survival of primary liver transplant recipients under tacrolimus: adults and children. *Transplantation.* 1998;65(suppl):S24.
105. Zheng SS, Yu ZY, Liang TB, et al. Prevention and treatment of hepatic artery thrombosis after liver transplantation. *Hepatobiliary Pancreat Dis Int.* 2004;3:21-25.
106. Quian YB, Lui CL, Lo CM, Fan ST. Risk factors for biliary complications after liver transplantation. *Arch Surg.* 2004;139:1101-1105.
107. Nakamura N, Nishida S, Neff GR, et al. Intrehepatic biliary strictures without hepatic artery thrombosis after liver transplantation: an analysis of 1,113 liver transplantations at a single center. *Transplantation.* 2005;79:427-432.
108. Wiesner RH, Demetris AJ, Belle SH, et al. Acute hepatic allograft rejection: incidence, risk factors, and impact on outcome. *Hepatology.* 1998;28:638-645.
109. Ghobrial RM, Rosen HR, Martin P. Long term issues in liver transplantation. In: Norman DJ, Turka LA, eds. *Primer of Transplantation.* American Society of Transplantation. 2001;581-590.
110. Charlton M. Hepatitis C infection in liver transplantation. *Am J Transplant.* 2001;1:197-203.
111. Berenguer M. Natural history of recurrent hepatitis C. *Liver Transpl.* 2002;8(suppl):S4-S18.
112. Charlton M, Ruppert K, Belle SH, et al. Long-term results and modeling to predict outcomes in recipients with HCV infection: results of the NIDDK liver transplantation database. *Liver Transpl.* 2004;10:1120-1130.
113. Charlton M. Natural history of hepatitis C and outcomes following liver transplantation. *Clin Liver Dis.* 2003;7:585-602.
114. Berenguer M, Ferrell L, Watson J, et al. HCV-related fibrosis progression following liver transplantation: increase in recent years. *J Hepatol.* 2000;32:637-684.
115. Berenguer M, Prieto M, San Juan F, et al. Contribution of donor age to the recent decrease in patient survival among HCV-infected liver transplant recipients. *Hepatology.* 2002;36:202-210.
116. Everson GT. Impact of immunosuppression therapy on the recurrence of hepatitis C. *Liver Transpl.* 2002;8(suppl 1):S19-S27.
117. Burak KW, Kremers WK, Batts KP, et al. Impact of cytomegalovirus infection, year of transplantation, and donor age on outcomes for liver transplantation for hepatitis C. *Liver Transpl.* 2002;8:362-369.
118. Shiffman ML, Stravitz RT, Contos MJ, et al. Histologic recurrence of chronic hepatitis C virus in patients after living donor and deceased donor liver transplantation. *Liver Transpl.* 2004;10:1248-1255.
119. Ghobrial RM. Retransplantation for recurrent hepatitis C. *Liver Transpl.* 2002;8(suppl):S38-S43.
120. Roayaie S, Schiano TD, Thung SN, et al. Results of retransplantation for recurrent hepatitis C. *Hepatology.* 2003;38:1428-1436.
121. Rosen HR. Retransplantation for hepatitis C: implications of different policies. *Liver Transpl.* 2000;6(suppl 2):S41-S46.
122. Abdelmalek MF, Firpi RJ, Soldevila-Pico C, et al. Sustained viral response to interferon and ribavirin in liver transplant recipients with recurrent hepatitis C. *Liver Transpl.* 2004;2:199-207.
123. Kim WR, Poterucha JJ, Kremers WK, Ishitani MB, Dickson ER. Outcome of liver transplantation for hepatitis B in the United States. *Liver Transpl.* 2004;8:968-974.
124. Marzano A, Gaia S, Ghisetti V, et al. Viral load at the time of liver transplantation and risk of hepatitis B virus recurrence. *Liver Transpl.* 2005;4:402-409.
125. Neff GW, O'Brien CB, Nery J, et al. Outcomes in liver transplant recipients with hepatitis B virus: resistance and recurrence patterns from a large transplant center over the last decade. *Liver Transpl.* 2004;11:1372-1378.
126. Roche B, Samuel D. Evolving strategies to prevent HBV recurrence. *Liver Transpl.* 2004;10(suppl 2):S74-S85.
127. Roayaie S, Schwartz JD, Sung MW, et al. Recurrence of hepatocellular carcinoma after liver transplant: patterns and prognosis. *Liver Transpl.* 2004;10:534-540.

Intestinal Transplantation

Laurel Williams, RN, MSN, CCTC
Deborah Andersen, RN, BSN, CCTC

Before 1970, patients who were unable to maintain nutrition through their gastrointestinal tract died of severe malnutrition, weight loss, or dehydration.[1] When total parenteral nutrition (TPN) was introduced, this therapy saved many lives and was the recommended treatment for patients with intestinal failure. However, although a lifesaving treatment for many patients, for others, TPN caused complications such as frequent catheter sepsis, cholestatic liver disease, and the loss of vascular access.[2] These complications resulted in death for many patients suffering from intestinal failure. Thus, the need to develop a lifesaving procedure such as intestinal transplantation remained urgent.

Almost 2 decades ago, intestinal transplant researchers wrote, "the small intestine is more complex than other organs that are transplanted because it is a bulky, highly immunocompetent organ that is colonized with micro-organisms and supported by relatively small main blood vessels," and concluded that the challenges to successful small bowel transplantation were more formidable than even Drs Lilllehei and Wangenstten considered in 1959.[3] Intestinal transplant pioneers remained diligent in their efforts, but until the early 1990s, long-term survival was rare.[4,5]

Throughout the past 15 years, numerous advancements have been made in patient and donor selection, surgical techniques, immunosuppressive regimens, graft surveillance protocols, and management of postoperative complications.[6,7] In 2000, the Center for Medicare and Medicaid Services approved intestinal, liver, intestinal and multivisceral transplantation as a standard of care for patients with irreversible intestinal failure and complications of TPN.[8] As of May 2003, The International Intestinal Transplant Registry reported 61 centers that performed intestinal transplantation worldwide.[9] These centers have provided data on 989 intestinal grafts in 923 patients. The 1-year patient survival rate was 81% at experienced transplant centers using induction immunosuppression; 61% of the patients were under 18 years of age, and there were more intestinal combined with liver transplantations performed overall. More than 80% of all the current survivors were able to stop TPN and resume normal daily activities; and, in 2003, the longest survivor had been alive more than 15 years after transplantation.[9]

Indications for Intestinal Transplantation

Intestinal transplantation has become the accepted treatment for patients with permanent intestinal failure and life-threatening complications of TPN. Intestinal failure has been described as the inability of the gastrointestinal tract to maintain nutrition, electrolytes, and fluid balance over an extended period.[10] Often, the causes of intestinal failure are divided into 2 major categories, structural and functional.[11,12]

Structural intestinal failure, often known as short-bowel syndrome (SBS), is the direct result of loss of a significant portion of the small intestine caused by surgical resection. This loss decreases the surface area of the small intestine and thus the ability of the small intestine to absorb adequate nutrition, fluid, and electrolytes.[13,14] In infants, structural intestinal failure is most often caused by surgical repair of congenital defects such as gastroschisis, intestinal atresia, or mid-gut volvulus. SBS may also be the result of massive resection for removal of necrotic bowel in infants who have necrotizing enterocolitis. In adults, trauma to the abdomen causing damage to the intestine or disruption of blood flow to the intestine may require substantial resection of the small intestine. Diseases such as Crohn's disease may necessitate removal of all or significant amounts of small intestine. Patients with desmoid tumors may have removal of the intestine and other visceral organs for treatment (Table 1).

Functional intestinal failure is caused by disorders of the small intestine that impair the motility or absorptive capacity of the small intestine. With functional intestinal failure, the entire bowel is present but unable to adequately perform the functions of digestion and absorption.[12] There may be loss of muscle or nerve function of the intestine as in intestinal pseudo-obstruction or there may be loss of nerve innervation to the muscle as is the case with Hirschsprung's disease or total intestinal aganglionosis. Other diseases such as microvillous inclusion disease or tufting enteropathy do not allow for absorption of adequate nutrition or fluids (Table 2).[6]

Not all patients with irreversible structural or functional intestinal failure require evaluation for intestinal transplantation. Many patients who receive TPN do not have life-threatening complications. In fact, only about 20% of patients receiving long-term TPN experience significant complications. Survival rates for patients dependent on TPN at 1 year are 90% and 86% at 4 years. These survival rates are still better than those published by the International Intestinal Transplant Registry in 2003. Therefore, patients who are doing well on TPN are not yet considered candidates for intestinal transplantation.[2]

Currently, to be considered for intestinal transplantation, patients must have irreversible intestinal failure and a life-threatening complication of TPN. These complications include liver disease, loss of venous access, repeated episodes of life-threatening catheter sepsis, and severe dehydration despite intravenous fluid replacement.[15] As survival rates continue to improve, other indications for intestinal transplantation may be related to the quality of life (QOL) of patients receiving daily TPN, as well as the costs that are associated with TPN and central catheter maintenance.

Many complex factors influence the development of TPN-associated liver disease, and not all of these factors are well understood. TPN-associated liver disease is more common in premature or low-birth-weight infants, which may be related to the immaturity of the neonatal liver. Prolonged enteral starvation decreases the release of bile and creates abnormal bile acid metabolism within the liver. Patients who are unable to tolerate even minimal amounts of enteral feedings are at much higher risk for developing liver disease because of this factor. Often, patients with short bowel syndrome or motility disorders have intestinal stasis, which may lead to bacterial overgrowth, bacterial translocation, and sepsis. The presence of a permanent indwelling central venous catheter may cause bacteremia and sepsis. Sepsis, in turn, is associated with progression of liver disease. Also, direct hepatotoxicity may be related to the components of TPN.[16,17] Elevation of bilirubin and any sequela of liver disease should prompt referral to a center that performs intestinal transplantation.

Thrombosis of central veins with loss of central venous access is associated with placement of multiple central venous catheters for long-term TPN. There are 6 central catheter sites most commonly used for infusion of TPN, including the 2 internal jugulars veins, 2 subclavian veins, and 2 femoral veins. Transhepatic and translumbar access may be considered in extreme cases. The use of sophisticated vascular procedures for placement of stents has made it possible for patients with superior vena cava syndrome to be considered for transplantation.[16] However, referral for intestinal transplantation should occur before exhausting all available catheter access sites. Referral for intestinal transplantation is appropriate when 2 of 6 available standard access sites are lost to thrombosis.[2] Central catheter access is important because patients must have adequate venous outflow to drain the transplanted intestine and have adequate central venous access to help them through the operative and perioperative period until they are weaned from TPN. Complete lack of venous access is considered a contraindication for transplantation.[6]

Central venous catheter sepsis presents considerable risks to the patient. Central venous catheter infections are thought to be related to the presence of an indwelling central catheter, translocation of enteral organisms, and the loss of gut-associated lymphoid tissue.[6] The evolution, frequency, and severity of central catheter infections seem random. Infections with various bacterial organisms are most common, and fungal infections are the most severe and life-threatening.[16] There is no consistent way to prevent central catheter infections, although meticulous attention to aseptic techniques and patient-centered training and support can improve outcomes and prolong the length of use of central catheters.[18] Central

Table 1. STRUCTURAL CAUSES OF INTESTINAL FAILURE

SYNDROME	DEFINITION	CLINICAL MANIFESTATIONS	DIAGNOSIS	PRIMARY TREATMENT
Gastroschisis	Herniation of variable lengths of intestine and sometimes liver without a peritoneal sac through an abdominal wall defect	Defects situated on the right of the umbilicus with evisceration of bowel or other organs	Prenatal ultrasonography Clinical presentation at birth	Staged operative repair of abdominal wall defect with replacement of intestine
Omphalocele	Herniation of abdominal viscera into the base of the umbilical cord	Abdominal contents enclosed within membranous sac outside the abdominal wall 75% present with other birth defects	Prenatal ultrasonography Clinical presentation at birth	Primary closure of abdominal wall defect
Mid-gut volvulus	Failure of the intestine to achieve normal anatomic position during embryonic development; may lead to twisting or obstruction of the intestine, causing vascular compromise resulting in necrosis of the intestine	Bilious vomiting Abdominal distention with tenderness Anorexia	Plain abdominal radiography Upper gastrointestinal series and small bowel follow through Barium enema	Surgical resection of necrotic bowel
Intestinal atresia	Absence or stenosis of portions of the duodenum, jejunum, or ileum	Jaundice Bilious vomiting Generalized abdominal distention Failure to pass meconium stool	Plain abdominal radiography Upper gastrointestinal series and small bowel follow through	Surgical resection of atretic or stenotic portion of the small intestine with restoration of intestinal continuity
Necrotizing enterocolitis	Ulceration and necrosis of gastrointestinal tract Associated with prematurity Associated with feeding intolerance Associated with vascular insufficiency Associated with colonization of the gut with gram-negative bacteria	Lethargy Bilious vomiting Abdominal distention Anorexia Fever Portal venous gas	Clinical presentation Plain abdominal radiography Metrizamide gastro-intestinal series Portal vein ultrasonography	Conservative medical management Broad-spectrum antibiotics Surgical resection if severe
Crohn's disease	Chronic transmural inflammation that may involve any part of the gastrointestinal tract Autoimmune disease of the gastrointestinal system	Mild cramps Postprandial pain Mucous and blood in stools Poor growth and weight loss before intestinal symptoms	Barium contrast studies: upper gastrointestinal series and barium enema Endoscopy Laparoscopy Laboratory studies	Drug therapy with antibiotics, corticosteroids, nonsteroidal anti-inflammatory drugs, immunosuppressive drugs Restricted oral intake Surgical resection
Trauma to the abdomen	Anything that causes massive trauma to the abdominal cavity	Gunshot wound, automobile accident, falls, blunt or sharp force trauma	Clinical presentation Plain abdominal radiography Computed tomography scan	Surgical resection
Superior mesenteric thrombosis (venous or arterial)	Blood clot in the blood vessel that leads to or drains the small intestine	Abdominal distention Fever Bowel obstruction	Plain abdominal radiography Venous angiogram Magnetic resonance imaging, venogram	Surgical resection of the ischemic small bowel
Desmoid tumors of the abdominal cavity	Benign fibrous neoplasm arising in skeletal muscle of the abdominal wall, may cause compromise of visceral organs		Computed tomography scan of abdomen Biopsy of tumor	Surgical removal of tumor, which may include abdominal visceral organs

(11, 28, 25)

Table 2. FUNCTIONAL CAUSES OF INTESTIAL FAILURE

SYNDROME	DEFINITION	CLINICAL MANIFESTATIONS	DIAGNOSIS	PRIMARY TREATMENT
Chronic intestinal pseudo-obstruction	Ineffective intestinal propulsion associated with myopathic or neuropathic disorder of the intestinal muscle wall	Bowel obstruction Abdominal distention Vomiting	Upper gastrointestinal and small bowel contrast series Enteroclysis Transmural intestinal muscle wall biopsy	Broad-spectrum antibiotics to treat bacterial overgrowth in dilated loops Dietary management, enteral feedings Surgical removal of portion of bowel that is not functioning
Hirschsprung's disease	Congenital absence of ganglion cells in submucosal and myenteric plexuses of distal intestine	Constipation Vomiting Abdominal distention Rectal impaction	Distention of colon on plain abdominal films Barium enema Anal manometry Transmural intestinal biopsy	Surgical removal of colon and bowel that is not functioning
Total aganglionosis	Congenital absence of ganglion cells in submucosal and myenteric plexuses of entire intestine	Constipation Vomiting Abdominal distention Rectal impaction	Distention of colon on plain abdominal films Barium enema Anal manometry Transmural intestinal biopsy	Surgical removal of colon and bowel that is not functioning
Microvillous inclusion disease	Rare autosomal recessive disorder in which there is a disorder of the brush border or microvilli of the intestinal lumen	Severe diarrhea resulting in dehydration	Biopsy of the small intestine with electron microscopy	Parenteral nutrition
Tufting enteropathy	Chronic mal-absorptive syndrome in which diarrhea is refractory to any treatment	Severe diarrhea resulting in dehydration	Biopsy of the small intestine, electron microscopy	Parenteral nutrition
Radiation enteritis	Radiation injury to intestine	Vomiting Diarrhea Strictures Fistulas Malabsorption and weight loss Abdominal pain Pelvic abscess	Upper gastrointestinal and small bowel contrast series Intestinal biopsy endoscopy Computed tomography	Nutritional support, low-fat diet, antispasmodic agents, sulfasalazine, Corticosteroids, cholestyramine, Ineffective intestinal

(Williams[11], Kosmach Park[28], Goulet[25])

catheter sepsis is an indication for referral for transplantation because of its life-threatening nature, impact on liver disease, and effect on sites for central venous access.

The inability of the intestine to absorb any enteral hydration leading to severe dehydration should be considered an indication for referral for intestinal transplantation. Patients with microvillous inclusion disease or tufting enteropathy, which is generally diagnosed shortly after birth, are at greater risk for developing significant liver disease due to the inability of the gut to tolerate even minute amounts of enteral feedings. Even in the absence of life-threatening complications of intestinal failure, these patients should be considered for intestinal transplantation early because of the rapid progression of their liver disease and decreased chance of survival.[6]

Patient Referral

The evaluation of the patient begins with the initial referral. A patient may be referred for evaluation for intestinal transplantation by self, family members, physicians, or third-party payors. Detailed information is taken at the time of the initial referral to assist the clinical transplant coordinator in assessing the appropriateness of the referral for evaluation for intestinal transplantation.[19] After release of medical information is obtained, more detailed reports are requested from multiple sources, including operative, radiology, and laboratory reports; current enteral and parenteral nutrition formulas; medications; history and physical examinations; discharge summaries; and any liver or intestinal biopsy slides (Table 3). All reports are thoroughly reviewed with the physician to determine if evaluation for intestinal transplantation is appropriate and/or if there is any additional information that may be needed during the evaluation.

Insurance information is also obtained during this initial patient referral. Although most third-party payors including Medicaid and Medicare acknowledge intestinal transplantation as an acceptable treatment for patients with intestinal failure, insurance coverage for the intestinal transplant evaluation must be verified and precertified before the time of evaluation. This is done by a dedicated financial coordinator who is familiar with the insurance contracts developed by the institution and previous encounters with insurance carriers. The financial coordinator also assists the family in understanding their insurance policies and resources for travel and lodging benefits.[20]

Evaluation for Intestinal Transplantation

The main goals of the intestinal transplant evaluation are to confirm the cause and the extent of intestinal failure, determine the potential for intestinal adaptation with medical and/or surgical intervention, identify any other organ system dysfunction, determine which type of transplantation is to be performed, and educate and provide support to the patient and family considering intestinal transplantation. The gastroenterologist and transplant surgeon confirm the cause and extent of intestinal failure through history and physical examination, radiologic procedures, nutritional history, and assessment and review of histology.

The extent of intestinal failure and the potential for intestinal adaption is based on the amount and segment of bowel remaining, the function of the remaining bowel, the presence of the ileocecal valve, the continuity of the intestine with the colon, and the amount of colon remaining.[21,22] The segment of bowel remaining is important because of the differences in the digestive and absorptive qualities of each segment of intestine.[17]

The intestine has 3 segments. The first segment is the duodenum, which is approximately 25 cm long in adults and connects to the stomach at the pylorus and continues to the duodenojejunal flexure. The main function of the duodenum is to carry food from the stomach, bile from the liver and pancreatic enzymes from the pancreas to the jejunum. Some digestion but little absorption takes place in the duodenum. The second section of the intestine is the jejunum. The jejunum begins at the duodenojejunal flexure. There are no landmarks where the jejunum ends and the ileum begins, but their appearance is different. The diameter of the jejunal wall is greater and it is thicker and more muscular than the ileum. The major function of the jejunum is digestion, which is the breaking down of foods in preparation for absorption. The jejunum makes up two fifths of the remaining intestine after the duodenum. The ileum extends from the jejunum to the ileocecal valve; it makes up the remainder of the intestine. It is smaller in diameter and less muscular than the jejunum, and provides for the majority of absorption of the nutrients that are a result of the breakdown of carbohydrates, proteins, and fats. The ileum has a much greater ability to adapt and can increase its absorptive capacity more efficiently than the jejunum. The ileocecal valve is the valve between the ileum of the intestine and the cecum or first section of the colon. The ileocecal valve is responsible for slowing down and stopping the passage of digested nutrients. The colon provides for absorption of water and electrolytes and helps maintain hydration. It cannot do this if an ileostomy or jejunostomy has been created as a result of bowel resection. The more colon remaining, the better the ability of the colon to reabsorb water and minerals. The length of the entire bowel in adults is

Table 3. INITIAL REFERRAL FOR INTESTINAL TRANSPLANTATION

Current date _____ Person taking referral _____ Date of Evaluation _____
Diagnosis _____
Name _____ Age _____ Date of birth _____
Parent's name _____ Social security number _____
Emergency contact: _____ Medical registration number _____
Address _____
City _____ State _____ Zip Code _____ Local hospital _____
Home phone _____ Phone number _____
Work phone _____ City and state _____
Cell phone _____ Contact person _____
E-mail address _____ Social worker _____

Referring physician _____ other physician _____
Address _____ Address _____
City and state _____ City and state _____
Phone number _____ Phone number _____
Fax number _____ Fax number _____
E-mail address _____ E-mail address _____
Contact person _____ Contact person _____

Insurance carrier: _____ Policy number _____
Phone number _____ Group number _____
Contact person _____ Person insured _____

Allergies: _____
Medical _____
_____
_____

Surgical history _____
_____
_____

Central venous catheter history _____
_____

Cultures _____
_____

Nutritional information
TPN rate _____ # of hours _____
Enteral feeding _____ rate _____ # of hours _____
Oral intake _____

Current medications:
_____   _____
_____   _____
_____   _____
_____   _____

Home infusion company _____ Nursing care company _____
Phone number _____ Phone number _____
Contact person _____ Contact person _____

Consent to release medical records _____ Requested medical records _____
Requested surgical records _____ Requested radiology CD _____
Requested liver biopsy slides _____ Requested intestinal biopsy slides or EMs _____
Lodging request: _____
Crib _____ # of persons _____
Flying _____ Driving _____
Arrival _____ Arrival _____
Airline _____
Flight number _____
Need volunteer _____
Send educational packet _____

approximately 600 cm and in children is roughly half that size, although the length of bowel varies greatly from one person to another.[23]

Several variables have been recognized to predict intestinal failure in patients with massive resection of the intestine. Both Wilmore[24] and Goulet et al,[25] in studies in children, found that full enteral nutrition was possible in children with greater than 40 cm of intestine without an ileocecal valve and greater than 15 cm of intestine with an ileocecal valve. Pharaon et al[21] and Vargas et al,[22] in studies in children, associated failure of enteral feedings with less than 30 cm of jejunum and ileum, lack of enterocolonic continuity, and lack of feeding tolerance after birth. Messing and colleagues,[26] in a larger study in adults, found that permanent intestinal failure was related to jejunal remnant length of less than 100 cm, end jejunostomy, and the absence of terminal ileum.

According to Abu-Elmagd and Bond,[15] Irreversibility of intestinal failure should be declared only after all optimal medical and surgical interventions have been utilized in an attempt to adapt the bowel and remove TPN. "Intestinal adaptation is the progressive recovery from intestinal insufficiency that follows a loss of intestinal length." Intestinal adaption may occur for up to 2 years following intestinal resection.[27] Manipulations in formula, treatment of bacterial overgrowth, and slow increase in enteral feedings have been used in selected patients to decrease or discontinue TPN.[7,15] In addition, surgical interventions such as tapering and lengthening; serial transverse enteroplasty (S.T.E.P.); repair of obstructions, dysmotility, and enteroenteric fistulas; and other surgical procedures may be helpful in achievement of enteral autonomy.[1] A few established intestinal transplant programs also have intestinal rehabilitation programs that are accessible to patients who are evaluated for transplantation. Comprehensive medical and surgical intestinal rehabilitation programs are challenging the previously held beliefs regarding permanent intestinal failure by providing medical and surgical interventions that allow for adaption and weaning of TPN.[1] Patients may be referred to these programs if there is any hope that bowel adaptation might be possible.

Evaluation for intestinal transplantation requires a dedicated team of care providers who specialize in intestinal transplantation. This team should include the gastroenterologist, transplant surgeon, transplant coordinator, psychologist, psychiatrist, social worker, financial coordinator, dietician, child-life specialist, staff nurse, occupational therapist, physical therapist, and developmental specialist. Each member of the team has a role in obtaining medical and social information and providing necessary education and support to the patient and his or her family. The evaluation process for intestinal transplantation is generally conducted over a 3- to 5-day period. This can be done on an inpatient or outpatient basis depending on the patient's medical condition.[17,28] The laboratory tests needed for transplantation are listed in Table 4. For small children or infants, laboratory tests may be ordered over several days to prevent extensive blood loss from laboratory work being drawn in one day. Radiology tests needed for transplantation are listed in Table 5.

Other procedures that may be done during the evaluation include endoscopies and biopsies. An upper and lower endoscopy with biopsy may be indicated to determine presence of bacterial overgrowth, identify strictures, assess length of bowel and mucosal integrity, and diagnose certain motility disorders. A liver biopsy may be done to determine the presence or extent of liver disease.[17]

Evaluating the function of other organ systems is necessary in determining potential problems that could occur after transplantation or that might provide a contraindication to transplantation. Consultations from other specialists are indicated for patients with any history of neurological, renal, pulmonary, cardiac, or immunologic disorders. Contraindications for intestinal transplantation are similar to those for other organ transplantations. The patient must have the potential ability to derive such benefit from the procedure that it would significantly improve the QOL (Table 6).[29] Tests and consultations may vary depending on medical symptoms and institutional protocols.

The organs to be transplanted are determined at the time of evaluation. For patients with irreversible intestinal failure and no liver disease or reversible liver disease, intestinal transplantation alone may be considered. For patients with irreversible intestinal failure, who also have irreversible liver failure, liver and intestinal transplantation is warranted. This type of transplantation may also be referred to as a multivisceral or composite graft. Most often, the composite graft includes the small intestine, liver, and the head of the pancreas. In some centers, multivisceral transplantation refers to transplantation of the

Table 4. LABORATORY TESTING FOR EVALUATION FOR INTESTINAL TRANSPLANTATION

Complete blood count with differential and platelet count	Detect presence of anemia and infection May indicate liver dysfunction portal hypertension and splenomegaly
Prothrombin time and internormal ratio:	Prolongation of the prothrombin time indicates the presence of liver disease Required for listing for liver transplantation
Type and cross-match:	Blood typing required by United Network for Organ Sharing (UNOS) x 2 for UNOS listing May require blood transfusion during evaluation
Cultures: blood, urine, stool	May be done if there is any concern of current infection
Liver function tests Total and direct bilirubin Alanine aminotransferase Asparate aminotransferase γ–glutamyl transpeptidase Alkaline phosphatase Total protein Albumin	May indicate the presence of liver disease. Total bilirubin is required for listing for liver transplantation Albumin is required for listing for liver transplantation
Nutritional evaluation Electrolytes: sodium, potassium, chloride, bicarbonate, glucose Calcium, magnesium, phosphorous Vitamin levels: vitamin A and E, vitamin D 25 OH Carnitine, zinc, selenium, copper Cholesterol and triglycerides D-xylose Fecal fat collection Creatinine and serum, urea nitrogen	Evaluate fluid status and general state of nutrition, determine appropriate parenteral nutrition formulas. D-xylose and feccal fat collection help evaluate gastrointestinal absorption Evaluate renal function and hydration status. Creatinine is required for listing for liver transplantation
Viral studies Human immunodeficiency virus Hepatitis B surface antibody Hepatitis B surface antigen Hepatitis B core antibody Hepatitis C antibody Cytomegalovirus DNA by PCR Cytomegalovirus IGG and IGM Epstein-Barr virus DNA by PCR Epstein-Barr virus antibodies Herpes zoster antibody Measles mumps rubella antibody	Determines the presence of current infection or past infection. Presence of HIV may be contraindication to transplantation. Positive HBsAb may indicate presence of past infection or vaccination Positive test for cytomegalovirus and Epstein-Barr virus help determine donor status, prophylaxis, or treatment plan following transplantation Positive measles mumps rubella antibody determines presence of immunity
Miscellaneous testing A-fetoprotein (AFP)	Elevation of AFP may indicate presence of malignancy (hepatocellular carcinoma) Quantitative immunoglobulins Test is indicated for patients with intestinal atresias. Intestinal atresia has been associated with immunodeficiency

Laboratory tests may vary from center to center.
DNA by PCR: deoxyribonucleic acid by Polymerase chain reaction
IGG: immunoglobulin G IGM; Immunoglobulin M

stomach, the pancreas, and/or the colon in addition to the liver and small intestine.[15,30] For those rare patients with irreversible liver disease in which intestinal adaptation has been accomplished and TPN can be weaned, liver transplantation has been shown to be an appropriate therapy option.[31]

Providing education and support to the patient and his or her family considering intestinal transplantation is an important goal of the intestinal transplant evaluation. Educational material may be provided in different formats, including written material, video tapes, group sessions, and one-on-one

Table 5. RADIOLOGY TESTS REQUIRED FOR INTESTINAL TRANSPLANT EVALUATION

Chest radiograph	Determine underlying pulmonary status
Barium enema	Determine length of colon, may also demonstrate presence of dilation or stricture in colon
Upper gastrointestinal and small bowel series	Determine length of small intestine, may demonstrate gastric reflux, may provide information on the motility of intestine and the presence of dilation or stricture
Echocardiogram	Determine any cardiac abnormalities
Abdominal ultrasound	Used to assess liver size, presence and flow of blood vessels, presence of splenomegaly, portal hypertension, ascites, and portal vein thrombosis
Doppler scan for vascular access	Provides information on blood vessel anatomy and indicates occlusions of blood vessels that are necessary for vascular access
Bone age scan (pediatrics)	Determines any delay in bone growth
Mammogram (adult women)	May reveal presence of malignancy

Table 6. CONSULTATIONS REQUIRED FOR EVALUATION FOR INTESTINAL TRANSPLANTATION

Clinical transplant coordinator	Provides written and oral information on the transplant process, acts as liaison between patient and other members of the transplant team and hospital
Nutritionist	Provides assessment and recommendations regarding current nutritional status, obtains diet and feeding history
Gastroenterologist	Obtains history and physical, determines medical plan of care, discusses the short-term and long-term risks and benefits of transplantation
Transplant surgeon	Obtains history and physical, discusses the short-term and long-term risks and benefits of transplantation, explains the operative procedure, determines if the patient is a surgical candidate
Psychologist	Provides developmental assessment for children, determines patient and family physical and emotional resources for transplantation
Psychiatrist	Provides assessment and recommendations for patients who are noncompliant or who are dealing with addiction or psychiatric problems
Social work	Assesses family and patient support system, provides information to the family regarding transportation, pagers and support services at the time transplantation and during recovery in area
Business office liaison	Provides information to patient and family on current insurance reimbursement and out-of-pocket expenses during transplantation and recovery in area
Child life specialist	For pediatric patients – becomes acquainted with the patient, provides coping strategies for the patient
Child development	Determines level of development and feeding issues for children
Nephrology (as indicated)	consulted any patient with history of congenital renal complications or elevation of creatinine and Blood, Urea, Nitrogen (BUN)
Cardiology (as indicated)	Consulted for any patient abnormality on echocardiogram or electroencephalogram, consulted for patients with history of cardiac complications or diabetes
Neurology (as indicated)	Consulted for children with history of ventricular bleeding secondary to prematurity or history of seizure disorder or history of other neurological complication
Pulmonology (as indicated)	Consulted for any patient with history of prolonged ventilator dependence, reactive airway disease, or bronchopulmonary dysplasia
Immunology (as indicated)	For any patient with history of immune deficiencies such as intestinal atresia
Infectious disease (as indicated)	For any patient with history of persistent organisms, tuberculosis, Cryptococcus, etc.

meetings. One-on-one time with the clinical transplant coordinator allows for individualized education on the entire transplant process and for answering specific patient and family questions. It is imperative that the family understands the risks while waiting for a transplant, the length of the recovery period, the numerous possible postoperative complications, and the necessary long-term follow-up.[17] People suffering from intestinal failure have endured multiple hospitalizations, been in life-threatening circumstances, and are often quite ill. Providing support services such as social work, psychology, or psychiatry, and developing a rapport with patients and family through trust and open communication will help patients and families through the long waiting and recovery process.[32]

After the evaluation is completed, all cases are reviewed at a multidisciplinary conference. Team members who have seen the patient and family provide their assessments. A team consensus is reached and the team decision is relayed to the patient and/or family. Results of the evaluation along with the team's recommendations are sent to the referring physician and to the third-party payors.

Listing for Intestinal Transplantation and Waiting Times

Information needed to test patients for intestinal transplantation includes blood type, body size, and medical necessity. Most patients requiring intestinal transplantation have loss of peritoneal domain; therefore, they may require transplantation with a graft from a donor who is only 50% to 60% of their weight.[33] Patients are listed for intestinal transplant by 1 of 2 medical status. Status 1 is a patient who has abnormal liver function tests and/or limited vascular access sites or other medical indications that warrant urgent transplantation such as repeated episodes of uncontrollable fluid and electrolyte imbalance. Status 2 is for all patients awaiting intestinal transplantation who do not meet the criteria for status 1. Patients may be made a status 7 after listing if they are considered temporarily unsuitable for transplantation. For example, a patient listed for intestinal transplantation who has a fever or culture-positive central catheter infection would be made a staus of until the fever and infection have resolved. Then the patient would resume his or her previous status.

Patients who are listed for combined liver and intestinal transplantation are listed on both the liver and intestinal transplant waiting lists. Adults are listed according to their MELD score and pediatric patients are listed according to their PELD score. **(See chapter on liver transplantation.)** In November 2004, a new policy was developed by the United Network for Organ Sharing (UNOS), which took into consideration the increased risk of dying while waiting for a combined liver and intestinal transplantation. UNOS policy 3.6.4.7 states that patients awaiting a combined liver-intestine transplant who are registered on both waiting lists will automatically receive an additional increase in their MELD/PELD score equivalent to a 10% risk of 3-month mortality rates.

According to the most recent data published from the Organ Procurement and Transplantation Network (OPTN), there were 199 patients listed for intestinal transplantation with or without liver transplantation as of May 2005. One hundred and five of these patients were in the pediatric age group. In 2002, OPTN documented median waiting times of 82 days for adults over age 50 and 438 days as age decreases for infants of 1 year or younger. Both adults and children with blood type O waited longer for transplantation than did patients with other blood types. There were 1518 patients listed for intestinal transplantation between January 1995 and February 2005. Of these, 453 (29%) were removed from the transplant waiting list because they were medically unsuitable for transplantation, too sick to undergo transplantation, or died.[34]

The transplant center must remain in frequent contact with the patient, family, and local physician during the waiting period. Obtaining frequent laboratory results for rescoring and recertifying PELD and MELD scores and updating current height and weights are vital for providing the best possible opportunity for organ transplantation. Patients who have been listed for isolated intestinal transplantation may develop further liver disease. A liver biopsy should be done when progressing liver disease is suspected so that the patient can then be listed for a composite graft, if necessary.[17]

Donor Selection

According to Jan and Renz,[33] the "intestines are exquisitely sensitive to ischemia from hypotension, sepsis, or vasopressors. Intestinal ischemia exacerbates ischemia/reperfusion injury that can lead to allograft dysfunction, impaired mucosal defense, and enhanced bacterial translocation... therefore, donor selection for intestinal transplantation has been limited to optimal candidates". Size matching is an important criterion in donor selection. Because of the loss of abdominal domain found in the majority of patients awaiting intestinal transplantation, the donor size may be smaller than the recipient.

Recipient Operations

Transplantation of an isolated intestinal graft is usually a more straightforward procedure than the composite grafts, which require extensive dissection and removal of major organs.[16] However, many of these patients have had multiple previous abdominal operations for intestinal resections, lengthening, tapering, or treatment of surgical complication or infections.[8,12] Previous operations and subsequent adhesions combined with problems of portal hypertension, splenomegaly, and coagulopathy can create significant surgical challenges.[12,35] There are reports of graft reduction of both liver and intestine to facilitate abdominal wound closure.[12,35] Also, reports have been made of abdominal wall transplantation to achieve skin closure when the organs were significantly larger than the abdominal cavity.[36]

All intestinal transplantations begin with a midline or subcostal incision. The failed organs are removed. The vascular anatomy for arterializations and venous drainage are identified, as is the proximal small bowel remnant, and finally the allograft, the entire small bowel from the ligament of Trietz to the ileal valve, is implanted. A loop ileostomy is created for endoscopic surveillance of graft function (Table 7 and Figures 1, 2, and 3).

There has been long-standing debate about the benefits of intestinal transplantation compared with composite grafts.[38] There are a greater number of isolated intestinal grafts for transplantation. Patients in need

Table 7. SURGICAL INTESTINAL TRANSPLANTATION

Isolated Intestinal Transplantation
- Midline or transverse incision
- Removal of diseased/nonfunctioning intestine
- Anastomosis of donor superior mesenteric artery (SMA) to recipient aorta
- Anastomosis of donor superior mesenteric vein (SMV) to recipient portal vein (PV), SMV, splenic vein (SV), or inferior vena cava (IVC)
- Establish intestinal continuity with native proximal and distal bowel
- Loop or end ileoscopy for endoscopic surveillance

Liver/Intestinal Transplantation
- Midline or subcostal incision
- Removal of liver and diseased/nonfunctioning intestine
- En bloc implantation of liver, intestine, duodenum, and head of pancreas
- Hepatic veins to IVC or retrohepatic vena cava replacement
- Arterial conduit of donor thoracic aorta divided distal to SMA
- Proximal donor aorta anastomosed end to side with recipient aorta (supraceliac or infrarenal)
- Establish proximal and distal bowel continuity
- Loop ileostomy for endoscopic surveillance

Multivisceral Transplantation
- The procedure for multivisceral transplantation is the same as for liver/intestinal transplantation with the addition of the stomach, colon, and/or the entire pancreas

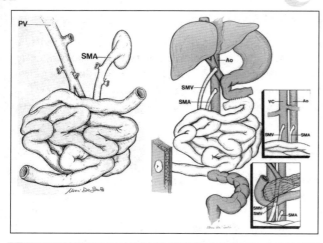

Figure 1. Isolated intestinal transplantation. Published with permission.[37]

of an isolated intestinal transplant are often less sick at the time of the operation compared with patients requiring composite grafts. If an isolated intestinal graft fails, the patient has the ability to return to TPN. However, patients undergoing isolated intestinal transplantation seem to experience more graft loss from acute and chronic rejection than do patients with combined liver-intestinal transplantation, from presumed immunologic protection by the liver. The literature also shows that the 1-year survival rate is better with isolated intestinal transplantation, but the long-term survival rate is better with combined liver-intestinal transplantation. The indication for multivisceral transplantation is rare and most often used with benign tumors such as desmoid tumors that have extensive intra-abdominal involvement.

Living Donor Intestinal Transplantation

Currently, the experience with living intestinal donation is small and somewhat controversial. As the numbers of living donors increase and outcomes are documented for both donors and recipients, there will be more agreement within the transplant community about the use of living donors for intestinal transplantation.

The International Transplant Registry has data on 989 intestinal transplantations, 957 from deceased donors and 32 from living donors.[39] No significant differences in patient or graft survival rates are noted in these 2 groups. However, because of the small numbers of living donor transplantations, there is no in-depth analysis of this cohort of patients in regards to graft function, rejection, HLA matching or cross-matching, donor/recipient age, or length of intestinal grafts.[40] Reports of case studies and small series of living intestinal transplantation do exist in the literature.[41-43]

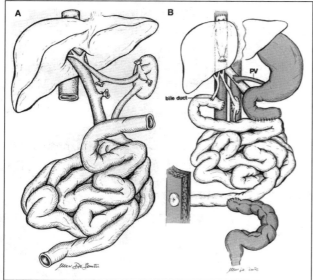

Figure 2. Liver-intestine enbloc graft before (A) and after (B) implantation. Published with permission.

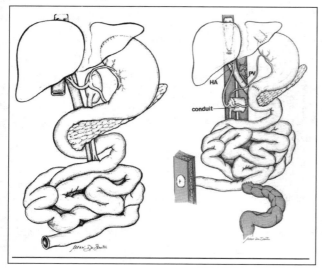

Figure 3. Multivisceral transplantation involves enbloc transplantation at the stomach, pancreas, liver, and intestine. Published with permission.

A CLINICIAN'S GUIDE TO DONATION AND TRANSPLANTATION

Selection of Living Donors

Donor selection involves providing comprehensive information to the donor regarding the evaluation, operation, and inherent risks, as well as other treatment options for the recipient. These risks may include some of the following:

Medical – Change in bowel habits (acute/chronic diarrhea); dehydration/electrolyte imbalance; and alterations in diet, vitamin deficiencies, pain, and discomfort; intestinal failure due to lack of adequate intestine; and donor death

Financial – Lack of coverage for complications/medication, loss of wages, inability to obtain additional health and/or life insurance (preexisting condition)

Psychological – Inadequate graft length, graft loss or death of recipient, ongoing medical issues for the donor, time away from family, pain, depression and anxiety[40]

Donors and recipients are matched by blood type and size. ABO-compatible combinations may be considered but may lead to greater potential for graft versus host disease in the recipient.[40] Segmental grafts are used from living donors and there may be a weight discrepancy of 5:1 between the donor and the recipient. Segmental graft lengths have been reported to be between 100 cm to 200 cm depending on the size of the recipient.[36,44,45]

The donor must be in good mental and physical health, with no health issues or contraindications to surgery or anesthesia. The medical workup may include blood values plus serologies, chest radiology, electrocardiogram, MRA of the mesenteric vessels, liver biopsy, endoscopy, and angiography if indicated. A physician who is not a member of the transplant team should be involved to determine medical suitability and act as a patient advocate while avoiding any conflict of interest. Adequate time should be allowed for the patient to give informed consent.[44]

The debates about the use of live intestinal donation have to do with the inherent need for living donation in this patient population. Few patients die awaiting isolated intestinal transplantation, so the risk to a healthy donor and possibly to the recipient may not be necessary.[40,43]

Segmental grafts from living donors may be significantly shorter than grafts from deceased donors, increasing the possibility of malabsorption and prolonged use of TPN in the recipient. There is also greater potential for the recipient to have vascular problems because of the small vascular anastomosis that may lead to thrombosis and graft loss.

The benefits to the donor are altruistic. The benefits to the recipient include the fact that they will not get sicker while waiting for transplantation. If the intestine is transplanted before the need for a composite graft, more patients will have access to liver transplantation. There may be some benefits in shorter cold ischemia times and HLA matching. Shorter cold ischemia times and HLA matching has been shown to improve graft survival in other organs. More studies will be needed to see the effects with intestinal transplantation.[40]

Other issues to consider include the cost/benefit ratio of long-term use of TPN versus intestinal transplantation. With survival rates improving for intestinal transplant recipients, QOL issues may factor into the decision to proceed with transplantation. As more people are placed on the list for intestinal transplantation, the accompanying donor organ availability issues may also come into play.

Surgical Complications

Reyes and Abu-Elmagd[12] note that 47% of recipients experience some type of surgical complication, including biliary and intestinal anastomotic leaks, intestinal perforations, abscesses, and intraabdominal infection. These types of complications may present with signs and symptoms of infection such as fever, elevated white blood cell counts, and abdominal distension with tenderness, and usually require surgical intervention. Vascular compromise to the intestine due to arterial or venous thrombosis/stenosis requires revascularization or partial resection of the damaged intestine. Any change in the color of the stoma or prolapse that does not easily reduce also requires prompt surgical intervention.[12]

Immediate Postoperative Care

The management of patients undergoing intestinal transplantation is challenging and requires meticulous attention to detail.[29,46] The massive lymphocyte content and bacterial load within the intestine intensifies postoperative problems of infection and rejection. The function of the transplanted bowel affects fluid and electrolyte balance and nutritional status. Surgical complications such as bowel perforations and intra-abdominal abscess are not uncommon. The patient's premorbid condition also tends to necessitate intensive rehabilitative support to return the patient to a functional status. The postoperative care therefore revolves around the prevention of rejection, avoidance of infection (management of immunosuppressant), maintenance of fluid and nutrition (graft function), and long-term rehabilitation.[46]

Rejection

Rejection is a common complication following intestinal transplantation. The use of induction therapy has helped to lower the rate of rejection,[12,29] and new combinations of maintenance immunosuppressive medications may also help to reduce the incidence of rejection.[47] Currently, there are no laboratory tests that indicate rejection. Rejection is diagnosed through routine endoscopic small bowel mucosal biopsies. Transplant centers have different surveillance biopsy protocols. In general, biopsies are done more

Table 8. NURSING CONSIDERATIONS – INTESTINAL TRANSPLANTATION

Rejection
  Administration of immunosuppressive medications
  Observe for signs and symptoms of rejection
    High stomal outputs (>50 mL/kg)
    Blood or tissue is stomal output
    Significant decrease in stoma outputs
    Decreased or absent bowel sounds
    Fever
    Abdominal pain
    Distention
  Preparation/education for endoscopic biopsy
  Radiologic monitoring of gastric emptying and intestinal transit time
Infection
  Monitor for signs and symptoms of infection
    Fever
    Rash
    Diarrhea
    Hemodynamic instability
  Meticulous catheter care
  Meticulous wound and skin care
  Change in size of lymph nodes
  Cultures obtained as ordered
  Administration of anti-infective agents as ordered
  Prophylaxis per center protocol
    Pneumocystis
    Cytomegalovirus, Epstein-Barr virus
    Fungal infections
Fluid and electrolyte balance
  Strict measurement of intake and output
  Daily weights
  Frequent biochemical monitoring and subsequent adjustment of fluids and replacement electrolytes
  Close monitoring of immunosuppression and antibiotic levels
	Nutrition
	  Strict intake and outputs
	  Calorie counts and nutritional consults
	  Oral stimulation/occupational therapy Consult
	  Enteral and parenteral nutrition as ordered
	  Long-term care
	  Vaccinations – center specific
	  Biochemical monitoring
	  Nutritional management including vitamin supplementation
	  Reverse ileostomy (3-12 months depending on center and disease process)
	  Monitor growth in pediatric patients
	  Monitor for infection and rejection
	    Persistent fever
	    Sudden change in ostomy output
	    Sudden change in color of stoma
	    Stomal prolapse
	    Blood in stomal output
	    Inability to tolerate feedings
	    Inability to maintain nutritional status
	    New onset snoring
	    Lymphadenopathy
	    Persistent headaches
	  Patient unwell without obvious cause

Table 9. REASONS FOR GRAFT REMOVAL

Reason	% of pediatric patients (n=93)	% of adult patients (n=67)	% of total no. of patients (N=160)
Rejection	62.4	47.8	56.3
Thrombosis, ischemia, bleeding	15.1	28.4	20.6
Sepsis	6.5	11.9	8.8
Lymphoma	2.2	0	1.2
Other	14.0	11.9	13.1

35

Table 10. CAUSES OF DEATH

Lymphoma	27	Respiratory causes	29
Rejection	49	Cardiac	14
Sepsis	202	Cerebral	15
Multisystem organ failure	11	Thrombosis/ischemia/bleeding	14
Other	27	Hepatitis C	2
Renal failure	5	Liver failure	10
Technical	27	Pancreatitis	3
		Total	439

Intestinal Transplant Registry, May 31, 2003.

frequently in the early postoperative course and diminish with time and are performed as indicated by clinical status.[5,6,48]

Rejection may be patchy in distribution. Acute rejection is usually characterized histologically by a combination of crypt injury, mononuclear mucosal infiltrates, and an increase in cell apoptosis.[49,50] Chronic rejection is less well understood and harder to diagnose. It is associated with obliterative arteriopathy and loss of mucosal integrity.[50,51] Some clinical signs of graft rejection that may trigger an intestinal biopsy are changes in stool quality or quantity, blood in the stoma output, abdominal distension, pain or cramping, fever, or stoma changes. Rejection is usually treated with intravenous steroid boluses, higher maintenance levels of tacrolimus, and/or addition of a secondary immunosuppressive medication or antibody therapy (Table 8).[12] Refractory rejection may require enterectomy (graft removal). Other reasons for graft removal are presented in Table 9.

Performing retransplantation when graft loss has already occurred has been met with high rates of failure. Retransplantation should be considered in selected, stable patients who have preferably not taken immunosuppressant medications for some time.[29,52]

Infection

The most common cause of death in intestinal transplant recipients is sepsis and multiorgan system failure (Table 10).[16,48] Higher incidence of infectious complications in intestinal transplant recipients correlates with an increased need for immunosuppression as compared to recipients of other organ transplants.[28,53] An infection considered routine in a person with a normal immune system may become rapidly fatal in an intestinal transplant recipient and requires prompt identification and therapy. Although any type of infection may be seen at any time after transplantation, bacterial infections are most frequently seen in the first month. These infections include wound infections, pneumonia, and central catheter infections. Bacterial or viral enteritis and acute rejection may be related as one can lead to the other and clinical manifestations are similar.[54] Increases in immunosuppression may precipitate opportunistic infections.[52] To prevent infections, some transplant programs use intestinal decontamination protocols in both donors and recipients. Broad-spectrum antibiotics may also be used for the first 5 to 7 days.[38]

Viral infections are more commonly seen after the first month after post-intestinal transplantation. Cytomegalovirus virus (CMV) and Epstein-Barr virus (EBV) are 2 types of the herpes virus that may range in severity from asymptomatic to life-threatening illness. Both donors and recipients are screened for CMV and EBV. Ideally, CMV-negative recipients receive CMV-negative donor organs. The incidence of CMV infections has been reported to be between 16% and 40%. CMV prophylaxis is widely practiced, with protocols varying among transplant centers.[6,29]

EBV is associated with mononucleosis in the general public. In immunocompromised patients, EBV is associated with posttransplant lymphoproliferative disorder (PTLD). PTLD ranges in severity from a benign polyclonal lesion to a malignant monoclonal lymphoma.[52] Historically, the incidence of PTLD in bowel transplantation has been higher than in recipients of other solid-organ transplants because of the necessary higher levels of immunosuppressant medications. High-dose acyclovir and cytomegalovirus immune globulin in the immediate postoperative period has been used to decrease the incidence of EBV and other viral infections in intestinal transplant recipients.[29]

Adenovirus in intestinal transplant recipients is manifested in mild forms as diarrhea. It can progress to more invasive forms such as life-threatening pneumonias, enterocolitis, and septicemia.[6,48] Treatment of milder forms of adenovirus consists of bowel rest with TPN and fluid replacement, plus symptomatic support.[55] With more invasive disease, the use of intravenous cidofovir and immunoglobulins and lowering of immunosuppression has been reported to improve survival. Opportunistic infections such as Cryptosporidium and Microsporidium can cause diarrhea in intestinal transplant recipients. Treatment consists of lowering immunosuppression and military antimicrobial agents. Significant morbidity has also been seen with respiratory syncytial virus, influenza, Norwalk virus, and rotavirus.[12,56]

Fungal infections such as *Candida* and aspergillus may occur at any time after transplantation.[28] Fungal translocation across the intestinal mucosa may be a source of endogenous contamination with *Candida albicans*. Colonization of *Candida* may be found in endotracheal tubes, gastric and nasogastric feeding tubes, urinary catheters, and central catheters (Table 8).[48,57]

Fluid Balance

Fluid shifts are not uncommon in the first few postoperative days because of surgical stress. Fluid status is affected by the use of colloids, high-dose steroids, and nephrotoxic drugs such as Prograf (tacrolimus) and antibiotics. Fluid shifts between the graft, lungs, and peripheral tissue may result in overall fluid retention while leaving the patient intravascularly depleted. Intense hemodynamic monitoring is necessary, as is meticulous measurement of fluid losses, including losses from abdominal drains and nasogastric, stoma, and urine output. IV or enteral replacement fluids may be required for a period of time to maintain fluid balance.[48] Frequent monitoring of serum electrolytes, proteins, and minerals helps ensure appropriate use of replacement fluids (Table 8).[46]

Nutrition

Once the patient is hemodynamically stable, usually within the first 24 to 48 hours, TPN is restarted for nutrition. TPN is gradually tapered off as caloric intake is advanced through enteric routes. Calculated caloric goals are based on endotracheal intubation, postoperative complications, pretransplant nutritional status, rejection, and renal function.[2,48]

Continuous enteral feedings are started once bowel sounds and ostomy output are present, normally within the first 4 to 5 days.[2,46,58] Enteral feedings are started at a low rate and are slowly advanced on the basis of patient tolerance and stoma outputs (<40-50 mL/kg). Intestinal adaptation is a slow process. Changes in enteral and oral intake reflect this slow process. Malabsorption of fat is a common posttransplant problem because of the disruption of the lymphatic channel to the intestine during surgery.[59] Fat-free or low-fat, low osmolar, elemental formulas are given in the early postoperative course,[28,48,60] and patients may start with diluted concentrations of formula. The volume of the feedings may be increased before increasing the concentration to maintain a low osmolar balance. Some centers have reported acceptable stool outputs with high or medium chain triglyceride peptide-based formulas. Excessive stomal outputs (>50 mL/kg) may respond to dietary fiber or antidiarrheal medications that decrease intestinal transit time. Before the first year after transplantation, patients may transition to a whole-protein, cows milk formula, and after a year has passed after transplantation, patients may transition to a fiber-containing, whole-protein formula. Concentrated sweets and dairy products may be limited as patients are susceptible to osmotic and secretory diarrhea. In adults, oral diets start with clear liquids and are advanced as tolerated by the patient.[58]

Rejection and intercurrent infection may contribute to problems with diarrhea. Pancreatic insufficiency and chylous ascites have been reported after intestinal transplantation and appear to respond to supplemental pancreatic enzymes, temporary return to full TPN, and/or use of a nonfat enteral formulas.[60] Fat-soluble vitamins and minerals must be monitored once patients are removed from TPN as they may be wasted in stoma output.[28]

Oral aversion is seen frequently in children who have never eaten by mouth or had oral stimulation before transplantation. Overcoming these aversions is a long and tedious process and requires a multidisciplinary team approach, including psychological support to the child and parents (Table 8).[12,46]

Long-Term Management

Survival rates are improving for intestinal transplant recipients (Table 11). However, patients continue to have complex and life-threatening problems even 10 years after transplantation. Therefore, they should have close follow-up and rapid access back to the transplant center if needed. A retrospective study by Andersen et al[61], showed that patients continue to need hospitalization for infection, gastrointestinal complications (diarrhea without rejection, stoma prolapsed, colitis, constipation), dehydration, rejection, pulmonary, renal and hematology/oncology problems (most commonly PTLD), and other surgical procedures (bowel obstruction, lyses of adhesions, fistula repair, ileostomy stoma take down). The length of stay decreases over time; however, the number of admissions remained between 2 and 4 each year.[61]

The majority of intestinal transplant recipients are not dependent on TPN. Some children require supplemental enteral feedings because of inadequate intake and/or oral aversions. Linear growth in children is maintained; however, there is often no "catch up" growth. QOL studies are limited in number and somewhat subjective. In adult studies, QOL has been reported similar to the QOL in patients who are TPN dependent and stable, and better than those waiting for intestinal transplantation.[62] In studies in children, QOL assessment is quite different depending on who is responding: the child or parent. Children have reported QOL scores essentially the same as normal children. The parents in the same study reported lower scores for their children in physical functioning and impact on the family.[63] The literature on QOL after intestinal transplantation will be enhanced as more transplantations are performed and better long-term graft function is achieved (Table 8).

Future

We have seen many advances in the field of intestinal transplantation over the past 20 years. It is clear that the clinical successes and applications of intestinal transplantation will continue to evolve with expected improvements in patient and graft survival and QOL. Early referral for isolated intestinal transplantation may decrease the need for composite organ replacement and save substantial cadaveric donor livers for patients with liver failure. Ongoing research includes looking at serum or tissue markers to better diagnosis rejection.[64] Centers are also looking at the mechanism and sequelae of injury to the gut from reperfusion, cold ischemia, and denervation of the intestine and disruption of the lymphatic channel to further improve patient care. With time, there should be improvement in both patient and graft survival and cost-effectiveness.[64] With improved patient survival and an increased number of intestinal transplantations, we will not only have better patient management strategies but also better interventions to help families adjust to the inherent changes after transplantation. The future is promising; however, much remains to be answered through ongoing research, the persistence and creativity of the healthcare professions, and the determination and commitment of patients and their families to this endeavor.

Acknowledgements:
Thank you to Tina Rackley for secretarial support and Dr. Windy Grant for editorial assistance.

Figure 4.

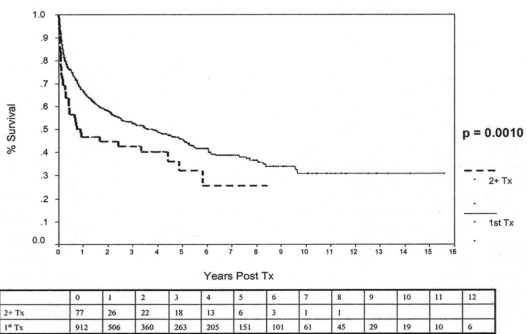

Intestinal Transplant Registry, May 31, 2003

References

1. Sudan D, Dibase J, Torres C, et al. A multi-disciplinary approach to the treatment of intestinal failure. *J Gastrointest Surg.* 2005;9:165-176.
2. Iyer K, Iverson A, DeVoll-Zabrocki A, Buckman S, Horslen S, Langnas A. Pediatric intestinal transplantation: review of current practice. *Nutr Clin Pract.* 2002;17:350-360.
3. Schwartz M. Small intestine transplantation. In: MW Fley, ed. *Principles of Organ Transplantation.* Philadelphia, Pa: W.B. Saunders Co; 1989;500-515.
4. Horslen S, Sudan D. Long term outcomes in small bowel transplantation: survival, nutrition, growth and quality of life. *Curr Opin Organ Transplant.* 2004;8:202-208.
5. Abu-Elmagd K, Reyes J, Bond G, et al. Clinical intestinal transplant: a decade of experience at a single center. *Ann Surg.* 2001;24:404-417.
6. Mittal K, Tzakis A, Kato T, Thompson J. Current status of intestinal transplantation in children: update 2003. *Pediatr Clin North Am.* 2003;50:1419-1433.
7. Caicedo J, Iyer K. Recipient selection for intestinal transplantation. *Curr Opin Organ Transplant.* 2005;10:116-119.
8. Abu-Elmagd K, Bond G, Reyes G, Fung J. Intestinal transplantation: a coming of age. *Adv Surg.* 2002;36:65-101.
9. Grant D, Abu-Elmagd K, Reyes J, et al. 2003 report of the intestinal transplant registry: a new era has dawned. *Ann Surg.* 2005;241:607-613 (Figure 4).
10. Reyes J. Intestinal transplantation for children with short bowel syndrome. *Semin Pediatr Surg.* 2001;10:99-104.
11. Williams L, Horslen S, Langnas A. Intestinal transplantation. In: Linda Ohler, ed. *Solid Organ Transplantation.* Springer Publishing Company, Inc. 2002 New York, NY
12. Reyes J, Abu-Elmagd K. Small bowel and liver transplantation in children. In: Kelly D, ed. *Diseases of the Liver and Hepatobiliary System.* London, England: Blackwell Science; 1998:313-331.
13. Vanderhoof J, Langnas A, Pinch L, Thompson J, Kaufman S. Short bowel syndrome. *J Pediatr Gastroenterol.* 1992;14:359-370.
14. Wease G. Short bowel syndrome: an overview. *Contemp Surg.* March-April 1995;2:16-19.
15. Abu-Elmagd K, Bond G. Gut failure and abdominal visceral transplantation. *Proc Nutr Soc.* 2003;62:727-737.
16. Reyes J, Mazariegos G, Bond G, et al. Pediatric intestinal transplantation: historical notes, principles, and controversies. *Pediatr Transplant.* 2002;6:193-207.
17. Andersen D, DeVoll-Zabrocki A, Brown C, Iverson A, Larsen J. Intestinal transplantation in pediatric patients: a nursing challenge. Part one: evaluation for intestinal transplantation. *Gastroenterol Nurs.* 2000;23(1):3-9.
18. Forbes A. Achieving and maintaining venous access for home parenteral nutrition. *Curr Opin Clin Nutr Metabol Care.* 2005;8:285-289.
19. Robinson J, Spencer R. Intestinal transplantation: the evaluation process. *Prog Transplant.* 2005;15:45-53.
20. Chaney M. Financial considerations insurance and coverage issues in intestinal transplantation. *Prog Transplant.* 2005;14:312-320.
21. Pharon I, Depres C, Aigrain Y, et al. Long-term parenteral nutrition in children who are potentially candidates for small bowel transplantation. *Transplant Proc.* 1994;26:1442.
22. Vargas JH, Ament ME, Berquist WE. Long-term parenteral nutrition in pediatrics: ten years of experience in 102 patients. *J Pediatr Gastroenterol Nutr.* January-February 1987;6:24-32.
23. Hole J. Human anatomy and physiology. In: *The Digestive System.* Dubuque, Iowa: William C. Brown, Publisher; 1987.
24. Wilmore DW. Factors correlating with a successful outcome following extensive intestinal resection in newborn infants. *J Pediatr.* January 1972;80:88-95.
25. Goulet O, Ruemmele F, Lacaille F. Irreversible intestinal failure. *J Pediatr Gastroenterol Nutr.* 2004;38:250-269.
26. Messing B, Crenn P, Beau P, et al. Long-term survival and parenteral nutrition dependence in adult patients with short bowel syndrome. *Gastroenterology.* 1999;117:1043-1050.
27. Torres C. Intestinal failure: is it permanent? *Curr Opinion Organ Transplant.* 2005;10:132-136.
28. Kosmach Park B. Intestinal transplantation in pediatric patients. *Prog Transplant.* 2002;12:97-113.
29. Grant W, Langnas A. Pediatric small bowel transplantation: techniques and outcomes. *Curr Opin Organ Transplant.* 2002;7:202-207.
30. Florman S, Kaufman S, Fishbein T. Decision making in intestinal transplantation. *Prog Transplant.* 2005;15:65-68.
31. Horslen S, Kaufman S, Sudan D, Fox I, Shaw B, Langnas A. Isolated liver transplantation in infants with total parenteral nutrition associated end-stage liver disease [abstract]. *Transplantation.* 1999;76:S589.
32. Samela K, Fennelly E, Brosnan M, et al. Interdisciplinary approach to the management of intestinal transplant recipients: evaluation, discharge and lifetime management. *Prog Transplant.* 2005;15:54-59.
33. Jan D, Renz J. Donor selection and procurement of multivisceral and isolated intestinal allografts. *Curr Opin Organ Transplant.* 2005;10:137.
34. Organ Procurement and Transplantation Network. New technology allows electronic sharing of recipient information and OPTN policies. Available at: http://www.OPTN.org. Accessed May 13, 2005.

35. Pirenne J. Advances in intestinal transplantation. Report from VII International Small Bowel Transplant Symposium. Medscape Transplantation. Available at: http://www.medscape/medscape/transplnataion/journal/2002/vol03.no1/myt0114.pire/mt01114pre-01.ntml. May 2005
36. Levi DM, Tzakis AG, Kato T, et al. Transplantation of the abdominal wall. *Lancet*. 2003;361:2173-2176.
37. Kato T, Tzakis A, Selvaggi G, et al. Surgical techniques used in intestinal transplantation. *Curr Opin Organ Transplant*. 2004;9:207-213.
38. Sudan DL, Kaufman SS, Shaw BW Jr, et al. Isolated intestinal transplantation for intestinal failure. *Am J Gastroenterol*. 2000;95:1506-1515.
39. Intestinal Transplant Registry. Available at: http://www.IntestinalTranpslantRegistry.org. Accessed May 2003.
40. Fryer JP, Angelos P. Is there a role for living donor intestine transplant? *Prog Transplant*. 2004;14:321-328.
41. Jaffe BM, Beck R, Flint L, et al. Living-related small bowel transplantation in adults: a report of two patients. *Transplant Proc*. 2000;32:1238.
42. Cicalase l, Baum C, Brown M, et al. Early living related segmental intestinal transplantation for trauma-induced ultra-short gut syndrome. *Transplant Proc*. 2002;34:914.
43. Abecassis M, Adams M, Adams P, et al. Consensus statement on the live organ donor. *JAMA*. 2002;284:2919-2926.
44. Bueno J, Abu-Elmagd K, Mazariegos G, Madariaga J, Fung J, Reyes J. Composite liver-small bowel allografts with preservation of donor duodenum and hepatic biliary system in children. *J Pediatr Surg*. 2000;69:555-559.
45. DeVille de Goyet J, Mitchell A, Mayer AD, et al. En bloc combined reduced liver and small bowel transplants: from large donors to small children. *Transplantation*. 2000;69:555-559.
46. Reyes J, Bueno J, Kocoshis S, et al. Current status of intestinal transplantation in children. *J Pediatr Surg*. 1998;33:243-254.
47. Sudan DL, Chinnakotla S, Horslen S, et al. Basiliximab decreased the incidence of acute rejection after intestinal transplantation (abstract). Presented at: The 2nd International Congress in Immunosuppression. December 2001; San Diego, Calif.
48. Andersen D, DeVoll-Zabrocki A, Brown C, Iverson A, Larsen J. Intestinal transplantation in pediatric patients: a nursing challenge. Part 2: intestinal transplantation in the immediate post operative period. *Gastroenterol Nurs*. 2000;23:201-205.
49. Garau P, Orenstein S, Neigut D, et al. Role of endoscopy following small intestinal transplantation in children. *Transplant Proc*. 1994;26:136-137.
50. Lee R, Tsamandas A, Abu-Elmagd K, et al. Histologic spectrum of acute cellular rejection in human intestinal allografts. *Transplant Proc*. 1996;28:2767.
51. Iyer KR, Srinath C, Horslen S, et al. Late graft loss and long-term outcomes after isolated intestinal transplantation in children. *Pediatr Surg*. 2002;37:151-154.
52. Langnas AN, Iyer K. Liver/Small bowel Transplantation. In: *Transplantation of the Liver*. 3rd ed. Philadelphia, Pa: Lippincott Williams and Wilkins; 1999. Willis Madrey, Eugene Schiff, Michael F. Sorrell editors
53. Sia I, Paya C. Infection complications following renal transplantation. *Surg Clin North Am*. 1998;78:95-112.
54. Damotte D. Pathology of intestinal transplantation. *Curr Opin Organ Transplant*. 1999;4:355-360.
55. McLaughlin GE, Delis S, Kashmawo L, et al. Adenovirus infection in pediatric liver and intestinal transplant recipients: utility of DNA detection by PCR. *Am J Transplant*. 2003;3:224-228.
56. Delis SG, Tector J, Kaito T, et al. Diagnosis and treatment of cryptosporidium infection in intestinal transplant recipients. *Transplant Proc*. 2002;34:951-952.
57. Paya C. Fungal infection in solid organ transplantation. *Clin Infect Dis*. 1993;16:677-688.
58. Strohm S, Koehler AN, Mazariegos GV, Reyes J. Nutrition management in pediatric small bowel transplantation. *Nutr Clin Pract*. 1999;14:58-63.
59. Funovits M, Altieri KA, Kovalak JA, Staschak-Chico S. Small intestine transplantation: a nursing perspective. *Crit Care Nurs Clin North Am*. 1993;5:203-213.
60. Silver H, Hastellanos V. Nutritional complications and management of intestinal transplantation. *Am Dietary Assoc*. 2002;680-689. Vol 100
61. Andersen D, Horslen S. An analysis of the long-term complications of intestinal transplant recipients. *Prog Transplant*. 2004;14:277-282.
62. Cameron E, Binnie J, Jamison N, et al Quality of life in adult patients following small bowel transplantation. *Transplant Proc*. 2002;34:965-966.
63. Sudan D, Iyer K, Horslen S, et al. Assessment of quality of life after pediatric intestinal transplantation by parents and pediatric recipients using the Child Health Questionnaire. *Transplant Proc*. 2002;34:963-964.
64. Sudan D. Small bowel transplantation: current status and new developments in allograft monitoring. *Curr Opin Organ Transplant*. 2005;10:124-127.

Islet Cell Transplantation

Barbara DiMercurio, RN, BS

Introduction

The morbidity and mortality associated with diabetes are well described, and healthcare costs incurred in caring for individuals with diabetes are growing rapidly each year. The Diabetes Control and Complications Trial (DCCT) Research Group have demonstrated that intensive therapy can reduce the long-term complications of type 1 diabetes.[1,2] Islet cell transplantation has the potential to restore normal islet cell function and maintain production of insulin, which could significantly improve the prognosis for metabolic control of diabetes and reduce long-term complications.

Islet cell transplantation has been investigated for more than a decade as a treatment for type 1 diabetes in patients with inadequate glucose control despite intensive insulin management. Early results reported by the International Islet Transplant Registry between 1990 and 1998 were quite discouraging; of 267 transplanted allografts, only 12.4% have resulted in insulin independence for periods of more than 1 week, and only 8.2% for periods of more than 1 year.[3] In the majority of these studies, the immunosuppression regimen consisted of an antibody induction, cyclosporine, azathioprine, and glucocorticoids. Researchers at the University of Alberta in Edmonton, Canada, reported a dramatic improvement in successful islet cell transplantation in 7 consecutive patients in July 2000. Their procedure has contributed to improvements in the islet isolation technique, the use of multiple pancreata to increase the total islet mass transplanted, and use of a glucocorticoid-free immunosuppressive protocol.[4]

Indications for Islet Cell Transplantation

- Type 1 diabetes > 5 years
- Brittle diabetes, as defined by one of the following:
  - Hypoglycemia unawareness, that is, the absence of adequate autonomic symptoms at plasma glucose levels of <54 mg/dL
  - Two or more episodes of severe hypoglycemia, defined as requiring the assistance of another person
  - Progressive secondary complications despite intensive insulin management, that is, retinopathy, neuropathy, and nephropathy

Contraindications to Transplantation

- Significant cardiac disease
- Active alcohol or substance abuse, including cigarette smoking
- Active infection, including hepatitis C, hepatitis B, human immunodeficiency virus, or tuberculosis (or under treatment for suspected tuberculosis)
- History of nonadherence to medical regimens
- Psychiatric disorder making the participant unsuitable for transplantation

- Inability to provide informed consent for an experimental study
- History of active malignancy
- Evidence of residual islet cell function, demonstrated by a positive C-peptide response (c-peptide >0.3 ng/mL)
- Age older than 65 years
- Creatinine clearance less than 70 mL/min/1.73 m^2
- Liver disease or structural liver abnormalities
- Pregnancy or breastfeeding
- Insulin requirement greater than 0.7 iU/kg/day
- Obesity, as defined by median body mass index greater than 28 kg/m^2
- Use of coumadin or other anticoagulant therapy (except aspirin) or prothrombin time-international normalized ratio greater than 1.5
- Medical treatment for a condition requiring chronic use of steroids

Evaluation Process

Islet cell transplantation, as described in this chapter, remains experimental. Thus, islet cell transplantation is not approved as an insurance reimbursable procedure in the United States. It is recommended that each center create and conduct a telephone or survey screening tool to decrease the overall cost of screen failures. Most institutions receive their funding by some form of government, institutional, industry, or private research funding. An example of screening tools can be found in Table 1. Table 2 outlines common tests performed during a candidate evaluation for islet cell transplantation.

Once the evaluation process has been completed and the patient is determined to be a good candidate for islet cell transplantation, the patient is listed with the local organ procurement organization (OPO) and with the United Network for Organ Sharing according to blood type. Only a few OPOs have begun registering islet cell transplant candidates. Table 3 outlines OPOs, regions, and number of candidates registered for an islet cell transplant as of November 11, 2005.

Table 1. COMMON SCREENING ELIGIBILITY QUESTIONS FOR ISLET CELL TRANSPLANTATION

Each institution should create questions to determine the following before conducting a full evaluation:

- Body mass index
- History of renal dysfunction
- History of cardiac disease
- Pregnancy or breastfeeding
- Insulin resistance
- History of malignancy
- Medication history

Table 2. COMMON TESTS PERFORMED DURING THE EVALUATION PROCESS FOR ISLET CELL TRANSPLANTATION

Comprehensive physical and medical examinations

Medical consultations
- Endocrinology
- Psychology*
- Social work*
- Dental

Laboratory screening tests
- Complete blood cell count with differential and platelet count
- Prothrombin time, partial thromboplastin time
- Stimulated C-peptide, hemoglobin A1C
- Lipid panel: total cholesterol, high-density lipoprotein cholesterol, low-density lipoprotein cholesterol, and triglycerides
- Chemistry panel: electrolytes, serum urea nitrogen, total bilirubin, creatinine, magnesium, phosphorus, and calcium
- Liver function tests: aspartate transaminase, alanine aminotransferase, total protein, total bilirubin, albumin, and alkaline phosphatase
- Urine tests: creatinine clearance corrected for body surface area, microalbumin, 24-hour protein, microalbumin/creatinine ratio, urinalysis, beta-human chorionic gonadotrophin (serum beta-human chorionic gonadotrophin test may substitute)

Infectious disease screening tests
- Human immunodeficiency virus
- Hepatitis C virus
- Hepatitis B virus
- Cytomegalovirus
- Epstein-Barr virus
- Varicella titer

Immunological screening tests
- Blood type and antibody screen
- Panel reactive antibody
- Human leukocyte antigen typing

Diagnostic tests
- Abdominal ultrasound to verify portal vein patency and to rule out gallstones and hemangioma
- Chest radiograph
- Electrocardiogram

ISLET CELL TRANSPLANTATION

Table 3. REGIONS, ORGAN PROCUREMENT ORGANIZATIONS, AND NUMBER OF REGISTERED ISLET CELL TRANSPLANT CANDIDATES

Region	Organ procurement organization	Number of islet cell registrations
5	California Transplant Donor Network	3
5	OneLegacy	10
8	Donor Alliance	2
2	Washington Regional Transplant Consortium	23
3	Life Alliance Organ Recovery Agency	27
3	LifeLink of Georgia	3
7	Gift of Hope Organ & Tissue Donor Network	90
10	Indiana Organ Procurement Organization	29
1	New England Organ Bank	21
7	LifeSource Upper Midwest Organ Procurement Organization	11
11	Lifeshare of the Carolinas	3
2	New Jersey Organ and Tissue Sharing Network	1
9	New York Organ Donor Network	9
10	LifeCenter Organ Donor Network	17
2	Gift of Life Donor Program	33
11	Mid-South Transplant Foundation	11
4	LifeGift Organ Donation Center	6
4	Southwest Transplant Alliance	7
11	LifeNet	3
6	LifeCenter Northwest Donor Network	7
7	Organ Procurement Organization at the University of Wisconsin	2
	Total	318

Data from the Organ Procurement and Transplantation Network, as of November 11, 2005.

Risks and Potential Benefits of Islet Cell Transplantation

As global experience has increased, the risks and potential benefits of islet cell transplantation are better defined. Table 4 outlines procedural risks of islet cell transplantation.

Risks

- Long-term immunosuppression
- Transplantation of allogeneic tissue
- Infection
- Death

Benefits

- Insulin independence
- Improvements to glycemic control (demonstrates partial graft function)
- Prevention of further secondary diabetic complications
- Improvements in quality of life

Table 4. PROCEDURAL RISKS OF ISLET CELL TRANSPLANTATION

Potential risk	Preventive measures	Treatment options
Liver hemorrhage Intra-abdominal bleeding	Sealing portal tract • Gelfoam • Collagen/thrombin paste (Floseal, D-stat) • Endovascular coils	Blood products (whole blood, packed red blood cells, fresh frozen plasma, platelets) Laparoscopy/Surgical intervention
Portal hypertension Portal vein thrombosis	Infuse only highly purified islet preparations Infuse >10 mL of packed tissue volume Coadministration of heparin with islet cells Administration of low-molecular-weight heparin (subcutaneous enoxaparin sodium [Lovenox] 30 mg twice a day, for 7 days) after transplantation Doppler ultrasound 7 days after transplantation	If portal hypertension is suspected during infusion of islet cells, suspend infusion until resolved If portal vein thrombosis is suspected during the islet cell infusion, the infusion is aborted If portal vein thrombosis is detected after transplantation, anticoagulation or surgical removal of the clot may be required

- Diminished hypoglycemia unawareness
- Lower surgical complications than whole pancreas transplantation

Islet Cell Transplantation Procedure

Isolated human islets of Langerhans may be administered fresh (immediately after the isolation) or placed in culture for 24 to 72 hours before administration. Once the preliminary islet yield is determined to be sufficient and of good quality (center specific), the patient is brought to the hospital. When the final islet yield is determined to be acceptable and all product release criteria have been met, the patient is prepared for the procedure. Before being sent to interventional radiology to begin the procedure, the patient receives daclizumab, tacrolimus, sirolimus, and prophylactic antibiotics. Table 5 outlines recommended product release testing.

Table 5. PRODUCT RELEASE TESTING

Product release test	Criteria
Islet enumeration	≥ 5000 IE/kg recipient body weight
Purity	≥ 30%
Viability	≥ 70%
Packed cell volume	≤ 10 mL
Endotoxin	≤ 5 EU/kg
Microbiological assessment	
Gram stain	
Aerobic culture*	
Anaerobic culture*	
Fungal culture*	
Mycoplasma*	Negative
Potency stimulation index (insulin secretion) *	≥ 1.0

*Final results reported after islet cell transplantation when cells are administered fresh.

Portal Vein Access

1. Access to the portal vein is achieved by either percutaneous transhepatic access under fluoroscopic, ultrasonographic, or real-time computed tomography guidance or by transjugular intrahepatic portosystemic shunt (TIPS). The most common approach for this procedure is the percutaneous transhepatic approach.
2. Before the portal vein is accessed, conscious sedation may be required for patient comfort.
3. Using the percutaneous approach, a 3- to 6-French catheter (center specific) is used to gain access to the main portal vein under fluoroscopic guidance. The larger sizes of catheters may increase the risk for bleeding.
4. The portal pressure is monitored at baseline, during the infusion, and after the completion of the islet transplantation.
5. Elevated absolute intraportal pressures (>18 mm Hg) before beginning the infusion or (>22 mm Hg or double baseline value) during the infusion should be a contraindication for continuing with the islet transplant infusion.

Route of Islet Administration

1. The islet cell infusion is delivered slowly either by a closed gravity-fed bag system into the portal vein (most common method) or via a syringe attached to a catheter hub.[5]
2. The sterile intravenous infusion tubing set is connected to the tip of the portal vein catheter via a 3-way stopcock.[5]
3. In a retrograde fashion, the tubing is flushed with isotonic sodium chloride solution.[5]
4. The islet cell infusion bag is then spiked with the sterile infusion tubing.
5. During the gravity infusion, the bag and tubing are slightly agitated as the islet cells infuse into the portal vein.[5]
6. After completion of the islet cell infusion, the catheter and islet container will be rinsed with an additional 50 mL of transplant media.[5]

Procedure Care After Islet Transplantation

1. Frequent vital sign monitoring
2. Frequent blood sugar checks
3. Close monitoring of hemoglobin and hematocrit levels
4. Ultrasound evaluation within 24 hours after transplantation and approximately 1 week after transplantation.
5. Close monitoring of the immunosuppressive regimen.

Many patients may require sequential islet transplants to be performed before they can become insulin independent. Studies have shown that multiple sequential islet transplants can be safely performed if the islet preparations are highly purified and transplanted in small packed cell volumes.[6] Sequential islet transplantations follow the same procedures and medication regimen as the initial transplantation.

Medications

Researchers at the University of Alberta contribute their success to the use of a glucocorticoid-free immunosuppressive regimen,[4] consisting of dacluzimab, tacrolimus, and sirolimus. Although this glucocorticoid-free immunosuppressive regimen remains to be the most commonly used today, many researchers worldwide are beginning to study novel immunosuppressive regimens. Table 6 outlines commonly used medications in islet cell transplantation.

Table 6. MOST COMMONLY USED MEDICATION REGIMENS FOR ISLET CELL TRANSPLANTATION

Medication category	Regimen
Immunosuppression	Dacluzimab 1.0 mg/kg every 2 weeks for a total of 5 doses. Therapy begins immediately before the first infusion. The dacluzimab regimen is repeated for subsequent islet transplantations. Tacrolimus initially at 1.0 mg twice a day, then titrate dose to desired trough levels. • Maintain trough levels between 3.0-6.0 ng/mL Sirolimus initially at 0.2 mg/kg, then 0.1 mg/kg titrate dose to desired trough levels. • Maintain trough levels between 8.0-12.0 ng/mL
Infection prophylaxis	*Pneumocystis carinii* pneumonia • Sulfamethoxazole-trimethoprim (Bactrim) or • Inhaled pentamidine Cytomegalovirus • Valganciclovir or • Ganciclovir
Anticoagulation prophylaxis	Low-molecular-weight heparin (enoxaparin sodium, Lovenox, 30-mg twice a day) for 7 days

Signs and Symptoms of Rejection

Currently, no definitive way to determine rejection following islet cell transplantation exists. Researchers worldwide are looking into mechanistic assays to better understand the mechanisms of islet rejection. The following tests and clinical history reported by the patient are used to determine the status of the islet graft:

- Elevated blood glucose levels
- C-peptide levels
- Hemoglobin A1C
- Glucose tolerance test, mixed meal tolerance test, and arginine stimulation test
- Hypoglycemic episodes

Conclusions

Islet cell transplantation has become a rapidly growing field. Researchers are continuing to study new, improved methods for islet isolation, islet cell transplantation, and immunosuppressive regimens. Organizations such as Medicare, Medicaid (CMS), Health Resources and Services Administration, the United Network for Organ Sharing, the Food and Drug Administration, and many international health authorities are closely monitoring this field.

References

1. The Diabetes Control and Complications Trial Research Group. The effect of intensive treatment of diabetes on the development and progression of long-term complications in insulin-dependent diabetes mellitus. *N Engl J Med.* 1993;329:977-986.
2. The Diabetes Control and Complications Trial/Epidemiology of Diabetes Interventions and Complications Research Group. Retinopathy and nephropathy in patients with type 1 diabetes four years after a trial of intensive therapy. *N Engl J Med.* 2000;342:381-389.
3. Brendel M, Hering B, Schulz A, Bretzel R. *International Islet Transplant Registry Report.* Giessen, Germany: University of Giessen; 1999:1-20.
4. Shapiro AM, Lakey JR, Ryan EA, et al. Islet transplantation in seven patients with type 1 diabetes mellitus using a glucocorticoid-free immunosuppressive regimen. *N Engl J Med.* 2000;343:230-238.
5. Baidal D, Froud T, Ferreria J, Khan A, Alejandro R, Ricordi C. The bag method for islet cell infusion. *Cell Transplant.* 2003;12:809-813.
6. Casey J, Lakey J, Ryan E, et al. Portal venous pressure changes after sequential clinical islet transplantation. *Transplantation.* 2002;74:913-915.

The Ethics of Living Organ Donation

Sheldon Zink, PhD
Stacey Wertlieb, MBe

Introduction

As the disparity between the number of people in need of a transplant and the number of deceased organs available for transplantation continues to increase annually, the greater the demand becomes for living donors. In 2001, the number of living donors surpassed the number of deceased donors for the first time.[1] Living donation continues to become an increasingly popular and realistic means by which to remove individuals from the transplant waiting list and offer more patients a life-saving transplant; however, this benefit is accompanied by a number of difficult ethical questions that transplant professionals must be aware of as the criteria for the use of living donors rapidly expand.

Ethical dilemmas are especially pervasive in the field of transplantation. Living donation is one of the more nuanced of the ethical controversies. Each type of living donor has a very different context in which ethical questions arise and issues of risk versus benefit are evaluated. The following section describes some of the guiding principles of medical ethics, which are the foundation of all contemporary issues in bioethics. (Also see Chapter 4, "Ethical Issues in Donation and Transplantation.")

Guiding Principles of Contemporary Medical Ethics

In the past, the principle now known as nonmaleficence guided a physician's code of ethics. Above all else, physicians were to do no harm to their patients. This principle serves as the foundation of the Hippocratic Oath, which is the ethical imperative for clinicians. Coupled with this negative principle of not doing harm is the positive principle of beneficence: Clinicians are to act in such a way that improves the welfare of their patients. Historically, this principle was interpreted as improving a patient's impaired medical or physical well-being. At times when these principles conflict, practitioners weigh the risks and expected benefits to determine if the action in question is likely to increase their patient's well-being to a great enough extent to subject him or her to the risk of the medical intervention.[2]

Contemporary medical ethics has been unnecessarily dominated by the principle of respect for autonomy. In the past, physicians were heavily critiqued, and rightfully so, for being paternalistic and often disempowering their patients. There exists a severe power imbalance between the physician who possesses medical expertise and the patient who is sick and vulnerable. This imbalance allowed physicians to invoke their power to make decisions on behalf of their patients, often without consultation or consideration of views of the patients, which may differ from those of physicians. In the post-Internet era, patients have access to information that has begun to challenge the authority of the clinical establishment. Patients demand to be part of the decision-making process; they are no longer willing to just be the recipients of clinical intervention. However, merely allowing patients to be part of the process can be a complicated and time-consuming endeavor. One aspect of informed consent is collaborative decision making in which all of the patient's options are examined and ideally the one that is in the best interest of the patient is selected.

Informed consent is the most common means by which respect for patient autonomy is carried out in modern-day medicine. Consent must be obtained from the patient or appropriate surrogate before a patient undergoes any medical procedure or participates in research. Consent must be completely voluntary. The physician must inform the patient of all risks and benefits as well as all realistic alternatives.[3] The patient has the ultimate decision-making power to determine what will happen to his or her body.

Many of the conflicts in contemporary medical practice are between respecting a patient's autonomy and following what the physician believes to be the best course of action for the patient's care. In these cases, the patient is generally permitted to choose, but the physician is free not to perform any action that he or she believes will cause undue harm to the patient. While patients do have the ethical and legal right to refuse any medical treatment, they do not have the absolute right to demand unnecessary treatment. This conflict becomes even more complicated when trying to apply these ethical principles to living donation.

Differences Among Living Donors

When thinking about the ethics of living donation, each potential donor must be considered primarily as an individual patient, not as one of a group of persons that is an opportunity to provide a life-saving transplant to someone on the waiting list. The risks and benefits for each individual vary greatly; it is imperative to evaluate each living donor as an individual in the context of what is generally a complex situation. Living donors consider giving an organ or organ segment to improve and potentially save the life of another, most often the life of someone with whom the potential donor has a close relationship. However, living donation imposes various degrees of physical demands; emotional stress; vulnerability; and the potential for extreme societal, familial, and commercial pressure on the donor.[4] The risks and benefits of living donation vary greatly depending on the organ in question, the relationship between the donor and recipient, the probability of success of the transplant, and a number of additional external factors.[5,6] Such medical and social variables contribute to the way the donor views the donation decision.

Living kidney donation is by far the most common. To date, there have been 75,263 living kidney donations; 6,565 of these transplantations were performed in 2005.[7] Kidney donation and transplantation is unique compared with the donation and transplantation of other organs because replacing kidney function can be achieved with dialysis. However, transplantation is the superior treatment option when considering the quality of life of the recipient. Additionally, graft survival from a living donor kidney is known to be greater than that of an organ from a deceased donor.[8,9] Medical complications for living kidney donors are low.[8,9] A retrospective study of 114 living kidney donations completed in 2003 found that 6% of donors had bleeding and 2% had lymphatic cysts postoperatively. Of those 114 donors, 3 patients required an operation because of bleeding and one patient developed acute renal failure after donation.[10] Other literature has estimated the mortality rate of living kidney donors to be 0.03% and the morbidity rate to be less than 10%; most of these morbidities were considered to be minor.[11]

When a living donor donates a kidney, it is often done to improve the quality of life of the recipient. A donor who is contemplating donating part of a liver is doing so in order to save the life of the recipient, for whom transplant is the only option.[12] However, living liver donation is a much newer and complicated procedure. In the United States, only 3,009 living liver transplants have been performed to date. In 2005, there were 323 living liver donations.[7] The graft survival rates from living donated livers are about 80% at 1 year after transplantation and 65% after 5 years.[13,14] Complications are also more common in living liver transplant donors because he or she is donating a segment of the liver rather than one of a pair of organs. Historically, adult to pediatric living liver transplant has been a much more common practice than adult to adult living liver transplant, and data regarding outcomes of the latter is sparse. Potential complications include hemorrhage, bile duct injury, infection, and pulmonary embolus in addition to the risks of general anesthesia.[15] Studies have reported a wide range of complication rates for living liver donors, from no significant complications to a complication rate greater than 50%.[12,15,16] Results of a survey of 30 transplant centers where 208 adult to adult living liver transplants were performed indicated a donor complication rate of 10%; the most common complication was a postoperative biliary leak. Re-operation due to complications of living donation was necessary in at least 3 of the patients.[15]

Other transplantations are possible using a graft from a living donor; however, they are comparatively much more rare. Living lobar lung transplantation accounts for a small fraction of lung transplants,[17] but the need to consider donor safety is heightened in this procedure because the health and lives of 2 donors are put at risk for each recipient. In living lobar lung transplantation, the right lower lobe is removed from 1 donor and the left lower lobe from another. These lobes are implanted and serve as the whole right and left lungs for the recipient. In a 2003 study[18] of 253 living lobar lung donors during the last decade, no perioperative or long-term mortalities occurred, but this is predicted to change as the procedure becomes more widespread; physicians estimate a potential mortality rate of 0.5% to 3%.[19] Additionally, the rates of intra-operative and postoperative complications for the donors is nearly 20%, with the most common complications being the unanticipated sacrifice of the right middle lobe, bleeding, pericarditis, arrhythmias, persistent air leaks, and increased duration of a necessary thoracostomy tube.[18,19]

Living small bowel transplantation is a relatively new and exceedingly rare procedure; therefore, data on morbidity and mortality are scarce. Although morbidity rates are not available, potential complications for the donor include bleeding, shortened intestinal transit time, onset of food intolerences, malabsorption of nutrients, and intestinal adhesions.[20] Additionally, no precise method exists by which to measure the length of the available small bowel before the operation, which means that the percentage of bowel donors retain is subject to variation.[20]

The risks and benefits for a donor are determined in part by the organ being donated, but there are several types of living donors. The benefit derived from organ donation is influenced by the relationship the donor has with the recipient [6] and the acceptability of the donation must be considered in this context. Living donors are often first-degree relatives of the recipient, usually siblings, parents, or children. Living related donors also can be cousins, nieces, nephews, and others who are genetically related to the donor. Some donors have an emotional relationship, such as marriage or friendship, with the recipient. In most cases, people who volunteer to be living donors because of an emotional relationship have the relationship before donation, not because of it. Unrelated living donors have been called altruistic donors, good Samaritans, or non-designated living donors; these are people who choose to donate one of their organs to someone they do not know and with whom they have no genetic or emotional attachment. The term "organ vendor" is used to describe individuals who receive payment for their organs. Payment for organs is currently illegal in the United States, but periodically a policy change is considered as a possible option for increasing organ supply.[21] A person who swaps or participates in organ matching is an individual whose organ is not compatible to a recipient who is genetically or emotionally related; this person is willing to donate his or her organ in exchange for another that is compatible with the desired recipient.[22]

Living Donors Are Not Patients

In the case of living donation, the principles of nonmaleficence, beneficence, and autonomy conflict in a way that is unique in contemporary medicine. Living donors volunteer to undergo an invasive procedure and subject themselves to risks that include a variety of complications, including death, without the possibility of therapeutic benefit for themselves. This indisputable fact underlies every discussion regarding living donation. Many physicians are uncomfortable subjecting their patients to a surgery for which there is great risk and no potential benefit.

Autonomous Decision Making

In terms of the medical risks to healthy living donors, it is difficult to make an ethical argument in favor of living donation. However, there is a clear argument that donors have the power to make autonomous decisions. If donors understand the risks of donation and make an informed choice, the donation is permissible. Yet, there are limits to an individual's autonomy and the obligation of a medical professional to respect it.[23] Traditionally, restrictions on a person's autonomy are to protect the rights and interests of others[24]; the same restrictions apply to protect an individual from harming himself or herself. A medical professional is not obligated to perform any procedure that he or she believes will do unnecessary harm to the patient. Normally, the patient's right to informed consent gives the patient the right to decide which medically appropriate treatment, if any, to undergo. However, it is the physician's responsibility to decide on the appropriate treatment options.[25] While living donation falls outside of standard medical practice, a healthcare provider's obligation to respect a patient's autonomy in no way obligates the healthcare provider to remove an organ or organ segment from an otherwise healthy individual. The final decision for a live organ donation should be that of the living donor, the recipient of the organ, and the medical team. The medical team should never feel pressured into performing a living donation.[26]

Informed consent, the medical hallmark of autonomy, is extremely complicated in cases of living donation. Living donation is different from other interventions in which informed consent serves as the basis for autonomy. The living donor often decides to donate before the informed consent process. For many living donors, being told the risks of donation generally do not affect the decision, especially when the potential donor is committed to helping a recipient with whom he or she has an emotional relationship. Additionally, many donors report that they felt they had no option but to donate to save a loved one. Familial and societal pressure can make it nearly impossible for a living donor to make a completely voluntary decision to donate. Separating such strong potential internal and external coercion from the decision to donate is difficult, if not impossible. In most circumstances, warning flags signal if a consent is not completely informed or voluntary.[24,26,27] While this is not to say that living donors cannot make autonomous and voluntary decisions, it is essential to keep these conflicts in mind when discussing the possibility of living donation. Autonomy does not give a donor the right to make a risky decision regarding his or her health. Informed decision making can happen only after the donor has preliminarily decided to donate.

These issues regarding autonomous decision making are further complicated by the scarcity of organs; living donation is often the only hope for a recipient to receive an organ in time. Healthcare providers in the transplant field often believe they have a dual responsibility to advocate for their patients and to serve as the gatekeeper of organs to ensure fair allocation. Physicians with multiple patients in need of a transplant are often prioritizing by basing them on the national allocation system rather than on the individual patient. In this context, living donation is then justified because it removes a recipient off the transplant waiting list and provides a greater chance for other patients to receive a transplantable organ from a deceased donor. A consequentialist argument can be made that a living donor provides a benefit for a greater number of people compared with the risk to one person (the donor) and therefore should be allowed; in this way of thinking, one person's risk is balanced with the benefit of many. However, this is not an acceptable argument because it devalues the living donor, and individuals become the means for an organ, ie, objects to be traded for the larger common good.

Conflicts of Interest

The most prevalent ethical issues for transplantation are outlined in Chapter 4. Living donation has a very specific set of ethical conflicts. The conflict of interest for parties involved in a living donation is perhaps one of the most problematic ethical concerns for living donation.

Patients on the transplant waiting list often have been in the care of a transplant team for many years. Strong bonds of friendship and a sense of professional obligation develop between transplant patients, their families, and the medical team. As a result, transplant care teams become advocates for their patients, who are often close to dying and in desperate need of organs, rather than for the potential living donors.

Potential living donors are, or should be, healthy individuals able to withstand the donation surgery with minimal risk of complications from pre-existing comorbidities. When a transplant team is treating both the donor and the recipient, the team is placed in the difficult position of advocating for 2 individuals with completely different needs.

The clinical needs of the patient or transplant recipient are clear. He or she needs an organ and/or medical support until an organ is found. Living donors, who are often treated by the same clinical team as the transplant recipient, often are not thought of as patients. After all, donors are not sick. Donors are possible resources, a means to an end, and an opportunity to save a life. Because donors are healthy and motivated to donate, clinical and social risks often are not taken completely into consideration. The medical team wants an organ to save a life; it is easy to rationalize that a healthy person who agrees to donate should be permitted to make an independent and autonomous decision. It is the obligation of the transplant team to establish a framework for understanding all of the aforementioned factors regarding the clinical, psychological and social details of each case and how the circumstances may cloud the consent process. Donors must be thought of independently from recipients and the larger issues of a growing transplant waiting list. Because the unfortunate reality is that too often donors are not considered independently from transplant recipients, it is essential for transplant teams to establish independent donor advocate teams to protect the interests of donors as well as transplant recipients.

Independent Donor Advocates

Independent donor advocates may make it possible to balance the needs of the recipient and the autonomous choice of the living donor. The donor would be assigned a separate clinical team for the medical evaluation, and eligibility for donation would be determined separately from consideration of the recipient's needs. In this way, the clinical evaluation is focused primarily on the fitness and informed choices of the donor. National medical criteria to determine the suitability of potential living donors have not yet been agreed upon. The threshold for allowable medical risk for living donation has no boundaries and is left largely unchecked and undocumented.

An independent donor team creates a buffer between the transplant team, whose first priority is and should be finding a donor organ for their patient, and the potential living donor. Donor advocates evaluate, independent of the recipient's needs, whether the donation is possible or in the best interests of the donor. The risk to the donor is then considered in terms specifically focused on the donor and not in the context of benefit to the recipient. The donor advocate team is responsible for ensuring that informed consent has been obtained before allowing the donation to move forward.

Organ Procurement Organization as Donor Advocates

There is a significant void of transplant programs throughout the country with the means to provide living donors the independent and objective evaluations necessary to qualify living donors. Organ procurement organizations (OPOs) in several states have taken some of the responsibility to perform preliminary evaluations on living donors, especially in cases of nondirected living donation. For example, nondirected living donors (NDLD), people who want to do donate but have no one in particular in mind, often contact a specific hospital or make contact through specific practitioners to inquire if there is someone in need of an organ. Some hospitals will refer the potential donor to the OPO for initial screening as a way to ensure objectivity. The OPO evaluation often entails an interview, waiting periods, education, psychological evaluation, and preliminary laboratory work. Unfortunately, there are no set standards for OPO evaluations, and this creates inconsistencies among OPOs; it is possible for a donor to be rejected by one OPO and accepted by another. If the OPO believes the donor is qualified for donation he or she will be referred to the appropriately matched recipient hospital for further clinical evaluation.

One of the main goals of OPOs is to obtain organs; they are less compelled by their obligation to a particular patient than they are to the entire procurement system, creating an inherent conflict of interest when an OPO serves as the primary advocate for living donors. Historically, OPOs have served the interests of donors and their families. However, the top priority of the transplant community is shifting to one primarily focused on increasing the number of transplantable organs. In this political environment, OPOS are no more capable than any other organization that might participate in this process to serve as third-party advocates for potential living donors.

Informed Consent

Living donors, at the very least, must know specific information to provide informed consent. Necessary elements of informed consent for living donation include knowledge of the risks and benefits to the donor; alternative treatments and potential complications for the recipient; risk of disease and chance of survival for the recipient; freedom from coercion and voluntary donation of the organ; possible financial costs to the donor; and acknowledgement of no personal financial gain.

Balancing the risks and benefits for donors is a complex and often confusing process. One rarely discussed and controversial issue in the field of transplantation is whether a donor has the right to know the clinical condition of the recipient. This issue is especially pertinent when recipients have the human immunodeficiency virus, Hepatitis C, or cancer. Many transplant programs are hesitant to disclose a recipient's medical information because of confidentiality issues. Because it is impossible for a potential donor to understand the risks and benefits of donation or the alternative treatment options for the recipient without knowing the recipient's clinical condition, transplant teams may feel that the recipient's medical information should be disclosed. In these cases, it might be prudent to ask the recipient to sign a consent form to release the necessary information. It is not ethically permissible to conceal or withhold information that might influence the donor's decision. If a recipient refuses to allow the information to be disclosed, a living donation should not be permitted.

Confirming that a donor is not being coerced and is voluntarily donating his or her organ is another difficult aspect of informed consent. Ideally, a social worker or psychologist should speak to the living donor to determine if the donor is voluntarily donating his or her organ. It may be difficult for potential donors to confide in medical staff for fear of retribution from family and friends if the potential donor does not want to donate and the potential recipient is unable to get a transplant. These situations are especially complicated in cases of living related donors. The medical team has an ethical obligation to protect the potential living donor from pressure to donate. If the potential living donor reveals to the medical team that he or she does not want to be a living donor and is fearful of retribution from others, the donor's advocacy team should help the donor explain this to the recipient. Some current practices allow the transplant team to create an excuse on behalf of the donor as to why the donation cannot proceed. Such practice may jeopardize the recipient's trust in the medical team and should not be the primary course of action. However, it violates all codes of medical ethics to proceed with a living donation when the donor is not donating his or her organ voluntarily or is being coerced. In cases in which all other possible solutions have been exhausted, creating an excuse on behalf of the donor to not donate may be permissible.

Ideally, donating an organ should be cost neutral for the donor. In many areas, there are programs to assist donors with incidental expenses; however, it is not always feasible for all of the donor's expenses to be paid. Therefore, it is important to outline the range of expenses that might be incurred. Expenses can include travel for donor and companion, lodging, food, parking, gasoline, and follow-up medical costs. It is also important to help potential donors think through ways their donation may effect their employment and possible ways to handle their specific circumstances, including medical leave, performance capability, whether they have a donation benefit in place and other insurance issues. If this information is not available to the transplant center, it is the transplant team's responsibility to obtain it.

Balancing the Risks and Benefits for Living Donors

When a person is considering whether to undergo a surgical procedure or enter a clinical trial, he or she should make the decision after considering the risks and potential benefits of the intervention as well as the possible outcome without it. Weighing the risks and benefits for a living donor is quite different from calculating the risks and benefits of a medical intervention for someone who is ill. For example, in the case of someone who needs a transplant, undergoing the surgery if possible is more beneficial than to go without the transplant. For the living donor this is not the case.

Donors generally have a greater health-related quality of life than the general population.[28] Without a doubt this should continue to be the norm, as the risk to a living donor is increased if the donor's health is already compromised shifting the risk/benefit ratio; living donation may not be the best option. In thinking about the ethics of living donation and the acceptability of a specific living donation, the donor and recipient must always be thought of as separate individuals. A minimal or even significant risk to the donor will always seem acceptable when compared to the enormous benefit of a transplant for the recipient. However, this is not an acceptable way to consider risk and benefit, the risk for the donor must be compared to the benefit the donor will gain from the transplant. This comparison is incredibly complex as much of the risk is medical while the benefit is generally psychological and often intrinsically linked the benefit of the recipient. Thinking about the risks and benefits in this light is among the most difficult challenges faced by the medical team.

It is essential that living donors clarify what they expect to gain from donating their organ. In the donation system, donors are expected to donate their organs altruistically (ie, without the expectation of personal gain). Altruistic donation of organs is the most fundamental concept of the deceased donation system. Families of deceased donors and those who give first-person consent do so willingly and without the expectation of personal gain. It should not be the case that most living donors are expected to give altruistically; it is acceptable to consider a personal gain and even appropriate when thinking of the risk and benefit for the donor.

Living donors do reap some benefits. Donors who give their organs to a close friend or relative may be saving the life or improving the life of a loved one. It is ethically permissible to allow a close friend or family member to donate an organ because the personal gain can balance the desire to give with the risk of surgery and potential complications. Evaluating the risks and benefits for a NDLD is more difficult.

Nondirected Living Donors

Nondirected living donation is a contested aspect of living donation. With public education programs highlighting the need for organs and the media showcasing NDLD success stories as acts of heroism, it is possible that more NDLDs will come forward as organ donors. Although many transplant centers accept organs from NDLDs, the debate regarding the ethical implications of nondirected living donation continues.

Although few transplant centers keep accurate records of all inquiries regarding nondirected living donation, one study[29] estimates that the number of inquiries is increasing and most centers are willing to consider the possibility of NDLD. In the past, this kind of donation was unacceptable because it was difficult to evaluate the NDLD's level of competence to make decisions. People who wanted to donate to strangers were automatically considered suspect, as the benefits seemed remote and not worth the risk.

Today, the acceptability of nondirected living donation is increasing largely due to the desperation of people on the transplant waiting list and the willingness of physicians to accept organs for their patients. However, this practice is ethically suspect and should be undertaken with caution.

Psychosocial Evaluations

One major concern of many healthcare practitioners in the field of transplantation is how to evaluate the psychosocial suitability of healthy people willing to donate their organs. Currently, psychosocial evaluations are conducted on patients who are being considered for listing. Evaluations are usually conducted by social workers and, when necessary, by psychologists or psychiatrists.

The most common psychosocial characteristics evaluated in living donors are informed consent, motivation for donation, signs of coercion, financial and emotional support, and overall psychological well-being.[30] One problem raised by psychosocial evaluations is that potential donors have an emotional attachment to the recipient that may prohibit them from making a clear and informed decision. While this emotional connection does not preclude individuals from making rational choices, it may affect the way in which information is perceived or understood. A significant aspect of the psychosocial evaluation is to give the potential donor information to assist him or her in making informed decisions. It may be necessary to clarify information given by other members of the medical team. Information should be given at a rate in which the potential donor is able to comprehend; several meetings and conversations may be necessary. By tailoring the psychosocial evaluation and education portion of the donation plan to each individual donor, the social worker or clinical transplant coordinator may be able to more accurately understand whether a donor is making an informed decision and whether the psychological needs of the donor will be met throughout the process.

Family members who are tested and not found to be a suitable donor for whatever reason also may have important psychosocial needs that should be addressed by the clinical team. Asking family and friends to be donors and exposing them to testing for compatibility can cause unexpected strain on relationships whether the individual becomes a donor or not. Disruptions in social networks can weaken support systems that are necessary for both the donor and recipient to recover from the surgery. Special attention must be paid to minimize the amount of stress throughout in the process of locating a living donor. After the donation has occurred, the restructuring of relationships, both positive and negative, must be monitored because both have an impact of psychological outcomes.[31]

An important and often overlooked aspect of the overall psychological health evaluation is a realistic description of the risks and possible outcomes of living donation. Transplant teams are usually so optimistic and motivated by the potential donor's good will that the risk of failure may not even be a factor in the decision-making process. One significant risk rarely discussed is the possibility that the donated organ will be rejected by the recipient's body. Although this surgical outcome is mentioned as a possibility, it often is not addressed in a way that makes the issue a real concern. Postsurgical complications and lengthy recovery process are also not discussed in a way that would make a potential donor reconsider. As a result, many donors who experience less than optimal outcomes are often plagued by depression and extended recovery periods, and they feel unprepared and frustrated by the decision to be a living donor.[32] When the medical team meets with the donor to explain the risks of morbidity and mortality for the donor, it is absolutely essential that the risks of graft failure and complication rates for the recipient are described as well.

Solicitation

Unrelated living donation has increased in recent years because of solicitation for living as well as deceased donors. Individuals in need of an organ or with a loved one in need of an organ make a public request for donation. Solicitation can take many forms: billboards, Web sites, postings in community newspapers, and the use of influential connections. Solicitors are not appealing for organ donors in general; they are making a personal plea to meet the need of one specific individual. What began as a few isolated incidents of organ solicitation has become an alarming trend. Web sites and advertising campaigns have become increasingly common. While this approach doesn't break any laws, solicitors are able to legally thwart the intention of the equitable waiting list and unfairly increase their chances of getting an organ at the expense of others. In the current system, organs are predominantly allocated to the highest ranking suitable recipient, but an organ solicitor can effectively take an organ away from the individual in greatest need of the organ. Solicitation, especially on a commercial scale, is unethical as it subverts the current allocation system, giving unfair advantage to those with financial means.

Individuals who decide to become living donors in response to a solicitation campaign are unique in that the relationship with the donor is formed because of the donation. The benefits derived from the donation are more abstract than for the typical donor, who has an emotional relationship with the individual receiving the transplant; therefore, the risks and benefits must be considered in a completely different context for donors who have been solicited. The concept that a healthy individual is willing to put himself or herself at risk for a stranger is often difficult to understand and can create suspicion of coercion, financial or otherwise, for the medical team. Furthermore, coercion in this population is more difficult to determine than the emotional coercion that may exist in cases when the donor and recipient have an emotional relationship, because both parties enter into the donation willingly. Especially, if the donor-recipient pair may have been turned down at another transplant center, the pair may be adept at hiding any monetary exchange from the transplant team. Additionally, unrelated donations that result from solicitation place the recipients at risk for future payment, as the donor could pressure the recipient for compensation after the donation. Again, this is not to say that unrelated and nondirected donation cannot occur, but when a donor wants to donate in response to a solicitation campaign, it is imperative that the donor undergo a thorough examination to ensure that he or she has no underlying motive and that the donor and recipient are fully informed of the ramifications of the donation.

Financial Incentives

Financial incentives for donors, a proposed method by which to increase the number of organs available for transplantation and a highly debated topic, is currently illegal on a state and federal level as a result of 2 pieces of legislation.

The Uniform Anatomical Gift Act (UAGA) was originally passed in 1968 and adopted by all states by 1973. At that time, the act did not specifically address payment for organ donation, but many states enacted such laws in addition to adopting the UAGA. When the UAGA was amended in 1987, the purchase and sale of cadaveric organs was explicitly prohibited; however, this ban did not cover organ sales by living donors.[21]

The National Organ Transplant Act (NOTA) was enacted in 1984; part of this act makes it a federal crime to "knowingly acquire, receive, or otherwise transfer any human organ for valuable consideration for use in human transplantation." NOTA defines "valuable consideration" in such a way as to allow for "reasonable payments associated with the removal, transportation, implantation, processing, preservation, quality control, and storage of a human organ or the expenses of travel, housing, and lost wages incurred by the donor of a human organ in connection with the donation of the organ."[33] Monetary exchange for a living donation is both unethical and illegal. However, living donors should not incur expenses for their donation.

A number of ethical issues make financial gain for living donation problematic. The intention of NOTA was to prevent commercialization of organs and thereby the commodification of the body. Placing a monetary value on various parts of the body, including organs, goes against fundamental values of our society.[34] Currently, the national allocation and transplant system is based on the concepts of altruism and equity; allowing financial incentives or permitting the selling of organs would destroy both principles.[35] For an individual with financial trouble, the ability to profit from the sale of an organ can be considered coercive and, at the very least, an "unrefusable offer."[36] As a market system becomes the established norm, indigent people may be expected to donate their organs as a viable option to make money. Live organ donors would no longer be donated to help save the life of another person, but to help improve their financial circumstances. Furthermore, a shift to a market in which the buying of organs is acceptable would place people of low socioeconomic status in an unethical position in which they are pressured to donate their organs, thereby creating a system of inequitable access to organs.

While it is unethical for living donors to financially profit from their donation, their act of altruism should not come at extreme personal financial cost. There should be a system in place to reimburse living donors for expenses incurred as a result of their donation. Solutions such as paid medical leave to offset potential loss of wages and reimbursement for life insurance or disability insurance would serve to offset much of the financial responsibility that a living donor assumes. While these solutions are financial in nature, they are not a direct payment, such as a tax credit for donors.[34]

Conclusion

Living donation might appear to be an easy solution to the mounting need for organ donors. As the transplant waiting list grows, so does the desperation to find willing donors. The limited number of deceased organ donors will never be enough to significantly reduce the organ donor waiting list. However, it is imperative that individuals willing to donate an organ or organ segment to save the life of another individual are thought of as more than just means to reducing the organ shortage. Transplant teams are responsible for ensuring that donors are not only medically appropriate but also psychologically and socially capable of handling the donation and any possible complications that result from the donation. The development of standard protocols and criteria, including a possible waiting time between the decision to donate and the donation, a thorough psychological evaluation, and the appointment of an independent donor advocate for all living donors, is an important step to protecting the donor. The risks and benefits for each potential living donor must be evaluated on a case-specific basis, and the transplant team must ensure that each donor gives a proper informed consent and that the donation is voluntary.

Acknowledgment:

We would like to thank Benjamin Grunwald and John Catalano for their valuable contributions to this chapter.

This work was supported in part by Health Resources and Services Administration contract 231-00-0115. The content is the responsibility of the authors alone and does not necessarily reflect the views or policies of the Department of Health and Human Services, nor does mention of trade names, commercial products, or organizations imply endorsement by the U.S. Government.

References

1. United Network of Organ Sharing Donors Recovered in the US by Donor Type: OPTN Data Report. http://www.optn.org/latestData/rptData.asp Accessed May 30, 2006.
2. Beauchamp T, Childress J. *Principles of Biomedical Ethics*. 5th ed. New York, NY: Oxford University Press; 2001.
3. Moreno JD, Caplan AL, Wolpe PW. Informed consent. In: Chadwick R, ed. The *Encyclopedia of Applied Ethics*. Vol 2. San Diego, Calif: Academic Press; 1998.
4. Dunstan GR The ethics of organ donation. *Br Med Bull*. 1997; 53:921-939.
5. Cotler SJ, McNutt R, Patil R, et al. Adult living donor liver transplantation: preferences about donation outside the medical community. *Liver Transpl*. 2001; 7:335-340.
6. Franklin PM, Crombie AK. Live related renal transplantation: psychological, social, and cultural issues. *Transplantation*. 2003; 768:1247-1252.
7. The Organ Procurement and Transplantation Network. Donors Recovered in the US by Donor type: OPTN Data Report. Available at: http://www.optn.org/latestData/rptData.asp Accessed May 30, 2006.
8. Nolan MT, Walton-Moss B, Taylor L, Dane K. Living kidney donor decision making: state of the science and direction for future research. *Prog Transplant*. September 2004; 14:201-209.
9. Cecka JM. Kidney transplantation from living unrelated donors. *Annu Rev Mede*. 2000; 51:393-406.
10. Sandmann W. Living donor kidney transplantation: pitfalls of the donor and recipient operation. *Transplant Proc*. 2003; 35:930.
11. Matas AJ, Garvey CA, Jacobs CL, Kahn JP. Nondirected donation of kidneys from living donors. *New Engl J Med*. 2000; 3436:433-436.
12. Karliova M, Malago M, Valentin-Gamazo C, et al. Living-related liver transplantation from the view of the donor: a 1-year follow-up survey. *Transplantation*. 2002; 73:1799-1804.
13. 2004 Annual Report of the U.S. Organ Procurement and Transplantation Network and the Scientific Registry of Transplant Recipients: Transplant Data 1994-2003. Department of Health and Human Services, Health Resources and Services Administration, Healthcare Systems Bureau, Division of Transplantation, Rockville, MD; United Network for Organ Sharing, Richmond, VA; University Renal Research and Education Association, Ann Arbor, MI. Available at: http://www.optn.org/AR2004/508c_can-gender_ki.htm. Accessed September 1, 2005.
14. Miller CM, Gondolesi GE, Florman S, et al. One hundred nine living donor liver transplants in adults and children: a single-center experience. *Ann Surg*. 2001; 234:301-312.
15. Renz JF, Busuttil RW. Adult-to-adult living-donor liver transplantation: a critical analysis. *Semin Liver Dis*. 2000; 204:411-424.
16. Ilkegami T, Nishizaki T, Yanaga K, et al. The impact of donor age on living donor liver transplantation. *Transplantation*. 2000; 7012:1703-1707.
17. Date H, Aoe M, Sano Y, et al. Improved survival after living-donor lobar lung transplantation. *J Thorac Cardiovasc Surg*. 2004; 1286:933-940.
18. Bowdish M, Barr ML, Schenkel FA, et al. A decade of living lobar lung transplantation: perioperative complications after 253 donor lobectomies. *Am J Transplant*. 2004; 4:1283-1288.
19. Veeken C, Palmer SM, Davis RD, Grichnik KP. Living-related lobar lung transplantation. *J Cardiothoracic Vas Anesth* 2004; 18:506-511.
20. Testa G, Panaro F, Schena S, Holterman M, Abcarian H, Benedetti E. Living related small bowel transplantation donor surgical technique. *Ann Surg*. 2004; 240:779-784.
21. National Conference of Commissioners on Uniform State Laws. Uniform Anatomical Gift Act (1987). Available at: http://www.law.upenn.edu/bll/ulc/fnact99/uaga87.htm. Accessed April 27, 2006.
22. Veatch R. *Transplantation Ethics*. Washington, DC: Georgetown University Press; 2000.
23. LaPointe Rudow D, Brown RS. Role of the independent donor advocacy team in ethical decision making. *Prog Transplant*. September 2005; 15:298-302.
24. Sauder R, Parker LS. Autonomy's limits: living donation and health-related harm. *Camb Q Healthc Ethics*. 2001; 10:399-407.
25. Minkoff H, Powderly KR, Chervenak F, McCullough LB. Ethical dimensions of elective primary cesarean delivery. *Obstet Gynecol*. 2004; 103:387-392.
26. Abecassis M, Adams M, Adams P, et al. Consensus statement on the live organ donor. *JAMA*. 2000; 28422:2919-2926.
27. Kallich JD, Merz JF. The transplant imperative: protecting living donors from the pressure to donate. *J Corp Law*. Fall 1994; 20:139-145.
28. Cotler SJ, Cotler S, Gambera M, Benedetti E, Jensen DM, Testa G. Adult living donor liver transplantation: perspectives from 100 liver transplant surgeons. *Liver Transpl*. 2003; 9:637-644.

29. Crowley-Matoka M, Switzer G. Nondirected living donation: a survey of current trends and practices. *Transplantation.* 2005; 79:515-519.
30. Olbrisch ME, Benedict S, Haller DL, Levenson JL Psychosocial assessment of living organ donors: clinical and ethical considerations. *Prog Transplant.* March 2001; 11:40-49.
31. Jacobs C, Johnson E, Anderson K, Gillingham K, Matas A. Kidney transplants from living donors: how donation affects family dynamics. *Adv Ren Replace Ther.* April 1998; 5:89-97.
32. Halijamae U, Nyberg G, Sjostrom B. Remaining experiences of living kidney donors more than 3 yr after Early recipient graft loss. *Clin Transplant.* 2003; 17:503-510.
33. National Organ Transplantation Act. Public Health Service Act. 1984. Available at: http://www.hpolicy.duke.edu/cyberexchange/Regulate/CHSR/HTMLs/F8-National%20Organ%20Transplant%20Act.htm Accessed May 30, 2006.
34. Delmonico FL, Arnold R, Scheper-Hughes N, Siminoff LA, Kahn J, Youngner SJ. Ethical incentives—not Payment—for organ donation. *N Engl J Med.* 2002; 346:2002-2005.
35. Dossetor JB. Financial and other incentives in post-mortem and living donor organ transplantation—Which are ethically acceptable? In: Gutmann T, Daar AS, Sells RA, Land W, eds. *Ethical, Legal, and Social Issues in Organ Transplantation.* Lengerich, Germany: Pabt Science Publishers; 2004:318-28.
36. Thiel G. Financial temptations for and against live organ donations. In: Gutmann T, Daar AS, Sells RA, Land W, eds. *Ethical, Legal, and Social Issues in Organ Transplantation.* Lengerich, Germany: Pabt Science Publishers; 2004:182-190.

Living Lobar Lung Transplant Donors

Ann M. Doyle, RN, CCRC

History and Introduction

In 1990 the first living donor lung transplant (LDLT) was performed at Stanford University by Vaughn Starnes, MD and colleagues. The first to receive this type of transplant were neonatal/pediatric patients. This has now evolved and expanded to selected patients with rapidly progressive illnesses such as cystic fibrosis and pulmonary hypertension. As recipient lists for patients in need of lung transplantation continue to grow, donor availability remains static. The end result is that many patients with end-stage pulmonary disease due to cystic fibrosis will die while waiting for lungs. Evidence suggests that lobar transplantation is technically feasible and can provide adequate pulmonary function in selected patients.[1,2]

The number of transplants performed can be dependant on variables such as staffing, operating room availability, and can vary from center to center. Not all programs are able to support a specific, separate coordinator as a donor advocate. The recipients in the Washington University living donor program are pediatric, adolescent and young adults and are under the care and evaluation of the pediatric transplant team. The Washington University program provides for a separate donor evaluation with a coordinator to act as an advocate to screen and evaluate adult donors with an independent team. This adult team is not involved with the recipient's health care, decisions, family conferences or medical treatment. We feel this provides an important marker, a confidential place for potential donors to withdraw their consent, despite their relationship to the recipient or family.

Selection Criteria/Screening Phase

The initial contact is made by the recipient's care team with the family and when appropriate, the recipient. This option is discussed with family during the transplant referral evaluation process. The family is given written information about the generalities of the living donor process, dates, time involved, costs etc. The family, not the transplant center or coordinator, is responsible for identifying potential donors to be screened. Families generally resist early referral to living donation. Many families struggle with the emotional burden of asking another family member, neighbor or stranger to become a donor for their child or loved one. This decision can lead to poor outcome and survival when the recipient rapidly deteriorates and donors have not been identified.[3]

There are general considerations when deciding on living donor transplant. This kind of program places more demand on resources. The surgery involves 3 surgeons and OR staff in the same location or in close proximity. Testing is performed so that resources are best utilized. For instance, the most expensive or consuming tests are placed later in the evaluation process.

There are psychosocial issues that need to be dealt with on an ongoing basis. Most frequently recipients carry the diagnosis of Cystic Fibrosis (CF). There is a high mortality rate of 10%-20% 'while waiting' for cadaver organs; these numbers are published on the waitlist by the Organ Procurement and Transplant Network (OPTN). Families are devoted to the care of the affected individual and the opportunity for 'further heroic action' may be more appealing.

There are timing issues that depend a great deal on the condition of the recipient. Experience has shown improved outcomes when a preference of LDLT is performed before frank respiratory failure occurs.[2] As previously stated, CF is not a disease with a predictable clinical scenario and many times a patient can have a rapid progression of disease. Therefore, the goal is to initiate the referrals as soon as transplant is discussed while the individual is still at a baseline level of functioning and not in a critical or decompensated state.

There are ethical issues to consider, as well. As a foundation for living donor transplant, a biologic relationship was required. Empiric evidence suggests marginal advantage beyond human leukocyte antigen (HLA) identical twins. We have used a variety of family members and also unrelated/no prior relationship donors.

The issue of motivation being altruistic and clear should be closely examined by the adult team. Most times if compatible, the parents are the first to respond. Careful consideration must be given to parents as they tend to be extremely enthusiastic about doing anything to help their child without consideration to the potential poor outcomes for the recipient and /or donor. A discussion with the parents is important regarding some benefit to the child by avoiding having both parents as donors, so that one may be available during the critical early days of recovery. Many times this is left to other family members such as grandparents or aunts and uncles. During this crucial time it can be of benefit to have one parent at the bedside.

Many times the family has to go outside of their immediate familial circle and look elsewhere such as church, hometown, workplace and media outlet. Donors without medical or life insurance are strongly encouraged to obtain adequate coverage prior to being screened. Non-coverage does not eliminate the potential donor, but the implications must be made clear. When donors return home, they are then under the care of their local physician / healthcare system and can experience post-operative complications requiring additional testing or interventions that are not covered by the recipient's insurance coverage. The donors then become financially responsible for their healthcare.

The disproportionate risks and benefits should be examined and discussed with the family and potential donors. The principal risk is borne by the donor and the main benefit goes to the recipient. An emotional relationship with the recipient can maximize the psychological benefit for the donor and can be justifiable.

The recipient's family is given 1 page 'donor information forms'. These forms are given to all potential donors and contain general information including demographics, relationship to recipient, medical history including blood type, height and weight, surgical history, smoking status, any medications, marital status, children and ages. The recipient family has no responsibility other than to give the form to those who may inquire. Information about the procedure, process, and commitment is the responsibility of the living donor coordinator. This can take some of the burden or guilt from the family. This form is faxed or mailed to the living donor coordinator for review. Table 1 is an example of a screening assessment tool for living donors.

Table 1. DONOR CONSIDERATIONS FOR SCREENING

AGE	Minimum age for donation is 18 years old. As a guideline, the maximum age for donation is 55, however our oldest donor was a healthy father at age 59
ABO Compatible	Donors must be same blood type or compatible; confirmation documented prior to evaluation
Non-Smoker	Former smokers can be considered with <20pk/year history and must have quit for at least 5 years prior to evaluation
Height & Weight	Donors must be at least 4 inches taller than the recipient; weight cannot exceed 20% over ideal body weight
Marital Status	Single parents and mothers of young children are excluded
Thoracic Surgery	Potential donors are not suitable if they have had any previous thoracic surgery, trauma or infection on donor side; previous organ donors are excluded
Medications	Certain medications and conditions may exclude donors
Biologic Relationship	We prefer to evaluate donors with a previous relationship with the recipient/family, but an unrelated donor with no prior relationship can still be considered

Potential donors need to be in a healthy state with no significant co-morbidities. Once the adult team receives the donor form and reviews it, the potential donor should be contacted to confirm the information that was provided is accurate and to further explore the medical / surgical history with intentional questioning. Every attempt should be made to get a concise picture of the health and psychological status of the individual and to determine suitability. This needs to be an objective assessment despite the donor's commitment to donate.

Educating Potential Donors to Ensure an Informed Decision

The initial contact / discussion with the potential donor should include an overall introduction to the process, the surgeons, the medical team, recipient coordinators and the role of the donor coordinator or advocate. Question the candidate regarding how they came to find out about the need. This can identify possible coercion by the family, as some families can be aggressive. Take the opportunity to assess what the candidate knows about the process/procedure and assure the candidate that the information shared is confidential, and will not be shared with the recipient family. The potential donors need to be informed of the practical considerations such as time off work, travel, recovery and financial responsibility.

The basic physiology of the lungs is explained in terms the candidate understands; the surgery is a lobectomy not a pneumonectomy and donation is one lobe per donor. One donor provides a right lower lobe and one donor provides a left lower lobe. A brief discussion of the recipient's disease needs to be included. A misconception of potential donors is a belief that the transplant will always cure the disease. A statement to clarify that the lung does not regenerate and the donor has the potential to lose 15-20% lung function after surgery should be disclosed.[6] A candid discussion of the survival rates, morbidity and mortality of recipients and donors should always be included so the candidate can be more informed regarding the risk/ benefit for them.

The donors are given time to reconsider their decision and consult with their family and friends about proceeding to the evaluation phase. To avoid being perceived as recruiting, the donor advocate should allow the potential donor to contact the site for confirmation of the wish to proceed and/ or clarify any concerns and ask further questions. Refer to figure 1.

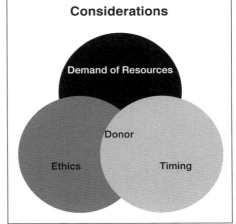

Figure 1. Demonstrates the complicated nature of the decision process.

Evaluation Phase

Once the potential donor has been identified as suitable for evaluation, the following tests and procedures will be scheduled in a 2-3 day period at the transplant center. If the donor must travel, arrangements need to be made for arrival the day prior to the evaluation visit. Each potential donor undergoes diagnostic testing including complete pulmonary function test (PFT) with arterial blood gas (ABG), if the donor is over the age of 45, an echocardiogram; radiological testing including standard chest x-ray PA and lateral and ventilation-perfusion scan (V-Q) which can identify any abnormalities not detected by radiographic findings is done. Laboratory testing includes comprehensive metabolic and electrolyte panel, IgE and IgG immunoglobulin, rapid plasma regain (RPR), acute hepatitis panel, complete blood count with differential, coagulation studies, type and screen, serologies human immunodeficiency virus (HIV), Epstein-Barr Virus (EBV), cytomegalovirus (CMV), and human chorionic gonadotropin (HCG) if the donor is a female of child bearing potential. An HLA is performed after the donors have been identified.

All donors undergo a formal psychological evaluation and testing. The final component is the medical evaluation with the pulmonary and/or cardio-thoracic physicians. This will include a review of the testing, a complete history and physical exam, and a repeated explanation of risks and benefits of this type of donation and the ability to confidentially withdraw. If any abnormality is found, further follow-up testing should be obtained at the transplant site, depending on time, or in the donor's home area.

The reason a donor withdraws or is excluded from evaluation should be kept confidential. The donor advocate protects the donor from any possible recrimination or personal guilt from the potential recipient and family.

Surgical considerations are discussed individually during the clinic visit. By using donors 4 inches or greater than the height of the recipient brings a variety of choices. Typically the shorter donor is identified as the left donor, as the left lower lobe is larger than the right, consequently the taller donor is identified as the right donor. This decision is based on lung mass and size matching to the recipient. Another consideration is the donor's 'handedness'. This however, is not a determining factor for candidacy.

All donor PFT's must have a forced expired volume, 1 second (FEV1) result >85% predicted. The ideal donor has a high FEV1 (> 92%) pre-operatively with the consideration of a 15-20% loss. Considering this, the individual with an FEV1 of 80% will have a post-op FEV1 of a marginal 60%.

The psychological evaluation is an opportunity for the potential donor to discuss with an objective professional, their motivation and their understanding of poor outcomes as well as their coping skills, detection of any underlying psychological conditions and a Mini Mental State Examination.

The anticipation for the donors is that the reviews of the examinations reveal nothing out of the normal ranges, that the donors are fit and the risk to them is kept to a minimum. Once the evaluation is completed, the donors return home for a 48-hour cooling-off period to reflect on their decision and possibly withdraw.[7,8,9,11]

The decision to become a donor can be difficult and traumatic. The more information that is given to the potential donors the easier it is to make an informed decision either for donation or against. Families need to feel supported and made comfortable with their decisions of who donates and who stays at the bedside during the critical post-operative period.

The education of the donors is a constant evolving process of repetition, reinforcement and support. The donors are healthy, so discussions of disease, therapies and treatments are usually directed to the recipient's disease process.

Confirmation of the donor's ability to withdraw their consent is reinforced throughout the process. As the donor's knowledge base expands, more details are added and the donor's questions and comments become more relevant and insightful.

Surgical Procedure

The ultimate decision regarding timing of transplant is guided by the condition of the recipient and the assessment of the pediatric team. The date for transplant may be indefinite. One of the advantages to living donor transplantation is the ability to plan the surgery in advance, becoming an elective vs. emergent procedure. Another advantage is the short ischemic time from procurement to transplantation. Once the date for transplant is determined, the donors need to be at the transplant site 2 days prior to the set date. During this time the donors meet with the surgeons, giving the donor opportunity for questions regarding the details of the specific procedure, surgical risks and complications to anesthesia. Potential donors are made aware that there may be unknown long-term risks due to lack of data. These unknown risks may impact on their future health. Donors undergo a standard pre operative evaluation including but not limited to, lab work, chest x-ray and electrocardiogram (ECG). This also allows for any follow-up testing that may be required. A tour of the pre and post-operative areas is given to the donor and families.

The thoracotomy lobectomy surgical procedure for each donor takes about 2-3 hours with no complications. Lumbar epidural catheters are placed routinely. The pulmonary resection is completed and the thoracotomy is closed in a standard manner after placement of two chest tubes. The patients are extubated in the operating room prior to transfer to the post-anesthesia care unit. Median length of stay in the hospital is 5 days.[10]

Follow-up Care

Donors are requested to stay at the transplant site up to an additional 7 days for a post operative visit with the surgeon for an inspection of the surgical incision and a repeat chest x-ray is done to confirm a fully expanded lung on the affected side. Donors are assessed for signs or symptoms of an infection and are provided with instructions for resuming regular activities or work. Most donors require a 4-6 week recuperation period prior to resuming regular activities.

Once the donors return home, we request a follow-up PFT, chest x-ray in 3-6 months and, if not performed at our site that the results are forwarded to us. Many donors live far away from the transplant center and are reluctant to return for routine follow-up evaluation. The compliance with this is, at times, determined by the outcome of the recipient transplant. Compliance tends to be better if the outcome is good for the recipient.[12] If the donor(s) is a family member, follow-up tends to be better as the recipient is at the transplant center/ area for at least 3 months postoperatively in rehabilitation.

The Washington University program makes an attempt to contact donors at yearly intervals to inquire about their health, problems and perceptions regarding donation.

Outcomes for Donors

Short- term complications tend to be surgery related. The complications can be post operative hemorrhage, airway complications including bronchial fistula stump and bronchial stricture, pleural effusions, phrenic nerve paralysis, dysrhythmias, pneumonia and atelectasis, pericarditis and the most common noted are persistent air leaks. Donors report persistent non-productive cough with resolution involving no treatment. The resolution times can be as prolonged as 4-6 months after surgery.[10] Other miscellaneous complications occur, such as ileus from narcotic administration, urinary tract infection, subcutaneous emphysema or contact dermatitis secondary to adhesive tape. Some of these complications may evolve into long term conditions and require subsequent intervention as medically directed.

The psychological effects of donation are harder to track due to the small numbers of living lobar donors. Donors and recipients are best situated to appraise the risks and benefits and for the donor the physical risk is balanced against the psychological benefit. There is always the potential for the donor to struggle with the phenomenon of cognitive dissonance, meaning the donor has conflicting thoughts or beliefs about what they are doing (altruistic donation or gift) as opposed to the outcomes (recipient death or donor complications) they experience. Interestingly, most donors, when questioned, would donate again.

Donors often reported a heightened feeling of well-being in connection with a successful transplantation for the recipient.[11] Data shows that donation includes a moderate psychosocial impact on the donor that appears to strengthen the bond between donor and recipient.

Prior to surgery donors scored their quality of life (QoL) better than the general public. Six months after living donor transplant, they rated the domains of 'physical health' and 'living conditions' significantly lower than prior to surgery; however, the QoL scores remained higher than the general population.[13,14]

The overall impression is that the short term as well as the long term donor risk is rather small and that the positive aspects associated with the donation dominate.

Conclusion

Living donation presents a viable option for motivated donors. Donors can be blood related, with an emotional relationship and even unrelated donors and should be allowed to donate, provided that they are carefully screened, evaluated and informed. On the basis of present findings, routines should be established by the transplant center to maintain contact with the donors after transplant for post-operative follow-up, including any complications and psychological support.[15,16]

References

1. Barr ML, Schenkel FA, Cohen RG, Barbers RG, Fuller CB, Hagen AJ, Wells WJ, Starnes VA: Recipient and donor outcomes in living related and unrelated lobar transplantation. *Transplantation Proceedings.* 1998;30:2261-2263
2. Starnes VA, Bowdish ME, Woo MS et al; A decade of living lobar lung transplantation: recipient outcomes. *J Thorac Cardiovasc Surg.* 2004;127:114-122
3. Bowdish ME, Barr ML, Starnes VA: Living lobar transplantation. *Chest Surg N Am.* 2003;13:505-524
4. Burroughs TE, Hong BA, Kappel DF, Freedman BK; The stability of family decisions to consent or refuse organ donation. *Psychosomatic Medicine.* 1998;60:156-162
5. Mallory GB, Cohen AH; Donor considerations in living-related donor lung transplantation. *Clinics in Chest Medicine.* 1997;18:239-243
6. Sritippayawan S, Keena TG, Horn MV, MacLaughlin EF, Barr ML, Starnes VA, Woo MS; Does lung growth occur when mature lobes are transplanted into children? *Pediatric Transplantation.* 2002;6:500-504
7. Shaw, LR, Miller JD, Slutsky AS, Maurer JR, Puskas JD, Patterson GA, Singer PA; Ethics of lung transplantation with live donors. *The Lancet.* 1991;338:678-681
8. Reyes-Acevedo R Ethics in organ transplantation; continuous search for defining what is acceptable. *Rev Invest Clin.* 2005;2:177-186
9. Hilhorst MT, Directed altruistic living organ donation: partial but not unfair. *Ethical Theory Moral Practice.* 2005; 8:197-215
10. Battafarano RJ, Anderson RC, Myers BF, Gutherie TJ, Cooper JD, Patterson GA; Perioperative complications after living donor lobectomy. *J Thorac Cardiovasc Surg.* 2000;5:909-915
11. Wells WJ, Barr ML; The ethics of living donor lung transplantation. *Thorac Surg Clin.* 2005;4:519-525
12. Heck G, Schweitzer J, Seidel-Weisel M; Psychological effects of living related kidney transplantation- risks and chances. *Clinical Transplantation.* 2004;18:716-723
13. Walter M, Dammann G, Papachristou C, pascher A, Neuhaus P, Danzer G, Klapp BF; Quality of life of living donors before and after living donor liver transplantation. *Transplant Proc.* 2003;35: 961-2963
14. Johnson EM, Anderson JK, Jacobs et al; Long term follow-up of living kidney donors; quality of life after donation. *Transplantation.* 1999;67:717-725
15. Kozower BD, Sweet SC, de la Morena M, Schuler P, Gutherie TJ, Patterson GA, Gandi SK, Huddleston CB; Living donor lobar grafts improve pediatric lung retransplantation survival. *J Thorac Cardiovasc Surg.* 2006;9:1142-1147
16. Barr ML, Schenkel FA, Bowdish ME, Starnes VA; Living donor lung transplantation: current status and future directions. *Transplant Proc.* 2005;9:3983-3986

Living Kidney Donors

Catherine A. Garvey, RN, BA, CCTC

Introduction

Kidney transplantations using living donors have been performed for 50 years. The first kidney transplantation using a living donor was performed in Boston in 1954 with twin brothers. The success of that kidney transplantation allowed physicians and scientists to continue to refine kidney transplantation for both recipients and living donors. In 2004, more than 16, 000 kidney transplantations, greater than 6000 of which involved living donors, were performed in the United States at more than 200 transplant centers.[1]

Kidney transplantation is the standard of care for patients with end-stage renal disease, and the transplantations performed using living donors provide the best long-term outcome for these patients. Currently, the biggest challenge in the field of transplantation is the lack of donor organs for the many people who need transplants. Increasingly, living donors have been used, especially in kidney transplantation. Many transplant centers have performed living donor kidney transplants and have a long experience in evaluation of and surgery for kidney donors.

In previous years, biologically related family members were viewed as the preferred organ donors. However, since the introduction of more potent immunosuppressive medications, the match between a donor and recipient has become less important. Potential living kidney donors now include spouses, friends, acquaintances, and coworkers. Some donors offer to donate to a particular recipient because they are members of the same church, social club, or association. A small number of centers now allow nondirected kidney donation, in which a person volunteers to donate to anyone awaiting a kidney transplant.[2,3] With the success of kidney transplantation and the fact that there are a growing number of possible recipients and not enough deceased donor organs, more transplant centers are offering and promoting living kidney donation. In 2001, for the first time ever, the number of living kidney donors outnumbered the number of deceased donors.

Living kidney donation must be a well-considered decision by the donor, recipient, and transplant center, as living donors receive no physical benefit from the procedure and yet they assume the risks of the surgery and general anesthesia.

Selection Criteria

Any healthy person between the ages of 18 and 70 years old may be considered as a kidney donor. It is possible for donors to be older than 70, but each of these donors must be evaluated on an individual basis. Prospective kidney donors must be in good health and understand the risks of undergoing a surgery that is not indicated for their physical benefit. Because organ transplantation and organ donation in the United States are based on altruism, the offer to donate must be made without expectation of any reward, financial or otherwise.

Contraindications to Donation

Living kidney donors must be in excellent health. Contraindications to becoming a kidney donor are listed in Table 1. Medical issues that prevent a person from becoming a donor include kidney disease or a family history of kidney disease, especially diseases with a strong genetic link such as polycystic kidney disease, Alport's syndrome, and diabetes mellitus. Other medical problems such as heart, lung, and liver disease also prevent donation. Donors are screened for viral infections and, despite treatment and a donor's absence of disease, positive results will rule out donation because of the risk of transmission with the donated kidney. Alcohol and substance use and dependence as well as psychosocial reasons for denying a donor must be investigated carefully, as these issues may not be obvious or shared at the first offer of donation.

Table 1. KIDNEY DONOR EXCLUSION CRITERIA

- Uncontrolled Hypertension
- Diabetes mellitus
- HIV or history of HIV high-risk behaviors
- Viral infections (e.g., hepatitis B or C, Lyme disease)
- History of recurrent kidney stones
- History of thrombosis or thromboembolism
- History of malignancy/cancer (exception: skin cancer)
- Heart and lung disease requiring medications
- Obesity (body mass index greater than 30)
- Proteinuria or microalbuminuria
- Low glomerular filtration rate (less than 80 mL/min)
- Active alcohol or substance abuse
- Current psychiatric illness, unstable psychosocial situation or impaired mental status that may influence judgment or compromise recovery
- Inappropriate motivations for donation

Recently, a small number of transplant programs began considering people with hypertension as possible kidney donors. Some programs have created definitions of levels of acceptable hypertension for certain age groups but are committed to doing long-term follow up on these donors.[4] Mortality due to kidney donation is low at 0.03%,[5] with the most frequent cause of mortality being pulmonary embolus. Donors with a history of thrombosis are considered to be at higher risk and should not donate. In addition, certain anatomical abnormalities (most commonly, multiple renal arteries) prevent a potential donor from donating an organ; these abnormalities may not be discovered until the potential donor undergoes a medical evaluation.

Evaluation of Living Donors

The first phase of donor evaluation is screening by the transplant center. Anyone interested in becoming a living donor must initiate contact with the transplant center. The donor is screened for obvious contraindications and is provided with educational materials describing the process, surgery, hospitalization, and recovery. Ideally, this screening is performed by a clinical transplant coordinator who is dedicated to the care of the living donor. Despite the need for transplant candidates, it is vital to ensure the well-being of potential living donors throughout the process of evaluation and surgery. Guidelines for the care of living organ donors have been issued by many healthcare practitioners in the transplant field and by professional societies, including the National Kidney Foundation, and the American Society of Transplantation.[1,6]

The next step in the screening process is a blood sample to determine donor and recipient compatibility. This includes ABO and immunologic compatibility, including crossmatch and tissue typing. This testing is usually performed at the intended recipient's transplant center. Often, multiple donors have offered to be considered, which means there may be more than one compatible donor. If no clear medical reason exists for choosing one potential donor instead of another, the donors decide among themselves who will go forward with the full medical evaluation. The transplant center and the clinical transplant coordinator are often called upon to assist potential donors in this decision-making process.

The full medical evaluation of a potential kidney donor is directed by the transplant center where the transplant surgery will be performed, as this allows the donor to meet the team and become familiar with the facility and caregivers. If distance from the donor's residence to the center is an issue, most centers arrange for evaluation testing to be performed where the donor is located. The cost of the donor evaluation is borne by the transplant center and recovered after the transplant surgery is performed. The recipient's medical insurance provider builds the cost of the donor evaluation into the coverage for the transplant surgery. It is reasonable to proceed through the evaluation performing the least invasive and least costly tests first. This insures that the donor does not undergo invasive tests unnecessarily and helps the transplant center control costs. It may be necessary to perform medical evaluations on multiple people before an appropriate donor is identified; of course, performing the evaluation on one person limits unnecessary testing and helps control costs.

Medical Evaluation

Once compatibility has been determined, the identified donor begins the medical and psychosocial evaluation tests (Table 2). Transplant centers may perform these tests in different sequences or change the order of the parts of the evaluation based on a particular donor situation. The evaluations should be performed by a medical team not involved in the intended recipient's care. Ideally, a medical team is dedicated to the evaluation, care, and follow up of living donors and collaborates in determining the suitability of the living kidney donor.[7]

Laboratory Testing

In addition to a thorough medical and family history and a complete physical examination, a potential donor undergoes laboratory testing, diagnostic studies, and consults with members of the donor team.

Routine cancer screening appropriate to age and sex of the donor should be current and normal. Results of these tests can be obtained from the donor's primary physician or performed at the time of donor evaluation.

Diagnostic Testing

Donors undergo an electrocardiogram and chest radiographs (posteroanterior and lateral) as well as visualization of renal anatomy and vasculature either by computerized tomography or magnetic resonance angiograph and urography.

Consultations

Any type of specialist can be consulted during the donor evaluation, but most donors meet with a transplant nephrologist, transplant surgeon, clinical transplant coordinator, clinical social worker, and psychologist. As the donor progresses through this evaluation, each of these consultants educates the donor about donation and the significance of the evaluation results, and any questions and issues raised by the donor or donor family are answered and addressed. These consultations provide the donor with the information needed to make a final decision about proceeding with the donation and allow the consultants time to gather information from the donor. If at any time during this evaluation the donor

Table 2.

Screening tests
- ABO Type
- Immunology testing crossmatch and HLA tissue typing

Medical tests
- Complete metabolic panel: electrolytes, blood urea nitrogen, creatinine
- Hemogram and platelet count
- Liver function and uric acid tests
- Fasting lipid levels
- International normalized ratio and partial thromboplastin time
- Viral serology for hepatitis B and C, and human immunodeficiency virus
- Rapid plasma reagin
- Urine for alb/cr ratio
- Urinalysis
- Serum pregnancy test (all females less than 55 years old)

Diagnostic tests
- Electrocardiogram
- Chest radiograph (posteroanterior and lateral)
- Computerized tomography angiogram and urography
- Complete history and physical examination

Cancer screening tests
- Pelvic examination, breast examination, and Pap smear (for women more than 18 years old)
- Mammogram (for women more than 40 years old)
- Prostate-specific antigen level (for men more than 55 years old)
- Colonoscopy/flexible sigmoidoscopy (for people more than 50 years old)

Consultations
- Transplant nephrologists
- Transplant surgeons
- Clinical psychosocial worker
- Psychologist
- Clinical transplant coordinator
- Specialists as indicated by evaluation results

expresses a hesitancy to continue, the consultant and/or team is able to stop the evaluation. The reason for not continuing with the donor evaluation is confidential, but the donor team will inform the intended recipient of the reason if that is the donor's wish.

The results of the evaluation and the consultants' findings are compiled and reviewed by all members of the team, and then a decision is made whether the donor is acceptable or not. A potential donor may express a willingness to assume a higher risk than the transplant team recommends, and this should be discussed. Usually, a mutually acceptable decision is reached.

Psychosocial Evaluation

A potential donor will meet with a clinical social worker for a confidential interview. In this interview, information about the donor's motivation for wanting to donate an organ, psychological status, and current life situation will be examined. This information helps the donor team assess the circumstances that prompted the donor to volunteer to donate. The decision to donate must be made freely by the donor and to obtain informed consent, the donor must demonstrate an understanding of the risks and possible complications of donation. The interview allows the team to help the donor make a plan for surgery and recovery. Issues that are addressed during the interview include financial ramifications, family situation, and donor support system. Potential donors and their medical insurance providers are not financially responsible for costs related to the evaluation, surgery, or hospitalization. Financial costs related to travel and lodging at the time of evaluation and surgery as well as costs related to lost wages during the donor's recovery are the responsibility of the donor. Some donors may have disability insurance or some type of paid time off from his or her employer. Some private employers and individual state employers are now providing paid time off to living organ donors based on the federal government's policy of 30 days paid time off for federal employees for organ donation, but this varies and must be discussed with each potential donor. There are also some transplant programs that have some funds available to assist donors.

Educational Needs: Donor and Family

Transplant programs are obligated to educate potential donors about kidney donation and transplantation (Table 3). Transplant centers are required to provide donors with information on the timing and process of becoming a donor and the risks and possible complications of donor nephrectomy, as well as other treatments and therapies that are available to the intended recipient. Centers fulfill this requirement with the use of written materials, videotapes, and DVDs. Transplant centers can also provide names of previous kidney donors who have volunteered to speak with people considering donation. Many professional societies and transplant organizations, as well as the US government, have developed different types of readily available educational materials. The Internet is an excellent source of information and has become widely used; however, potential donors should be cautious about accepting this information as the only source of information.

Table 3. DONOR EDUCATION TOPICS

- Evaluation process and timing
- Surgical risks
- Surgical complications
- Recovery period, postoperative follow up, and lifting restrictions
- Effect on family
- Financial issues
- Alternative treatment available to recipient
- Expected outcome for recipient, complications, and postoperative follow up

In some centers, the clinical transplant coordinator may assume the role of donor advocate or participate on the team that functions as advocate for the potential donor. Donor advocacy has become more widely discussed and recommended because of increased living donation of kidneys as well as livers and lungs. The donor advocate is responsible for ensuring that each living donor's interests are foremost as the donor makes decisions regarding whether to proceed as a donor and the medical team decides whether to accept an individual donor.[6] The topic of donor advocacy is covered in greater detail in another chapter.

Surgical Considerations

The mortality and morbidity risks of donor nephrectomy are low. The two main ways that a kidney can be removed are an open surgery using a flank incision and laparoscopic surgery. Since the early 1990s when laparoscopic donor nephrectomy was introduced, most transplant centers use the laparoscopic approach because of its benefits to the donor. The operative field for performing a hand assisted laparoscopic nephrectomy is seen in Figure 1. In a study by Wolf and colleagues,[13] donors who underwent laparoscopic nephrectomy reported that they returned to normal activities and used fewer pain medications compared with donors who had an open nephrectomy. Nephrectomy can be performed via pure laparoscopy or hand-assisted laparoscopy. A healed incision from a hand assisted laparoscopic donor nephrectomy is seen in Figure 2. Transplant centers surveyed in 2001 after the introduction of laparoscopic nephrectomy confirmed that mortality associated with donor nephrectomy remains at 0.03%. Complications occur in fewer than 1% of all donors, rates unchanged from when most donor nephrectomies were performed using the traditional open approach.[5]

Laparoscopic donor surgery usually takes 3 to 4 hours and can be performed in an operating room adjacent to the room where the recipient is located. Some centers use one operating room, performing the donor nephrectomy first and then performing the recipient's surgery.

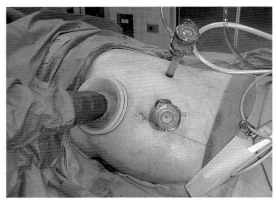

Figure 1. Photograph of the operative field for hand assisted laparoscopic nephrectomy.

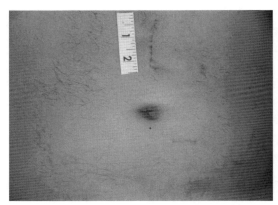

Figure 2. Photograph of a healed incision after laparoscopic donor nephrectomy.

Hospitalization, Restrictions, and Activities

Donors undergo preoperative testing and pre-operative instructions before transplantation. The instructions include an explanation of what to expect while hospitalized including pain management. The testing includes current laboratory tests and radiography as well as a final immunologic crossmatch to verify compatibility and is usually performed several days before the surgery. During the preoperative visit, donors also may meet with anesthesiologists, sign consent forms, and obtains instructions about surgical scrubs and bowel preparation.

Donors are admitted to the hospital on the same day as the surgery and are usually hospitalized for 2 to 4 days. Postoperative care for donors can be provided on the transplant ward or a general surgery ward and can vary at different transplant programs. Donors return to the general floor unit with a catheter, and intravenous access for fluid replacement, and pain control measures. Many centers use patient-controlled analgesia pumps for postoperative pain control. Postoperative complications include all the risks of general surgery and therefore precautions are taken to prevent the risk of pneumonia, thrombosis, and infection. Once bowel function returns and donors are able to ingest food and fluids by mouth, they can be discharged. All donors, whether they undergo open or laparoscopic surgery, have a lifting restriction of 10 or fewer pounds for 6 weeks after surgery. The recovery period varies among donors. Job duties may dictate the recovery time, but most donors will need assistance once they are home and should refrain from driving for a period of time, especially when still taking pain medications.

Donors should see their physicians for any problem and also should have scheduled follow-up clinic appointments. The timing of these follow-up appointments can be center specific but should include an early visit to evaluate the incision site, pain control, and bowel function as well as a later visit to assess kidney function. Long-term donor follow up is now being promoted as necessary to ensure that there is information on long-term outcome for living kidney donors. United Network for Organ Sharing regulations require information on kidney donors for one year postoperatively, and many transplant programs are initiating or developing long-term donor studies to obtain information on donor outcomes.

Outcomes of Donors

Problems that can occur in the immediate postoperative period include bleeding, infection, nausea, and bowel problems (Table 4). Pain control is usually achieved, but some donors may experience nerve pain or numbness or pain and/or injuries from positioning on the operating room table. Occasionally, a patient may have referred shoulder pain from retained carbon dioxide used during a laparoscopic nephrectomy. Gastrointestinal complaints are the most common and include nausea, vomiting, and constipation. Bowel obstruction is possible and has been reported after both laparoscopic and open nephrectomy. Most often, these problems are time limited but may require additional outpatient visits and treatment by the center after surgery. When donors are discharged, they are reminded to maintain regular medical care as appropriate for their age and health history.

Long-term problems that can occur include incisional hernia and risk of living with a solitary kidney. Donors are at risk if they develop kidney stones and associated infection in their remaining kidney. A solitary kidney can cease to function or be damaged due to trauma, renal cell cancer, or other causes, leaving the donor with no kidney. These risks are not increased in the donor population but must be explained to the donor during the evaluation.[5,15] A very small number of kidney donors develop kidney disease and receive a kidney transplant due to end-stage kidney disease. According to data from the United Network of Organ Sharing, about 100 previous kidney donors have been listed for kidney transplant.[1,17]

The psychological effects of kidney donation and donor quality of life have been examined retrospectively by surveying previous kidney donors. Most donors report that the donation was a positive experience, that they have experienced an increased feeling of self-esteem, and that they would make the decision to donate again.[10]

Donors can be negatively affected by the donation if they experience complications and if their recipient's outcome after transplantation is not what was expected. A few donors report mild depressive symptoms and a feeling of being ignored or forgotten after the surgery. These problems usually subside as

Table 4. COMPLICATIONS OF DONOR NEPHRECTOMY

Short-term complications
- Infection
- Urinary tract infection
- Pneumonia
- Deep vein thrombosis
- Pain
- Numbness
- Diarrhea, constipation, ileus, and bowel obstruction

Long-term complications
- Hernia
- Bowel obstruction
- Trauma or disease affecting one kidney

donors recover, but they should be reminded that the transplant donor social worker and donor team are available if the donors experience emotional distress.[11,12]

In the past few years, transplant programs have developed methods for recognizing the great gift that all living donors make. To recognize and thank these donors, some centers organize receptions and dinners, award pins or certificates, and provide small gifts or flowers. These efforts could help prevent the feelings of letdown reported by some donors. Donors should also be instructed to contact the transplant center with any issues or questions after donation.

References

1. United Network for Organ Sharing. Transplants by Donor Type, Center. Available at:http://www.optn.org/latestData/rptData.asp Accessed May 14, 2006.
2. Matas AJ, Garvey CA, Jacobs CL, Kahn JP. Nondirected donation of kidneys from living donors. *N Engl J Med.* 2000;343:433-436.
3. Gilbert JC, Brigham L, Batty DS Jr, Veatch RM. The nondirected living donor program: a model for cooperative donation, recovery and allocation of living donor kidneys. *Am J Transplant.* 2005;5:167-174.
4. Textor S, Taler S, Larson TS, et al. Blood pressure evaluation among older kidney donors. *J Am Soc Nephrol.* 2003;14:2159-2167.
5. Matas AJ, Bartlett AT, Leichtman AB, Delmonico F. Morbidity and mortality after living kidney donation in 1999-2001: a survey of United States transplant centers. *Am J Transplant.* 2003;3:830-834.
6. New York State Transplant Council. Report of the Committee on Quality Improvement in Living Liver Donation. Available at http://www.health.state.ny.us. Accessed May 14, 2006
7. Abecassis M, Adams M, Adams P, et al, for Live Organ Donor Consensus Group. Consensus statement on the live organ donor. *JAMA.* 2000;284:2919-2926.
8. Spital A, Spital M. Living kidney donation: attitudes outside the transplant center. *Arch Intern Med.* 1988;148:1077-1080.
9. Adams PL, Cohen DJ, Danovitch GM, et al. The nondirected live-kidney donor: ethical considerations and practice guidelines: A National Conference Report. *Transplantation.* 2002;74:582-589.
10. Johnson EM, Anderson JK, Jacobs CJ, et al. Long-term follow-up of living kidney donors: quality of life after donation. *Transplantation.* 1999;67:717-721.
11. Jacobs C, Johnson E, Anderson K, Gillingham K, Matas A. Kidney transplants from living donors: how donation affects family dynamics. *Adv Ren Replace Ther.* 1998;5:89-97.
12. de Graaf Olson W, Bogetti-Dumlao A. Living donors; perception of their quality of health after donation. *Prog Transplant.* 2001;11:108-115.
13. Wolf JS Jr, Merion RM, Leichtman AB, et al. Randomizedcontrolled trial of hand-assisted laparoscopic versus open surgical live donor nephrectomy. *Transplantation.* 2001;72:284-290.
14. Najarian JS, Chavers BM, McHugh LE, Matas AJ. 20 years or more of follow up of living kidney donors. *Lancet.* 1992;340:807-810.
15. Johnson EM, Remucal MJ, Gillingham KJ, Dahms RA, Najarian JS, Matas AJ. Complications and risks of living donor nephrectomy. *Transplantation.* 1997;64:1124-1128.
16. Spital A. Life insurance for kidney donors–an update. *Transplantation.* 1988;45:819-820.
17. Ellison MD, McBride MA, Taranto SE, Delmonico FL, Kauffman HM. Living kidney donors in need of kidney transplants: a report from the organ procurement and transplantation network. *Transplantation.* 2002;74:1349-1351.
18. Davis CL . Evaluation of the living kidney donor: current perspectives. *Am J Transplant.* 2004;43:508-530.
19. Kasiske B, Ravenscraft M, Ramos EL, Gaston RS, Bia MJ, Danovitch GM. The evaluation of living renal transplant donors: clinical practice guidelines. *J Am Soc Nephrol.* 1996;7:2288-2313.
20. Asolati M, Matas A . Risks versus benefits of living kidney donation. *Curr Opin Organ Transplant.* 2003;8:155-159.
21. Gritsch HA, Rosenthal, JT, Danovitch,GM. Living and cadaveric kidney donation. In: Danovitch G, ed. *Handbook of Kidney Transplantation.* 3rd ed. Philadelphia, Pa: Lippincott 2201.

The Living Liver Donor

Dianne LaPointe Rudow, DrNP, CCTC

Introduction and History of Living Donor Liver Transplantation

The high mortality rate for patients on the liver transplant waiting list has led to the use of living donors to expand the donor pool. Pioneers in the field first used living donor liver transplantation (LDLT) in the late 1980s to alleviate the long waiting times for pediatric liver transplant candidates[1] and today the procedure is routinely considered for this patient population. Typically, the left lateral segment of the donor liver is used for the pediatric transplant recipient. Outcomes are excellent and donor morbidity and mortality are low.[1]

In 1997, the first adult-to-adult living donor liver transplantation (aLDLT), using the right lobe of the liver, was performed in the United States.[2,3] Factors that led to the demand for aLDLT included increases in (1) number of patients meeting criteria for liver transplantation, (2) rates of hepatocellular carcinoma, and (3) waiting list mortality. The progressive inequity between supply and demand motivated centers to offer aLDLT to patients; shortly thereafter, a rapidly increasing number of transplant programs began performing aLDLT. In 2001, 408 procedures were performed, with a total of 1409 by the end of 2003.[4] The evaluation process, surgical experience, and team composition vary markedly from center to center.[5,6] Initially, 49 transplant programs performed aLDLT, but this number has declined to 36 in 2003.[7]

In January 2002, a highly publicized death of a living donor resulted in scrutiny of aLDLT both from the medical community and the lay public.[8] Consequently, because of increased oversight by New York State, restrictions were imposed on centers performing aLDLT in the state until further study. In addition, New York State developed a committee that submitted a report on quality improvement in living liver donation to the New York State Department of Transplant.[9] The recommendations became regulation in New York in February 2004. The regulations require that each program have an informed consent, donor selection, and education and evaluation process centralized around an independent donor advocacy team (IDAT); specified facility support including 2 surgeons in the donor hepatectomy procedure, separate anesthesia teams, and defined nurse-to-patient ratios in the postanesthesia care unit and surgical nursing unit; and a discharge plan that includes written referrals, short- and long-term follow-up plans, and abdominal imaging after donation.

The Advisory Committee on Organ Transplantation (ACOT) has made similar recommendations on the ethics of living donation to the Department of Health and Human Services. These recommendations focused on informed consent, donor advocacy, minimum standards for transplant centers, and tracking of long-term data.[10] These changes have been developed into guidelines by the Living Donor Committee of the United Network for Organ Sharing and are being implemented by many aLDLT programs across the United States. In 2005, Center for Medicare and Medicaid has also required that transplant centers seeking Medicare approval have protocols in place for donor and recipient selection, donor evaluation, and preoperative and postoperative care and follow-up. In addition, they recommend that transplant centers follow ACOT's recommendations to ensure informed consent.[11]

Success of LDLT is primarily due to the liver's natural ability to regenerate after insult or injury, and the anatomical structure of the liver that allows for surgical division of the liver while preserving portal blood flow and biliary drainage to all segments of the liver. Regeneration occurs rapidly in both the donor and the recipient; within the first 7 days, significant regeneration has occurred.[12]

The main advantage of LDLT is that it provides immediate organ availability to those awaiting transplantation, allowing for a planned procedure that potentially avoids the progression of the recipient's liver disease. In hepatocellular cancer, the transplantation can be performed before the increase in size of the lesion outside acceptable criteria for transplantation or the threat of metastasis.[13] Additional advantages are adequate time to evaluate the donor for viruses, malignancies, and chronic health problems to ensure an optimal liver segment for transplantation, as well as a decrease in the cold ischemic time that potentially compromises posttransplant function.

Because the risk for complications is great, the main disadvantage of LDLT is the risk a healthy person must be subjected to without any personal physical gain. Early results of donor and recipient safety are favorable. To date, 2680 procedures have been performed, of which 1718 have been for adult recipients.[4] A study sponsored by the National Institutes of Health is underway to investigate adult recipient and donor outcomes (Adult to Adult Living Donor Liver Transplant Cohort Study –[A2ALL]).[14]

Living Donor Selection Criteria

The donor evaluation, ideally, needs to be performed outside the evaluation of the recipient, with a team dedicated to and released from the responsibilities of the recipient but with knowledge and expertise in LDLT. Any adult who has an emotional relationship to the recipient can be considered as a living donor. Most centers do not consider nondirected donation in liver transplantation at this time.[15] Potential donors must be between 18 to 60 years old (although this may vary from center to center), have a compatible blood type to the recipient, and be medically and psychologically well. Generally, nonemancipated minors under the age of 18 years are not candidates for donation because they are not able to freely consent to surgery. Some centers consider emancipated minors as candidates for their children who require transplantation, but not for aLDLT. Younger patients between the ages of 18 to 21 years old may be more susceptible to even subtle family coercion, especially when donating to a parent or younger sibling. Young adults often lack the maturity to grasp the scope of the risk and therefore are often declined as donors. Older adults (>60 years), on the other hand, may have comorbidities that increase their surgical risk and likelihood of exclusion. Older age may also influence regeneration and the functional reserve of the remnant liver after hepatectomy.[16] Although older age is associated with longer recovery after major abdominal surgery, there have been no data implicating donor age as an independent factor in morbidity, likely because of the careful screening that excludes individuals with underlying risk factors for surgery. Additional selection criteria are shown in Table 1.

Table 1. LIVING DONOR SELECTION CRITERIA

1. Age 18 to 60 years
2. Emotional relationship to the recipient
3. Compatible blood type
4. Absence of significant medical illness
5. Absence of liver disease
6. Absence of moderate to severe psychological disorders or active substance abuse
7. Not overweight (body mass index <35)
8. Absence of payment or material compensation
9. Absence of coercion

Contraindications to Living Donation

Donor exclusion criteria may vary between centers depending on their experience and comfort with the technical aspect of the surgeries. Potential donors may be excluded at any stage of the evaluation. Potential absolute contraindications include uncontrolled chronic medical illness, latent or chronic infection, donor and recipient size incompatibility, abnormal liver biopsy result, and unresolved psychological issues. Relative contraindications include age, obesity, smoking, hypercholesterolemia, hypertension, previous abdominal surgery, anatomical abnormalities, sole wage earner status, lack of health insurance, and substance abuse history (Table 2).[15,17,18,19] Transplant professionals must consider donors individually and evaluate each donor carefully to ensure safety.

Table 2. CONTRAINDICATIONS TO LIVING DONATION

Absolute	Relative
Uncontrolled medical Illness	Age
Latent/chronic infection	Overweight/obesity
Donor/recipient size incompatibility	Smoking
Consistent abnormal laboratory values	Previous upper abdominal surgery
Abnormal liver biopsy	Anatomic abnormality
Cancer	Sole family wage earner
Unresolved psychiatric issues	Substance abuse history
	Hypercholesterolemia
	Hypertension
	Absence of health insurance

Role of the IDAT

Many in the transplant community have suggested that transplant programs provide a donor advocate to ensure informed consent and ethical practice on behalf of the donor. An independent donor advocate is critical to provide an objective assessment of potential donors.[7,9,10,17] This person(s) is typically a hepatologist or internist not involved in the care of the recipient, a psychiatrist, or a physician outside the team; however, it can be any member of the team that is involved only in the care of the donor. The goal of the advocate is to ensure that the potential donor is informed of all risks, procedures, and alternatives.

The New York State Committee on Quality Improvement in Living Liver Donation requires that the donor advocate be a team of people (not an individual) that make up the IDAT.[9] ACOT does not make recommendations regarding a team versus individual approach, but also recommends an advocate.[10] The main role of the advocate/team is to protect the interest and well being of the donor; structure process of informed consent; discuss care with the transplant team; educate the donor about the medical, psychosocial, and financial implications of donation; explain the evaluation process; determine donor suitability; discuss formal conclusions with the donor; and ensure continuity of care.[9]

Transplant centers using the team approach include an internal medicine physician, a transplant coordinator/nurse practitioner, a medical social worker, and a psychiatrist in the team.[20] In addition, an ethicist should be available for consultation. The team may also include a hepatologist, a surgeon, and a financial coordinator. It is beneficial to use an advocate team because each member brings his or her own areas of expertise and personal experiences to the group.[20] It is important the team members understand liver disease and the transplant process so they can accurately depict the process to the donor. Roles and responsibilities need to be delineated ahead of time, so that each member knows the boundaries from which to function.

The IDAT carefully evaluates the potential donor and attempts to give the donor all the information required to make an informed choice. This information includes the evaluation process; tests required; surgical procedure; risks; benefits; psychiatric effects; financial implications; long-term outcomes; and recipient issues such as chance of survival, disease process, and alternative sources of organ allocation.[9] However, all donors are informed that if the IDAT, in collaboration with the donor surgeon, believes the donor's risk is greater than what is currently medically acceptable (most centers estimated mortality risk >~1%, although the actual mortality rate reported is lower),[6] the team will decline the donor regardless of the donor's wishes.

Evaluation of Living Liver Donors

Initial Screening

The biggest concern for living donation is coercion.[21] Coercion exists on many levels and varies from obvious coercion of a recipient to a prospective donor to the coercive nature of having a loved one sick and feeling obligated to help him or her. To prevent the perception of coercion of donors by the transplant center, once a transplant candidate is listed at a transplant center and amenable to LDLT, potential donors must make the initial contact with the center. Some centers ask the transplant candidate to sign a consent form to have donors evaluated because confidential information about the candidate's medical condition will be relayed in the donor evaluation. The transplant coordinator should speak with each interested potential donor to give a brief description of the risks and benefits of the surgery, inclusion and exclusion criteria, and medical history. This information may be enough to eliminate many donors and eliminate unnecessary evaluation with its attendant costs. At least 20% of all donors are estimated to be excluded in this initial interaction.[22] If a potential donor clears the preliminary medical questionnaire and wants to be evaluated, consent for evaluation should be signed.[10] The content of the consent document should include information to ensure that all persons understand the donation process, know they can stop at any time, and that the transplant team has a right to determine donor suitability.

Medical Evaluation

Although there is no particular order to the evaluation, the workup begins with a comprehensive history and physical examination to rule out any medical contraindications to hepatectomy or surgery in general (Table 3). The laboratory and radiological examinations usually begin from least expensive and least invasive and proceed in logical progression. Presented here is an overview of a basic evaluation. Additional tests and consults are ordered as medical history and evaluation dictate. Certain uncontrolled chronic illness or previous major abdominal surgery may increase the risk to the donor and preclude donation. Patients with a personal or family history of coronary artery disease or those older than age 50 need a more thorough cardiovascular assessment, often including an echocardiogram and stress test.

As part of the medical history, alcohol and drug use as well as sexual history (promiscuity, homosexual behavior, prostitution), tattoos, body piercing, incarceration, exposure to infectious diseases, and foreign travel help to determine potential risk of transmission of infectious disease.

A surgical evaluation is performed to identify any surgical risk that would preclude donation and allow the potential donor and his or her family the opportunity to discuss with the surgeon any questions or concerns they may have.

Laboratory Evaluation

Comprehensive laboratory testing is required to rule out medical diseases that would increase the donor's risk or make the quality of the organ less suitable (Table 3).[15,17] Detailed explanation of laboratory tests are discussed in chapter 24: Understanding Laboratory Values. A donor who is considered high risk because of social behavior may have a second set of serologies after a period of time. If a laboratory value is abnormal, it may require repeating or additional testing.

Cancer Screening

Before donation, the transplant center needs to be certain that the donor is free of malignancy. Each patient should be assessed for age-appropriate cancer risks, that is, those older than 50 years of age need a serum carcinoembryonic antigen test and colonoscopy. All female patients need to have a PAP smear performed within 1 year of donation. In addition, women 40 years of age and older require a recent mammography. Male patients should have a prostate-specific antigen test. Any suspicious skin lesions should be assessed by dermatology and biopsied accordingly. Patients with a history of cancer (except perhaps for distant history of nonmelanoma skin cancer) should be ruled out for donation.

A CLINICIAN'S GUIDE TO TRANSPLANTATION AND DONATION

Table 3. THE DONOR EVALUATION

	Universal donor	Evaluation	Center specific*

Consent process	**Consultations**
	Donor surgeon
	Hepatologist
	Nurse practitioner
	  Social work
	  Psychiatric evaluation
	  Specialist consults as needed
	  Education
	  Financial counseling
			Medical internist: independent of transplant team

	Medical evaluation *Medical history* • Family • Social *Physical examination* • Height • Weight • Vital signs		
	Laboratory evaluation *Hematology* ABO and antibody screen • Complete blood cell count with differential • Coagulation profile *Chemistry* • Basic metabolic panel • Hepatic function panel • Lipids • Thyroid function *Urine* • Urinalysis • Urine toxicology *Serologies* • Hepatitis A total, immunoglobulin M • Hepatitis C antibody • Hepatitis B core antibody • Hepatitis B surface antigen • Cytomegalovirus immunoglobulin G • Rapid plasma reagin • Human immunodeficiency virus *Other markers for liver disease* • Anti Nuclear Antibody • Iron, ferritin, iron-binding capacity • Ceruloplasm *Tumor markers* • Carcinoembryonic antigen • Prostate-specific antigen	**Additional medical evaluation** • Chest radiograph • Electrocardiogram • Echocardiogram† • Stress test† • Mammography • Pap smear • Colon cancer screening • Sonogram (BMI >30)† • MRI/MRA	**Optional Laboratory tests:** • Factor 5 Leiden • Protein S • Protein C • α_1- antitrypsin • Anticardiolipin antibodies **Optional radiological tests†** ERCP Computed tomography of abdomen Liver biopsy MRCP Angiography
	Living donor liver transplant consent *Surgical consent*		IDAT donor selection meeting

Abbreviations: BMI, body mass index; ERCP, endoscopic retrograde cholangiopancreatography; IDAT, independent donor advocate team; MRCP, magnetic resonance cholangiopancreatography, MRI, magnetic resonance imaging; MRA, magnetic resonance angiography.

*Items in this column represent components of evaluation that vary from center to center and consensus is not met in terms of importance.

†Determined on a case-by-case basis.

Screening for Infectious Disease

It is important that not only the safety of the donor is considered in the evaluation but also the safety of the recipient. Therefore, donors need to be screened for infectious diseases that could affect recipient safety. A detailed history of the donor should include history of fevers, recurrent colds or flu, night sweats, abnormal blood cell counts, childhood illnesses, tuberculosis exposure, sexually transmitted diseases, and hepatitis exposure.

Antibodies to hepatitis C and positive hepatitis B surface antigen are absolute contraindications to donation. Donors who are hepatitis C or hepatitis B positive are at risk for liver disease themselves, thus making the hepatectomy an unacceptable risk. Hepatitis B core antibody positive living donors are considered at certain centers,[15] but this remains controversial because it is unknown what effect viral hepatitis has on the regeneration process and whether it could accelerate the donor developing active hepatitis.

Radiological Evaluation

The goal of the radiological evaluation is to assess hepatic volume, liver parenchyma, anatomy of the vasculature, and the biliary system (Table 3). When assessing hepatic volume, it is important to make sure the right lobe of the liver is large enough to support the size of the recipient and also leave the donor with adequate mass to avoid liver dysfunction. A 30% functional residual volume is a proposed minimum threshold in the donor, although some centers use calculated remnant volume in relation to donor weight. Remnant volumes less than 30% have been associated with prolonged cholestasis, portal hypertension, normal or near normal enzymes and synthetic function after hepatectomy ("small for size syndrome"), especially in the presence of moderate steatosis. In the transplant candidate, a graft-to-body-weight ratio of 0.8 g/kg of body weight is desirable for optimal outcomes. Less than 0.8 g/kg is associated with increased incidence of hepatic dysfunction, prolonged cholestasis, and increased mortality in the recipient;[15,18,19] therefore, careful assessment of the size differences between donor and recipient is crucial. Furthermore, small for size remnants tolerate additive complications poorly. The presence of concomitant complications such as bile leak, infection, or bleeding may exacerbate the poor recovery in a small for size liver.

The functional status of the recipient must also be considered. Critically ill patients with MELD (Model for End-Stage Liver Disease) scores greater than 26 may not have the functional reserve to receive a partial transplant and may benefit from the volume of a whole graft. This is also true of transplant candidates with fulminant hepatic failure. LDLT in adults with fulminant hepatic failure has been met with great controversy in the transplant community and is not considered at many centers.

The radiological studies used to assess the liver vary from center to center, largely because of technology of the radiological equipments at each center and the comfort level of the transplant team and radiologist with the technology. Many choose magnetic resonance imaging[18,19,23,24] because this noninvasive test can be used to measure the venous and arterial structures as well as liver volumes. Magnetic resonance cholangiography can be used to look at the biliary system with great detail at the same time. Other options for evaluation include a computed tomography scan, an endoscopic retrograde cholangiopancreatography, hepatic angiography, liver sonography, and liver biopsy.[25]

Surgical Considerations

To determine suitability, a detailed evaluation of the liver anatomy is critical. The purpose of the detailed liver and structural assessment is to evaluate the liver parenchyma for anatomical or functional abnormalities. These abnormalities may consist of adenomas, nodules, and hemangiomas, as well as aberrant biliary structures or venous and arterial abnormalities. Of great importance is the detection of steatosis that may require further evaluation. Patient's who have a body mass index (BMI) of greater than 30 are more likely to have significant steatosis.[20] In addition, patients with hypercholesterolemia, diabetes, and a history of increased alcohol intake have increased prevalence of steatosis in the liver. Steatosis has been associated with primary nonfunction both in deceased and living donor grafts. Studies indicate that selective donors with a BMI of greater than 30 can be used safely with good graft function in the recipient and slightly higher risk of wound complications in the donor.[26] These donors may require liver biopsy before clearance for hepatectomy. The exact percentage of fat that is acceptable is unknown and varies from center to center. One must consider percentage of fat in relation to functional liver volume in the recipient graft as well as the donor remnant.

Consultations

Any abnormal results of the evaluation may require additional testing or consultation on a case-by-case basis. Because the ultimate goal is to provide a transplant candidate with a viable organ without harming the donor, consultations may result to determine organ viability or donor risk. The donor team needs to be prudent to refer when even a slight abnormality is found in the evaluation.

Psychosocial Evaluation

It is recommended that centers require that both a social worker and a psychiatrist separately evaluate each potential living donor alone as well as with a member of his or her support system who is not the potential transplant recipient. This evaluation focuses on issues of informed consent, motivation for donation, the decision-making process, financial and emotional support, history of psychological illness, substance abuse, and the relationship with the recipient.[27] The donor must demonstrate adequate decision-making capabilities and be able to appreciate the risks and benefits of the procedure. Any suspicion of coercion needs to be explored and excluded as well.

The social worker interview explores the emotional and financial issues in detail, and prepares the donor and family for the process in terms of discharge planning and recovery. This interview should also determine what support systems are in place or need to be put in place to adequately advocate for and care for the donor after the surgery. The donor and recipient should have different care partners or care teams so that the needs of both are met. A healthcare proxy and living will are encouraged so that the donor is prepared and has fully appreciated the risks, including the risk of death.

The psychiatrist takes a complete mental health history and assesses for current illness including depression and anxiety. These conditions may not be enough to exclude a donor but treatment may be indicated before considering donation. Donors with active alcohol or substance abuse problems are excluded; however, a donor with a history of addiction that is in remission may be considered on a case-by-case basis. The psychiatrist makes a careful evaluation and discusses risks of recidivism so that the donor can make an educated decision about donation.

The role of the social worker and psychiatrist is not complete when the donor is cleared for donation. Many psychological and family stressors develop before, during, and after the surgery. Counseling remains available to donors and families whenever needed.

Educational Needs of Donor and Family

Education of the donor and his or her care partner is an essential part of the evaluation process and needs to be given in multiple forms. The crucial components of the education topics are shown in Table 4. Education should begin at the recipient's initial evaluation, when the concept of LDLT is introduced. Potential donors are encouraged to attend support/education groups offered at many transplant centers, use the Internet for professional living donor-specific Web sites, and talk with donors who have gone through the process.

Table 4. CRUCIAL COMPONENTS OF DONOR AND FAMILY EDUCATION[17]

- Elements of donation process
- Participation is voluntary and confidential
- Components of evaluation
- Surgical procedure
- Recuperation period
- Short- and long–term follow-up
- Alternatives to living donation and transplantation
- National and center-specific statistics
- Meet a donor who went through living liver donation
- Prohibition of receiving monetary gain from donation
- Short- and long-term complications of donation
- Chance of unforeseen risk
- Quality of life after donation
- Lack of long-term follow-up studies after donation
- Potential psychiatric effects of donation
- Financial impact of donation
- Recipient's disease, chance of survival, and risk of recurrent disease
- Explanation of feelings about recipient outcome and chance of graft failure
- Potential risk of future problems ascertaining health and life insurance due to preexisting condition

At the time of the donor evaluation, the transplant nurse practitioner or coordinator presents one-on-one education that is reinforced by each additional team member. Written information is used as a supplement and the donor has the opportunity to meet individually with a former donor.

Donor education must focus on the risks of the operation, including a risk of death, bleeding, need for blood products, infection, reaction to anesthesia, pulmonary emboli, hernia, bile leak, prolonged hospital stay, scar formation, adhesions, and allergic reaction to medications.[2,3,6,7,10,17,19,28,29,30,31] Donors are instructed that although the liver does regenerate, it may not regenerate to 100% of the original size, and living donation is only possible once.[28] Donors also need to know that long-term follow-up data of living liver donation are currently not available.

Surgical Procedure

In pediatric LDLT, the left lateral segment is typically used because of the small size of the potential recipient. Initial experience in aLDLT began with the use of the left lobe; however, because of the small size and less favorable anatomic positioning after transplantation, difficulty performing biopsy of the graft, and increased risk for graft failure, many centers in the United States currently only use the right lobe for aLDLT.[18] In Asia, however, centers have experience using the left lobe and extended right lobe for aLDLT. The surgery takes between 4 to 6 hours to perform; the incision and surgical procedure will vary slightly depending on the surgery.

Left lateral hepatectomy typically requires a midline incision and dissection of the left lateral segment. Approximately 20% of the liver volume is removed, as are portions of the left hepatic vein, left hepatic artery, and a portion of the left bile duct. The gallbladder remains intact.

Left hepatectomy requires a midline incision and dissection of the entire left lobe. The left hepatic vein, left hepatic artery, and left bile duct are ligated. Approximately 40% of the liver volume is removed. Typically, this surgery is reserved for large pediatric patients and small adults with donors whose size is significantly greater than the recipient.

Right hepatectomy begins with a subcostal incision and midline extension (inverted L-shaped) and dissection of the right lobe of the liver. The right lobe, which comprises approximately 60% of the liver mass, is removed and transplanted in the recipient with the right hepatic vein, right hepatic artery, right branch of the portal vein, and right bile duct. Before division of the hepatic parenchyma, intraoperative ultrasound is frequently used for identification of the middle hepatic vein. Transection of the parenchyma to the right or left of the middle hepatic vein remains an active controversy worldwide because of potential risk to the donor. During the removal of the right lobe of the liver, the gallbladder is also removed. All or most of segment 4 and the left lateral lobe remain intact within the donor, 40% of the liver, along with the main hepatic artery, portal vein, and common bile duct (see the Figure). Technical difficulties can arise when there are vascular or biliary variations or anomalies, many of which require the surgical team to vary the operation according to the anomaly.

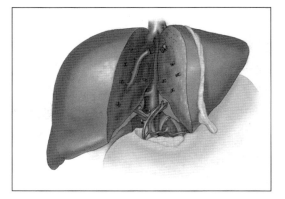

Figure. Donor Hepatectomy

Follow-Up Care

Success of LDLT is primarily due to the liver's natural ability to regenerate after insult or injury. Regeneration occurs rapidly in both the donor and recipient [12]; typically, significant regeneration in both the donor and recipient has occurred by 6 weeks after transplantation. Recent reports, however, suggest that regeneration continues throughout the first year after donation and that 83% ±9% of total volume is achieved at 1 year.[28] Some experts recommend radiological imaging of donors at 3 months and 1 year to determine the degree of regeneration.[9,14] Others feel that invasive testing is not necessary as long as the donors are clinically well.

Liver function in the donor returns to normal within 2 weeks. The international normalized ratio and total bilirubin level typically are normal at the end of week 1 after surgery, with 45% of donors having complete normalization of liver function tests by day 14.[28] The alkaline phosphatase and γ-glutamyl transpeptidase are the last to resolve, as they remain elevated during intense regeneration. By 6 weeks after donation, most donors have normal liver chemistry values.

A donor is typically hospitalized for 5 to 7 days after the partial hepatectomy and is unable to return to work for 4 to 6 weeks. The goal for donor management during the initial postoperative phase is (1) to assess liver function, (2) to observe for bleeding or bile leak, (3) pain management, (4) phosphorous supplementation, (5) return of bowel function, and (6) to prevent blood clots and deep venous thrombosis.

Patients are discharged taking oral pain medication and are followed closely by the medical team for the first 6 weeks. Donors usually report feeling moderately fatigued for several weeks after surgery. Most report returning to work by 6 weeks, but not feeling fully recovered for 6.6 months.[33] Donors are strongly encouraged to avoid alcohol and any medications or herbal remedies that can be toxic to the liver during regeneration, which typically lasts for 6 months. Donors should seek annual follow-up care at the transplant center for at least 5 years[9] to monitor for long-term complications of this innovative procedure. In practice, this is quite difficult, with a 32% 1-year follow-up rate by donors reported.[29] In addition, the donor should be reintroduced to his or her community physician with detailed records from the donation so that continuity of care is provided.

Living Donor Outcomes

Data on long-term outcomes of liver donation are limited because of small clinical experience, especially in adults; variability in defining and tracking morbidity across centers; and poor long-term compliance with follow-up by the living donors. Donor complications appear to be more frequent in centers performing fewer procedures,[6] and in single center reports there is an inverse correlation between experience and donor morbidity. Studies report early morbidity ranging from 0% to 67%, varying from simple quality of life changes to serious medical complications such as bile leaks.[30]

Donor deaths have occurred in pediatric and adult liver donors, with mortality reported as 0.13% and 0.2%, respectively. In the United States, 2 donor deaths have been reported related to pulmonary emboli in women who donated to children;[31] both donors were smokers. Two donors of right lobes have died of surgical complications early after donation and 1 has required a liver transplant for liver failure.[6] The transplant community speculates that there have been between 9 and 14 donor deaths worldwide. Actual mortality figures are difficult to establish because most of the donor deaths are not actually published but obtained by personal communication and through lay press. Therefore, additional deaths may have been unreported and unpublicized. Public analysis of the causes of death in both pediatric and adult donors has led to meaningful adjustments in clinical practice. After the 2 deaths related to thromboembolism were reported in lateral segment donors, preoperative health of the donor has been more carefully scrutinized and preoperative intervention (weight loss, discontinuation of smoking, and oral contraception) recognized as a means of reducing risk. Unfortunately, only 1 right lobe donor death has been published in the medical literature. In this case, death was the result of late postoperative liver failure and portal hypertension caused by underlying steatohepatitis not appreciated during preoperative screening of the donor.[34] The Organ Procurement and Transplantation Network/United Network for Organ Sharing (OPTN/UNOS) has recently made mortality reporting mandatory so that accurate mortality can be tracked and studied, and future deaths prevented.

Short-Term Complications

Morbidity after living donor hepatectomy is influenced by the extent of resection because of the influence of functional residual hepatic reserve in postoperative recovery. Right lobe donors experience increased morbidity compared to left lobe or lateral segment donors and complications tend to be more serious. Short-term complications vary within the literature. Table 5 lists common donor complications of right and left lobe donation. Bile leaks, prolonged ileus, and wound problems were the most frequently reported complications, although interpretation of the data is limited by the lack of standardized definitions of complications in different published reports. Serious, life-threatening complications are much less frequent. Liver failure in the absence of an early technical complication such as arterial or portal venous thrombosis is likely to be caused by a small for size remnant liver. Again, data on serious complications are limited.

Table 5. DONOR COMPLICATIONS

Death	Wound complications
Liver failure	• Infection
Aborted procedure	• Hernia
Nonautologous blood transfusion	Other
Biliary complications	• Anesthesia complications
• Leak	• Catheter/intravenous complications
• Stricture	• Transient nerve injury
Vascular complications	• Illeus
• Portal vein thrombus	Psychiatric
• Hepatic vein thrombus	• Chronic pain
• Hepatic artery thrombosis	• Depression
• Pulmonary emboli	• Suicide
• Deep venous thrombosis	
Pulmonary complications	
• Pleural effusion	
• Pneumonia	

Liver-Related Complications

Biliary leaks are the most commonly reported liver complication in pediatric and adult living donors. Although the incidence is low in left lateral segment donation, the incidence can be up to 8% in some studies of right lobe donation.[18] The leak can occur in the cut surface of the remnant or from the biliary stump (suture line from where the bile duct was ligated for donation). Often, external drainage through a Jackson Pratt drain or biliary tube will be sufficient to allow the leak to seal itself. More serious bile leaks can require percutaneous cholangiogram, endoscopic retrograde cholangiopancreatography, or surgical repair. Strictures are less commonly reported as an early complication but may require dilatation and stent placement or surgery.[3,6,18,19,28,29,30,31]

Vascular thrombus within the liver is possible but rare and requires immediate surgical intervention. Complex anatomy, such as portal vein trifurcation, may increase the potential for vascular compromise of the remnant by increasing the technical challenge of removing the graft. Clinical findings may be subtle, such as increased ascitic drainage suggestive of portal hypertension or mild encephalopathy. Overt signs include evidence of liver ischemia with rising enzymes, synthetic dysfunction, and progressive encephalopathy. Prompt attention to symptoms is crucial.

Bleeding from the cut surface of the liver and suture line may require additional interventions and transfusion. The incidence of postoperative bleeding requiring transfusion is low, less than 5%,[6,29] but because a postoperative bleeding event can be unpredictable and life threatening, surveillance for bleeding in the initial postoperative period is a routine feature of care and includes frequent clinical examinations and serial hemoglobin assessments. Drains are commonly inserted during the initial surgery and kept in place for 48 hours. Although drains are useful for early diagnosis of bile leaks, they are less effective in diagnosis of acute hemorrhage because of their tendency to become obstructed by clot. Therefore, the absence of bloody drainage should not exclude the diagnosis of hemorrhage when other signs are present, including tachycardia, hypotension, or abdominal distension.

Pulmonary Complications

Donors are at risk for pulmonary complications as a result of major abdominal surgery. Atelectasis is quite common and may not always be viewed as a complication, but pneumonia requiring treatment and pleural effusion resulting in external drainage with a pigtail catheter is associated with significant morbidity.[29]

Wound Complications

Wound complications such as infection, wound dehiscence, and hernia can be associated with delayed recovery and additional surgery. A higher incidence of wound complications has been reported in donors with a BMI greater than 30.[26] Typical risk factors for wound complications are usually not present in living donors, who are excluded from donation if they are diabetic, exhibit nutritional or systemic constitutional signs, or are taking steroids. Nevertheless, hernia is the most common reason for reoperation following living donor hepatectomy;[29] even in a carefully screened population, wound complications can occur and seem to occur more frequently in the presence of obesity. Potential donors who are dependent on physical activity for livelihood or those who are overweight should be counseled preoperatively about the possibility of prolonged recovery related to wound complications and the impact of such complications on return to work, and they should be encouraged to lose weight before surgery.

Additional Risks

Other complications reported in the literature that should be included in the informed consent process of potential donors are risk of aborted procedures, anesthesia allergy, catheter complication, prolonged ileus, dyspepsia, chronic pain, and transient brachial nerve injury.[3,6,18,19,28,29,30,31] It is important to note that there may be some inherent unknown risks related to partial hepatectomy, and as donors are followed longer these will become apparent.

Psychological Effects of Donation

The psychological impact of donation should not be minimized. Often, donors feel overwhelmed after the surgery. Documented cases of depression have been reported regardless of the outcome in the recipient, and antidepressant medications are sometimes required.[35] Insomnia, anxiety, and somatic pain may exist as well.[36] In addition, certain donors report marital adjustment after interspouse liver donation as a result of unrealistic expectations from the donation.[37] Trotter et al[38] recently reported suicide in 2 patients as a late complication of donation in the 390 donors in the A2ALL study. Two other patients died, 1 in a train accident and 1 because of surgical complications. Eleven patients (2.8%) experienced severe psychiatric complications. This important preliminary survey suggests that there is much work to be done in the assessment of psychiatric risk of living donation. Donors need to be educated about these psychological stressors before donation and monitored during the postoperative phase for evidence of psychosocial disorders and referred for counseling as needed. In addition, ongoing counseling and support are required if the donor's expectations of the donation were not met, including issues such as altered relationship with the recipient, declining recipient health, or recipient death.

Financial Effects of Donation

Most donors will underestimate the potential financial impact of donation. For donors of modest means, out-of-pocket expenses such as travel costs to the center, hotel stay if travel is from a long distance, parking, cost of prescription drugs, and unpaid leave from work are all significant potential factors in postoperative financial stress. At this point, it is not clear whether the act of donation will influence future insurability of the donor, especially if there is a complication. This is a greater issue in the United States, where there is no guarantee of universal healthcare coverage, as compared to nations such as Canada, where donors will always have access to care irrespective of economic status. A recent survey of several insurance carriers in the United States suggested that there may be a negative impact of donation on the access and/or cost of future insurance for the donor.[39] Not all centers require active health insurance in potential donors, because the initial hospitalization costs are reimbursed through the recipient's insurance in the United States. However, the area of greatest concern for donors is complications requiring healthcare resource utilization after discharge from the hospital. In these cases, it is not clear who has primary responsibility for payment of services: the recipient, the donor, or the transplant center. Most recipient insurance carriers will have specific policies for coverage of the donor, which are generally restricted to coverage of the hospitalization itself and possibly 90 days of perioperative coverage of treatment-related complications, although even this cannot be assumed, and there are generally no provisions for prescription medications. Donors with limited economic means may find it impossible to pay for prescriptions for even pain medication or acid suppression therapy upon discharge. Centers are generally unwilling to ask the donor or his or her insurance to be responsible for care related to the donation in the immediate postoperative period. Most centers will therefore provide perioperative services without charge for a specified period when the services are provided for complications of the donation. It is crucial that the center has a clear written policy that is acceptable to hospital administration, and that the donor be educated about the center's policies regarding financial responsibility for postoperative care.

Long-Term Complications

Because of a lack of standardization for donor follow-up in the transplant community, the incidence of long-term complications is limited but believed to be low. Donors are currently strongly encouraged to comply with long-term follow-up so that data can be collected. A single center report of 1-year follow-up indicated a 22% incidence of persistent thrombocytopenia. A clearly operative factor was identified in only 1 donor with thrombocytopenia; in the remaining 4 donors, no technical complication could be identified, suggesting that right hepatectomy alone can result in this finding. However, the significance of this finding is not clear at this time.[29] Future studies such as the A2ALL study will hopefully define the true incidence of long-term complications. Until then, donors need to be educated that there are unknown risks to donation.

Quality of Life

Few studies are available regarding donors who underwent partial hepatectomy for living donation, but those available report a positive experience following donation surgery. Liver donors who donated to children overwhelmingly endorse living donation regardless of recipient outcome and reported minor physical symptoms, including pain and surgical wound problem.[40] Right lobe donors reported no significant change in physical or social activities.[41] In addition, donors scored higher than the general public on SF-36, a measure of health-related quality of life.[42] The flaw in some quality-of-life studies is that there was no predonation survey done to assess any variation between the time periods before and after donation. A majority of donors state that they believe they benefited from donation and would donate again if needed.[33] Improved relationships with the recipient as well as with the donor's significant other are also reported.[33]

Conclusion

Current studies only superficially examine the true donor experience. Living liver donation, although believed to be safe by many but criticized by others, is still in its infancy. Controlled clinical trials are warranted to examine the medical and psychological factors that affect the donor before and after donation. With such data, future potential donors will have the information necessary to decide if the benefits to the recipient outweigh the risks to the donor.

References

1. Broelsch CE, Emond JC, Whillyton PF, Thistethwaife JR, Baker AL, Lichton JC. Application of reduced-size liver transplants as split grafts, auxiliary orthotopic grafts, and living related segmental transplants. *Ann Surg.* 1998;212:368-377.
2. Wachs ME, Bak TE, Karrer FM, et al. Adult living donor liver transplantation using the right hepatic lobe. *Transplantation.* 1998;66:1313-1316.
3. Marcos A, Ham JM, Fisher RA, Olziniski AT, Posner MP. Single center analysis of the first 40 adult-to-adult living donor liver transplantation using the right lobe. *Liver Transplant.* 2000;6:296-301.
4. United Network for Organ Sharing. Available at: http://www.unos.org. Accessed May 14, 2005.
5. Beavers KL, Cassara JE, Shrestha R. Practice patterns for long-term follow-up of adult-to-adult right lobe donors at US transplant centers. *Liver Transplant.* 2003;9:645-648.
6. Brown RS, Russo MW, Lai M, et al. A survey of liver transplantation from living adult donors in the United States. *N Engl J Med.* 2003;348:818-825.
7. Russo MW, Brown RS. Adult living donor liver transplantation. *Am J Transplant.* 2004;4(4):458-465.
8. Grady D. Healthy give organs to dying, raising issues of risk and ethics. *New York Times.* June 24, 2001:A1-16.
9. New York State Committee on Quality Improvement in Living Liver Donation. A report to New York State Transplant Council and New York State Department of Health. Available at: http://www.health.state.ny.us. Accessed April 21, 2004.
10. Consensus Report: Secretary Tommy G. Thompson's Advisory Committee on Organ Transplantation (ACOT). Available at: http://www.hrsa.gov. Accessed January 2004.
11. Transplant Center Conditions of Participation, United States Department of Health and Human Services, Centers for Medicare and Medicaid Services. Available at: http://www.cms.hhs.gov/CFCsAndCoPs/11_transplantcenter.asp#TopOfPage May 8, 2006.
12. Marcos A, Fisher RA, Ham JM, et al. Right lobe living donor liver transplantation. *Transplantation.* 1999;6:798-803.
13. Sarasin FP, Majno PE, Llovet JM, Mentha G, Hadengue A. Living donor liver transplantation for early hepatocellular carcinoma: a life-expectancy and cost-effectiveness perspective. *Hepatology.* 2001;33:1073-1079.
14. Adult to Adult Living Donor Liver Transplantation Cohort Study. Available at: http://www.nih-a2all.org. Accessed May 27, 2005.
15. Troter JF. Selection of donors for living donor liver transplantation. *Liver Transplant.* 2003;9(10 suppl 2):S2-S7.
16. Makuuchi M, Miller CM, Olthoff K, et al. Adult-adult living donor liver transplantation. *J Gastrointest Surg.* 2004;8:303-312.
17. LaPointe Rudow D, Brown RS Jr. Evaluation of living liver donors. *ProgTransplant.* 2003;13:110-116.
18. Shiffman ML, Brown RS, Olthoff KM, et al. Living donor liver transplantation: summary of a conference at the national institutes of health. *Liver Transplant.* 2002;8:174-188.
19. Renz JF, Busuttil RW. Adult-to-adult living-donor liver transplantation: a critical analysis. *Semin Liver Dis.* 2000;20:411-424.
20. LaPointe Rudow D, Brown RS Jr. The role of the independent donor advocate team in ethical decision making. *Prog Transplant.* 2005;15:298-302.
21. Abecassis M, Adams M, Adams P, et al. Consensus statement on the live organ donor. JAMA. 2000;284:2919-2926.
22. Samstein B, Emond J. Liver transplants from living related donors. *Annu Rev Med.* 2000;52:147-160.
23. Trotter JF, Wachs M, Everson GT, Kam I. Adult-to-adult transplantation of the right hepatic lobe from a living donor. *N Engl J Med.* 2002;346:1074-1082.
24. Cheng YF, Chen CL, Huang TL, et al. Single imaging modality evaluation of living donors in liver transplantation: magnetic resonance imaging. *Transplantation.* 2001;72:1527-1533.
25. Schroeder T, Malago M, Debatin JF, et al. Multidetector computer tomographic cholangiography in the evaluation of potential living liver donors. *Transplantation.* 2002;73:1972-1973.
26. Moss J, LaPointe Rudow D, Renz JF, et al. Select utilization of obese donors in living donor liver transplantation: implications for the donor pool. *Am J Transplant.* 2005;5:2974-2981.
27. Olbrisch ME, Benedict SM, Haller DL, Levenson JL. Psychosocial assessment of living organ donors: clinical and ethical considerations. *Prog Transplant.* 2001;11:40-49.
28. Pomfret EA, Pomposelli JJ, Gordon FD, et al. Liver regeneration and surgical outcomes in donors of right-lobe liver grafts. *Transplantation.* 2003;76:5-10.
29. LaPointe Rudow D, Brown RS Jr, Emond JC, Marratta D, Bellemare S, Kinkhabwala M. One-year morbidity after donor right hepatectomy. *Liver Transplant.* 2004;10:1428-1431.
30. Beavers KL, Sandler RS, Shrestha R. Donor morbidity associated with right lobectomy for living donor liver transplantation to adult recipients: a systematic review. *Liver Transplant.* 2003;8:110-117.
31. Renz JF, Roberts JP. Long term complications of living donor liver transplantation. *Liver Transplant.* 2000;6:S73-S76.
32. Russo MW, LaPointe Rudow D, Teixeira A, et al. Interpretation of liver chemistries in adult donors after living donor liver transplantation. *J Clin Gastroenterol.* 2004;38:810-814.
33. LaPointe Rudow D, Charlton M, Sanchez C, Chang S, Serur D, Brown RS Jr. Kidney and liver donors: a comparison of experiences. *Prog Transplant.* 2005;15:1-7.

34. Akabbayashi A, Slingsby BT, Fujita M. The first donor death after living related liver transplantation in Japan. *Transplantation*. 2004;77:634-639.
35. Kita Y, Fukunishi I, Harihara M, et al. Psychiatric disorders in living relate liver liver transplantation. *Transplant Proc*. 2001;33:1350-1352.
36. Fukunishi I, Sugawara Y, Makuuchi M, Surman OS. Pain in liver donors. *Psychosomatics*. 2003;44:172-173.
37. Lam BK, Lo CM, Fung AS, Fan ST, Liu CL, Wong J. Marital adjustment after interspouse living donor liver transplant. *Transplant Proc*. 2000;32:2095-2096.
38. Trotter JF, Hill-Callahan M, Gillespie BW, et al. Deaths due to psychiatric complications in right hepatic lobe donors for adult to adult living donor liver transplantation. *Hepatology*. 2005;42(suppl 1):451A.
39. Nissing MH, Hayashi PH. Right hepatic lobe donation adversely affects donor life insurability up to one year after donation. *Liver Transplant*. 2005;11:843-847.
40. Diaz GC, Renz JF, Mudge C, et al. Donor health assessment after living-donor liver transplantation. *Ann Surg*. 2002;236:120-126.
41. Hunt KK, Chandra A, Smith K, LaPointe Rudow D, Emond J, Brown RS Jr. Predictors of living liver donation: faith, education and close relationship to the recipient. *Am J Transplant*. 2003;3(suppl 5):1409.
42. Trotter JF, Talamantes M, McClure M, et al. Right hepatic lobe donation for living donor liver transplantation: impact on donor quality of life. *Liver Transplant*. 2001;7:485-493.

Education and the Transplant Patient

Marian Charlton, RN, CCTC
Kara Ventura, CPNP

Improvements in surgical technique, immunosuppression management, and prevention of complications have led to the success of solid-organ transplantation. Patients are living longer and more fulfilled lives. This success is largely due to the commitment on the part of the transplant program to inform and educate their patients before and after transplantation, as well as the patient's ability for self-care. The transplant professional plays a critical role in this education. This chapter will identify strategies to educate transplant patients and discuss crucial components of transplant education.

The Basics

The first step in providing information about a medical diagnosis to a patient includes basic education. Level of education cannot always be used as a measure of the patient's ability to understand the information being presented to him or her.[1] Clinical transplant coordinators can ensure optimal patient outcomes by establishing a secure and trusting relationship with their patients, allowing for the process of learning to begin. Initially, needs and skills of the patient must be assessed. The clinical transplant coordinator can then develop more specific individualized distribution of information, which is essential to patient education.

Assessment of Learning Needs and Skills

Patient education is the most commonly used strategy for guiding patients to increase health promotion behaviors and to manage lifestyle problems.[2] It is essential to instruct patients about their specific illnesses, treatment, and available health services. The clinical transplant coordinator needs to determine the patient's style of learning, level of knowledge and competency, readiness, physical and developmental capabilities, attitudes, and feelings.[3] Health literacy is a constellation of skills, including the ability to perform basic reading and numerical tasks required to function in the healthcare environment. Patients with adequate literacy can read, understand, and act on healthcare information.[3]

To determine the most effective way to provide individualized patient education, at the appropriate level, the clinical transplant coordinator needs to evaluate the patient's knowledge base by asking encouraging questions. Often, transplant centers use psychological and social evaluations to assess patients' overall understanding of their disease process and treatment options. Functional health illiteracy is a disability, and patients may be reluctant to disclose this problem because they fear discrimination and stigmatization.[4] Some centers use questionnaires to gain an understanding of patients' knowledge deficit and have one-on-one consultations during which patient awareness can be assessed.

Illiteracy should not be a barrier to achieving favorable post transplant education. Collaboration between the clinical transplant coordinator and the patient and his or her family can overcome this barrier.[5] Alternative educational methods are crucial when formulating a plan in these circumstances. Video presentations, oral one-on-one presentations, and picture-orientated educational material are tools provided to patients so that they can receive the necessary education. Additional tools are presented in Table 1.

Table 1. EDUCATION TOOLS

- Speak slowly and start with context
- Provide a quiet environment with minimal distractions
- Start with the most important information and limit new information
- Provide no more than 1 or 2 instructions at a time
- Use repetition and reinforcement
- Ask the patient to repeat the information
- Include several family members in each session

Patient Education

Initially, it is important to establish a trusting relationship with the patient so the clinical transplant coordinator will be perceived as a credible source. The use of open-ended questions allows the provider to assess the patient's comprehension. Providing written and verbal instruction, preferably in the patient's native language, is the first step in this process. Some centers recommend developing a written patient curriculum (Table 2), including information that addresses protocols.[6]

Time is a factor when educating a patient. Short educational sessions with frequent repetition allow for greater understanding of the information. It is helpful to use interpreters during education sessions; however, the transplant coordinator must ensure the interpreter is familiar with medical terminology so that miscommunication can be avoided. Use of family members as interpreters is discouraged because the translated information can be filtered at the discretion of the family member.[7]

The inclusion of family members and friends in the education process is encouraged, as some patients may need others present to enhance the reception of the information. Therefore, it is essential family members are educated also. Cultural diversity awareness is the norm in healthcare today; therefore, providers need to understand cultural differences to effectively educate patients. Cultural competency extends beyond understanding values, beliefs, and needs associated with patients' age or gender or with racial, ethical, and religious backgrounds. Providers hold numerous simultaneous cultural associations and each have implications for the care process.[8]

Roles are important in families; they define who the individuals are, and education needs to be tailored to acknowledge these society roles.[9] For example, if a provider is educating an Islamic woman about activity restriction after transplantation, they cannot just say to the woman to cease her current activity, which will diminish her role in the family as the person who takes care of all the domestic needs.

Table 2. PATIENT CURRICULUM

- Comply with office visits and requested laboratory studies
- Attend educational sessions provided by transplant center
- Know medication names, dosages, appearance, timing, storage, and medication form (ie, pills, liquid)
- Accordance with activity restriction, if indicated
- Accordance with dietary restriction, if indicated
- Comply with medication, and be aware of side effects
- Comply with health promotion (skin protection, smoking cessation, weight maintenance) and routine care
- Attend support groups for emotional health
- Know when it is necessary to call the transplant team or go to the emergency department

The educator needs to teach activity restriction, but incorporate certain tasks that are routine for the woman and will not interfere with healing.[9] Also, it is important for the educator to not assume that entire ethnic groups such as Hispanic Americans have the same beliefs; providers should recognize differences in beliefs among various nationalities.[9] Under Castro's rule in Cuba, all citizens are expected to comply with health promotion suggestions such as getting an annual physical examination. Cubans feel that complying with health recommendations makes them a good citizen. Focus on health maintenance is important because Cubans respect health maintenance as a good characteristic. In all of these situations, if the patient is offended, his or her trust for the provider will be diminished, completely impeding education and learning.

Methods of Education

When initiating the education process, the healthcare provider should determine the best environment conducive to the individual patient's needs. Various teaching methods may be implemented. One-on-one settings, group discussions, and video or slide presentations are effective. Many transplant pharmaceutical companies have educational resources available through their Web sites as well as in written and audiovisual form. The clinical coordinator should review these materials carefully before using them to ensure they reflect the philosophy of the transplant center.

The educator must be able to provide information at the level of education the patient can understand. Providing written material to a patient who is illiterate is obviously not effective. Using terms and advanced vocabulary that may not be readily understood by a patient immediately puts a barrier up during the education periods. Conversely, using limited explanations may be frustrating to a patient who has a more intricate understanding of his or her disease process and the ability for greater comprehension.

Although all education methods need to be curtailed to the specific learning ability of the patient, it is important that the educator confirms the patient has been informed fully of his or her health status, future needs, and requirements. The expectation of the transplant team for the patient must be fully understood by the patient, despite his or her level of comprehension. Employing the use of translators and family members, although not always appropriate or effective, may be helpful in enhancing the learning of a patient. The greater number of family members present during education sessions may be helpful to patients later on when they are trying to recall certain points brought up in the session.

Essential Pretransplant Teaching

Educating patients at the time of evaluation for organ transplantation is critical to success. At this time, education alleviates fears associated with transplantation, assists candidates to determine if transplantation is for them, and clears up many misconceptions. It is also a means for the transplant team to get to know the candidate and develop a trusting relationship. Essential components of pretransplant education are presented in Table 3.

Table 3. ESSENTIAL COMPONENTS OF PRETRANSPLANT EDUCATION

1. Organ allocation system
2. Role of transplant team
3. Evaluation process
4. Waiting for a transplant
5. Options for end-stage organ disease
6. Transplant options
7. Risks and benefits of transplantation
8. Surgical procedures

Organ Allocation

Each day the number of patients on the waiting list for transplantation increases. Patients awaiting a transplant need to have a basic working knowledge of the organ allocation system. Patients must know their expected waiting time for an organ and their responsibility in maintaining their place on the list.

The United Network for Organ Sharing and the Organ Procurement and Transplantation Network (OPTN) collaborate to provide the transplant community with a means to regulate the field of transplantation. The OPTN is the Unified Transplant Network established by US Congress under the National Organ Transplant Act (NOTA) of 1984 [10]to be operated by a private, nonprofit organization under federal contact. OPTN is a unique public-private partnership that links all of the professionals involved in the donation and transplantation system.[10] Refer to chapter three). Although patients do not necessarily need to know the inner workings of these agencies, they do need to have a basic understanding. Often, there are myths surrounding the "list" and who gets priorities and it is therefore essential that patients understand how the waiting list is regulated and operated. Organ allocation policies are intended to ensure equitable distribution of organs on the basis of medical and regional criteria.

Patients and families should be aware of the Scientific Registry of Transplant Recipients (SRTR).[11] The SRTR supports the ongoing evaluation of the scientific and clinical status of solid-organ transplantation. The University Renal Research and Education Association at the University of Michigan administer this registry. Every 6 months, the SRTR publishes updated reports on activities at each transplant center and organ procurement organization in the United States. These reports include statistics about organ donation and recovery, wait list activity such as transplant rate, and post transplant outcomes such as graft and patient survival rates.[11]

Role of the Transplant Team

Many team members are involved in the care and education of the transplant recipient. From the transplant coordinator, physician, surgeon, social worker, and financial coordinator to the referring physician, each member has the responsibility of educating the patient and family throughout the entire process. The transplant coordinator begins the process during the initial evaluation, covering such topics as the evaluation, listing, maintenance on the wait list, waiting time, and the need to establish ongoing regular contact with the transplant center. The physicians and surgeons discuss the medical and surgical implications and risks associated with transplantation. During the initial psychosocial evaluation, the social worker and/or the transplant psychiatrist evaluates the patient's and the family understands of transplantation and their ability to process the material being presented to them.

Once the patient is listed for transplantation, the role of the transplant team shifts from the evaluation phase to the waiting phase. During this waiting phase, patients need to continue to follow with the transplant center according to the center's protocol. However, the referring physician again assumes the role of the primary caregiver and works in conjunction with the transplant center. A clear delineation of the role of the transplant center and the primary physician needs to be established so that patients may comply with requirements and to ensure adequate medical follow-up

Options for End-Stage Organ Disease

Current science in the field of regenerative medicine and tissue engineering is working on applying cell transplantation, material science, and bioengineering principles to create biological substitutes that will restore and maintain normal function in diseased and injured tissues. Stem cell research is also looking for new options for therapy.[12] Currently, transplantation is the optimal choice for patients with end-stage organ disease; however, other treatment options are available that patients need to be aware of.

For patients with end-stage organ disease and with cardiac or respiratory failure, the best treatment option is transplantation. For patients with renal, liver, or intestinal failure, other long-term treatment options are available. Patients need to understand these options so that they can decide if transplantation is an appropriate treatment option for them.

Kidney

For patients with end-stage kidney disease, many dialysis options such as hemodialysis, peritoneal dialysis, and, most recently, nocturnal and home dialysis, are used.

Liver

Although there are no permanent options for end-stage liver disease other than transplantation, some treatments can provide adequate liver function for some period of time. Patients with hepatocellular carcinoma may opt for resection of local regional therapy. Patients may also receive an auxiliary liver transplant, that is, a segment or lobe of the liver is implanted in the hopes it will provide adequate liver mass for function or regenerate into enough mass. The controversy in this type of transplantation is whether this could be misusing a liver portion that could have been sufficient for another recipient such as a child. In addition, clinical trials are underway for bioartificial liver devices.

Heart

A few alternative therapeutic strategies have been developed to treat advance heart failure. Xenotransplantation, mechanical support devices, and cell transfer and tissue engineering protocols are used in end-stage heart disease.[13]

Intestine

Although there is a high morbidity associated with patients on home total parenteral nutrition (TPN), including cholestasis of the liver, patients can survive long term with proper TPN management and close attention to prevention of liver disease.[14] Recently, patients have been undergoing surgical intestinal lengthening procedures, such as the Bianchi and Serial transverse enteroplasty. In some cases, the additional intestinal length obtained after these surgeries has allowed for adequate nutritional support through enteral feedings solely.

Transplantation Options

Patients have choices regarding their organ transplantation. Therefore, education about the options for organ transplantation, including standard criteria donation, living donation, expanded criteria donors (ECDs), and multiple listing, must be included in the initial discussions.

Standard Criteria Donation

The standard criteria for organ donors are deceased donors between the age of 18 and 60, with no medical history of hypertension and diabetes, normal creatinine level, and death not caused by cerebral vascular accident.[10]

Living Donation

At many centers, living donation is an option for all organs but heart transplantation. However, some types of transplantations involving living donors are more common than others; for example, kidney transplantation is more routine than pancreas or intestinal transplantation. Transplant candidates need to be informed of the efficacy of living donor organ transplantation, who can be a donor, and how they can approach a potential donor. In addition, they need to be aware of donor risks and outcomes. In living donation, both the recipient and the donor must meet specific medical requirements. It is important for both the donor and recipient to fully understand the evaluation process for living donation, because it is quite comprehensive with a significant commitment required from both the patient and the donor. Chapters 9, 10 and 11 provide more information about this subject. For a more detailed discussion of process and education of living donors, refer to the organ-specific chapters.

Expanded Criteria Donors

Because of the limited availability of organs, some transplant centers are using organs from ECDs.[16] Kidneys from ECDs are helping ease the organ shortage. In some areas in the United States, liver programs are also using organs from ECDs because of long time on waiting lists and increased pretransplant mortality. Who among the many waiting list candidates are most likely to benefit from these organs, which are characterized by a higher risk of graft failure? A new SRTR study, published in the *Journal of the American Medical Association*, shows that ECD transplants should be offered principally to candidates who are older than 40 years in organ procurement organizations with long waiting times.[15] The definition of ECDs in kidney transplantation is well defined, but these donors are less defined in liver transplantation. Regardless of the type of organ received, transplant recipients must sign a consent form to receive an organ from an ECD. Topics for education when discussing ECD transplantation should include types of ECDs, risk or donor-acquired infections and cancers, risk of primary nonfunction or slow graft function, risk of retransplantation, and unknown risks. In addition, a discussion of the risk of waiting for a standard criteria organ needs to be part of the education. The provider must ensure the patient understands the definition of an ECD and which option is best for his or her particular situation.

Multiple Listing

During the initial evaluation, the option and requirements of multiple listing should be explored and reviewed with the patient. According to OPTN policy, patients may be listed as transplant candidates at multiple centers, as long as the centers are not within the same region.[10] This multiple listing may increase patients' chances of receiving an organ offer. However, patients must be aware of the commitment necessary with multiple listing. First, they should speak with their insurance carriers to determine if they will reimburse the cost of an additional evaluation at another center. Also, they need to consider other costs associated with multiple listing not covered by insurance, including travel and lodging. They will need to maintain current laboratory results and contact with each center, and they will need to consider their post transplant care. Due to differences in past operative protocols transplant centers may not accept patients transplanted at other centers.

Risks and Benefits of Transplantation

Although the above mentioned treatment options can sometimes sustain life, transplantation is thought to offer improved quality of life and benefits to the patient.[15-17] However, the risks associated with transplantation must be clearly and precisely addressed with both the patient and family members. It is essential that they understand not only the short-term risks such as donor-acquired infections and disease, but long-term risks as well, including immunosuppression, cardiovascular disease, renal insufficiency, and cancer. Although the risks and benefits of organ transplantation have been reviewed in previous chapters, it is important to address how to deliver this information for the most optimal patient education and understanding.

Surgical Procedures

Although most surgeons perform transplantations using similar procedures, individual centers may employ different techniques. Also, there may be different methods of surgical implantation for each organ. It is important for patients to know what will be happening to their body; however, the provider must use discretion based on their assessment of the patient's coping ability and literacy when providing specific surgical detail to avoid overwhelming or confusing the patient.

The postoperative course should be reviewed in great detail with the patient and their family to avoid the unexpected. Addressing specific issues such as pain, presence of intravenous catheters, intubation tubes, drains, dietary restrictions, and duration of hospital stay, as well as expected recovery time is imperative. Research has shown that patients forget aspects of their preoperative education after transplantation.[18] Providers need to be prepared to review the teaching already given.

Essential Posttransplant Education

The post transplant phase of a patient's education begins on the first day after surgery. Despite extensive pretransplant education, when faced with the reality of receiving a transplant, both the patient and his or her family often forget most of the previous education. In the pretransplant period, patients may have barriers to education such as encephalopathy, hypoxia, or uremia, or they may have been on the waiting list for an extended period of time. Education at this stage is more in-depth and focused on getting patients discharged and returning to their normal environment.

Discharge Planning

Patients are often excited yet nervous about caring for themselves when it is time to be discharged after transplantation. Essential components of discharge teaching are presented in Table 4.

Table 4. ESSENTIAL COMPONENTS OF POSTTRANSPLANT EDUCATION

- Medication review
- Adherence and compliance
- When to call the transplant team
- Team's expectations for follow-up appointments and laboratory studies
- Health promotion requirements such as personal hygiene; including wound care and dental visits; cancer screening; weight management and exercise routine.
- Resumption of social and physical activities and any limitations such as when to restrict contact with others, lifting restrictions, and changes in pretransplant everyday jobs such as restricting animal care and specific household chores

Medications

The primary focus of posttransplant education is directed toward medication, including side effects and need for compliance. Before discharge, patients and their caregivers need to demonstrate a certain level of understanding of their posttransplant care.[19]

They should have a good understanding of their medication regime (how, when, and what to take; side effects; drug interactions; and increase risk of infection). In terms of education, it is imperative that the patient understands the importance of adherence to his or her prescribed regimen. Lacking awareness of these factors affects a patient's ability to comply fully with the discharge plan of care.[20]

Patients should be provided with written material, preferably in their native language. If this is not available, family members and/or interpreters should be present during educational sessions. The content will vary depending on the type of organ transplant and is usually center specific. Centers need to reevaluate their patient population on a regular basis and ensure they have education material available to meet their needs. Refer to chapter 16 for more specific information about posttransplant medications.

Adherence and Compliance

Adherence is the joint responsibility of the patient and his or her transplant team. Open, nonjudgmental discussions must occur with all patients regarding adherence. Team members must convince patients that benefits of compliance include prevention of rehospitalization, rejection of graft, disruption of newly acquired "normal life," and, ultimately, loss of the transplanted organ. Although it may seem obvious to the healthcare team that a patient would not want to jeopardize their "gift of life," patients are often noncompliant, especially the adolescent population or transplant recipients who have recovered and resumed a normal life. Unfortunately, as adverse events associated with the drug regime increase, the likelihood of patient noncompliance also increases. Adverse events or side effects that are visible to the patient may be particularly problematic-that is, cosmetic or side effects that alter the physical appearance of the patient-and may tempt the patient to discontinue the medication.[21]

Factors affecting adherence are outlined in Table 5 and can be divided into 3 major categories: patient-specific, medication-related, and transplant-related factors.

Table 5. FACTORS AFFECTING ADHERENCE[22,23]

Patient-specific factors	Medication-related factors	Transplant-related factors
Age	Complexity of medication regimen	Time since transplantation
Ethnicity	Number of medications	Rejection episodes
Gender	Adverse effects	Quality of interactions and relationship between patient and physician/other healthcare professionals
Education	Cost of medications	Knowledge of disease
Marital status	Readability of education materials	
Social economic status		
Employment status		

Patient-Specific Factors

There are several factors that have been found to contribute to patients' nonadherence and noncompliance. Younger adult recipients are less likely to be compliant than older, more mature recipients. White recipients appear to be more adherent than those of foreign descent which suggests, presence of a language barrier for non-white patients may be a contributing factor.[22,23] Married recipients and those with a strong family and social support system in place are more adherent than recipients without close family members or support system. Recipients with low socioeconomic status are less adherent than those of higher status because of low self-efficacy, a poor understanding of their health condition, and sometimes a lack of health insurance.[22,23] However, those with higher levels of education are not necessarily more adherent than those with elementary school education. Employment status in it self does not necessarily contribute to nonadherence, but some studies show that recipients who have leadership roles are more likely to be nonadherent[22] In addition, some underlying psychological issues such as depression and increased stress can contribute to nonadherence.

Medication-Related Factors

Complexity of medication regimen including number of medications, cost of medication, and quality of education material provided to the patient all play an important role in determining whether a recipient will be adherent. Most posttransplant medication regimens include numerous medications at various time points throughout the day. It is therefore not surprising that patients may get confused. Complicated regimens further add to the patient's confusion. Unfamiliarity with generic versus brand names may also add to the confusion.

Many immunosuppressive agents have adverse effects such as weight gain, alopecia, insomnia, and gum hyperplasia. To minimize these adverse effects, patients may decrease their doses, contributing to their nonadherence[21]

During the initial phase of the pretransplant processes, patients are evaluated and screened by either a financial coordinator or social worker to determine their insurance coverage for transplant and posttransplant prescription coverage.

Medicare is one of the leading prescription plans for the majority of transplant patients. Many patients may find that they are unable to pay their copays on a long-term basis and this may contribute to noncompliance. With the new Medicare reimbursement under Medicare part D, established in 2006, patients may find they will need to contribute a large amount on a regular basis. Transplant recipients' inability to return to work, which limits their access to private health insurance, must be considered.

If a patient cannot obtain medication because of inability to pay or obtain insurance, adherence is not possible.

Transplant-Related Factors

Patients who have had their transplants for a long period show an increased likelihood of nonadherence.[21] They may become less attentive to their medication regimens and follow-up appointments with their transplant center. The further from transplantation the patient is, the less frequent the visits to their own physician or the transplant center, thus decreasing the opportunity to monitor for nonadherence. However, once a rejection episode occurs, patients are more compliant and less likely to be nonadherent.[22] Patients who lack a basic understanding of their disease and need for a transplant often have difficulty understanding the need for strict adherence to their prescribed medication regimen. Therefore, it is important to ensure that patients receive adequate education during the initial pretransplant phase to allow them to achieve a basic understanding of their disease and need for a transplant.

Team members must incorporate practical solutions to minimize disruption of patients' return to a "normal" routine. Adherence is not only based on psychological theories of individual behavior, it is influenced by the patient's social setting. Identifying social constraints can improve adherence behavior.[23]

The chapter on medications describes management strategies, which can be used in medication teaching and to achieve optimal patient understanding thus resulting in improved compliance.

When to Call the Transplant Team

Patients who maintain contact with their transplant team have decreased morbidity and improved psychological health.[24] These benefits are related to the team's ability to evaluate patients for medical changes. Although it is imperative centers identify predictors of patient noncompliance and use prevention strategies such continued education and support services, patients must be taught to partner with the transplant team in their long-term care to sustain their improved quality of life and graft function.[16] Patients must comply with screening evaluations and being aware of signs and symptoms of recurrent disease, infection, and rejection and what necessitates an immediate call to the transplant center.

Health Promotion: Long Term

Although the initial focus of posttransplant education is on the above mentioned topics, long-term education needs to focus on promoting self care and the resumption of normal activities.

Long-term health promotion needs to include limiting sun exposure, continuing cessation of smoking and alcohol use, and maintaining primary care visits.

Women must continue their routine gynecological care. Often following transplantation, patients have the desire to return to sexual activity, necessitating the need for disease prevention and birth control while still taking certain medications.

Education concerning sexual activity should be discussed with all patients. It should be done for all women of child bearing age, beginning with teens who have begun menses. Men who have had impotence secondary to kidney failure should be reminded that they may once again be able to enjoy sexual activity.

Growth and development in the pediatric population must be closely monitored to ensure patients reach their developmental and growth potential. Patients must also preserve their psychological health through support groups, education sessions, and provision of psychosocial services, as needed, by the transplant team.

Conclusion

Education for transplant patients must begin at the first contact patients have with the transplant center. The transplant process is overwhelming, with extensive available information and patient responsibility. Ensuring an open trusting relationship with patients and their family can prevent obtaining inaccurate and false information from noncredible sources, which can negatively affect patient care, experience, and results. Education is a continuing process that must occur at every encounter with the transplant patient.

References

1. Gazmararian JA, Baker DW, Williams MV, et al. Health literacy among Medicare enrollees in a managed care organization. JAMA. 1999;281:545-551.
2. Burns C, Brady M, Dunn A, Starr N. *Pediatric Primary Care*. 2nd ed. Philadelphia, PA: WB Saunders. 2000.
3. Ad Hoc Committee on Health Literacy for the Council on Scientific Affairs. Health Literacy: Report of the Council on Scientific Affairs. JAMA. 1999;281:552-557.
4. Erlen JA. Functional health illiteracy. Ethical concerns.*Orthop Nurs*. 2004;2 3:150-153.
5. Blanchard WA. Teaching an illiterate transplant patient. *Anna J*. February 1998;25:69-70, 76.
6. Behar-Horenstein LS, Guin P, Gamble K, Hurlock G, Leclear E, Philipose M, Shellnut D, Ward M, Weldon J. Improving patient care through patient-family education programs. *Hosp Top*. Winter 2005;83:21-27.
7. Rollins G. Translation, por favor. *Hosp Health Netw*. December 2002;76:46-50, 51.
8. Eddey GE, Robey KL.Considering the culture of disability in cultural competence education. *Acad Med*. 2005;80:706-712.
9. Lipson JG, Dibble SL. *Culture in Clinical Care*. San Francisco, Calif: UCSF Publishing Press; 2005.
10. United Network for Organ Sharing Web site. Available at: http://www.unos.org. Accessed January 13,2006.
11. The Scientific Registry of Transplant recipients. Available at: http://www.ustransplant.org. Accessed January 13, 2006.
12. Atala A. Tissue engineering, stem cells and cloning: current concepts and changing trends. *Expert Opin Biol Ther*. 2005;5:879-892.
13. Garry DJ, Goetsch SC, McGrath AJ, Mammen PP. Alternative therapies for orthotropic heart transplantation. *Am J Med Sci*. August 2005;330:88-101.
14. Cavicchi M, Beau P, Crenn P, Degott C, Messing B. Prevalence of liver disease and contributing factors in patients receiving home parenteral nutrition for permanent intestinal failure. *Ann Intern Med*. 2000;132:525-532.
15. Keitel E, Michelon T, dos Santos AF, et al. Renal transplants using expanded cadaver donor criteria. *Ann Transplant*. 2004;9:23-24.
16. Merion, RM, Ashby, VB, Wolfe, RA, Distant, DA, et al. Decreased-donor characterics and the survival benefit of kidney transplantation. JAMA. 2005;2726-33.
17. Madan AK, Tichansky DS. Patients postoperatively forget aspects of preoperative patient education. *Obes Surg*. 2005;15:1066-1069.
18. Galbraith CA, Hathaway D. Long-term effects of transplantation on quality of life. *Transplantation*. 2004;77(suppl): S84-S87.
19. Cupples SA, Ohler L. *Transplantation Nursing Secrets*. Philadelphia, Pa: Hanley & Belfus; 2003.
20. Makaryus AN, Friedman EA. Patients' understanding of their treatment plans and diagnosis at discharge. *Mayo Clin Proc*. 2005;80:991-994.
21. Cramer JA. Practical issues in medication compliance. *Transplant Proc*. June 1999;31(4A):7S-9S.
22. Chisholm MA. Issues of adherence to immunosuppressant therapy after solid-organ transplantation. *Drugs*. 2002;62:567-575.
23. Bunzel B. Solid organ transplantation: are there predictors for posttransplant noncompliance? A literature overview. *Transplantation*. 2000;70:711-716.
24. Williams AB, Burgess JD, Danvers K, Malone J, Winfield SD, Saunders L. Kitchen table wisdom: a Freudian approach to medication adherence. *Assoc Nurses AIDS Care*. January-February 2005;16:3-12.
25. Jowsey G, Taylor ML, Schneekloth TD, Clark MM. Psychosocial challenges in transplantation. *J Psychiatr Pract*. 2001;7:404-414

Long-term Complications Following Solid Organ Transplantation

Jamie Blazek, FNP-C, MPH, CCTC, CCTN

Introduction

In the early days of transplantation, emphasis was placed on the immediate and acute problems surrounding surgery, finding the "magic bullet" that would prevent all rejection, and dealing with the sequelae of drug side effects, especially infections. Today recipients of solid organ transplants are surviving longer thanks to advances in surgical techniques, preservation, and medical management as well as improvements in drug therapy and immunosuppression. No one can predict how long an individual transplant recipient will live or how long a graft will survive. Table 1 reviews published data on the longest functioning graft survival for solid organs in North America.[1]

As successes in transplantation have evolved, criteria for candidacy have been expanded to include older patients and patients with comorbidities that were once considered contraindications. Now more than ever, emphasis is placed on preventing and managing long-term complications. Comorbidities are common because of medication side effects, aging recipients, lifestyle choices, and preexisting diseases. Cardiovascular events are the third most common cause of death in liver recipients who survive longer than 1 year.[2] Cardiovascular disease can also diminish graft survival in recipients with renal, heart, or liver transplants.[3]

Quality of life for long-term survivors of solid-organ transplants depends on early recognition and management of diseases that negatively impact cardiovascular health, such as hypertension, diabetes mellitus, hyperlipidemia, and renal insufficiency. Other conditions, such as recurrent disease (Table 2) and osteoporosis can also diminish quality of life for transplant recipients.[4-9] Although some diseases can recur in a transplanted allograft, patients with these diseases can still be considered candidates for transplantation. In some cases, the disease may take decades to recur. But it is still important to monitor for recurrence and treat if possible. Organ-specific chapters of this book discuss recurrence of disease in more detail.

Table 1. DURATION OF CONTINUOUS FUNCTIONING OF ALLOGRAFTS AS OF 2002*

Allograft Type	Transplant Date	Years of Function
Renal (deceased donor)	March 30, 1966	36 years, 9 months
Pancreas only	May 21, 1983	19 years, 7 months
Liver	January 22, 1970	32 years, 11 months
Heart	August 30, 1978	24 years, 4 months
Double lung	November 26, 1986	16 years, 1 month
Single Lung	September 15, 1987	15 years, 3 months

*Taken from Cecka and Terasaki[1]

Table 2. DISEASES THAT CAN RECUR IN A SOLID ORGAN TRANSPLANT

Allograft	Recurrent Disease
Renal	Focal segmental glomerulosclerosis Membranoproliferative glomerulonephritis Types I and II Membranous nephropathy IgA nephropathy Henoch-Schönlein purpura Anti-basement membrane nephritis Hemolytic uremic syndrome Diabetic nephropathy Wegener granulomatosis Amyloidosis Oxalosis

Liver	Hepatitis B
	Hepatitis C
	Autoimmune hepatitis
	Primary sclerosing cholangitis
	Primary biliary cirrhosis
	Cryptogenic cirrhosis
	Hemochromatosis
	Budd-Chiari syndrome
	Metastatic hepatic malignant neoplasm
	Primary liver tumors
	   Cholangiocarcinoma
	   Hepatocellular carcinoma with large-vessel vascular invasion and/or extrahepatic metastasis

Heart	Amyloidosis Hemochromatosis Ischemic heart disease Sarcoidosis
Lung	Sarcoidosis Lymphangioleiomyomatosis Diffuse panbronchiolitis Pulmonary alveolar proteinosis Desquamative interstitial pneumonia Pulmonary Langerhans histiocytosis Bronchioalveolar carcinoma Idiopathic pulmonary hemosiderosis Giant cell interstitial pneumonitis α_1-antitrypsin deficiency

Hypertension

Hypertension is a common complication after transplantation. In renal transplant recipients, the incidence can be as high as 60% to 80%,[10] in liver transplant recipients 65%,[2] in lung transplant recipients 66%,[11] and in heart transplant recipients 70%.[8] Hypertension even occurs in pediatric transplant recipients at as high a rate as 65% to 80%.[12,13] Risk factors for hypertension after transplantation are summarized in Table 3.[11]

The seventh report of the Joint National Committee on Prevention, Detection, Evaluation, and Treatment of High Blood Pressure (JNC7) defines hypertension as systolic blood pressure greater than 140 mm Hg and diastolic blood pressure greater than 90 mm Hg taken on 2 or more occasions in an adult 18 years or older.[14] According to JNC7, morbidity and mortality increased in diabetic patients when systolic pressure was greater than 130 mm Hg.[14] Left untreated, hypertension can lead to target organ disease in the heart (left ventricular hypertrophy, angina, myocardial infarct, heart failure, coronary arteriopathy), the brain (stroke), the eyes (retinopathy), and the kidneys (chronic renal disease) as well as peripheral vascular disease. It has been documented that hypertension can decrease long-term allograft survival and lead to premature death in transplant recipients. Hypertension is a risk factor for chronic rejection in all solid-organ transplants.[11]

The cause of hypertension in transplant recipients is multifactorial. One important factor is immunosuppression, which can have an adverse effect on blood pressure. Steroids and calcineurin inhibitors (cyclosporine and tacrolimus) have been associated with the greatest increase in blood pressure. Steroids increase total blood volume through sodium retention. Steroids are also associated with increased body weight, which can adversely affect blood pressure. Of the calcineurin inhibitors, cyclosporine appears to have the greatest adverse effect on blood pressure. The exact mechanism is unknown. But systemic vasoconstriction and vasoconstriction of the afferent arteriole of the renal vascular bed do occur, causing subsequent impairment of glomerular filtration and sodium excretion.[15] Tacrolimus also appears to be associated with the development of hypertension. The mechanism is thought to be similar to cyclosporine, but the effect less so. Studies comparing the effect of tacrolimus versus cyclosporine on hypertension have yielded conflicting results. The effects of maintenance immunosuppression on blood pressure are summarized in Table 4.

Numerous studies have been published on treatment of hypertension after transplantation in all solid-organ recipients. Most of these studies involve renal transplant recipients and compare only 1 or 2 specific drug regimens. No definitive study has been done that is applicable to all patient circumstances. Therefore, the recommendations for the general population made by JNC7 have been used as guidelines for treating patients after transplantation. A blood pressure of 135/85 mm Hg or less is the goal for many adults. JNC7 also recommends that patients who have diabetes, proteinuria greater than 500 mg/24 hour, 2 risk factors for cardiovascular disease, or damage to target organs should have a blood pressure goal of 125/75 mm Hg or lower.[14] Those risk factors for cardiovascular disease identified by JNC7 include smoking, dyslipidemia, diabetes, age greater than 60 years, male gender, and family history of premature heart disease.[14]

Choosing a treatment regimen for the patient with hypertension after transplantation requires consideration of the patient's specific needs and comorbidities. Calcium channel blockers can be effective in reducing the vasoconstriction caused by calcineurin inhibitors. But calcium channel blockers may also affect blood levels of immunosuppressants because both are metabolized through the cytochrome P450 system. Although it is not within the scope of this chapter to review all antihypertensive drugs, Table 5[11,16-18] lists some commonly used drugs and transplant considerations. As with the general population, 1 drug may be initiated, but multiple drugs may ultimately be needed to treat hypertension adequately, especially in renal transplant recipients. One treatment strategy is switching patients from a calcineurin inhibitor to a sirolimus- or mycophenolate-based immunosuppression regimen which may reduce hypertension, renal insufficiency, and diabetes.[19] This strategy, however, must be weighed against risk of rejection.

The cornerstone of treatment of hypertension is education that engages the patient in becoming a participant in self-care. The patient or a family member should be taught to monitor blood pressure and pulse. Requests for vital signs logs at clinic visits and during telephone consultations should continue throughout the patient's long-term care. Table 6 includes other important aspects of patient education and hypertension.

Table 3. RISK FACTORS FOR HYPERTENSION AFTER TRANSPLANTATION

Preexisting hypertension
Renal insufficiency
Immunosuppression: steroids, cyclosporine, tacrolimus
Obesity
In renal transplant recipients
    Stenosis of renal artery
    Delayed graft function
    Increased cold and warm ischemia time
    Elderly donor
    Female donor
    Early acute rejection
    Poor HLA match
    Grafting of right kidney

Table 4. EFFECTS OF IMMUNOSUPPRESSION ON BLOOD PRESSURE

Drug	Effect on Blood Pressure
Steroids	Increase
Tacrolimus	Increase
Cyclosporine	Increase
Mycophenolate mofetil	No direct effect
Azathioprine	No direct effect
Sirolimus	No direct effect

Renal Disease

Renal insufficiency and chronic renal failure are significant complications seen after transplantation even in nonrenal solid-organ transplant recipients. Common causes include renal disease before transplantation, nephrotoxic drugs (especially the calcineurin inhibitors, tacrolimus and cyclosporine), hypertension, diabetes mellitus, perioperative hemodynamic injury to the kidneys, and dyslipidemia. Table 7 lists some of the agents commonly used that may cause nephrotoxic effects after transplantation. The incidence of chronic kidney disease (CKD) has been reported between 10% and 83% in recipients of solid-organ transplants.[20] The longer a transplant recipient survives, the greater the risk of renal disease due to increased exposure to nephrotoxic conditions. Add to that the natural decline of renal function that occurs as patients age beyond the fourth decade of life. The 5-year risk of CKD after transplantation of a nonrenal organ ranges from 7% to 21%.[20] In one study of heart transplant recipients taking cyclosporine,

Table 5. ANTIHYPERTENSIVE MEDICATIONS AND TRANSPLANT CONSIDERATIONS

Drug	Transplant Considerations
Omega-3 fatty acids and fish oils	May help with cyclosporine-induced hypertension. Cyclosporine increases thromboxane synthesis, which causes an imbalance between vasodilatative and vasoconstrictive prostaglandins. Omega-3 fatty acids and fish oils inhibit thromboxane synthesis.
Diuretics: bumetanide, ethacrynic acid, furosemide, torsemide	Higher doses reduce blood pressure by increasing sodium and water loss. May be helpful in patients taking steroids. Lower doses probably lower blood pressure by changing intracellular calcium levels, causing vasodilatation. Potassium-wasting side effects may help in patients with hyperkalemia due to calcineurin inhibitors. May cause increase in serum creatinine and urea nitrogen levels in patients with renal impairment, especially at higher doses.
Diuretics: chlorothiazide, chlorthalidone	Higher doses reduce blood pressure by increasing sodium and water loss. May be helpful in patients taking steroids. Lower doses probably lower blood pressure by changing intracellular calcium levels, causing vasodilatation. May increase blood glucose levels. Monitor closely in diabetics. May exacerbate lupus and gout. Potassium-wasting side effects may help in patients with hyperkalemia due to calcineurin inhibitors. May cause increase in serum creatinine and urea nitrogen levels in patients with renal impairment, especially at higher doses.
β-blockers: atenolol, propranolol, nadalol, metoprolol, timolol	Can cause bronchospasm. May increase triglyceride levels. Use with caution in diabetics. May affect the release of insulin, requiring dose adjustments of antihyperglycemics. Also may mask premonitory signs of hypoglycemia. Slows the heart rate: not indicated in patients with bradycardia or overt cardiac failure. β-blockers decrease cardiac contractility. Dose adjustment is needed in patients with renal impairment. Most β-blockers are excreted through the kidneys.
Angiotensin-converting enzyme (ACE) inhibitors: quinapril, ramipril, captopril, benazepril, fosinopril, lisinopril, enalapril, trandolapril, perindopril	In diabetics, may improve microalbuminuria and slow progression of renal disease. Improves left ventricular hypertrophy. Can cause hyperkalemia, especially in patients taking tacrolimus. Renal transplant patients and patients taking loop diuretics should be monitored for nephrotoxic effects when starting an ACE inhibitor. Can cause elevated levels of alanine aminotransferase (AST) and aspartate aminotransferase (ALT). Decreases number of red blood cells: can worsen anemia, but useful in treating polycythemia. Can cause leukopenia and thrombocytopenia. Use with caution in patients with hepatitis or liver transplant. Monitor complete blood count in these patients and in patients taking mycophenolate, sirolimus, or azathioprine when starting treatment with an ACE inhibitor. Risk of angioedema.
Angiotensin II receptor blocker: candesartan, irbesartan, olmesartan, losartan, valsartan	Improves microalbuminuria. Can cause pedal edema. Can cause hyperkalemia, especially in patients taking tacrolimus
Calcium channel blocker (CCB) Nondihydropyridine type: diltiazem, verapamil Dihydropyridine type: nifedipine, isradipine, nicardipine, amlodipine, felodipine, nisoldipine	Nondihydropyridine types may increase tacrolimus and cyclosporine levels as much as 3 times. Dihydropyridine types may have less of an effect. Monitor levels when starting or stopping a CCB. Nondihydropyridine types may potentiate effects of steroids by decreasing metabolism via cytochrome P-450 system isoenzymes. Conversely can decrease effectiveness if discontinued. This has implications for acute allograft rejection. May worsen gingival hyperplasia caused by cyclosporine. All CBB may reduce nephrotoxic effects of calcineurin inhibitors by lessening vasoconstriction.

Table 5. ANTI-HYPERTENSIVE MEDICATIONS AND TRANSPLANT CONSIDERATIONS (continued)

Drug	Transplant Considerations
α-Blockers: doxazosin, prazosin, terazosin	Useful in men with benign hypertrophy of the prostate. Can cause orthostatic hypotension. Use with caution in diabetics.
α/β-Adrenergic blocker: carvedilol	Concomitant use with β-blockers causes synergistic effect. Can increase cyclosporine levels by 20% to 30%. Monitor levels when starting or stopping.

Table 6. EDUCATION ISSUES FOR TRANSPLANT PATIENTS WITH HYPERTENSION

Routine monitoring of blood pressure and pulse; reporting of abnormalities
Dietary: high fiber
      low saturated fats, reduced total fats
         sodium restriction: especially in African Americans and patients taking steroids
            or calcineurin inhibitors
Exercise
Weight reduction
Cessation of smoking
Control of blood sugar in diabetics to prevent nephropathy
Control of lipid levels through exercise, diet, and when needed, medications
Compliance with medication regimen

Table 7. MEDICATIONS THAT CAN CAUSE NEPHROTOXIC EFFECTS AFTER TRANSPLANTATION

Calcineurin inhibitors: cyclosporine, tacrolimus
Nonsteroidal anti-inflammatory drugs: ibuprofen, naproxen, indomethacin, fenoprofen, ketoprofen, diclofenac
Cox-2 inhibitors: celecoxib, rofecoxib, valdecoxib (some have been withdrawn from the US market, but patients may have past exposure)
Antimicrobials: Aminoglycosides (gentamycin, amikacin), systemic amphoterican, foscarnet, ganciclovir, adefovir, cidofovir, vancomycin (when used with aminoglycosides), systemic pentamidine
Intravenous contrast dye
Diuretics: furosemide, torsemide, bumetanide
Any drug that may increase cyclosporine or tacrolimus levels, therefore increasing nephrotoxic side effects

55% of patients had normal renal function at 6 months, 17% at 12 months, only 4% at 24 months, and none had normal renal function at 36 months after transplantation.[21] Renal function can become severely depressed in the first few months after liver transplantation. In some patients, renal function improves and remain relatively stable for years, whereas in others it may progress to end-stage renal disease.[22]

Many risk factors are associated with renal dysfunction. One risk factor that is not widely appreciated is smoking. Smoking increases blood pressure, increases intra-glomerular pressure, and can even cause chronic renal endothelial cell dysfunction.[23] These effects are accelerated in elderly persons, those with hypertension, those with diabetes mellitus type 1, and those who already have some renal impairment. Graft survival is decreased in renal transplant recipients who smoke.[24] Other risk factors for chronic renal dysfunction in transplant recipients include increasing age, female gender, hepatitis C, diabetes mellitus, hypertension, acute renal failure after transplantation, and use of a calcineurin inhibitor. Proteinuria is a sign of renal dysfunction, and may also be injurious to the renal allograft in and of itself.[4]

The effects of immunosuppressants on renal function are varied. The most deleterious effects are associated with the use of calcineurin inhibitors, tacrolimus and cyclosporine. In the early postoperative period, initial effects of calcineurin inhibitors are correlated with higher doses and can be reversed by decreasing the dose or withdrawing the drug.[25] Over longer periods of time, though, these effects result in the irreversible loss of functioning renal cells. Reported pathology of kidneys chronically damaged by the toxic effects of calcineurin inhibitors shows loss of renal cells and tubules, basement membrane thickening, and focal segmental sclerosis of glomeruli with interstitial fibrosis.[5]

Renal toxicity of calcineurin inhibitors can cause renal arteriolopathy, seen as intimal thickening and narrowing of the lumen.[26] The nephrotoxic effect is thought to be dose dependent: the higher the dose, the greater the toxic effects. But there doesn't appear to be a dose low enough to avoid all nephrotoxic damage. Cyclosporine has a direct effect on the kidney, causing vasoconstriction in the afferent arteriole of the glomerulus that results in decreased glomerular filtration. It increases vascular resistance and thus increases blood pressure. Prednisone and sirolimus have no direct nephrotoxic effects. But prednisone can have an indirect adverse effect on renal function by causing hypertension, diabetes, or dyslipidemia. Sirolimus can also cause dyslipidemia and therefore indirectly adversely affect renal function. Mycophenolate and azathioprine appear to have no direct adverse affect on renal function.

Strategies to improve renal function after transplantation include withdrawing calcineurin inhibitors and switching to a sirolimus- or mycophenolate-based regimen. Renal function appears to improve after conversion.[25,27,28] This strategy, however, must be weighed against the risk of rejection. In patients with hypertension and renal dysfunction after transplantation, certain antihypertensive drugs regimens may improve renal function. These are reviewed in the section on hypertension.

Mortality rates are increased in recipients of nonrenal transplants in whom end-stage renal disease develops. Renal replacement therapy options include hemodialysis or renal transplantation. Peritoneal dialysis is not the best option for treatment because of the increased risk of infection. Patients who wish to pursue renal transplantation must fulfill the same eligibility requirements as any other patient with end-stage renal disease being considered for a renal transplant. If the nonrenal transplant recipient subsequently receives a renal allograft, for the first 4 months after surgery, the mortality risk is higher than cohorts who are still on the list awaiting a renal transplant. But after 4 months, the risk of death is lower.[20]

Education of patients can positively impact renal function after transplantation. Topics that include nephrotoxic risks should be introduced and periodically reinforced. These can even be included in education sessions and literature given to patients during evaluation for transplantation. Candidates being evaluated for transplantation should be advised of their risk for renal dysfunction, even renal failure, as complications following transplantation. Table 8 lists other patient education topics to optimize renal function after transplantation.

Table 8. EDUCATION ISSUES FOR TRANSPLANT PATIENTS TO OPTIMIZE RENAL FUNCTION

Discontinuance of smoking
Control of hypertension
Control of diabetes mellitus
Control of dyslipidemia
Avoidance of nonsteroidal anti-inflammatory drugs
Adequate oral fluid intake
Lifestyle behavior modifications: heart healthy diet and exercise
Reporting to transplant center any newly prescribed drug (including over-the-counter medications)

Diabetes Mellitus in Transplant Recipients

The diagnosis of diabetes mellitus has been defined by the American Diabetes Association (ADA) as a fasting plasma glucose level greater than 126 mg/dL (7.0 mmol/L), or a random (or 2 hour postprandial glucose) level greater than 200 mg/dL (11.1 mmol/L).[29] Diabetes mellitus is common in recipients of a solid organ transplant. Many patients may be diabetic before transplantation, whereas others become diabetic only after transplantation. Two terms are described in the literature and are used synonymously for persons in whom posttransplant diabetes mellitus (PTDM) develops: de novo diabetes and new-onset diabetes.

A review of the literature yields differing rates of PTDM. Sometimes the difference is due to center or study specific definitions of diabetes and not the ADA definition, so rates may be underreported. Some rates are as high as 53% in certain populations.[30] The longer a transplant recipient survives, the greater the risk of developing PTDM. Thus ongoing monitoring for impaired glucose metabolism is important.

Diabetes can have an adverse affect on survival of both patient and graft.[2,31] The incidence of infections, cardiovascular disease, renal failure, and bone disease is increased. Early detection and appropriate treatment can improve graft function, patient survival and quality of life. Frequent screening in the first year after transplantation by checking fasting plasma glucose level is recommended.[32]

Immunosuppression is a strong risk factor for PTDM. Many recipients, especially those taking steroids, have impaired glucose metabolism that requires insulin therapy in the early months after transplantation. Then as immunosuppression is tapered, insulin requirements decrease and these patients can be managed with oral agents or diet alone. PTDM is more likely to develop in African Americans, and they are less likely to be able to be weaned off insulin.[33] Even pediatric recipients are at increased risk for PTDM. Use of tacrolimus appears to increase that risk.[34-36] Table 9 lists the risk factors for PTDM .

The effects of immunosuppression on PTDM are well documented. Steroids have the most deleterious effect. Steroids decrease insulin secretion, decrease glucose uptake by the liver, increase glucogenesis, and can cause insulin resistance by adversely affecting insulin receptor sensitivity.[33] Cyclosporine and tacrolimus both inhibit insulin secretion. Tacrolimus may also induce insulin resistance. Tacrolimus appears to be more diabetogenic than cyclosporine. Both have an additive affect on development of PTDM when used with steroids. Azathioprine, mycophenolate, and antithymocyte globulins appear to have no diabetogenic effect.[33,37] Sirolimus had toxic effects on the islet cells of the pancreas in animal studies,[38] but studies in humans[37] have not shown this effect.

Treatment of PTDM generally follows the ADA guidelines. In the first few months, when steroid doses are being tapered, caution must be exercised to avoid overtreating hyperglycemia. Fasting plasma glucose levels must be followed closely. Steroid avoidance, rapid reduction, and/or withdrawal protocols have been advocated. The risk of diabetes must be weighed against the risk of rejection requiring higher doses of steroids for longer periods. Reduction of steroid doses, as soon as possible, should be considered. Another option would be switching to a non-diabetogenic regimen of immunosuppression.[36] Glucose-lowering agents have been used in transplant recipients. Table 10 lists some of these agents and some transplant considerations. Combination therapies have been used but not studied extensively. It is important to monitor and treat diabetic transplant recipients for other cardiovascular risk factors, such as dyslipidemia, hypertension, and anemia. Periodic screening for microalbuminuria and renal dysfunction is recommended in these patients as well.

Even if patients develop PTDM and are able to be weaned off of antihyperglycemic therapy, they should continue to self-monitor peripheral blood glucose levels frequently. Healthy lifestyle habits such as exercise, weight control, and smoking cessation are encouraged. Table 11 includes other topics for patient education as related to impaired glucose metabolism..

Hyperlipidemia

Abnormalities in lipid metabolism, such as increased levels of total serum cholesterol, low-density lipid cholesterol (LDL-C), and very low density lipid cholesterol (VLDL-C), decreased levels of high-density lipid cholesterol (HDL-C), and high serum levels of triglycerides occur frequently after transplantation.

Table 9. RISK FACTORS FOR DIABETES MELLITUS AFTER TRANSPLANTATION

Immunosuppression: steroids, tacrolimus, cyclosporine
Ethnicity: African American, Hispanic, American Indian
Age greater than 40 years
History of impaired glucose metabolism
Family history of diabetes mellitus
Obesity > 20% above ideal body weight (especially intra-abdominal obesity)
Metabolic syndrome
Hepatitis C
Use of beta blockers (in the general population, but not conclusive in transplant)
Certain HLA antigens have been associated (A28, A30, Bw42, Dw16)

Table 10. ORAL ANTIHYPERGLYCEMIC MEDICATIONS AND TRANSPLANT CONSIDERATIONS

Antihyperglycemic Medications	Transplant Considerations
α-glucosides: acarbose, miglitol	Gastrointestinal side effects may interfere with absorption of oral immunosuppressants. Monitor levels. Give 2 to 3 hours after immunosuppressant dose. Contraindicated in patients with malabsorption syndromes and colitis. Use with caution in patients with impaired renal function. Can cause elevations of liver enzyme levels. Monitor liver function closely, especially in liver transplant recipients.
Biguanide: metformin	Dose adjustment required in patients with renal dysfunction. Inhibits hepatic glucose metabolism. Use with caution in patients with liver dysfunction. Contraindicated in patients with congestive heart failure. Use with caution in the elderly and patients taking β-blockers.
Meglitinide: repaglinide	Use with caution in patients with liver dysfunction and renal impairment. When used in combination with an "azole" antifungal agent, hypoglycemic effects may be decreased.
Sulfonylureas: glyburide, glypizide, glimepiride	Renal excretion. In patients with renal dysfunction, severe hypoglycemia may occur.
Thiazolidinediones: rosaglitazone, proglitazone, troglitazone	Troglitazone was withdrawn from the US market because of liver toxicity. Decreases tacrolimus and cyclosporine levels in the P450 system. Rosaglitazone and proglitazone are also metabolized in the P450 system, but use a different enzyme from cyclosporine and tacrolimus. Should not affect levels. Hepatotoxic: monitor liver enzyme levels. Avoid use in liver transplant patients. Avoid use in patients with congestive heart failure. Can cause fluid retention and edema.

TABLE 11. PATIENT EDUCATION ISSUES AND DIABETES AFTER TRANSPLANTATION

Self-monitoring of blood glucose level even if no longer taking antihyperglycemics
Routine exercise: 30 minutes 3 to 5 times a week
Weight control
Dietary intervention
Relationship of blood glucose level and increased doses of steroids, cyclosporine, or tacrolimus
Importance of routine examinations for complications of diabetes (eye, heart, kidneys, feet, etc)
Smoking cessation
Foot care instructions
Signs of hyperglycemia: polydypsia, polyuria, weight loss, blurred vision, frequent dermatologic infections
   in children: fatigue, weakness, listlessness, nocturnal enuresis

Hyperlipidemia is an important risk factor for the development of cardiovascular disease. Hyperlipidemia has also been associated by biopsy with chronic allograft nephropathy and is an independent risk factor for graft loss in renal transplant recipients.[16] Incidence rates vary depending on the type of solid organ transplant. Rates of dyslipidemia are greater than 60% in renal transplant recipients,[39] 58% in liver recipients,[40] and 80% in cardiac recipients.[31] Deleterious changes in lipid metabolism can be observed as early as 3 to 6 months after transplantation. The most consistent change observed is increased levels of total cholesterol, LDL-C, VLDL-C, and triglycerides. Changes in HDL-C levels are more variable.[40]

Risk factors for hyperlipidemia include older age, male gender, obesity, dyslipidemia before transplantation, proteinuria, hyperglycemia, insulin resistance, family history, and alcohol comsumption. In renal transplant patients, diet and sedentary lifestyle have also been associated with hyperlipidemia.[4] Drugs that can adversely affect lipid metabolism include loop diuretics, β-blockers, steroids, cyclosporine, tacrolimus, and sirolimus. Among liver transplant patients, those treated with tacrolimus have better lipid profiles than do patients treated with cyclosporine. Those treated with tacrolimus have a significantly lower incidence of cardiovascular disease.[41] Tacrolimus is also associated with less dyslipidemia in cardiac transplant recipients.[21] Cyclosporine increases levels of total cholesterol, LDL-C, and triglycerides and decreases levels of HDL-C. Its effects appear to be dose dependent[16]: the higher the dose, the greater the degree of dyslipidemia. Cyclosporine may also increase homocysteine levels. High homocysteine levels have been associated with increased risk of cardiovascular disease and graft loss in renal transplant patients.[42]

The effect of steroids on lipid metabolism also appears to be dose dependent. Patients who have been weaned off steroids can sometimes see improvements in lipid profiles. Sirolimus, of all the immunosuppressants, appears to have the most deleterious effect on lipid metabolism.[40] The effects are dose dependent: the higher the dose, the worse the dyslipidemia. As sirolimus trough levels decrease over time, lipid profiles may improve. Mycophenolate and azathioprine do not seem to adversely affect lipid metabolism. Other comorbidities, such as diabetes and renal impairment, can further impair lipid metabolism in transplant recipients and increase the risk of cardiovascular disease.

Treatment strategies for dyslipidemia include withdrawal of steroids,[43] reduction or elimination of cyclosporine, and reduction of sirolimus. Patients should also be on a heart-healthy diet consisting of low saturated fats and decreased total fats. Increased exercise, elimination or reduction of alcohol use, and weight reduction should be encouraged. Omega-3 fish oils and use of plant stanols can also be incorporated into these lifestyle modifications. The National Cholesterol Education Program of the National Institutes of Health has established an Adult Treatment Panel III (ATP-III).[44] Although these guidelines are for the general population they are also useful in managing transplant recipients. The ATP-III guidelines stratify individuals into low, moderate, and high risk for developing cardiovascular events. The aggressiveness of treatment depends on the risk stratification. It has been recommended that renal transplant recipients be considered in the highest risk category.[4] In the high-risk category, LDL-C levels should be less than 100 mg/dL (2.59 mmol/L).[45]

Often lifestyle behavior modification measures are not enough to reach goal levels, even in the most highly motivated patients. Recommendations on treatment of hyperlipidemia in transplant recipients have included use of statins, fibrates, and other drugs to improve lipid profiles.[10,31] Some patients may require combination drug therapy to control lipid levels. In heart transplant recipients, use of pravastatin or simvastatin has been associated with improved mortality rates, improved rejection rates, and decreased coronary artery vasculopathy.[31] Table 12 includes some of the drugs commonly used to treat dyslipidemia and some transplant considerations.[46,47] Patients must always be monitored closely for side effects such as rhabdomyolysis, especially when combination therapies are used. As always, risks of treatment must be weighed against risks of cardiovascular events such as myocardial infarction, peripheral vascular disease, retinopathy, renal disease, and stroke. Every transplant recipient should be periodically screened for lipid abnormalities and other cardiovascular health risks.

Osteoporosis

Loss of bone density, osteopenia and osteoporosis, has been documented in recipients of each solid organ transplant.[9,13,31,48,49] The most rapid loss of bone density appears to occur in the first 3 months after transplantation.[16] The cause is multifactorial, but it has been well associated with use of high doses of glucocorticoids. Many patients have low bone density before transplantation and so are at even higher risk after transplantation. Other risk factors are listed in Table 13. Rates of fractures after transplantation have been reported to be around 30% to 50%. In some populations, such as caucasian women with biliary cirrhosis who have received a liver transplant, fracture rates can be as high as 65%.[2] The vertebrae and ribs are the most common sites for fractures.[48]

Bone mineral density is measured by dual-energy x-ray absorptiometry (DEXA) scans. Table 14 lists other radiographic and laboratory tests used to detect abnormalities in bone mineral density and to guide treatment. Bone mineral density is usually measured in terms of the standard deviation (SD) from normal. T scores compare the patient's bone mineral density with that of a normal young healthy population representing peak bone density. Z scores compare the bone mineral density with that of an average age-matched group. The World Health Organization has defined normal DEXA scores as negative one to positive one (-1 to 1 SD).[50,51] Osteopenia is a T score between -1 to -2.5 SD. Osteoporosis is any T score

Table 12. MEDICATIONS USED TO TREAT DYSLIPIDEMIA AND TRANSPLANT CONSIDERATIONs

Medications	Transplant Considerations
Niacin	Poorly tolerated in some patients because of side effects such as flushing. Glucose intolerance may worsen if used in combination with steroids, cyclosporine, or tacrolimus. Use with caution in diabetics and monitor blood glucose level closely. Can elevate uric acid levels. May worsen gout. Can be hepatotoxic. Use with caution in patients taking cyclosporine, which can also cause hepatotoxic effects. Monitor results of liver function tests closely.
Fibrates: fenofibrate, gemfibrozil, clofibrate	Use with caution in patients taking statins, cyclosporine, or tacrolimus due to increase in myopathies and rhabdomyolysis. May potentiate oral anticoagulants, such as warfarin. Monitor prothrombin times and international normalized ratio closely when a patient also taking warfarin starts or stops taking a fibrate. Renal excretion. Dose adjustment required in patients with renal dysfunction. Can be nephrotoxic when used in conjunction with cyclosporine or tacrolimus. Can cause pancreatitis.
HMG-CoA reductase inhibitors (statins): atorvastatin, lovastatin, pravastatin, rosuvastatin, simvastatin, fluvastatin, cerivastatin	Cyclosporine and tacrolimus may increase the serum concentration of all statin drugs to 3 to 11 times normal. The serum level of cyclosporine or tacrolimus is usually not affected. Elevation of serum statin levels can cause increased myopathies and rhabdomyolysis. Use of cyclosporine with fluvastatin and pravastatin results in increased levels of the statin, but does not appear to have clinical side effects. Start statin dose low and monitor patient closely for elevations of serum level of creatine phosphokinase, muscle aches, and rhabdomyolysis. Can be hepatotoxic. Monitor results of liver function tests closely, especially in liver transplant recipients. Gastrointestinal side effects may worsen in patients also taking mycophenolate.
Bile acid sequestrants: cholestyramine, colestipol, colesevelam	May cause increase in serum level of triglycerides. Because fat absorption is decreased, levels of fat-soluble vitamins A, D, E, and K may also be decreased, resulting in bleeding tendencies and bone disorders. Use with caution in patients with liver disease and malabsorption syndromes. May interfere with the absorption of other drugs, including immunosuppressants, if given at the same time. Take at least 1 to 2 hours after and 2 to 3 hours before any other drug. Monitor immunosuppressant drug levels when starting or stopping. A patient who is taking any sustained release formulation of any drug may have decreased absorption of that drug through the gastrointestinal tract. Gastrointestinal side effects may worsen in patients taking mycophenolate.
Cholesterol absorption inhibitor: ezetimibe	Use in transplant patients very limited. Appears to have fewer side effects. Usually used in combination with another lipid-lowering agent. Acts by inhibiting absorption of cholesterol in the gut.

below -2.5 SD. At T scores this low, the risk of fracture increases significantly. It is important to determine which patients are at high risk so that interventions can be offered before a fracture occurs. Each transplant center should develop protocols to assess patients for risk of fracture before and after transplantation.

Numerous studies in solid organ transplantation have evaluated differing treatment protocols for minimizing loss of bone density. One study in renal patients documented that in the first 3 months after transplantation, patients who were given oral calcium and vitamin D supplements lost bone density at rates similar to the rates in patients who received no supplementation. Between 3 and 6 months, however, the group receiving supplements had a slight recovery of bone density whereas the group receiving no supplementation continued to lose bone density.[52] As with other long-term complications following

Table 13. RISK FACTORS FOR OSTEOPOROSIS AFTER TRANSPLANTATION

Caucasian race
Female gender
Age greater than 50 years
Low gonadal hormone levels (estrogen, testosterone)
Small body habitus (low body weight)
History of personal fracture
Family history of osteoporosis
Smoking history
Reduced mobility or sedentary lifestyle
Nutrition related issues
    Low dietary intake of calcium
    Inadequate intake or impaired metabolism of vitamin D
    Excess alcohol ingestion
    Eating disorder such as anorexia or bulimia
Malabsorption syndromes such as inflammatory bowel disease, colitis, or gastrectomy
Disease related
    Hyperparathyroidism
    Hyperthydoidism
    Hypo phosphatemia or hyperphosphatemia
    Diabetes mellitus type 1
    Primary biliary cirrhosis
    Sclerosing cholangitis
    Cystic fibrosis
    Chronic renal disease
Medication related
    Glucocorticoids
    Long-term use of heparin
    Use of calcineurin inhibitors (cyclosporine or tacrolimus): strong evidence in animal models, but in human transplant recipients, study results are inconclusive

Table 14. TESTS FOR DETECTION OF ABNORMALITIES IN BONE MINERAL DENSITY

Dual-energy x-ray absorptiometry usually done on lumbar spine, hip, femur, and/or wrist
Thoracic and lumbar spine radiographs (evidence of fracture)
Quantitative computed tomography and magnetic resonance imaging used in research to assess trabecular versus cortical bone
Ultrasound has been correlated with fracture risk, but results have not been standardized
Laboratory tests
    Serum and urinary calcium levels
    Serum phosphorus levels
    Vitamin D levels
    Osteocalcin
    Intact parathyroid hormone
    Alkaline phosphatase (bone specific)
    Chemistry panel to detect underlying renal or hepatic disease
    Urinary pyridinoline crosslink
    N- or C-teleopeptides
    Thyroid function studies
    Testosterone levels in men
    Estrogen levels in women

transplantation, no general consensus has been reached as to specific treatment protocols for loss of bone density.

Several studies in solid organ transplant recipients reported that patients whose bone mineral density T scores were -1 SD or below benefited from use of such agents as calcitriol, etidromate, alendronate,

Table 15. DRUG THERAPY FOR TRANSPLANT PATIENTS WITH OSTEOPOROSIS AND OSTEOPENIA

Medications	Transplant Considerations
Calcium	1000 to 1500 mg per day for nonhypercalcemic patients. Caution in patients with renal stones. Start early after transplantation
Vitamin D	400 to 800 U per day. In patients with renal disease, vitamin D analogues, such as calcitriol, are used. These can cause hypercalcemia and hypercalcuria.
Calcitonin	Can be given subcutaneously or by inhalation. Alternate nostril every other day. Inhibits osteoclast activity. May also be helpful in osteoporotic patients to manage bone pain. Tolerance can be developed as early as 6 months of use.
Estrogen for women	Controversial in postmenopausal women because of risk of cardiovascular mortality and cancer. Women with an intact uterus also need progesterone.
Testosterone for men	Testosterone use in men is also controversial because of risk of cancer. Beneficial in increasing hematocrit in anemic patients. Patients who are also taking cyclosporine must be monitored for increase risk of hepatotoxic effects.
Selective estrogen receptor modulators: reloxifene, tamoxifen	Can also reduce total cholesterol and low-density lipid cholesterol. Used in general population for women who cannot take estrogen. Have not been adequately studied in the transplant population.
Bisphosphonates: alendronate, risedronate, etidronate, pamidronate, ibandronate	Contraindicated in patients with glomerular filtration rate lower than 30 mL/min. Use with caution in patients with low bone turnover. Monitor urinary peptide levels for bone turnover. Gastric irritation may be worse in patients taking mycophenolate. Oral forms can be taken daily, weekly or monthly. Must be taken on an empty stomach. Patient must stay upright and take no food, drink, or other medications for 30 to 60 minutes after taking oral drug. Sitting up helps avoid gastrointestinal irritation. Fasting increases absorption of oral drug. Patient should immediately report symptoms of gastrointestinal reflux or heartburn.
Parathyroid hormone: teriparatide	Can cause hypercalcemia. Long-term excess parathyroid hormone can lead to bone loss, but studies of intermittent use have demonstrated improvement in bone density in certain patients with osteoporosis.

pamidronate, and ibandronate.[53-57] Those researchers reported either a decrease in the rate of bone loss compared with the control group or an increase in bone density in the treatment group. In at least 1 study, researchers observed that at 6 months of treatment with pamidronate, all patients in the treatment group had adynamic bone disease compared with the control group, of which only 50% had adynamic bone disease.[58] Bone resorption was stopped, but new bone was not being laid down. In transplant recipients with normal serum levels of calcium, adequate dietary intake of calcium and vitamin D should be encouraged. In patients at high risk of fracture, anti-resorptive treatment should be considered with close monitoring for side effects and effectiveness of treatment. Patients with osteopenia fall into the gray area. Risks of treatment must always be balanced against risks of side effects of the drug. Table 15 lists the drugs commonly used to treat osteoporosis.

Management of immunosuppression and other drug therapies after transplantation should be reviewed in patients at risk for and patients with osteoporosis. Reduction of steroid doses must be balanced against risk for rejection. Treatment for rejection may lead to even higher doses of steroids for longer periods, putting the patient at greater risk of bone disease. Steroid avoidance protocols are being studied for long-term benefits to bone health. Another class of drugs that can adversely affect bone health is loop diuretics, such as furosemide, torsemide, and bumetamide. These diuretics increase calcium excretion by the kidneys, whereas thiazide diuretics can increase calcium absorption by the kidneys. Patients with osteopenia or osteoporosis who need diuretic therapy would benefit from use of a thiazide type instead of a loop diuretic.

All patients should also receive education on lifestyle measures to minimize bone loss. These measures include weight-bearing and resistive exercise several times a week. Walking is a great inexpensive exercise for most. Muscle strengthening and balance training is important in patients who have become debilitated. Dietary consultation can be done to evaluate adequacy of calcium and vitamin D intake. Home health services can evaluate the patient's environment for tripping and fall hazards, such as small floor mats. Patients who smoke should be strongly encouraged to stop for many reasons, including bone health.

Conclusion

Increased survival rates after transplantation have brought to the forefront the deleterious effects of long-term use of immunosuppressant medications. Long-term complications that adversely affect patients' morbidity, mortality, and quality of life have been well documented. Many choices and combinations of immunosuppressants are available today. No one protocol can be applied to all cases. But drug therapies tailored to each patient are a reality now more than ever. Better use of immunosuppressants, new medications to treat complications, and early intervention are giving patients and transplant centers options they never had before. Early recognition and aggressive modification of causative factors of common complications after transplantation are crucial for managing long-term survivors of solid organ transplantation.

References

1. Cecka JM, Terasaki PI. *Clinical Transplants 2002*. Los Angeles, Calif: UCLA Immunogenetics Center; 2003.
2. Brown AS, Williams R. Long term postoperative care. In: Maddrey WC, Schiff ER, Sorrell MF, eds. *Transplantation of the Liver*. 3rd ed. Philadelphia, Pa: Lippincott Williams & Wilkins; 2001;163-175.
3. Wheeler DC, Steiger J. Evolution and etiology of cardiovascular disease in renal transplant recipients. *Transplantation*. December 15, 2000;70(suppl):ss40-43.
4. Kasiske B. Long-term post transplant management of complications. In Danovitch GM, ed. *Handbook of Kidney Transplantation*. 3rd ed. Philadelphia, Pa: Lippincott Williams & Wilkins; 2001.
5. Tolkoff-Rubin N, Langhoff E. Renal considerations of organ transplantation. In: Ginns LC, Cosimi AB, Morris PJ, eds. *Transplantation*. Malden, Mass: Blackwell Science; 1999.
6. Crippin JS. Late onset complications and recurrent nonmalignant disease. In: Busuttil RW, Klintmalm GB, eds. *Transplantation of the Liver*. Philadelphia, Pa: WB Saunders Co; 1996.
7. McDiarmid SV. Current status of liver transplantation in children. *Pediatr Clin North Am*. 2003;50:1335-1374.
8. Anderson AS. Prognosis after orthotopic heart transplantation, uptodate online Version 13.1, data taken from the 16th Official Report–1999 of the Registry of the International Society for Heart and Lung Transplantation. Available at: www.uptodate.com. Accessed March 1, 2005.
9. Trulock EP. Miscellaneous complications following lung transplantation. UpToDate Online version 12.3. Available at: www.uptodate.com. Accessed February 1, 2005.
10. Magee C, Pascual M. Update of renal transplantation. *Arch Intern Med*. 2004;164:1373-1388.
11. Midtvedt K, Neumayer H. Management strategies for posttransplant hypertension. *Transplantation*. December 15, 2000; 70(suppl)11:ss64-ss69.
12. Bostom AD, Chavers BM, Cosio FG, et al. Prevention of posttransplant cardiovascular disease: report and recommendations of an ad hoc group. *Am J Transplant*. 2002;2:491-500.
13. Cohen D, Galbraith C. General health management and long term care of the renal recipient. *Am J Kidney Dis*. 2001;38(6 suppl):s10-s25.
14. Chobanian AV, Bakris GL, Black HR, et al. Seventh report of the Joint National Committee on Prevention, Detection, Evaluation, and Treatment of High Blood Pressure. Hypertension. 2003;42:1206-1252.
15. Cotler S. Nonimmunologic complications of liver transplantation. UpToDate Online version 13.1. Available at: www.uptodate.com. Accessed March 1, 2005.
16. Rodino MA, Schacter N, Shane E. Endocrine and metabolic considerations of organ transplantation. In: Ginns LC, Cosimi AB, Morris PJ, eds. *Transplantation*. Malden, Mass: Blackwell Science; 1999.
17. Jardine AG. Pretransplant management of end-stage renal disease to minimize posttransplant risk. *Transplantation*. December 15, 2000;70(11 suppl):ss46-ss50.
18. Lexi-Comp Online Interaction Monograph: Corticosteroids (systemic)/Calcium Channel Blockers. Available at: www.lexi-comp.com. Accessed March 1, 2005.
19. McDonald AS. Impact of immunosuppressive therapy on hypertension. *Transplantation*. December 15, 2000;70(11 suppl): ss70-ss76.
20. Ojo AO, Held PJ, Port FK, et al. Chronic renal failure after transplantation of a non-renal organ. *N Engl J Med*. September 4, 2003;349:931-940.
21. Parry G, Meiser B, Bago GR. The clinical impact of cyclosporine nephrotoxicity in heart transplantation. *Transplantation*. 2000;69(12 suppl):ss23-ss26.
22. Fisher NC, Malag M. The clinical impact of nephrotoxicity in liver transplantation. *Transplantation*. June 27, 2000;69(12): ss18-ss22.

23. Orth SR. Effects of smoking on systemic and intrarenal hemodynamics: influence on renal function. *J Am Soc Nephrol.* 2004;15:58-63.
24. Orth SR. Smoking and the kidney. *J Am Soc Nephrol.* 2002;13:1663-1672.
25. Sayegh MH, Bennett WM. Cyclosporine and tacrolimus nephrotoxicity-I. UpToDate Online version 13.1. Available at: www.uptodate.com. Accessed March 1, 2005.
26. Davies DR. Histopathology of calcineurin inhibitor induced nephrotoxicity. *Transplantation.* 2000;69(12 suppl):ss11-ss13.
27. Groth CG. Sirolimus (Rapamycin) based therapy in human renal transplantation: similar efficacy and different toxicity compared with cyclosporine. *Transplantation.* 1999;67:1036-1042.
28. MacDonald AS. Management strategies for nephrotoxicity. *Transplantation.* 2000;69(12 suppl):ss31-ss36.
29. American Diabetes Association. All about diabetes. Available at: http://www.diabetes.org/about-diabetes.jsp Accessed May 20, 2006.
30. Montori VM, Velosa JA, Basu A, et al. Posttransplant diabetes: a systematic review of the literature. *Diabetes Care.* 2002;25:583-592.
31. Lindenfeld J, Page, RL, Ronald MD, et al. Drug therapy in heart transplant recipient: III. Common medical problems. *Circulation.* 2005;111:113-117.
32. Gaston R, Howard A, Macauley J, et al. *Diabetes and Kidney Transplantation: Maximizing Long Term Health.* Birmingham, Ala: Transplant Community Outreach Program, University of Alabama School of Medicine; April 2003.
33. Reisaeter AV, Hartmann A. Risk factors and incidence of post transplant diabetes mellitus. *Transplant Proc.* 2001;33(S5A):85-185.
34. Paolillo JA, Boyle GJ, Law YM, et al. Post transplant diabetes mellitus in pediatric thoracic organ recipients recipients receiving tacrolimus-based immunosuppression. *Transplantation.* January 27, 2001;71:232-256
35. Greenspan LC, Gitelman SE, Leung MA, et al. Increased incidence in post transplant diabetes mellitus in children: a case controlled analysis. *Pediatr Nephrol.* 2002;17:1-5.
36. Davidson J, Wilkinson A, Dantal J, et al. New onset diabetes after transplantation: 2003 international consensus guidelines. *Transplantation.* 2003;75(10 suppl):ss3-ss24.
37. Jindal RM, Hjelmesaeth J. Impact and management of post transplant diabetes mellitus. *Transplantation* 2000;70(11 suppl):58-63.
38. Fabian ML, Lakely JR, et al. The efficacy and toxicity of rapamune in murine islet transplantation. *Transplantation* 1993;56:1137-1142.
39. Hricik DE. Non-immunologic complications of kidney transplantation. *Am J Kidney Dis.* 2004;43:1135-1137.
40. Fellstrom B. Impact and management of hyperlipidemia in post transplantation. *Transplantation.* 2000;70(11 suppl):ss51-ss57.
41. Robkin JM, Corless CC, Rosen HR, et al. Immunosuppression impact on long term cardiovascular complications post liver transplantation. *Am J Surg.* 2002;183:595-599.
42. Bostom AG. Homocysteine: expensive creatinine or important modifiable risk factor for arteriosclerotic outcomes in renal transplant recipients? *J Am Soc Nephrol.* 2000;11:149-151.
43. Abtahi PZ. Management of hyperlipidemia in the stable solid organ transplant recipient. *Graft.* 2001;4(suppl 4):266-275.
44. National Cholesterol Education Program, National Heart Lung and Blood Institute. Detection, evaluation, and treatment of high cholesterol in adults. Available at: www.nhlbi.nih.gov/guidelines/cholesterol. Accessed May 20, 2006.
45. Gotto AM. *Contemporary Diagnosis and Management of Lipid Disorders.* 3rd ed. Newtown, Pa: Handbooks in Health Care Co; 2004.
46. Lexi-Comp Online Interactive Monograph: HMG-CoA reductase inhibitors and cyclosporine. Available at: www.lexi-comp.com. Accessed March 2005.
47. Page RL, Miller G, Lindenfeld J. Drug therapy in the heart transplant recipient: part iv: drug-drug interactions. *Circulation.* January 18, 2005;8:230-239.
48. Rosen HN. Osteoporosis After Solid Organ Transplantation. UpToDate Online version13.1. Available at: www.uptodate.com. Accessed March 1, 2005.
49. Sheiner P, Magliocca JF, Bodian CA, et al. Long-term medical complications in patients surviving >5 years after liver transplant. *Transplantation.* 2000;69:781-789.
50. Brown SA, Clifford JR. Osteoporosis. *Med Clin North Am.* 2003;87:1039-1063.
51. World Health Organization practice guidelines on the use of bone mineral density measurements. Available at: http://www.emro.who.int/ncd/publications/osteoporosis-guidelines.pdf. Accessed May 20, 2006.
52. De sevaux RG, Hoitsma AJ, Corstens FH, et al. Treatment with vitamin D and calcium reduces bone loss after renal transplantation: a randomized study. *J Am Soc Nephrol.* 2002;13:1608-1614.
53. Sambrook P, Henderson NK, Keogh A, et al. Effects of calcitriol on bone loss after cardiac or lung transplantation. *J Bone Miner Rev.* 2002;15:1818-1824.
54. Arlen DJ, Lambert K, Ioannidis G, et al. Treatment of established bone loss after renal transplantation with etidronate. *Transplantation.* 2001;71:669-673.
55. Fan SL, Almond MK. Pamidronate therapy as prevention of bone loss following renal transplantation. *Kidney Int.* 2000;57:684-690.
56. Shane E, Addesso V, Namerow PB, et al. Alendronate vs calcitriol for the prevention of bone loss following cardiac transplantation. *N Engl J Med.* 2004;350:767-776.
57. Grotz W, Nagle C, Poeschel D, et al. Effect of ibandronate on bone loss and renal function after kidney transplantation. *J Am Soc Nephrol.* 2001;12:1530-1537.
58. Coco M, Glicklich D, Faugere M, et al. Prevention of bone loss in renal transplant recipients: bone loss in renal transplant recipients: a prospective, randomized trial of intravenous pamidronate. *J Am Soc Nephrol.* 2003;14:2669-2676.

Infection in Solid Organ Transplant Recipients

Meredith J. Aull, PharmD
Rudina Odeh-Ramadan, PharmD

Introduction

The occurrence of infection after transplantation is a significant determinant of transplant outcome.[1] The incidence of infections after solid-organ transplantation is dependent on several factors, including the degree of immunosuppression, the type of organ transplanted, technical or surgical complications, the need for additional antirejection therapy, environmental exposures, and the time frame after transplantation. The occurrence of infection after transplantation usually falls within 3 general time frames: the first month, the second through the sixth month, and more than 6 months after transplantation.[2]

Infections that occur during the first month after transplantation are generally the same nosocomial infections seen in nonimmunosuppressed patients after surgery. These infections include bacterial and candidal wound infections, pneumonia, urinary tract infection (UTI), and sepsis due to intravascular or drainage catheters.

The period from the second to sixth month after transplantation is the time during which opportunistic infections "classically" associated with transplantation occur.[1] The most common infections during this period include cytomegalovirus (CMV), *Pneumocystis (carinii) jiroveci*, *Aspergillus* species, *Nocardia* species, *Toxoplasmosis*, *Listeria monocytogenes*, and fungal infections. In addition, reactivation of immunomodulating viruses will begin to manifest a clinically significant effect. These viruses include Epstein Barr virus (EBV), CMV, hepatitis B virus (HBV), hepatitis C virus (HCV), human herpesvirus type 6 (HHV-6), and human immunodeficiency virus (HIV).[1,2]

More than 6 months after transplantation, most transplant recipients (80%) are doing well, and the most common infections seen during this period mimic those seen in the general community.[2] Such infections include influenza virus, UTIs, and pneumococcal pneumonia. Although opportunistic infections are rarely observed during this time period, reactivation of varicella zoster virus (VZV) or CMV can occur. In addition, transplant recipients who have had multiple rejection episodes requiring additional antirejection may be predisposed to opportunistic infections more commonly seen 2 to 6 months after transplantation. Transplant recipients experiencing chronic infection due to HBV, HCV, CMV, EBV, or HIV, resulting in a greater degree of morbidity, are subsequently at an increased risk for other infections.[1,2]

In patients who undergo retransplantation, the typical timetable of infections may be altered. Infections characteristic of 1 of the 3 conventional time periods may occur simultaneously and with an increased severity.[3]

Bacterial Infection

Some of the most prevalent microbial pathogens observed after organ transplantation are bacteria. Bacterial infections occur in 33% to 68% of liver, 21% to 30% of heart, 54% of lung, 35% of pancreas, and 47% of kidney transplant recipients.[3-5]

The specific bacterial infections that occur after transplantation can be divided into 4 categories[6]:
- Infections due to surgical or technical complications,
- Infections related to prolonged hospitalization (nosocomial infections),
- Infections associated with the degree of immunosuppression (opportunistic infections), and
- Infections occurring months after transplantation when the transplant recipient resumes normal activity (community-acquired infections).

Although transplant recipients are susceptible to common bacterial pathogens observed in normal hosts, the immunosuppressed state of the recipient after transplantation predisposes the patient to bacterial pathogens not commonly observed in the normal host. These opportunist pathogens include *Legionella* species, *Nocardia* species, *Rhodococcus* species, *L monocytogenes*, and *Mycobacteria* species.[7]

Following transplantation, disruption of anatomic barriers is commonly associated with bacterial infections. For instance, the upper airway is normally colonized with bacteria, and the lower respiratory tract is normally sterile. Endotracheal intubation creates a conduit between the upper and lower respiratory tract, introducing bacteria to the lower respiratory tract and resulting in disease of the bronchial tubes or lung parenchyma.[7] Bacteria most commonly associated with these infections include *Streptococcus pneumoniae*, *Haemophilus influenzae*, *Neisseria meningitides*, group A streptococci, and *Klebsiella pneumoniae*.[8] Associated with endotracheal intubation, the most common pathogens to colonize the oropharynx and spread to the lower respiratory tract are nosocomial bacteria. Such pathogens include gram-negative facultative anaerobic bacteria (primarily species of the Enterobacteriaceae family, such as *Escherichia coli*, *Klebsiella* species, *Enterobacter* species, *Proteus* species, *Serratia* species); gram-negative obligate aerobic bacteria (*Pseudomonas* species, *Stenotrophomonas maltophilia*, *Burkholderia cepacia*); or gram-positive facultative anaerobic bacteria (methicillin-resistant *Staphylococcus aureus*, methicillin-resistant coagulase-negative staphylococci, vancomycin-resistant *Enterococcus* species).[8] Indwelling vascular catheters may become colonized with nosocomial bacteria or cutaneous flora and introduce these pathogens into the bloodstream, resulting in sepsis. Pathogens commonly implicated in these infections include *Staphylococcus* species, coagulase-negative bacteria; *Streptococcus* species, viridans group, and *Corynebacterium* species.[9,10]

Renal and Pancreatic Transplantation

Overview

The most common infections occurring after kidney transplantation are UTIs. The reported incidence of UTI in kidney recipients is 83% to 90%.[11,12] Predisposing factors include renal insufficiency, ischemic changes of the graft, decreased urine flow through the urinary epithelium, prolonged urinary catheterization, and underlying medical conditions such as diabetes mellitus. The most common pathogens implicated in UTIs include enteric gram-negative bacilli, staphylococci, enterococci, and *Pseudomonas aeruginosa*.[13] In addition, surgical wound infections and catheter-related bacteremias are commonly observed.

The most common bacterial infections observed after pancreatic transplantation are wound and intraabdominal infections. The most common pathogens implicated in such infections include enteric bacteria.[14] Bladder infections may also readily occur after pancreatic transplantation because of the change in urinary pH due to the drainage of exocrine pancreatic secretions into the bladder.

Prophylaxis

Trimethoprim/sulfamethoxazole (cotrimoxazole; Septra, Bactrim) has proven efficacy in reducing the incidence of UTIs, as well as bacteremias after transplantation. Trimethoprim/sulfamethoxazole is also effective in preventing infections by *P (carinii) jiroveci*, *L monocytogenes*, *Nocardia* species, and *Toxoplasmosis gondii*. Therapy should continue for at least 6 months after transplantation, although the duration varies from center to center. In sulfa-allergic patients, alternatives may include atovaquone, pentamidine, and dapsone.

To prevent surgical wound and abdominal infections, the appropriate perioperative antibacterial prophylaxis should be instituted in the operating room and continue postoperatively for more than 24 hours and less than 72 hours.[15] The prophylactic antibiotic of choice should be determined by the resident flora of the transplanted, the prevalent bacterial flora identified in wound infections and the institutional antibiotic susceptibility pattern.[15] In kidney transplant recipients, the target pathogens include uropathogens and staphylococci; hence either a first-generation cephalosporin or ampicillin/sulbactam is an appropriate prophylactic agent. For pancreatic transplantation, coverage should be extended to prevent against gram-negative bacteria.[15]

Treatment

The antibiotic of choice for the treatment of infection after renal or pancreatic transplantation is largely dependent on the susceptibility of the bacteria identified in the urine, blood, or wound culture. Fluoroquinolones, cephalosporins, or penicillins are commonly used to treat UTIs. For infections due to coagulase-negative staphylococci or ampicillin-resistant enterococci, vancomycin is the drug of choice.[16] Treatment duration depends on the origin and severity of infection. Wound infections and most UTIs require treatment for 5 to 7 days, whereas pyelonephritis usually requires 2 weeks of therapy or longer. Imaging to rule out obstruction or anatomic abnormalities should be considered in cases of recurrent UTIs. In addition, wound infections may require debridement with an adjunctive antibiotic regimen.

Liver Transplantation

Overview

The most commonly observed infection after liver transplantation is intra-abdominal infection (30%).[13,17] Other commonly occurring infections include intrahepatic and extrahepatic abscesses, cholangitis, bacteremia, surgical wound infection, and lower respiratory tract infection. The majority of these infections occur within the first 2 months after transplantation and are associated with a mortality rate of 4%.[17] Predisposing factors include prolonged surgical time, high transfusion requirements, repeat abdominal surgery, CMV infection, and choledochojejunostomy (Roux-en-Y) biliary anastomosis instead of a choledochostomy (duct to duct).[18-21] The sphincter of Oddi is maintained in a duct-to-duct anastomosis and is therefore associated with less infection. However, a Roux-en-Y anastomosis provides a free-flowing communication between the intestinal contents and the biliary system and is therefore associated with a higher incidence of cholangitis after transplantation as well as infection after liver biopsy.[13,22]

The predominant organisms causing infection in liver transplant recipients are enteric gram-negative bacilli like *E coli*, Enterobacteriaceae, and *Pseudomonas* species. Additional pathogens include enterococci, staphylococci, and anaerobes.[18-21,23-25] Infections by vancomycin-resistant enterococci are particularly problematic.[15]

Prevention

Because of the high degree of morbidity and mortality associated with gram-negative infections after hepatic transplantation, it is imperative to enable appropriate means of prevention. A crucial prophylactic measure is to ensure appropriate surgical technique. It is also essential to initiate perioperative antimicrobial prophylaxis and continue it for 24 to 48 hours after transplantation, to prevent surgical wound infections. Prophylactic antimicrobials commonly selected include an extended-spectrum cephalosporin or penicillin.

Another effective means of prevention is eradication of oral and gut flora, known as selective bowel decontamination. This is done to prevent colonization of the oral cavity and gastrointestinal tract with gram-negative aerobic bacteria and fungi, while sparing the protective anaerobic flora.[26] Selective bowel decontamination is achieved by initiating nonabsorbable oral antibiotics. However, selective bowel decontamination spares gram-positive and anaerobic organisms that have an antagonistic effect on the growth of gram-negative pathogens. Selective decontamination is most effective when initiated 1 week before transplantation and continued for 1 to 3 weeks after transplantation.[15,27-29] Selective decontamination has decreased the overall incidence of infections after liver transplantation. The incidence of gram-negative bacteremias, which carry a high degree of mortality, has decreased significantly. Nevertheless, an increase in infections caused by pathogens (ie, *Lactobacillus* species) not covered by selective bowel decontamination has been reported.[30] In addition, a substantial increase in the incidence of infections due to vancomycin-resistant enterococci and methicillin-resistant *S aureus* has been observed. However, an association between the use of selective bowel decontamination and the increase in vancomycin-resistant enterococci and methicillin-resistant *S aureus* has not been characterized.[15,16]

Treatment

Pathogen identification and antimicrobial susceptibility testing are essential to achieve optimal treatment. Fluid collections, purulent secretions, and blood should be cultured when infection is suspected. If an abscess has been identified, drainage may be necessary to achieve optimal therapeutic response. While culture results are pending, empiric antimicrobial therapy should be initiated in the seriously ill. Empiric therapy should be selected on the basis of known colonizing flora. Once the pathogen has been identified and susceptibility patterns reported, antibiotic therapy should be tailored appropriately. Cholangitis should be treated with intravenous antimicrobials in the absence of an obstruction. In the case of a biliary obstruction, endoscopic retrograde cholangiopancreatography with dilatation may be necessary.[16]

Heart Transplantation

Overview

The most common bacterial infection occurring after heart transplantation is nosocomially acquired ventilator-associated pneumonia. The most prevalent pathogens include gram-negative bacteria like *P aeruginosa*, *K pneumoniae*, and other Enterobacteriaceae.[31-34] Other infections commonly observed include wound infections, mediastinitis, vascular access device bacteremias, and UTIs.

Prophylaxis

Aggressive efforts to wean patients from ventilation should be employed to prevent the occurrence of pneumonia. Also, perioperative antimicrobial therapy should be instituted to target gram-positive organisms and prevent sternal wound infections. Antibiotics selected may include first-generation cephalosporins or penicillins. However, vancomycin may be used if methicillin-resistant *S aureus* is a concern. In addition, to prevent endocarditis, standard antibiotic prophylaxis should be initiated in heart transplant recipients undergoing any high-risk procedure.[34]

Treatment

Treatment of pneumonia should be guided by culture and susceptibility testing. Infections of the sternum and mediastinitis may require surgical debridement followed by adjunctive antimicrobial therapy.[16]

Lung Transplantation

Overview

The most common bacterial infection occurring in a lung transplant recipient is pneumonia, with an overall prevalence rate of 60%.[16] Pneumonias in lung recipients typically occur within the first 2 weeks after transplantation. Factors predisposing lung transplant recipients to pneumonia include impaired cough reflex of the lung allograft, poor mucociliary clearance, ischemia to the explanted lung, disruption of lymphatic drainage, reperfusion injury, and rejection-mediated airway inflammation resulting in bacterial colonization.[16] The most common causative pathogens are gram-negative bacteria including *Enterobacter cloacae*, *P aeruginosa*, *E coli*, and *K pneumoniae*. Other infecting organisms include *S aureus*, *H influenzae*, and *S pneumoniae*.[8] Unfortunately, shortly after transplantation, patients with cystic fibrosis who have colonization of the airways with *B cepacia* are at an increased risk of morbidity and mortality.[35]

Prevention

Aggressive prophylactic antibiotic therapy is required for lung transplant recipients. The prophylactic antibiotic of choice should be selected on the basis of growth of cultures of respiratory tract secretions from the donor and the recipient. Patients colonized with *B cepacia* or other multidrug-resistant gram-negative bacteria may require treatment with inhaled aminoglycosides as well. To prevent postoperative wound infections, perioperative prophylaxis should be directed against gram-positive organisms.[16]

Treatment

Pneumonia should be treated aggressively, and antibiotic selection should be based on antimicrobial susceptibilities of the bacteria isolated. Infections with *P aeruginosa, B cepacia,* or Enterobacteriaceae may require a regimen consisting of 2 antimicrobials. Postoperative wound infections and mediastinitis may require debridement and antibiotic therapy.

Fungal Infection

Invasive fungal infections are a significant infectious complication among solid-organ transplant recipients and remain a major cause of morbidity and mortality. Although the incidence of fungal infections varies with the specific type of organ transplanted, the overall incidence ranges from 5% among kidney transplant recipients to 40% among liver transplant recipients.[36] *Aspergillus* and *Candida* are the most common fungal pathogens in solid-organ transplantation. Invasive *Aspergillus* infections are associated with the highest mortality rate (70%), whereas *Candida* infections are associated with a 30% mortality rate in renal transplant recipients.[37] The most common cause of opportunistic pneumonia is *P (carinii) jiroveci,* occurring in approximately 10% of transplant recipients. *Pneumocystis* pneumonia usually occurs within the first 6 months after transplantation.

Kidney and Pancreas Transplantation

Among all solid-organ transplant recipients, renal transplantation is currently associated with the lowest rate (5%) of fungal infections. However, the urinary tract is the most prevalent site for fungal infections in these recipients. The most common pathogen is the *Candida* species, mostly *Candida albicans.*[38] The majority of these infections occur within the first 2 months after transplantation. However, infections due to endemic fungi occur in the mid to late posttransplantation period. Endemic fungal infections are associated with pathogens like *Histoplasma capsulatum, Blastomyces dermatitidis,* and *Coccidioides immitis.*

Intraabdominal fungal infections have been reported in 9% to 19% of pancreas transplant recipients.[39] *Candida* species are the most common organisms associated with fungal infections among these patients. The predominant risk factors associated with pancreas transplant recipients that predisposes them to fungal infections include (1) the presence of diabetes mellitus and (2) pancreas transplantation into patients with preexisting renal grafts who are therefore already immunosuppressed.

Liver and Small-Bowel Transplantation

The incidence of fungal infections in liver transplant recipients ranges from 4% to 50%. The majority of the infections are due to *Candida* species (77% to 83%), with more *Candida* fungal infections occurring in liver transplant recipients than recipients of any other organ. The high incidence of *Candida* fungal infections in these patients may be attributed to the disruption and surgical manipulation of the gut and biliary tree during transplantation, resulting in disseminated gastrointestinal candidiasis. Infections due to *Candida* usually occur within the first 2 months after transplantation, with the majority occurring within the first 2 weeks.[40] Documented risk factors for invasive fungal infection after transplantation include retransplantation, prolonged initial surgery time (>11 hours), high intraoperative transfusion requirement, preoperative steroid use, preoperative antibiotic therapy, treatment of rejection, bacterial infections, and renal insufficiency (serum level of creatinine >265 μmol/L [>3 mg/dL]).[41-44] However, fungal colonization detected by postoperative day 3 is the greatest risk factor for early infection.

Aspergillus infection occurs in 1% to 8% of liver transplant recipients. Unfortunately, most *Aspergillus* infections in these patients occur soon after transplantation. Independent risk factors for *Aspergillus* infection in liver recipients include renal dysfunction and use of muromonab CD3 (OKT3).[41, 45,46]

Relative to the frequency of other solid-organ transplantations, small-bowel transplantation is rare. However, from estimates based on the number of cases of fungal infections reported in bowel recipients, *Candida* species are the most common pathogens, followed by *Aspergillus* species. The candidal infections most commonly described include candidal esophagitis followed by intraabdominal infections and candidemia with dissemination. The incidence of *Aspergillus* infections in small-bowel transplant recipients is similar to that reported in kidney recipients.[47,48]

Several factors put small-bowel recipients at an increased risk of fungal infection, including poor gastrointestinal function before transplantation with an increased risk of fungal colonization, bowel surgery, and ischemic injuries.[49]

Lung Transplantation

Airway colonization with *Aspergillus* is common in lung transplant recipients owing to direct communication of the transplanted lung with the environment and impaired host defenses. The bronchial arteries are disrupted at the site of the anastomosis during surgery. Until collaterals from bronchial circulation form, the anastomotic healing is dependent on the blood supply from pulmonary circulation of the transplanted lung. Therefore, the anastomotic site with transient devascularization remains susceptible to ischemic injury, necrosis, and infection with *Aspergillus*.[50,51]

Aspergillus is reported to be isolated from airway cultures in 9% to 68% of lung transplant recipients.[52-56] Tracheobronchitis is observed only in lung transplant recipients and can be characterized by endobronchial lesions ranging from mild bronchitis to ulcers and pseudomembranes. Tracheobronchitis may be early or locally invasive disease and can progress to disseminated infection.[57] Lesions involving or located near the anastomotic site can result in fatal bronchopleural fistulas.[58]

Lung recipients with airway colonization with *Aspergillus* tend to have a higher risk of invasive infection. It has been reported that an invasive *Aspergillus* infection is 11 times more likely to develop in patients who have respiratory cultures positive for *Aspergillus* within 6 months after transplantation than in patients who do not.[59] Most *Aspergillus* invasive infections in lung transplant recipients are due to *Aspergillus fumigatus*.[53] However, colonization with *Aspergillus* before transplantation does not predispose cystic fibrosis patients to invasive *Aspergillus* infections after transplantation.[59] Additional risk factors for invasive *Aspergillus* infections in lung recipients include CMV infection, obliterative bronchiolitis, rejection, and high-dose immunosuppression therapy.[59-62] The reported mortality rate associated with invasive *Aspergillus* infections in these patients is 68%.[63]

Although *Candida* is commonly isolated from the respiratory tract of lung transplant recipients, *Candida* pneumonia is rare. However, candidal colonization of the anastomotic site can cause tracheobronchitis that may lead to potentially fatal mediastinitis.

Heart Transplantation

Fungal infections in heart transplant recipients are reported less frequently then in heart-lung or lung transplant recipients.[36] Nevertheless, *Aspergillus* infection is the most commonly occurring mycosis in heart recipients. Of all fungal infections occurring in heart recipients, *Aspergillus* accounts for 69.8% of infections.[64] Although the incidence of *Aspergillus* infection is greater than the incidence of *Candida* infection in heart recipients, this patient population is considered to be at far less risk for invasive aspergillosis than are liver or lung transplant recipients.[63] Nevertheless, *Aspergillus* is detected in approximately 10% of heart recipients after transplantation.[65] *Aspergillus* infection in heart recipients usually manifests as pulmonary infection with subsequent dissemination and typically has an earlier onset than *Candida* infection. Onset of invasive *Aspergillus* infections has been reported to occur between 36 and 52 days after transplantation, with approximately 75% of the cases having occurred within 90 days after transplantation.[66]

Isolating *Aspergillus*, especially *A fumigatus*, has proven to be highly predictive of invasive aspergillosis infection.[65] The risk factors for invasive aspergillosis infection in heart recipients includes reoperation, CMV infection, hemodialysis after transplantation, and the occurrence of an episode of invasive *Aspergillus* infection within the heart transplant program at the same institution 2 months before or after the date of transplantation.[67] The mortality rate of invasive aspergillosis in heart recipients is reported to be 53% to 78%. However, the mortality rate has been reported to be as high as 90% for disseminated infections and 100% for disseminated infections involving the central nervous system.[68]

Candida infections have been associated with the occurrence of mycotic aneurysm, resulting in rupture of the aortic anastomosis and sudden death. Candida mediastinitis should be suspected with the occurrence of sternal instability and a failure to heal.

Treatment of Fungal Infections

Multiple options are available for the treatment of invasive fungal infections in solid-organ transplantation. The optimal regimen should be based on antifungal susceptibility testing. The antifungal agents available today can be categorized into 3 primary classes including the polyenes, azole antifungals, and the echinocandins.

Polyenes

The polyene antifungals include amphotericin B and nystatin. However, this segment reviews only amphotericin B in detail because nystatin is used for prevention of oral thrush after transplantation and not for the treatment of systemic fungal infections.

Mechanism of Action

The mechanism of action for amphotericin B focuses on the fungal cytoplasmic membrane and binding of sterols, specifically ergosterol. Amphotericin B increases cell membrane permeability via pore and channel formation, resulting in fungal cell death from loss of intracellular molecules.

Spectrum of Activity

Amphotericin B is a broad-spectrum antifungal agent with activity against Candida species (with the exception of Candida lusitaniae, which is resistant to amphotericin B), H capsulatum, Cryptococcus neoformans, Aspergillus species (with the exception of Trichosporon beigelii, Aspergillus terreus, Pseudallescheria boydii, Malassezia furfur, and Fusarium species), B dermatitidis, Candida glabrata, and C immitis, mucormycosis, Sporothrix schenkii and Penicillium.[69] Due to its broad spectrum of activity and clinical effectiveness, amphotericin B is generally considered the "gold standard" for many fungal infections, including aspergillus infections.

Pharmacokinetics

Amphotericin B is available only as an intravenous formulation. Following a 4- to 6-hour intravenous administration, peak plasma levels are achieved in 1 hour. The initial elimination half-life is approximately 15 to 48 hours; however, because of extensive tissue binding, the terminal half-life can extend to 15 days and the drug can be detected in the blood for up to 4 weeks and in urine for 4 to 8 weeks after discontinuation of treatment.[69] Only minimal amounts of amphotericin penetrate the cerebrospinal fluid (inflamed or noninflamed meninges), brain, aqueous humor, amniotic fluid, pleural fluid, and synovial fluid. The highest concentrations of amphotericin are in the liver and spleen.

Formulations

There are two formulations of amphotericin B, one formulation is amphotericin B deoxycholate also known as "conventional" amphotericin B. The other is the lipid formulation of amphotericin B. Three lipid formulations are currently available on the market. These include amphotericin B colloidal dispersion (ABCD, Amphotec), amphotericin B lipid complex (ABLC, Abelcet), and liposomal amphotericin B (Ambisome). The lipid formulations differ from the conventional amphotericin in that they are less nephrotoxic; however, no difference in efficacy has been shown between the 2 formulations.

Tolerability

The primary toxicity associated with amphotericin B is nephrotoxicity. Although nephrotoxicity can be seen to some degree with all of the amphotericin agents, the lipid formulations are associated with less nephrotoxicity. Nephrotoxicity generally manifests as a dose-dependent decrease in glomerular filtration rate through a direct vasoconstrictive effect on afferent renal arterioles.[70] However, permanent renal failure can occur and is related to the total dose of amphotericin B and is caused by destruction of renal tubular cells, disruption of tubular basement membrane, and loss of functioning nephron units. The risk factors for nephrotoxic effects include the use of concomitant nephrotoxic agents, hypotension, intravascular volume depletion, renal transplantation, and other preexisting renal conditions.[71] Saline hydration before and after amphotericin infusion has been used in an effort to reduce the incidence of nephrotoxic effects.

Electrolyte abnormalities may also occur during treatment with amphotericin B. The most commonly occurring include renal tubular acidosis and renal wasting of potassium, magnesium, and phosphate. Daily monitoring and electrolyte replacement are generally necessary.

Infusion-related reactions are also common during early treatment with amphotericin B. The reactions usually manifest as chills, fever, and tachypnea during the infusion. Although such reactions can occur with every dose of amphotericin B, the most severe reactions are usually observed during the first 3 to 5 infusions. Premedication with diphenhydramine and acetaminophen is recommended and should be administered with every dose of amphotericin B to reduce the occurrence of such infusion-related reactions. If rigors occur, then the dose of amphotericin B should be interrupted or discontinued and a dose of meperidine may be administered (caution: meperidine should not be administered to patients with renal insufficiency). Infusion-related reactions can occur with all of the amphotericin B products, although they appear to be less common with liposomal amphotericin B.

Flucytosine

Flucytosine is currently the only antifungal in the pyrimidine class of antifungals. This agent has activity against cryptococcosis, candidiasis, and chromomycosis. Because its clinical efficacy is inferior to that of amphotericin B, flucytosine is usually not the drug of choice for treatment of such fungal infections. However, flucytosine may used in combination with amphotericin B for treatment of cryptococcal meningitis. The most common toxic effects include dose- and duration-dependent toxic effects on the bone marrow and gastrointestinal tract. Monitoring of serum levels and adjustment of dosing for azotemia are required. Unfortunately, since this agent is highly toxic, flucytosine has limited clinical use.

Azoles

The most commonly used systemic triazole antifungals include fluconazole, itraconazole, and voriconazole. The triazoles have less of an effect on human sterol synthesis, resulting in fewer adverse effects as compared with the imidazoles (ketoconazole). Unfortunately, with prolonged use, azole resistance has emerged and has been associated with treatment failure.

Mechanism of Action

The azoles inhibit C-14 alpha demethylation of lanosterol in fungi by binding to one of the cytochrome P-450 enzymes. This results in an accumulation of C-14 alpha methylsterols and reduced concentrations of ergosterol. Ergosterol is a sterol necessary for a normal fungal cytoplasmic membrane.[71]

Fluconazole

Spectrum of Activity

As a result of its low toxicity and ease of use, fluconazole is the most commonly used triazole antifungal. Its spectrum of activity includes most *Candida* species (with the exception of *Candida krusei* and *C glabrata*, which are intrinsically resistant to fluconazole), *C neoformans*, and coccidiodomycosis. Fluconazole has some activity against sporotrichosis, ringworm, histoplasmosis, and blastomycosis. However, fluconazole has no activity against *Aspergillus* species or mucormycosis.[69]

Pharmacokinetics

Fluconazole is available as both an oral and an intravenous formulation. The oral formulation is very well absorbed and has a bioavailability of greater than 90%. Fluconazole is widely distributed with good penetration in the cerebral spinal fluid, eye, peritoneal, fluid, sputum, skin, and urine.[69] Fluconazole is hepatically metabolized by, and an inhibitor of, CYP3A4.

Tolerability

Fluconazole is very well tolerated, and adverse effects are relatively uncommon. The most common toxic effects include nausea, vomiting, diarrhea, anorexia, and headache. In less than 1% of patients, an increase in liver enzyme levels may be observed.[69]

Itraconazole

Itraconazole has a broader spectrum of activity, a more desirable pharmacokinetic profile, and less toxicity than ketoconazole. Also, unlike fluconazole, itraconazole has activity against aspergillosis. However, its use is limited because of its variable pharmacokinetic profile and its wide range of toxic effects.

Spectrum of Activity

The spectrum of activity for itraconazole includes *Candida* species, blastomycosis, histoplasmosis, coccidiodomycosis, paracoccidiodomycosis, sporotrichosis, ringworm, tinea versicolor, and aspergillosis.[69]

Pharmacokinetics

Itraconazole is available in an oral and an intravenous formulation. However, concentrations achieved after oral administration are variable and associated with treatment failure; therefore, use of the oral formulation is limited. Itraconazole is metabolized in the liver by CYP3A4 and is also an inhibitor of CYP3A4. The half-life is 30 to 40 hours and can be prolonged in patients with severe liver disease. The intravenous formulation of itraconazole is coformulated with hydroxypropyl-β-cyclodextrin to improve solubility. In patients with renal dysfunction, cyclodextrin may accumulate. Therefore, in patients with a creatinine clearance of less than 30 mL/min, intravenous itraconazole is not recommended.[69]

Toxic Effects

Itraconazole is associated with dose-dependent nausea, diarrhea, and abdominal discomfort. In addition, hepatotoxic effects have been observed in 3% of patients with systemic fungal infections and 1% of patients with nonsystemic infections.[69] The intravenous formulation is associated with thrombophlebitis when administered peripherally. To prevent thrombophlebitis, an increased fluid dilution volume may be necessary. In addition, a negative inotropic effect has been observed with the intravenous administration of itraconazole. Therefore, an alternative antifungal should be considered in patients with congestive heart failure or ventricular dysfunction.[69]

Voriconazole

Voriconazole is structurally related to fluconazole but expands on fluconazole's clinical activity to include fluconazole-resistant *Candida* species, *Aspergillus* species, and rare molds (*Scedosporium* species, *Fusarium* species). In addition, voriconazole is fungicidal against molds and fungistatic against yeast.[69] Voriconazole has a more favorable pharmacokinetic profile than itraconazole and has a greater spectrum of activity (primarily its fungicidal activity against *Aspergillus* species) than the other azoles. In addition, voriconazole is available not only in an intravenous formulation but also as an oral tablet and oral suspension. The bioavailability of the oral formulation is greater than 90%, making it a good option for long-term maintenance therapy for mold infections like *Aspergillus* in immunosuppressed patients.[69]

Spectrum of Activity

Voriconazole's spectrum of activity includes the *Candida* species (including most fluconazole-resistant strains), *Aspergillus* species, *B dermatitidis*, *C immitis*, and *H capsulatum*. Voriconazole also has activity against some strains of *P boydii*, *Scedosporium apiospermum*, *Fusarium* species, *Paecilomyces* species, *Bipolaris* species, and *Alternaria* species.[69]

Pharmacokinetics

Voriconazole exhibits nonlinear pharmacokinetics in adults due to saturation of metabolism. A significant degree of interpatient variability in serum concentrations has been observed. In children, elimination is linear and higher doses are required to attain similar concentrations as in adults. Voriconazole is metabolized in the liver via the CYP450 system, specifically CYP2C9, CYP3A4, CYP2C19.[69] As with all of the other triazoles, voriconazole is an inhibitor of CYP3A4 and therefore has the potential for multiple drug-drug interactions.

When treating patients with hepatic dysfunction, dosage adjustment may be necessary. The intravenous formulation is formulated with sulfobutyl ether β-cyclodextrin sodium (SBECD) to increase the solubility of voriconazole. SBECB is eliminated renally and may accumulate in patients with renal dysfunction. Therefore, voriconazole is not recommended in patients with a creatinine clearance less than 50 mL/min.[69]

Tolerability

Visual disturbances have been reported to occur in approximately 30% of patients but rarely result in discontinuation of therapy. Symptoms occur early in therapy with the first few doses, usually begin within 30 minutes of a dose, and last for about 30 minutes. Visual effects include altered color discrimination, blurred vision, appearance of bright spots, and photophobia. In addition, these effects are associated with changes in electroretinogram tracings, which normalize upon discontinuation of treatment. Elevations in hepatic enzyme levels may occur with voriconazole. Although most patients experience asymptomatic elevations, life-threatening hepatitis has been described. Hepatotoxic effects with voriconazole are dose-dependent and resolve with discontinuation of therapy. In addition, skin reactions (in the form of photosensitivity reactions) and prolongation of QT interval have been reported rarely with voriconazole.[69]

Drug-Drug Interactions (Fluconazole, Itraconazole, Voriconazole)

The azole antifungals are all metabolized by cytochrome P-450 3A4 and also inhibit the metabolic activity of CYP3A4. As a result, azole antifungals may increase plasma concentrations of other drugs metabolized by CYP3A4. Common immunosuppressants administered after transplantation include cyclosporine, tacrolimus, and sirolimus. Each of these agents is also metabolized via CYP 3A4. Therefore, the concomitant administration of the azole antifungals with the described immunosuppressants can result in a pharmacokinetic interaction. The result can be an increase in the plasma concentration of the immunosuppressant (cyclosporine, tacrolimus, or sirolimus). Therefore, the immunosuppressant drug level requires frequent monitoring and adjustment of the immunosuppressant dose to achieve the desired drug level.

Concomitant use of voriconazole with sirolimus is contraindicated by the manufacturer. When initiating voriconazole therapy in patients receiving cyclosporine or tacrolimus, it is recommended that the dose of cyclosporine or tacrolimus be empirically decreased by half or one third, respectively.[69]

Echinocandins

Before the advent of the echinocandins, antifungal therapy was primarily limited to polyenes, amphotericin, and azoles. Although amphotericin B has been considered the gold standard in the treatment of invasive fungal infections, its use is hampered by severe collateral toxic effects (ie, nephrotoxic effects, infusion reactions). The introduction of azole antifungals offered a less toxic antifungal option, but was hampered by drug-drug interactions and tolerability issues. Drug resistance has also been of concern with the existing antifungals.

Echinocandins are a new and unique class of antifungal agents that act by inhibiting production of β(1,3)-D-glucan, a component of the fungal cell wall. In addition, the development of resistance to echinocandins is rare. Currently, 3 echinocandin antifungal agents are available: caspofungin, micafungin, and anidulafungin

Mechanism of Action

β(1,3)-D-Glucan synthase is an enzyme responsible for formation of the polysaccharide, β(1,3)-D-glucan, an essential cell wall component in many fungi and *P (carinii) jiroveci* cysts, but not in mammalian cells.[72-74] Caspofungin and micafungin are noncompetitive inhibitors of this enzyme, resulting in disruption of cell wall integrity and osmotic stability, and cell lysis.

Caspofungin

Spectrum of Activity

Caspofungin has concentration-dependent fungicidal activity against *Candida* species, including azole-susceptible and resistant strains.[75] Caspofungin is most active against *C albicans, C glabrata, Candida tropicalis, Candida kefyr,* and *Candida pelliculosa*. Caspofungin is fungistatic against *Aspergillus* species.[75]

The indications for caspofungin approved by the Food and Drug Administration include the following:

- Treatment of candidemia and the following candidal infections: intra-abdominal abscesses, peritonitis, and pleural space infections
- Treatment of esophageal candidiasis
- Treatment of invasive aspergillosis in patients refractory to or intolerant of other therapies (ie, amphotericin, itraconazole). Caspofungin has not been studied as initial therapy for invasive aspergillosis

Pharmacokinetics

Caspofungin is only available in the intravenous formulation because the oral bioavailability is poor. Accumulation of caspofungin occurs with multiple doses and steady state is achieved between 14 and 21 days. Trough plasma concentrations exceeding the required target concentration of 1 µg/mL (the concentration necessary to inhibit ≥90% of *Candida* strains in vitro) cannot be achieved on day 1 with a standard dose of 50 mg/kg.[76] Therefore, when dosing caspofungin, a loading dose of 70 mg/kg is required. Caspofungin is 97% bound to plasma proteins.[77]

Caspofungin is slowly metabolized in the liver by nonenzymatic peptide hydrolysis and/or N-acetylation.[78] Current studies suggest that caspofungin does not inhibit any enzyme in the CYP450 system.[79]

Tolerability

Caspofungin is generally well tolerated. The most frequent adverse events reported include phlebitis/thrombophlebitis (13%), fever, chills, headache (11%), nausea, vomiting, abdominal pain, diarrhea, rash, and flushing. The most common laboratory abnormalities reported for caspofungin include hypokalemia (10%), hypoalbuminemia, decreased hemoglobin/hematocrit (12%), neutropenia (3%), thrombocytopenia (3%) increased urinary protein level, hypercalcemia, leukopenia, and elevated creatinine (1.5%). Hepatotoxic effects manifesting as increased aminotransferases has also been reported in up to 11% of patients treated with caspofungin. Elevation in alkaline phosphatase level has also been observed in 3% to 10% of patients treated.[75,79] In addition, the concurrent use of cyclosporine and caspofungin in 3 of 4 healthy volunteers has been associated with transient increases (≥2 to 3 times the upper limit of normal) in levels of liver transaminases.[75] Although subsequent retrospective analysis indicates that the risk of clinically significant hepatotoxic effects is low, caution should be taken when using the combination in patients with hepatic dysfunction.[80-82] Histamine-mediated symptoms including rash, facial swelling, pruritus, and sensations of warmth have occurred in less than 5% of patients. Anaphylaxis has been reported in less than 2% of patients treated with caspofungin.[75]

Drug-Drug Interactions

As with the other antifungals discussed, this section explores only the potential for drug-drug interactions between caspofungin and transplant immunosuppressant agents. Caspofungin does not inhibit or induce any enzyme in the CYP450 system. However, pharmacokinetic interactions between caspofungin and cyclosporine or tacrolimus have been documented. When cyclosporine and caspofungin are administered concomitantly, cyclosporine increased the area under the curve of caspofungin. This combination has resulted in increased plasma levels of caspofungin and an increased risk of elevations of hepatic enzyme levels. Although the mechanism of this interaction is unknown, levels of liver transaminases should be monitored during concomitant therapy.[75]

In addition, when concomitantly administered, caspofungin can reduce the trough blood concentration of tacrolimus by 26% and the maximum concentration by 16%. Although, the mechanism of this interaction is unknown, when tacrolimus is coadministered with caspofungin, tacrolimus blood levels should be monitored and the dosage adjusted as needed.[75,79]

Micafungin

Spectrum of Activity

Micafungin has activity against a range of *Candida* species including *C albicans, C glabrata, C guillermondii, C tropicalis, C krusei,* and *C parapsilosis*. In vitro micafungin is also active against azole-resistant clinical isolates of *C albicans*, as well as clinical isolates of *A fumigatus, Aspergillus flavus, Aspergillus niger,* and *A terreus*. With respect to pathogenic dimorphic fungi, micafungin has also demonstrated activity against *B dermatidis, H capsulatum,* and *C immitis*.[83]

The indications for micafungin approved by the Food and Drug Administration include treatment of esophageal candidiasis, and prophylaxis of *Candida* infections in patients undergoing hematopoietic stem cell transplantation.

Pharmacokinetics

Micafungin is available only in the intravenous formulation. Micafungin is highly protein bound with a distribution half-life of 14 to 17.2 hours. In HIV-positive patients with esophageal candidiasis receiving daily doses of 150 mg daily, the mean half-life was 15.2 hours and steady state was achieved at day 14 to 21.[84]

Micafungin is metabolized to M-1 (catechol form) by arylsulfatase, with further metabolism to M-2 (methoxy form) by catechol-O-methyltransferase. M-5 is formed by hydroxylation at the omega-1 position side chain of micafungin. This metabolism is catalyzed by cytochrome P-450 enzymes. Although micafungin is a substrate for and a weak inhibitor of CYP3A4 in vitro, hydroxylation by CYP3A4 in vivo is a minor pathway for metabolism of micafungin. Also, micafungin is not a P-glycoprotein substrate or inhibitor.[84]

In patients with renal impairment, no dosage adjustment of micafungin is necessary. In addition, because it is so highly protein bound, micafungin is not dialyzable and supplementary dosing after hemodialysis is not required. In patients with moderate hepatic insufficiency, the dose of micafungin does not need to be adjusted. However, the pharmacokinetics in patients with severe hepatic insufficiency has not been studied.[85]

Tolerability

Micafungin is generally well tolerated. In a double-blind trial, micafungin prophylaxis was tolerated as well as fluconazole. The most common adverse events included bilirubinemia, nausea, and diarrhea.[85] Infusion-related side effects like rigors occurred in 1% of patients treated with micafungin, and phlebitis has been documented at a rate of 1.6%. Other commonly noted adverse effects in micafungin treated patients include rash, delirium, headache, and leukopenia. Liver function abnormalities, hepatocellular damage and hepatic disorder have been reported in postmarketing surveillance.[84]

Drug-Drug Interactions

Drug-drug interaction studies were conducted in healthy volunteers between micafungin and mycophenolate mofetil, cyclosporine, tacrolimus, prednisolone, sirolimus, nifedipine, fluconazole, ritonavir, and rifampin. However, this review is focused on the potential for drug-drug interactions between micafungin and immunosuppressant agents only. In each of the studies conducted, no interactions were noted to alter the pharmacokinetics of micafungin. In addition, micafungin had no effect on the pharmacokinetics of mycophenolate mofetil, cyclosporine, tacrolimus, and prednisolone.

However, the concomitant use of micafungin and sirolimus caused an increase in sirolimus exposure as evidenced by a 21% increase in area under the curve. No effect on maximal concentration was noted. Hence, patients receiving sirolimus in combination with micafungin should be monitored for toxic effects of sirolimus. Dosages of sirolimus should be adjusted as needed.[84]

Anidulafungin

Spectrum of Activity

Anidulafungin has demonstrated in vitro activity against a broad range of *Candida* species including *C albicans*, *C glabrata*, *C parapsilosis*, and *C tropicalis*.[86] Anidulafungin also showed activity in vitro against species of *C krusei* (intrinsically resistant to azoles) and *C lusitaniae* (intrinsically resistant to amphotericin B).[87-90] In addition, anidulafungin has demonstrated activity against *C albicans* resistant to fluconazole.[86] In vitro, anidulafungin also demonstrates activity against *A fumigatus* and other *Aspergillus species*.[91,92] Additive effects have been reported in vitro for anidulafungin in combination with amphotericin B for use against *Aspergillus* and *Fusarium* isolates.[93] Also, when anidulafungin was combined with itraconazole or voriconazole, synergistic activity was demonstrated against *Aspergillus*.[94,95]

Pharmacokinetics

Anidulafungin is available only in the intravenous formulation. It is 84% bound to plasma proteins with a short distribution half-life of 0.5 to 1 hour and a terminal elimination half-life of 40 to 50 hours.[86] Anidulafungin is not a clinically relevant substrate, inducer, or inhibitor of CYP450 isoenzymes. Therefore, it is unlikely that anidulafungin will have a clinically relevant effect on the metabolism of medications metabolized by CYP450 isoenzymes like calcineurin inhibitors.[86]

In patients with hepatic insufficiency, no dosage adjustments are required. In addition, anidulafungin has negligible renal clearance; therefore, no dosage adjustments are necessary in patients with renal impairment. Anidulafungin is not dialyzable and supplementary dosing after hemodiaysis is not required.[86]

Tolerability

Like the other echinocandins, anidulafungin is generally well tolerated. Histamine-mediated signs and symptoms have been reported, including rash, urticaria, flushing, pruritus, dyspnea, and hypotension. However, when administered at a rate less than 1.1 mg/min, the histamine-mediated signs and symptoms are infrequent. Adverse events reported in greater than or equal to 2% of subjects include diarrhea, elevations in hepatic enzyme levels, hypokalemia, and deep vein thrombosis. Other adverse events reported in greater than or equal to 1% of subjects include neutropenia, leukopenia, nausea, vomiting, headache, and pyrexia.[86]

Drug-Drug Interactions

As discussed previously, since anidulafungin is not a clinically relevant substrate, inducer, or inhibitor of CYP450 isoenzymes, drug-drug interactions are not expected with calcineurin inhibitors. Drug interaction studies conducted with anidulafungin and tacrolimus or cyclosporine indicated that no dosage adjustment is necessary for anidulafungin or the calcineurin inhibitors.[86] Although drug interaction studies have not been conducted with sirolimus and anidulafungin, as with the calcineurin inhibitors an interaction is unlikely. Drug interaction studies have also been conducted with anidulafungin and amphotericin B, voriconazole, and rifampin. No dosage adjustment was necessary for anidulafungin or the other agents tested.[86]

Viral Infection

Many factors affect the development of viral infection after solid-organ transplantation. These factors include recipient and donor serostatus, recipient comorbidities (eg, diabetes mellitus), immunosuppression regimen, organ(s) transplanted, ischemia-reperfusion injury to graft, and community-acquired infection. Viral infection can be particularly devastating to transplant recipients because of the immunosuppressive properties of the viral pathogens themselves, which may increase the patients' susceptibility to other opportunistic infection (particularly fungal infection), or posttransplant lymphoproliferative disease (PTLD).

Cytomegalovirus

Cytomegalovirus (CMV), a herpesvirus, is the most important viral infection in solid-organ transplantation because of its broad effects on immunocompromised patients.[2] Active infection produces not only signs and symptoms associated with the viral syndrome itself, but also has other widespread effects associated with cytokine-mediated inflammatory response and generation of cross-reactive T cells.[96] These effects, including cytokine-mediated inflammation and generation of cross-reactive T cells, may lead to allograft injury and/or acute rejection, systemic immunosuppression from the virus, and EBV-associated PTLD.[2]

Risk factors for CMV infection/disease include CMV donor-positive/recipient-negative (D+/R-) serostatus pairs, recent treatment for acute rejection[97] and recent completion of prophylactic antiviral therapy.[98] In CMV D+/R- pairs, there may be an association between the use of CMV prophylaxis and improved graft survival and lower acute rejection rates.[99] Kidney, lung, heart, and heart/lung recipients were found to have improved graft survival if they had received CMV prophylaxis, and kidney and heart transplant recipients also had lower rates of acute rejection. An association was not found in liver transplant recipients.[99]

Clinical Manifestations

Differentiation between CMV infection and CMV disease is important when assessing a patient for CMV. A patient with CMV infection has active viral replication in the blood or other body fluids, but does not necessarily experience systemic signs and symptoms such as malaise, fever, and pancytopenia. Patients with CMV disease, however, have an invasive infection that has affected an organ system, most commonly manifesting as colitis, hepatitis, or pneumonitis in recipients of solid-organ transplants.[98]

Diagnosis and Monitoring

CMV serology of the donor and recipient are useful for estimating the recipient's risk of CMV developing after transplantation.[100] Serology is generally not useful for diagnosing CMV infection/disease because seroconversion often does not occur until after symptoms are resolved. Rather, methods that quantify the extent of the CMV infection are necessary to make the diagnosis. Two common methods include CMV antigenemia (stain circulating neutrophils for CMV antigen) and CMV DNA polymerase chain reaction (PCR) (viral load).[101] A major limitation of antigenemia, however, is the need for sufficient quantities of neutrophils to perform the test, which is often not possible because of the neutropenia caused by the CMV virus itself. Therefore, the CMV viral load is a key diagnostic tool; trends in viral loads are more valuable than individual levels.[100] Viral load assays vary between laboratories, however, and assay standardization is needed. Another limitation includes the fact that often no peripheral viral load is detectable in patients with invasive CMV disease, particularly when the gastrointestinal tract and lungs are sites of infection. In these cases, biopsy of the infected tissue and/or bronchial alveolar lavage are often necessary to confirm diagnosis.[100]

Prevention

Several strategies have been used to prevent and treat CMV. Some centers routinely provide antiviral prophylaxis to patients at risk for CMV (particularly D+/R- pairs), whereas others employ preemptive strategies, in which patients are routinely monitored and receive prophylaxis only if laboratory markers become positive. Each method has benefits and drawbacks. Benefits of universal prophylaxis include preventing both CMV and other herpes viruses and lack of need for intensive monitoring. Drawbacks include the risk of developing ganciclovir-resistant CMV (although a small risk), adverse effects of the medications, the fact that late CMV disease may occur despite early prophylaxis (delayed onset), and the fact that the disease may have atypical features.

For preemptive strategies, benefits include decreasing the use of antivirals and their associated adverse effects and costs. However, the logistically demanding monitoring schedule, requirement for strict compliance to the costly surveillance methods, potential to develop CMV disease before detection, and development of drug resistance are disadvantages of preemptive strategies.[100] CMV-related morbidity is also a significant risk when adherence to monitoring guidelines is poor.[102] Drug resistance can occur if ganciclovir is used in a patient with active viral replication, owing to its poor oral bioavailability.[103]

Table 1 contains recommended CMV prophylactic strategies for several organ transplant populations.[100,103] With the introduction of valganciclovir, a prodrug of ganciclovir with superior oral bioavailability, recent interest has focused on use of this agent to prevent and treat CMV infection and disease. However, its use is not yet routinely recommended.[100,103] Pharmacokinetic studies show that oral valganciclovir administration at 450 mg (given once daily) gives exposure that is equivalent to the standard oral regimen of ganciclovir (1 g administered 3 times a day).[104] The manufacturer-recommended dose of valganciclovir for CMV prophylaxis is 900 mg/day, and this dose appears to be equivalent in efficacy to oral ganciclovir, with an increased incidence of neutropenia compared with ganciclovir.[98]

Table 1. RECOMMENDED GUIDELINES FOR PREVENTION OF CYTOMEGALOVIRUS (CMV) INFECTION[100,103]

Therapeutic Options	Duration of Prophylaxis	PATIENT POPULATION		
		Heart/Kidney/Liver/Pancreas High Risk (D+/R-)	Heart/Kidney/Liver/Pancreas Intermediate Risk (D+/R+ or D-/R+)	Lung/Heart-Lung High Risk (All patients)
Ganciclovir (oral)	3 months	√	√	
Valganciclovir* (oral)	3 months	√	√	√ (up to 6 months if D+/R-)
Ganciclovir (intravenous)	1 to 3 months	√	√	√ (minimum 3 months) (up to 6 months if D+/R-)
Valacyclovir (oral)	3 months	√ (kidney only)	√ (kidney only)	
CMV immune globulin	Variable	√		√
Preemptive therapy	N/A		√	
Clinical Observation	N/A		√	

* Precautions exist regarding use of valganciclovir in liver recipients (Food and Drug Administration).

In several studies,[105,106] researchers have retrospectively evaluated the efficacy of low-dose valganciclovir (450 mg daily) as prophylaxis for CMV in liver and kidney transplant recipients. In liver transplant recipients, 3 months of low-dose valganciclovir was as effective as standard ganciclovir (1 g orally 3 times a day) in preventing CMV disease.[105] An analysis comparing 3 months of standard ganciclovir versus low-dose valganciclovir in the prophylaxis of CMV in 129 kidney or pancreas transplant recipients revealed a 14% incidence of CMV disease at 1 year after transplantation (10% noninvasive and 4% invasive).[106] The incidence was similar between patients receiving ganciclovir and valganciclovir, and risk factors for development of CMV disease included CMV D+/R- serostatus and use of thymoglobulin as part of immunosuppression regimen (incidence 25% in patients receiving thymoglobulin). The same investigators later reported outcomes in 37 kidney or pancreas recipients who received thymoglobulin induction and an extended course (6 months) of CMV prophylaxis with low-dose valganciclovir.[107] The incidence of CMV disease decreased in thymoglobulin-treated patients from 25% when 3 months of prophylaxis was employed to 8% when 6 months was employed.

The duration of CMV prophylaxis also remains controversial; current recommendations suggest a minimum of 3 months of therapy.[100,103] Several studies have demonstrated a lower incidence of CMV disease after transplantation in patients receiving prophylaxis for 6 months, particularly in patients at highest risk for developing CMV.[107-110]

Treatment

Patients with CMV infection/disease should be treated with intravenous ganciclovir.[100,103] Ganciclovir (intravenous) is the gold standard for treatment due to the large body of experience with it and its lack of nephrotoxicity, which limits the use of other antiviral agents such as cidofovir and foscarnet. The treatment dose of 5 mg/kg intravenously every 12 hours must be adjusted for renal function; this adjustment should be done carefully, as subtherapeutic ganciclovir exposure in the setting of high CMV viral load may promote the development of resistance.[100,103] Because the bone marrow–suppressive effects of ganciclovir may further compound the neutropenia caused by the CMV virus itself, care should be exercised in adjusting the dose of ganciclovir to avoid these effects. Rather, use of white blood cell growth factors may be preferable in order to avoid the subtherapeutic ganciclovir exposure.[100]

At a dose of 900 mg, valganciclovir provides exposure similar to that of 5 mg/kg body weight of intravenous ganciclovir.[104] Thus, the cost of treating active CMV infection could be substantially lowered by its potential to treat with oral valganciclovir in the outpatient setting. Another key component of managing patients with CMV disease includes careful reduction in immunosuppression, taking into consideration patient and organ-specific factors. CMV immunoglobulin may also have a role in treatment of CMV disease, particularly as adjunct therapy in patients with severe CMV disease.[100,103]

Close monitoring of viral load is necessary to assess response to therapy; monitoring should begin 1 week after initiation of therapy and treatment should be continued until the viral load has been undetectable for 1 week.[100] The role of secondary prophylaxis after treatment is not clearly defined. When secondary prophylaxis is employed, viral load should be monitored for potential development of resistance and use of valganciclovir may be preferable owing to its superior bioavailability.[100]

CMV disease recurs in approximately 15% to 35% of patients. Recurrence is due to incomplete suppression of CMV rather than the development of resistance. Patients at higher risk for recurrence include seronegative recipients of seropositive grafts, patients with multisystem CMV disease, those who receive treatment for acute rejection, patients with high viral loads at the time of initial diagnosis of the infection, and those who had a detectable viral load at the end of therapy for the initial infection.[100]

Ganciclovir-resistant stains of CMV have developed in recent years.[111] Patients at highest risk for developing ganciclovir-resistant CMV include donor-seropositive/recipient-seronegative pairs, as well as lung and kidney-pancreas transplant recipients.[100] The resistance is most likely related to poor bioavailability of ganciclovir, as resistance has not yet been reported in patients receiving valganciclovir.[112] The apparent lack of resistance may also be a result of improved adherence of patients to valganciclovir's once-daily regimen. Treatment for ganciclovir-resistant strains includes high-dose intravenous ganciclovir, combination therapy with ganciclovir plus foscarnet, and CMV hyperimmunoglobulin.[100,113] Increasing the ganciclovir dose (up to 10 mg/kg every 12 hours) with careful monitoring for toxic effects may also be useful in these patients.[100] For patients who do not respond to an increased dose of ganciclovir, reduced-dose ganciclovir plus reduced-dose foscarnet or full-dose foscarnet alone may be used; cidofovir is usually reserved for last-line therapy.[100] As with ganciclovir-sensitive CMV, viral load should be monitored on a weekly basis and treatment should continue for 1 week after an undetectable viral load.[100]

Table 2 summarizes information about the various antiviral agents used in the prevention and treatment of CMV.

Varicella Zoster Virus

The adult seroprevalence rate for VZV (herpes zoster) in the United States is greater than 90%.[114] In an analysis of herpes zoster (shingles) infection in the setting of modern immunosuppression, researchers evaluated 869 solid-organ transplants performed between 1994 and 1999. Overall incidence of varicella zoster was 8.6%; the lowest incidence occurred in liver (5.7%), followed by kidney (7.4%), lung (15.1%), and heart (16.8%) transplant recipients. Herpes zoster infection occurred at a median of 9.0 months after transplantation (range 0.6-69.3 months after transplantation) and resulted in significant morbidity. Herpes zoster developed in most patients (62.7%) within 1 year of transplantation. Independent risk factors for infection included induction therapy and antiviral therapy (other than >6 weeks of CMV prophylaxis with acyclovir or ganciclovir). Among liver transplant recipients, female gender and use of mycophenolate mofetil were independent risk factors for herpes zoster.[115]

Table 2. ANTIVIRAL AGENTS USED IN THE PREVENTION AND TREATMENT OF CYTOMEGALOVIRUS (CMV) INFECTION

Antiviral Agent	Usual Dosing	Pharmacokinetic Considerations	Tolerability/ Adverse Effects	Comments
Ganciclovir	Prophylaxis: 1000 mg by mouth 3 times a day or 5 mg/kg intravenously daily Treatment: 5 mg/kg intravenously every 12 hours	• Dose must be adjusted in renal impairment • Oral formulation should be taken with food • Poor oral bioavailability (<10%)	• Neutropenia • Thrombocytopenia • Anemia • Diarrhea • Nausea • Vomiting • ↑Serum creatinine level • ↑ Liver transaminase levels • Neuropathy • Paresthesias	• Teratogenic and carcinogenic; do not open capsules
Valganciclovir	Prophylaxis: 450-900 mg by mouth daily	• Dose must be adjusted in renal impairment • Valine ester prodrug ganciclovir with of improved bioavailability (~60%)	• Neutropenia • Thrombocytopenia • Anemia • Diarrhea • Nausea • Vomiting • Abdominal pain • Headache • Insomnia • Fever	• Not approved by the Food and Drug Administration (FDA) for treatment of active CMV infection in solid-organ-transplant recipients • FDA-approved dose for prophylaxis is 900 mg/day • FDA cautions against use in liver transplant recipients • Teratogenic and carcinogenic; do not crush tablets
CMV Immune Globulin	Prophylaxis: Heart, liver, pancreas, lung: 150 mg/kg intravenously within 72 hours of transplantation and weeks 2, 4, 6, and 8, then 100 mg/kg weeks 12 and 16 Kidney: 150 mg/kg intravenously within 72 hours of transplantation, then 100 mg/kg weeks 2, 4, 6, and 8, then 50 mg/kg weeks 12 and 16	• Risk of acute renal failure with administration of immunoglobulin preparations	• Nausea • Vomiting • Fever • Chills • Flushing • Diaphoresis • Wheezing • Aseptic meningitis	• Adjunctive therapy in high risk patients only; treatment dose not clearly defined • At times, product may be in short supply due to manufacturing and/or human immune globulin shortages
Valacyclovir	Prophylaxis: 8 g/day	• Dose must be adjusted in renal impairment • Valyl ester of acyclovir	• Nausea • Vomiting • Diarrhea • Headache • Neutropenia • Thrombocytopenia • ↑ Liver transaminase levels	• Recommended for prophylaxis in kidney transplant recipients only
Foscarnet	Treatment: Doses not clearly defined; depends on concomitant therapy	• Dose must be adjusted in renal impairment	• Nephrotoxicity • Fever • Headache • Nausea • Vomiting • Diarrhea • Anemia • Electrolyte abnormalities	• Adverse effects (nephrotoxicity) limits use • Use limited to rescue therapy (ganciclovir-resistant strains or nonresponders)

Table 2. ANTIVIRAL AGENTS USED IN THE PREVENTION AND TREATMENT OF CYTOMEGALOVIRUS (CMV) INFECTION (continued)

Antiviral Agent	Usual Dosing	Pharmacokinetic Considerations	Tolerability/ Adverse Effects	Comments
Cidofovir	Treatment: Doses not clearly defined; depends on concomitant therapy	• Dose must be adjusted in renal impairment	• Nephrotoxicity • Fever • Headache • Nausea • Vomiting • Diarrhea • Anemia • Neutropenia • Rash	• Adverse effects (nephrotoxicity) limits use • Use limited to rescue therapy (ganciclovir-resistant strains or nonresponders) if all other therapies fail

Clinical Manifestations

Cutaneous scarring, defined as skin disfigurement (scarring or hypopigmentation), occurred in 18.7% of patients with herpes zoster. Postherpetic neuralgia, defined as pain persisting more than 30 days after rash development, occurred in 42.7% of patients.[115] More serious manifestations of VZV infection may include pneumonitis, hepatitis, or encephalitis.[114] This is especially true in primary infections (manifesting as chickenpox), where morbidity and mortality may be high.

Diagnosis and Monitoring

Diagnosis of VZV infection typically involves clinical examination of skin lesions. Viral cultures or direct fluorescent antibody assays may be used to confirm diagnosis when necessary.[114]

Prevention

CMV prophylaxis with ganciclovir will most likely prevent VZV, although acyclovir is effective for those patients not receiving ganciclovir.[114] Patients who are VZV seronegative before transplantation should be vaccinated against varicella whenever possible. According to the Advisory Committee on Immunization Practices of the Centers for Disease Control and Prevention, the vaccine should not be administered to patients receiving immunosuppressants, because the varicella vaccine is a live, attenuated vaccine that may cause infection in immunocompromised patients.[116] After transplantation, seronegative patients exposed to VZV should receive postexposure prophylaxis, although this is not guaranteed to prevent infection.[114] Postexposure prophylaxis consists of varicella zoster immunoglobulin if the patient arrives for treatment within 96 hours of initial exposure (preferred), or antiviral therapy if that 96-hour window has passed.[114] Although some centers have reported administration of the varicella vaccine after transplantation with minimal adverse effects,[117] others have reported development of infection.[118] Therefore, this practice remains controversial[119] and is not supported by existing guidelines.[116]

Treatment

Patients with active, serious VZV infection should be treated with intravenous acyclovir, whereas less serious infections may be treated with oral acyclovir, valacyclovir, or famciclovir. In rare cases of acyclovir resistance, foscarnet may be used.[114]

Herpes Simplex Virus 1 and 2

Adult seroprevalence rates for herpes simplex virus 1 and 2 in the United States are 62% and 22%, respectively. Most infections after transplantation are due to reactivation of latent virus.[114]

Clinical Manifestations

Infection with herpes simplex virus generally is manifested by orolabial lesions or genital/perianal lesions, although more serious systemic infection can result in esophagitis, hepatitis, or pneumonitis.[114]

Diagnosis and Monitoring

Diagnosis of infection with herpes simplex virus 1 or 2 typically involves clinical examination of skin lesions. Culture of scrapings/tissue from lesions may be necessary to confirm diagnosis in some cases.[114]

Prevention and Treatment

CMV prophylaxis with ganciclovir will most likely prevent HSV; acyclovir is effective for those patients not receiving ganciclovir.[102] HSV infections are usually treated with oral acyclovir, valacyclovir, or famciclovir. In more serious infections, intravenous acyclovir may be employed.[114]

Human Herpesvirus 6, 7 and 8

Human herpesvirus (HHV) 6 and 7 are viral pathogens that can cause significant morbidity and mortality in transplant recipients. Although HHV 6 infection has been most commonly reported among stem cell transplant recipients, several cases have also been reported in solid-organ transplant recipients.[120-125] As with CMV, HHV 6 and 7 appear to have immunomodulatory effects and may predispose patients to secondary infection. Indeed, the mortality associated with HHV 6 appears to be related primarily to the development of secondary fungal infection.[122,123,125] HHV 8 is also know as Kaposi sarcoma–associated herpesvirus because development of Kaposi sarcoma is driven by this virus.[114] The seroprevalence of HHV 8 exhibits geographic variation; it is most common in the Mediterranean, Middle East, and some areas of Africa.

Clinical Manifestations

Transplant recipients with HHV 6 infection commonly have fever, bone marrow suppression, interstitial pneumonitis, and/or encephalitis. In addition, fever, hepatitis, and cutaneous rash have also been found in patients infected with HHV 6. Severe cases may progress to aplastic bone marrow and secondary infection with fungal and/or other viral pathogens. Symptoms associated with HHV 7 are not as well documented.[114] Patients with HHV 8 may have cutaneous lesions, fever, and evidence of bone marrow suppression.[114]

Diagnosis and Monitoring

Patients who are HHV 6–negative before transplantation appear to have a higher incidence of infection, although most cases are reactivations because more than 90% of patients are seropositive by adulthood.[114] As with other viral illnesses, quantitative PCR is useful in diagnosis and in monitoring patients with this infection. HHV 8 serostatus of the donor and recipient may be assessed on the basis of geographic location. Patients who are seropositive before transplantation, who are at risk for primary infection, or who have Kaposi sarcoma can then be monitored after transplantation by means of HHV 8 viral loads.[114]

Prevention and Treatment

Similar to CMV prophylaxis and treatment, ganciclovir appears to provide protection against HHV 6 infection and may be used to treat active infection; however, HHV 7 does not appear to be responsive to ganciclovir.[114] In some cases, foscarnet has successfully been used to treat severe infections, particularly in patients not responding to ganciclovir. Symptomatic patients may be treated with ganciclovir, foscarnet, or cidofovir, in combination with immunosuppression reduction.[114] CMV prophylaxis may also offer protection in the development of HHV 8 infection. For patients with Kaposi sarcoma, reduction and/or withdrawal of immunosuppression is first-line therapy[114]; antiviral agents, irradiation, chemotherapy, and anti-CD20 monoclonal antibody have been used as adjunctive therapy.[114,126,127]

Epstein Barr Virus

EBV is a herpesvirus that infects most people at a young age and causes infectious mononucleosis. In immunocompromised patients, primary EBV infection or reactivation of latent infection can cause PTLD, a feared consequence of immunosuppressive therapy. Risk factors for the development of PTLD include EBV seronegativity at the time of transplantation (leaving children at higher risk than adults), type of organ transplanted, type and degree of immunosuppression, CMV donor/recipient mismatch, and CMV disease.[128,129] The highest rate of PTLD occurs in small-bowel transplant (up to 32%), followed by moderate risk in pancreas, heart, lung, and liver transplantation (rates of 3% to 12%), and lowest risk in kidney transplantation (~1%).[130] PTLD affects the transplant allograft in approximately 30% of cases. Lesions in the central nervous system are the most difficult to treat. In general, early occurrence of PTLD is polyclonal and easier to treat, whereas late PTLD is often monoclonal, and infected B cells may lose CD20 expression, making treatment difficult.

Clinical Manifestations

Signs and symptoms of PTLD may include those of a primary EBV infection/infectious mononucleosis, specifically fever, malaise, and swollen lymph nodes in the neck, tonsils, axilla, and/or groin. In addition, patients may have other nonspecific symptoms, depending on the type of organ transplanted.

Diagnosis and Monitoring

Pathological examination of tissue is the gold standard for the diagnosis of PTLD; excisional biopsies are preferred over needle biopsies. No specific staging system exists for PTLD; however, the current recommendation is to use the Ann Arbor staging classification system with Cotswold's modifications, which is used to stage non-Hodgkin lymphoma. Diagnosis is based on morphological classification, origin cell type, presence of EBV, and presence of CD20+ cells.[128,129]

Prevention

Because no definitive methods to prevent PTLD are known, diligent monitoring of high-risk patients is needed; this is done by performing serial EBV PCR. Risk is defined as high in D+/R- pairs, children, small-bowel transplant recipients, and patients receiving high dose and/or intensity immunosuppression.[128,129] Utilization of ganciclovir/valganciclovir for CMV prophylaxis may give some protection, as ganciclovir has greater in vitro activity against EBV than acyclovir.

Treatment

Unfortunately, controlled trials in the treatment of PTLD are generally lacking. Key strategies for the management of patients with PTLD include reduction in immunosuppression, surgical resection, and local irradiation.[128] Secondary treatments may include antivirals, immunoglobulin, and monoclonal antibodies against B cells.[128] Anti-CD20 antibody (rituximab) is promising as first-line therapy after immunosuppression reduction because of its high specificity for B cells with a low adverse event profile. Cytotoxic chemotherapy (such as CHOP) is often used when first- and second-line therapies fail. Patients with CNS lesions may be treated with local radiotherapy, intrathecal anti-CD20 antibody, and/or interferon α.[128] EBV-specific cytotoxic T lymphocytes (CTL) may also have a role in the treatment of PTLD.[131] Patients may receive another transplant after successful treatment of PTLD; however, careful examination of patient-specific factors must occur.

Adenovirus

A concern mostly in children, adenovirus is a virus with many different serotypes that may cause diverse signs and symptoms during acute illness. Adenovirus is transmitted through respiratory secretions, fecal-oral route, and fomites; donor transmission has also been postulated in several reported cases. Adenovirus infection may occur in transplant recipients of any age; however, complications occur more commonly, and infections may be more severe in children.[132]

Clinical Manifestations

Symptomatic disease can vary greatly, ranging from self-limiting febrile illness, to cystitis or gastroenteritis, to severe infection with necrotizing hepatitis or pneumonia.[132]

Diagnosis and Monitoring

The gold standard for diagnosis of adenovirus is by culture or antigen detection (shell vial assay gives more rapid diagnosis). In patients with invasive disease, tissue specimens can be examined for histology ("smudge cells" signaling cytopathic inclusions) or adenovirus PCR may be performed on the specimen.[132]

Prevention and Treatment

No specific preventative measure is available, other than avoiding the spread of the virus via droplet and contact precautions for infected patients.[132] Supportive care, in conjunction with a decrease in immunosuppression is the standard of care for these patients. The use of antiviral agents such as ribavirin, ganciclovir, cidofovir, and respiratory syncytial virus immunoglobulin have been reported.[132]

Human Parvovirus B19

By adulthood, 30% to 60% of people are seropositive for parvovirus B19, an infection that usually is asymptomatic or manifests as a mild illness called erythema infectiosum in school-aged children and is commonly acquired through infected respiratory secretions. Parvovirus infects erythroid precursor cells, causing areticulocytic anemia in patients with severe infection.[133]

Clinical Manifestations

Parvovirus infection develops in approximately 1% to 2% of transplant recipients, resulting in a pure red cell aplasia with a low or absent reticulocyte count.[133] Other manifestations of the infection may include fever, rash, pancytopenia, and hepatitis.

Diagnosis and Monitoring

In transplant recipients, parvovirus B19 immunoglobulin M is a marker for ongoing infection, and parvovirus B19 DNA PCR may also be useful. Both have limitations, however, because transplant recipients may not be able to mount a response, making the serologic findings a less than ideal marker, whereas PCR may remain positive for up to 9 months after the initial infection. Therefore, the best diagnostic tool appears to be a positive PCR in a patient with pure red cell aplasia.[133]

Prevention and Treatment

No strategies are available to prevent parvovirus B19 infection in transplant recipients.[133] The treatment of choice for parvovirus B19 infection is intravenous immunoglobulin, although the optimal dosing regimen and duration of therapy are not clear.[133]

Human Papilloma Virus

The incidence of skin cancer in solid organ transplant recipients is 50 to 100 times higher than that in the general population, and patients with anogenital human papillomavirus (HPV) infection have a 20 to 100 times higher risk of cervical and anogenital cancers.[134] HPV appears to play an important role in the development of skin cancers in transplantation. The virus, in combination with exposure to ultraviolet radiation (the most significant risk factor) and the degree and length of immunosuppression are important factors in the development of squamous cell carcinoma, and to a lesser extent, basal cell carcinoma. Viral warts may progress to these cancers in immunocompromised patients, with HPV DNA being found in 70% to 90% of cutaneous tissue in patients with squamous cell carcinoma. Many strains of HPV exist, with HPV 5 and HPV 8 appearing to have a higher prevalence in transplant recipients with skin cancers.[135]

Clinical Manifestations

Infected patients have cutaneous and anogenital warts (verruca vulgaris).[135] Although less common, HPV may also manifest as a respiratory tract infection. [134]

Diagnosis and Monitoring

Diagnosis is made by examination of cutaneous warts during physical examination. Warts that look suspicious (eg, discolored) should be sampled by biopsy because of the known risk of malignant transformation of these lesions. In addition, suspicious anogenital warts should also be sampled, particularly as these lesions may be clinically indistinguishable from squamous epithelial lesions.

Prevention

Patients with preexisting lesions should receive treatment before transplantation. An HPV vaccine has been developed, although its potential role before transplantation remains to be determined. After transplantation, high-risk patients (those with a history of warts, keratoses, skin cancer, or long-term immunosuppression) should be followed up by a dermatologist every 3 to 6 months. Patients must be educated to avoid excessive sun exposure, to wear protective clothing when in the sun, and to use sunscreen to protect them. For those patients (or their partners) with anogenital lesions, sexual transmission should be avoided by abstinence or condoms (although condoms do not provide complete protection).[134,135]

Treatment

It is recommended that warts causing physical and/or psychological signs or symptoms be treated with cytotoxic agents that destroy the infected epidermis. In addition, surgical removal and physical ablation are often employed; a more rare treatment includes stimulation of the local immune response in the infected area.[134,135]

Polyomavirus

Polyomavirus nephropathy (PVN) is a significant cause of morbidity in renal transplant recipients. PVN is caused by BK virus (BKV), or less commonly, by JC or SV40 virus. BKV infects most people in childhood and becomes latent in the genitourinary tract. In renal transplant recipients, the latent virus becomes reactivated under immunosuppression and causes asymptomatic viruria. However, invasive infection of the transplanted kidney develops in a small percentage of patients; this infection is termed PVN. BKV infection becomes latent in renal and uroepithelial cells, and evidence shows that the virus may be donor-transmitted in some cases.[136,137] Although most cases occur in kidney transplant recipients, PVN has also been documented in native kidneys of other solid-organ and stem cell transplant recipients.[138,139] In 1 series, PVN was the leading cause of kidney graft loss within 2 years of simultaneous pancreas-kidney transplantation; BKV infection had no effect on pancreas graft function.[140]

Clinical Manifestations

PVN is characterized by tubulointerstitial nephritis that manifests as a progressive increase in serum creatinine level. Ureteral stenosis or stricture also develops in some patients, and hemorrhagic cystitis develops in bone marrow transplant recipients. Graft loss occurs in 30% to 40% of renal transplant recipients with PVN. Risk factors for PVN in renal transplantation include older age, male gender, degree of HLA mismatch, and treatment for acute rejection. In addition, use of corticosteroids and newer immunosuppressive agents (tacrolimus, mycophenolate mofetil, sirolimus) appears to convey risk.

In a series of 200 renal transplant patients who were prospectively monitored for BK viruria and viremia, viruria developed in 35% of patients by year 1, whereas viremia developed in 11.5%. The immunosuppression regimen with the highest rates of viruria was tacrolimus-mycophenolate mofetil (46%), and the regimen with the lowest rates was cyclosporine-mycophenolate mofetil (13%).[141]

Diagnosis and Monitoring

The gold standard for diagnosis of BKV nephropathy is biopsy of the transplanted kidney.[136] However, BKV nephropathy/PVN may be misinterpreted as acute rejection; therefore, immunohistochemistry nucleic acid detection assays or electron microscopy should be used to detect BKV infection.[136] Other adjunctive diagnostic tools include measurement of "decoy" cells in the urine (suggestive of viruria) and BKV DNA PCR to measure BKV replication in the blood.[136] Use of serum and urine BKV DNA PCR may provide the best monitoring tools for viral clearance during treatment[142] and is also recommended to be routinely monitored at months 1 through 6, 9, and 12 after transplantation in kidney transplant recipients enrolled in clinical trials.[143]

Treatment

Although no standard treatment for PVN is available, reduction in immunosuppression appears to be a key component of management. In the series mentioned earlier, reduction in immunosuppression (withdrawal of antimetabolite) caused 95% of viremia to resolve with no increase in acute rejection, allograft dysfunction, or graft loss.[141] In addition, overt BKV nephropathy did not develop in any patients. As with other viral diseases, reduction in immunosuppression must be performed cautiously, with close monitoring for acute rejection.[136]

Antiviral agents are also useful adjunctive agents in the management of patients with PVN. Despite its nephrotoxicity, low-dose cidofovir may help to successfully clear BKV and stabilize renal function.[144] In addition, leflunomide, an immunosuppressive agent with activity against BKV effectively clears BKV when kept at therapeutic blood levels. In a series of 26 renal transplant recipients with biopsy-proven BKV nephropathy, treatment with leflunomide was dosed by using measurements of the active metabolite (A77 1726) (target level 50-100 µg/mL) and patients were monitored via serial blood and urine PCR, serum creatinine levels, and repeat biopsy.[145] All patients were followed up for at least 6 months, with graft loss occurring in 15% of patients. BK viral load in blood and urine was significantly reduced with leflunomide (+/- cidofovir), and BKV in the renal biopsy specimen either decreased or disappeared in patients maintained within the targeted range.

Intravenous immunoglobulin may also have a role in the management of patients with BKV nephropathy when combined with reduction in immunosuppression.[146] In 1 study, intravenous immunoglobulin was given at a dose of 2 g per kilogram body weight as a divided dose over 2 to 5 days. Seven of 8 patients maintained stable, although impaired graft function at a mean of 15 months after diagnosis.

Hepatitis B

The risk of recurrence of hepatitis B is very high in patients who are surface antigen–positive at the time of transplantation. For patients who are positive for hepatitis B before transplantation, it is important to reduce the viral load as much as possible before transplantation.[147] Unfortunately, the natural course of hepatitis B is accelerated after transplantation because of the effects of immunosuppressants, particularly corticosteroids and azathioprine.[147]

Diagnosis and Monitoring

Hepatitis B–positive patients should be monitored monthly after transplantation, specifically for viral load (HBV DNA), hepatitis B early antigen, and antibody to hepatitis B early antigen and hepatitis B surface antigen.[147]

Prevention and Treatment

In order to prevent recurrence of hepatitis B, treatment regimens have been developed, including hepatitis B immunoglobulin and antiviral agents such as lamivudine.[147] Liver transplant recipients are recommended to receive 10,000 IU of hepatitis B immunoglobulin daily for 7 days after transplantation, followed by redosing every 3 to 4 weeks; the goal is to maintain serum hepatitis B immunoglobulin levels above 100 or 500 IU/mL for life.[147,148] In addition, patients with HBV viremia before transplantation should receive oral lamivudine (100 mg daily) until viremia is resolved, and again if viremia returns.[147] Lamivudine resistance is a concern; the role of newer antiviral agents such as adefovir and entecavir is yet to be defined.

Hepatitis C

Hepatitis C is the leading indication for liver transplantation in the United States, and recurrence after liver transplantation is very common, with cirrhosis developing in up to 25% of patients within 5 years of transplantation. As with hepatitis B, it is important to decrease viral load as much as possible before transplantation.[147] Risk factors for HCV recurrence after liver transplantation include genotype 1b, corticosteroid use, OKT3 use, and treatment of acute rejection.

Diagnosis and Monitoring

Patients should be monitored monthly for an increase in hepatitis C viral load (HCV DNA PCR).[101,147,148]

Prevention and Treatment

In liver transplant recipients, treatment is often not given to patients with viral replication by itself, but rather when histological evidence is found upon liver biopsy.[147] Interferon/ribavirin has been used to treat patients with hepatitis C after transplantation, particularly liver transplant recipients; however, caution must be used because of interferon's ability to induce acute rejection.[148]

Rare Viral Infections After Transplantation

West Nile Virus

West Nile Virus (WNV) is a single-stranded RNA virus of the Flaviviridae family that is transmitted to humans by mosquitoes. Since 1999, an increasing number of cases have occurred in North America. In general, healthy individuals are asymptomatic, although approximately 20% may have a self-limiting febrile illness. Morbidity and mortality from WNV have occurred mostly in elderly persons. A limited number of severe cases have been reported in solid-organ transplant recipients. Kumar and colleagues[149] reported 4 cases of WNV in kidney (n = 2), liver (n = 1), and heart (n = 1) transplant recipients. Cases occurred a mean of 3.8 years after transplantation (range 2 months to 8 years), and all patients with WNV infection had identifiable occupational or recreational risk factors for acquiring it. Compared with the general population, where the infection rate for WNV was 5 per 100,000, the rate in transplant recipients was 200 per 100,000 ($P < .001$).[149] The same authors performed a seroprevalence study and found a 0.25% seroprevalence and a resultant 40% risk of meningoencephalitis in a transplant patient with community-acquired WNV.[150] Similar studies of immunocompetent persons estimate the risk of meningoencephalitis to be less than 1%.

Clinical Manifestations

Initial signs and symptoms of WNV may be nonspecific, with more severe symptoms developing later in the course of the infection. In the cases reported by Kumar, clinical signs and symptoms of infection included fever (100%), confusion (75%), headache (100%), weakness (50%), encephalitis (75%), and meningitis (25%).[149] Cerebrospinal fluid showed pleocytosis (100%) and elevated protein level (75%). Outcomes included death, lower limb paralysis, mild neurological sequelae, and full recovery (25% each).

Diagnosis and Monitoring

Based on the limited number of cases of WNV infection in transplant recipients, it appears that delayed seroconversion due to immunosuppression may occur, leading to delayed diagnosis. Other diagnostic methods such as PCR may be used, although that method is not useful in all patients.[149]

Prevention and Treatment

Transplant recipients should be educated about the risks of WNV infection, particularly in endemic areas. Patients should be encouraged to use insect repellant and to avoid the outdoors during the periods of dawn and dusk, when mosquitoes are most active. Treatment of WNV in recipients of solid-organ transplants has generally been empiric and supportive. Both interferon and ribavirin have in vitro activity against WNV,[151] but available data are not sufficient to associate use of these agents with clinical outcome. In addition, intravenous immune globulin may be useful.[152] Reduction or discontinuation of immunosuppression, based on the clinical situation, is most likely important adjunct treatment.[149]

Lymphocytic Choriomeningitis Virus

Lymphocytic choriomeningitis virus (LCMV) is a rodent-borne, Old World arenavirus. Two clusters of LCMV infection in solid-organ transplant recipients have been reported, with one specifically linked to donor transmission of the virus.[153, 154]

Clinical Manifestations

Liver function and coagulation abnormalities, transplant organ dysfunction, fever, rash, diarrhea, hyponatremia, thrombocytopenia, hypoxia, and renal failure developed in 4 transplant recipients of infected organs.[153] Three patients died; hepatocellular necrosis was an autopsy finding in all 3 patients.

Diagnosis and Monitoring

LCMV is very rare; no routine screening is performed on organ donors. LCMV antibodies, immunohistochemistry, PCR, and viral culture may be used for diagnosis in suspected cases.[153]

Treatment

Treatment with intravenous ribavirin, in combination with reduction in immunosuppression, may have been beneficial in the 1 surviving patient of the outbreak mentioned earlier.[153]

Vaccination in Solid-Organ Transplant Candidates and Recipients

Because of the likelihood of poor response to vaccines after transplantation due to inability to mount an effective response, it is very important to have all vaccinations up to date before transplantation.[155,156] In addition, influenza and pneumococcal vaccines should be given at their recommended schedules after transplantation, in order to confer as much protection to the patient as possible. Household contacts of transplant patients should also receive the influenza vaccine on an annual basis.[155,156] Live vaccines should be avoided in transplant recipients, their household contacts, and healthcare professionals caring for these patients.[155]

Table 3 outlines the recommended vaccination schedule for solid-organ transplant candidates and recipients.[155,156]

Conclusion

In summary, infectious complications after solid-organ transplantation can lead to significant morbidity and mortality if not promptly diagnosed and treated. However, the growing armamentarium of knowledge and therapeutic agents available for the prevention and treatment of these infections will continue to improve the quality of care for these patients.

Table 3. RECOMMENDATIONS FOR VACCINATION OF TRANSPLANT CANDIDATES AND RECIPIENTS[155, 156]

Vaccine	Patients	Before Transplantation	After Transplantation	Comments
Pneumococcal	All	√	√	Revaccinate every 2 to 3 years
Hepatitis A	Liver transplant candidates	√		
Hepatitis B	All seronegative patients	√	√	Check titers annually; give booster if antibody falls to < 10 mIU/mL
Influenza	All	√	√	Revaccinate yearly (including household contacts)
Varicella	All seronegative patients	√		
Tetanus-diphtheria toxoid	All children and booster for adults	√		Booster if not given within 5 years
Mumps, measles, rubella (MMR)	All seronegative patients	√		
Poliovirus vaccine inactivated (IPV)	All seronegative patients	√		Also use in household contacts and healthcare workers
Haemophilus influenzae b conjugate (H flu B)	All children and adults with low titers	√		
Meningococcal	Patients who will be entering college within 1 to 2 years	√		

References

1. Snydman DR. Infection in solid organ transplantation. *Transpl Infect Dis.* 1999;1:21-28.
2. Fishman JA, Rubin RH. Infection in organ-transplant recipients. *N Engl J Med.* 1998;338:1741-1751.
3. Patel R, Paya CV. Infections in solid-organ transplant recipients. *Clin Microbiol Rev.* 1997;10:86-124.
4. Rubin RH, Tolkoff-Rubin NE. Antimicrobial strategies in the care of organ transplant recipients. *Antimicrob Agents Chemother.* 1993;37:619-624.
5. Wagener MM, Yu VL. Bacteremia in transplant recipients: a prospective study of demographics, etiologic agents, risk factors, and outcomes. *Am J Infect Control.* 1992;20:239-247.
6. Paya C, Hermans PE. Bacterial infections after liver transplantation. *Eur J Clin Microbiol Infect Dis.* 1989;8:499-534.
7. Cockerill FR. *Diagnosis of Bacterial and Parasitic Infection.* Philadelphia, Pa: Lippincott-Raven Publishers; 1998.
8. Deusch E, End A, Grimm M, Graninger W, Klepetko W, Wolner E. Early bacterial infections in lung transplant recipients. *Chest.* 1993;104:1412-1416.
9. Groeger JS, Lucas AB, Thaler HT, et al. Infectious morbidity associated with long-term use of venous access devices in patients with cancer. *Ann Intern Med.* 1993;119:1168-1174.
10. Raad, II, Bodey GP. Infectious complications of indwelling vascular catheters. *Clin Infect Dis.* 1992;15:197-208.
11. Peterson PK, Balfour HH Jr, Fryd DS, Ferguson RM, Simmons RL. Fever in renal transplant recipients: causes, prognostic significance and changing patterns at the University of Minnesota Hospital. *Am J Med.* 1981;71:345-351.
12. Wyner LM. The evaluation and management of urinary tract infections in recipients of solid-organ transplants. *Semin Urol.* 1994;12:134-139.
13. Villacian JS, Paya CV. Prevention of infections in solid organ transplant recipients. *Transpl Infect Dis.* 1999;1:53-64.

14. Lumbreras C, Fernandez I, Velosa J, Munn S, Sterioff S, Paya CV. Infectious complications following pancreatic transplantation: incidence, microbiological and clinical characteristics, and outcome. *Clin Infect Dis*. 1995;20:514-520.
15. Soave R. Prophylaxis strategies for solid-organ transplantation. *Clin Infect Dis*. 2001;33(suppl 1):S26-S31.
16. Stosor V. Infections in transplant recipients. In: Stuart FP AM, Kaufman DB, eds. *Organ Transplantation*. Georgetown, Tex: Landes Bioscience; 2003:399-425.
17. Kibbler CC. Liver transplantation. In: Berry C, ed. *Transplantation Pathology*. Heidelberg, Germany: Springer; 1999:27-29.
18. Winston DJ, Emmanouilides C, Busuttil RW. Infections in liver transplant recipients. *Clin Infect Dis*. 1995;21:1077-1089; quiz 1090-1071.
19. Paya CV, Wiesner RH, Hermans PE, et al. Risk factors for cytomegalovirus and severe bacterial infections following liver transplantation: a prospective multivariate time-dependent analysis. *J Hepatol*. 1993;18:185-195.
20. Bubak ME, Porayko MK, Krom RA, Wiesner RH. Complications of liver biopsy in liver transplant patients: increased sepsis associated with choledochojejunostomy. *Hepatology*. 1991;14:1063-1065.
21. Hadley S, Samore MH, Lewis WD, Jenkins RL, Karchmer AW, Hammer SM. Major infectious complications after orthotopic liver transplantation and comparison of outcomes in patients receiving cyclosporine or FK536 as primary immunosuppression. *Transplantation*. 1995;59:851-859.
22. Kibbler CC. Infections in liver transplantation: risk factors and strategies for prevention. *J Hosp Infect*. 1995;30(suppl):209-217.
23. Wade JJ, Rolando N, Hayllar K, Philpott-Howard J, Casewell MW, Williams R. Bacterial and fungal infections after liver transplantation: an analysis of 284 patients. *Hepatology*. 1995;21:1328-1336.
24. George DL, Arnow PM, Fox AS, et al. Bacterial infection as a complication of liver transplantation: epidemiology and risk factors. *Rev Infect Dis*. 1991;13:387-396.
25. Lumbreras C, Lizasoain M, Moreno E, et al. Major bacterial infections following liver transplantation: a prospective study. *Hepatogastroenterology*. 1992;39:362-365.
26. Stoutenbeek CP, van Saene HK, Miranda DR, Zandstra DF. The effect of selective decontamination of the digestive tract on colonisation and infection rate in multiple trauma patients. *Intensive Care Med*. 1984;10:185-192.
27. Ledingham IM, Alcock SR, Eastaway AT, McDonald JC, McKay IC, Ramsay G. Triple regimen of selective decontamination of the digestive tract, systemic cefotaxime, and microbiological surveillance for prevention of acquired infection in intensive care. *Lancet*. 1988;1(8589):785-790.
28. Arnow PM, Carandang GC, Zabner R, Irwin ME. Randomized controlled trial of selective bowel decontamination for prevention of infections following liver transplantation. *Clin Infect Dis*. 1996;22:997-1003.
29. Arnow PM, Furmaga K, Flaherty JP, George D. Microbiological efficacy and pharmacokinetics of prophylactic antibiotics in liver transplant patients. *Antimicrob Agents Chemother*. 1992;36:2125-2130.
30. Patel R, Cockerill FR, Porayko MK, Osmon DR, Ilstrup DM, Keating MR. Lactobacillemia in liver transplant patients. *Clin Infect Dis*. 1994;18:207-212.
31. Smart FW, Naftel DC, Costanzo MR, et al. Risk factors for early, cumulative, and fatal infections after heart transplantation: a multiinstitutional study. *J Heart Lung Transplant* 1996;15(4):329-341.
32. Walker R. *Gram-Negative Infections*. Philadelphia, Pa: Lippincott-Raven; 1998.
33. Waser M, Maggiorini M, Luthy A, et al. Infectious complications in 100 consecutive heart transplant recipients. *Eur J Clin Microbiol Infect Dis*. 1994;13:12-18.
34. Grossi P, De Maria R, Caroli A, Zaina MS, Minoli L. Infections in heart transplant recipients: the experience of the Italian heart transplantation program. Italian Study Group on Infections in Heart Transplantation. *J Heart Lung Transplant*. 1992;11:847-866.
35. Ramirez JC, Patterson GA, Winton TL, de Hoyos AL, Miller JD, Maurer JR. Bilateral lung transplantation for cystic fibrosis. The Toronto Lung Transplant Group. *J Thorac Cardiovasc Surg*. 1992;103:287-293; discussion 294.
36. Paya CV. Fungal infections in solid-organ transplantation. *Clin Infect Dis*. 1993;16:677-688.
37. Paya CV. Prevention of fungal infection in transplantation. *Transpl Infect Dis*. 2002;4(suppl 3):46-51.
38. Cohen J, Hopkins J, Kurtz J. *Infectious Complications After Renal Transplantation*. Philadelphia, Pa: WB Saunders; 1988.
39. Hesse UJ, Sutherland DE, Simmons RL, Najarian JS. Intra-abdominal infections in pancreas transplant recipients. *Ann Surg*. 1986;203:153-162.
40. Collins LA, Samore MH, Roberts MS, et al. Risk factors for invasive fungal infections complicating orthotopic liver transplantation. *J Infect Dis*. 1994;170:644-652.
41. Wajszczuk CP, Dummer JS, Ho M, et al. Fungal infections in liver transplant recipients. *Transplantation*. 1985;40:347-353.

42. Castaldo P, Stratta RJ, Wood RP, et al. Clinical spectrum of fungal infections after orthotopic liver transplantation. *Arch Surg.* 1991;126:149-156.
43. Tollemar J, Ericzon BG, Barkholt L, Andersson J, Ringden O, Groth CG. Risk factors for deep candida infections in liver transplant recipients. *Transplant Proc.* 1990;22:1826-1827.
44. Tollemar J, Ericzon BG, Holmberg K, Andersson J. The incidence and diagnosis of invasive fungal infections in liver transplant recipients. *Transplant Proc* 1990;22(1):242-244.
45. Kusne S, Dummer JS, Singh N, et al. Infections after liver transplantation: an analysis of 101 consecutive cases. *Medicine (Baltimore).* 1988;67:132-143.
46. Nadeem I, Yeldani, V, Sheridan, P, et al. Efficacy of itraconazole prophylaxis for aspergillosis in lung transplant recipients. Paper presented at: annual meeting of Infectious Diseases Society of America, 1994; Orlando, Fla.
47. Kusne S, Abu-Elmagd K, Hutson W, et al. Invasive fungal infections after adult small bowel transplantation (SBTX). Presented at: Fifth International Symposium on Small Intestinal Transplantation; July 31-August 2, 1997; Cambridge, UK. Abstract 034.
48. Reyes J, Abu-Elmagd K, Tzakis A, et al. Infectious complications after human small bowel transplantation. *Transplant Proc.* 1992;24:1249-1250.
49. Tollemar JG. Fungal infections. In: Bowden RA, Ljungman P, Paya CV, eds. *Transplant Infections.* Philadelphia, Pa: Lippincott-Raven;1998:339-350.
50. Kramer MR, Marshall SE, Starnes VA, Gamberg P, Amitai Z, Theodore J. Infectious complications in heart-lung transplantation: analysis of 200 episodes. *Arch Intern Med.* 1993;153:2010-2016.
51. Higgins R, McNeil K, Dennis C, et al. Airway stenoses after lung transplantation: management with expanding metal stents. *J Heart Lung Transplant.* 1994;13:774-778.
52. Kanj SS, Welty-Wolf K, Madden J, et al. Fungal infections in lung and heart-lung transplant recipients: report of 9 cases and review of the literature. *Medicine (Baltimore).* 1996;75:142-156.
53. Cahill BC, Hibbs JR, Savik K, et al. Aspergillus airway colonization and invasive disease after lung transplantation. *Chest.* 1997;112:1160-1164.
54. Yeldandi V, Laghi F, McCabe MA, et al. Aspergillus and lung transplantation. *J Heart Lung Transplant.* 1995;14:883-890.
55. Westney GE, Kesten S, De Hoyos A, Chapparro C, Winton T, Maurer JR. Aspergillus infection in single and double lung transplant recipients. *Transplantation.* 1996;61:915-919.
56. Hamacher J, Spiliopoulos A, Kurt AM, Nicod LP. Pre-emptive therapy with azoles in lung transplant patients. Geneva Lung Transplantation Group. *Eur Respir J.* 1999;13:180-186.
57. Kramer MR, Denning DW, Marshall SE, et al. Ulcerative tracheobronchitis after lung transplantation: a new form of invasive aspergillosis. *Am Rev Respir Dis.* 1991;144(3 Pt 1):552-556.
58. Nunley DR, Ohori P, Grgurich WF, et al. Pulmonary aspergillosis in cystic fibrosis lung transplant recipients. *Chest.* 1998;114:1321-1329.
59. Paradowski LJ. Saprophytic fungal infections and lung transplantation—revisited. *J Heart Lung Transplant.* 1997;16:524-531.
60. Husni RN, Gordon SM, Longworth DL, et al. Cytomegalovirus infection is a risk factor for invasive aspergillosis in lung transplant recipients. *Clin Infect Dis.* 1998;26:753-755.
61. Tazelaar HD, Baird AM, Mill M, Grimes MM, Schulman LL, Smith CR. Bronchocentric mycosis occurring in transplant recipients. *Chest.* 1989;96:92-95.
62. Scott JP, Fradet G, Smyth RL, et al. Prospective study of transbronchial biopsies in the management of heart-lung and single lung transplant patients. *J Heart Lung Transplant.* 1991;10(5 Pt 1):626-636; discussion 636-627.
63. Singh N. Antifungal prophylaxis for solid organ transplant recipients: seeking clarity amidst controversy. *Clin Infect Dis.* 2000;31:545-553.
64. Grossi P, Farina C, Fiocchi R, Dalla Gasperina D. Prevalence and outcome of invasive fungal infections in 1,963 thoracic organ transplant recipients: a multicenter retrospective study. Italian Study Group of Fungal Infections in Thoracic Organ Transplant Recipients. *Transplantation.* 2000;70:112-116.
65. Munoz P, Alcala L, Sanchez Conde M, et al. The isolation of *Aspergillus fumigatus* from respiratory tract specimens in heart transplant recipients is highly predictive of invasive aspergillosis. *Transplantation.* 2003;75:326-329.
66. Montoya JG, Chaparro SV, Celis D, et al. Invasive aspergillosis in the setting of cardiac transplantation. *Clin Infect Dis.* 2003;37(suppl 3):S281-S292.
67. Munoz P, Rodriguez C, Bouza E, et al. Risk factors of invasive aspergillosis after heart transplantation: protective role of oral itraconazole prophylaxis. *Am J Transplant.* 2004;4:636-643.
68. Montoya JG, Giraldo LF, Efron B, et al. Infectious complications among 620 consecutive heart transplant patients at Stanford University Medical Center. *Clin Infect Dis.* 2001;33:629-640.

69. McEvoy GK e. *AHFS: Drug Information*. Bethesda, Md: American Society of Health-System Pharmacists; 2005:519-531.
70. Sawaya BP, Weihprecht H, Campbell WR, et al. Direct vasoconstriction as a possible cause for amphotericin B-induced nephrotoxicity in rats. *J Clin Invest*. 1991;87:2097-2107.
71. Stevens DA BJ. Antifungal agents. In: Mandell GL BJ, Dolin R, ed. *Principles and Practice of Infectious Diseases*. Philadelphia, Pa: Churchill Livingstone; 2000:448-459.
72. Bartizal K, Gill CJ, Abruzzo GK, et al. In vitro preclinical evaluation studies with the echinocandin antifungal MK-0991 (L-743,872). *Antimicrob Agents Chemother*. 1997;41:2326-2332.
73. Ernst EJ, Klepser ME, Ernst ME, Messer SA, Pfaller MA. In vitro pharmacodynamic properties of MK-0991 determined by time-kill methods. *Diagn Microbiol Infect Dis*. 1999;33:75-80.
74. Pfaller MA, Marco F, Messer SA, Jones RN. In vitro activity of two echinocandin derivatives, LY303366 and MK-0991 (L-743,792), against clinical isolates of *Aspergillus, Fusarium, Rhizopus*, and other filamentous fungi. *Diagn Microbiol Infect Dis*. 1998;30:251-255.
75. Product Information: Cancidas [R], Caspofungin. Whitehouse Station, NJ: Merck & Co; 2001.
76. Stone JA, Holland SD, Wickersham PJ, et al. Single- and multiple-dose pharmacokinetics of caspofungin in healthy men. *Antimicrob Agents Chemother*. 2002;46:739-745.
77. Stone JA, Xu X, Winchell GA, et al. Disposition of caspofungin: role of distribution in determining pharmacokinetics in plasma. *Antimicrob Agents Chemother*. 2004;48:815-823.
78. Balani SK, Xu X, Arison BH, et al. Metabolites of caspofungin acetate, a potent antifungal agent, in human plasma and urine. *Drug Metab Dispos*. 2000;28:1274-1278.
79. McCormack PL, Perry CM. Caspofungin: a review of its use in the treatment of fungal infections. *Drugs*. 2005;65:2049-2068.
80. Marr KA, Hachem R, Papanicolaou G, et al. Retrospective study of the hepatic safety profile of patients concomitantly treated with caspofungin and cyclosporin A. *Transpl Infect Dis*. 2004;6:110-116.
81. Sanz-Rodriguez C, Lopez-Duarte M, Jurado M, et al. Safety of the concomitant use of caspofungin and cyclosporin A in patients with invasive fungal infections. *Bone Marrow Transplant*. 2004;34:13-20.
82. Morrissey CO, Slavin, MA, O'Reilly MA, et al. Caspofungin as salvage therapy for invasive aspergillosis: results of the Australian Compassionate Access Program. Paper presented at: 44th Interscience Conference on Antimicrobial Agents and Chemotherapy, 2004 Oct 30-Nov 2; Washington, DC83. Jarvis B, Figgitt DP, Scott LJ. Micafungin. *Drugs*. 2004;64:969-982; discussion 983-964.
84. Product Information: Mycamine [R], micafungin. Deerfield, Ill: Astellas Pharma US I; 2005.
85. Van Burik J, Ratanatharathorn V, Lipton J, et al. Randomized, double-blind trial of micafungin (MI) versus fluconazole (FL) for prophylaxis of invasive fungal infections inpatients (pts) undergoing hematopoietic stem cell transplant (HSCT), NIAID/BAMSG protocol 46. Paper presented at: Proceedings of the 42nd Interscience Conference on Antimicrobial Agents and Chemotherapy, 2002 Sep 27-30; San Diego, Calif.
86. Product Information: Eraxis®, Anidulafungin. New York, NY: Roerig Division of Pfizer Inc; 2006.
87. Marco F, Pfaller MA, Messer SA, et al. In vitro susceptibilities of clinical yeast isolates to a new echinocandin derivative, LY303366, and other antifungal agents. *Antimicrob Agents Chemother*. 1997;41:763-766.
88. Cuenca-Estrella M, Mellado E, Diaz-Guerra TM, et al. Susceptibility of fluconazole-resistant clinical isolates of *Candida* spp. To echinocandin LY303366, itraconazole and amphotericin B. *J Antimicrob Chemother*. 2000;46:475-477.
89. Moore CB, Oakley KL, Denning DW. In vitro activity of a new echinocandin, LY303366, and comparison with fluconazole, flucytosine and amphotericin B against *Candida* species. *Clin Microbiol Infect*. 2001;7:11-16.
90. Zhanel GG, Karlowsky JA, Harding GA, et al. In vitro activity of a new semi-synthetic echinocandin, LY-303366, against systemic isolates of *Candida* species, *Cryptococcus neoformans, Blastomyces dermatitidis*, and *Aspergillus* species. *Antimicrob Agents Chemother*. 1997;41:863-865.
91. Serrano Mdel C, Valverde-Conde A, Chavez MM, et al. In vitro activity of voriconazole, itraconazole, caspofungin, anidulafungin (VER002, Ly303366) and amphotericin B against *Aspergillus* spp. *Diagn Microbiol Infect Dis*. 2003;45:131-135.
92. Petraitis V, Petraitiene R, Groll AH, et al. Antifungal efficacy, safety, and single-dose pharmacokinetics of LY303366, a novel echinocandin B, in experimental pulmonary aspergillosis in persistently neutropenic rabbits. *Antimicrob Agents Chemother*. 1998;42:2898-2905.
93. Ostrosky-Zeichner L, Matar M, Paetznich VL, Rodriguez JR. In-vitro synergy testing of anidulafungin (AFG) and micafungin (MFG) in combination with amphotericin B (AMB) against *Aspergillus* spp. and *Fusarium* spp. In: Program and Abstracts of the 42nd Interscience Conference on Antimicrobial Agents and Chemotherapy; September 27-30, 2002; San Diego, Calif. Monograph M-1816.

94. Philip A, Odabasi Z, Rodrigues JR, et al. In vitro synergy testing of anidulafungin (ANID) with itraconazole (ITR) and voriconazole (VOR) against *Aspergillus* spp. and *Fusarium* spp. In: Program and Abstracts of the 43rd Interscience Conference on Antimicrobial Agents and Chemotherapy; September 14-17, 2003; Chicago, Ill. Monograph M-988.
95. Odabasi Z, Paetznick VL. Rodriguez JR, et al. In vitro activity of anidulafungin against selected clinically important mold isolates. *Antimicrob Agents Chemother.* 2004;48:1912-1915.
96. Kotton CN, Fishman JA. Viral infection in the renal transplant recipient. *J Am Soc Nephrol.* 2005;16:1758-1774.
97. Razonable RR, Rivero A, Rodriguez A, et al. Allograft rejection predicts the occurrence of late-onset cytomegalovirus (CMV) disease among CMV-mismatched solid organ transplant patients receiving prophylaxis with oral ganciclovir. *J Infect Dis.* 2001;184:1461-1464.
98. Paya C, Humar A, Dominguez E, et al. Efficacy and safety of valganciclovir vs. oral ganciclovir for prevention of cytomegalovirus disease in solid organ transplant recipients. *Am J Transplant.* 2004;4:611-620.
99. Opelz G, Dohler B, Ruhenstroth A. Cytomegalovirus prophylaxis and graft outcome in solid organ transplantation: a collaborative transplant study report. *Am J Transplant.* 2004;4:928-936.
100. Preiksaitis JK, Brennan DC, Fishman J, Allen U. Canadian society of transplantation consensus workshop on cytomegalovirus management in solid organ transplantation final report. *Am J Transplant.* 2005;5:218-227.
101. Snydman DR. Posttransplant microbiological surveillance. *Clin Infect Dis.* 2001;33(suppl 1):S22-S25.
102. Kunzle N, Petignat C, Francioli P, et al. Preemptive treatment approach to cytomegalovirus (CMV) infection in solid organ transplant patients: relationship between compliance with the guidelines and prevention of CMV morbidity. *Transpl Infect Dis.* 2000;2:118-126.
103. Cytomegalovirus. *Am J Transplant* 2004;4(suppl 10):51-58.
104. Pescovitz MD, Rabkin J, Merion RM, et al. Valganciclovir results in improved oral absorption of ganciclovir in liver transplant recipients. *Antimicrob Agents Chemother.* 2000;44:2811-2815.
105. Park JM, Lake KD, Arenas JD, Fontana RJ. Efficacy and safety of low-dose valganciclovir in the prevention of cytomegalovirus disease in adult liver transplant recipients. *Liver Transpl.* 2006;12:112-116.
106. Akalin E, Sehgal V, Ames S, et al. Cytomegalovirus disease in high-risk transplant recipients despite ganciclovir or valganciclovir prophylaxis. *Am J Transplant.* 2003;3:731-735.
107. Akalin E, Bromberg JS, Sehgal V, Ames S, Murphy B. Decreased incidence of cytomegalovirus infection in thymoglobulin-treated transplant patients with 6 months of valganciclovir prophylaxis. *Am J Transplant.* 2004;4:148-149.
108. Gabardi S, Magee CC, Baroletti SA, Powelson JA, Cina JL, Chandraker AK. Efficacy and safety of low-dose valganciclovir for prevention of cytomegalovirus disease in renal transplant recipients: a single-center, retrospective analysis. *Pharmacotherapy.* 2004;24:1323-1330.
109. Taber DJ, Ashcraft E, Baillie GM, et al. Valganciclovir prophylaxis in patients at high risk for the development of cytomegalovirus disease. *Transpl Infect Dis.* 2004;6:101-109.
110. Doyle AM, Warburton KM, Goral S, Blumberg E, Grossman RA, Bloom RD. 24-week oral ganciclovir prophylaxis in kidney recipients is associated with reduced symptomatic cytomegalovirus disease compared to a 12-week course. *Transplantation.* 2006;81:1106-1111.
111. Limaye AP, Corey L, Koelle DM, Davis CL, Boeckh M. Emergence of ganciclovir-resistant cytomegalovirus disease among recipients of solid-organ transplants. *Lancet.* 2000;356:645-649.
112. Boivin G, Goyette N, Gilbert C, et al. Absence of cytomegalovirus-resistance mutations after valganciclovir prophylaxis, in a prospective multicenter study of solid-organ transplant recipients. *J Infect Dis.* 2004;189:1615-1618.
113. Mylonakis E, Kallas WM, Fishman JA. Combination antiviral therapy for ganciclovir-resistant cytomegalovirus infection in solid-organ transplant recipients. *Clin Infect Dis.* 2002;34:1337-1341.
114. Other herpesviruses: HHV-6, HHV-7, HHV-8, HSV-1 and -2, VZV. *Am J Transplant.* 2004;4(suppl 10):66-71.
115. Gourishankar S, McDermid JC, Jhangri GS, Preiksaitis JK. Herpes zoster infection following solid organ transplantation: incidence, risk factors and outcomes in the current immunosuppressive era. *Am J Transplant.* 2004;4:108-115.
116. Prevention of varicella: Recommendations of the Advisory Committee on Immunization Practices (ACIP). Centers for Disease Control and Prevention. *MMWR Recomm Rep.* 1996;45(RR-11):1-36.
117. Khan S, Erlichman J, Rand EB. Live virus immunization after orthotopic liver transplantation. *Pediatr Transplant.* 2006;10:78-82.
118. Levitsky J, Te HS, Faust TW, Cohen SM. Varicella infection following varicella vaccination in a liver transplant recipient. *Am J Transplant.* 2002;2:880-882.
119. Neu AM. Indications for varicella vaccination post-transplant. *Pediatr Transplant.* 2005;9:141-144.
120. Singh N, Paterson DL. Encephalitis caused by human herpesvirus-6 in transplant recipients: relevance of a novel neurotropic virus. *Transplantation.* 2000;69:2474-2479.

121. Paterson DL, Singh N, Gayowski T, Carrigan DR, Marino IR. Encephalopathy associated with human herpesvirus 6 in a liver transplant recipient. *Liver Transpl Surg.* 1999;5:454-455.
122. Rossi C, Delforge ML, Jacobs F, et al. Fatal primary infection due to human herpesvirus 6 variant A in a renal transplant recipient. *Transplantation.* 2001;71:288-292.
123. Rogers J, Rohal S, Carrigan DR, et al. Human herpesvirus-6 in liver transplant recipients: role in pathogenesis of fungal infections, neurologic complications, and outcome. *Transplantation.* 2000;69:2566-2573.
124. Singh N, Carrigan DR. Human herpesvirus-6 in transplantation: an emerging pathogen. *Ann Intern Med.* 1996;124:1065-1071.
125. Benito N, Ricart MJ, Pumarola T, Marcos MA, Oppenheimer F, Camacho AM. Infection with human herpesvirus 6 after kidney-pancreas transplant. *Am J Transplant.* 2004;4:1197-1199.
126. Verucchi G, Calza L, Trevisani F, et al. Human herpesvirus-8-related Kaposi's sarcoma after liver transplantation successfully treated with cidofovir and liposomal daunorubicin. *Transplant Infect Dis.* 2005;7:34-37.
127. Thaunat O, Mamzer-Bruneel MF, Agbalika F, et al. Severe human herpesvirus-8 primary infection in a renal transplant patient successfully treated with anti-CD20 monoclonal antibody. *Blood.* 2006;107:3009-3010.
128. Epstein-Barr virus and lymphoproliferative disorders after transplantation. *Am J Transplant.* 2004;4(suppl 10):59-65.
129. Preiksaitis JK, Keay S. Diagnosis and management of posttransplant lymphoproliferative disorder in solid-organ transplant recipients. *Clin Infect Dis* 2001;33(suppl 1):S38-S46.
130. Cockfield SM. Identifying the patient at risk for post-transplant lymphoproliferative disorder. *Transpl Infect Dis.* 2001;3:70-78.
131. Davis JE, Moss DJ. Treatment options for post-transplant lymphoproliferative disorder and other Epstein-Barr virus-associated malignancies. *Tissue Antigens.* 2004;63:285-292.
132. Adenovirus. *Am J Transplant.* 2004;4(suppl 10):101-104.
133. Human parvovirus B19. *Am J Transplant.* 2004;4(suppl 10):92-94.
134. Human papillomavirus infection. *Am J Transplant.* 2004;4(suppl 10):95-100.
135. Stockfleth E, Nindl I, Sterry W, Ulrich C, Schmook T, Meyer T. Human papillomaviruses in transplant-associated skin cancers. *Dermatol Surg.* 2004;30:604-609.
136. BK virus. *Am J Transplant* 2004;4 Suppl 10:89-91.
137. Bohl DL, Storch GA, Ryschkewitsch C, et al. Donor origin of BK virus in renal transplantation and role of HLA C7 in susceptibility to sustained BK viremia. *Am J Transplant.* 2005;5:2213-2221.
138. Limaye AP, Smith KD, Cook L, et al. Polyomavirus nephropathy in native kidneys of non-renal transplant recipients. *Am J Transplant.* 2005;5:614-620.
139. Menahem SA, McDougall KM, Thomson NM, Dowling JP. Native kidney BK nephropathy post cardiac transplantation. *Transplantation.* 2005;79:259-260.
140. Lipshutz GS, Mahanty H, Feng S, et al. BKV in simultaneous pancreas-kidney transplant recipients: a leading cause of renal graft loss in first 2 years post-transplant. *Am J Transplant.* 2005;5:366-373.
141. Brennan DC, Agha I, Bohl DL, et al. Incidence of BK with tacrolimus versus cyclosporine and impact of preemptive immunosuppression reduction. *Am J Transplant.* 2005;5:582-594.
142. Tong CY, Hilton R, MacMahon EM, et al. Monitoring the progress of BK virus associated nephropathy in renal transplant recipients. *Nephrol Dial Transplant.* 2004;19:2598-2605.
143. Humar A, Michaels M. American Society of Transplantation recommendations for screening, monitoring and reporting of infectious complications in immunosuppression trials in recipients of organ transplantation. *Am J Transplant* 2006;6(2):262-274.
144. Kadambi PV, Josephson MA, Williams J, et al. Treatment of refractory BK virus-associated nephropathy with cidofovir. *Am J Transplant.* 2003;3:186-191.
145. Josephson MA, Gillen D, Javaid B, et al. Treatment of renal allograft polyoma BK virus infection with leflunomide. *Transplantation.* 2006;81:704-710.
146. Sener A, House AA, Jevnikar AM, et al. Intravenous immunoglobulin as a treatment for BK virus associated nephropathy: one-year follow-up of renal allograft recipients. *Transplantation.* 2006;81:117-120.
147. Paya CV. Prevention of fungal and hepatitis virus infections in liver transplantation. *Clin Infect Dis.* 2001;33(suppl 1):S47-S52.
148. Viral hepatitis guidelines in hemodialysis and transplantation. *Am J Transplant.* 2004;4(suppl 10):72-82.
149. Kumar D, Prasad GV, Zaltzman J, Levy GA, Humar A. Community-acquired West Nile virus infection in solid-organ transplant recipients. *Transplantation.* 2004;77:399-402.
150. Kumar D, Drebot MA, Wong SJ, et al. A seroprevalence study of West Nile virus infection in solid organ transplant recipients. *Am J Transplant.* 2004;4:1883-1888.

151. Anderson JF, Rahal JJ. Efficacy of interferon alpha-2b and ribavirin against West Nile virus in vitro. *Emerg Infect Dis.* 2002;8:107-108.
152. Hamdan A, Green P, Mendelson E, Kramer MR, Pitlik S, Weinberger M. Possible benefit of intravenous immunoglobulin therapy in a lung transplant recipient with West Nile virus encephalitis. *Transpl Infect Dis.* 2002;4:160-162.
153. Lymphocytic choriomeningitis virus infection in organ transplant recipients: Massachusetts, Rhode Island, 2005. *MMWR Morb Mortal Wkly Rep.* 2005;54:537-539.
154. Paddock C, Ksiazek, T, Comer, JA, et al. Pathology of fatal lymphocytic choriomeningitis virus infection in multiple organ transplant recipients from a common donor. *Mod Pathol.* 2005;18(suppl):263A-264A.
155. Avery RK, Ljungman P. Prophylactic measures in the solid-organ recipient before transplantation. *Clin Infect Dis.* 2001;33(suppl 1):S15-S21.
156. Guidelines for vaccination of solid organ transplant candidates and recipients. *Am J Transplant.* 2004;4(suppl 10):160-163.

Transplant Immunology

Linda Ohler, MSN, RN, CCTC, FAAN

Introduction

The immune system is one of the most complex systems in the human body. Working in the field of transplantation requires that both procurement and clinical coordinators have a basic knowledge of how immunology may affect recipients and donors. Although most information has been focused on clinical applications of immunology to mechanisms of rejection and suppression of the immune system, recent studies are suggesting that cytokines released in traumatic brain injury influence the function of donated organs. Laboratory tests that measure various aspects of immune function are important tools for procurement and clinical coordinators to use to evaluate clinical situations. The immune system holds a key to many disease processes, and we are learning more about this complex system each day. In the past 5 decades of transplantation, we have used many therapies designed to minimize or prevent rejection. Many of the therapies used to suppress the immune system have resulted in long-term complications for recipients. With newer immunosuppressive agents, we are now able to individualize therapies and minimize some of these complications.

The immune system provides the body with a complex structure of cells that communicate with one another in ways we are still trying to understand. Communication networks provide the body with protection against foreign entities such as infectious agents, dangerous environmental elements, and even transplanted organs. But a new organ is neither infectious nor should it be considered dangerous. After all, it is just an organ that has been removed from one individual and kept in preservation solution before being transplanted. So why is it dangerous? The answer lies in understanding the cells of the immune system, inflammation, and a rather complex network of communication.

This chapter provides readers with an overview of immunology as it pertains to transplantation. Donor characteristics, pretransplantation clinical issues for potential recipients, and posttransplantation management of immune function are addressed in this chapter. After a description of the cells of the immune system, details about laboratory testing are provided.

Cells of the Immune System

Cells of the immune system reside in the spleen, tonsils, Peyer patches of the intestines, thymus, and bone marrow and circulate in the blood and lymphatic systems. Lymphocytes possess a basic instinct to react against potentially damaging foreign agents and tissues. An understanding of Human Leukocyte Antigens (HLA) will lay the framework for understanding reactions by immune cells to non-self. Several types of lymphocytes are involved in transplantation: T and B cells are those discussed in this chapter.

Other significant cells of the immune system include neutrophils, eosinophils, basophils, monocytes, and macrophages. These cells have a variety of roles that range from recognition of invading antigens to communication with other cells and destruction of the invader. Lymphocytes are white blood cells; thus they do not possess the characteristic Rh factor found on red blood cells. In transplantation, we carefully ensure that donors and recipients have compatible blood types but we do not concern ourselves with the Rh factor because the cells of the immune system are within the white blood cell network.

Antigens

Antigens are molecules or tissues that can be recognized by the immune system as self or nonself.[1] These antigens can be infectious agents, pollens, or transplanted organs and tissues. They possess characteristics that enable them to react with components of the immune system such as lymphocytes or antibodies. An essential feature of the immune system is its ability to distinguish self antigens from antigens that are non-self. In most cases, the host's own antigens are recognized as self and are considered tolerogenic. Antigens that are not self are able to activate lymphocytes and antibodies in an immune response.

It is the same immune response that protects us from infections that is activated against transplanted organs. Thus in our attempts to suppress rejections with immunosuppressive agents, we also suppress the immune response that protects our patients from infections. Finding that balance between protection from infection and avoidance of rejection is currently an art that needs scientific applications. Research protocols are focused on evaluating methods for inducing tolerance, understanding chimerism, blocking signaling pathways, and studying drugs that deplete lymphocytes in an attempt to trick the immune system when a new organ is slipped in.

Each of us carries a set of antigens that we receive from our parents. These are called HLA antigens, a set of proteins located on the surface of most cells and responsible for discriminating self from non-self. You may also see this system of personal identifiers referred to as major histocompatibility complex or MHC. When we transplant an organ, HLA antigens carried by the donor organ are recognized by the recipient's immune system as non-self. This recognition sets off an immune response that is not influenced by the fact that the new kidney, liver, heart, or lungs is intended to improve the health of the recipient. This fact poses several challenges to us as transplant professionals. How can we teach the immune system to be more tolerant and accepting of a transplanted organ? First, we must understand how the immune system functions. This understanding will allow us to begin to think of ways to induce tolerance, to block communication pathways, and prevent rejection of these vital organs.

HLA antigens are divided into 2 classes. Class I molecules are found on most nucleated cells and seem to be most involved in cellular rejection. Each individual has 3 sets of class I molecules: HLA-A, HLA-B, and HLA-C. Class II molecules are encoded by genes in the HLA-D region of chromosome 6 and seem to influence the humoral or chronic rejection that limits long-term graft survival in many cases. HLA-DR is most commonly referenced in solid organ transplantation. In bone marrow transplantation, matching of class II molecules such as HLA-DQ and HLA-DP goes beyond those antigens we evaluate for solid organ transplantation. Six antigen matches (HLA-A, B, and DR) are highly valued in renal transplantation, especially for those individuals with preformed antibodies. In addition to its use in solid organ and bone marrow or stem cell transplantation, HLA testing can also be used to determine paternity and in recent years has been applied to forensics.

Initially, HLA typing or tissue typing was accomplished via serology testing methods that required 6 to 8 tubes of blood. This test can now be performed with a simple drop of blood, a hair follicle, or a swab from mucous membranes by using DNA technology. In heart, lung, and liver transplantation, HLA evaluation is done retrospectively without considerations for matching.[2] If a candidate has preformed antibodies, specificity tests (described later) are done to determine to which of the HLA antigens the candidate may have developed sensitivities. The time it would take to match antigens between donors and recipients would increase the ischemic times for hearts or lungs. In retrospective analyses of HLA compatibility on organs such as the heart, outcomes have been evaluated in terms of rejection and allograft survival. Findings from longitudinal retrospective studies have demonstrated that graft survival is significantly influenced by the extent of HLA compatibility.[2] Class II antigens seem to be particularly useful in determining outcomes. However, it remains impractical at this time to match thoracic organs prospectively before transplantation.

Preformed Antibodies and Specificities Against HLA

In the early days of transplantation, hyperacute rejections confronted clinicians with serious problems that usually resulted in allograft failure and, in some cases, death of the recipient. Today hyperacute rejections are rare, and our knowledge of immune function has been enhanced through laboratory testing of preformed antibodies, specificities, and crossmatching. Individuals may have preformed antibodies against specific donor antigens through blood transfusions and previous transplants. Women have the added risk of developing preformed antibodies through pregnancy and autoimmune diseases.

A panel of reactive antibodies (PRA) is performed by mixing serum from a transplant candidate with lymphocytes from a select panel of donors whose HLA antigens are known. If there is no reactivity between donor antigens and the antibodies of the transplant candidate, the PRA is reported as 0%. If, however, the candidate's serum reacts to half of the donor lymphocytes, the PRA is reported as 50%. This percentage serves as an index, telling us that the potential transplant candidate may have antibodies against 50% of all possible donor organs.[3] Patients with elevated PRA often have longer wait times for a suitable donor organ because of the probability that there will be a positive crossmatch with the prospective donor antigens. Candidates who have an elevated PRA are sensitized and should be tested for any changes in the antibody titers on a regular basis while awaiting a suitable donor organ. Recent protocols have been described by physicians whereby therapies that use plasmapheresis and immunoglobulins have successfully decreased PRA in sensitized individuals and allowed transplantation.[4]

In thoracic transplantation, only individuals with elevated levels of preformed antibodies are prospectively crossmatched against potential donors. Immunology laboratories have been able to identify specific antigens to which a potential recipient may have developed preformed antibodies. For example, in a potential candidate with preformed antibodies, immunology laboratories can identify HLA antigens to which an individual is sensitive. These specificities alert clinicians to serious antibody-antigen reactivity that could lead to a hyperacute rejection of the transplanted organ. When specificities are identified, they are entered into a computer as unacceptable antigens for a particular transplant candidate. When potential donors are identified, the donor HLA antigens are entered into the computer to identify potential recipients. Any patients possessing specific antibodies against the donor HLA will be excluded from consideration as a candidate to receive that donor organ. This process has eliminated the need for time-consuming crossmatches in many cases because individuals with antibodies against specific donor antigens will have a positive crossmatch.

The Crossmatch

A crossmatch is performed prospectively on all potential kidney recipients and any transplant candidate with an elevated PRA for whom specificities have not been identified. Crossmatch results are reported retrospectively on all other transplants. Without an elevated PRA or specificities, the retrospective crossmatches are usually negative. Results should always be documented in the recipient's chart. Positive results always should be reported directly to the transplanting physician. Reporting such results to the physician is often the responsibility of transplant coordinators. Crossmatch testing requires a peripheral blood specimen, lymph node, or spleen from the donor. Donor cells are then mixed with the recipient's serum. If a reaction occurs, recipient antibodies will bind to and attack the donor's cells.[3] In most cases, a positive crossmatch would be a contraindication for the transplant to proceed. However, methods to desensitize candidates by using immune-modulating therapies including plasmapheresis, cyclophosphamide, and immunoglobulin are decreasing the risk of transplanting across positive crossmatches.[4,5]

If a retrospective crossmatch is positive, the immunology laboratory determines the class of antibodies as either IgG or IgM. IgM antibodies are less threatening, but IgG antibodies can be detrimental to long-term outcomes of the new organ. The immunology laboratory also can identify whether the crossmatch reactivity is targeting B or T cells. This information helps clinicians determine appropriate therapeutic interventions to mediate the situation.

Understanding Immune Responses

T cells

In the most simplistic terms, T cells attack foreign antigens, and B cells produce antibodies that attach to specific antigens that have activated the B cells. Early in our studies of biology and the human body, we learned that this antigen-antibody reactivity is the hallmark of the immune system's protection of self. T cells are lymphocytes that mature in the thymus and account for about 15% of circulating white blood cells. Each T cell has molecules on its surface that recognize antigens through a T-cell receptor site. This recognition is an important step in eliciting an immune response to a perceived dangerous microbe or tissue. Receptor sites can be likened to the eyes of a lymphocyte in that they can see the dangerous microbe and respond by attaching to the epitope of a specific antigen.

There are several types of T cells and, to make it a bit more confusing, they each have several names. This situation could be compared to reading a Tolstoy novel where the characters have various nicknames. Helper T cells are also called immune regulators or CD4 cells. CD stands for cluster of differentiation. In a military analogy, the helper T cell is the army general who will activate the reserves, develop a strategic plan of attack, and communicate that plan to the proliferating army of lymphocytes. This army contains a variety of T cells, including the ominous CD8 or cytotoxic T lymphocytes. As you read on in this chapter, you will learn how the CD8 cells function in an immune response. Most of the time, the immune system is strictly a surveillance system that awaits a signal to activate.

HLA molecules play a significant role in T-cell activation when antigen-presenting cells recognize the danger of non-self. The transplanted organ or tissue sends a signal of non-self and provides the immune system with a continuous source of antigens to which it naturally responds. Reducing the responsiveness of the immune system is the role of many of our immunosuppressive agents such as calcineurin inhibitors and monoclonal or polyclonal antibodies.

Antigens contain epitopes that serve as binding sites for immune cell receptors when an appropriate recognition of non-self or danger occurs. Epitopes may be compared to a docking station in terms of connection and fit with specific receptor sites. Chemical signals serve as a communication network within the immune system. Antigens give off such signals that actually attract cells of the immune system such as macrophages. It is this signaling that begins the immune response.[6]

Antigen-Presenting Cells

Antigen-presenting cells start this signaling process by recognizing tissue stress/necrosis, foreign antigens, or vascular disruption. The cells engulf and digest these factors, sending a chemical message with protein fragments that indicate danger to the helper T cell.[7,8] This process is referred to as signal 1 and is the first step in initiating an immune response.

Antigen-presenting cells include dendritic cells, macrophages and monocytes that are found throughout the body and circulate in a surveillance type of mode. They sample and test potentially damaging antigens by ingesting them. Dangerous microbes are then displayed on the cell surface with HLA molecules that can be recognized by T cells.[9] Once this alarm from signal 1 has been recognized by the helper T cell, a second signal (signal 2) is initiated through production and release of chemical messengers called cytokines.[7] This co-stimulatory signal is responsible for further proliferation of the immune response. Transplanted organs contain antigen-presenting cells and are sites of an inflammatory response that attracts additional antigen-presenting cells from the recipient. This immune response at the graft site is both complex and powerful.[9]

Most of our current therapies for preventing or decreasing the risk of rejection are blocking neither signal 1 nor signal 2. Rather, we are suppressing the proliferation of T and B cells after they have been stimulated. It is believed that research aimed at blocking the co-stimulatory response may provide improved protection against rejection and may even induce tolerance.[7] Research is currently underway to evaluate methods of preventing signal 1 from communicating with signal 2 in an effort to attenuate the immune response.

Cytokines

Cytokines are great communicators that induce T- and B-cell proliferation. The different families of cytokines are categorized according to their source, target cell, or effects on a target cell.[10] Two cytokines play an important role in transplantation: interleukin-2 and interferon-γ. Because they are produced by lymphocytes they are most accurately referred to as lymphokines. Interleukin-2 receptors control T-cell division through a process known as clonal expansion. Additional T cells, especially CD8 or cytotoxic T cells, are cloned in response to messages sent by interleukin-2. Cytotoxic T cells divide and multiply. In transplantation, this proliferation may lead to an acute rejection episode.

Interferon-γ is another cytokine that produces havoc in solid organ transplantation. Cytotoxic T cells are also activated and proliferate along with macrophages in response to this substance. When cytotoxic T cells and macrophages proliferate, they focus on the HLA antigens of the transplanted organ and attack it as non-self. Once proliferation of the immune system has begun, it is challenging to control or stop unless the initiating antigen is destroyed.

B cells

B cells are produced daily in the bone marrow. Because the immune system has such specificity for antigens, a large number of B cells are needed to protect the body from dangerous microbes. B cells have 3 receptor sites: 2 that bind with specific antigens and 1 that binds with phagocytic cells such as macrophages. Figure 1 shows the "Y" shaped antibody with its 3 receptor sites. The arms or forked ends of the antibody attach to specific antigens and the tail binds to the macrophages. The tail of an antibody molecule contains properties that determine the class of antibody such as IgG, IgM, IgE, and so on. Each class of antibody is able to interact with a specific type of effector cell.

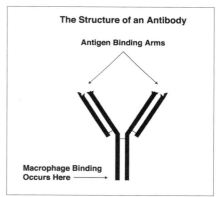

Figure 1. Antibody Structure

B cells are descendants of stem cells and play an important role in immune function. When the helper T cell alerts the defending lymphocytes to a danger, the B cells respond by proliferating in a process known as mitosis. Once a B cell binds to an antigen, the cell enlarges and divides into an identical antibody molecule designed to react to the same problematic antigen. These cloned B cells each contain numerous receptor sites but all recognize only the antigen for which they were reproduced. Antibodies can attach to a virus and prepare it for destruction by macrophages through a process known as phagocytosis. Undetected viruses that are able to sneak by the immune system can, unfortunately, invade a cell and begin to replicate themselves.[2] Once this process begins, the antibodies have no recourse against the virus and relinquish their control to the cytotoxic T cells.

Cells of Phagocytosis

Phagocytosis is a process whereby specific cells of the immune system engulf and digest foreign antigens that are perceived as dangerous. The most well known phagocytes are macrophages and neutrophils. Macrophages are basically considered garbage collectors of dying or killed cells in the body. Most of the time, they are in a resting state, doing their job of removing cellular debris. They can, however, be activated or primed by a signal that the body's barrier of defense has been breached. In this primed state, the macrophage serves as an antigen-presenting cell, displaying foreign HLA antigens and presenting them to helper T (CD4+) cells to elicit an immune response. During this immune response, macrophages proliferate and continue communicating danger signals to the immune system. They are providing the immune system with information from the battlefield, detailing the need for reinforcements from T cells and B cells.

Macrophages begin life as monocytes. They migrate from blood to tissues, where they mature into macrophages. It is not unusual for transplant clinicians to monitor monocyte repopulation immediately after surgery. They are watching this migration to determine the influx of this army of immune cells that mature and transform into macrophages that could attack the new organ. When the cells begin repopulation, it is time for additional immunosuppression to halt the invasion.

In addition to removing debris and serving as an antigen-presenting cell, macrophages can also kill invaders. Once primed, macrophages can become "hyperactive". In this state they have several functions:

1. Produce and secrete a cytokine called tumor necrosis factor that can further active the immune system,
2. Kill ingested invaders,
3. Increase production of reactive oxygen species such as hydrogen peroxide, a killer of bacteria.

Inside an activated macrophage, the number of lysosomes increases, which allows the macrophage to begin destruction of invading foreign organisms.

Neutrophils are often the first responders to a breach in immune function. About 55% to 65% of our white blood cells are neutrophils. They have a short life span of about 5 days and are programmed to die in a process known as apoptosis or programmed death.[11] Cells of the immune system do not respond to debris from cells that die an apoptotic death; they react only to cells that have been destroyed and presented to the immune system by antigen-presenting cells. Neutrophils are activated once they enter the circulation. They are very phagocytic but do not function as antigen-presenting cells. Neutrophils contain powerful chemicals that destroy ingested cells. Because neutrophils have such powerful phagocytic action, there can be collateral damage to normal tissue. Thus, their short life may be well planned.

Role of the Transplantation Process in Upregulating the Immune Response: Donor and Surgical Factors

Numerous donor factors can influence the outcomes of allograft function. Mode of death, age of donor, and cytokines released during brain death are just a few of the factors. For example, a large number of cytokines are produced with the inflammatory response in ischemic or traumatic brain injury in potential donors and have been associated with intense systemic effects.[12] Cytokines may affect the donor's cardiac output and may be sensitizing donor organs, thus adding to the challenge of graft function after transplantation and rejection in the recipient.[12]

Acute ischemia, such as that seen in brain injury, can also be seen in other clinical situations. Ischemia causes the endothelium to become more permeable and express more adhesion molecules. This process causes the endothelium to lose its antiadhesive properties and develop a susceptibility to leukocyte and platelet adhesion. Leukocytes that adhere to the endothelium then release reactive oxygen species and cytokines, which increase the inflammatory reaction and result in ischemic reperfusion injury.[13] This process has a profound effect on early graft function.[13] Tumor necrosis factor-α causes decreased left ventricular contractility.[14] This cytokine has been found in elevated levels in donor hearts that have been unsuccessfully transplanted.[15] It is thought that the influence of the inflammatory response and cytokine release following traumatic brain injury may be transported with the organ when transplanted. This influence could add to the immune response and should be considered a factor in the overall immune burden following organ transplantation.

Organs that are transplanted are often procured from donors being cared for in cities far from the recipient. Once organs are removed from the donor and put on ice, they are immersed in a preservation solution. This process creates a cold ischemic time. For thoracic organs, ischemic time is relatively short and attempts are made not exceed 4 hours to ensure optimal function after transplantation. Even with the best preservation solution and care of the donor organ, however, reperfusion injury occurs, creating yet another opportunity for an inflammatory response and upregulation of the immune system.

Reperfusion injury is the result of blood flow being returned to an organ or tissues after a period of ischemia. A good example of reperfusion injury is a donor heart that has been implanted and reperfused once the aorta is unclamped. The interruption of blood flow may last 4 to 6 hours in a thoracic organ. During cold ischemic times, proinflammatory agents accumulate in the graft. Once blood flow is restored, free radicals and cytokines rush through the graft vasculature, creating widespread inflammation. This inflammatory process can significantly compromise graft function.[7] Cells of the immune system are also used in the inflammatory response. Thus chemotactic substances attract leukocytes to the inflamed site, and cells of the immune system are upregulated. Of course, reperfusion injury is not limited to transplantation; it can also occur in clinical situations such as circulatory shock, myocardial infarction, and stroke.[16]

Surgery itself can create an immune response with the break in the skin, the body's first line of defense. The body recognizes the breach in the defense system and reacts with an inflammatory response. This inflammatory response upregulates many of the cells of the immune system, including macrophages, T cells, and B cells. Protocols that deplete lymphocytes before transplantation often are hampered by this postoperative inflammatory response, which seems to activate and upregulate the immune system, despite immune suppression before transplantation.

Rejection

Once the new organ has survived the effects of donor factors, preservation, and reperfusion injury, it will meet the recipient's immune system. You can see how the processes the new organ has encountered up to this point may have made it more vulnerable to the onslaught of cells it is about to encounter. As mentioned earlier in the chapter, hyperacute rejection seldom occurs because we are able to identify preformed antibodies and specificities in advance. By identifying these high-risk transplants, we have been able to prevent hyperacute rejections.

Today if hyperacute rejection occurs, it is usually associated with an error whereby a patient receives an organ with the incorrect blood type. Hyperacute rejection occurs in minutes to hours after transplantation and results in immediate graft damage. Neutrophils, the first responders, attack the new organ and destroy it. Hyperacute rejection results in loss of the organ and, in most cases of thoracic transplants, results in death of the recipient. Acute rejection can occur weeks to months after implantation of a new organ. Graft damage is usually the result of cytotoxic T cell infiltration and is treated with antirejection medications that target T-cell proliferation. Chronic rejection often displays an inflammatory process within the endothelial cells of the organ vasculature. This process is often referred to as vascular rejection and appears to be mediated by class II antigens. You will also hear this referred to as humoral rejection. This form of rejection is more difficult to treat and limits long-term graft survival.

Over time, the smoldering inflammation of endothelial cells causes vascular diseases such as coronary artery disease and obliterative bronchiolitis in thoracic organs. Hepatic artery disease may develop in liver recipients and stenosis of the renal artery may develop in kidney recipients. Loss of blood supply to the organ usually results in loss of the transplant, with retransplantation being considered an option for some recipients.

Conclusions

We are still learning about the immune system and its reaction to nonself. In our process of learning, we are also attempting to teach the immune system to respond only to dangerous microbes as opposed to those that are nonself HLA antigens transplanted with a donor organ. To do this, we will require an excellent understanding of the immune system along with the development of pharmacological agents that can block the communication network involved in the immune and inflammatory responses. We also need to develop a better understanding about how to control the release of cytokines during brain death and how to prevent their damaging effects on organs we hope to procure and transplant. Controlling oxygen free radicals and the effects they have on reperfusion injury is another step in the process that affects the cells of an organ being transplanted. You see, it is not just the recipient's immune system that we should worry about. The donor's mode of death, cytokine release in brain death, donor management issues, procurement, preservation, and reperfusion injury all affect the organ being transplanted . . . and that process occurs before the transplanted organ meets the macrophages, neutrophils, and antibodies of the recipient's immune system. We still have a lot to learn.

References

1. Kirk AD. Immunology of transplantation. In: Norton JA, Bollinger RR, Change AE, eds. *Surgery: Basic Science and Clinical Evidence.* New York, NY: Springer-Verlag; 1998.
2. Opelz G, Wujciak T. The influence of HLA compatibility on graft survival after heart transplantation: The Collaborative Transplant Study. N Engl J Med. 1994;330:816-819.
3. Ohler L, Bray R. Transplant immunology. In: Cupples S, Ohler L. *Transplantation Nursing Secrets.* Philadelphia, Pa: Hanley Belfus/Elsevier Publishing; 2003.
4. Warren DS, Simpkins CE, Cooper M, Montgomery RA. Modulating immune responses with plasmapheresis and IVIG. *Curr Drug Targets Cardiovasc Haematol Disord.* 2005;5:215-222.
5. Davidson BT, Donaldson TA. Immune system modulation in the highly sensitized transplant candidate. *Crit Care Nurs Q.* 2004;27:1-9.
6. Sompayrac L. *How the Immune System Works.* Malden, Mass: Blackwell Science; 2003.
7. Kirk AD. Immunosuppression without immunosuppression? How to be a tolerant individual in a dangerous world. *Transplant Infect Dis.* 1999;1:65-75.
8. Matzinger P. Graft tolerance: a duel of two signals. Nature Med. 1999;5:616-617.
9. Van Den Berghe L. *Introduction to Transplant Immunology and Immunosuppression.* London: Mosby-Wolfe Medical Communications; 1999.
10. VanBuskirk A, Pidwell DJ, Adams, PW, Orosz CG. Transplantation immunology. JAMA. 1997;278:1993-1999.
11. McCance KL. Structure and function of the immune system. In: McCance KL, Heuther S, eds. Pathophysiology, 4th ed. St. Louis, Mo: Mosby; 2002.
12. Powner DJ. Effects of gene induction and cytokine production in donor care. Progr Transplant. 2003;1 3:9-16.
13. Boros P, Bromberg JS. New cellular and molecular immune pathways in ischemia reperfusion injury. *Am J Transplant.* 2006;6:652-658.
14. Birks EJ, Burton PBJ, Owen VJ, Latif N, Nyawo B, Yacoub M. Molecular and cellular mechanisms of donor heart dysfunction. Transplant Proc. 2001;33:2749-2751.
15. Birks EJ, Burton PBJ, Owen VJ, et al. Elevated tumor necrosis factor α and interleukin 6 in myocardium and serum of malfunctioning donor hearts. *Circulation.* 2000;102 (suppl III):352-358.
16. Li C, Jackson R. Reactive species mechanisms of cellular hypoxia-reoxygenation injury. *Am J Physiol Cell Physiol.* 2002;282:C227-C241.

Pharmaceutical Care

Steven Gabardi, PharmD, BCPS
Steven A. Baroletti, PharmD, BCPS
Lisa M. McDevitt, PharmD, BCPS
Sarah B. Saxer, PharmD
Fallon M. Vaughan, PharmD
Christin C. Rogers, PharmD

Introduction

The optimal management of organ transplant recipients, in order to achieve long-term survival of patients and allografts, should be the major focus of transplantation practitioners. Short-term outcomes (ie, acute rejection rates, 1-year graft survival) of transplantation have improved considerably since the first successful transplantation more than 50 years ago. This improvement is due in large part to a better understanding of the immune system and improvements in surgical techniques, organ procurement, immunosuppression, and care after transplantation. Despite the success in improving short-term outcomes, the frequency of late graft loss remains high.

In order to improve all outcomes of organ transplantation, it is critical that the knowledge base of practitioners of transplantation be expanded beyond understanding the basics of immunosuppressive therapies. It is imperative that clinicians be aware of the specific advantages and disadvantages of the available immunosuppressants, as well as the potential for adverse drug reactions and drug-drug interactions (DDI) commonly seen with these agents. Proper management of solid-organ transplant recipients also involves the treatment of other common medical manifestations, such as infectious and cardiovascular diseases.

This chapter reviews the currently available immunosuppressive agents used for induction and maintenance of immunosuppression. Also, the authors address other issues associated with the pharmaceutical care of patients after transplantation, including DDI, medications used for the prevention and treatment of infectious complications and hypertension, and the appropriate selection of available nonprescription and complementary and alternative medicines (CAM).

Immunosuppressive Therapies—Induction Therapy

The introduction of highly potent and selective agents for the initiation of immunosuppression has reduced the frequency of acute rejection. However, acute rejection is still a concern in organ transplantation, and its impact on chronic rejection is undeniable. In this situation, induction immunosuppressive strategies with monoclonal (ie, OKT-3, basiliximab, daclizumab) or polyclonal (antithymocyte globulin equine and rabbit) antibodies play an important role.

The goal of induction therapy is to provide a high level of immunosuppression at the time of transplantation, when the risk of acute rejection is highest.[1-5] This type of therapy is often initiated intraoperatively or immediately postoperatively and is generally concluded within the first 1 to 2 weeks after transplantation. Induction therapy is not a mandatory stage of recipient immunosuppression; however, it is often considered essential to optimize outcomes, particularly in high-risk individuals such as highly sensitized patients, recipients with a history of previous transplantation, or those receiving calcineurin inhibitor or corticosteroid withdrawal regimens.[1-13]

Induction therapy in used for several important reasons. First, the currently available induction therapies are highly immunosuppressive, with some trials demonstrating significant reductions in acute rejection rates and improved 1-year graft survival, especially in renal transplant recipients.[1-13] Second, because of their pharmacological effect on the immune system, these agents are often considered vital in patients at high risk for poor short-term outcomes, such as those patients with preformed antibodies, history of previous organ transplants, multiple HLA mismatches, or transplantation of organs with prolonged cold ischemic time or from expanded criteria donors.

Induction therapy in renal transplant recipients also plays a vital role in helping to prevent nephrotoxic effects induced by calcineurin inhibitors immediately after transplantation.[3] By using induction therapy, initiation of a calcineurin inhibitor can often be delayed until the graft regains some degree of function. This strategy may help reduce the risk of nephrotoxic effects from either cyclosporine or tacrolimus.[2,3,5]

The improved short-term outcomes seen with induction therapies come with a high degree of risks. By using these highly potent immunosuppressive agents, particularly the antilymphocyte antibodies (ALA; OKT-3, and the antithymocyte antibodies), the body loses much of its innate ability to mount an immune response, which increases the risk of opportunistic infections or the development of certain types of cancer.[3,5] Also, some of these agents are associated with severe adverse events.

Currently Available Induction Therapies

A list of the currently available immunosuppressive agents can be found in Table 1.

Table 1. CURRENTLY AVAILABLE INDUCTION THERAPIES[6]

Generic (Trade) Name	Manufacturer	Monoclonal or Polyclonal	Route of Administration
Daclizumab (Zenapax)	Roche	Monoclonal	- Intravenous infusion (15 min)
Basiliximab (Simulect)	Novartis	Monoclonal	- Intravenous infusion (20–30 min) Intravenous bolus
Lymphocyte immune globulin, antithymoglobulin equine (Atgam)	Pfizer	Polyclonal (ALA)	- Intravenous infusion (4–6 h)
Antithymocyte globulin rabbit (Thymoglobulin)	Genzyme	Polyclonal (ALA)	- Intravenous infusion (4–6 hours)
Muromonab-CD3 (Orthoclone-OKT3)	Ortho-Biotech	Monoclonal (ALA)	- Intravenous bolus (<1 min)
Alemtuzumab (CamPath)	Berlex	Monoclonal (ALA)	- Intravenous infusion (2 h)

Abbreviation: ALA, antilymphocyte antibody.

Daclizumab and Basiliximab

Mechanism of Action

Both daclizumab and basiliximab are monoclonal antibodies produced by recombinant DNA technology.[2,5,6] Daclizumab is a humanized antibody that is approximately 10% murine and 90% human, whereas basiliximab is a chimeric antibody that is approximately 30% murine and 70% human.[2,6] These agents have a high affinity for the alpha subunit of the interleukin-2 (IL-2) receptor that is also known as CD25. These receptors are present on almost all activated T cells. Their role in induction therapy involves inhibiting IL-2–mediated activation of lymphocytes, which is an important step for the clonal expansion of T cells. Clonal expansion of this cell line is a critical pathway in the activation of cell-mediated allograft rejection.[2,5,6]

Dosing

The dose of basiliximab is 20 mg intravenously given within 2 hours before transplantation, followed by a second dose of 20 mg on postoperative day 4.[2,5,6] This dosing schedule can be used for both children of 35 kg or more and adults. Two doses of 10 mg intravenously with the same dosing schedule should be used for children less than 35 kg. No specific dosage adjustments are needed in renal or hepatic impairment.[2,5,6]

The dose of daclizumab approved by the Food and Drug Administration (FDA) is 1 mg/kg infused for 15 minutes within 24 hours of transplant surgery and then 1 mg/kg administered every 14 days after surgery for a total of 5 doses.[2,5,6] No dose adjustment is needed for renal impairment, and no data are available for dose adjustment in hepatic impairment. Some trials in renal transplantation have shown that a shorter dosing regimen of daclizumab may be as safe and effective as the full, 5-dose course.[7,8]

Adverse Drug Reactions

The most evident benefit of induction therapy with the IL-2 receptor antibodies is their safety. The most common adverse reaction with daclizumab is hyperglycemia.[2,6] Studies show that hyperglycemia developed in a total of 16% of placebo-treated patients versus 32% of patients treated with daclizumab. The majority of the high glucose levels occurred the day after transplantation or in patients with preexisting diabetes. All other adverse events in the clinical trials did not differ significantly between patients treated with daclizumab and patients given a placebo. The incidence of all adverse reactions with basiliximab was similar to the incidence seen with placebo in clinical trials.[2,6] One of the possible advantages of the IL-2 receptor antibodies is their apparent low risk of infectious complications and malignant neoplasms when compared with the ALAs. This finding is difficult to elucidate because few head-to-head studies between the 2 groups of agents have been completed and for the studies that are available, the evaluation period was often 12 months or less.

Antithymoglobulin Equine (ATG)

Mechanism of Action

This agent is a lymphocyte-specific immunosuppressant that contains antibodies against several T-cell surface markers, including CD2, CD3, CD4, CD8, CD11a, and CD18.[1,5,6] After binding to these antigens, ATG promotes T-cell depletion through opsonization and complement-mediated T-cell lysis. The spleen, liver, and lungs subsequently clear the damaged T cells.[1,5,6]

Dosing

The common dosing strategy for ATG when used for induction therapy is 15 to 30 mg/kg per day intravenously for 3 to 14 days. The first dose usually begins within 24 hours before or after the transplantation procedure.[1,5,6] A test dose (0.1 mL of 0.05 mg/mL solution in isotonic sodium chloride solution) given intradermally is recommended. The patient and injection site should be examined every 15 to 20 minutes for 1 hour after the administration of the test dose. A negative test does not guarantee a reaction-free administration.

Adverse Drug Reactions

Because of T-cell lysis and a subsequent cytokine release, ATG is associated with several infusion-related reactions.[1,5,6] The most common of these include fever (63%), chills (43.2%), headache (34.6%), back pain (43.2%), nausea (28.4%), diarrhea (32.1%), dizziness (24.7%), and malaise (3.7%). Premedication with an antihistamine and acetaminophen is recommended to lower the incidence of these potential infusion-related reactions. Myelosuppression is also a frequent adverse event, with a high incidence of leukopenia (29.6%) and thrombocytopenia (44.4%). The overall incidence of infection is 27.2%, with cytomegalovirus (CMV) disease occurring in 11.1% of patients. Some institutions choose to monitor T-cell subsets to gauge the degree of immunosuppression provided by ATG.

Antithymocyte Globulin Rabbit (RATG)

Mechanism of Action

RATG induces T-cell clearance, but, more importantly, it alters T-cell activation, homing, and cytotoxic activities.[1,6] This agent seems to have a more specific mechanism of action when compared with ATG, which results in less T-cell lysis. It is believed that RATG may also play a role in inducing T-cell apoptosis.[1,5,6]

Dose

RATG has been dosed between 1 and 2.5 mg/kg per day and is usually administered for 3 to 10 days after transplantation.[1,5,6] Many renal transplant centers aim to initiate the first dose intraoperatively to help reduce organ reperfusion injury. The manufacturer does not recommend a test dose.

Adverse Reactions

Adverse reactions are common and may include fever (63.4%), chills (57.3%), headache (40.2%), nausea (36.6%), diarrhea (36.6%), malaise (13.4%), dizziness (8.5%), leukopenia (57.3%), thrombocytopenia (36.6%) and generalized pain (46.3%).[1,5,6] In order to lower the incidence of fever and chills during the infusion, premedication with an antihistamine and acetaminophen is recommended. The incidence of infection is 36.6%, with the rate of CMV disease being 13.4%. Some institutions choose to monitor T-cell subsets to gauge the degree of immunosuppression provided by RATG.

Muronomab-CD3 (OKT3)

Mechanism of Action

OKT3 is a murine monoclonal antibody that targets the CD3 receptor, which is found only on T cells and medullary thymocytes.[3,6,9] After binding with the CD3 receptor, complement-mediated T-cell lysis occurs rapidly.

Dosing

For induction therapy, the general dose is 5 mg/day given as an intravenous bolus.[6] This dose is given daily for 10 to 14 days. Lower doses (2.5 mg/day for 5-10 days) of this agent have been used successfully in adult liver transplant recipients.[9] Test doses are not routinely recommended. Some centers may require that a physician administer the first few doses because of the severity of the adverse reaction associated with the initiation of OKT3.

Adverse Drug Reactions

Because of its ability to cause lysis of nearly 95% of all activated T cells after the first dose, OKT3 has several severe adverse effects that can be seen within 1 to 3 hours after administration.[3,6,9] These adverse reactions are often referred to as the "first-dose effect" and are usually associated with cytokine release after T-cell lysis. The adverse reaction profile of OKT3 includes fever (77%), chills (43%), dyspnea (16%), nausea (32%), vomiting (25%), diarrhea (37%), and tachycardia (26%). Because of these types of reactions, the FDA strongly advises that methylprednisolone be administered 1 to 4 hours before using OKT3 and also states that acetaminophen and antihistamines may aid in decreasing infusion-related reactions. One of the major complications of OKT3 is the development of severe pulmonary edema following the first dose.[6,10,11] In all reported cases of this complication, patients were fluid overloaded at the time of the initial dose. No cases of pulmonary edema have been reported in individuals who were euvolemic. The use of diuretics or hemodialysis may be warranted before initiation of OKT3 therapy in order to achieve euvolemia or minimize volume overload. Another problematic adverse reaction is the development of nephropathy after the initial OKT3 dose.[6,12] The cause of the nephropathy is not fully understood, however, the changes in renal function are usually reversible. Some centers choose to monitor quantitative T-lymphocyte (ie, CD3, CD4, CD8) levels (target CD3-positive T-cells <25 cells/mm^3) in order to gauge the overall level of immunosuppression.

Alemtuzumab

Mechanism of Action

Alemtuzumab is a recombinant DNA-derived monoclonal antibody that binds to the 21- to 28-kD cell surface glycoprotein, CD52.[6,13,14] CD52 is present on the surface of almost all B and T lymphocytes, many macrophages, NK cells, and a subpopulation of granulocytes. This agent's mechanism of action is believed to be antibody-dependent cell lysis following its binding to CD52 cell surface markers.[6,13,14]

Dosing

At the time of this publication, alemtuzumab has not been approved by the FDA for use in solid-organ transplant recipients. It is currently FDA approved for the treatment of B-cell chronic lymphocytic leukemia.[6] However, clinical trials have demonstrated a dose of 20 to 30 mg on day 0 and either day 1 or 4 to be effective in preventing acute rejection.[13,15-18]

Adverse Drug Reactions

Some of alemtuzumab's serious adverse reactions include anemia (47%), neutropenia (70%), thrombocytopenia (52%), headache (24%), dysthesias (15%), dizziness (12%), nausea (54%), vomiting (41%), diarrhea (22%), autoimmune hemolytic anemia (rare), infusion-related reactions (15%-89%), and infection (37%; CMV viremia occurred in 15% of patients).[6,13-18] The FDA has recommended that premedication with acetaminophen and oral antihistamines may be advisable to reduce the incidence of infusion-related reactions.

Immunosuppressive Therapies—Maintenance Therapy

The goals of maintenance immunosuppression are to further aid in preventing acute rejection episodes and to optimize survival of patients and grafts. Antirejection medications require careful selection and adjustment of dosage to balance the risks of rejection and toxic effects.

During the early years of organ transplantation, few choices were available for maintenance immunosuppression, with azathioprine and corticosteroids being the cornerstones of therapy. In the early 1980s, the development of cyclosporine revolutionized organ transplantation by dramatically reducing rejection rates and improving 1-year graft survival. The evolution of maintenance immunosuppressants in the 1990s saw several new options become available to further prevent rejection and improve outcomes. These agents have made it possible to attain acute rejection rates at or below 10% and increase 1-year graft survival to greater than 80% for most transplanted organs.[4,5,19]

Common maintenance immunosuppressive agents can be divided into 4 basic medication classes:
- Calcineurin inhibitors (cyclosporine and tacrolimus),
- Antiproliferatives (azathioprine and the mycophenolic acid [MPA] derivatives),
- Target of rapamycin inhibitors (sirolimus), and
- Corticosteroids (prednisolone derivatives and dexamethasone).

Please refer to Table 2 for a list of the available maintenance immunosuppressive agents.

Table 2. CURRENTLY AVAILABLE MAINTENANCE THERAPIES[6]

Generic (Trade) Name	Manufacturer	Generic Availability?	Route of Administration
Calcineurin Inhibitors			
Cyclosporine USP (Sandimmune)	Novartis	Yes	Intravenous, oral capsules and solution
Cyclosporine modified USP (Neoral, Gengraf)	Novartis	Yes. Gengraf (Abbott) is a brand name, generic medication	Oral capsules and solution
Tacrolimus (Prograf)	Astellas	No	Intravenous, oral capsules
Antimetabolites			
Azathioprine (Imuran)	Prometheus	Yes	Intravenous, oral tablets
Mycophenolate mofetil (CellCept)	Roche	No	Intravenous, oral capsules, tablets and suspension
Enteric-coated mycophenolic acid (Myfortic)	Novartis	No	Oral tablets
Target of Rapamycin Inhibitors			
Sirolimus (Rapamune)	Wyeth	No	Oral tablets and solution
Corticosteroids			
Prednisone (Deltasone)	Upjohn	Yes	Intravenous, oral tablets and solution
Methylprednisolone (Solumedrol, Medrol)	Pfizer	Yes	Intravenous, oral tablets and solution
Dexamethasone (Decadron)	Merck	Yes	Intravenous, oral tablets, suspension and solution

Maintenance immunosuppression is generally achieved by combining 2 or more medications from the different classes to maximize efficacy by specifically targeting unique components of the immune system responsible for rejection. This method of selecting medication also helps to minimize toxic effects by choosing agents with different adverse event profiles. Immunosuppressive regimens vary between organs types and transplant centers, but most often they include a calcineurin inhibitor with an adjuvant agent, plus or minus corticosteroids. Selection of appropriate immunosuppressive regimens should be patient-specific. When selecting immunosuppressants, the transplant practitioner must take into account the patient's concomitant disease states and the associated treatments.

Calcineurin Inhibitors

Cyclosporine and tacrolimus belong to a class of immunosuppressants called the calcineurin inhibitors. These agents are considered by many to be the backbone of clinical immunosuppression.

Mechanism of Action

The calcineurin inhibitors work by complexing with cytoplasmic proteins (cyclosporine with cyclophylin and tacrolimus with tacrolimus-binding protein 12).[5,6,20,21] These complexes then inhibit the enzyme calcineurin phosphatase. Inhibition of this enzyme results in reduced transcription of the *IL-2* gene. The end result is a decrease in IL-2 synthesis and a subsequent reduction in T-cell activation.[5,6,20,21]

Cyclosporine

It should be noted that cyclosporine USP (Sandimmune) was first approved by the FDA in 1983 but was associated with a variable oral absorption. The development of a newer formulation, cyclosporine microemulsion USP, introduced as Neoral in 1994, allowed for a more consistent drug exposure due to a decrease in intrapatient pharmacokinetic variability.[22] Most transplant centers that use cyclosporine initiate maintenance immunosuppression with the microemulsion formulation because of the aforementioned benefit. The 2 formulations are not interchangeable.

Dosing and Therapeutic Drug Monitoring

The typical oral adult dose of cyclosporine ranges from 4 to 18 mg/kg per day given in 2 divided doses.[6] The appropriate selection of the starting dose usually depends on the organ type, the patients' preexisting disease states, and other concomitant immunosuppressive agents used. Cyclosporine microemulsion is available as 25- and 100-mg individually blister-packed capsules and an oral solution. Patients should be advised not to remove the capsules from their blister packs any more than 7 days before the pills are consumed. The liquid formulation may be mixed with milk or orange juice to improve flavor; however, it should never be mixed in polystyrene plastic (Styrofoam) containers. An intravenous formulation is also available, but it is used less frequently because of its high risk of nephrotoxic effects and potential incompatibilities with other intravenous infusions. The incidence of nephrotoxic effects with the intravenous formulation may be higher that what is seen with oral dosing because of the inherent poor bioavailability of oral cyclosporine. If used, the intravenous formulation must be diluted before administration and should be infused over at least 2 hours or may be given as a continuous infusion. Cyclosporine solutions should be diluted in 5% dextrose in water and contained in glass bottles to maximize stability. When converting a patient from oral to intravenous administration, the dosage should be reduced to approximately one third of the oral dose and given as a continuous infusion.[6]

Cyclosporine whole blood trough concentrations have traditionally been obtained to help monitor for efficacy and safety. Therapeutic trough levels (C_0) may range from 50 to 400 ng/mL. Target levels should be individualized for each patient, usually depending on the organ transplanted and the time elapsed since the transplantation. Unfortunately, cyclosporine C_0 does not correlate well with efficacy or toxicity. Newer studies suggest that cyclosporine blood concentration at 2 hours after the dose is administered (C_2) correlates better with toxicity and efficacy than does C_0.[23-26] Because blood samples for assessment of C_2 levels are obtained shortly after the administration of the medication, the whole blood concentrations are much higher than the trough levels (range 800-2000 ng/mL).

Tacrolimus

Tacrolimus (FK-506, Prograf) is the second calcineurin inhibitor and was FDA approved in 1997. Even though cyclosporine and tacrolimus both belong to the same general medication class, the two have several differences. Most importantly, looking at efficacy, some studies suggest that tacrolimus-based regimens are associated with less acute rejections when compared with cyclosporine-based regimens.[27-31] However, newer data suggest that there is no significant difference in acute rejection rates between cyclosporine with C_2 monitoring and tacrolimus with C_0 monitoring.[32] In recent years, tacrolimus has become the workhorse calcineurin inhibitor in many transplant centers, owing in large part to its more favorable adverse drug reaction profile.[21]

Dosing and Therapeutic Drug Monitoring

Oral starting doses of tacrolimus range from 0.1 to 0.3 mg/kg per day in 2 divided doses. Tacrolimus is available in 0.5-, 1-, and 5-mg capsules and as an injectable.[6] The intravenous formulation is usually avoided because of the risk of anaphylaxis due to its castor oil component.[6] In rare instances, oral tacrolimus may also be given sublingually to avoid the first-pass metabolism commonly seen after oral administration.[33,34] Tacrolimus C_0 blood levels should be monitored (12 hours after the last administered dose) and maintained between 5 and 20 ng/mL, again depending on the organ type, concomitant immunosuppressants, and the time since transplantation.[6]

Adverse Drug Reactions

One of the major drawbacks of the calcineurin inhibitors is their ability to cause acute and chronic nephrotoxic effects. Acute nephrotoxic effects have been correlated with high doses and are usually reversible. Chronic toxic effects, however, are typically irreversible and are linked to chronic drug exposure. Table 3 expands upon the more common adverse events induced by calcineurin inhibitors.

Table 3. MANAGEMENT OF COMMON ADVERSE EFFECTS OF CALCINEURIN INHIBITORS[5,6]

Adverse Event	Most Likely Offending Calcineurin Inhibitor	Monitoring Parameters	Therapeutic Management Options
Nephrotoxic effects	Either	- Serum creatinine - Serum urea nitrogen - Urine output - Biopsy-proven nephrotoxic effects induced by calcineurin inhibitor	- Reduce dose of calcineurin inhibitor (if possible) - Use of calcium channel blocker for control of hypertension - Modify regimen (add or change to regimen containing no calcineurin inhibitors) - Avoid use of other potential nephrotoxins
Hypertension*	Cyclosporine	- Blood pressure - Heart rate	- Initiate patient-specific antihypertensive therapy - Reduce dose of cyclosporine (if possible) - Change from cyclosporine to tacrolimus or sirolimus
Hyperlipidemia*	Cyclosporine	- Fasting lipid panel	- Initiate patient-specific cholesterol-lowering therapy - Reduce dose of cyclosporine (if possible) - Change from cyclosporine to tacrolimus or sirolimus
Hyperglycemia†	Tacrolimus	- Blood glucose (fasting and nonfasting) - Hemoglobin A_{1c}	- Diet modifications - Reduce tacrolimus dose (if possible) - Reduce steroids (if patient is taking them and if possible) - Initiate patient-specific glucose-lowering therapy (insulin or oral therapy) - Change from tacrolimus to cyclosporine or sirolimus
Toxic effects on central nervous system†	Tacrolimus	- Fine hand tremor - Headache - Changes in mental status	- Reduce dose of tacrolimus (if possible) - Change from tacrolimus to cyclosporine or sirolimus
Hematological	Either	- White blood cell count - Platelets - Hemoglobin - Hematocrit - Symptoms of anemia	- Reduce dose of calcineurin inhibitor (if possible) - Modify regimen (add or change to regimen containing no calcineurin inhibitors; although hematological risks are high for all medications except steroids)

Table 3. MANAGEMENT OF COMMON ADVERSE EFFECTS OF CALCINEURIN INHIBITORS[5,6], continued

Adverse Event	Most Likely Offending Calcineurin Inhibitor	Monitoring Parameters	Therapeutic Management Options
Hepatotoxic effects	Either	- Liver function tests	- Reduce dose of calcineurin inhibitor (if possible) - Modify regimen (add or change to regimen containing no calcineurin inhibitors) - Avoid additional hepatotoxins
Electrolyte Imbalance	Either	- Potassium (usually ↑) - Magnesium (usually ↓) - Phosphate (usually ↓)	- Treat electrolyte imbalance (ie, magnesium replacement) - Reduce dose of calcineurin inhibitor (if possible) - Modify regimen (add or change to regimen containing no calcineurin inhibitors) - Dietary modification
Hirsutism	Cyclosporine	- Patient complaints of excessive hair growth or male-pattern hair growth	- Reduce dose of cyclosporine (if possible) - Cosmetic hair removal - Change from cyclosporine to tacrolimus or sirolimus
Alopecia	Tacrolimus	- Patient complaints of excessive hair loss	- Reduce dose of tacrolimus (if possible) - Hair growth treatments (ie, minoxidil [topically], finasteride [orally] – males only) - Change from tacrolimus to cyclosporine or sirolimus
Gingival hyperplasia	Cyclosporine	- Patient complaints of excessive gum growth - Recommendations for therapy from the patient's dentist	- Reduce dose of cyclosporine (if possible) - Oral surgery (gum resection) - Change from cyclosporine to tacrolimus or sirolimus

* Tacrolimus is also associated with hypertension and hyperlipidemia, but to a lesser extent than cyclosporine.

† Cyclosporine is also associated with hyperglycemia and toxic effects on central nervous system, but to a lesser extent than tacrolimus.

Antiproliferatives

These agents are generally considered to be adjuvant to the calcineurin inhibitors or possibly sirolimus. The most common medications used in transplantation from this class are azathioprine and the MPA derivatives.

Azathioprine

Azathioprine was originally approved by the FDA in 1968 as an adjunct immunosuppressant for use in renal transplant recipients. It is available in oral and intravenous forms.[6] Before the advent of cyclosporine, the combination of azathioprine and corticosteroids was the mainstay of immunosuppressive therapy. In the past 10 years, the use of azathioprine has declined markedly, due in large part to the success of the MPA derivatives, which are more specific inhibitors of T-cell proliferation.

Mechanism of Action

Azathioprine is a prodrug for 6-mercaptopurine (6-MP), a purine analog. 6-MP acts as an antimetabolite and inhibits T-cell proliferation.[6]

Dosing and Therapeutic Monitoring Parameters

The typical oral dose of azathioprine for organ transplantation is 3 to 5 mg/kg once a day.[6] Data are available to support a 1:2, intravenous-to-oral conversion[35]; however, others believe that the intravenous and oral doses of azathioprine are equivalent (1:1 conversion).[6] The maintenance dose is usually reduced to 1 to 2 mg/kg per day within a few weeks after transplantation. Dose reductions due to severely impaired renal function may be necessary because 6-MP and its metabolites are renally eliminated.[6] Trough concentrations of 6-MP are not monitored; however, most clinicians often monitor for signs of myelosuppression and liver dysfunction.

Adverse Drug Reactions

Myelosuppression (mainly leukopenia and thrombocytopenia) is a frequent, dose-dependent, and dose-limiting complication (>50% of patients) that often prompts dose reductions.[6] Other common adverse events include hepatotoxic effects (2%-10%) and gastrointestinal problems (10%-15%, mostly nausea and vomiting). Importantly, pancreatitis and venoocclusive disease of the liver occurs in less than 1% of patients receiving long-term azathioprine therapy.[6] This medication should be stopped in the case of serious adverse reactions, especially if venoocclusive disease is suspected.[6,36] However, some patients may respond to a reduction in the dose.[6]

Mycophenolic Acid Derivatives

Mycophenolate mofetil (MMF) was FDA approved in 1995 and enteric-coated MPA (EC-MPA) was FDA approved in 2004. Both agents are considered to be adjunctive immunosuppressants when used in combination with the calcineurin inhibitors.

Mechanism of Action

Both MMF and EC-MPA are prodrugs for MPA.[5,6,37-39] MPA acts by inhibiting inosine monophosphate phosphate dehydrogenase, a vital enzyme in the de novo pathway of purine synthesis. Inhibition of this enzyme prevents the proliferation of most cells that are dependent upon the de novo pathway for purine synthesis, including T cells.[5,6,37-39] This mechanism of action makes the inhibition of replication more specific to lymphocytes when compared with azathioprine.

Dosing and Therapeutic Drug Monitoring

MMF is available in 250- and 500-mg capsules, an oral suspension (100 mg/mL, in cherry syrup), and as an injectable.[6] Usual doses of MMF range from 1000 to 3000 mg/day in 2 to 4 divided doses. The conversion between oral and intravenous MMF is 1:1. EC-MPA is available in 180- and 360-mg tablets. The appropriate equimolar conversion between MMF and EC-MPA is as follows: 1000 mg of MMF is equivalent to 720 mg of EC-MPA.[37,40] The recommended starting dose of EC-MPA is 720 mg given twice daily.[6] Studies have demonstrated that EC-MPA and MMF have similar efficacy and safety in renal transplant recipients.[37] It appears that conversion of MMF to EC-MPA is safe, but more studies are needed to determine its exact role of EC-MPA in the immunosuppressive armamentarium. MPA trough concentrations can be monitored; however, they are not routinely recommended.

Adverse Drug Reactions

The most common adverse events associated with these agents are gastrointestinal (18%–54%; diarrhea, nausea, vomiting, and gastritis) and myelosuppression (20%–40%).[5,6,37-39] Despite being enteric-coated, EC-MPA has shown no benefit in terms of reduction in gastrointestinal adverse events when compared with MMF in renal transplant recipients.[37]

Target of Rapamycin Inhibitors

Sirolimus

Sirolimus is currently the only FDA-approved target of rapamycin inhibitor. One of its derivatives, everolimus, is in phase 3 clinical trials and been approved for use in some European countries.[41] Sirolimus is a macrolide antibiotic derivative that has no effect on calcineurin activity.[6,42,43] Studies have shown that sirolimus may be used safely and effectively with either cyclosporine or tacrolimus.[44] Sirolimus can also be used as an alternative agent for patients who do not tolerate calcineurin inhibitors because of the nephrotoxic effects or other adverse events.[45] At this time, some of the most exciting data for sirolimus point to its ability to prevent long-term renal allograft dysfunction when used as a substitute for the calcineurin inhibitors and also to slow the progression of cardiac vasculopathy in heart transplant recipients.[42,44-46]

Mechanism of Action

Sirolimus inhibits T-cell activation and proliferation by binding to and inhibiting the activation of the mammalian target of rapamycin, which suppresses cellular response to IL-2 and other cytokines (ie, IL-4, IL-15).[6,42] This mechanism is unique in comparison to the other immunosuppressants.

Dosing and Therapeutic Drug Monitoring

Available in a 1- and 2-mg tablet and a 1 mg/mL oral solution, the current FDA-approved dosing regimen for sirolimus is a 6-mg loading dose followed by a 2 mg/day maintenance dose.[6] It was recommended that this agent does not require therapeutic drug monitoring. However, most centers do check trough concentrations and adjust doses to reach goal concentrations.[47] Most clinicians who use sirolimus use a loading dose of 5 to 15 mg/day for 1 to 3 days to more rapidly achieve adequate immunosuppression.[42,44,45] Maintenance doses of sirolimus usually range from 1 to 6 mg/day given once daily. Sirolimus blood C_0 levels should be obtained and maintained between 5 and 20 ng/mL, depending on the institution-specific protocols.[47] Of note, sirolimus has a half-life of approximately 62 hours, which means that it will not reach steady state after dosage changes for several days.[6]

Adverse Drug Reactions

The most common adverse events reported with sirolimus are leukopenia (20%), thrombocytopenia (13%-30%), and hyperlipidemia (38%-57%).[6,42] Other adverse effects include delayed wound healing, anemia, diarrhea, arthralgias, rash, and mouth ulcers. Sirolimus has an FDA black box warning in recent recipients of liver transplants (hepatic artery thrombosis) and lung transplants (bronchial anastomotic dehiscence).[6]

Corticosteroids

Traditional triple-therapy immunosuppressive regimens have consisted of a calcineurin inhibitor, an antiproliferative or target of rapamycin inhibitor, and corticosteroids. In recent years, many protocols have focused on corticosteroid sparing or avoidance. Avoidance or sparing of corticosteroids have been supported in the literature, although more studies are needed to help better characterize which patients should follow these protocols.[48-51]

Mechanism of Action

Corticosteroids have various effects on immune and inflammatory response systems, although their exact mechanism in the prevention of rejection is not fully understood. It is generally believed that at high doses, the agents are directly lymphotoxic and at lower doses, the corticosteroids act by inhibiting the production of various cytokines that are necessary to amplify the immune response.[6]

Dosing and Therapeutic Drug Monitoring

The most commonly used corticosteroids are methylprednisolone (IV and oral) and prednisone (oral), although prednisolone and dexamethasone have also been shown to be effective for organ transplantation. Corticosteroids doses vary by center-specific protocols, organ type, and characteristics of patients. A typical dosage would include an intravenous bolus of methylprednisolone 100 to 500 mg at the time of transplantation then tapered over 5 to 7 days to a maintenance dose of prednisone 20 mg/day or completely stopped (renal transplant recipients).[4,5,52-55] It is important for practitioners to know that approximately 4 mg of methylprednisolone is equivalent to 5 mg of prednisone and 0.75 mg of dexamethasone.[6] At most transplant centers, therapeutic drug monitoring of corticosteroids is not used.

Adverse Drug Reactions

Corticosteroids are associated with a variety of acute and chronic toxic effects. The most common adverse events are summarized in Table 4.

Table 4. COMMON ADVERSE EVENTS ASSOCIATED WITH CORTICOSTEROIDS[6]

Body System	Adverse Event
Cardiovascular	- Hyperlipidemia - Hypertension
Central nervous system	- Anxiety - Insomnia - Mood changes - Psychosis
Dermatological	- Acne - Diaphoresis - Ecchymosis - Hirsutism - Impaired wound healing - Petechiae - Thin skin
Endocrine/metabolic	- Cushing syndrome - Hyperglycemia - Sodium and water retention
Gastrointestinal	- Gastritis - Increased appetite - Nausea, vomiting, diarrhea - Peptic ulcers
Hematological	- Leukocytosis
Neuromuscular/skeletal	- Arthralgia - Impaired growth - Osteoporosis - Skeletal muscle weakness
Ocular	- Cataracts - Glaucoma
Respiratory	- Epistaxis

Immunosuppressive Therapies—Treatment of Acute Rejection Episodes

Acute rejection is generally treated with a course of high-dose methylprednisolone (250 – 1000 mg/day IV for 3 days) (5), which is usually sufficient to ameliorate the rejection episode. If the acute rejection episode is resistant to the initial course of steroids, a second course may be administered or the patient may begin therapy with antithymocyte globulin (1.5 mg/kg/day for three to 14 days) (4-6). Acute rejection refractory to these treatments may require OKT-3. However, the use of this agent has fallen out of favor due to the severe short- and long-term adverse events associated with its use.

Immunosuppressive Therapies—Drug-Drug Interactions

As the number of medications that a patient takes increases, so does the potential for DDI. Disease severity, the patient's age, and renal and hepatic dysfunction are all risk factors for increased DDI. In general, DDI have a prevalence of 5% to 9% among the general population.[56] More alarming is the fact that approximately 7% of all hospitalizations are caused by these interactions.[56]

In general, DDI can be broken down into 2 categories:
- *pharmacokinetic interactions*: DDI where 1 medication alters the pharmacokinetic profile (absorption, distribution, metabolism, or excretion) of another medication (ie, phenytoin decreasing whole blood concentrations of cyclosporine or tacrolimus), and
- *pharmacodynamic interactions*: use of medications that share a common mechanism of action, therapeutic effect, or adverse event profile (ie, cyclosporine or tacrolimus and gentamicin causing nephrotoxic effects). Because of the breadth of interpretation of this type of DDI, it will not be discussed in great detail here.

Given the abundance of medications taken by transplant recipients, it is not surprising that transplant recipients are at high risk for DDI. Pharmacokinetic DDI are often considered a major problem with some of the agents used for maintenance immunosuppression. Most pharmacokinetic interactions may result in increased concentrations of one or more agent with a potential to lead to toxic effects or reduced concentrations of one or more agents that may lead to subtherapeutic decreased efficacy, possibly leading to rejection in the transplant setting.

Induction Therapies

No pharmacokinetic DDI have currently been reported with any of the induction therapy agents; however, the ALA do have pharmacodynamic interactions with other medications that cause myelosuppression.[1,5,6] The manufacturer of OKT3 has the herbal medicinal echinacea listed as the only agent that has been found to interact with OKT3, because of echinacea's potential to stimulate the immune system.[6]

Corticosteroids, Cyclosporine, Tacrolimus, and Sirolimus

Cyclosporine, tacrolimus, and sirolimus are substrates of the cytochrome P-450 (CYP) 3A isozyme system and P-glycoprotein transport protein.[6,57-59] The CYP isozyme system is responsible for the oxidative biotransformation of many medications. The majority of the CYP-mediated metabolism takes place in the liver, however CYP is also expressed in other areas, such as the intestine, lungs, kidneys, and brain. Two types of interactions usually occur with medications metabolized via the CYP enzyme system: inhibitory interactions and inducing interactions. Enzyme inhibition occurs when there is enzyme inactivation or mutual competition of substrates at a catalytic site. This usually results in an inhibition of drug metabolism, leading to increased whole blood trough concentrations and a prolonged half-life of all medications involved. Enzyme induction interactions are just the opposite and occur when there is increased synthesis or decreased degradation of CYP enzymes. This can lead to decreased plasma concentrations of medications and a decreased pharmacodynamic effect.[6,57-59]

The metabolic pathways of the maintenance immunosuppressants are illustrated in Table 5. Cyclosporine, tacrolimus, and sirolimus are all metabolized via the CYP3A4 pathway; therefore, it would be anticipated that they would experience similar pharmacokinetic DDI. Table 6 details the clinically relevant DDI that occur with the calcineurin inhibitors and sirolimus as a result of inhibition or induction of the CYP enzyme system. One of the most overlooked DDIs in transplant recipients is the effect that corticosteroids have on other immunosuppressants.[60] Corticosteroids are CYP3A enzyme inducers, meaning they may reduce the whole blood trough concentrations of cyclosporine, tacrolimus, and sirolimus.[6,60] This interaction is usually not clinically

Table 5. METABOLIC PATHWAYS OF THE MAINTENANCE IMMUNOSUPPRESSANTS[6]

Immunosuppressant	Metabolic Pathway
Cyclosporine	- Metabolized by CYP3A4 in the gut and liver
Tacrolimus	- Metabolized by CYP3A4 in the gut and liver
Azathioprine	- Azathioprine: metabolized by hepatic xanthine oxidase to 6-MP - 6-mercaptopurine: requires detoxification by thiopurine methyltransferase
Mycophenolate mofetil	- MMF: hydrolyzed by esterases in the plasma, liver, and kidneys to MPA - MPA: undergoes conjugation in the liver to MPAG - MPAG: may be deglucuronidated in the gut back to MPA if it is enterohepatically recirculated
Enteric-coated mycophenolic acid	- MPA: undergoes conjugation in the liver to MPAG - MPAG: may be deglucuronidated in the gut back to MPA if it is enterohepatically recirculated
Sirolimus	- Metabolized by CYP3A4 in the gut and liver
Corticosteroids	- Metabolized in the liver from prednisone/methylprednisolone (inactive) to prednisolone (active)

Abbreviations: CYP3A4, cytochrome P 3A4 isozyme; MMF, mycophenolate mofetil; MPA, mycophenolic acid; MPAG, mycophenolic acid glucoronide.

Table 6. EXAMPLES OF MEDICATIONS WITH DOCUMENTED INTERACTIONS OR POTENTIAL FOR DRUG-DRUG INTERACTIONS WITH CYCLOSPORINE, TACROLIMUS, OR SIROLIMUS MEDIATED THROUGH THE CYP3A4 ISOZYME[6]

Substrates*		Inducers†	Inhibitors‡
Alfentanil	Lidocaine	Carbamazepine	Cimetidine
Alprazolam	Loratadine	Dexamethasone	Clarithromycin
Amiodarone	Lovastatin	Ethosuximide	Clotrimazole
Amlodipine	Nevirapine	Isoniazid	Delavirdine
Atorvastatin	Nicardipine	Nevirapine	Diltiazem
Cilostazol	Nifedipine	Phenobarbital	Erythromycin
Cisapride	Omeprazole	Phenytoin	Fluconazole
Chlorpromazine	Paclitaxel	Prednisone	Fluoxetine
Clonazepam	Propafenone	Rifabutin	Fluvoxamine
Cocaine	Progesterone	Rifampin	Grapefruit juice
Cortisol	Quetiapine		Indinavir
Cyclophosphamide	Quinidine		Itraconazole
Dantrolene	Sertraline		Ketoconazole
Dapsone	Simvastatin		Miconazole
Diazepam	Tamoxifen		Nefazodone
Disopyramide	Testosterone		Nelfinavir
Enalapril	Triazolam		Ritonavir
Estradiol	Venlafaxine		Saquinavir
Estrogen	Vinblastine		Troleandomycin
Etoposide	Warfarin		Verapamil
Felodipine	Zolpidem		Voriconazole
Flutamide			Zafirlukast

* Substrates of the cytochrome P 3A4 (CYP3A4) isozyme will compete with cyclosporine, tacrolimus, and sirolimus for metabolism; therefore, concentrations of both medications will be increased (usually by ≤20%).

† Inducers of the CYP3A4 isozyme will enhance the metabolism of cyclosporine, tacrolimus, and sirolimus; therefore, concentrations of cyclosporine, tacrolimus, and sirolimus will be decreased.

‡ Inhibitors of the CYP3A4 isozyme will decrease the metabolism of cyclosporine, tacrolimus, and sirolimus; therefore, concentrations of cyclosporine, tacrolimus, and sirolimus will be increased.

significant, because the doses of cyclosporine, tacrolimus, and sirolimus can be adjusted to achieve target trough concentrations. However, this DDI has been problematic during steroid withdrawal protocols and is evidenced by an increase in trough concentrations of cyclosporine, tacrolimus, and sirolimus after the steroids have been completely withdrawn.

The majority of pharmacokinetic interactions that occur with these agents occur because of interactions with the CYP enzyme system; however, a few other interactions occur via alternative mechanisms. One of the most notable is the interaction seen with the prokinetic agents, cisapride, and metoclopramide. Both of these agents have been shown to increase the absorption of tacrolimus by enhancing gastric emptying.[61]

P-glycoprotein is a plasma membrane transport protein that is present in the gut, brain, liver, and kidneys.[62] This transport protein provides a biological barrier to these organs by extruding toxic substances and xenobiotics out of cells. P-glycoprotein plays a significant role in drug absorption and distribution. Medications that are CYP3A4 substrates, inhibitors, or inducers are also often affected by P-glycoprotein; therefore, the potential for even more DDIs exists.[62]

Azathioprine and the Mycophenolic Acid Derivatives

Azathioprine, MMF, and EC-MPA are not metabolized by the CYP isozyme system, thus, these agents do not experience the common interactions shared by cyclosporine, tacrolimus, and sirolimus. Azathioprine has a very small DDI profile, with the major offending agents being allopurinol, angiotensin-converting enzyme (ACE) inhibitors, aminosalicylates (ie, mesalamine, sulfasalazine) and warfarin.[6,63,64] Of these interactions, allopurinol is the most significant. Allopurinol inhibits xanthene oxidase, which is the enzyme that is responsible for metabolizing azathioprine. Combination of these agents can result in severe toxic effects, especially myelosuppression. It is recommended to avoid using these 2 agents in combination, but if necessary to reduce the azathioprine dose to one third or one quarter of the normal dose.[63,64] Concomitant use of azathioprine and ACE inhibitors or the aminosalicylates can result in enhanced myelosuppression.[6] Some case reports[65-67] indicate that warfarin's therapeutic effects may be decreased by azathioprine.

Most interactions that occur with MMF and EC-MPA are due to alterations in their intestinal absorption. The concomitant use of aluminum-, magnesium-, or calcium-containing antacids results in a decrease in the peak level and overall exposure of MPA from either of the preparations.[6] If liquid antacids are used in combination with these agents, their administration should be separated by at least 4 hours. Cholestyramine given in combination with the MPA derivatives decreases the overall MPA exposure.[68,69] This interaction is thought to be due to the ability of cholestyramine to inhibit the enterohepatic recirculation of MPA glucuronide. MPA glucuronide is an inactive metabolite of both MMF and EC-MPA that is converted back to the active component, MPA, via enterohepatic recirculation. A similar interaction has been identified with the concomitant use of cyclosporine and the MPA derivatives.[70-72] Recent studies[70,71] have shown a lower MPA exposure in cyclosporine-based immunosuppression regimens than in tacrolimus-based regimens.

In addition to the numerous pharmacokinetic interactions that may occur with the maintenance immunosuppressive agents, there exists the possibility for pharmacodynamic interactions as well. An in-depth review of pharmacodynamic interactions with maintenance immunosuppressive agents goes beyond the scope of this chapter. However, some common pharmacodynamic DDIs are discussed. The addition of nephrotoxic agents such as amphotericin B, aminoglycosides (ie, gentamicin, tobramicin, amikacin) and nonsteroidal anti-inflammatory drugs (NSAIDs; ie, naproxen, ibuprofen, ketorolac) may potentiate the known nephrotoxic effects of the calcineurin inhibitors. The use of myelosuppressive agents such as cotrimoxazole, valganciclovir, and ganciclovir could also potentiate the myelosuppression from azathioprine or the MPA derivatives.

The potential exists for several DDIs in the transplant setting, owing to the complexity of current immunosuppressive regimens. Practitioners must be diligent in reviewing all concomitant and new medications for potential DDIs. In addition to reviewing prescribed medications with patients, it is essential to question patients about the use of nonprescription medications and CAM, as these products also have the potential for substantial interactions. Unfortunately, clear-cut guidelines are not available as to how to dose adjust immunosuppressants with the concomitant use of interacting medications. Acquiring the knowledge of the primary metabolic pathways of commonly used immunosuppressants, as well as the common inducers and inhibitors of those pathways is essential in being able to anticipate DDIs that can occur in transplant recipients.

Anti-infectives

Transplant recipients are at increased risk of infection, and these complications are an important cause of early morbidity and mortality. The incidence of infection after transplantation depends on a combination of clinical risk factors, environmental exposures, and the net state of immunosuppression. Antimicrobial agents are universally prescribed in this population, and their use can be split into 3 different categories: prophylactic therapy refers to antimicrobials given to prevent an infection; preemptive therapy refers to antimicrobials given because of clinical suspicion of an active infection; and treatment refers to antimicrobials given to manage a documented infection.

Infections after transplantation generally occur in a predictable pattern, and prevention is a key management strategy. The information in this section is not designed to be a comprehensive review of antimicrobials, but rather to highlight prophylactic medications that are routinely used in organ transplant recipients.

Antibiotics

Surgical prophylaxis refers to antibiotics administered before the initial incision to prevent infections at the surgical site. The choice of antibiotic depends on the type of surgical procedure, likely pathogens, institutional susceptibility patterns, and the patient's tolerance. Penicillins or first-generation cephalosporins (particularly cefazolin) are generally the preferred choice in most surgical procedures because of their good gram-positive coverage.[73] Gram-positive organisms are common skin flora and are frequently implicated in infections at the surgical site. Vancomycin and clindamycin are common alternatives for patients who are allergic to penicillin.[73] Additional gram-negative and anaerobic coverage may be required in certain procedures (ie, small-bowel transplantation) and medications should be redosed, as needed, to ensure adequate serum and tissue concentrations throughout long procedures.

Without prophylactic treatment, *Pneumocystis jiroveci* (formerly *Pneumocystis carinii*) pneumonia occurs in 5% to 15% of transplant recipients.[74] Prophylaxis for *Pneumocystis* pneumonia is extremely effective and is generally used in all organ transplant recipients for at least 6 months after transplantation. The duration may be prolonged in patients who have intensified immunosuppression (ie, active CMV disease, treatment for rejection) and those who are liver or lung recipients.[75] A summary of medications used for *Pneumocystis* prophylaxis and their doses and adverse events are listed in Table 7. Sulfamethoxazole-trimethoprim (Bactrim, SMZ-TMP, cotrimoxazole) is the preferred agent. One of its major advantages is that it offers prophylaxis against *Pneumocystis* pneumonia, toxoplasmosis, and other common bacterial infections. Patients who are sulfa allergic, deficient in glucose-6 phosphate dehydrogenase, or are unable to tolerate SMZ-TMP should receive one of the second-line therapies.[6] These second-line agents are antiparasitics and have no meaningful activity against common bacteria. For this reason, an appropriate antibiotic may be added if prophylaxis against bacterial infections is desired. The common second-line agents include dapsone, atovaquone, and pentamidine.

Table 7. PROPHYLACTIC OPTIONS FOR PNEUMOCYSTIS JIROVECI PNEUMONIA[6,50,51]

Medication	Dosing	Common Adverse Events
First-Line Therapy		
Sulfamethoxazole-trimethoprim (Bactrim, Septra, SMZ-TMP, cotrimoxazole)	One single-strength (400 mg SMZ, 80 mg TMP) tablet orally every day* One double-strength (800 mg SMZ, 160 mg TMP) tablet orally every day* One double-strength (800 mg SMZ, 160 mg TMP) tablet orally every Monday, Wednesday, and Friday*	Hyperkalemia Myelosuppression Nephrotoxic effects Neutropenia Photosensitivity Rash
Second-Line Therapy		
Pentamadine (NebuPent)	300 mg inhaled every 3-4 weeks	Bronchospasm Cough Hypoglycemia or hyperglycemia
Dapsone (Avlosulfon)	50- to 100-mg tablet orally every day	Hepatotoxic effects Myelosuppression Nephritis
Atovaquone (Mepron)	1500 mg suspension orally every day	Elevated levels of liver transaminases Nausea Rash

*Dose adjustment required in renal insufficiency.

Antivirals

CMV is considered the most important opportunistic pathogen in solid-organ transplantation because of its association with poor outcomes for patients and allografts.[76] CMV seropositivity is present in 30% to 97% of the general population, but CMV disease is typically restricted to immunocompromised hosts.[77] The risk of CMV disease is highest among CMV-naive recipients who receive an allograft from CMV-positive donors (D+/R-).[76]

Other factors that increase the risk of CMV disease include the organ type (lung and pancreas recipients are considered high risk) and immunosuppressive regimen (ALA use increases risk). CMV infection typically occurs within the first 3 to 6 months after transplantation, but the incidence can be delayed even further in patients receiving prophylaxis.[76]

Whether used for prophylaxis or preemptive therapy, certain antivirals have proven efficacy in preventing and/or treating CMV.[76] A list of these agents can be seen in Table 8. Valacyclovir and valganciclovir are prodrugs of acyclovir and ganciclovir, respectively.[6] These prodrugs have improved bioavailability compared with their parent compounds and offer the advantage of less frequent administration. CMV prophylaxis typically extends for the first 100 days, or longer, after transplantation and may be continued or reinstated if ALA are administered.[77,78] Intravenous ganciclovir or oral valganciclovir may be used for preemptive therapy or for treatment of established CMV disease. The adverse events are similar among these agents and include myelosuppression and gastrointestinal effects.[6]

Table 8. PROPHYLACTIC AND TREATMENT OPTIONS FOR CYTOMEGALOVIRUS DISEASE[6,52-54]

Medication	Prophylactic Dose	Teatment Dose	Common Adverse Events
Valganciclovir (Valcyte)	450-900 mg orally every day*	900 mg orally twice a day for 3 weeks, followed by 900 mg orally every day for 2-3 months*	Stomach upset (8%-41%) Myelosuppression (2%-27%) Headache (9%-22%)
Ganciclovir (Cytovene)	5 mg/kg intravenously every day; or 1000 mg orally 3 times a day*	5 mg/kg intravenously twice a day for 3 weeks, followed by 5 mg/kg intravenously every day for 2-3 months*	Stomach upset (13%- 40%) Myelosuppression (5%-40%) Rash (10%-15%)
Valacyclovir (Valtrex)	1-2 g orally 4 times a day*	Not approved for treatment	Stomach upset (1%-15%) Myelosuppression (<1%) Headache (14%-35%)
Cytomegalovirus immunoglobulin (CytoGam) and polyvalent intravenous immunoglobulin	The maximum recommended total dosage per infusion is 150 mg/kg beginning within 72 hours of transplantation Follow-up doses and time intervals depend on the type or organ transplanted	Not approved for treatment	Stomach upset (1%-6%) Fevers and chills (1%-6%) Flushing (1%-6%)

*Dose adjustment required in renal insufficiency.

Antifungals

Fungal infections are an important cause of morbidity and mortality in solid-organ transplant recipients. Immunological factors (ie, immunosuppressants, CMV infection), anatomic factors (ie, tissue ischemia and damage), and surgical factors (ie, duration of surgery, transfusion requirements) contribute to the risk for fungal infections. Treatment of established fungal infections can be challenging.[79] Mucocutaneous candidal infections are associated with corticosteroids and ALA induction therapy. Oral nystatin or clotrimazole troche are effective prophylactic options for the prevention of oral thrush. However, clotrimazole does inhibit the CYP3A system in the gut and can alter cyclosporine, tacrolimus, and sirolimus levels.[6] The use of systemic fungal prophylaxis, such as oral fluconazole, is controversial because of the potential for DDI and the risk of developing fungal resistance. However, the American Society of Transplantation and the American Society of Transplant Surgeons have recommended the use of antifungals for prophylaxis in liver, lung, and small-bowel transplant recipients.[80] The agent of choice depends on the most common fungus in that particular population. For example, liver and small-bowel transplant recipients are at high risk for candidiasis; therefore, the use of medications that cover *Candida* spp is important, such as the triazole antifungals (ie, fluconazole, itraconazole) or the echinocandins (ie, caspofungin, micafungin). In lung transplant recipients, who are at high risk for aspergillosis, it is imperative to use antifungal prophylaxis with agents that cover *Aspergillus* spp, such as the echinocandins or polyenes (ie, amphotericin B, lipid-based amphotericin B products).[80]

Vaccinations

Every effort should be made to ensure appropriate vaccination of transplant candidates and recipients, their household contacts, and healthcare workers. A brief summary of recommended vaccinations for adult transplant recipients can be found in Table 9. The response to vaccines may be blunted or diminished in immunosuppressed patients. After transplantation, routine vaccinations should be delayed for about 6 months and live vaccines should be avoided indefinitely.[81]

Table 9. RECOMMENDED VACCINATIONS FOR ADULT TRANSPLANT CANDIDATES AND RECIPIENTS[57]

Vaccine	Vaccine Type	Safe to Administer to Transplant Candidates?	Safe to Administer to Transplant Recipients?
Influenza	Inactivated	Yes	Yes
Hepatitis B	Inactivated	Yes	Yes
Hepatitis A	Inactivated	Yes	Yes
Tetanus	Inactivated	Yes	Yes
Polio, inactivated	Inactivated	Yes	Yes
Streptococcus pneumoniae	Inactivated	Yes	Yes
Neisseria meningitidis	Inactivated	Yes	Yes
Rabies	Inactivated	Yes	Yes
Varicella	Live attenuated	Yes	No
BCG	Live attenuated	Yes	No
Smallpox	Live attenuated	No	No*
Anthrax	Inactivated	No	No

*Transplant recipients who are face-to-face contacts of a patient with smallpox should be vaccinated.

Some published reports reveal a trend toward higher rates of rejection in heart transplant recipients around the time of influenza vaccination.[82,83] However, newer data indicate that vaccination with influenza does not affect rejection rates among cardiac transplant recipients.[84-86]

Hypertension

The increase in early graft survival has revealed several long-term morbidities that accompany solid-organ transplantation. Cardiovascular disease has been identified as one of the leading causes of death in transplant recipients.[87] Hypertension after transplantation, perhaps the most concerning of the comorbidities, is associated with an increase in cardiac morbidity and patient mortality across the transplant population.[88,89] Hypertension after transplantation is also an independent risk factor for chronic allograft dysfunction and loss.[90] Based on all of the available data on morbidity and mortality after transplantation, it is imperative that hypertension be identified and managed appropriately. Antihypertensive therapy is associated with a 35% to 40% mean reduction in stroke incidence, 20% to 25% in myocardial infarction, and more than 50% in heart failure.[91]

Epidemiology

The incidence of hypertension following transplantation varies with organ type, although hypertension has been reported to affect at least half of all transplant patients and as many as 95% of renal and cardiac allograft recipients.[90] This high prevalence is uniform throughout transplant recipients because it is the immunosuppressive medications that are mainly responsible for hypertension. As immunosuppressive agents continue to improve graft survival, the incidence and need for treatment of hypertension in these patients increases.

Pathophysiology

Several underlying mechanisms are responsible for hypertension after transplantation. The most easily recognized is the administration of corticosteroids and the calcineurin inhibitors.[92,93] Other causes of hypertension may be impaired renal function, caused directly by rejection of the kidneys or indirectly by decreased cardiac function and chronic allograft nephropathy. Even a minor decrease in renal function is associated with an increase in the number of antihypertensive agents a patient requires.[94] Other postulated mechanisms include increased sensitivity to endothelin-1 and angiotensin, increased density of glucocorticoid receptors in the vascular smooth muscle and decreased production of vasodilatory prostaglandins.[95]

Cyclosporine administration is associated with a number of effects that may result in hypertension. The most pronounced actions involve a reduction in glomerular filtration rate and renal blood flow, an increase in systemic and intrarenal vascular resistance, and increased sodium retention.[96] Cyclosporine administration has also been associated with a reduction in the vasodilators prostacyclin and nitric oxide and an increase in the vasoconstrictor thromboxane.[97] Additionally, during corticosteroid therapy, sodium retention occurs that will often further increase blood pressure.[95] Tacrolimus has less dramatic effects on afferent arteriolar resistance in the kidneys, and thus it is less likely to produce an increase in blood pressure. When compared with cyclosporine in clinical trials, tacrolimus displayed significantly less severe hypertension and required significantly fewer antihypertensive medications at both 24 and 60 months after transplantation.[98-100]

Treatment

Control of hypertension in transplant recipients is essential in preventing cardiac morbidity and mortality and in prolonging graft survival. Lifestyle modifications, including diet, exercise, sodium restriction, and smoking cessation are recommended as initial treatment of hypertension.[100] Restricting dietary sodium intake to less than 1 g daily can modify hypertension due to sodium retention from both glucocorticoids and calcineurin inhibitors.[101] Although diet and exercise are major components of lifestyle for the general population, transplant recipients may be limited in the quantity and quality of exercise they can perform initially. Patients should be encouraged to maintain a low-fat, low-sodium diet and perhaps incorporate exercise slowly into their life once complete recovery from transplantation has occurred. Lifestyle modifications alone are often inadequate to control hypertension in this high-risk population, and antihypertensive medication should be initiated soon after transplantation.

No single class of antihypertensive medications is recognized as the ideal treatment of hypertension after transplantation. Numerous factors must be considered when determining appropriate treatment for a given patient, including the type of organ transplanted, the safety and efficacy data of the available agents, patient-specific situations and potential comorbidities, and medication cost. The underlying causes of hypertension described in the preceding section should be a target of therapy. Although efficacy data from large randomized control studies are limited to the general population, these results may help guide the choice of the most appropriate antihypertensive therapies.

A large majority of patients often require multiple medications to achieve their target blood pressure. This conclusion is supported by the recommendations of JNC-VII, where combination therapy is regarded as an appropriate first-line treatment in patients with a blood pressure greater that 20/10 mm Hg above the target blood pressure (140/90 mm Hg or 130/80 for patients with diabetes or renal disease).[102] The remainder of this section reviews the characteristics of the various antihypertensive medication options for transplant recipients, a summary of which can be found in Table 10.

Table 10. REVIEW OF SELECTED ANTIHYPERTENSIVE TREATMENT OPTIONS IN SOLID-ORGAN TRANSPLANT RECIPIENTS[6,58]

Medication Class	Drug Name Generic (Brand)	Daily Dose Range	Advantages	Disadvantages
Thiazide diuretics	Chlorothiazide (Diuril) Hydrochlorothiazide Metolazone (Zaroxolyn) Chlorthalidone (Thalitone*)	250-1000 mg 12.5-50 mg 2.5-5 mg 25-100 mg	Strong efficacy data to prevent cardiovascular events in general population No known pharmacokinetic interactions with immunosuppressive medications	Not effective with a glomerular filtration rate <30 mL/min May cause hyperglycemia, hypokalemia, hypomagnesemia, hypercalcemia, and hyperuricemia
β-Blockers	Metoprolol tartate (Lopressor) Metoprolol succinate (Toprol XL) Atenolol (Tenormin) Carvedilol (Coreg) Bisoprolol (Zebeta) Propranolol (Inderal) Labetalol (Trandate*) Pindolol (Visken) Nadolol (Corgard)	75-450 mg 50-400 mg 25-100 mg 6.25-50 mg 5-20 mg 40-480 mg 100-2400 mg 20-60 mg 20-120 mg	Compelling indications for coronary artery disease, after myocardial infarction or heart failure No known negative effect on glomerular filtration rate No known pharmacokinetic interactions with immunosuppressive medications	Mask the signs and symptoms of hypoglycemia Pharmacodynamic interactions: dyslipidemia, skeletal muscle weakness Concerns about excessive heart rate and blood pressure reductions soon after heart transplantation
Angiotensin-converting enzyme inhibitors	Benazepril (Lotensin) Captopril (Capoten) Enalapril (Vasotec) Lisinopril (Prinivil*) Fosinopril (Monopril) Perindopril (Aceon) Quinapril (Accupril) Ramipril (Altace) Trandolapril (Mavik)	5-40 mg 12.5-100 mg 10-40 mg 10-40 mg 5-40 mg 3.75-60 mg 10-80 mg 2.5-20 mg 1-8 mg	Beneficial in maintaining glomerular filtration rate in the long term Beneficial effects in patients with concomitant diabetes mellitus, proteinuria, and polycythemia No known pharmacokinetic interactions with immunosuppressive medications	Acute, but reversible, decrease in glomerular filtration rate and renal blood flow Use caution if preexisting renal dysfunction Pharmacodynamic interactions: nephrotoxic effects, hyperkalemia, and anemia\
Angotensin-receptor blocker	Irbesartan (Avapro) Candesartan (Atacand) Losartan (Cozaar) Valsartan (Diovan) Telmisartan (Micardis) Olmesartan (Benicar) Eprosartan (Tevetan)	150-300 mg 8-32 mg 50-100 mg 80-320 mg 20-80 mg 20-40 mg 400-800 mg	Same as angiotensin-converting enzyme inhibitors Use in patients with bradykinin-specific angiotensin-converting enzyme inhibitor side effects	Acute, but reversible, decrease in glomerular filtration rate and renal blood flow Use caution if preexisting renal function Pharmacodynamic interactions: nephrotoxic effects, hyperkalemia, and anemia

Table 10. REVIEW OF SELECTED ANTIHYPERTENSIVE TREATMENT OPTIONS IN SOLID-ORGAN TRANSPLANT RECIPIENTS[6,58], continued

Medication Class	Drug Name Generic (Brand)	Daily Dose Range	Advantages	Disadvantages
Calcium-channel blockers, dihydropyridines	Amlodipine (Norvasc) Nifedipine (Adalat*) Isradipine (DynaCirc) Felodipine (Plendil) Nicardipine (Cardene) Nisoldipine (Sular)	2.5-10 mg 30-180 mg 5-20 mg 2.5-20 mg 60-120 mg 10-60 mg daily	May counteract cyclosporine-induced nephrotoxic effects and hypertension Initiate in patients unable to tolerate thiazide diuretics and angiotensin-converting enzyme inhibitors	Peripheral edema, gingival hyperplasia, skeletal muscle weakness
Calcium-channel blockers, nondihydropyridines	Diltiazem (Cardizem*) Verapamil (Calan*)	90-360 mg daily 120-480 mg daily	Patients with hypertension and tachycardia Diltiazem has potentially beneficial effects in preventing allograft coronary artery disease in heart transplant recipients	Pharmacokinetic drug interactions with most immunosuppressant agents Constipation and heart block
α-Blockers	Terazosin (Hytrin) Prazosin (Minipress) Doxazosin (Cardura)	1-20 mg daily 6-15 mg /day (twice a day) 1-16 mg daily	May be effective for treating patients with benign prostatic hypertrophy (although newer specific $α_{1a}$-antagonists are preferred)	May increase cardiovascular events in patients with cardiac risk factors Causes orthostatic hypotension, edema, somnolence, and sexual dysfunction

* May have additional brand names.

Diuretics

Diuretics are excellent agents in transplant recipients for treatment of hypertension caused by excess fluid and sodium retention due to cyclosporine and corticosteroids.[103] The data demonstrating the ability of thiazide diuretics to prevent cardiovascular events and mortality associated with hypertension in the general population are unquestionable.[104] However, no comparative trials have been conducted to demonstrate any benefit of diuretics for controlling hypertension after transplantation. Careful monitoring of electrolytes is warranted in renal transplant recipients receiving diuretic therapy, because of the inconsistency of renal function and the potential for adverse reactions. Common adverse reactions of concern include dyslipidemia, hyperglycemia, hyperuricemia, and precipitation of gout.[105]

Diuretics are generally avoided if renal dysfunction exists after transplantation because of their potential effects on serum levels of creatinine. For long-term use, thiazide diuretics should be implemented as antihypertensive therapy, either as monotherapy or in conjunction with other agents. Thiazide diuretics are ineffective in patients with poor renal function (glomerular filtration rate < 35 mL/min).[6]

β-Blockers

β-Blockers antagonize the action of catecholamines at β-adrenergic receptors in the sympathetic nervous system, slowing the heart rate and decreasing blood pressure.[89] Overwhelming evidence shows the benefit of β-blockers in reducing morbidity and mortality in patients with coronary artery disease (CAD), following acute myocardial infarction and heart failure.[106,107] β-Blockers should be used cautiously in the early posttransplantation phase in cardiac transplant recipients, because transplanted hearts are very dependent on catecholamine stimulation to maintain heart rate and cardiac output owing to the lack of vagal connection postoperatively. Overall, these agents show no clinically important effect on glomerular filtration rate, renal perfusion, or renal vascular resistance in patients who have not undergone transplantation.

Two common adverse effects associated with β-blockers may be detrimental to transplant recipients. β-Blockers blunt several clinical signs and symptoms of hypoglycemia, which may complicate treatment in a large percentage of renal transplant recipients with diabetes mellitus.[108] Dyslipidemia is an independent risk factor for graft survival, and therapy with β-blockers may further complicate a patient's lipid profile.[109]

Angiotensin-Converting Enzyme Inhibitors

Reduction in blood pressure with ACE inhibitors is mediated through the suppression of angiotensin II production and the inhibition of bradykinin inactivation. The benefits of ACE inhibitors in high-risk patients who have not undergone transplantation is proven. The Heart Outcomes Prevention Evaluation (HOPE) trial demonstrated that patients at high-risk for cardiovascular disease who received ACE inhibitors had a significant decrease in all cardiovascular events.[110] It is believed that ACE inhibitors have additional benefits in blood pressure reduction via a positive effect on endothelial dysfunction.[111]

Much controversy has centered on determining the role of ACE inhibitors in transplant recipients, especially after renal transplantation. These agents may cause an acute decrease in glomerular filtration rate.[112] Although this change is a reversible physiological effect caused by decreased glomerular capillary pressure, the initial elevation in serum level of creatinine is often a source of anxiety among practitioners. ACE inhibitors slow the progression of renal dysfunction in both diabetic and nondiabetic patients. In clinical studies in the general population, ACE inhibitors have had success in reducing proteinuria, glomerular hypertension, and hyperfiltration.[113] The renal protective effects of both the ACE inhibitors and angiotensin-receptor blockers (ARBs) have been demonstrated in one study of renal transplant recipients.[114] Several studies have also demonstrated the beneficial effects of ACE inhibitors in cardiac transplant recipients in terms of reducing coronary allograft vasculopathy and potentially having a long-term vasculoprotective effect.[115,116]

ACE inhibitors can cause significant hyperkalemia, particularly in patients with multiple risk factors for high potassium levels (ie, calcineurin inhibitors, β-blockers, uremia, diabetes mellitus, dietary noncompliance). Chronic cough can also limit the use of these agents in up to 10% of patients.[6]

ACE inhibitors have a number of advantages over other agents for the chronic management of hypertension after transplantation. They should be used with caution in the early postoperative period when acute uremia can confound the diagnosis of rejection and when the risk of hyperkalemia is greatest.

Angiotensin-Receptor Blockers

The ARBs have been theorized to possess benefits similar to those of ACE inhibitors. To date, very few studies of ARBs in transplant recipients have been completed. One of the studies using ARBs in transplant recipients exhibited tolerability and blood pressure control comparable to those of other agents and improved surrogate markers of renal dysfunction.[117] A second study showed similar efficacy and safety results for ARB losartan and amlodipine.[118]; however, the ability of ARB to retard the progression of chronic allograft nephropathy remains unproven.

Several large-scale randomized, double-blinded, placebo-controlled trials have demonstrated the benefits of ARB use in patients with diabetic nephropathy from type 2 diabetes.[119,120] These studies using either irbesartan or losartan, concluded that ARBs are effective in protecting against the development and progression of nephropathy in patients with type 2 diabetes. The use of an ARB in all of these trials exhibited a renoprotective effect independent of its effect on blood pressure. No trials have been conducted to date to compare ACE inhibitors with ARBs in preventing proteinuria in patients with diabetes. Thanks to the wealth of available studies in both the general population and renal transplant recipients, ACE inhibitors should be used before ARBs, unless bradykinin-specific adverse effects (ie, chronic cough) have been experienced with prior use of an ACE inhibitor.

Calcium Channel Blockers

Calcium channel blockers (CCBs) can be separated into 2 subtypes: the nondihydropyridines (ie, diltiazem, verapamil) and the dihydropyridines (ie, amlodipine, nifedipine). The nondihydropyridines are more advantageous for control of heart rate than blood pressure and are associated with several DDIs that were discussed in detail earlier in this chapter. Diltiazem has found a niche among heart transplant recipients despite its DDI potential, as some studies have demonstrated its abilities to help prevent coronary artery disease in the allograft.[121,122] Throughout the rest of this section, the term CCB will be used to refer to the dihydropyridines. These CCBs reduce blood pressure through vasodilatation of the peripheral vessels mediated by the inhibition of calcium entering the smooth muscle of vasoconstricted arterioles.[123]

CCBs may be effective in alleviating nephrotoxic effects induced by calcineurin inhibitors, controlling hypertension, and preventing acute tubular necrosis (ATN) after transplantation.[124] CCBs promote dilatation of the afferent arterioles, which counteracts the vasoconstriction induced by cyclosporine and tacrolimus, resulting in improved renal function.[125-127] However, when weighed against other antihypertensive agents in other clinical trials, this benefit was not clinically significant.[128,129]

As a class, CCBs are relatively well tolerated, but they are not devoid of adverse events, especially among transplant recipients. Some common adverse events seen with CCBs are similar to those produced by standard immunosuppression. This situation, therefore, predisposes transplant recipients to pharmacodynamic interactions that occur between these 2 classes of medications, including peripheral edema (corticosteroids), gingival hyperplasia (cyclosporine), and skeletal muscle weakness (corticosteroids).[130]

Although CCBs provide adequate control of hypertension, patients may receive additional benefit from maintenance therapy with β-blockers and/or ACE inhibitors in lieu of or in addition to CCBs.

α-Blockers

One class of antihypertensives that have endured considerable criticism lately is the α-blockers (doxazosin, prazosin, and terazosin). This class of medications lowers blood pressure by causing a peripheral postsynaptic blockade of α-receptors, which results in a decrease in arterial tone. In a recent study[131] of cardiovascular events in patients receiving various antihypertensive agents, researchers found an increase in cardiovascular events in high-risk patients taking α-blocking agents. The Antihypertensive and Lipid Lowering Treatment to Prevent Heart Attack Trial (ALLHAT), a multicentered, randomized control trial including 42,448 patients 55 years old and older, halted the doxazosin arm prematurely when it was determined that these patients were 25% more likely to experience a cardiovascular event.[131]

Some of the more common adverse reactions associated with the use of α-blockers include postural hypotension, edema, somnolence, and sexual dysfunction. With increasing data showing detrimental effects associated with use of α-blockers, it would be wise to reserve the use of these agents as add-on therapy in patients with hypertension after transplantation that is difficult to control.

Key points for treatment of hypertension in solid-organ transplant recipients:

- Proper blood pressure control with diet and pharmacological intervention is essential for preventing cardiac morbidity and mortality and for prolonging graft survival.
- Most patients require multiple medications to achieve their target blood pressure.
- In most patients, β-blockers (potential exception in heart transplant recipients) and dihydropyridine CCB (diltiazem in heart transplant recipients) should be used after transplantation until patients can tolerate other agents.
- Thiazide diuretics and ACE inhibitors (ARBs if intolerant to ACE inhibitors) offer advantages as long-term therapy and should be initiated whenever tolerated.
- Careful monitoring of agent-specific adverse events is required.

Nonprescription Medications

Between 43% and 90% of organ transplant recipients will survive 5 years after their transplantation procedure, depending on the organ type and various other factors.[19] As more patients live longer lives with transplanted organs, common maladies such as aches and pains, flulike symptoms, diarrhea, constipation, and several other nagging conditions are likely to develop. Healthcare professionals should anticipate questions regarding the safety of over-the-counter (OTC) products in transplant recipients; therefore, we briefly address some of the more commonly used nonprescription medications and evaluate their potential for harm in organ transplant recipients.

Nonprescription Analgesics

Nonprescription analgesics (ie, aspirin, choline salicylate, magnesium salicylate, sodium salicylate, ibuprofen, ketoprofen, naproxen sodium, acetaminophen) are the most commonly purchased nonprescription agents in the United States.[132,133] These agents are generally considered to be safe; however, most are associated with some important adverse events. A closer look at the nonprescription analgesics reveals their potential for harm when used by solid-organ transplant recipients.

Salicylates

The salicylates (ie, aspirin, choline salicylate, magnesium salicylate, sodium salicylate) are associated with gastrointestinal damage, hematological changes, electrolyte imbalance, liver and kidney dysfunction, and breathing difficulties.[6,132,133] In organ transplant recipients, the salicylates should be avoided if possible, because of these potential toxic effects, especially renal dysfunction. Low-dose aspirin used for the prevention of cardiovascular and cardiocerebral events appears to be safe, but patients must still be followed up carefully.

NSAIDs

The NSAIDs (ie, ibuprofen, ketoprofen, naproxen), generally considered the OTC drugs of choice for inflammatory conditions, have an adverse event profile similar to that for the salicylates.[6,133] In addition, these agents worsen hypertension. As with the salicylates, these agents should be avoided, if at all possible, in solid-organ transplant recipients.

Acetaminophen

Acetaminophen is generally considered the nonprescription analgesic and antipyretic of choice in transplant recipients because of its favorable toxicity profile. However, acetaminophen induces hematological changes and liver and renal dysfunction.[6,132] It is imperative that patients and transplant practitioners are aware that this agent is not without toxic effects and proper monitoring is advised, especially soon after liver transplantation.[133] Acetaminophen does not have any appreciable anti-inflammatory effects.[132]

Nonprescription Laxatives

Constipation can be characterized by 2 distinct colorectal motility disorders: slow-transit constipation (slow movement of fecal contents) and pelvic floor dysfunction (storage of fecal contents for prolonged time in the rectum).[132,134] Causes of constipation are numerous and can be linked to various medical conditions and/or medications, lifestyle characteristics, psychological conditions, and physiological complications. In addition, specific populations of patients are more susceptible to constipation and its associated complications (eg, the elderly).[132,134,135]

Many drugs may induce or complicate constipation. Calcium or aluminum-containing antacids, narcotic analgesics, some tricyclic antidepressants, certain CCBs, and medications with anticholinergic activity, for example, can all cause constipation.[6,132,134] Narcotic analgesics are notoriously associated with constipation and can lead to a condition known as narcotic bowel syndrome characterized by chronic constipation and abdominal pain. This problem is very common immediately after transplantation. All of the maintenance immunosuppressants have been associated with some degree of constipation.[6,132]

Nonprescription laxatives are generally considered safe; however, these medications can be harmful if overused. Laxatives have a number of adverse effects that should be closely monitored in order to prevent drug-induced toxic effects.

Bulk-Forming Laxatives

Bulk-forming laxatives (ie, methylcellulose, carboxy methylcellulose sodium, malt soup extract, polycarbophil, plantago seeds) are not generally used as frequently as emollient and lubricant laxatives in patients after abdominal surgery.[6,132,134] Nevertheless, they closely mimic the physiological method of fecal evacuation and can be used in patients longer than other laxatives. Their adverse drug reaction profile is limited only to gastrointestinal effects, although additive gastrointestinal effects may occur with the maintenance immunosuppressants.[6,132] The bulk-forming laxatives can decrease the oral absorption of several prescription medications (ie, anticoagulants, salicylates, antibiotics),[6,132] and an interaction does exist between calcium polycarbophil and mycophenolate, where MPA absorption in decreased after co-administration of MPA and this bulk-forming laxative.[136]

Emollient Laxatives

Emollient laxatives (ie, docusate sodium, calcium, and potassium) may be useful for the treatment of constipation in solid-organ transplant recipients. These agents are very useful in preventing or treating short-term constipation. These agents may not be of benefit in patients with slow-transit constipation, because of their lack of stimulation of the gastrointestinal tract. Docusate causes nausea, vomiting, and diarrhea and can worsen these effects in patients on maintenance immunosuppression.[6,132] Caution should be given when docusate calcium is used in transplant recipients, because of the potential for chelation interactions between calcium and MPA, and when docusate potassium is used, because of the potential for additive hyperkalemia with the calcineurin inhibitors, although these interactions are based solely in theory.

Lubricant Laxatives

Lubricant laxatives (ie, mineral oil) should be used carefully in solid-organ transplant recipients. As are stool softeners, lubricant laxatives are useful in treating patients with constipation after abdominal surgery.[6,132] Moreover, they are also used to treat constipation in hypertensive patients. Because a number of renal transplant recipients have underlying hypertension, this therapy may be a practical choice for these patients. However, mineral oil is not as useful in preventing constipation as stool softeners. It is also important to consider the possibility of lipid pneumonia with these laxatives because some transplant recipients may be bedridden after surgery. Coadministration of docusate with mineral oil may facilitate absorption or cellular uptake of the mineral oil and result in inflammation of intestinal mucosa, liver, spleen, and lymph nodes.[6,132]

Saline Laxatives

Saline laxatives (ie, magnesium citrate, magnesium hydroxide, magnesium sulfate, dibasic sodium phosphate, monobasic phosphate, sodium biphosphate) should generally be avoided in organ transplant recipients. Many saline laxatives contain high levels of magnesium and are associated with 20% systemic absorption of magnesium. In healthy persons, this absorbed magnesium is cleared renally with no complications.[6,132] However, in renally impaired patients, magnesium can accumulate and cause hypotension, muscle weakness, central nervous system disturbances, and electrocardiographic changes. Additionally, these laxatives are also contraindicated in patients with dehydration syndromes and restricted salt intake or with delicate fluid balances. Several case reports of acute renal failure following the use of saline laxatives as bowel preparations have been published, adding to the mounting evidence for avoidance of saline laxatives in transplant recipients.[137,138]

Osmotic Laxatives

Osmotic laxatives (ie, glycerin) should be used with caution in transplant recipients with a history of diabetes mellitus because glycerin can increase plasma insulin levels.[6,132] If glycerin is used, clinicians should advise their patients to closely monitor their plasma glucose regularly. Use of this agent in liver transplant recipients should be monitored closely as transient hepatomegaly may occur as a result of glycogen storage.[6,132]

Stimulant Laxatives

Stimulant laxative (ie, anthraquinones, aloe, cascara sagrada, senna alkaloids, bisacodyl, castor oil) are often used before radiological or endoscopic examinations or in situations where evacuation is necessary.[6,132] These agents, in particular senna alkaloids, have long been considered the laxatives of choice for narcotic-induced constipation. Bisacodyl is also effective in patients with colostomies. Stimulant laxatives may also be used as initial therapy for simple constipation, but they should not be used for more than 1 week. Stimulant laxatives are highly effective but should be recommended with caution; overuse can lead to "cathartic colon" or a poorly functioning colon. Chronic use can also lead to reversible melanotic pigmentation of colonic mucosa. The most common adverse events associated with stimulant laxatives are electrolyte and fluid deficiencies, malabsorption, and hypokalemia.[6,132] In solid-organ transplants, imbalances in electrolytes caused by these agents could be problematic. Additionally, nausea and diarrhea have also been associated with use of stimulant laxatives.

Nonprescription laxatives are generally considered safe in treating constipation. However, these agents have several adverse effects, especially if used long-term, which might be dangerous in solid-organ transplant recipients. Therefore, it is important for healthcare practitioners to consider patient-specific factors in choosing the most appropriate laxatives and to closely monitor the patients for potential adverse events when combining OTC laxatives with maintenance immunosuppressants. Clinicians should also take an active role in educating patients on the proper use of these agents, their common adverse effects, and the potential for laxative abuse.

Nonprescription Antidiarrheals

Diarrhea is a common problem among transplant recipients.[139] Most often it is induced by the immunosuppressants or intestinal pathogens. Currently, data on the appropriate management of diarrhea in solid-organ transplant recipients are scarce. Often times, in cases of excessive gastrointestinal motility, the nonprescription antidiarrheal agents are the easiest and fastest way to relieve some of these bothersome signs and symptoms. However, infectious causes of diarrhea must be ruled out before the recommendation of an antidiarrheal.

Loperamide

Loperamide is the most common OTC antidiarrheal used in the United States. It is primarily metabolized by liver enzymes and only minimally excreted in the urine.[6,132] Because of its metabolic pathway, patients with liver dysfunction should use this agent with caution. Loperamide does not appear to affect the pharmacokinetics of maintenance immunosuppressive agents, although one in vitro analysis[140] shows that cyclosporine appears to increase intestinal absorption of loperamide (interaction mediated by P-glycoprotein). Some of loperamide's more common adverse reactions include urinary retention, dysuria, toxic effects on the gastrointestinal tract, and hyperglycemia. Because of these adverse events, this agent should be used in caution in renal transplant recipients and any patient with diabetes mellitus.[6,132] In cases of diarrhea induced by an intestinal pathogen, the antiperistaltic activity of loperamide will not allow excretion of the bacterial pathogen or its toxic by-products, which may result in toxic megacolon.[132,141]

Bismuth Subsalicylate

Bismuth subsalicylate is inferior to loperamide in terms of antidiarrheal activity. In general, bismuth subsalicylate is well tolerated, with adverse effects on the gastrointestinal system being the most common.[6,132] The tablet formulation of this product has a high calcium content; therefore, this agent should be avoided in patients with hypercalcemia or hyperphosphatemia and should never be given concomitantly with the MPA derivatives because of the potential for chelation interactions in the gut.[6,132]

Polycarbophil

Technically, polycarbophil is classified as a bulk-forming laxative (as described above), but this agent is also used for treatment of constipation.[6,132] Polycarbophil has the ability to absorb up to 60 times its original weight in water. This agent's adverse event profile and DDI potential with MPA derivatives are outlined in the laxative section.

Lactobacillus

Lactobacillus is an anaerobic bacterium, and several of its species make up part of the normal flora of the intestine and vagina.[6,132] This agent has demonstrated effectiveness in preventing and treating antibiotic-induced diarrhea, which may be important because both tacrolimus and sirolimus are macrolide antibiotic derivatives. The benefit of using this agent is that it reestablishes a normal gastrointestinal environment and is associated with a good safety profile and no known DDIs.[6,132]

The appropriate management of diarrhea in solid-organ transplant recipients will not only improve the patient's quality of life, but it may also contribute to better compliance with immunosuppressive medications, such as the MPA derivatives. More research should be done to establish the safety and effectiveness of nonprescription antidiarrheals in patients who have undergone solid-organ transplantation.

Nonprescription Antihistamines

Antihistamines have been available OTC for more than 60 years. They are popular largely because they are generally safe medications.[132,142] In the United States, antihistamines are used as sleep-aids and for the treatment of seasonal allergy symptoms, nausea, and motion sickness.[6,132,142] The currently available nonprescription antihistamines include brompheniramine, chlorpheniramine, clemastine, dexbrompheniramine, diphenhydramine, doxylamine, loratadine, and triprolidine.

Although no direct contraindication exists for use of antihistamines in transplant recipients, many factors should be considered before therapy with these agents is started. All of the available agents are hepatically metabolized, and clemastine is considered a weak inhibitor of CYP3A4. Both chlorpheniramine and loratadine are substrates for this same hepatic isozyme. For that reason, any patient with hepatic dysfunction should use these agents with caution. To date, no DDIs between the nonprescription antihistamines and any of the maintenance immunosuppressive agents have been documented. Lung transplant recipients should use these agents with extreme caution, as they have all been shown to have a suppressive effect on the respiratory system. Finally, OTC antihistamines all have anticholinergic adverse events, some worse than others. Given this fact, patients should be warned about the potential for urinary retention and constipation when self-medicating with these agents.[6,132,142]

Nonprescription Cough Suppressants and Expectorants

A cough is a sign often associated with respiratory infections, asthma, and chronic respiratory conditions.[132,143] Nonprescription oral agents available for treating cough include codeine, dextromethorphan, diphenhydramine, and guaifenesin. Diphenhydramine was discussed earlier in the antihistamine section. Often, cough suppressants are not considered desirable in transplant recipients. The major reason for this is the belief that suppressing a cough in a patient with a respiratory infection may lead to worsening of the infection. However, primary literature in support of this claim does not exist.

Codeine

Although not available without a prescription in all states, codeine is considered by many to be the gold standard antitussive. For this indication, codeine requires lower dosing than when used as an analgesic (10-20 mg every 4-6 hours: maximum daily antitussive dose is 120 mg).[6,132] At antitussive doses, risks of adverse events are low, but such events may include nausea, vomiting, sedation, dizziness, and constipation. This agent does have some pharmacodynamic interactions with central nervous system depressants, but no known interactions with immunosuppressive medications. One important note is that codeine is hepatically metabolized to morphine. Morphine metabolites can accumulate in patients with renal dysfunction; therefore, this product should be used cautiously in patients with renal dysfunction.[6,132]

Dextromethorphan

Dextromethorphan is likely to provide a safe option for the treatment of cough in transplant recipients. Additional caution may be warranted in patients who have hepatic dysfunction, because dextromethorphan is metabolized by CYP2D6. The most common adverse events include drowsiness, dizziness, respiratory depression, nausea, gastrointestinal upset, constipation, and abdominal discomfort.[6,132]

Guaifenesin

Guaifenesin is also likely to be a safe treatment option in transplant recipients. It has few documented DDIs and no DDIs are known of between it and the maintenance immunosuppressants.[6,132] Additional caution should be exercised when using guaifenesin in patients who have undergone renal transplantation because the metabolite of guaifenesin may contribute to the formation of kidney stones.[144,145] Some of the more common adverse effects include dizziness, drowsiness, headache, rash, and abdominal pain.[6,132]

It is likely that most transplant recipients will experience episodes of the common cold and its associated symptom, a cough. Based on the characteristics of each patient, carefully selected oral OTC cough preparations can safely provide relief of signs and symptoms in solid-organ transplant recipients.

Complementary and Alternative Medicine

CAM is a multibillion dollar industry in the United States. Almost half of the population uses some form of CAM, including herbs, nonherbal supplements, and vitamins.[132,146] In a study[147] published in 1997, researchers reported that 20% of transplant recipients were using CAM.[132] More recently, a survey[148] of liver transplant recipients showed that 35% of those surveyed admitted to continuous use of vitamins and 19% admitted to using both vitamin and herbal remedies, with the most commonly used products consisting of milk thistle and green tea.[132] Many people use CAM in addition to prescription medications, but the majority fail to inform their healthcare providers of their use.[132,149] Physicians rarely inquire about the use of CAM, and many patients assume that these agents are innocuous. In contradiction to this belief, however, is the observation that thousands of adverse events induced by dietary supplements are reported yearly to the American Association of Poison Control Centers. Importantly, manufacturers of dietary supplements, as classified by the FDA, are not responsible for proving the safety and efficacy of these agents.[132,150] Nephrotoxicity, hepatotoxicity, and DDIs are commonly associated with many conventional medications, and it is highly likely that dietary supplements are no different.

When evaluating CAM for the potential for harm in transplant recipients, several factors must be evaluated. The first should be the potential for interactions with immunosuppressive agents. Next, the potential for CAM-induced hepatotoxic and nephrotoxic effects must also be evaluated. Finally, the potential immunomodulatory effects of CAM must be considered.

Drug-Drug Interactions

The importance of DDIs in transplant recipients was discussed in detail earlier in this chapter. There is a true potential for CAM products to interact with maintenance immunosuppressants.[151-166] Please refer to Table 11 for a list of documented DDIs between CAM products and immunosuppressive agents.

Table 11. DOCUMENTED DRUG-DRUG INTERACTIONS BETWEEN AGENTS USED IN COMPLEMENTARY AND ALTERNATIVE MEDICINE AND MAINTENANCE IMMUNOSUPPRESSIVE AGENTS [113-128]

Scientific Name (Common Name) of Agent Used in Complementary and Alternative Medicine	Documented Interaction
Citrus paradisi (grapefruit juice)	Inhibition of both cytochrome P 3A4 isozyme system (CYP3A4) and P-glycoprotein causes accumulation of cyclosporine, tacrolimus, and sirolimus, resulting in increased drug levels with the potential for toxic effects of drug or excessive immunosuppression
Hypericum perforatum (St. John's wort)	Induces activity of both CYP3A4 and P-glycoprotein, resulting in decreased levels of cyclosporine, tacrolimus, and sirolimus Numerous case reports published on increased rejection rates in transplant patients taking St. Johns wort
Monascus purpureus (red yeast rice)	Single case report of rhabdomyolysis induced by an herbal preparation in a stable renal-transplant recipient, attributed to the presence of red yeast rice Theorized interaction of cyclosporine and red yeast rice through the cytochrome P-450 system resulted in the rhabdomyolysis associated with increased serum concentrations of constituents of the red yeast rice

Hepatotoxic Effects

Reports of hepatotoxic effects induced by CAM products are accumulating rapidly. Several case reports have demonstrated liver injury from CAM agents, ranging from mild elevations of liver enzyme levels to fulminant liver failure requiring transplantation.[167-183] Please refer to Table 12 for a list of CAM products that have been associated with hepatotoxic effects.

Table 12. AGENTS USED IN COMPLEMENTARY AND ALTERNATIVE MEDICINE WITH DOCUMENTED HEPATOTOXICITY[129-145]

Scientific Name	Common Name
Chelidonium majus	Greater celandine
Ephedra sinica	Ma-huang
Hedeoma pulegioides	Pennyroyal
Hydrazine sulfate	
Larrea tridentate	Chaparral
Lycopodium serratum	Jin bu huan
Piper methysticum	Kava
Rhamnus purshiana	Cascara sagrada
Symphytum officinale	Comfrey
Teucrium chamaedrys	Germander

Nephrotoxic Effects

Drug-induced nephrotoxic effects account for approximately 7% of all medication-related toxic effects nationwide.[184] The kidneys are highly susceptible to injury because of their intrinsic functions of filtration, reabsorption, metabolism, and concentration. It is reasonable to expect that, as with conventional medications, some CAM agents may also have nephrotoxic potential. Please refer to Table 13 for a list of CAM agents that show either direct nephrotoxic effects, nephrolithiasis, or nephrotoxic effects due to rhabdomyolysis.[159,183,185-250]

Table 13. AGENTS USED IN COMPLEMENTARY AND ALTERNATIVE MEDICINE THAT HAVE DOCUMENTED NEPHROTOXICITY[121,145,147-212]

Scientific Name	Common Name
Aristolochia serpentaria	Snakewood
Artemisia absinthium	Wormwood
Ascorbic acid	
Chromium picolinate	
Creatine monohydrate	
Echinacea angustifoli	Echinacea
Ephedra sinica	Ma-huang
Fucus vesiculosis	Bladderwrack
Germanium	
Glucosamine	
Glycyrrhiza glabra	Licorice
Hedeoma pulegioides	Pennyroyal
Hydrazine sulfate	
L-Lysine	
Larrea tridentate	Chaparral
Rumex crispus	Yellow dock
Salix daphnoides	Willow bark
Taxus celebica	Yew
Thevetia peruviana	Yellow oleander
Tripterygium wilfordii	Thunder God vine
Uncaria tomentosa	Cat's claw
Vaccinium macrocarpon	Cranberry
Valeriana officinalis	Valerian

Immunomodulation

In organ transplantation, the purpose of immunosuppressive therapy is to decrease the undesirable immunologic activity of the host toward the allograft. Conversely, it is also important that the host's defense mechanisms continue to function. There is often a fine line between too little and too much immunosuppression. This balancing act can be disrupted by CAM agents that promote immunomodulation. Several CAM products have shown immunomodulatory effects either in vitro or in vivo[251-288] (Table 14).

Table 14. AGENTS USED IN COMPLEMENTARY AND ALTERNATIVE MEDICINE THAT HAVE IN VIVO OR IN VITRO IMMUNOMODULATING PROPERTIES[213-250]

Scientific Name	Common Name
Apis mellifera	Royal jelly
Arnica montana	Wolf's bane
Ascorbic acid	
Astragalus membranaceus	Tragacanth
Baptista tinctoria	Wild indigo
Boswellia serrata	Frankincense
Curcuma longa	Tumeric
D-α-Tocopherol	
Echinacea angustifoli	Echinacea
Eleutherococcus senticosus	Siberian ginseng
Eupatorium perfoliatum	Feverwort
Ganoderma lucidum	Reishi mushroom
Ginseng quinquefolius	American ginseng
Glycyrrhiza glabra	Licorice
Grifola frondosa	Maitake
Hydrastis canadensis	Goldenseal
Matricaria chamomilla	Chamomile
Medicago sativa	Alfalfa
Oenothera biennis	Evening primrose oil
Panax ginseng	Asian ginseng
Spirulina platensis	Spirulina
Tripterygium wilfordii	Thunder God vine
Viscum album	Mistletoe
Zinc	

It is essential that transplant recipients be informed about the dangers of CAM products. In general, it would be best to discourage the use of such agents after transplantation; however, with the increasing popularity of alternative medicine, it is unrealistic to assume all patients will adhere to this recommendation. It is imperative that healthcare practitioners take an active role in identifying patients who use CAM products and be willing and open to providing appropriate and prudent education to those patients.

References

1. Beiras-Fernandez A, Thein E, Hammer C. Induction of immunosuppression with polyclonal antithymocyte globulins: an overview. *Exp Clin Transplant*. 2003;1:79-84.
2. Berard JL, Velez RL, Freeman RB, Tsunoda SM. A review of interleukin-2 receptor antagonists in solid organ transplantation. *Pharmacotherapy*. 1999;19:1127-1137.
3. Nashan B. Antibody induction therapy in renal transplant patients receiving calcineurin-inhibitor immunosuppressive regimens: a comparative review. *BioDrugs*. 2005;19:39-46.
4. Halloran PF. Immunosuppressive drugs for kidney transplantation. *N Engl J Med*. 2004;351:2715-2729.

5. Hardinger KL, Koch MJ, Brennan DC. Current and future immunosuppressive strategies in renal transplantation. *Pharmacotherapy.* 2004;24:1159-1176.
6. Micromedex(r) Healthcare Series (electronic version). Greenwood Village, Colo: Thomson Healthcare, Inc; 2006.
7. Vincenti F, Pace D, Birnbaum J, Lantz M. Pharmacokinetic and pharmacodynamic studies of one or two doses of daclizumab in renal transplantation. *Am J Transplant.* 2003;3:50-52.
8. Soltero L, Carbajal H, Sarkissian N, et al. A truncated-dose regimen of daclizumab for prevention of acute rejection in kidney transplant recipients: a single-center experience. *Transplantation.* 2004;78:1560-1563.
9. Whiting JF, Fecteau A, Martin J, Bejarano PA, Hanto DW. Use of low-dose OKT3 as induction therapy in liver transplantation. *Transplantation.* 1998;65:577-580.
10. Hooks MA, Wade CS, Millikan WJ Jr. Muromonab CD-3: a review of its pharmacology, pharmacokinetics, and clinical use in transplantation. *Pharmacotherapy.* 1991;11:26-37.
11. Wilde MI, Goa KL. Muromonab CD3: a reappraisal of its pharmacology and use as prophylaxis of solid organ transplant rejection. *Drugs.* 1996;51:865-894.
12. Abramowicz D, De Pauw L, Le Moine A, et al. Prevention of OKT3 nephrotoxicity after kidney transplantation. *Kidney Int Suppl.* 1996;53:S39-S43.
13. Ferrajoli A, O'Brien S, Keating MJ. Alemtuzumab: a novel monoclonal antibody. *Expert Opin Biol Ther.* 2001;1:1059-1065.
14. Dumont FJ. Alemtuzumab (Millennium/ILEX). Curr Opin Investig Drugs. 2001;2:139-160.
15. Knechtle SJ, Fernandez LA, Pirsch JD, et al. Campath-1H in renal transplantation: The University of Wisconsin experience. *Surgery.* 2004;136:754-760.
16. Knechtle SJ, Pirsch JD, H. Fechner JJ, et al. Campath-1H induction plus rapamycin monotherapy for renal transplantation: results of a pilot study. *Am J Transplant.* 2003;3:722-730.
17. Watson CJ, Bradley JA, Friend PJ, et al. Alemtuzumab (Campath 1H) induction therapy in cadaveric kidney transplantation-efficacy and safety at five years. *Am J Transplant.* 2005;5:1347-1353.
18. Friend PJ, Hale G, Waldmann H, et al. Campath-1M—prophylactic use after kidney transplantation: a randomized controlled clinical trial. *Transplantation.* 1989;48:248-253.
19. Scientific Registry of Transplant Recipients. 2006. Available at: http://www.ustransplant.com Accessed June 14, 2006.
20. Braun WE. Renal transplantation: basic concepts and evolution of therapy. *J Clin Apheresis.* 2003;18:141-152.
21. Shapiro R, Young JB, Milford EL, Trotter JF, Bustami RT, Leichtman AB. Immunosuppression: evolution in practice and trends, 1993-2003. *Am J Transplant.* 2005;5(4 Pt 2):874-886.
22. Cyclosporine microemulsion (Neoral) absorption profiling and sparse-sample predictors during the first 3 months after renal transplantation. *Am J Transplant.* 2002;2:148-156.
23. Citterio F, Scata MC, Romagnoli J, Nanni G, Castagneto M. Results of a three-year prospective study of C2 monitoring in long-term renal transplant recipients receiving cyclosporine microemulsion. *Transplantation.* 2005;79:802-806.
24. Mathias HC, Ozalp F, Will MB, et al. A randomized, controlled trial of C0- vs C2-guided therapeutic drug monitoring of cyclosporine in stable heart transplant patients. *J Heart Lung Transplant.* 2005;24:2137-2143.
25. Barnard JB, Thekkudan J, Richardson S, et al. Cyclosporine profiling with C2 and C0 monitoring improves outcomes after heart transplantation. *J Heart Lung Transplant.* 2006;25:564-568.
26. Kyllonen LE, Salmela KT. Early cyclosporine C0 and C2 monitoring in de novo kidney transplant patients: a prospective randomized single-center pilot study. *Transplantation.* 2006;81:1010-1015.
27. Mayer AD, Dmitrewski J, Squifflet JP, et al. Multicenter randomized trial comparing tacrolimus (FK506) and cyclosporine in the prevention of renal allograft rejection: a report of the European Tacrolimus Multicenter Renal Study Group. *Transplantation.* 1997;64:436-443.
28. Treede H, Klepetko W, Reichenspurner H, et al. Tacrolimus versus cyclosporine after lung transplantation: a prospective, open, randomized two-center trial comparing two different immunosuppressive protocols. *J Heart Lung Transplant.* 2001;20:511-517.
29. O'Grady JG, Burroughs A, Hardy P, Elbourne D, Truesdale A. Tacrolimus versus microemulsified ciclosporin in liver transplantation: the TMC randomised controlled trial. *Lancet.* 2002;360:1119-1125.
30. Wang CH, Ko WJ, Chou NK, Wang SS. Efficacy and safety of tacrolimus versus cyclosporine microemulsion in primary cardiac transplant recipients: 6-month results in Taiwan. *Transplant Proc.* 2004;36:2384-2385.
31. Meiser BM, Groetzner J, Kaczmarek I, et al. Tacrolimus or cyclosporine: which is the better partner for mycophenolate mofetil in heart transplant recipients? *Transplantation.* 2004;78:591-598.
32. Levy G, Villamil F, Samuel D, et al. Results of lis2t, a multicenter, randomized study comparing cyclosporine microemulsion with C2 monitoring and tacrolimus with C0 monitoring in de novo liver transplantation. *Transplantation.* 2004;77:1632-1638.
33. Reams BD, Palmer SM. Sublingual tacrolimus for immunosuppression in lung transplantation: a potentially important therapeutic option in cystic fibrosis. *Am J Respir Med.* 2002;1:91-98.
34. Reams D, Rea J, Davis D, Palmer S. Utility of sublingual tacrolimus in cystic fibrosis patients after lung transplantation. *J Heart Lung Transplant.* 2001;20:207-208.
35. Chan GL, Canafax DM, Johnson CA. The therapeutic use of azathioprine in renal transplantation. *Pharmacotherapy.* 1987;7:165-177.

36. Romagnuolo J, Sadowski DC, Lalor E, Jewell L, Thomson AB. Cholestatic hepatocellular injury with azathioprine: a case report and review of the mechanisms of hepatotoxicity. *Can J Gastroenterol.* 1998;12:479-483.
37. Gabardi S, Tran JL, Clarkson MR. Enteric-coated mycophenolate sodium. *Ann Pharmacother.* 2003;37:1685-1693.
38. Sollinger HW. Mycophenolates in transplantation. *Clin Transplant.* 2004;18:485-492.
39. Sollinger HW. Mycophenolate mofetil. *Kidney Int Suppl.* 1995;52:S14-S17.
40. Sollinger H. Enteric-coated mycophenolate sodium: therapeutic equivalence to mycophenolate mofetil in de novo renal transplant patients. *Transplant Proc.* 2004;36(2 suppl):517S-520S.
41. Gabardi S, Cerio J. Future immunosuppressive agents in solid-organ transplantation. *Prog Transplant.* 2004;14:148-156.
42. Vasquez EM. Sirolimus: a new agent for prevention of renal allograft rejection. *Am J Health Syst Pharm.* 2000;57:437-448; quiz 449-451.
43. Hong JC, Kahan BD. Sirolimus-induced thrombocytopenia and leukopenia in renal transplant recipients: risk factors, incidence, progression, and management. *Transplantation.* 2000;69:2085-2090.
44. MacDonald AS. A worldwide, phase III, randomized, controlled, safety and efficacy study of a sirolimus/cyclosporine regimen for prevention of acute rejection in recipients of primary mismatched renal allografts. *Transplantation.* 2001;71:271-280.
45. Kreis H, Oberbauer R, Campistol JM, et al. Long-term benefits with sirolimus-based therapy after early cyclosporine withdrawal. *J Am Soc Nephrol.* 2004;15:809-817.
46. Mancini D, Pinney S, Burkhoff D, et al. Use of rapamycin slows progression of cardiac transplantation vasculopathy. *Circulation.* 2003;108:48-53.
47. Holt DW. Therapeutic drug monitoring of immunosuppressive drugs in kidney transplantation. *Curr Opin Nephrol Hypertens.* 2002;11:657-663.
48. Ahsan N, Hricik D, Matas A, et al. Prednisone withdrawal in kidney transplant recipients on cyclosporine and mycophenolate mofetil: a prospective randomized study. Steroid Withdrawal Study Group. *Transplantation.* 1999;68:1865-1874.
49. Liu CL, Fan ST, Lo CM, et al. Interleukin-2 receptor antibody (basiliximab) for immunosuppressive induction therapy after liver transplantation: a protocol with early elimination of steroids and reduction of tacrolimus dosage. *Liver Transpl.* 2004;10:728-733.
50. Laftavi MR, Stephan R, Stefanick B, et al. Randomized prospective trial of early steroid withdrawal compared with low-dose steroids in renal transplant recipients using serial protocol biopsies to assess efficacy and safety. *Surgery.* 2005;137:364-371.
51. Kaufman DB, Leventhal JR, Koffron AJ, et al. A prospective study of rapid corticosteroid elimination in simultaneous pancreas-kidney transplantation: comparison of two maintenance immunosuppression protocols: tacrolimus/mycophenolate mofetil versus tacrolimus/sirolimus. *Transplantation.* 2002;73:169-177.
52. Kumar MS, Heifets M, Moritz MJ, et al. Safety and efficacy of steroid withdrawal two days after kidney transplantation: analysis of results at three years. *Transplantation.* 2006;81:832-839.
53. Matas AJ, Ramcharan T, Paraskevas S, et al. Rapid discontinuation of steroids in living donor kidney transplantation: a pilot study. *Am J Transplant.* 2001;1:278-283.
54. Boots JM, Christiaans MH, Van Duijnhoven EM, Van Suylen RJ, Van Hooff JP. Early steroid withdrawal in renal transplantation with tacrolimus dual therapy: a pilot study. *Transplantation.* 2002;74:1703-1709.
55. Vincenti F, Monaco A, Grinyo J, Kinkhabwala M, Roza A. Multicenter randomized prospective trial of steroid withdrawal in renal transplant recipients receiving basiliximab, cyclosporine microemulsion and mycophenolate mofetil. *Am J Transplant.* 2003;3:306-311.
56. Preskorn SH. How drug-drug interactions can impact managed care. *Am J Manag Care.* 2004;10(6 suppl):S186-S198.
57. Page RL 2nd, Miller GG, Lindenfeld J. Drug therapy in the heart transplant recipient: part IV: drug-drug interactions. *Circulation.* 2005;111:230-239.
58. Gaston RS. Maintenance immunosuppression in the renal transplant recipient: an overview. *Am J Kidney Dis.* 2001;38(6 suppl 6):S25-S35.
59. Lake KD, Canafax DM. Important interactions of drugs with immunosuppressive agents used in transplant recipients. *J Antimicrob Chemother.* 1995;36(suppl B):11-22.
60. van Duijnhoven EM, Boots JM, Christiaans MH, Stolk LM, Undre NA, van Hooff JP. Increase in tacrolimus trough levels after steroid withdrawal. *Transplant Int.* 2003;16:721-725.
61. Prescott WA Jr, Callahan BL, Park JM. Tacrolimus toxicity associated with concomitant metoclopramide therapy. *Pharmacotherapy.* 2004;24:532-537.
62. Aszalos A. P-glycoprotein-based drug-drug interactions: preclinical methods and relevance to clinical observations. *Arch Pharm Res.* 2004;27:127-135.
63. Kennedy DT, Hayney MS, Lake KD. Azathioprine and allopurinol: the price of an avoidable drug interaction. *Ann Pharmacother.* 1996;30:951-954.
64. Cummins D, Sekar M, Halil O, Banner N. Myelosuppression associated with azathioprine-allopurinol interaction after heart and lung transplantation. *Transplantation.* 1996;61:1661-1662.
65. Walker J, Mendelson H, McClure A, Smith MD. Warfarin and azathioprine: clinically significant drug interaction. *J Rheumatol.* 2002;29:398-399.
66. Singleton JD, Conyers L. Warfarin and azathioprine: an important drug interaction. *Am J Med.* 1992;92:217.
67. Rivier G, Khamashta MA, Hughes GR. Warfarin and azathioprine: a drug interaction does exist. *Am J Med.* 1993;95:342.

68. Bullingham RE, Nicholls AJ, Kamm BR. Clinical pharmacokinetics of mycophenolate mofetil. *Clin Pharmacokinet.* 1998;34:429-455.
69. Mignat C. Clinically significant drug interactions with new immunosuppressive agents. *Drug Saf.* 1997;16:267-278.
70. Cattaneo D, Merlini S, Zenoni S, et al. Influence of co-medication with sirolimus or cyclosporine on mycophenolic acid pharmacokinetics in kidney transplantation. *Am J Transplant.* 2005;5:2937-2944.
71. Cremers S, Schoemaker R, Scholten E, et al. Characterizing the role of enterohepatic recycling in the interactions between mycophenolate mofetil and calcineurin inhibitors in renal transplant patients by pharmacokinetic modelling. *Br J Clin Pharmacol.* 2005;60:249-256.
72. Gregoor PJ, de Sevaux RG, Hene RJ, et al. Effect of cyclosporine on mycophenolic acid trough levels in kidney transplant recipients. *Transplantation.* 1999;68:1603-1606.
73. Bratzler DW, Houck PM. Antimicrobial prophylaxis for surgery: an advisory statement from the National Surgical Infection Prevention Project. *Am J Surg.* 2005;189:395-404.
74. Fishman JA. Prevention of infection caused by Pneumocystis carinii in transplant recipients. *Clin Infect Dis.* 2001;33:1397-1405.
75. Pneumocystis jiroveci (formerly Pneumocystis carinii). *Am J Transplant.* 2004;4(suppl 10):135-141.
76. Cytomegalovirus. *Am J Transplant.* 2004;4(suppl 10):51-58.
77. Gabardi S, Magee CC, Baroletti SA, Powelson JA, Cina JL, Chandraker AK. Efficacy and safety of low-dose valganciclovir for prevention of cytomegalovirus disease in renal transplant recipients: a single-center, retrospective analysis. *Pharmacotherapy.* 2004;24:1323-1330.
78. Paya C, Humar A, Dominguez E, et al. Efficacy and safety of valganciclovir vs. oral ganciclovir for prevention of cytomegalovirus disease in solid organ transplant recipients. *Am J Transplant.* 2004;4:611-620.
79. Golan Y. Overview of transplant mycology. *Am J Health Syst Pharm.* 2005;62(8 suppl 1):S17-S21.
80. Fungal infections. *Am J Transplant.* 2004;4(suppl 10):110-134.
81. Guidelines for vaccination of solid organ transplant candidates and recipients. *Am J Transplant.* 2004;4(suppl 10):160-163.
82. Beyer WE, Diepersloot RJ, Masurel N, Simoons ML, Weimar W. Double failure of influenza vaccination in a heart transplant patient. *Transplantation.* 1987;43:319.
83. Wagner CR, Hosenpud JD. Enhanced lymphocyte proliferative responses to donor-specific aortic endothelial cells following influenza vaccination. *Transpl Immunol.* 1993;1:83-85.
84. Kimball P, Verbeke S, Flattery M, Rhodes C, Tolman D. Influenza vaccination does not promote cellular or humoral activation among heart transplant recipients. *Transplantation.* 2000;69:2449-2451.
85. Magnani G, Falchetti E, Pollini G, et al. Safety and efficacy of two types of influenza vaccination in heart transplant recipients: a prospective randomised controlled study. *J Heart Lung Transplant.* 2005;24:588-592.
86. Kobashigawa JA, Warner-Stevenson L, Johnson BL, et al. Influenza vaccine does not cause rejection after cardiac transplantation. *Transplant Proc.* 1993;25:2738-2739.
87. Baroletti SA, Gabardi S, Magee CC, Milford EL. Calcium channel blockers as the treatment of choice for hypertension in renal transplant recipients: fact or fiction. *Pharmacotherapy.* 2003;23:788-801.
88. Jarowenko MV, Flechner SM, Van Buren CT, Lorber MI, Kahan BD. Influence of cyclosporine on posttransplant blood pressure response. *Am J Kidney Dis.* 1987;10:98-103.
89. Psaty BM, Smith NL, Siscovick DS, et al. Health outcomes associated with antihypertensive therapies used as first-line agents: a systematic review and meta-analysis. *JAMA.* 1997;277:739-745.
90. Taylor DO, Edwards LB, Mohacsi PJ, et al. The registry of the International Society for Heart and Lung Transplantation: twentieth official adult heart transplant report—2003. *J Heart Lung Transplant.* 2003;22:616-624.
91. Neal B, MacMahon S, Chapman N. Effects of ACE inhibitors, calcium antagonists, and other blood-pressure-lowering drugs: results of prospectively designed overviews of randomised trials. Blood Pressure Lowering Treatment Trialists' Collaboration. *Lancet.* 2000;356:1955-1964.
92. Taler SJ, Textor SC, Canzanello VJ, et al. Role of steroid dose in hypertension early after liver transplantation with tacrolimus (FK506) and cyclosporine. *Transplantation.* 1996;62:1588-1592.
93. Curtis JJ. Hypertension following kidney transplantation. *Am J Kidney Dis.* 1994;23:471-475.
94. Charnick SB, Nedelman JR, Chang CT, et al. Description of blood pressure changes in patients beginning cyclosporin A therapy. *Ther Drug Monit.* 1997;19:17-24.
95. Whitworth JA. Mechanisms of glucocorticoid-induced hypertension. *Kidney Int.* 1987;31:1213-1224.
96. Kaskel FJ, Devarajan P, Arbeit LA, Partin JS, Moore LC. Cyclosporine nephrotoxicity: sodium excretion, autoregulation, and angiotensin II. *Am J Physiol.* 1987;252(4 Pt 2):F733-F742.
97. Perico N, Benigni A, Zoja C, Delaini F, Remuzzi G. Functional significance of exaggerated renal thromboxane A2 synthesis induced by cyclosporin A. *Am J Physiol.* 1986;251(4 Pt 2):F581-F587.
98. Macleod AM, Thomson AW. FK 506: an immunosuppressant for the 1990s? *Lancet.* 1991;337(8732):25-27.
99. Jensik SC. Tacrolimus (FK 506) in kidney transplantation: three-year survival results of the US multicenter, randomized, comparative trial. FK 506 Kidney Transplant Study Group. *Transplant Proc.* 1998;30:1216-1218.

100. Sacks FM, Svetkey LP, Vollmer WM, et al. Effects on blood pressure of reduced dietary sodium and the Dietary Approaches to Stop Hypertension (DASH) diet. DASH-Sodium Collaborative Research Group. *N Engl J Med.* 2001;344:3-10.
101. Curtis JJ, Luke RG, Jones P, Diethelm AG. Hypertension in cyclosporine-treated renal transplant recipients is sodium dependent. *Am J Med.* 1988;85:134-138.
102. Chobanian AV, Bakris GL, Black HR, et al. The Seventh Report of the Joint National Committee on Prevention, Detection, Evaluation, and Treatment of High Blood Pressure: the JNC 7 report. *JAMA.* 2003;289:2560-2572.
103. Cusi D, Barlassina C, Azzani T, et al. Polymorphisms of alpha-adducin and salt sensitivity in patients with essential hypertension. *Lancet.* 1997;349:1353-1357.
104. Major outcomes in high-risk hypertensive patients randomized to angiotensin-converting enzyme inhibitor or calcium channel blocker vs diuretic: The Antihypertensive and Lipid-Lowering Treatment to Prevent Heart Attack Trial (ALLHAT). *JAMA.* 2002;288:2981-2997.
105. Baroletti S, Bencivenga GA, Gabardi S. Treating gout in kidney transplant recipients. *Prog Transplant.* 2004;14:143-147.
106. Dargie HJ. Effect of carvedilol on outcome after myocardial infarction in patients with left-ventricular dysfunction: the CAPRICORN randomised trial. *Lancet.* 2001;357:1385-1390.
107. Hjalmarson A, Goldstein S, Fagerberg B, et al. Effects of controlled-release metoprolol on total mortality, hospitalizations, and well-being in patients with heart failure: the Metoprolol CR/XL Randomized Intervention Trial in congestive heart failure (MERIT-HF). MERIT-HF Study Group. *JAMA.* 2000;283:1295-1302.
108. Giugliano D, Acampora R, Marfella R, et al. Metabolic and cardiovascular effects of carvedilol and atenolol in non-insulin-dependent diabetes mellitus and hypertension: a randomized, controlled trial. *Ann Intern Med.* 1997;126:955-959.
109. Kasiske BL, Ma JZ, Kalil RS, Louis TA. Effects of antihypertensive therapy on serum lipids. *Ann Intern Med.* 1995;122:133-141.
110. Yusuf S, Sleight P, Pogue J, Bosch J, Davies R, Dagenais G. Effects of an angiotensin-converting-enzyme inhibitor, ramipril, on cardiovascular events in high-risk patients. The Heart Outcomes Prevention Evaluation Study Investigators. *N Engl J Med.* 2000;342:145-153.
111. Piana RN, Wang SY, Friedman M, Sellke FW. Angiotensin-converting enzyme inhibition preserves endothelium-dependent coronary microvascular responses during short-term ischemia-reperfusion. *Circulation.* 1996;93:544-551.
112. Zeier M, Mandelbaum A, Ritz E. Hypertension in the transplanted patient. *Nephron.* 1998;80:257-268.
113. Remuzzi G, Ruggenenti P, Perico N. Chronic renal diseases: renoprotective benefits of renin-angiotensin system inhibition. *Ann Intern Med.* 2002;136:604-615.
114. Montanaro D, Gropuzzo M, Tulissi P, et al. Renoprotective effect of early inhibition of the renin-angiotensin system in renal transplant recipients. *Transplant Proc.* 2005;37:991-993.
115. Steinhauff S, Pehlivanli S, Bakovic-Alt R, et al. Beneficial effects of quinaprilat on coronary vasomotor function, endothelial oxidative stress, and endothelin activation after human heart transplantation. *Transplantation.* 2004;77:1859-1865.
116. Erinc K, Yamani MH, Starling RC, et al. The effect of combined angiotensin-converting enzyme inhibition and calcium antagonism on allograft coronary vasculopathy validated by intravascular ultrasound. *J Heart Lung Transplant.* 2005;24:1033-1038.
117. del Castillo D, Campistol JM, Guirado L, et al. Efficacy and safety of losartan in the treatment of hypertension in renal transplant recipients. *Kidney Int Suppl.* 1998;68:S135-S139.
118. Formica RN Jr, Friedman AL, Lorber MI, Smith JD, Eisen T, Bia MJ. A randomized trial comparing losartan with amlodipine as initial therapy for hypertension in the early post-transplant period. *Nephrol Dial Transplant.* 2006;21:1389-1394.
119. Brenner BM, Cooper ME, de Zeeuw D, et al. Effects of losartan on renal and cardiovascular outcomes in patients with type 2 diabetes and nephropathy. *N Engl J Med.* 2001;345:861-869.
120. Lewis EJ, Hunsicker LG, Clarke WR, et al. Renoprotective effect of the angiotensin-receptor antagonist irbesartan in patients with nephropathy due to type 2 diabetes. *N Engl J Med.* 2001;345:851-860.
121. Schroeder JS, Gao SZ. Calcium blockers and atherosclerosis: lessons from the Stanford Transplant Coronary Artery Disease/Diltiazem Trial. *Can J Cardiol.* 1995;11:710-715.
122. Schroeder JS, Gao SZ, Alderman EL, et al. A preliminary study of diltiazem in the prevention of coronary artery disease in heart-transplant recipients. *N Engl J Med.* 1993;328:164-170.
123. Droogmans G, Declerck I, Casteels R. Effect of adrenergic agonists on Ca^{2+}-channel currents in single vascular smooth muscle cells. *Pflugers Arch.* 1987;409:7-12.
124. Wagner K, Albrecht S, Neumayer HH. Prevention of posttransplant acute tubular necrosis by the calcium antagonist diltiazem: a prospective randomized study. *Am J Nephrol.* 1987;7:287-291.
125. Textor SC, Canzanello VJ, Taler SJ, et al. Cyclosporine-induced hypertension after transplantation. *Mayo Clin Proc.* 1994;69:1182-1193.
126. Luke RG. Pathophysiology and treatment of posttransplant hypertension. *J Am Soc Nephrol.* 1991;2(2 suppl 1):S37-S44.
127. Venkat-Raman G, Feehally J, Elliott HL, et al. Renal and haemodynamic effects of amlodipine and nifedipine in hypertensive renal transplant recipients. *Nephrol Dial Transplant.* 1998;13:2612-2616.
128. Sennesael J, Lamote J, Violet I, Tasse S, Verbeelen D. Comparison of perindopril and amlodipine in cyclosporine-treated renal allograft recipients. *Hypertension.* 1995;26:436-444.

129. Mourad G, Ribstein J, Mimran A. Converting-enzyme inhibitor versus calcium antagonist in cyclosporine-treated renal transplants. *Kidney Int.* 1993;43:419-425.
130. Abernethy DR, Schwartz JB. Calcium-antagonist drugs. *N Engl J Med.* 1999;341:1447-1457.
131. Major cardiovascular events in hypertensive patients randomized to doxazosin vs chlorthalidone: the antihypertensive and lipid-lowering treatment to prevent heart attack trial (ALLHAT). ALLHAT Collaborative Research Group. *JAMA.* 2000;283:1967-1975.
132. Berardi R, DeSimone E, Newton G, et al. *Handbook of Nonprescription Drugs.* 14th ed. Washington, DC: APhA Publications; 2004.
133. Gabardi S, Luu L. Nonprescription analgesics and their use in solid-organ transplantation: a review. *Prog Transplant.* 2004;14:182-190.
134. Locke GR 3rd, Pemberton JH, Phillips SF. American Gastroenterological Association Medical Position Statement: guidelines on constipation. *Gastroenterology.* 2000;119:1761-1766.
135. De Lillo AR, Rose S. Functional bowel disorders in the geriatric patient: constipation, fecal impaction, and fecal incontinence. *Am J Gastroenterol.* 2000;95:901-905.
136. Kato R, Ooi K, Ikura-Mori M, et al. Impairment of mycophenolate mofetil absorption by calcium polycarbophil. *J Clin Pharmacol.* 2002;42:1275-1280.
137. Markowitz GS, Nasr SH, Klein P, et al. Renal failure due to acute nephrocalcinosis following oral sodium phosphate bowel cleansing. *Hum Pathol.* 2004;35:675-684.
138. Orias M, Mahnensmith RL, Perazella MA. Extreme hyperphosphatemia and acute renal failure after a phosphorus-containing bowel regimen. *Am J Nephrol.* 1999;19:60-63.
139. Rao VK. Posttransplant medical complications. *Surg Clin North Am.* 1998;78:113-132.
140. Crowe A, Wong P. Potential roles of P-gp and calcium channels in loperamide and diphenoxylate transport. *Toxicol Appl Pharmacol.* 2003;193:127-137.
141. Brown JW. Toxic megacolon associated with loperamide therapy. JAMA. 1979;241:501-502.
142. Simons FE. H1-receptor antagonists. Comparative tolerability and safety. *Drug Saf.* 1994;10:350-380.
143. Fuller RW, Jackson DM. Physiology and treatment of cough. *Thorax.* 1990;45:425-430.
144. Bennett S, Hoffman N, Monga M. Ephedrine- and guaifenesin-induced nephrolithiasis. *J Altern Complement Med.* 2004;10:967-969.
145. Assimos DG, Langenstroer P, Leinbach RF, Mandel NS, Stern JM, Holmes RP. Guaifenesin- and ephedrine-induced stones. *J Endourol.* 1999;13:665-667.
146. Kessler RC, Davis RB, Foster DF, et al. Long-term trends in the use of complementary and alternative medical therapies in the United States. *Ann Intern Med.* 2001;135:262-268.
147. Crone CC, Wise TN. Survey of alternative medicine use among organ transplant patients. *J Transpl Coord.* 1997;7:123-130.
148. Neff GW, O'Brien C, Montalbano M, et al. Consumption of dietary supplements in a liver transplant population. *Liver Transpl.* 2004;10:881-885.
149. Astin JA. Why patients use alternative medicine: results of a national study. JAMA. 1998;279:1548-1553.
150. Clinical practice guidelines in complementary and alternative medicine: an analysis of opportunities and obstacles. Practice and Policy Guidelines Panel, National Institutes of Health Office of Alternative Medicine. *Arch Fam Med.* 1997;6:149-154.
151. Knuppel L, Linde K. Adverse effects of St. John's Wort: a systematic review. *J Clin Psychiatry.* 2004;65:1470-1479.
152. Izzo AA. Drug interactions with St. John's wort (Hypericum perforatum): a review of the clinical evidence. *Int J Clin Pharmacol Ther.* 2004;42:139-148.
153. Bauer S, Stormer E, Johne A, et al. Alterations in cyclosporin A pharmacokinetics and metabolism during treatment with St John's wort in renal transplant patients. *Br J Clin Pharmacol.* 2003;55:203-211.
154. Bolley R, Zulke C, Kammerl M, Fischereder M, Kramer BK. Tacrolimus-induced nephrotoxicity unmasked by induction of the CYP3A4 system with St John's wort. *Transplantation.* 2002;73:1009.
155. Moschella C, Jaber BL. Interaction between cyclosporine and *Hypericum perforatum* (St. John's wort) after organ transplantation. *Am J Kidney Dis.* 2001;38:1105-1107.
156. Barone GW, Gurley BJ, Ketel BL, Abul-Ezz SR. Herbal supplements: a potential for drug interactions in transplant recipients. *Transplantation.* 2001;71:239-241.
157. Barone GW, Gurley BJ, Ketel BL, Lightfoot ML, Abul-Ezz SR. Drug interaction between St. John's wort and cyclosporine. *Ann Pharmacother.* 2000;34:1013-1016.
158. Turton-Weeks SM, Barone GW, Gurley BJ, Ketel BL, Lightfoot ML, Abul-Ezz SR. St John's wort: a hidden risk for transplant patients. *Prog Transplant.* 2001;11:116-120.
159. Prasad GV, Wong T, Meliton G, Bhaloo S. Rhabdomyolysis due to red yeast rice (Monascus purpureus) in a renal transplant recipient. *Transplantation.* 2002;74:1200-1201.
160. Egashira K, Fukuda E, Onga T, et al. Pomelo-induced increase in the blood level of tacrolimus in a renal transplant patient. *Transplantation.* 2003;75:1057.
161. Hermann M, Asberg A, Reubsaet JL, Sather S, Berg KJ, Christensen H. Intake of grapefruit juice alters the metabolic pattern of cyclosporin A in renal transplant recipients. *Int J Clin Pharmacol Ther.* 2002;40:451-456.

162. Bistrup C, Nielsen FT, Jeppesen UE, Dieperink H. Effect of grapefruit juice on Sandimmun Neoral absorption among stable renal allograft recipients. *Nephrol Dial Transplant.* 2001;16:373-377.
163. Brunner LJ, Munar MY, Vallian J, et al. Interaction between cyclosporine and grapefruit juice requires long-term ingestion in stable renal transplant recipients. *Pharmacotherapy.* 1998;18:23-29.
164. Brunner LJ, Pai KS, Munar MY, Lande MB, Olyaei AJ, Mowry JA. Effect of grapefruit juice on cyclosporin A pharmacokinetics in pediatric renal transplant patients. *Pediatr Transplant.* 2000;4:313-321.
165. Ameer B, Weintraub RA. Drug interactions with grapefruit juice. *Clin Pharmacokinet.* 1997;33:103-121.
166. Hollander AA, van Rooij J, Lentjes GW, et al. The effect of grapefruit juice on cyclosporine and prednisone metabolism in transplant patients. *Clin Pharmacol Ther.* 1995;57:318-324.
167. Singh YN. Potential for interaction of kava and St. John's wort with drugs. *J Ethnopharmacol.* 2005;100:108-113.
168. Jorge OA, Jorge AD. Hepatotoxicity associated with the ingestion of Centella asiatica. *Rev Esp Enferm Dig.* 2005;97:115-124.
169. Aniya Y, Koyama T, Miyagi C, et al. Free radical scavenging and hepatoprotective actions of the medicinal herb, Crassocephalum crepidioides from the Okinawa Islands. *Biol Pharm Bull.* 2005;28:19-23.
170. Myagmar BE, Shinno E, Ichiba T, Aniya Y. Antioxidant activity of medicinal herb Rhodococcum vitis-idaea on galactosamine-induced liver injury in rats. *Phytomedicine.* 2004;11:416-423.
171. Bielory L. Complementary and alternative interventions in asthma, allergy, and immunology. *Ann Allergy Asthma Immunol.* 2004;93(2 suppl 1):S45-S54.
172. Anke J, Ramzan I. Kava hepatotoxicity: are we any closer to the truth? *Planta Med.* 2004;70:193-196.
173. Schiano TD. Hepatotoxicity and complementary and alternative medicines. *Clin Liver Dis.* 2003;7:453-473.
174. Abebe W. Herbal medication: potential for adverse interactions with analgesic drugs. *J Clin Pharm Ther.* 2002;27:391-401.
175. Dourakis SP, Papanikolaou IS, Tzemanakis EN, Hadziyannis SJ. Acute hepatitis associated with herb (*Teucrium capitatum* L.) administration. *Eur J Gastroenterol Hepatol.* 2002;14:693-695.
176. Stedman C. Herbal hepatotoxicity. *Semin Liver Dis.* 2002;22:195-206.
177. Cheng B, Hung CT, Chiu W. Herbal medicine and anaesthesia. *Hong Kong Med J.* 2002;8:123-130.
178. Miller LG. Herbal medicinals: selected clinical considerations focusing on known or potential drug-herb interactions. *Arch Intern Med.* 1998;158:2200-2211.
179. Batchelor WB, Heathcote J, Wanless IR. Chaparral-induced hepatic injury. *Am J Gastroenterol.* 1995;90:831-833.
180. Lin SC, Lin CC, Lin YH, Shyuu SJ. Hepatoprotective effects of Taiwan folk medicine: *Wedelia chinensis* on three hepatotoxin-induced hepatotoxicity. *Am J Chin Med.* 1994;22:155-168.
181. Kassler WJ, Blanc P, Greenblatt R. The use of medicinal herbs by human immunodeficiency virus-infected patients. *Arch Intern Med.* 1991;151:2281-2288.
182. Ridker PN, McDermont WV. Hepatotoxicity due to comfrey herb tea. *Am J Med.* 1989;87:701.
183. Sullivan JB, Jr., Rumack BH, Thomas H, Jr., Peterson RG, Bryson P. Pennyroyal oil poisoning and hepatotoxicity. *JAMA.* 1979;242:2873-2874.
184. Leape LL, Brennan TA, Laird N, et al. The nature of adverse events in hospitalized patients: Results of the Harvard Medical Practice Study II. *N Engl J Med.* 1991;324:377-384.
185. Lord GM, Cook T, Arlt VM, Schmeiser HH, Williams G, Pusey CD. Urothelial malignant disease and Chinese herbal nephropathy. *Lancet.* 2001;358:1515-1516.
186. Lord GM, Tagore R, Cook T, Gower P, Pusey CD. Nephropathy caused by Chinese herbs in the UK. *Lancet.* 1999;354:481-482.
187. Katz SA, Salem H. The toxicology of chromium with respect to its chemical speciation: a review. *J Appl Toxicol.* 1993;13:217-224.
188. Fristedt B, Lindqvist B, Schuetz A, Ovrum P. Survival in a case of acute oral chromic acid poisoning with acute renal failure treated by haemodialysis. *Acta Med Scand.* 1965;177:153-159.
189. van Heerden PV, Jenkins IR, Woods WP, Rossi E, Cameron PD. Death by tanning: a case of fatal basic chromium sulphate poisoning. *Intensive Care Med.* 1994;20:145-147.
190. Cerulli J, Grabe DW, Gauthier I, Malone M, McGoldrick MD. Chromium picolinate toxicity. *Ann Pharmacother.* 1998;32:428-431.
191. Wasser WG, Feldman NS, D'Agati VD. Chronic renal failure after ingestion of over-the-counter chromium picolinate. *Ann Intern Med.* 1997;126:410.
192. Mullins RJ, Heddle R. Adverse reactions associated with echinacea: the Australian experience. *Ann Allergy Asthma Immunol.* 2002;88:42-51.
193. Conz PA, La Greca G, Benedetti P, Bevilacqua PA, Cima L. Fucus vesiculosus: a nephrotoxic alga? *Nephrol Dial Transplant.* 1998;13:526-527.
194. Walkiw O, Douglas DE. Health food supplements prepared from kelp--a source of elevated urinary arsenic. *Clin Toxicol.* 1975;8:325-331.
195. Luck BE, Mann H, Melzer H, Dunemann L, Begerow J. Renal and other organ failure caused by germanium intoxication. *Nephrol Dial Transplant.* 1999;14:2464-2468.
196. Schauss AG. Nephrotoxicity in humans by the ultratrace element germanium. *Ren Fail.* 1991;13:1-4.

197. Takeuchi A, Yoshizawa N, Oshima S, et al. Nephrotoxicity of germanium compounds: report of a case and review of the literature. *Nephron.* 1992;60:436-442.
198. Bakerink JA, Gospe SM Jr, Dimand RJ, Eldridge MW. Multiple organ failure after ingestion of pennyroyal oil from herbal tea in two infants. *Pediatrics.* 1996;98:944-947.
199. Mack RB. "Boldly they rode ... into the mouth of hell." Pennyroyal oil toxicity. *N C Med J.* 1997;58:456-457.
200. Anderson IB, Mullen WH, Meeker JE, et al. Pennyroyal toxicity: measurement of toxic metabolite levels in two cases and review of the literature. *Ann Intern Med.* 1996;124:726-734.
201. Black M, Hussain H. Hydrazine, cancer, the Internet, isoniazid, and the liver. *Ann Intern Med.* 2000;133:911-913.
202. Hainer MI, Tsai N, Komura ST, Chiu CL. Fatal hepatorenal failure associated with hydrazine sulfate. *Ann Intern Med.* 2000;133:877-880.
203. Sotaniemi E, Hirvonen J, Isomaki H, Takkunen J, Kaila J. Hydrazine toxicity in the human: report of a fatal case. *Ann Clin Res.* 1971;3:30-33.
204. Sheikh NM, Philen RM, Love LA. Chaparral-associated hepatotoxicity. *Arch Intern Med.* 1997;157:913-919.
205. Smith AY, Feddersen RM, Gardner KD Jr, Davis CJ Jr. Cystic renal cell carcinoma and acquired renal cystic disease associated with consumption of chaparral tea: a case report. *J Urol.* 1994;152(6 Pt 1):2089-2091.
206. Evan AP, Gardner KD Jr. Nephron obstruction in nordihydroguaiaretic acid-induced renal cystic disease. *Kidney Int.* 1979;15:7-19.
207. Goodman T, Grice HC, Becking GC, Salem FA. A cystic nephropathy induced by nordihydroguaiaretic acid in the rat: light and electron microscopic investigations. *Lab Invest.* 1970;23:93-107.
208. Schmid B, Kotter I, Heide L. Pharmacokinetics of salicin after oral administration of a standardised willow bark extract. *Eur J Clin Pharmacol.* 2001;57:387-391.
209. D'Agati V. Does aspirin cause acute or chronic renal failure in experimental animals and in humans? *Am J Kidney Dis.* 1996;28(1 suppl 1):S24-S29.
210. Schwarz A. Beethoven's renal disease based on his autopsy: a case of papillary necrosis. *Am J Kidney Dis.* 1993;21:643-652.
211. Lin JL, Ho YS. Flavonoid-induced acute nephropathy. *Am J Kidney Dis.* 1994;23:433-440.
212. Samal KK, Sahu HK, Kar MK, Palit SK, Kar BC, Sahu CS. Yellow oleander (*Cerbera thevetia*) poisoning with jaundice and renal failure. *J Assoc Physicians India.* 1989;37:232-233.
213. Chou WC, Wu CC, Yang PC, Lee YT. Hypovolemic shock and mortality after ingestion of Tripterygium wilfordii hook F: a case report. *Int J Cardiol.* 1995;49:173-177.
214. Hilepo JN, Bellucci AG, Mossey RT. Acute renal failure caused by "cat's claw" herbal remedy in a patient with systemic lupus erythematosus. *Nephron.* 1997;77:361.
215. Boniel T, Dannon P. [The safety of herbal medicines in the psychiatric practice]. *Harefuah.* 2001;140:780-783, 805.
216. Goldberg SH, Von Feldt JM, Lonner JH. Pharmacologic therapy for osteoarthritis. *Am J Orthop.* 2002;31:673-680.
217. Morelli V, Naquin C, Weaver V. Alternative therapies for traditional disease states: osteoarthritis. *Am Fam Physician.* 2003;67:339-344.
218. Pavelka K, Gatterova J, Olejarova M, Machacek S, Giacovelli G, Rovati LC. Glucosamine sulfate use and delay of progression of knee osteoarthritis: a 3-year, randomized, placebo-controlled, double-blind study. *Arch Intern Med.* 2002;162:2113-2123.
219. Guillaume MP, Peretz A. Possible association between glucosamine treatment and renal toxicity: comment on the letter by Danao-Camara. *Arthritis Rheum.* 2001;44:2943-2944.
220. Danao-Camara T. Potential side effects of treatment with glucosamine and chondroitin. *Arthritis Rheum.* 2000;43:2853.
221. Bastian HP, Vahlensieck W. [Renal function under parenteral application of aescinat (author's transl)]. *Med Klin.* 1976;71:1295-1299.
222. Sandler B, Aronson P. Yohimbine-induced cutaneous drug eruption, progressive renal failure, and lupus-like syndrome. *Urology.* 1993;41:343-345.
223. Hatch M, Mulgrew S, Bourke E, Keogh B, Costello J. Effect of megadoses of ascorbic acid on serum and urinary oxalate. *Eur Urol.* 1980;6:166-169.
224. Alkhunaizi AM, Chan L. Secondary oxalosis: a cause of delayed recovery of renal function in the setting of acute renal failure. *J Am Soc Nephrol.* 1996;7:2320-2326.
225. Friedman AL, Chesney RW, Gilbert EF, Gilchrist KW, Latorraca R, Segar WE. Secondary oxalosis as a complication of parenteral alimentation in acute renal failure. *Am J Nephrol.* 1983;3:248-252.
226. Lawton JM, Conway LT, Crosson JT, Smith CL, Abraham PA. Acute oxalate nephropathy after massive ascorbic acid administration. *Arch Intern Med.* 1985;145:950-951.
227. Mashour S, Turner JF Jr, Merrell R. Acute renal failure, oxalosis, and vitamin C supplementation: a case report and review of the literature. *Chest.* 2000;118:561-563.
228. Ono K. The effect of vitamin C supplementation and withdrawal on the mortality and morbidity of regular hemodialysis patients. *Clin Nephrol.* 1989;31:31-34.
229. Ponka A, Kuhlback B. Serum ascorbic acid in patients undergoing chronic hemodialysis. *Acta Med Scand.* 1983;213:305-307.
230. Pru C, Eaton J, Kjellstrand C. Vitamin C intoxication and hyperoxalemia in chronic hemodialysis patients. *Nephron.* 1985;39:112-116.

231. Swartz RD, Wesley JR, Somermeyer MG, Lau K. Hyperoxaluria and renal insufficiency due to ascorbic acid administration during total parenteral nutrition. *Ann Intern Med*. 1984;100:530-531.
232. Wong K, Thomson C, Bailey RR, McDiarmid S, Gardner J. Acute oxalate nephropathy after a massive intravenous dose of vitamin C. *Aust N Z J Med*. 1994;24:410-411.
233. Powell T, Hsu FF, Turk J, Hruska K. Ma-huang strikes again: ephedrine nephrolithiasis. *Am J Kidney Dis*. 1998;32:153-159.
234. Blau JJ. Ephedrine nephrolithiasis associated with chronic ephedrine abuse. *J Urol*. 1998;160(3 Pt 1):825.
235. Farre M, Xirgu J, Salgado A, Peracaula R, Reig R, Sanz P. Fatal oxalic acid poisoning from sorrel soup. *Lancet*. 1989;2:1524.
236. Terris MK, Issa MM, Tacker JR. Dietary supplementation with cranberry concentrate tablets may increase the risk of nephrolithiasis. *Urology*. 2001;57:26-29.
237. Weisbord SD, Soule JB, Kimmel PL. Poison on line--acute renal failure caused by oil of wormwood purchased through the Internet. *N Engl J Med*. 1997;337:825-827.
238. Kraemer WJ, Volek JS. Creatine supplementation. Its role in human performance. *Clin Sports Med*. 1999;18:651-666, ix.
239. Kuklo TR, Tis JE, Moores LK, Schaefer RA. Fatal rhabdomyolysis with bilateral gluteal, thigh, and leg compartment syndrome after the Army Physical Fitness Test: a case report. *Am J Sports Med*. 2000;28:112-116.
240. Robinson SJ. Acute quadriceps compartment syndrome and rhabdomyolysis in a weight lifter using high-dose creatine supplementation. *J Am Board Fam Pract*. 2000;13:134-137.
241. Sandhu RS, Como JJ, Scalea TS, Betts JM. Renal failure and exercise-induced rhabdomyolysis in patients taking performance-enhancing compounds. *J Trauma*. 2002;53:761-763; discussion 3-4.
242. Koshy KM, Griswold E, Schneeberger EE. Interstitial nephritis in a patient taking creatine. *N Engl J Med*. 1999;340:814-815.
243. Pritchard NR, Kalra PA. Renal dysfunction accompanying oral creatine supplements. *Lancet*. 1998;351:1252-1253.
244. Poortmans JR, Auquier H, Renaut V, Durussel A, Saugy M, Brisson GR. Effect of short-term creatine supplementation on renal responses in men. *Eur J Appl Physiol Occup Physiol*. 1997;76:566-567.
245. Poortmans JR, Francaux M. Long-term oral creatine supplementation does not impair renal function in healthy athletes. *Med Sci Sports Exerc*. 1999;31:1108-1110.
246. Robinson TM, Sewell DA, Casey A, Steenge G, Greenhaff PL. Dietary creatine supplementation does not affect some haematological indices, or indices of muscle damage and hepatic and renal function. *Br J Sports Med*. 2000;34:284-288.
247. Conn JW, Rovner DR, Cohen EL. Licorice-induced pseudoaldosteronism. Hypertension, hypokalemia, aldosteronopenia, and suppressed plasma renin activity. *JAMA*. 1968;205:492-496.
248. Saito T, Tsuboi Y, Fujisawa G, et al. An autopsy case of licorice-induced hypokalemic rhabdomyolysis associated with acute renal failure: special reference to profound calcium deposition in skeletal and cardiac muscle. *Nippon Jinzo Gakkai Shi*. 1994;36:1308-1314.
249. Ishikawa S, Kato M, Tokuda T, et al. Licorice-induced hypokalemic myopathy and hypokalemic renal tubular damage in anorexia nervosa. *Int J Eat Disord*. 1999;26:111-114.
250. Lo JC, Chertow GM, Rennke H, Seifter JL. Fanconi's syndrome and tubulointerstitial nephritis in association with L-lysine ingestion. *Am J Kidney Dis*. 1996;28:614-617.
251. Melchart D, Linde K, Worku F, et al. Results of five randomized studies on the immunomodulatory activity of preparations of echinacea. *J Altern Complement Med*. 1995;1:145-160.
252. Stimpel M, Proksch A, Wagner H, Lohmann-Matthes ML. Macrophage activation and induction of macrophage cytotoxicity by purified polysaccharide fractions from the plant *Echinacea purpurea*. *Infect Immun*. 1984;46:845-849.
253. Rehman J, Dillow JM, Carter SM, Chou J, Le B, Maisel AS. Increased production of antigen-specific immunoglobulins G and M following in vivo treatment with the medicinal plants *Echinacea angustifolia* and *Hydrastis canadensis*. *Immunol Lett*. 1999;68:391-395.
254. See DM, Broumand N, Sahl L, Tilles JG. In vitro effects of echinacea and ginseng on natural killer and antibody-dependent cell cytotoxicity in healthy subjects and chronic fatigue syndrome or acquired immunodeficiency syndrome patients. *Immunopharmacology*. 1997;35:229-235.
255. Wustenberg P, Henneicke-von Zepelin HH, Kohler G, Stammwitz U. Efficacy and mode of action of an immunomodulator herbal preparation containing echinacea, wild indigo, and white cedar. *Adv Ther*. 1999;16:51-70.
256. Stein GM, Bussing A, Schietzel M. Activation of dendritic cells by an aqueous mistletoe extract and mistletoe lectin-3 in vitro. *Anticancer Res*. 2002;22:267-274.
257. Kovacs E. Serum levels of IL-12 and the production of IFN-gamma, IL-2 and IL-4 by peripheral blood mononuclear cells (PBMC) in cancer patients treated with Viscum album extract. *Biomed Pharmacother*. 2000;54:305-310.
258. Ribereau-Gayon G, Dumont S, Muller C, Jung ML, Poindron P, Anton R. Mistletoe lectins I, II and III induce the production of cytokines by cultured human monocytes. *Cancer Lett*. 1996;109:33-38.
259. Mannel DN, Becker H, Gundt A, Kist A, Franz H. Induction of tumor necrosis factor expression by a lectin from *Viscum album*. *Cancer Immunol Immunother*. 1991;33:177-182.
260. Pae HO, Seo WG, Shin M, Lee HS, Kim SB, Chung HT. Protein kinase A or C modulates the apoptosis induced by lectin II isolated from Korean mistletoe, *Viscum album* var. Coloratum, in the human leukemic HL-60 cells. *Immunopharmacol Immunotoxicol*. 2000;22:279-295.
261. Stein GM, Pfuller U, Schietzel M, Bussing A. Intracellular expression of IL-4 and inhibition of IFN-gamma by extracts from European mistletoe is related to induction of apoptosis. *Anticancer Res*. 2000;20:2987-2994.

262. Scaglione F, Ferrara F, Dugnani S, Falchi M, Santoro G, Fraschini F. Immunomodulatory effects of two extracts of *Panax ginseng* C.A. Meyer. *Drugs Exp Clin Res.* 1990;16:537-542.
263. Wang M, Guilbert LJ, Ling L, et al. Immunomodulating activity of CVT-E002, a proprietary extract from North American ginseng (*Panax quinquefolium*). *J Pharm Pharmacol.* 2001;53:1515-1523.
264. Gao H, Wang F, Lien EJ, Trousdale MD. Immunostimulating polysaccharides from *Panax notoginseng. Pharm Res.* 1996;13:1196-1200.
265. Mossad SB, Macknin ML, Medendorp SV, Mason P. Zinc gluconate lozenges for treating the common cold: a randomized, double-blind, placebo-controlled study. *Ann Intern Med.* 1996;125:81-88.
266. Keen CL, Gershwin ME. Zinc deficiency and immune function. *Annu Rev Nutr.* 1990;10:415-431.
267. Tanaka Y, Shiozawa S, Morimoto I, Fujita T. Zinc inhibits pokeweed mitogen-induced development of immunoglobulin-secreting cells through augmentation of both CD4 and CD8 cells. *Int J Immunopharmacol.* 1989;11:673-679.
268. Driessen C, Hirv K, Rink L, Kirchner H. Induction of cytokines by zinc ions in human peripheral blood mononuclear cells and separated monocytes. *Lymphokine Cytokine Res.* 1994;13:15-20.
269. Salas M, Kirchner H. Induction of interferon-gamma in human leukocyte cultures stimulated by Zn^{2+}. *Clin Immunol Immunopathol.* 1987;45:139-142.
270. Scuderi P. Differential effects of copper and zinc on human peripheral blood monocyte cytokine secretion. *Cell Immunol.* 1990;126:391-405.
271. Chandra RK. Excessive intake of zinc impairs immune responses. *JAMA.* 1984;252:1443-1446.
272. Duchateau J, Delespesse G, Vereecke P. Influence of oral zinc supplementation on the lymphocyte response to mitogens of normal subjects. *Am J Clin Nutr.* 1981;34:88-93.
273. Oka H, Emori Y, Kobayashi N, Hayashi Y, Nomoto K. Suppression of allergic reactions by royal jelly in association with the restoration of macrophage function and the improvement of Th1/Th2 cell responses. *Int Immunopharmacol.* 2001;1:521-532.
274. Sver L, Orsolic N, Tadic Z, Njari B, Valpotic I, Basic I. A royal jelly as a new potential immunomodulator in rats and mice. *Comp Immunol Microbiol Infect Dis.* 1996;19:31-38.
275. Carcamo JM, Borquez-Ojeda O, Golde DW. Vitamin C inhibits granulocyte macrophage-colony-stimulating factor-induced signaling pathways. *Blood.* 2002;99:3205-3212.
276. Sinclair S. Chinese herbs: a clinical review of *Astragalus, Ligusticum,* and *Schizandrae. Altern Med Rev.* 1998;3:338-444.
277. Zhao KS, Mancini C, Doria G. Enhancement of the immune response in mice by *Astragalus membranaceus* extracts. *Immunopharmacology.* 1990;20:225-233.
278. Chu DT, Wong WL, Mavligit GM. Immunotherapy with Chinese medicinal herbs. II. Reversal of cyclophosphamide-induced immune suppression by administration of fractionated *Astragalus membranaceus* in vivo. *J Clin Lab Immunol.* 1988;25:125-129.
279. Sharma ML, Khajuria A, Kaul A, Singh S, Singh GB, Atal CK. Effect of *Salai guggal ex-Boswellia serrata* on cellular and humoral immune responses and leucocyte migration. *Agents Actions.* 1988;24:161-164.
280. Kang BY, Song YJ, Kim KM, Choe YK, Hwang SY, Kim TS. Curcumin inhibits Th1 cytokine profile in $CD4^+$ T cells by suppressing interleukin-12 production in macrophages. *Br J Pharmacol.* 1999;128:380-384.
281. South EH, Exon JH, Hendrix K. Dietary curcumin enhances antibody response in rats. *Immunopharmacol Immunotoxicol.* 1997;19:105-119.
282. Shoskes DA, Jones EA, Shahed A. Synergy of mycophenolate mofetil and bioflavonoids in prevention of immune and ischemic injury. *Transplant Proc.* 2000;32:798-799.
283. Wang SY, Hsu ML, Hsu HC, et al. The anti-tumor effect of *Ganoderma lucidum* is mediated by cytokines released from activated macrophages and T lymphocytes. *Int J Cancer.* 1997;70:699-705.
284. Mayell M. Maitake extracts and their therapeutic potential. *Altern Med Rev.* 2001;6:48-60.
285. Suzuki I, Hashimoto K, Oikawa S, Sato K, Osawa M, Yadomae T. Antitumor and immunomodulating activities of a beta-glucan obtained from liquid-cultured Grifola frondosa. *Chem Pharm Bull (Tokyo).* 1989;37:410-413.
286. Okazaki M, Adachi Y, Ohno N, Yadomae T. Structure-activity relationship of (1-->3)-beta-D-glucans in the induction of cytokine production from macrophages, in vitro. *Biol Pharm Bull.* 1995;18:1320-1327.
287. Shibata S. A drug over the millennia: pharmacognosy, chemistry, and pharmacology of licorice. *Yakugaku Zasshi.* 2000;120:849-862.
288. Lemaire I, Assinewe V, Cano P, Awang DV, Arnason JT. Stimulation of interleukin-1 and -6 production in alveolar macrophages by the neotropical liana, *Uncaria tomentosa* (una de gato). *J Ethnopharmacol.* 1999;64:109-115.

Understanding Laboratory Values

Sharon M. Augustine, RN, MS, CRNP
Suzanne Lanks, RN, MS, CRNP
Carol Wade, RN, MS, CRNP

Transplant clinicians rely heavily on laboratory data to screen for, diagnose, and monitor disease and infection, to determine the effectiveness and side effects of medications, and to measure drug levels. The purpose of this chapter is to review laboratory tests, factors related to the procedures, and clinical implications that can be gleaned from the information the tests provide. Routine tests such as complete blood count, basic and comprehensive metabolic panels, serological tests, and cultures are reviewed. Normal levels for adults are printed in parentheses after each test but vary depending on the laboratory where the test is done and the patient's age.

The information regarding routine chemistries and complete blood count is straightforward. Information from LeFever Kee,[1] Nicoll et al,[2] and Chernecky and Berger[3] was used to synthesize a concise review.

Complete Blood Count

The complete blood count is an assessment of the red and white blood cell components done to evaluate for the presence of infection and anemia. Serial values are used to monitor the progress of various diseases and the side effects of medications that cause bone marrow suppression that leads to blood dyscrasias.

Red Blood Cell Count *(Males 4.6-6.0 mill/mcL and females 4.0-5.0 mill/mcL*

Most peripheral blood cells are red blood cells (RBCs). They have a life span of about 120 days, are formed by red bone marrow, and are removed from the blood by the liver, spleen, and bone marrow. They are involved in hemoglobin transport to deliver oxygen to tissues.

Mean corpuscular volume is the average size of RBCs. The mean corpuscular volume is elevated when RBCs are larger than normal (macrocytic), for example, in patients with anemia caused by vitamin B_{12} deficiency. When the mean corpuscular volume is decreased, RBCs are smaller than normal (microcytic), as occurs in iron deficiency anemia. Mean corpuscular hemoglobin is a calculation of the average amount of oxygen-carrying hemoglobin inside 1 RBC, usually given in picograms. Because macrocytic RBCs are larger than either normal or microcytic RBCs, they also tend to have higher mean corpuscular hemoglobin values. Mean corpuscular hemoglobin concentration is a calculation of the concentration of hemoglobin inside the RBCs, usually given in grams per liter. Red cell distribution width is a calculation of the variation in the size of RBCs. In some anemias, such as pernicious anemia, the amount of variation in RBC size (anisocytosis) along with variation in shape (poikilocytosis) causes an increase in the red cell distribution width.

Hemoglobin *(Males 13.5-17.0 g/dL, females 12.0-15.0 g/dL)*

Hemoglobin is the oxygen-carrying pigment of the RBCs. It is made up of amino acids that form the protein "globulin" and the compound "heme," which contains iron atoms and the red pigment porphyrin.

UNDERSTANDING LABORATORY VALUES

Hematocrit *(Males 0.40-0.52, females 0.35-0.47)*

Hematocrit is the proportion of RBCs in a volume of whole blood relative to plasma. Hematocrit and hemoglobin level may be decreased in patients who have mechanical ventricular assist devices, indicating a hemolytic anemia. Adjustment of device settings or of anticoagulation therapy may rectify this problem.

Reticulocyte Count *(25×10^9/L to 75×10^9/L, or 0.5%-1.5% of all RBCs)*

Reticulocytes are immature nonnucleated RBCs that are formed in the bone marrow and then passed into the circulation. Reticulocytes become matured RBCs 1 to 2 days later. Assessing reticulocyte count is helpful for diagnosing anemias. An increased level indicates that the marrow is responding. Total absolute reticulocyte count is calculated by multiplying the proportion of reticulocytes by the RBC count (eg, $0.005 \times 4.6 \times 10^{12}$/L).

White Blood Cell Count *(4,500 to 11,000/mm³)*

White blood cells (leukocytes) are either mononuclear (monocytes and lymphocytes) or polymorphonuclear (neutrophils, eosinophils, and basophils). White blood cells function as part of the body's defense system by responding immediately to foreign invaders. Assessment for leukopenia or leukocytosis is done to detect the presence of infection or inflammation. Aspirin, some antibiotics, streptomycin, and steroids can increase white blood cell count. Differential white blood cell count includes 5 types of leukocytes (Table 1).

Table 1. DIFFERENTIAL WHITE BLOOD CELL COUNT

Type	Percentage of White Blood Cells	Function
Granulocytes		
1. Neutrophils	50-70	Also known as polymorphonuclear leukocytes ("polys") or segmented neutrophils or ("segs")
Segments	50-65	Short-lived, respond rapidly to inflammation and tissue injury by phagocytosis
Bands	0-5	Immature neutrophils that multiply quickly during acute infection
2. Eosinophils	1-3	Suppression of inflammation and destruction of certain parasites; increased steroids (endogenous or exogenous) will decrease the number of eosinophils
3. Basophils	0.4-1.0	Have high concentrations of heparin and histamine; when released, result in vascular permeability, smooth muscle spasm, and vasodilatation. If release of histamines severe, anaphylaxis can result
Nongranulocytes		
4. Monocytes	4-6	Second line of defense against bacterial infection and foreign substances; slower but stronger than neutrophils; when monocytes mature, they leave cells and enters tissue as macrophages
5. Lymphocytes	25-35	Cells of acquired immunity (adaptive immunity)
B cells		Antigen-specific receptors on B cells are called membrane antibodies or membrane immunoglobulins; when activated, some differentiate into plasma cells, which secrete antibodies (vs. expressing on cell surface); secreted antibodies are soluble proteins called humoral factors
T cells		
Helper T		Secrete soluble proteins (humoral factors) called cytokines required for immune responses
Cytotoxic T		Kill virally infected host cells

Platelets *(150,000 to 400,000/mcL)*

Platelets (or thrombocytes) are cells in the blood that promote coagulation. Thrombocytopenia is associated with bleeding, and thrombocytosis is associated with increased clotting.

Coagulation Factors

Coagulation factors are important in patients with ventricular assist devices and in patients requiring anticoagulation for other disease processes (eg, pulmonary embolus, deep vein thrombosis) that are common in this transplantation population.

Prothrombin is synthesized in the liver and is an inactive precursor involved in clotting of blood. Prothrombin time is used predominately to monitor anticoagulation therapy. International normalized ratio is a way of reporting prothrombin time that is based on international standardization.

Partial thromboplastin time is used to detect deficiencies in all clotting factors except factors VII and XIII and also to detect platelet variation. Activated partial thromboplastin time (APTT) is more sensitive than partial thromboplastin time because the activator shortens the clotting time.

Coagulation times are the most sensitive laboratory indices of liver function. Abnormality in liver function is reflected by prolonged coagulation times. Postoperatively, especially in liver transplant recipients, values vary depending on preoperative levels and occurrences during surgery, but a steady downward trend toward normal levels is expected.[4]

Free Hemoglobin in Plasma

Hemoglobin that escapes from erythrocytes during hemolysis is referred to as free hemoglobin. Although small amounts of free hemoglobin are normal, elevated levels are seen in the blood and urine after massive hemolysis. In conjunction with measurement of levels of bilirubin and lactate dehydrogenase, measurement of free hemoglobin in the plasma is used to evaluate for the presence of hemolysis due to hemolytic anemia syndromes, medications, or as a direct result of shear force from mechanical blood pumping in patients with ventricular assist devices.

Basic and Comprehensive Metabolic Panel

Tests included in the basic metabolic panel are measurements of the level of sodium, potassium, chloride, carbon dioxide, urea nitrogen, creatinine, glucose, and calcium. The comprehensive metabolic panel further includes measurements of levels of protein, albumin, aspartate aminotransferase and alanine aminotransferase, total bilirubin, and alkaline phosphatase. Normal reference values for adults are reported in parentheses after each specific test.

Chemistries

Sodium, Na+ *(135-145 mmol/L)*

Sodium is the major cation of extracellular fluid. It primarily is involved with maintaining osmotic pressures and acid-base balance as well as transmitting nerve impulses. Normally, sodium content remains fairly constant despite wide variations in sodium intake. Sodium is absorbed from the small intestine and excreted in the urine. Decreases in sodium can be divided into hypovolemic, euvolemic, and hypervolemic hyponatremia (Table 2). In general, treatment of sodium imbalances relies on assessment of extracellular fluid volume rather than serum levels of sodium.

Table 2. THREE TYPES OF HYPONATREMIA AND THEIR FEATURES

Type	Features
Hypovolemic	Sodium and free water are lost and replaced by hypotonic fluids
Euvolemic	Normal sodium level with an excess of total body free water
Hypervolemic	Inappropriately increased sodium stores: this can result from acute or chronic renal failure when dysfunctional kidneys are unable to excrete dietary sodium load or when intravascular volume responses are ineffective

Hyponatremia in renal transplant recipients can result from the decreased concentrating abilities of the transplanted kidney immediately after transplantation.[4]

Potassium, K+ (3.5-5.0 mmol/L)

Potassium is the predominant intracellular cation. Potassium is obtained through dietary ingestion, and its plasma level is regulated by renal excretion. Plasma potassium concentration determines neuromuscular irritability and affects muscle contraction as well as acid-base balance. Increased levels are noted during massive hemolysis, severe tissue damage, rhabdomyolysis, acidosis, dehydration, and acute or chronic renal failure. Hyperkalemia seen in the liver transplant population indicates cell death with release of intracellular potassium into the circulation.[5] Increased levels of potassium may also be seen with delayed functioning in kidney transplant recipients, which may be compounded by administration of blood.[4] Care should be taken with administration of drugs that cause hyperkalemia, such as potassium salts, potassium-sparing diuretics (eg, spironolactone, triamterine), calcineurin inhibitors, nonsteroidal anti-inflammatory drugs, β-blockers, angiotensin-converting enzyme inhibitors, and high-dose sulfamethoxazole. Very high white blood cell counts or platelet counts can cause falsely high measurements of serum level of potassium when levels are normal. Low dietary intake, prolonged vomiting or diarrhea, and renal tubular acidosis commonly promote hypokalemia. It is not unusual for liver transplant recipients to experience hypokalemia during the early postoperative period. Potassium-rich preservation solution is used to flush the liver, which causes an osmotic shift from the interstitial space into the cell. Renal transplant recipients are at risk for hypokalemia when initial function occurs with rapid diuresis. Drugs such as adrenergic agents, diuretics, steroids, insulin, laxatives, and aspirin commonly cause hypokalemia as well.

Chloride (Cl-) (97-107 mmol/L)

As the predominant anion in extracellular fluid, it counterbalances cations such as sodium and is important in maintaining normal acid-base balance and osmolality. It is obtained through dietary ingestion, mostly in combination with sodium. Bicarbonate ingestion, steroids, and diuretics can reduce chloride levels

Carbon Dioxide, Total Bicarbonate (22-30 mmol/L)

Total carbon dioxide level refers to the total amount of carbon dioxide (in solution bound to proteins as bicarbonate, carbonate, and carbonic acid) and is a general reflection of the body's buffering capacity. Total carbon dioxide is a bicarbonate and base solution and is regulated by the kidneys. Carbon dioxide gas is acidic and regulated by the lungs. Approximately 80% of carbon dioxide is present in the form of bicarbonate, and this test is used as a surrogate for bicarbonate concentration. Carbon dioxide levels are elevated in primary metabolic alkalosis, compensated respiratory acidosis, and volume contraction. Diuretics, steroids, antacids, and sodium bicarbonate are common drugs that can contribute to elevated levels.

Carbon dioxide is decreased in metabolic acidosis and compensated respiratory alkalosis. Chlorothiazide diuretics may contribute to decreased levels of carbon dioxide.

Urea Nitrogen (1.8-8.9 mmol/L [5-25 mg/dL])

Although commonly referred to as blood urea nitrogen, this test is actually performed on either plasma or serum. The nitrogen portion of urea is formed in the liver through a process of protein breakdown. Normally, urea is filtered through the renal glomeruli and excreted in the urine. A small amount is reabsorbed in the tubules, and this amount is inversely related to the rate of urine formation. Thus, urea nitrogen is a less useful measure of glomerular filtration rate (GFR) than is serum level of creatinine. An elevated level of urea nitrogen in the blood is referred to as azotemia, but the cause should be further delineated into prerenal, renal, or postrenal (Table 3). Uremia refers to extremely high levels of urea in the blood (>71 mmol/L [200 mg/dL]). In severe hepatic disease, the liver may not be able to synthesize urea from protein breakdown. This results in low urea nitrogen levels and elevated ammonia levels, leading to hepatic encephalopathy.[3] Drugs that can affect levels include various nephrotoxic (eg, some antibiotics,

Table 3. DELINEATION OF AZOTEMIA

Type	Cause
Prerenal	Factors resulting in inadequate renal blood flow, or conditions causing high levels of protein in the blood
Renal	Impaired renal filtration and excretion
Postrenal	Problems in the lower urinary tract such as obstruction

nonsteroidal anti-inflammatory drugs). Nephrotoxic drugs are especially significant in transplant recipients because most are treated with a calcineurin inhibitor (eg, cyclosporine or tacrolimus). Serum urea nitrogen, in junction with creatinine, is important to monitor in transplant recipients because of the nephrotoxic effects of calcineurin inhibitors. Careful management of medications after transplantation can be very challenging.

Creatinine (44-133 µmol/L [0.5-1.5 mg/dL])

Creatinine is derived from the breakdown of muscle creatine and creatine phosphate. The amount of creatinine produced is proportional to muscle mass. Creatinine is consistently excreted by the renal system via glomerular filtration and tubular secretion; therefore, increased levels of creatinine indicate a slowing of glomerular filtration. Creatinine is therefore a very specific indicator of renal function. Females may be expected to have slightly lower levels of creatinine because of their lower muscle mass. For approximately every doubling in serum creatinine level, GFR is reduced approximately 50%. Drugs contributing to increases in creatinine level include some antibiotics, nonsteroidal anti-inflammatory drugs, and any drug that is nephrotoxic. As with urea nitrogen, calcineurin inhibitors have nephrotoxic effects and are synergistic with other nephrotoxic drugs.

Glucose (3.3-6.1 mmol/L [60-110 mg/dL]

Glucose is formed in the body by digestion of carbohydrates and conversion of glycogen by the liver. It is the main source of cellular energy and is essential for brain and erythrocyte function. Excess glucose is stored as glycogen in liver and muscle. Normally the glucose concentration in extracellular fluid is tightly regulated to maintain a ready source of energy and no glucose is excreted in urine. A fasting blood glucose level of greater than 7 mmol/L (126 mg/dL) on more than one occasion is diagnostic for diabetes mellitus.[6]

Hyperglycemia in a new liver transplant recipient is an indication that the liver is functioning well and able to convert glucose into glycogen.[5] Drug-induced hyperglycemia due to corticosteroids, tacrolimus, and cyclosporine is common in transplant recipients.

Calcium Total (Serum 2.25-2.75 mmol/L [9-11 mg/dL], ionized 1.1-1.3 mmol/L [4.25-5.25 mg/dL])

Calcium is absorbed into the bloodstream from dietary sources. The functions of calcium include bone formation, transmission of nerve impulses, contraction of myocardial and skeletal muscle, and blood clotting. Calcium is stored in the bones and teeth, and circulating calcium is filtered by the kidneys. Normally 46% to 50% of total calcium is ionized (free or unbound), and most of the remainder is in the form of calcium-ligand complexes. Only ionized calcium can be used by the body. Parathyroid hormone and vitamin D are hormones that control calcium levels. A decrease in free (ionized) calcium stimulates the release of parathyroid hormone, which causes a release of calcium from bone and decreases loss through kidneys. Parathyroid hormone in turn stimulates vitamin D, which increases calcium absorption in the intestines and also decreases loss through the kidneys. In general, as vitamin D levels increase, calcium levels increase and parathyroid hormone level decreases. Total calcium levels vary directly in association with serum albumin, but ionized calcium does not. The level of ionized calcium increases with a decrease in blood pH and decreases with an increase in pH and hypoalbuminemia. Thiazide diuretics are the most common drug-induced cause for hypercalcemia.

Protein (serum 60-80 g/L)

Serum proteins are important in the regulation of colloid osmotic pressure. They comprise mostly albumin and globulins.

Albumin (serum 35-50 g/L)

One of the 2 components of protein, albumin is synthesized by the liver and maintains oncotic pressure. A decrease in serum level of albumin causes fluid to shift into tissues and results in edema. Protein is normally essentially reabsorbed by the kidney.

Aspartate aminotransferase (20-48 U/L)

This intracellular enzyme is involved in amino acid metabolism. It is found mainly in the heart, liver, and skeletal muscle and is released into the bloodstream during tissue damage. In liver disease, serum levels increase 10-fold or more.

Alanine aminotransferase (10-40 U/L)

Alanine aminotransferase is an intracellular enzyme involved in amino acid metabolism, found mainly in liver cells but also in heart, kidneys, pancreas, and skeletal muscle. Levels of alanine aminotransferase may increase 50-fold in patients with liver damage. Alanine aminotransferase is generally assessed in conjunction with aspartate aminotransferase to evaluate degree of liver disease.

Increases in levels of transaminases are commonly seen in cases of liver dysfunction such as acute viral hepatitis (alanine aminotransferase > aspartate aminotransferase), biliary tract obstruction, alcoholic hepatitis, and cirrhosis (aspartate aminotransferase > alanine aminotransferase), and passive failure due to right-sided heart failure, ischemia, or hypoxia. In patients who have had organ transplants, calcineurin inhibitors (tacrolimus and cyclosporine) are hepatotoxic and thus may be synergistically damaging in combination with other hepatotoxic drugs. In liver transplant recipients, elevations in levels of liver transaminases may suggest hepatocellular necrosis. Mild dysfunction may be manifested by significant increases in transaminase levels postoperatively (>2500 U) as a result of preservation injury with a second peak within 24 hours, which may be due to reperfusion injury. If the trend is not downward after the first 24 hours after transplantation, further assessment should be provided.

Bilirubin (Total 2-21 µmol/L [0.1-1.2 mg/dL], direct 1.7-5.1 µmol/L [0.1-0.3 mg/dL], indirect 1.7-17.1 µmol/L [0.1-1.0 mg/dL]

Bilirubin, formed from the breakdown of hemoglobin, is carried to the liver and conjugated (directly) and excreted in the bile. Bilirubin occurs in 2 forms: direct or conjugated (soluble), which is primarily excreted through the intestinal tract, and unconjugated or indirect (protein bound), which primarily circulates intravascularly. Jaundice is often noticed if the total bilirubin level is greater than 51 µmol/L (3 mg/dL). When obstruction or hepatic jaundice occurs, increasing amounts of direct bilirubin remain in the circulation and are filtered and excreted by the kidneys. With hemolysis, increasing amounts of direct bilirubin accumulate in the bloodstream as a result of increased hemoglobin breakdown. Indirect bilirubin is a calculated number (total bilirubin minus direct bilirubin). Increased bilirubin may be a sign of rejection or biliary tract complications in liver transplant recipients. If the bilirubin level is greater than 51 µmol/L (3 mg/dL), the patient may appear jaundiced. Increased levels of direct bilirubin are usually the result of an obstruction, whereas increased levels of indirect bilirubin are associated with hemolysis.

Alkaline Phosphatase (42-136 U/L)

Alkaline phosphatase is an enzyme found mainly in bone and liver, but also produced in the intestines, kidney, and placenta. Its levels tend to increase during periods of bone disease, liver disease, and bile duct obstruction.

Magnesium 0.74-1.23 mmol/L [1.8-3.0 mg/dL])

Magnesium is the second most abundant intracellular cation. Most magnesium is concentrated in the bone, cartilage, and within cells. Magnesium absorbed through the intestines is excreted through stool, and the unabsorbed magnesium is eventually excreted through the kidneys, thus the concentration of magnesium is determined by intestinal absorption, renal excretion, and exchange with bone and intracellular fluid. Magnesium influences use of potassium, calcium, and protein. The potentiating effects of cyclosporine with other calcium-wasting drugs should be avoided or carefully monitored.

Transplant recipients, especially kidney transplant recipients, are prone to electrolyte imbalances due to the effects of cyclosporine and tacrolimus on the renal tubules. Sodium retention, hyperkalemia, acidosis, hypomagnesemia, and hypophosphatemia often occur and should be anticipated.

Miscellaneous

Creatinine Clearance/Urinary Protein

Creatinine is excreted via glomerular filtration and by tubular excretion. Assessment of creatinine clearance involves measurement of a blood sample and a urine sample to determine the rate at which creatinine is being cleared from the circulation. It is thus a common and acceptable measure of glomerular filtration, although it sometimes leads to overestimates of GFR. Creatinine clearance is decreased with decreased muscle mass and can be affected by several drugs, including steroids, thiazides, and cefoxitin. Creatinine clearance is also invalidated if the samples are not kept refrigerated or if an inaccurate volume is recorded. Therefore, the National Kidney Foundation recommends estimation of GFR by using prediction equations rather than traditional creatinine clearance because of problems associated with 24-hour creatinine clearance tests.[7,8] Levey et al[8] concluded that the equation developed from the Modification of Diet in Renal Disease Study provided a more accurate estimate of GFR in patients with chronic renal disease than did measured creatinine clearance or other commonly used equations such as the Cockroft-Gault equation:

$$GFR = \frac{(140 - age) \times body\ weight\ in\ kilograms}{Serum\ creatinine\ level\ in\ milligrams\ per\ deciliter \times 72}$$

The quadratic GFR equation (derived from the original equation from the Modification of Diet in Renal Disease Study) is recommended as the best equation because it is based on a combined sample of healthy patients and patients with chronic kidney disease.[9] Because of problems similar to the problems with use of 24-hour urine collection for assessment of creatinine clearance, assessment of proteinuria in an untimed urine specimen has replaced protein excretion in a 24-hour collection as the preferred method of measurement.[8] If 24-hour specimens are ordered, however, it is important to explain as clearly as possible the requirements for an accurate result. Specifically, ask the patient to empty his or her bladder upon waking and discard the urine. From that point forward, save all urine for the next 24 hours. The specimen should be refrigerated or kept on ice. If the patient mistakenly discards a portion of the urine output, the test must be restarted.

Glycosylated Hemoglobin

Glycosylated hemoglobin is blood glucose bound to hemoglobin. Three portions of hemoglobin exist: A_{1a}, A_{1b}, and A_{1c}. Hemoglobin A_{1c}, the predominant hemoglobin fraction, is formed as hemoglobin is glycosylated slowly over 120 days, the lifespan of the RBCs. The level of glycosylated hemoglobin is related to the amount of glucose available. In general, a hemoglobin A_{1c} of 7% or less indicates well-controlled diabetes.

Anion Gap (10-17 mmol/L)

An anion gap is calculated to determine the difference between positively charged and negatively charged ions and thus detect the presence of acidosis. The measured cations (sodium and potassium) and measured anions (chloride and bicarbonate) are used to determine the unmeasured cations and anions. Some centers disregard potassium because it is a relatively small number. Normal value ranges reflect this adjustment. The unmeasured ions are phosphates, sulfates, lactates, ketone bodies, and other organic acids that affect acid-base imbalances. The formula used to determine the anion gap is:

Anion gap = [sodium + potassium] − [chloride + bicarbonate]

An elevated gap is indicative of metabolic acidosis, and a decreased gap is indicative of metabolic alkalosis.

Antinuclear Antibodies

Antinuclear antibodies (ANA) is a measurement of antibodies to nuclear antigens (RNA, DNA, histones, chromatin). Used as a screening test in patients with clinical features suggestive of an autoimmune process, positive ANAs can be seen in systemic autoimmune diseases, organ-specific autoimmune diseases, and a variety of infections. Systemic autoimmune diseases associated with a positive ANA include lupus, scleroderma, mixed connective tissue disorders, rheumatoid arthritis, Sjogren syndrome, drug-induced lupus, and discoid lupus. Graves disease, Hashimoto thyroiditis, autoimmune hepatitis, and primary biliary cirrhosis also can cause a positive ANA. Infectious diseases associated with a positive ANA include mononucleosis, hepatitis C infection, subacute bacterial endocarditis, tuberculosis, and human immunodeficiency virus (HIV). Certain drugs can elicit a positive ANA, including carbamazepine, hydralazine, isoniazid, penicillin, phenytoin, procainamide, tetracycline, and thiazide diuretics. Positive low-titer ANAs are commonly found in the normal population. In those clinically well, ANA appears to have little use as a screening tool for connective tissue disorders.[10]

Anti-Smooth Muscle Antibody

Anti-smooth muscle antibody testing enables conditions that involve the liver, including autoimmune hepatitis, extrahepatic biliary obstruction, drug-induced liver disease, viral hepatitis, and others, to be differentiated. These antibodies found in the serum are autoantibodies against actin microfilaments and intermediate filaments found in smooth muscles. Anti–smooth muscle antibodies are not found in healthy persons.[1-3]

Higher titers of antibody (1:80 to 1:360) that persist over time are suggestive of chronic autoimmune active hepatitis. Titers below 1:80 that are transient are present in acute viral hepatitis or mononucleosis. Titers between 1:10 and 1:40 are present in primary biliary cirrhosis.[1-3]

α-Fetoprotein

α-Fetoprotein (AFP) is a glycoprotein normally produced during gestation by the fetal liver, yolk sac, and the gastrointestinal tract. Levels of AFP are elevated in infants but rapidly decline after birth to low levels. AFP is a commonly used tumor marker for hepatocellular carcinoma. AFP levels may also be elevated in patients with some testicular tumors. Normal levels of AFP are 10 to 20 μg/L in most laboratories.[11]

AFP level does not correlate with the size, stage, or prognosis of hepatocellular carcinoma; however, an increase in AFP level in those patients with cirrhosis (usually to levels > 500 μg/L) indicates the development of hepatocellular carcinoma. AFP level is also elevated in patients with other liver conditions such as viral hepatitis, drug hepatitis, cirrhosis, alcoholic liver, and extrahepatic biliary disease. Serum levels of AFP can decrease significantly in patients with hepatitis C treated with pegylated interferon plus ribavirin. Of note, some hepatocellular carcinoma tumors (eg, fibrolamellar carcinoma) are not producers of AFP.[11]

Serum Ceruloplasmin

Ceruloplasmin is a protein produced by the liver and secreted into the general circulation. It is the major carrier of copper within the blood. Each molecule of ceruloplasmin carries 6 copper atoms. In Wilson disease, an autosomal recessive genetic mutation of cellular copper export, excess copper is deposited in tissue because of a deficiency in ceruloplasmin that leads to hepatic, neurological, and renal impairment. Excess copper is also deposited in the cornea.[12]

Normal ceruloplasmin level is dependent on age. Ceruloplasmin levels are low during early infancy until approximately 6 months, peak in early childhood to levels higher than in adulthood (300 to 500 mg/L), then decline to adult ranges (200 to 350 mg/L). Serum levels of ceruloplasmin less than 200 mg/L accompanied by Kayser-Fleischer rings (gray-green rings that represent fine pigmented granular deposits found surrounding the cornea during slit-lamp examination) are diagnostic of Wilson disease.[12]

Other causes of low ceruloplasmin levels include the following:
- fulminant hepatic failure
- chronic active hepatitis in children
- normal neonates
- malnutrition
- intestinal malabsorption
- renal protein loss (nephrotic syndrome)[1-3]

Thyroid Function Studies

The release of thyroid hormones is controlled through a negative feedback loop linked with the pituitary gland and the hypothalamus. Secretion of thyroid hormones thyroxine (T_4) and triiodothyronine (T_3) is regulated by the release of thyroid-stimulating hormone (TSH) from the anterior pituitary gland. TSH is released as a result of the secretion of thyrotropin-releasing hormone by the hypothalamus. Small elevations in T_4 suppress the release of TSH from the pituitary gland by suppressing the release of thyrotropin-releasing hormone by the hypothalamus. Thus, the relationship between the levels of T_4 and TSH is reciprocal.

Thyroid diseases can by classified as primary or secondary. Primary hypothyroidism is directly related to dysfunction of the thyroid gland. Secondary hypothyroidism (a less common problem) is caused by pituitary dysfunction. A deficiency in thyroid hormone is called hypothyroidism, and an excess of thyroid hormone is called hyperthyroidism.[1-3]

Laboratory tests commonly used to assess thyroid function include the following measurements:

Serum TSH concentration

Serum total T_4 concentration

Serum total T_3 concentration

Serum free T_4 concentration

Measurement of TSH concentration is used as a tool to diagnose hypothyroidism and hyperthyroidism, screen for thyroid disease, and monitor for appropriate thyroid replacement therapy and antithyroid therapy. TSH level is elevated in hypothyroidism and low in hyperthyroidism. Today, most laboratories use third-generation studies that measure TSH to a low of 0.01 mIU/L. The reference range for TSH is 0.5 to 5.0 mIU/L.[1-3]

Total T_4 is a measurement of thyroid function. Total T_4 measures both protein-bound and free or unbound T_4. Of note, only the unbound T_4 is physiologically active. When thyroid hormone is released into the bloodstream, it is bound to thyroid-binding globulin and to a lesser extent prealbumin. Normal total T_4 levels are 64 to 167 nmol/L (5-13 µg/dL) in adults.[1-3]

Total T_3 concentration also measures both unbound and protein-bound T_3. It reflects the metabolically active form of thyroid hormone. It has little value in the diagnosis of hypothyroidism. T_3 is elevated in approximately 5% of patients with hyperthyroidism who have T_4 levels within normal limits (T_3 toxicosis). This test should be completed when hyperthyroidism is clinically suspected but when T_4 levels are normal.[1-3]

Serum level of free T_4 measures unbound, physiologically active T_4 concentrations. The free T_4 level is elevated in hyperthyroidism and reduced in hypothyroidism. It should not be used to determine the appropriateness of replacement therapy of levothyroxine for primary hypothyroidism. Measurement of TSH levels is the preferred method to avoid overreplacement of thyroid hormone. In secondary hypothyroidism (due to pituitary or hypothalamic disease), T_4 should be maintained in the upper 50% of normal. Normal free T_4 levels are 17 to 49 pmol/L (1.3-3.8 ng/dL).[1-3]

Factor V Leiden

Factor V Leiden is a genetically acquired trait that can result in a hypercoagulable state leading to activated protein C resistance, which was first described in 1993. The discovery and description of factor V Leiden followed in 1994.[13(p166-167)]

Factor V (proaccelerin) supports factor Xa activation of factor II (prothrombin) to factor IIa (thrombin), which splits fibrinogen into fibrin. Factor V (Leiden) mutation is a substitution leading to glutamine replacing arginine at a site where coagulation factor V is cleaved by activated protein C. This mutation causes factor V to be partially resistant to protein C, which participates in the inhibition of coagulation. Factor V mutations may be present in up to half of the cases of unexplained venous thrombosis and occur in the vast majority of patients with activated protein C resistance.[13(p166-167)]

Protein C

Protein C is a protein that prevents thrombosis. It is dependent on vitamin K and is produced in the liver and circulated in the plasma. It inactivates factors V and VII, thus functioning as an anticoagulant. Protein C also functions as a profibrinolytic, by enhancing fibrinolysis, and therefore prevents extension of intravascular thrombi.

Protein C is a proenzyme synthesized in the liver. Following its activation by thrombin, it exerts an anticoagulant effect through inactivation of factors Va and VIIa using protein S as a cofactor.

Deficiency is inherited in autosomal dominant fashion. Protein C deficiency may be manifested as a hypercoagulable state, with recurrent thrombophlebitis or pulmonary emboli.[2]

Protein S

Protein S is also dependent on vitamin K. A deficiency of either protein S or protein C is associated with a tendency toward thrombosis. Protein S serves as a cofactor to enhance the anticoagulant effects of activated protein C. Protein C, activated in the presence of protein S, promptly inactivates factor V and VII.[2]

Protein S is a vitamin K–dependent glycoprotein synthesized in the liver. It acts as a cofactor for protein C in producing an anticoagulant effect. Deficiency is associated with recurrent venous thromboid before the age of 40.[2]

Serological Tests Before Transplantation

Knowing a patient's exposure history assists with determining candidacy for transplantation, tailoring of immunosuppression, and finding probable causes of infections after transplantation. Interpreting most results of serological tests depends on knowing the humoral mediators produced during the course of an active infection.

Immunoglobulins (antibodies) either inactivate or remove parasites, bacteria, or other toxic substances recognized as potentially harmful to the body. Immunoglobulins G and M (IgG and IgM) are markers for chronic or acute infection.[14] IgM is the marker for primary antibody formation to a previously unknown agent and represents acute infection. IgG is activated when the host is rechallenged with a previously known antigen. Presence of IgG implies previous exposure to the antigen, but the patient does not have an acute or active infection.

Hepatitis B

Hepatitis B is caused by an infection with the hepatitis B virus (HBV), a DNA virus that is a member of the animal virus family known as hepadnaviruses (hepatotrophic DNA viruses).[15] Patients can be exposed to HBV through myriad routes. The infection is most efficiently transmitted via mucous membranes or percutaneous exposure from an infectious source, that is, sexual contact or intravenous routes.[15,16] Time from exposure to symptom onset is on average 6 weeks to 6 months, in which time the HBV can replicate and be transmitted to others virtually undetectably.[5,16]

Diagnostic tests detect different components of the HBV DNA's molecular structure and the body's immune response to its viral genomic material. The protein envelope expressed on the outer surface of the HBV is referred to as the hepatitis B surface antigen (HBsAg), which is the first virological detectable marker produced after infection with HBV.[15] Before elevations in serum transaminase levels or clinical symptoms are apparent, HBsAg is detectable and typically becomes undetectable 1 to 2 months after the icteric phase, with absolute resolution by 6 months. Antibodies to HBsAg (anti-HBs) are detectable indefinitely after the disappearance of the HbsAg.[15]

The hepatitis B core antigen (HBcAg) is expressed within the protein coat of the nucleocapsid and is undetectable in the serum. However, its corresponding antibody, anti-HBc, is detectable and appears in the serum 1 to 2 weeks after HBsAg appears and preempts detection of anti-HBs for anywhere from a few weeks to several months.[15] With lag times of several weeks to months between positive serological indicators, anti-HBc may be the only marker for active or remote exposure to HBV. In addition, the presence of anti-HBc and the absence of HBsAg and anti-HBs has been linked to transfusion-related transmission of hepatitis B.[11] The diagnosis of acute or chronic HBV infection cannot be made on clinical grounds; rather, it requires serological testing (Table 4).

Table 4. INTERPRETATION OF THE HEPATITIS B PANEL

Tests*	Results	Interpretation
HBsAg anti-HBc anti-HBs	Negative Negative Negative	Susceptible
HBsAg anti-HBc anti-HBs	Negative Positive Positive	Immune because of natural infection
HBsAg anti-HBc anti-HBs	Negative Negative Positive	Immune because of hepatitis B vaccination
HBsAg anti-HBc IgM anti-HBc anti-HBs	Positive Positive Positive Negative	Acutely infected
HBsAg anti-HBc IgM anti-HBc anti-HBs	Positive Positive Negative Negative	Chronically infected
HBsAg anti-HBc anti-HBs	Negative Positive Negative	Four interpretations possible†

* Definitions

Hepatitis B Surface Antigen (HBsAg): A serologic marker on the surface of HBV. It can be detected in high levels in serum during acute or chronic hepatitis. The presence of HBsAg indicates that the person is infectious. The body normally produces antibodies to HBsAg as part of the normal immune response to infection.

Hepatitis B Surface Antibody (anti-HBs): The presence of anti-HBs is generally interpreted as indicating recovery and immunity from HBV infection. Anti-HBs also develops in a person who has been successfully vaccinated against hepatitis B.

Total Hepatitis B Core Antibody (anti-HBc): Appears at the onset of symptoms in acute hepatitis B and persists for life. The presence of anti-HBc indicates previous or ongoing infection with hepatitis B virus (HBV) in an undefined time frame.

IgM Antibody to Hepatitis B Core Antigen (IgM anti-HBc): This antibody appears during acute or recent HBV infection and is present for about 6 months

† Four interpretations:

1. Might be recovering from acute HBV infection.
2. Might be distantly immune and test not sensitive enough to detect very low level of anti-HBs in serum.
3. Might be susceptible with a false positive anti-HBc.
4. Might be undetectable level of HBsAg present in the serum and the person is actually chronically infected.

Reprinted with permission from Centers for Disease Control.[17]

Table 5. HEPATITIS C INFECTION

Signs and Symptoms	80% of persons have no signs or symptoms.	
	• Jaundice • Fatigue • Dark urine	• Abdominal pain • Loss of appetite • Nausea
Cause	• Hepatitis C virus (HCV)	
Long-term effects	• Chronic infection: 55%-85% of infected persons • Chronic liver disease: 70% of chronically infected persons • Deaths from chronic liver disease: 1%-5% of infected persons may die • Leading indication for liver transplant	
Transmission Recommendations for testing based on risk for HCV infection	• Occurs when blood or body fluids from an infected person enters the body of a person who is not infected. • HCV is spread through sharing needles or "works" when "shooting" drugs, through needlesticks or sharps exposures on the job, or from an infected mother to her baby during birth. Persons at risk for HCV infection might also be at risk for infection with hepatitis B virus (HBV) or HIV. Recommendations for Testing Based on Risk for HCV Infection **Persons** **Risk of infection** **Testing recommended?** Injecting drug users High Yes Recipients of clotting factors made before 1987 High Yes Hemodialysis patients Intermediate Yes Recipients of blood and/or solid organs before 1992 Intermediate Yes People with undiagnosed liver problems Intermediate Yes Infants born to infected mothers Intermediate After 12-18 mos. old Healthcare/public safety workers Low Only after known exposure People having sex with multiple partners Low No* People having sex with an infected steady partner Low No* *Anyone who wants to get tested should ask their doctor.	

Table 5. HEPATITIS C INFECTION, continued

Prevention	• There is no vaccine to prevent hepatitis C. • Do not shoot drugs; if you shoot drugs, stop and get into a treatment program; if you can't stop, never share needles, syringes, water, or "works," and get vaccinated against hepatitis A and B. • Do not share personal care items that might have blood on them (razors, toothbrushes). • If you are a health care or public safety worker, always follow routine barrier precautions and safely handle needles and other sharps; get vaccinated against hepatitis B. • Consider the risks if you are thinking about getting a tattoo or body piercing. You might get infected if the tools have someone else's blood on them or if the artist or piercer does not follow good health practices. • HCV can be spread by sex, but this is rare. If you are having sex with more than one steady sex partner, use latex condoms* correctly and every time to prevent the spread of sexually transmitted diseases. You should also get vaccinated against hepatitis B. • If you are HCV positive, do not donate blood, organs, or tissue.
Treatment and Medical Management AASLD Practice Guideline: Diagnosis, Management, and Treatment of Hepatitis C	• HCV-positive persons should be evaluated by their doctor for liver disease. • Interferon and ribavirin are 2 drugs licensed for the treatment of persons with chronic hepatitis C. • Interferon can be taken alone or in combination with ribavirin. Combination therapy, using pegylated interferon and ribavirin, is currently the treatment of choice. • Combination therapy can get rid of the virus in up to 5 out of 10 persons for genotype 1 and in up to 8 out of 10 persons for genotypes 2 and 3. • Drinking alcohol can make your liver disease worse.
Statistics and trends	• Number of new infections per year has declined from an average of 240,000 in the 1980s to about 30,000 in 2003. • Most infections are due to illegal injection drug use. • Transfusion-associated cases occurred prior to blood donor screening; now occur in less than one per million transfused units of blood. • Estimated 3.9 million (1.8%) Americans have been infected with HCV, of whom 2.7 million are chronically infected.

Reprinted with permission from Centers for Disease Control.[19]

Hepatitis C

Hepatitis C (previously referred to as hepatitis non A–non B) is the most common chronic blood-borne infection in the United States; an estimated 2.7 million persons are chronically infected.[15,18] Hepatitis C virus (HCV) is primarily transmitted by direct percutaneous exposure to HCV-infected blood (eg, blood transfusion, needle stick, or sharing of needles; see Table 5).

Diagnosis

Current guidelines from the Centers for Disease Control and Prevention for detection of hepatitis C include testing for either antibody to HCV (anti-HCV) or HCV RNA (ribonucleic acid); both will result in a positive finding for HCV infection. Anti-HCV is recommended for first-line testing because of its high sensitivity; specificity depends on the presence of other clinical indicators such as elevated liver enzyme levels and positive history of risk factors.[20]

Routine testing of asymptomatic persons should include use of both enzyme immunoassay to test for anti-HCV and a confirmatory second-generation recombinant immunoblot assay for all positive anti-HCV results.[20,21] Polymerase chain reaction (PCR) is a laboratory technique that amplifies DNA sequences, making it possible to detect genetic information in a sample at very low numbers. PCR can be used to identify HCV RNA chains and is considered the gold standard confirmatory test for detecting the actual virus versus antibodies and differentiates prior exposure from current viremia.[20,21]

HIV Infection

In the United States alone, close to 1 million people are infected with the human immunodeficiency virus (HIV). Almost 25% of the infected population are unaware that they are infected and continue to engage in high-risk behaviors, exponentially increasing the spread of the disease.[22] There are 2 classes or strains of HIV: HIV-1 and HIV-2. Most infections occurring in the United States are due to HIV-1, whereas HIV-2 is endemic to West Africa. A high suspicion for exposure to the HIV-2 strain should be aroused if the patient has traveled to or had relations with someone from West Africa.[22,23] Initial presentation of HIV is referred to as acute retroviral syndrome; most common signs and symptoms include fever, malaise, lymphadenopathy, and skin rash.[19-21]

Diagnostic Testing

The enzyme-linked immunosorbent assay is 99.5% sensitive and is the standard initial screening for HIV-1 and HIV-2. One must keep in mind, however, that this is an antibody-dependent marker and it may take up to 4 to 8 weeks for antibodies to form,[19,20] so there is a 4- to 8-week period where a false-negative test result can occur. The Western blot is a confirmatory test to rule out false-positive results. Written informed consent is required before testing, and a positive test must be reported to the local Department of Health and Human Services.[22,23,24]

Toxoplasmosis

Toxoplasmosis is caused by the parasite *Toxoplasma gondii*. It is acquired from ingestion of contaminated undercooked meat or contact with soil containing *Toxoplasma gondii* spores.[25] The cysts can lay quiescent for years within an immunocompetent host's brain matrix until the host's immune system is compromised either iatrogenically or by an immune debilitating disease.[25]

Diagnosis

Detection of *Toxoplasma*-specific IgG antibodies is the primary diagnostic test to determine prior exposure.[26] On an epidemiological note, IgM antibodies remain present for up to 18 months. In turn, a positive IgM–capture enzyme immunoassay test on a seroconverted patient would plot the time course of the infection to within the past 18 months[26] (see Figure). Of note, current serological testing standards cannot be used to confirm active toxoplasmosis of the central nervous system in immunocompromised patients.[26]

Syphilis

Syphilis is a sexually transmitted disease caused by the spirochete *Treponema pallidum*.[27,28] Syphilis has 3 stages: primary, secondary, and latent. Detailed explanation of the different stages is beyond the scope of this chapter.

Diagnosis

Two types of antibodies are formed in a syphilitic infection: antilipid "reaginic" antibody and specific antitreponemal antibody that appears approximately 4 to 6 weeks after infection.[28,13] Rapid plasma reagin and Venereal Disease Research Laboratory are the 2 most common tests with similar sensitivity (70%/ 80% in primary stage and 99%/ 99% in secondary stage).[13(p580),28] A 4-fold or greater increase in titer is indicative of early syphilis evolution (eg, 1:8 to 1:32).[28] During the latent stage of syphilis, however, these tests have less than 1% sensitivity.[13(p580),28] Biologic false-positive results arise with both tests because of acute and chronic diseases. Therefore, specific treponemal testing with either fluorescent treponemal antibody absorption test or *Treponema pallidum* particle agglutination should be performed for confirmation. A biologic false-positive result should be investigated, as this may be indicative of another serious biologic infection (eg, malaria has a 100% biologic false-positive with both tests).[13(p581)].

Figure 1. Toxophasmosis Algorhythm
Abbreviations: IgG, immunoglobulin G; IgM, immunoglobulin M.
Reprinted with permission from Centers for Disease Control.[26]

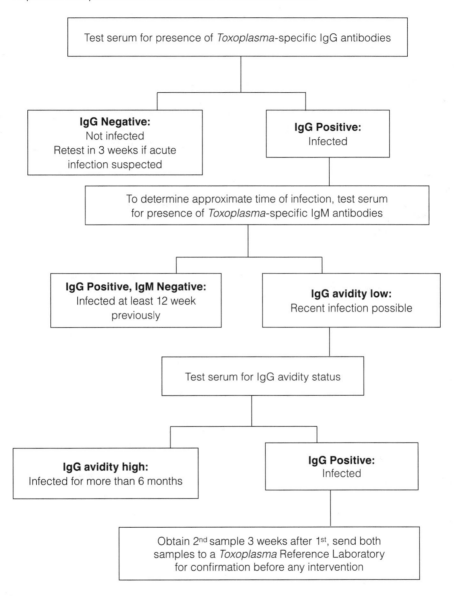

Epstein Barr Virus

One of the most common human viruses, the Epstein-Barr virus (EBV), is a member of the family Herpesviridae.[29,30] In the United States, as many as 95% of adults between 35 and 40 years of age have been infected, as this virus has 2 peaks of occurrence, one in early childhood and another in late adolescence.[29,30]

EBV-Specific Laboratory Tests

Current testing uses antibodies to measure 3 specific antigens: viral capsid, the early antigen, and the EBV nuclear antigen. If active or acute infection is suspected, then testing for IgM to the viral capsid antigen is first-line testing. IgM appears quickly and then disappears within 4 to 6 weeks.[30] However, IgG to the viral capsid antigen appears in the acute phase, peaks at 2 to 4 weeks, declines slightly, and then persists for life. IgG to the early antigen appears in the acute phase and generally decreases to undetectable levels after 3 to 6 months[30] (Table 6).

Table 6. SUMMARY OF INTERPRETATION

The diagnosis of EBV infection is summarized as follows:

Susceptibility
If antibodies to the viral capsid antigen are not detected, the patient is susceptible to EBV infection.

Primary Infection
Primary EBV infection is indicated if IgM antibody to the viral capsid antigen is present and antibody to EBV nuclear antigen, or EBNA, is absent. A rising or high IgG antibody to the viral capsid antigen and negative antibody to EBNA after at least 4 weeks of illness is also strongly suggestive of primary infection. In addition, 80% of patients with active EBV infection produce antibody to early antigen.

Past Infection
If antibodies to both the viral capsid antigen and EBNA are present, then past infection (from 4 to 6 months to years earlier) is indicated. Since 95% of adults have been infected with EBV, most adults will show antibodies to EBV from infection years earlier. High or elevated antibody levels may be present for years and are not diagnostic of recent infection.

Reactivation
In the presence of antibodies to EBNA, an elevation of antibodies to early antigen suggests reactivation. However, when EBV antibody to the early antigen test is present, this result does not automatically indicate that a patient's current medical condition is caused by EBV. A number of healthy people with no symptoms have antibodies to the EBV early antigen for years after their initial EBV infection. Many times reactivation occurs subclinically.

Chronic EBV Infection
Reliable laboratory evidence for continued active EBV infection is very seldom found in patients who have been ill for more than 4 months. When the illness lasts more than 6 months, it should be investigated to see if other causes of chronic illness or CFS are present.

Abbreviations: CFS, chronic fatigue syndrome; EBNA, antibody to EBV nuclear antigen; EBV, Epstein-Barr virus; IgM, immunoglobulin M.
Reprinted with permission from Centers for Disease Control and National Center for Infectious Diseases.[30]

Herpes Simplex Virus

A double-stranded DNA virus, the herpes simplex virus (HSV) belongs to the herpesvirus family and exists in 2 forms: HSV-1 and HSV-2, with HSV-2 predominantly encompassing genital herpes.[21,31] HSV is extremely tenacious, as it remains dormant for an extended time with periods of recurrence during the life of the host.

Diagnosis

Clinical diagnosis can be made from a simple physical examination, though this not recommended, because the multivesicular lesions can resemble other disorders. Lesions can be scraped and stained with Giemsa (Tzanck preparation), or Papanicolaou stain to reveal expected giant cells with intranuclear eosinophilic herpetic inclusions.[31]

Both type-specific and nonspecific antibodies to HSV develop during the first several weeks following infection and persist indefinitely. Indirect immunofluorescence assay and enzyme-linked immunosorbent assay can be used to detect reactivation by a 4-fold or greater increase in HSV IgG.[31,32] Other types of specific assays are complement fixation and radioimmunoassay.[31,32] Western blot assay is useful in detecting several types of specific proteins; it can differentiate between HSV-1 and HSV-2 if clinically indicated.[31,32] PCR is a laboratory technique that amplifies DNA sequences, making it possible to detect genetic information in samples at very low numbers. PCR can be used to detect HSV DNA. PCR is highly sensitive for detecting HSV in spinal fluid for diagnosis of active HSV CNS infection.[32] However, the sensitivity of PCR declines to 50% for detection of cervical and salivary HSV infection.[31]

Varicella

Varicella zoster virus is the root organism that causes 2 diseases, varicella (chickenpox) and herpes zoster (shingles).[33,34] Humans are the only known vectors for this highly contagious disease.[33,34]

Diagnosis

Tzanck smear, PCR, and direct immunofluorescent stain can all be used to confirm an active primary infection.[33,34] IgM and IgG serological assays are also available to confirm acute infection versus convalescent varicella zoster virus.

Cytomegalovirus

Characteristically producing enlarged cells, hence its namesake, cytomegalovirus (CMV) is a member of the herpesvirus family.[32] Once infected, the host carries the virus for life.[35]

Diagnosis

Detection of CMV IgG is confirmation of antibody formation against the virus.[36] Patients with CMV-negative IgG before transplantation should be monitored serially after transplantation for seroconversion. Increases in antibodies to CMV antigens can also be detected by several serological assays: complement fixation, indirect immunofluorescence assay, indirect hemagglutination, and enzyme-linked immunosorbent assay.[35] For best results, 2 samples should be obtained 2 weeks apart if suspicion is high for CMV to allow for seroconversion and the formation of IgM antibodies.[33]

CMV antigenemia testing has replaced several other assays for detecting CMV in peripheral blood.[16] The assay detects an early protein matrix (pp65) on polymorphonuclear leukocytes.[16] The number of positively stained polymorphonuclear leukocytes gives an estimate of CMV viral load.[16,35] PCR is the most sensitive for detecting antigens to CMV in any medium (tissue or fluid).[16] CMV antigenemia appears to have a slight advantage over PCR as it yields positive results approximately 7 days before the onset of the disease, that is 4 days sooner than with PCR.[16]

Tuberculosis

What used to be referred to as consumption, tuberculosis is in fact an infection with a member of the family Mycobacteriaceae.[37] *Mycobacterium tuberculosis* cannot be decolorized with acid alcohol, which gives it the distinction of being "acid fast."[37-39] People can either have active disease or be carriers, in which case a reactivation of the disease can occur during low immune states. European countries have a high prevalence of the disease, and most Europeans have been vaccinated with the *Mycobacterium bovis* (BCG) vaccine.[38,39]

Diagnosis

The American Thoracic Society guidelines define the following diagnostic criteria for a positive skin test (purified protein derivative, or PPD) after 48 to 72 hours.[39] Patients with known HIV infection, who have had close contact with someone with known tuberculosis, or who have fibrotic lesions on chest radiographs with a reaction with an induration of 5 mm or greater are considered positive for tuberculosis. In at-risk adults (eg, healthcare workers) and children (including children less than 4 years old), a reaction with an induration of 10 mm or greater is considered positive. In patients without any known risk factors, a reaction with an induration of 15mm or greater is considered positive.[38,39] Induration is measured in millimeters across the forearm and is the hardened raised area produced in response to the purified protein derivative (PPD) tuberculin, not the erythematous (reddened) area that accompanies the induration.[38]

Chest radiography may yield the initial suspicion for tuberculosis, as the typical presentation is an upper lobe infiltrate or cavitary lesion.[37-39] Confirmatory testing with acid-fast bacillus microscopy can be used for initial screening of a sputum sample. A follow up acid-fast bacillus culture should be performed as microscopy does not differentiate other *Mycobacterium* species from M *tuberculosis*.[37-39]

Geographic Distribution and Travel

Special notation should be made for transplant candidates who have lived or visited certain geographical locations that are known endemic areas of particular diseases. Histoplasmosis and coccidiomycosis are 2 pathogens with known endemic areas in the United States.

A fungal opportunistic infection with *Histoplasmosis encapsulatum* contaminates bird and bat droppings in the Mississippi and Ohio River Valleys, Puerto Rico, the Dominican Republic, and Central and South America.[40-43] Coccidioidomycosis, caused by *Coccidioides immitis*, is a mold that is mainly endemic to the desert southwest (Southern California, Texas, Arizona, and New Mexico).[40,43,44] Coccidioidomycosis is typically endemic to the Central Valley of California and is found mainly in desert areas.[40,43,44] However, natural shifts in wind patterns (eg, Santa Ana winds) can bring dry spore-laden soil to areas previously not contaminated with *Coccidioidomycosis* (eg, coastal region of California). A high level of suspicion should be raised if symptoms warrant testing for these disease states outside their known endemic area, especially when travel or environmental factors exist.

Diagnosis

Complement fixing antibody levels of 1:32 (or higher) or a 4-fold increase is diagnostic of active histoplasmosis.[41,42] Both IgM and IgG are activated in coccidiodomycosis.[43] The IgG level is indicative of intensity of the infection.[43] Otherwise, laboratory values that are diagnostically negative for histoplasmosis and coccidiomycosis are absence of fungal antibodies, IgM, and IgG; complement fixing titer less than 1:8; and negative result on immunodiffusion test.[13(p610),42,43]

Cultures and Gram Stains

Due to immunosuppression, transplant recipients are vulnerable to myriad bacterial, fungal, and viral infections. Within the first year after transplantation, two thirds of patients with solid organ transplants will acquire some infectious process.[45] Prompt identification of the offending organism and the site of infection is important to guide appropriate selection of an antimicrobial agent to prevent morbidity and mortality associated with infection.

The most rapid method of identifying infectious organisms is through the direct examination of the body fluids one suspects are infected.[12] These techniques permit the prompt initiation of empiric antibiotic coverage while results of cultures and sensitivities are pending.

Gram Stains

Gram stains are used to identify staining characteristics as well as the morphology associated with an organism. Of note, bacteria are invisible on light microscopy. Gram stains provide colorful stains that help visualize bacteria. To perform a Gram stain, a small amount of sample is smeared on the slide. The slide is heated to fix the bacteria to the slide. The staining material is then applied. Gram-positive bacteria stain blue whereas gram-negative bacteria stain red. The morphology of the organism is then identified. Table 7 provides a simplistic version of how bacteria are identified on the basis of stain and morphology.[46]

Table 7. COMPARISON OF GRAM-POSITIVE AND GRAM-NEGATIVE BACTERIA

Type of bacteria	Morphology	Specific organism
Gram-positive bacteria	Cocci: spherical	*Staphylococcus* and *Streptococcus*
	Bacilli: rods	*Bacillus, Clostridium, Corynebacterium, Listeria*
Gram-negative bacteria	Bacilli: rods	*Enterobacter sp., Escherichia coli, Klebsiella, Serratia, Proteus, Shigella, Pseudomonas, Bacteroides* sp.
	Cocci: spherical	*Neisseria*
	Spirochetes: spiral	*Treponema pallidum* (causes syphilis)
	Pleomorphic: jello, no shape	*Clostridium* species

Other Direct Examination Methods

Some bacteria and fungi are best identified microscopically via special stains, wet mounts, fixed slides, or specimens treated with fluorescent antibody specific for antigen found on a pathogen. DNA hybridization techniques allow direct examination of tissues with signal-emitting probes that are specific for the nucleic acids found in a variety of pathogens. RNA and DNA sequences of a pathogen may be identified via commercially available probes, which can be placed in culture or tissue specimens. These probe-based techniques use small segments of DNA or RNA segments that bind (hybridize) with the complementary sequence from a microorganism, allowing rapid, sensitive, and specific methods for identification of an organism. Probe hybridization has been used in a variety of clinical diseases. Probe methods have been used for slow-growing organisms such as mycobacteria and some fungi (*Histoplasma capsulatum, Coccidioides immitis,* and *Blastomyces dermatitidis*). Additionally, they can be used for the detection and quantification of viruses (HBV, HCV, HIV) but with less sensitivity than PCR.[12]

PCR has become useful in the detection of specific DNA or RNA from pathogens present in low numbers. Its principle lies in the ability to produce multiple copies of pathogen DNA or RNA in the laboratory without the need for probes.[12] The benefit of PCR over culture and serological methods of testing in immunosuppressed patients cannot be overlooked. PCR does not depend on immunological responses. Additionally, PCR can easily detect reactivation of a disease process, unlike serological methods, which cannot be used to detect reactivation in those patients who were previously seropositive. Last, PCR testing can be used to identify de novo infection and reactivation of disease earlier than culture.[47] This allows prompt identification and treatment of infection. Clinicians should analyze this exceedingly sensitive tool carefully as it can detect as little as 10 copies of DNA.[48] Individual transplant programs establish a threshold for treatment based on laboratory technique and clinical experience within the transplant center. PCR is used clinically in transplantation for therapeutic monitoring of HCV, HBV, EBV, BK virus, and CMV.[47]

Culture and Sensitivity

The gold standard for identification of infectious organisms is a culture. Body fluids that are suspected to be infected are placed in medium that enhances the growth of the organism. The laboratory is then able to identify the specific organism and test its susceptibility to various antibiotics through sensitivity testing. This testing allows the practitioner to narrow antibiotic coverage to only those agents that effectively eradicate an organism that is causing an infection.[46]

The time-tested method for evaluating sensitivity in vivo to antimicrobial agents is via the minimal inhibitory concentration (MIC). MIC is defined as the lowest concentration of antimicrobial agent that significantly interferes with bacterial growth. A drug with a high MIC is less effective in vivo because a greater concentration of the drug is required to inhibit microbial growth. A drug with a low MIC indicates a high level of antimicrobial activity against the targeted organism. An organism is considered if the drug's MIC is above a level that can be achieved through normal delivery routes or if the MIC is in the toxic range.[12,46]

On the basis of each drug's MIC, pathogens are classified as being susceptible, resistant, or of indeterminate susceptibility to that drug. Pathogens are classified as susceptible to antibiotics that have the lowest MICs; in such cases the organisms are most likely to be eradicated during treatment with "usual" drug doses. Organisms are resistant to drugs with high MICs, suggesting that clinical efficacy would be less than desirable even if high doses of the antibiotic were used. Intermediate susceptibility indicates that organisms are moderately susceptible to an antibiotic; the antibiotic is less likely to be effective than antibiotics testing within the susceptible range. Treatment of organisms in this range may be successful when maximum doses of the drug are used or if the drug is known to be concentrated at the site of infection.[46]

The MIC serves as a quantitative measure of drug activity against bacteria. Several studies in animal models as well as in humans demonstrate that the MIC correlates with clinical efficacy and with clinical improvement. Caution, however, should be used when interpreting this testing; the importance of the site

Testing for Viruses

Various techniques are used in viral laboratory diagnosis. These include immunological studies of sera, microscopic methods, and nucleic acid identification (molecular probes or PCR, see preceding section on PCR for a detailed discussion).

Immunological Studies of Sera

Levels of specific antibodies increase and decrease during the course of a viral illness, although the rise and persistence of the titer depend on the specific virus. Ideally, both acute and convalescent IgG blood specimens for antibodies are collected. The acute specimen is collected immediately upon presentation and the convalescent specimen is obtained 7 to 30 days after the acute serum. Generally, a 4-fold or greater rise in IgG antibody titer is considered evidence of disease. Care should be used when evaluating these studies in transplant recipients because significantly immunosuppressed patients may not mount a serological response.[45,48,49]

Antigenic testing for certain viruses may also be helpful and can be used to detect viral presence regardless of the disease duration or antibody response of the patient. Antigenic testing is helpful in detecting hepatitis (HbsAg), HCV, or cytomegalovirus.[12,48]

Microscopic Methods

Microscopic methods are used to evaluate and examine cells, body fluids, biopsy specimens, or aspirates in search of viral cytopathic effects (eg, multinucleated giant cells at the base of herpes lesions or the presence of inclusion bodies with CMV infections).[12] Viral culture should be completed using viral medium. Calling the laboratory to ensure use of proper medium, time restrictions, and technique for collection can yield accurate and prompt results.

The Tzanck test is a rapid and sensitive staining technique used to identify viral infections associated with blistering vesicles such as herpes simplex virus (HSV) or varicella zoster. The test is performed by gently rupturing a vesicle with a scalpel blade, scraping the base of the lesion with a cotton tip swab or the edge of the scalpel, and smearing the material obtained onto a glass slide. The laboratory then looks for the presence of multinucleated giant cells. This test cannot differentiate between HSV or varicella, because these viruses resemble each other microscopically.[5,6,48]

Immunofluorescent methods, direct immunofluorescent antibody staining, allow rapid detection of antigens in scraped cells infected with virus. Specimens for direct antigen testing may be obtained for respiratory virus detection or from vesicular lesions. Cells are stained by using monoclonal antibodies and examined under a fluorescence microscope looking for specific fluorescence of the cell cytoplasm or the nucleus. Such testing is used for varicella, HSV, or respiratory syncytial virus.[6,48]

References

1. LeFever Kee J. *Handbook of Laboratory and Diagnostic Tests*. 5th ed. Upper Saddle River, NJ: Pearson-Prentice Hall; 2004.
2. Nicoll D, McPhee SJ, Pignone M. *Pocket Guide to Diagnostic Tests*. New York, NY: Lange Medical Books/McGraw-Hill; 2004.
3. Chernecky CC, Berger BJ. *Laboratory Tests and Diagnostic Procedures*. 3rd ed. Philadelphia,. Pa: W B Saunders Co; 2001.
4. Holechek MJ, Agunod MO, Burrell-Diggs D, Darmody JK. Renal transplantation. In: Nolan MT, Augustine SM, eds. *Transplantation Nursing: Acute and Long Term Management*. Norwalk, Conn: Appleton-Lange; 1995.
5. Smith SL, Ciferni M. Liver transplantation. In: Smith S, ed. *Tissue and Organ Transplantation: Implications for Professional Nursing Practice*. St. Louis, Mo: Mosby–Year Book; 1990:273-300.
6. American Diabetes Association: Clinical Practice Recommendations 2001. *Diabetes Care*. 2002;25(suppl 1).

7. K/DOQI clinical practice guidelines for chronic kidney disease evaluation, classification, and stratification. Kidney Disease Outcome Quality Initiative. *Am J Kidney Dis.* 2002:39:S1-246.
8. Levey AS, Coresh J, Balk E, et al. National Kidney Foundation practice guidelines for chronic kidney disease: evaluation, classification, and stratification. *Ann Intern Med.* 2003;139:137-147.
9. Rule AD, Larson TS, Bergstralh EJ, et al. Using serum creatinine to estimate glomerular filtration rate; accuracy in good health and in chronic kidney disease. *Ann Intern Med.* 2004;141:929-937.
10. Measurement and clinical significance of antinuclear antibodies. Available at: www.uptodate.com. Accessed January 20, 2006.
11. Clinical features, diagnosis, and screening for primary hepatocellular carcinoma. Available at: www.uptodate.com. Accessed January 20, 2006.
12. Dudley MN. Use of laboratory tests in infectious diseases. In: Dipiro JT, Talbert RL, Yee GC, Matzke GR, Wells BG, Posey LM, eds. *Pharmacotherapy: A Pathophysiologic Approach.* 3rd ed. Stamford, Conn: Appleton & Lange; 1997: 1931-1951.
13. Fischback F. A *Manual of Laboratory and Diagnostic Tests.* 6th ed. Philadelphia, Pa: Lippincott; 2000.
14. Haynes BF, Fauci AS. Disorders of the immune system, connective tissue, and joints: introduction to the immune system. In: Fauci A, Braunwald E, Isselbacher K, et al, eds. *Harrison's Principles of Internal Medicine.* 14th ed. New York, NY: McGraw-Hill; 1998:1753-1776.
15. Dienstag, JL, Isselbacher KJ. Acute viral hepatitis. In: Fauci A, Braunwald E, Isselbacher K, et al. *Harrison's Principles of Internal Medicine.* 14th ed. New York, NY: McGraw-Hill; 1998:1677-1692.
16. Kirklin JK, Young JB, McGiffin DC. *Heart Transplantation.* Philadelphia, Pa: Churchill Livingstone; 2002.
17. Centers for Disease Control. Hepatitis B frequently asked questions. Available at: http://www.cdc.gov/ncidod/diseases/hepatitis/b/faqb.htm#serology. Accessed June 27, 2006.
18. Alter MJ, Kruszon-Moran D, Nainan OV, et al. The prevalence of hepatitis C virus infection in the United States, 1988 through 1994. *N Engl J Med.* 1999;341:556-562.
19. Centers for Disease Control. Hepatitis C fact sheet. Available at: http://www.cdc.gov/ncidod/diseases/hepatitis/c/fact.htm. Accessed June 27, 2006.
20. Centers for Disease Control. Sexually transmitted diseases treatment guidelines 2002 for hepatitis C. Available at: http://www.cdc.gov/STD/treatment/7-2002TG.htm#DiagnosisTreatment. Accessed May 18, 2005.
21. Barkley TW, Myers CM. *Practice Guidelines for Acute Care Nurse Practitioners.* Philadelphia, Pa: W B Saunders Co; 2001.
22. AidsInfo.org. Available at: www.AIDSinfo.org. Accessed May 18,2005.
23. Centers for Disease Control. Sexually transmitted diseases treatment guidelines 2002 for detection of HIV infection. Available at:: http://www.cdc.gov/STD/treatment/1-2002TG.htm#DetectionHIVInfectionDiagnosticTesting. Accessed May 18, 2005
24. Fauci AS, Lane HC. Human immunodeficiency virus (HIV) disease: AIDS and related disorders. In: Fauci A, Braunwald E, Isselbacher K, et al, eds. *Harrison's Principles of Internal Medicine.* 14th ed. New York, NY: McGraw-Hill; 1998:1791-1856.
25. Kasper LH. *Toxoplasma* infection. In: Fauci A, Braunwald E, Isselbacher K, et al, eds. *Harrison's Principles of Internal Medicine.* 14th ed. New York, NY: McGraw-Hill; 1998:1197-1202.
26. Centers for Disease Control. Diagnostic findings: toxoplasmosis. Available at: http://www.dpd.cdc.gov/dpdx/HTML/Toxoplasmosis.htm. Accessed May 18, 2005.
27. Centers for Disease Control. Sexually transmitted diseases treatment guidelines 2002 *diagnostic considerations and use of serologic tests for syphilis. Available at:* http://www.cdc.gov/STD/treatment/2-2002TG.htm#Syphilis. Accessed June 27, 2006.
28. Lukehart SA, Holmes KK. Spirochetal diseases: syphilis. In: Fauci A, Braunwald E, Isselbacher K, et al, eds. *Harrison's Principles of Internal Medicine.* 14th ed. New York, NY: McGraw-Hill; 1998:1023-1033.
29. Cohen JI. Epstein-Barr virus infections, including infectious mononucleosis. In: Fauci A, Braunwald E, Isselbacher K, et al, eds. *Harrison's Principles of Internal Medicine.* 14th ed. New York, NY: McGraw-Hill; 1998:1089-1091.
30. Centers for Disease Control, National Center for Infectious Diseases. Epstein-Barr virus and infectious mononucleosis. Available at: http://www.cdc.gov/ncidod/diseases/ebv.htm. Accessed May 18, 2005.
31. Corey L. DNA viruses: herpes simplex viruses. In: Fauci A, Braunwald E, Isselbacher K, et al, eds. *Harrison's Principles of Internal Medicine.* 14th ed. New York, NY: McGraw-Hill; 1998:1080-1086.
32. Centers for Disease Control. Sexually transmitted diseases treatment guidelines 2002 for genital herpes simplex virus. Available at: http://www.cdc.gov/STD/treatment/2-2002TG.htm#GenitalHerpes. Accessed May 18, 2005.
33. Whitley RJ. Varicella-zoster virus infections. In: Fauci A, Braunwald E, Isselbacher K, et al, eds. *Harrison's Principles of Internal Medicine.* 14th ed. New York, NY: McGraw-Hill; 1998:1086-1089.
34. Centers for Disease Control. Chapter 14, Varicella. VPD Surveillance Manual. 3rd ed. 2002. Available at: http://www.cdc.gov/nip/publications/surv-manual/chpt14_varicella.pdf. Accessed May 18, 2005.
35. Hirsch MS. Cytomegalovirus and human herpesvirus types 6,7, and 8. In Fauci A, Braunwald E, Isselbacher K, et al, eds. *Harrison's Principles of Internal Medicine.* 14th ed. New York, NY: McGraw-Hill; 1998:1092-1095.

36. Centers for Disease Control, National Center for Infectious Diseases. Cytomegalovirus. Available at: http://www.cdc.gov/ncidod/diseases/cmv.htm. Accessed May 18, 2005.
37. Raviglione MC, O'Brien RJ. Tuberculosis. In: Fauci A, Braunwald E, Isselbacher K, et al, eds. *Harrison's Principles of Internal Medicine*. 14th ed. New York, NY: McGraw-Hill; 1998:1004-1014.
38. Centers for Disease Control. Core Curriculum on Tuberculosis (2000). Available at: http://www.cdc.gov/nchstp/tb/pubs/corecurr/default.htm. Accessed May 18, 2005.
39. American Thoracic Society and Centers for Disease Control. Diagnostic standards and classification of tuberculosis in adults and children. *Am J Respir Crit Care Med*. 2000;161. Available at: www.thoracic.org/sections/publications/statements/pages/mtpi/tbadult1-20.html. Accessed June 27, 2006.
40. Bennett JE. Histoplasmosis. In: Fauci A, Braunwald E, Isselbacher K, et al, eds. *Harrison's Principles of Internal Medicine*. 14th ed. New York, NY: McGraw-Hill; 1998:1150-1151.
41. Centers for Disease Control, Division of Bacterial and Mycotic Diseases. Histoplasmosis. Available at: http://www.cdc.gov/ncidod/dbmd/diseaseinfo/histoplasmosis_t.htm. Accessed May 18, 2005.
42. Centers for Disease Control. National Institute for Occupational Safety and Health. Histoplasmosis: protecting workers at risk. Available at: http://www.cdc.gov/niosh/docs/2005-109/. Accessed June 27, 2006.
43. Bennett JE. Coccidioidomycosis. In: Fauci A, Braunwald E, Isselbacher K, et al, eds. *Harrison's Principles of Internal Medicine*. 14th ed. New York, NY: McGraw-Hill; 1998:1151-1152.
44. Coccidioidomycosis. Available at: http://www.cdc.gov/ncidod/dbmd/diseaseinfo/coccidioidomycosis_t.htm. Accessed June 27, 2006.
45. Rubin RH. Infection in organ transplant recipient. In: Rubin RH, Young LS, eds. *Clinical Approach to Infection in the Compromised Host*. 3rd ed. New York, NY: Plenum; 2004.
46. Galdwin M, Trattler B. *Clinical Microbiology Made Ridiculously Simple*. 3rd ed. Miami, Fla: Medmaster, Inc; 2004.
47. University of Pittsburgh School of Medicine, Department of Pathology. Molecular Diagnostics, Microbiology, Virology, and Infectious Diseases. Available at: http://path.upmc.edu/divisions/diagnostics/services/micro.html. Accessed August 30, 2005.
48. Bakerman S. *ABC's of Interpretive Laboratory Data*. 4th ed. Scottsdale, Ariz: Interpretive Laboratory Data; 2002.
49. Tierney LM, McPhee SJ, Papadakis MA. *Current Medical Diagnosis and Treatment*. 39th ed. New York, NY: Lange Medical Books/McGraw Hill; 2000.

Women's Health After Transplant

Lisa A. Coscia, RN, BSN, CCTC
Carolyn H. McGrory, RN, MS
John M. Davison, MD
Michael J. Moritz, MD
Vincent T. Armenti, MD, PhD

Introduction

Organ transplantation has improved the quality and length of life for transplant recipients, and in enhancing the health of women it has specifically empowered them to assume roles as sexual partners and mothers and to anticipate the prospect of a healthy life. Specific health issues for transplant recipients encompass special considerations regarding the potential for the return of fertility, the possibility for posttransplant pregnancies, the need for appropriate contraception, and recommendations for suitable hormone replacement therapy (HRT).

The issues faced by healthcare professionals in counseling those recipients who received the first organ transplants were very different from the issues facing practitioners today. Recipients have higher expectations and now look forward to a fulfilling life that includes the real possibilities of once again "being well," the ability to resume working, the possibility of motherhood, and a longer life. For example, healthcare professionals must determine the appropriateness of a myriad of medications necessary both for immunosuppression and to treat a variety of comorbidities, including potential interactions. This task is complicated by the fact that many medications have not been studied in pregnant women, and for numerous medications there is a paucity of pregnancy outcome data.

A major role of healthcare professionals, however, is as counselor, educator, and guide, providing an interface between recipients and the medical realm. This chapter provides information to the practitioner in counseling transplant recipients regarding contraception, pregnancy, and HRT.

Return of Fertility

Most women with end-stage organ failure develop irregular or absent menses and diminished fertility. Restoration of organ function usually leads to return to premorbid reproductive function, often quite rapidly.[1,2] Although pregnancies occurring early after transplantation can be successful, the fetus may be exposed to greater risks. Potential risks include higher doses of immunosuppression, higher risks of rejection, less stable graft function, a greater risk of fetal exposure to cytomegalovirus and other early posttransplant infections, exposure to potentially fetotoxic prophylactic medications (e.g., ganciclovir or valganciclovir), and labile, changing comorbid conditions (e.g., hypertension and diabetes). Thus it is recommended that women wait for a period after transplantation until the above factors and other individual circumstances result in lower risks for the fetus and the transplant. The general recommendation is to wait 1 to 2 years after transplantation before conceiving;[3,4] this recommendation is not based on clinical trials, but key case studies and common sense.

Contraception

There is little information available in the literature supporting specific recommendations regarding contraceptives for transplant recipients. No clear choice of an ideal contraceptive exists for this group of patients. It is generally agreed upon that contraceptive information is important and transplant recipients of childbearing age should be educated about the potential for a return of fertility and the need for appropriate birth control measures after transplantation. In determining which measures to advise, caretakers must assess each recipient individually, consider their health status, and allow for personal choice.[5] Because the rate of unplanned pregnancy in female transplant recipients is about 50% (National Transplantation Pregnancy Registry data), it is recommended that discussion of the return of fertility and the need for contraception should occur as early as at the initial transplant evaluation, then immediately after transplantation before discharge from the hospital, and again during the ensuing outpatient visits.[6,8]

Several transplant centers have surveyed the contraceptive methods used by their recipients.[9,10] Mattix-Kramer et al[9] reported results of an observational study among 107 women with kidney transplants who completed a questionnaire. Of 41 premenopausal women, 26% reported using no contraception. An article from Iran[10] reported that coitus interuptus was the predominant method of contraception, used by 56% of the female kidney transplant recipients surveyed. Other methods used were surgical sterilization (28%), condoms (14%), and oral contraceptives (2%).[10]

Because there are no medical contraindications to their use, the logical contraceptive of choice for transplant recipients would be barrier devices, including male and female condoms. These contraceptives prevent conception, while also providing protection from most sexually transmitted diseases. Other barrier devices include diaphragms with spermicidal creams, foams, tablets, or jellies.

Few publications exist regarding the use of oral contraceptives in transplant recipients.[8,11] Debate continues regarding this method of birth control, because these medications can cause or exacerbate hypertension, predispose to thromboembolism, and may cause subtle changes in the immune system. In addition, liver recipients taking oral contraceptives may be more susceptible to cholestatic drug reactions.[8] Although not specifically contraindicated for transplant recipients, close surveillance is warranted during the use of oral contraceptives, especially with regard to calcineurin inhibitor monitoring as oral contraceptives may affect drug levels.[8]

The use of an intrauterine contraceptive device (IUD) may cause menstrual problems, and with long-term use the risk of pelvic infections is increased.[12,13] Periprocedure antibiotic coverage should be considered for transplant recipients who choose to have an IUD placed. The efficacy of an IUD may potentially be decreased because of the possible modification of the leukocyte response associated with immunosuppressive and anti-inflammatory agents taken by these recipients.[1]

Pregnancy After Transplantation

It has been almost 50 years since the first pregnancy in a kidney transplant recipient occurred. The donor and recipient were identical twins, negating the need for immunosuppression. The pregnancy occurred in 1958 (reported in 1963) with the delivery of a healthy term infant.[14] The recipient also delivered another baby 2 years later. Since these events, there have been thousands of posttransplant pregnancies reported through case, center, and registry reports.[15-19]

In 1976, Davison and colleagues,[20] on the basis of a literature review and their own management of a case, published preconception guidelines for kidney transplant recipients. The criteria included (1) good general health for at least 2 years since the transplantation; (2) stature compatible with good obstetric outcome; (3) no proteinuria; (4) no significant hypertension; (5) no evidence of renal rejection; (6) no evidence of pelvicaliceal distension on a recent excretory urogram; (7) a plasma creatinine level of 2 mg/dL (180 µmol/L) or less; and (8) drug therapy at maintenance levels or with prednisone at 15 mg/day or less and azathioprine at 3 mg/kg/day or less.[20] Although these guidelines were written before the introduction of modern day immunosuppression, they are generally still applicable today and may also be extrapolated for use with nonrenal transplant recipients contemplating pregnancy.

In 1991, the National Transplantation Pregnancy Registry (NTPR) was established to gather information on female solid organ transplant recipients who have had pregnancies and male transplant recipients who have fathered pregnancies in North America. Tables 1 (women) and 2 (males, fathered pregnancies) show the total number of recipients enrolled in the registry as of January 2005.[21] The registry also follows the long-term outcomes of these recipients, their transplants, and their offspring. The registry continues an ongoing database, enrolling all pregnancies, and is also accessible as a resource for providing information to recipients and healthcare providers.

Overall, if patients enter pregnancy with adequate stable transplant function on maintenance levels of immunosuppression, the likelihood of a successful pregnancy outcome is enhanced. Although newborns to transplant recipients are often premature, the children in general are reported to be healthy and developing well. Each organ type has its own particular recipient issues; for example, chronic viral hepatitis present among some liver recipients. Other considerations for recipients contemplating pregnancy include the possible ramifications of their original diagnosis and familial or hereditary conditions.

Typically, transplant recipients are taking 1 or more immunosuppressive medications. As new medications and novel combinations of these medicines are developed, recommendations for their use during pregnancy become increasingly complex. There have been concerns raised regarding the use of mycophenolate mofetil (MMF; CellCept) during pregnancy. Outcomes of pregnancies of transplant recipients who are taking MMF are listed in Table 3. In the NTPR database, there were a total of 15 kidney recipients with 23 pregnancies reporting exposure to MMF. Among the liveborn of these pregnancies, the malformation rate was 33%, including hypoplastic nails and shortened fifth fingers (n=1), cleft lip, cleft palate, and microtia (ear deformity; n=1), microtia alone (n=1), and multiple malformations resulting in neonatal death (n=1).

In the literature, malformations after exposure to MMF during pregnancy after kidney transplantation have been reported twice.[22,23] The recipient reported by Pergola et al[22] is included in the NTPR data. The report by LeRay et al[23] (from France, and not included in the NTPR data) describes termination of a fetus with multiple malformations.

Table 1. PREGNANCIES REPORTED TO THE NATIONAL TRANSPLANTATION PREGNANCY REGISTRY (JANUARY 2005)

Organ	Recipients	Pregnancies	Outcomes*
Kidney	716	1097	1125*
Liver	111	187	189*
Liver-Kidney	4	6	7*
Pancreas-Kidney	38	56	58*
Heart	33	54	54
Heart-Lung	3	3	3
Lung	14	15	15
Total	**919**	**1418**	**1451***

*Include twins and triplets; all types of outcomes are included (live births, spontaneous abortions, therapeutic abortions, stillbirths, and ectopic pregnancies)

Tables 1-7 adapted and reprinted with permission from Clinical Transplants 2004[21]

Table 2. PREGNANCIES FATHERED BY MALE TRANSPLANT RECIPIENTS REPORTED TO THE NATIONAL TRANSPLANTATION PREGNANCY REGISTRY (JANUARY 2005)

Organ	Recipients	Fathered pregnancies	Outcomes*
Kidney	526	784	796*
Liver	54	71	76*
Liver-Kidney	2	4	4
Pancreas-Kidney	28	34	35*
Heart	91	123	125*
Heart-Lung	1	2	2
Lung	2	2	2
Total	**704**	**1020**	**1040***

*Include twins and triplets; all types of outcomes are included (live births, spontaneous abortions, therapeutic abortions, stillbirths, and ectopic pregnancies)

Table 3. EXPOSURE TO MYCOPHENOLATE MOFETIL DURING PREGNANCY IN KIDNEY TRANSPLANT RECIPIENTS: NATIONAL TRANSPLANTATION PREGNANCY REGISTRY DATA

Case No.	Regimen	Outcome	Birthweight (g)	Gestational age (weeks)
1	MMF, tacrolimus, prednisone	Live birth	2240	34*
2	MMF, tacrolimus, prednisone	SA	N/A	7
3	MMF, tacrolimus, prednisone	Live birth	822	31
4	MMF, tacrolimus, prednisone	Live birth	1701	35
5	MMF, Neoral (cyclosporine, USP, modified), prednisone	Live birth SA SA Live birth	2495 N/A N/A 2977	36 7 6 36
6	MMF, Neoral (cyclosporine, USP, modified), prednisone	SA Live birth	N/A 2240	8 35
7	MMF, tacrolimus, prednisone, sirolimus	Live birth	1531	31*
8	MMF, Neoral (cyclosporine, USP, modified), prednisone	Live birth	3118	39
9	MMF, tacrolimus, prednisone	SA Live birth	N/A 2211	4 33
10	MMF, tacrolimus, prednisone	SA	N/A	5
11	MMF, tacrolimus	SA SA	N/A N/A	4 5
12	MMF, tacrolimus	Live birth	3118	38
13	MMF, Gengraf (cyclosporine, USP, modified), prednisone	SA SA SA	N/A N/A N/A	9 6 7
14	MMF, tacrolimus, prednisone	Live birth	2886	39*
15	MMF, tacrolimus, prednisone	Live birth	2551	35†

Abbreviations: MMF, mycophenolate mofetil; N/A, not available; SA, spontaneous abortion.
*Birth defect reported; see text for details.
†Neonatal death at 1 day old due to multiple malformations.

Experience with MMF in nonrenal transplant recipients in the NTPR database includes 3 liver recipients with 3 pregnancies (2 live births and 1 fetal loss at 18 weeks)- with no malformations reported. In a recent article from Sweden[24] (not included in the NTPR data), researchers reported 1 liver recipient exposed to MMF during pregnancy with multiple malformations in the newborn, including esophageal atresia, cardiac defects (not specified), and an iris anomaly. In addition, in the NTPR database, 1 heart transplant recipient reported a spontaneous abortion.[25]

Although there have been successful outcomes among recipients taking MMF in combination with other immunosuppressive agents, to date there is a higher incidence of both malformations and spontaneous abortions reported among kidney transplant recipients. The true denominator of exposure to MMF during pregnancy, however, is not known. Regarding pregnancy and MMF, there is an array of treatment options including decreasing MMF, discontinuing MMF, changing MMF to azathioprine or another immunosuppressant, and when to time this change in maintenance immunosuppression. It is a serious matter to determine the best course in weighing the unknown risks of a birth defect when taking MMF, versus an unknown risk of rejection or graft dysfunction without MMF. Reproductive animal data indicate the possibility of adverse pregnancy events at doses in the therapeutic range.[26] When contemplating pregnancy, recipients should be apprised of the limited clinical outcome data available and that reproductive animal data do not always correlate to problems in humans. The package insert for MMF recommends effective contraception before beginning therapy, during therapy, and for 6 weeks after discontinuing the medication before attempting conception.[26] The European Best Practice Guidelines recommend not using MMF during pregnancy until more information is available.[27]

Five pregnancies in kidney transplant recipients with exposure to sirolimus (including case 7 from Table 3 in which the recipient was switched from MMF to sirolimus for rejection), have been reported to the NTPR.[26] These pregnancies resulted in 4 live births and 1 spontaneous abortion. In the 4 sirolimus cases without MMF, the sirolimus was discontinued in the first trimester and there were no malformations reported among the 3 newborn. There was 1 pancreas-kidney transplant recipient who reported a spontaneous abortion while taking sirolimus. In addition, there is a case report from Poland[28] of a liver recipient with sirolimus exposure during the first 6 weeks of gestation who delivered a healthy infant with no malformations. Similar to MMF, the package insert for sirolimus recommends that effective contraception must be initiated before sirolimus therapy, during sirolimus therapy, and for 12 weeks after sirolimus therapy has been discontinued.[29] Again, the European Best Practice Guidelines state that sirolimus use in pregnancy is contraindicated.[27] Recipients taking this medication who are planning a pregnancy must be made aware of the dilemma surrounding the unknown risk of birth defects versus the unknown risk of rejection and transplant dysfunction if sirolimus is discontinued.

Kidney Transplant Recipients

Pregnancies among kidney transplant recipients have been reported via case reports, center studies, and registry reports.[15-19] Pregnancy outcomes of female kidney recipients enrolled in the NTPR are listed in Table 4 and are divided by calcineurin inhibitor therapy; the largest recipient group in the NTPR are those who are taking cyclosporine (Sandimmune).[21]

Even though there is a high incidence of hypertension and preeclampsia among kidney recipients, overall outcomes are favorable for recipient, graft, and offspring. Most reported infections have been minor, for example, urinary tract infections, and very few infections have been life threatening.

Rejections have been reported in 2% to 4% of pregnancies (Table 4). Although infrequent, rejections may occur unexpectedly, and in recipients who are thought to be at low risk.[30] When rejection occurs during pregnancy, it can be treated and recovery of graft function is possible. If a rejection occurs, the chances are increased that the newborn infant will be more severely premature and have a low birth weight. Chronic rejection has been identified as a prepregnancy risk factor for potential problems during pregnancy by a study in Poland.[31]

Two case controlled studies[32,33] comparing pregnant and nonpregnant kidney transplant recipients have shown that pregnancy does not affect long-term graft survival, although minor deleterious effects cannot be excluded. Similarly, in NTPR data, a slight increase in the mean serum creatinine level has been shown from prepregnancy to postpregnancy, when all kidney transplant recipients entered in the database are compared.[21]

Offspring of Female Kidney Transplant Recipients

Numerous studies of the offspring of female kidney transplant recipients have reported a high incidence of prematurity and low birth weight, without an increased number of birth defects.[34-40] Di Paolo et al[34] showed that there was a delay in immune system development in offspring exposed to immunosuppressive agents, but that the immune system returned to normalcy by age 1.[31] These researchers concluded that it may be necessary to delay childhood vaccinations. In the NTPR database, however, the majority of kidney transplant recipients have reported that their children received their vaccinations on time and without obvious problems or complications, but a more detailed evaluation is warranted.

Cochat et al[41] hypothesized that in utero exposure to cyclosporine may result in nephrotoxic effects to the exposed fetus; however, preliminary results of renal function studies in these children were encouraging. These investigators also noted that continued studies are needed to determine the long-term effects of cyclosporine exposure in utero.[41] Giudice et al[36] reported comparable results in an earlier study.

Similarly, 133 children were assessed for developmental delays in an NTPR study[38]; the majority (84%) demonstrated no delay and did not require extra educational support. The 29 (16%) children with

Table 4. PREGNANCY OUTCOMES IN FEMALE KIDNEY TRANSPLANT RECIPIENTS REPORTED TO THE NATIONAL TRANSPLANTATION PREGNANCY REGISTRY

Maternal factors	Sandimmune (Cyclosporine)	Neoral (Cyclosporine USP, Modified)	Tacrolimus
Time from transplantation to conception, mean years	3.3	5.2	3.3
Hypertension during pregnancy	62%	72%	58%
Diabetes during pregnancy	12%	3%	10%
Infection during pregnancy	23%	22%	34%
Rejection episode during pregnancy*	4%	2%	4%
Pre-eclampsia	29%	31%	29%
Mean serum creatinine level, mg/dL			
Before pregnancy	1.4	1.4	1.2
During pregnancy	1.4	1.4	1.5
After pregnancy	1.6	1.5	1.5
Graft loss within 2 years of delivery	11%	4%	13%
Outcomes†	**n=496**	**n=154**	**n=71**
Therapeutic abortions	8%	1%	1%
Spontaneous abortions	12%	19%	24%
Ectopic pregnancies	1%	0%	0%
Stillbirth	3%	1%	3%
Livebirths	76%	79%	71%
Live births	**n=376**	**n=121**	**n=50**
Mean gestational age, weeks	36	36	35
Mean birth weight, g	2493	2448	2378
Premature (<37 weeks)	52%	54%	53%
Low birth weight (<2500 g)	46%	50%	50%
Cesarean section	51%	46%	55%
Newborn complications	41%	50%	54%
No. (%) of neonatal deaths (within 30 days of birth)	3 (1%)	0	1 (2%)

*Rejection for cyclosporine including chronic rejection; Neoral and tacrolimus biopsy proven acute rejection only
†Includes twins and triplets
Sandimmune brand cyclosporine (321 recipients, 486 pregnancies)
Neoral brand cyclosporine (109 recipients, 146 pregnancies)
Tacrolimus (56 recipients, 70 pregnancies)

developmental delay had a mean gestational age of 34 weeks, with 14 children delivered less than or equal to 33 weeks. Offspring follow-up is essential for this aspect of development.

    The long-term follow-up of the children born to transplant recipients remains one of the goals of the NTPR. Even though the majority of children have been reported as healthy and developing well, there could be subtle effects from in utero exposure to immunosuppression that may not be apparent until much later in life. The issue of in utero exposure affecting offspring later in life is illustrated in a case report by Scott et al, in which a child of a recipient later developed systemic lupus erythematosus.[42] In children of recipients taking Neoral (cyclosporine USP, modified) or tacrolimus in combination with prednisone and/or azathioprine there has been no increase in the number or pattern of malformations reported (3%-5%) when compared with malformations in the general population.[30,43]

Pancreas-Kidney Transplant Recipients

Pregnancy outcomes of pancreas-kidney transplant recipients are shown in Table 5. Recipients maintained euglycemia during pregnancy, with the exception of 1 case requiring sliding-scale regular insulin coverage during pregnancy only, with no rejection reported during pregnancy. There have been other reports in the literature of similar outcomes for pancreas-kidney transplant recipients with regard to glycemic control.[44-47]

According to NTPR data, 75% of pancreas-kidney transplant recipients reported hypertension during pregnancy, the highest incidence when compared to other recipient groups. Chronic hypertension can be associated with prematurity, low birth weight, and perinatal mortality for the fetus and newborn.[48]

Table 5. PREGNANCY OUTCOMES IN 38 FEMALE PANCREAS-KIDNEY RECIPIENTS WITH 56 PREGNANCIES (58 OUTCOMES, INCLUDING TWINS) REPORTED TO THE NATIONAL TRANSPLANTATION PREGNANCY REGISTRY

Maternal factors	
Time from transplantation to conception, mean years	3.7
Hypertension during pregnancy	75%
Diabetes during pregnancy	2%
Infection during pregnancy	55%
Rejection episode during pregnancy	6%
Preeclampsia	34%
Graft loss within 2 years of delivery	16%
Outcomes*	**n=58**
Therapeutic abortions	5%
Spontaneous abortions	14%
Ectopic pregnancies	2%
Stillbirth	0%
Live births	79%
Live births	**n=46**
Mean gestational age, weeks	34
Premature (<37 weeks)	78%
Mean birth weight, g	2096
Low birth weight (<2500 g)	63%
Cesarean section	57%
Newborn complications	57%
No. (%) of neonatal deaths† (within 30 days of birth)	1 (2%)
Immunosuppression by pregnancy	**No. (%) of recipients**
Cyclosporine, azathioprine, and prednisone	19 (34)
Cyclosporine and prednisone	6 (11)
Cyclosporine (Neoral), azathioprine, and prednisone	13 (23)
Cyclosporine (Neoral) and prednisone	3 (5)
Tacrolimus, azathioprine, and prednisone	5 (9)
Tacrolimus and azathioprine	2 (4)
Tacrolimus and prednisone	4 (7)
Tacrolimus and sirolimus	1 (2)
Tacrolimus	1 (2)
Gengraf (cyclosporine, USP, modified), azathioprine, and prednisone	2 (4)

*Includes twins.
†One neonatal death due to sepsis (26 weeks, 624 g)

In a previous NTPR report, pancreas-kidney transplant recipients with and without postpartum graft loss were analyzed.[47] Six recipients reported graft loss and 21 reported no graft loss. Recipients with graft loss had a mean prepregnancy serum creatinine level of 2.23 mg/dL versus 1.49 mg/dL for recipients with no graft loss (P=.013). Rejection episodes during pregnancy were also significant in the graft loss group (3 of 8 versus 0 of 28 in the no graft loss group, P=.008). It was concluded that prompt investigation and treatment of graft dysfunction is warranted, because a decrease in graft function may be associated with an increased risk of graft loss postpartum.

Overall, pancreas-kidney transplant recipients can carry a successful pregnancy, but the risk for more severe prematurity and lower birth-weight infants appears to be greater than for other organ recipients, perhaps because of the higher comorbidities among these recipients, including hypertension.

Liver Transplant Recipients

Pregnancy outcomes of liver transplant recipients reported to the NTPR are presented in Table 6.[21,49-52] The incidence of hypertension during pregnancy among liver transplant recipients is 35%, lower than among kidney transplant recipients (58%-72%). The incidence of preeclampsia in tacrolimus-treated liver transplant recipients is 13%, lower than that of cyclosporine-treated liver transplant recipients (25%-33%). The lower incidence of preeclampsia among tacrolimus-treated liver transplant recipients has also been reported by the Pittsburgh group.[49] Diabetes during pregnancy, however, has been shown to be more common in tacrolimus-treated liver transplant recipients (13%) compared to those treated with cyclosporine (0%-2%).[53]

Liver transplant recipients have reported acute rejection during 8% of pregnancies. In an earlier NTPR analysis of acute rejection during pregnancy, there was a significant difference in the mean gestational age of newborns in those recipients with rejection versus those without rejection. Fifty-nine recipients with 101 pregnancy outcomes without rejection were compared with 10 recipients with 11 pregnancy outcomes with rejection. The mean gestational age of the 77 live births in the group without rejection was 37.2 weeks and the mean birth weight was 2807g. These live births were compared to the 8 live births whose mothers reported rejections, with a mean gestational age of 33.8 weeks (P=.0014) and a mean birth weight of 1946 g (P=.006).[50]

In a subpopulation of liver transplant recipients with hepatitis C, there is concern with maternal survival especially with subsequent pregnancies.[50] Further comparison of recipients with hepatitis C versus those with other diagnoses would be beneficial to assess the risk of pregnancy in this population.

In a recent analysis of registry data, liver transplant recipients originally diagnosed with autoimmune hepatitis were compared to those with other diagnoses. There were no significant differences in the rate of rejection during pregnancy (autoimmune hepatitis, 10%; other diagnoses, 7%) or graft loss within 2 years (autoimmune hepatitis, 6%; other diagnoses, 8%).[54]

Overall, the offspring of liver transplant recipients have higher mean birth weights and gestational ages than those of kidney transplant recipients, and the children are reported as healthy and developing well. Birth defects were reported in 3 of 63 offspring of liver transplant recipients treated with cyclosporine (4.76%), which is similar to the rate in the general population.[43]

Thoracic Organ Transplant Recipients

Table 7 presents the outcomes of heart and lung transplant recipients in the NTPR. Additional reports have been noted in the literature.[55-60] The overall pregnancy outcomes of heart transplant recipients have been favorable, with no graft losses reported within 2 years of pregnancy. In an earlier NTPR report,[57] 10 rejections were diagnosed during pregnancy; 6 recipients received steroid-based treatment and 4 recipients required no treatment.

Newborns of heart transplant recipients have similar outcomes to those of liver transplant recipients, with a mean gestational age of 36 weeks and a mean birthweight of 2717 g. Again, overall these children are reported as healthy and developing well. There have been reports, however, of 3 offspring who have inherited diseases similar to those that had caused the illness for which their mothers had required a transplant.[57] Genetic counseling before pregnancy is essential for anyone who may have a disorder that could be inherited.

Table 6. PREGNANCY OUTCOMES IN FEMALE LIVER TRANSPLANT RECIPIENTS REPORTED TO THE NATIONAL TRANSPLANTATION PREGNANCY REGISTRY

Maternal factors	
Time from transplantation to conception, mean years	4.3
Hypertension during pregnancy	35%
Diabetes during pregnancy	5%
Infection during pregnancy	27%
Rejection episode during pregnancy	8%
Preeclampsia	23%
Graft loss within 2 years of delivery	7%
Outcomes*	**n=189**
Therapeutic abortions	6%
Spontaneous abortions	19%
Ectopic pregnancies	0%
Stillbirth	2%
Live births	73%
Live births	**n=138**
Mean gestational age, weeks	37
Premature (<37 weeks)	36%
Mean birth weight, g	2705
Low birth weight (<2500 g)	34%
Cesarean section	35%
Newborn complications	29%
No. (%) of neonatal deaths (within 30 days of birth)	0%
Immunosuppression by pregnancy†	**No. (%) of recipients**
No immunosuppression	5 (3)
Cyclosporine, azathioprine and prednisone	51 (27)
Cyclosporine and prednisone	40 (22)
Cyclosporine and azathioprine	1 (1)
Cyclosporine	3 (2)
Cyclosporine (Neoral), azathioprine, and prednisone	10 (5)
Cyclosporine (Neoral) and prednisone	15 (8)
Cyclosporine (Neoral) and azathioprine	2 (1)
Cyclosporine (Neoral)	7 (4)
Tacrolimus, azathioprine, and prednisone	7 (4)
Tacrolimus and azathioprine	2 (1)
Tacrolimus and prednisone	27 (15)
Tacrolimus, mycophenolate mofetil, and prednisone	1 (1)
Tacrolimus and mycophenolate mofetil	1 (1)
Tacrolimus	12 (7)
Gengraf (cyclosporine, USP, modified) and azathioprine	1 (1)
Gengraf (cyclosporine, USP, modified)	1 (1)

*Includes twins.
†One pregnancy in a recipient receiving an unknown regimen.

Table 7. PREGNANCY OUTCOMES IN 33 FEMALE HEART AND 14 FEMALE LUNG TRANSPLANT RECIPIENTS REPORTED TO THE NATIONAL TRANSPLANTATION PREGNANCY REGISTRY

Maternal factors	Heart (n=33)	Lung (n=14)
Time from transplantation to conception, mean years	4.1	3.1
Hypertension during pregnancy	46%	53%
Diabetes during pregnancy	4%	27%
Infection during pregnancy	11%	20%
Rejection episode during pregnancy	21%	27%
Preeclampsia	10%	13%
Graft loss within 2 years of delivery	0%	21%
Outcomes	**n=54**	**n=15**
Therapeutic abortions	9%	33%
Spontaneous abortions	17%	13%
Ectopic pregnancies	2%	0%
Stillbirth	2%	0%
Livebirths	69%	53%
Live births	**n=37**	**n=8**
Mean gestational age, weeks	37	35
Premature (<37 weeks)	32%	63%
Mean birth weight, g	2717	2285
Low birthweight (<2500 g)	32%	63%
Cesarean section	30%	38%
Newborn complications	22%	75%
No. (%) neonatal deaths (within 30 days of birth)	0%	0%
Immunosuppression by pregnancy	**No. (%) of recipients**	**No. (%) of recipients**
Cyclosporine, azathioprine and prednisone	32 (59)	6 (40)
Cyclosporine and prednisone	7 (13)	1 (7)
Cyclosporine and azathioprine	2 (4)	0
Cyclosporine (Neoral), azathioprine, and prednisone	5 (9)	2 (13)
Cyclosporine (Neoral) and prednisone	1 (2)	0
Cyclosporine (Neoral) and azathioprine	1 (2)	0
Tacrolimus, azathioprine, and prednisone	1 (2)	4 (27)
Tacrolimus and prednisone	2 (4)	1 (7)
Tacrolimus	2 (4)	1 (7)
Tacrolimus, mycophenolate mofetil, and prednisone	1 (2)	0

Successful pregnancies have been reported among lung transplant recipients.[59-60] This recipient group should approach pregnancy with caution, however, because there is a high rate of rejection during pregnancy (27%) as well as a high incidence of graft loss within 2 years of pregnancy (21%). The high rate of pregnancy terminations (33%) and the long-term impact of pregnancy on maternal graft survival in this population require further study. At this time, lung transplant recipients appear to be at higher risk compared to other solid-organ transplant recipients, and should be counseled accordingly when considering pregnancy.

Breast-feeding

There are a few published studies regarding breast-feeding while receiving immunosuppression after transplantation.[61-65] Thirty-three transplant recipients breast-feeding their 38 babies reported no problems to the NTPR registry, with their breast-feeding time varying from a few days to 2 years. One mother chose to stop breast-feeding after detectable but low levels of cyclosporine were found in her infant.[21] The decision to breast-feed remains controversial, with the known benefits of breast-feeding weighed against the unknown risks of immunosuppressive exposure, and continued studies in this area are needed.

Hormone Replacement Therapy

Although the use of HRT among transplant recipients has not been well studied, it has been recommended that postmenopausal transplant recipients be considered for HRT, on the basis of studies mostly in the liver transplant population.[66] Vo et al[67] found that HRT has been used among liver transplant recipients more often than in kidney transplant recipients. In another study[68] of 32 menopausal liver transplant recipients, researchers concluded that transdermal estradiol in combination with progestin (EstracombR-Ciba, 50 mcg/24h, 250 mcg/24h) if the uterus was intact and estradiol alone (EstradermR-Ciba, 50 mcg) if the uterus was removed, were safe and effective. These investigators published a 2-year follow-up, concluding that liver transplant recipients using HRT responded similarly to healthy postmenopausal women.[69] Other studies have also stated that HRTs can safely be prescribed after liver transplantation.[70]

Few randomized, case-controlled studies looking at HRT among female transplant recipients exist, and further study is required. With the more recent controversies surrounding the appropriateness of HRT use in general, use in any population should be questioned.

Summary

The transplant professional plays a vital role in counseling women both before and after transplantation about contraception, family planning, the advisability of becoming pregnant, and HRT. It is important for women of childbearing age to use contraception after transplantation because fertility often returns quickly and unexpectedly with the potential for pregnancy occurring within weeks after transplantation. Ultimately, the use of contraception is a personal choice and the responsibility of healthcare professionals is to provide information and guidance.

As transplant recipients are a high-risk group, prepregnancy planning should be an essential component and should include genetic counseling. With the newer medications such as MMF and sirolimus, and the novel combinations in use, prepregnancy counseling and planning become even more important, given the limited clinical pregnancy outcome data regarding the use of these medications.

Overall, pregnancy is well tolerated and successful outcomes have been reported in each solid-organ recipient group; however, each case must be considered individually on the basis of the health of the woman and her transplanted organ. Two areas where pregnancy safety is not clearly established are lung recipient pregnancies and the new immunosuppressant agents. Lung transplant recipients have reported higher graft loss rates after pregnancy and should approach pregnancy with caution. The newer immunosuppressives present challenges in assessing pregnancy risk given the small number of exposures and the complex milieu of the transplant recipient.

The care of the pregnant transplant recipient requires a coordinated effort among many specialists, including the transplant team and the high-risk obstetrical team. The transplant nurse can assist in coordinating this effort and referring recipients to existing resources, including the NTPR. Although there has been much learned in the area of pregnancy, additional studies are needed as well as the formation of organ-specific uniform practice guidelines for caring for these recipients. Continued study through entries to the NTPR, as well as case reports and center reports, will help the practitioner in the care of these unique pregnancies.

Acknowledgment:
The National Transplantation Pregnancy Registry gratefully acknowledges the cooperation of the many transplant recipients and more than 200 centers in the United States, Canada, and Puerto Rico who have contributed their time and information to the registry.

References

1. Davison JM. Pregnancy in renal allograft recipients: problems, prognosis and practicalities. In: Lindheimer MD, Davison JM, eds. *Balliere's Clin Obstet Gynaecol: Renal Disease in Pregnancy.* London, United Kingdom: Bailliere Tindall. 1994; 501-525.
2. Cundy TF, O'Grady JG, Williams R. Recovery of menstruation and pregnancy after liver transplantation. *Gut.* 1990; 31:337-338.
3. Davison JM. Dialysis, transplantation, and pregnancy. *Am J Kidney Dis.* 1991; 17:127-132.
4. Hou S. Pregnancy in transplant recipients. *Med Clin North Am.* 1989; 73:667-683.
5. McKay D, Josephson M, Armenti VT, et al. Reproduction and transplantation: report on the AST Consensus Conference on reproductive issues and transplantation. *Am J Transplant.* 2005; 5:1592-1599.
6. Riley CA. Contraception and pregnancy after liver transplantation. *Liver Transpl.* November 2001; 7(11 suppl 1):74-76.
7. Lessan-Pezeshiki M. Pregnancy after renal transplantation: points to consider. *Nephrol Dial Trans.* 2002; 17:703-704.
8. Coscia LA, McGrory CH, Philips LZ, et al. Pregnancy and transplantation. In: Cupples SA, Ohler L, eds. *Solid Organ Transplantation.* New York, NY: Springer Publishing; 2002:373-393.
9. Mattix-Kramer HJ, Tolkoff-Rubin NE, Williams WW, et al. Reproductive and contraceptive characteristics of premenopausal kidney transplant recipients. *Prog Transplant.* 2003; 13:193-196.
10. Lessan-Pezeshki M, Ghazizadeh S, Khatami MR, et al. Fertility and contraceptive issues after kidney transplantation in women. *Transplant Proc.* 2004; 36:1405-1406.
11. Dourkis SP, Tolis G. Sex hormonal preparations and the liver. *Eur J Contracept Reprod Health Care.* March 1998; 3(1):7-16.
12. Washington AE, Aral SO, Wolner-Hanssen P, et al. Assessing risk for pelvic inflammatory disease and its sequelae. *JAMA.* 1991; 266:2581-2586.
13. Steen R, Shapiro K. Intrauterine contraceptive devices and risk of pelvic inflammatory disease: standard of care in high STI prevalence settings. *Reprod Health Matters.* 2004; 12:136-143.
14. Murray JE, Reid DE, Harrison JH, et al. Successful pregnancies after human renal transplantation. *N Engl J Med.* 1963; 269:341-343.
15. Penn I, Makowski EL, Harris P. Parenthood following renal and hepatic transplantation. *Transplantation.* 1980; 30:397-400.
16. Toma H, Kazunari T, Tokumoto T, et al. Pregnancy in women receiving renal dialysis or transplantation in Japan: a nationwide survey. *Nephrol Dial Transplant.* 1999; 14:1511-1516.
17. Jimenez E, Gonzalea-Carabello Z, Morales-Otero L, et al. Triplets born to a kidney transplant recipient. *Transplantation.* 1995; 59:435-436.
18. Thompson BC, Kingdon EJ, Tuck SM, et al. Pregnancy in renal transplant recipients: the Royal Free Hospital experience. *Q J Med.* 2003; 96:837-844.
19. Armenti VT, Ahlswede KM, Ahlswede BA, et al. National Transplantation Pregnancy Registry: outcomes of 154 pregnancies in cyclosporine-treated female kidney transplant recipients. *Transplantation.* 1994; 57:502-506.
20. Davison JM, Lind T, Uldall PR. Planned pregnancy in a renal transplant recipient. *Br J Obstet Gynaecol.* 1976; 83:518-527.
21. Armenti VT, Moritz MJ, Radomski JS, et al. Report from the National Transplantation Pregnancy Registry (NTPR): outcomes of pregnancy after transplantation. In: Cecka JM, Terasaki PI, eds. *Clinical Transplants 2004.* Los Angeles, Calif: UCLA Immunogenetics Center; 2005:103-119.
22. Pérgola PE, Kancharla A, Riley DJ. Kidney transplantation during the first trimester of pregnancy: immunosuppression with mycophenolate mofetil, tacrolimus and prednisone. *Transplantation.* April 2000; 71(7):94-97.
23. Le Ray C, Coulomb A, Elefant E, et al. Mycophenolate mofetil in pregnancy after renal transplantaition: a case of major fetal malformations. *Obstet Gynecol.* 2004; 103:1091-1094.
24. Källén B, Westgren M, Åberg A, et al. Pregnancy outcomes after maternal organ transplantation in Sweden. *Br J Obstet Gynecol.* 2005; 112:904-909.
25. Gaughan WJ, Coscia LA, Hecker WP, et al. Pregnancy outcomes in female transplant recipients on newer adjunctive therapies. *Am J Transplant.* May 2005; 5(suppl 11):291.
26. Mycophenolate mofetil [package insert]. Nutley, NJ: Roche Laboratories; 2004.
27. EBPG Expert Group on Renal Transplantation. European best practice guidelines for renal transplantation. *Nephrol Dial Transplant.* 2002; 17(suppl 4):50-55.
28. Jankowska I, Oldakowska-Jednyak U, Jabiry-Zieniewicz Z, et al. Absence of teratogenicity of sirolimus used during early pregnancy. *Transplant Proc.* 2004; 36:3232-3233.
29. Sirolimus [package insert]. Philadelphia, Pa: Wyeth Laboratories; 2005.
30. Armenti VT, Radomski JS, Moritz MJ, et al. Report from the National Transplantation Pregnancy Registry (NTPR): outcomes of pregnancy after transplantation. In: Cecka JM, Terasaki PI, eds. *Clinical Transplants 2002.* Los Angeles, Calif: UCLA Immunogenetics Center; 2003:121-130.

31. Kozlowska-Boszko B, Lao M, Gaciong Z, et al. Chronic rejection as a risk factor for deterioration of renal allograft function following pregnancy. *Transplant Proc.* 1997; 29:1522-1523.
32. First MR, Combs CA, Weiskittel P, et al. Lack of effect of pregnancy on renal allograft survival or function. *Transplantation.* 1995; 59:472-476.
33. Sturgiss SN, Davison JM. Effect of pregnancy on the long-term function of renal allografts: an update. *Am J Kidney Dis.* 1995; 26:54-56.
34. Di Paolo S, Schena A, Morrone L, et al. Immunologic evaluation during the first year of life of infants born to cyclosporine-treated kidney transplant recipients: analysis of lymphocyte subpopulations and immunoglobulin serum levels. *Transplantation.* 2000; 69:2049-2054.
35. Schen FP, Stallone G, Schena A, et al. Pregnancy in renal transplantation: immunologic evaluation of neonates from mothers with transplanted kidney. *Transplant Immunol.* 2002; 9:161-164.
36. Giudice PL, Dubourg L, Hadj-Aïssa A, et al. Renal function of children exposed to cyclosporine in utero. *Nephrol Dial Transplant.* 2000; 15:1575-1579.
37. Willis FR, Findlay Ca, Gorrie MJ, et al. Children of renal transplant recipient mothers. *J Paediatr Child Health.* 2000; 36:230-235.
38. Stanley CW, Gottlieb R, Zager R, et al. Developmental well-being in offspring of women receiving cyclosporine post-renal transplant. *Transplant Proc.* 1999; 31:241-242.
39. Oz BB, Hackman R, Einarson T, et al. Pregnancy outcome after cyclosporine therapy during pregnancy: a meta-analysis. *Transplantation.* 2001; 71:1051-1055.
40. Kainz A, Harabacz I, Cowlrick IS, et al. Review of the course and outcome of 100 pregnancies in 84 women treated with tacrolimus. *Transplantation.* 2000; 70:1718-1721.
41. Cochat P, Decramer S, Robert-Gnansia E, et al. Renal outcome of children exposed to cyclosporine in utero. *Transplant Proc.* 2004; 36(suppl 2):208-210.
42. Scott JR, Branch DW, Holman J. Autoimmune and pregnancy complications in the daughter of a kidney transplant patient. *Transplantation.* 2002; 73:815-817.
43. Armenti VT, Radomski JS, Moritz MJ, et al. National Transplantation Pregnancy Registry (NTPR): outcomes of pregnancy after transplantation. In: Cecka JM, Terasaki PI, eds. *Clinical Transplants 2001.* Los Angeles, Calif: UCLA Immunogenetics Center; 2002:97-105.
44. Barrou BM, Gruessner AC, Sutherland DER, et al. Pregnancy after pancreas transplantation in the cyclosporine era. *Transplantation.* 1998; 65:524-527.
45. McGrory CH, Groshek MA, Sollinger HW, et al. Pregnancy outcomes in female pancreas-kidney recipients. *Transplant Proc.* 1999; 31:652-653.
46. Jain AB, Shapiro R, Scantlebury VP, et al. Pregnancy after kidney and kidney-pancreas transplantation under tacrolimus: a single center's experience. *Transplantation.* 2004; 77:897-902.
47. Wilson GA, Coscia LA, McGrory CH, et al. National Transplantation Pregnancy Registry: postpregnancy graft loss among female pancreas-kidney recipients. *Transplant Proc.* 2001; 33:1667-1669.
48. Barron WM. Hypertension. In: Barron WM, Lindheimer MD, eds. *Medical Disorders During Pregnancy.* St. Louis, Mo; 2000:1-38.
49. Jain A, Venkataramanan R, Fung JJ, et al. Pregnancy after liver transplantation under tacrolimus. *Transplantation.* 1997; 64:559-565.
50. Armenti VT, Herrine SK, Radomski JS, et al. Pregnancy after liver transplantation. *Liver Transpl.* 2000; 6:671-685.
51. Nagy S, Bush M, Berkowitz R, et al. Pregnancy outcome in liver transplant recipients. *Obstet Gynecol.* 2003; 102:121-128.
52. Wu A, Nashan B, Messner U, et al. Outcome of 22 successful pregnancies after liver transplantation. *Clin Transplant.* 1998; 12:454-464.
53. Armenti VT, Radomski JS, Moritz MJ, et al. Report from the National Transplantation Pregnancy Registry (NTPR): outcomes of pregnancy after transplantation. In: Cecka JM, Terasaki PI, eds. *Clinical Transplants 2002.* Los Angeles, Calif: UCLA Immunogenetics Center; 2003:121-130.
54. Coscia LA, Hecker WP, Moritz MJ, et al. Pregnancy outcomes in female liver transplant recipients with autoimmune hepatitis. *Am J Transplant.* May 2005; 5(suppl 11):179.
55. Branch KR, Wagoner LE, McGrory CH, et al. Risks of subsequent pregnancies on mother and newborn in female heart transplant recipients. *J Heart Lung Transpl.* 1998; 17:698-702.
56. Wagoner LE, Taylor DO, Olsen SL, et al. Immunosuppressive therapy, management, and outcome of heart transplant recipients during pregnancy. *J Heart Lung Transplant.* 1993; 13:993-1000.
57. Cowan SW, Coscia LA, Philips LZ, et al. Pregnancy outcomes in female heart and heart-lung transplant recipients. *Transplant Proc.* 2002; 34:1855-1856.
58. Miniero R, Tardivo I, Centofanti P, et al. Pregnancy in heart transplant recipients. *J Heart Lung Transplant.* 2004;23:898-904.
59. Gertner G, Coscia L, McGrory C, et al. Pregnancy in lung transplant recipients. *Prog Transplant.* 2000; 10:109-112.

60. Donaldson S, Novotny D, Paradowski L, et al. Acute and chronic lung allograft rejection during pregnancy. *Chest.* 1996; 110:293-296.
61. Thiru Y, Bateman D, Coulthard M. Successful breast-feeding while mother was taking cyclosporin. *BMJ.* 1997; 315:463.
62. Nyberg G, Haljamae U, Frisenette-Fich C. Breast-feeding during treatment with cyclosporine. *Transplantation.* 1998; 65:253-255.
63. Munoz-Flores KD, Easterling T, Davis C, et al. Breast-feeding by a cyclosporine–treated mother. *Obstet Gynecol.* 2001; 97:816-818.
64. Moretti ME, Sgro M, Johnson DW. Cyclosporine excretion into breast milk. *Transplantation.* 2003; 75:2144-2146.
65. French AE, Soldin SJ, Soldin OP, et al. Milk transfer and neonatal safety of tacrolimus. *Ann Pharmacother.* 2003; 37:815-818.
66. Pirsch JD, Douglas MJ. Liver transplantation. In: Cupples SA, Ohler L, eds. *Solid Organ Transplantation.* New York, NY: Springer Publishing; 2002:261-291.
67. Vo T, McKay D, King A, et al. Hormone replacement therapy (HRT) in female transplant recipients. *Am J Transplant.* May 2005; 5(suppl 11):291.
68. Appelberg J, Isoniemi H, Nilsson CG, et al. Safety and efficacy of transdermal estradiol replacement therapy in postmenopausal liver transplanted women. A preliminary report. *Acta Obstet Gynecol Scand.* 1998; 77:660-664.
69. Isoniemi H, Appelberg J, Nilsson CG, et al. Transdermal estrogen therapy protects postmenopausal liver transplant women from osteoporosis. *J Hepatol.* 2001; 34:299-305.
70. Dourkis SP, Tolis G. Sex hormonal preparations and the liver. *Eur J Contracep Reprod Health.* March 1998; 3(1):7-16.

Pediatric Transplantation

Patricia Harren, DrNP, CPNP, CANP, CCTC

Introduction

Pediatric transplantation is truly a world of small patients and small numbers. Large pediatric heart, liver, and kidney centers perform an average of 25 to 40 transplants for each organ group annually. In comparison, large adult programs perform 80 to 150 transplants for each organ group annually. Thus, pediatric programs have many more challenges: contracting issues due to low volumes and survival rates, patients' ages that range from birth to young adulthood, and having multiple "patients" per transplantation performed, that is, the entire family. Pediatric transplantation programs are geared to deal with multiple complex family issues and patients at various developmental stages, and the staff in pediatric programs accept the challenge willingly. It is important to remember that children are not small adults. They metabolize medications differently and are dosed truly by weight. Many of the medications we use in transplantation today do not have a Food and Drug Administration (FDA) label for pediatrics; however, such is the case most medications used in general pediatrics today. Only recently has the FDA required pharmaceutical companies to perform clinical trials in children. Children also differ from adults in the fact that they are still physically and mentally developing. When treating children, it is important to take into consideration what developmental stage the child should be experiencing. Doing so aids in assessing if any delays are present and also helps staff tailor their interactions to be appropriate for the child's level of understanding.

The purpose of this chapter is to review the different developmental stages from infancy to young adulthood as defined by developmental theorist Erickson. (1) The different issues and important interventions that are age appropriate are discussed, as are the methods ensuring a successful transition from pediatrics to an adult transplant team. Also covered are different ways to handle challenging family issues and the ethics of transplanting organs in children despite their family dysfunction.

Neonates and Infants: Birth to Age 1 Year

Normal Development

Developmental theorist Erik Erikson calls this period "basic trust versus mistrust."[1] Infants develop a sense of trust and dependency with the adult who meets their basic need of food, security, love, and shelter. Cognitively, infants understand the world through their senses and the movements around them. They are soothed through these senses and enjoy familiar touch, smell, sights, sounds, and tastes.[3] Infants express discomfort and that their needs are not being met in several ways. Crying is the most noticeable; however, they also communicate through stiffness or limpness, changes in skin color, change in sleep habits, and change in appetite.[2,3] Infant's social development continues to show the effects of individual personality and temperament. Stranger anxiety varies among infants, depending on the variety of caregivers they have experienced and their temperament. Infants use gestures such as stretched arms and tugging to get caregiver's attention and communicate their needs.[4] Infants' expressive language skills are limited; however, their receptive language can clearly be seen as they listen and respond to their caregiver's instructions and requests.[4] Emotional development with the expression of anger, jealousy, affection, and anxiety becomes more pronounced at around age 1 year.

Transplantation Issues

Interaction with infants should be aimed at fostering their contact with their primary caregiver, thus allowing the infants' trust to develop. Candidates for transplantation and transplant recipients in this age group often require hospitalizations for complex medical therapies such as surgery or interventions for feeding issues related to poor growth and development. They can become distrustful when their pain isn't eased quickly or when they are not fed for long periods because of radiologic studies or invasive procedures that are necessary.

Parents should be there to comfort and should not be used to help restrain the baby during procedures. Infants must feel safe and secure, so caregivers are encouraged to hold them whenever possibly, especially when the infants are hospitalized. Staff should help facilitate this even when the infant is connected to multiple intravenous catheters and monitoring wires. If parents cannot be handed their baby, they are encouraged to hold them in the crib or bed, making physical contact and talking to them. Staff contact with the baby should be limited because it is unfamiliar and makes the baby tense. Familiar items from home, such as a favorite blanket, doll, or stuffed animal can be used to comfort infants, and their parents' participation in care is encouraged as much as possible.[5]

Encourage families to stay with their infant and avoid separation whenever possible. If and when family members have to leave, they should have another familiar person take their place. Infants who are not held or whose cries are not attended to withdraw. They stop crying and become low tone, and they often do not develop good coordination because they spend much of their time lying in a crib with no stimulation. Because lack of stimulation can have such a detrimental effect on babies, hospitals often use volunteers to sit and hold babies and frequently nurses on duty take the babies into the nursing station so that the babies are continually stimulated by the interaction of the staff, lights, and sounds when their families are not present.

Interventions

Caregivers are also under extreme stress. They are often unfamiliar with the medical interventions that are needed and are anxious about whether they are making the correct decision for their child. Transplant teams should provide caregivers with a description of the sequence of events and what to expect and ease the caregivers' tensions.[3] Ways to reduce anxiety and make caregivers more cooperative include providing both verbal and written information, directing caregivers to appropriate resources where they can gather information, encouraging them to seek second and third opinions, and providing them with the records they need.

Child-life specialists, in addition to occupational and physical therapists, should be involved with these small patients early in the process. Infants should have large amounts of time dedicated to supervised play activities and should be encouraged to extend their range of motion and gross motor abilities as appropriate.[3]

Toddlers: Age 1 to 3 Years

Normal Development

Many of the same issues from infancy carry over into this age group. Toddlers have limited communication skills and are still dependent on adults. In addition, Erikson calls this phase "autonomy versus shame" because toddlers like to choose and decide for themselves. Toddlers understand the world around them through their senses and body movements. Parents are important to provide these children with a feeling of protection, and toddlers often need to see a parent to feel safe enough to act independently.[3] In this stage of development, language skills begin to emerge. Toddlers are often frustrated by their inability to communicate their wishes verbally because that skill is not yet well developed. Fine and gross motor skills are also being developed, as demonstrated by the ability to feed themselves and hold crayons and markers for art projects.

Transplantation Issues

Ill toddlers have difficulty with their loss of independence. They have an intense sense of stranger anxiety and insecurity, which they demonstrate through hyperactive tantrums and regression of skills they have already developed. Toddlers who have been chronically ill begin to withdraw and their stranger anxiety shifts to apathy, which they demonstrate by not eating well, being much less active, and crying less with interventions. They think that hospitalizations and painful procedures are punishments for bad behavior.[3]

Chronically ill toddlers may have to experience separation from caregivers because prolonged or multiple hospitalizations may place a financial burden on the family, and caregivers may need to work part of the day to ensure income to pay the bills and provide care and support for siblings. For toddlers, the time away from familiar caregivers can be very traumatic.[3] Parents also feel very guilty about their absence.

Interventions

Parents should be involved with care and procedures as much as possible. Staff members should be assigned to provide consistency in staffing so that the toddler can get used to them and be less fearful during interactions. Staff should also move slowly and deliberately to avoid frightening the child. Staff should direct communication with the toddler during history taking and physical examination. Doing so not only supplies information about the patient but gives the provider information about the child's cognitive skills and language development. Staff members should speak at eye level, adjusting their height to meet the gaze of the child.[3] When approaching toddlers, you should avoid direct eye contact with their caregivers and allow the toddlers to observe you while you gradually move closer to them. You should position yourself next to the toddler rather then directly in front of him or her because the child finds this less threatening. When you make eye contact with toddlers, you should smile briefly but continue to speak. Slowly integrate yourself into their play with cars, blocks, or similar toys. By taking your time, you've prepared for the predictable stranger anxiety and allowed the toddler to get used to you and your surroundings. Using these measures alleviates much anxiety for the child and makes interactions easier for the providers.

Many child life specialists who work with toddlers use dolls and role playing as a way to allow the children to become familiar with common procedures and as a way for the children to express their feelings. Staff members can simulate drawing blood from a teddy bear, placing an adhesive bandage on the bear's arm either before or after drawing the child's blood (let it be their choice who goes first: bear or child). Allowing toddlers to make choices is important, but make sure you give them an option only when it is truly an option. An example of a good choice is asking whether the child wants to go to the play room or watch a video. You wouldn't offer a choice of whether or not the child wants to get stuck with this needle to draw blood; that is not an option. When speaking with toddlers and children in general, it is better not to ask permission for a procedure that is needed. You can tell the toddler that "I am going to look for the crayons I lost before" when looking in their ears, but don't ask them "Can I look in your ears now?" If you need to do an assessment of a toddler's tympanic membranes and the toddler says no, what do you do? You do it anyway, and the child gets upset and angry. It is also important to allow toddlers to participate in their care as much as possible. Ways that toddlers can help include encouraging them to participate in bathing activities, feeding themselves (even though this can be very time consuming), holding equipment, and handing you non-sharp items such as a stethoscope or diaper. Making toddlers' care as fun and engaging an activity for them as you can is crucial for long-term cooperation and less traumatic for the toddlers.

Preschoolers: 3 to 6 Years Old

Normal Development

According to Erickson, the preschooler stage of development is known as "initiative versus guilt." In this stage, preschoolers are developing their own sense of identity but still need their parents to be close by. It is easier for preschoolers to establish trust with strangers, but they still need the support of adults.[3] In this stage, vocabulary increases and fine and gross motor skills develop. Preschoolers often like to pick out their clothes and dress themselves. Their fine motor skills have improved: they can easily feed themselves, and it is in this stage that they are toilet trained. Preschoolers are unable to see others' point of view; for example, John is holding a doll with its face toward Ann, and Ann thinks John can also see the doll's face.[4]

Fears and magical thinking also manifest in this stage. Preschoolers are afraid of monsters under the bed or in the closet. Learned fears can also begin, such as fear of the dark and of doctors or animals. Their understanding of the world is based on direct experience, and they cannot understand abstract concepts like time.[3]

Preschoolers are also very literal. When they hear healthcare providers on rounds saying that some organism is growing in the blood, they think that things like bugs are growing inside them, and they get very upset.

Transplantation Issues

Preschoolers face many of the same transplantation issues as children of other ages, such as loss of control, intense fear, and regression of developmental milestones. The magical thinking that predominates in this developmental stage leads preschoolers to have many misconceptions about their medical condition, and their limited verbal skills make it difficult for care providers to understand what the children perceive. That is why it is very important not to "round" in the patient's room, but rather to discuss laboratory values, radiology reports, and the overall plan of care in a place separate from the patient. Whenever possible, information should be discussed with the parents when the child is not present. Regressive behaviors are common and are often manifested in children of this age by actions like sucking a thumb again, soiling undergarments, and using "baby talk" even though these behaviors were stopped months to years prior.

Interventions

Any staff members interacting with preschoolers should provide them with age-appropriate information about what is being done. Preschoolers often grasp only part of the explanation; for example, the child who is told "this won't hurt" may hear only the "hurt" part. They are often very afraid despite what they say, so parents should be allowed to be present through as much of the procedure as possible, such as letting parents stay in the operating room until the patient is unconscious.

Humor is often very effective when dealing with preschoolers. During physical examinations, pretending to hear French fries or guessing what they had for breakfast engages them. Using equipment that is outfitted for use in children, such as an otoscope with an attachment that looks like an elephant, distracts children from procedures that so many dislike. It is also helpful to allow children in this age group to play with and explore the equipment so that they become more familiar with it.

Preschoolers can be empowered by holding their hands and closing their eyes to help them cope with difficult situations. Make them feel brave by telling them how strong they are and how much you can see they are trying to be brave, thus avoiding any low self-esteem that may follow a procedure during which they were difficult.

School Age: 6 to 12 Years

Normal Development

Children ages 6 to 12 years are considered school age. Erikson calls this developmental stage "industry versus inferiority." Children's image of themselves is based on their physical and mental abilities.[6,7] Typically this is a time when children are known to suppress their feelings and instead channel them into hobbies and skills.[3] School-age children can understand how their body functions, and they typically become very conscious of their body image and are modest. They are also afraid of body mutilation and injury and they begin to fear death.[3]

Socially, school-age children begin to develop strong peer relationships and migrate to groups of the same sex. They are very interested in fads and "fitting in." It is important to most children in this age group that they blend into the group, so it is common to see many wearing the same clothes and listening to the same music and belonging to the same team or after-school activities.

School-age children frequently want all information told to them to be backed up. They ask a lot of "how" and "why" questions, and their understanding of information regarding medical interventions is much more sophisticated than appreciated by most adults.

Transplantation Issues

Prolonged separation from their peer groups is a concern for school-age children. They need the support of their group, and they seek reinforcement that the transplantation will not make them so different that they will no longer fit into the group.[6] The physical changes that happen to their bodies as a result of the side effects of the medications greatly influence their self-image and often result in avoidance behaviors such delayed return to school or activities.[8]

The advanced interest and understanding of the medical aspects of the transplantation make explaining the procedures and medications easier for the transplant team, but children in this age group need more than explanations. They need concrete examples that use visual aids and video to enhance their learning and understanding.

Prolonged hospitalizations can further isolate these children and may lead to avoidance behaviors such as missing school days. Often the attention they receive when they return to school is counterproductive because it makes them stand out at a time when they so desperately want to blend in. Prolonged hospitalizations can cause regression in behavior, such as thumb sucking or crying when blood is being drawn.

Interventions

Preparing school-aged children by telling them what to expect and explaining the sequence of events enhances the outcome of what you are asking them to do or understand. This preparation reinforces and capitalizes on competencies during procedures, which in turn gives the child a greater feeling of success.[3,5] Allow the child to have some control over interventions; for example, let the child decide when to start or take a break if appropriate. Pay attention to the children's body language and listen to what they are saying during the procedures to minimize their anxiety.[3] If they are becoming upset or losing control, it is important to allow them to express their feelings without making them feel guilty for delaying or prolonging the procedure. Focus your commenting on the positive in the situation, offering praise for their efforts.[3]

It is easiest to get information from school-aged children while they are engaged in activities; they are more apt to express their feelings in this setting, often feeling safer thanks to the distraction of the activities. This intervention can make office visits longer and is usually reserved for situations when interventions need to occur or have occurred and you are looking for feedback from the child to help understand what he or she is thinking or experiencing.

Interactions with peers should be encouraged if they are medically safe for the patient. Going to the playroom or the computer center is helpful because patients can see other patients going through the same thing or in similar circumstances, and peer interactions provide them a peer group within the center to identify with. Staying in their room playing video games and watching movies is isolating, and such behavior should be minimized if possible.

Adolescence: 12 to 19 Years

Normal Development

The developmental phase in this age group is "identity versus role confusion." This is the stage of development when children start to become independent from their family; they form very strong peer relationships and are extremely influenced by their peer groups, and risk-taking behaviors are common. Cognitively, they are able to think in abstract forms. Teenagers can think about the future and give that future various outcomes. They question most of the information that is provided to them, and they have an advanced verbal ability to discuss these issues.[3]

Physically, adolescence is a time where both boys and girls are experiencing physical changes related to puberty. They develop a more defined body image and often become sexually active. Both the physical and emotional changes often cause adolescents to have an increased sensitivity toward their appearance, excessive modesty, mood swings, low self-esteem, and sometimes rebellion.[3]

Transplantation Issues

Pediatric transplantation programs note that high rates of nonadherence and risky behaviors are linked to morbidity and mortality among adolescents.[9] The transplant teams should approach these children in a manner that helps foster a relationship to achieve better outcomes. Hospitalization results in a loss of independence and a lack of control and privacy. Adolescents can develop fear, insecurity, and a low self-esteem because of the changes in their physical appearance resulting from side effects of medications, surgical incisions, and scarring. In their quest for independence, adolescents often argue and fight interventions, which frustrates staff and family members.[3] It is extremely important for adolescents to attain this milestone, which is often delayed for transplantation patients because of their complex medical regime and their need for assistance from their family support systems. It is not uncommon for adolescents to have 2 groups of peer support, one at the transplant center and one at home.[3,8]

The transplantation center and hospital inpatient units offer little to no privacy for these very sensitive patients. Adolescents often are embarrassed by questions and should be questioned alone and not in front of parents and other staff. They avoid answering questions if they do not trust the person asking them. They often experience shame if they become emotional in situations. Frequently adolescents feel invincible and take risks. They don't think that medication noncompliance will have any lasting bad effects on their life or their transplanted organ. Their cognition should allow them to understand the cause and effect you teach them; however, they just don't think the bad things will happen to them. But the opposite is true. Results of various studies support the findings that transplant recipients who are nonadherent to therapy have significantly more episodes of adverse outcomes.[10] Other risk-taking behaviors such as taking illicit drugs, unprotected sexual activity, or getting body piercing or tattoos are more common in adolescents with a chronic health problem.[11]

Interventions

The key to a successful relationship with an adolescent is honesty. Positive interactions with these children improves your ability to interact with them and obtain information from them. Although they are still children, it is very important for both patients and their parents that adolescents begin to foster independence. Transplant teams can see adolescents for a portion of the visit alone and then invite their parents into the room to address their questions and concerns. Speaking directly to patients even when their parents are present conveys to them that you see them as the persons involved and gives them a sense of control.

Seeing patients alone opens the door for truthful dialogue. Reminding the patient that you are obligated not to discuss anything they want kept private with their parents unless it poses a threat to them helps make them feel comfortable in confiding information that may be important. Body image and the need to be private are very important. Allow adolescent patients to cover up as much as possible and to wear their own clothing while in the hospital if appropriate. Staff should question patients alone to limit their perception of embarrassment and facilitate honesty in the answers. Coping strategies for patients to vent their frustrations and aggression are also important, and patients should not feel guilty and be reassured that their feelings are normal.[3]

Maintaining the ability to interact with their peers is important, and adolescents should be encouraged while hospitalized to contact their friends via phone or the Internet. Their time with friends should be respected, and they should not have multiple intrusions if possible. Roommates of similar age should be matched if possible, and patients should be encouraged to meet and interact with other patients and form new, supportive peer relationships.[3]

Transition from Pediatrics to Adult Transplant Teams

The transition of patients from pediatrics to adult transplant teams has long been a challenge for many programs. This transition is handled differently from transitions from program to program, and often much stress is associated with the transfer of care. The stress is experienced by the practitioners, who have long cared for the patient (often since infancy), and by the patient and the patient's family, who now are leaving providers with whom they have a long-term relationship and whose judgment they trust.

The age when this transfer of care occurs depends on the program, and most pediatric programs tend to hold onto patients for as long as possible. It is the responsibility of the pediatric transplant team to prepare patients for this transition, and the process should start well before the patients 18th birthday. It is advisable to start the process when the patient enters adolescence. Starting at age 14 years, a written plan for transition should be made. This plan would include the creation of a portable medical record, a checklist of needed services, plans for insurance coverage, and identification of adult-oriented providers.[11]

Dealing directly with adolescent patients is usually the best way to work with them. One approach is to call the adolescent patient into the room, do the examination, question the patient about the issues that relate to the visit, and allow the patient time to ask questions. Then invite the patients' parents or caregivers to join you and summarize your findings to them and allow them time to voice any concerns and ask questions. When you need to contact a patient regarding results of laboratory tests or changes in medication, speak with the patient and relate the pertinent information, but then also speak with the parents to ensure they are aware of the changes and that they can contact the pharmacy if needed. Encouraging the parents or caregivers to participate with these types of interactions is paramount to success, and if they can carry this process over to home responsibilities, it will prove to be more successful.

Often the way to know when a patient is ready for the transition to the adult team is when you can consistently hear the patient take responsibility for his or her actions. An example is "I woke up late and didn't take my medication on time," instead of "My mother didn't wake me up on time so I didn't take my medications when I was supposed to." Patients transferring to the adult team must be independent and responsible. Adult transplant teams deal with many more patients, and the team members will not call to remind patients to get laboratory tests, keep appointments, or go to referral appointments. If the patient is not mature enough and does not comply with the transplant team's recommendations, the patient's long-term outcome can suffer.

Occasionally the pediatric transplant team may come in contact with a family that is more challenging. These challenges include lack of resources that other families may possess in the way of housing, benefits, or support. The psychosocial requirements that adult transplant teams require, such as a place to live, insurance benefits, and compliance with medical appointments, are also important for the pediatric program but are not mandatory. Children receive transplants even if those requirements are not met. Transplant centers will not allow a child to miss the opportunity for an available organ because of their caregiver's difficulties or dysfunctions. The transplant teams have access to children rehabilitation hospitals, which can offer a transitional setting for a child while their parents can learn to care for them and or obtain adequate housing. Removal of the child by making a report of medical neglect to authorities and the child being placed in medical foster care is the last option a center will use, but many centers have needed to make a report to ensure the safety of the child.

Conclusion

Pediatric transplantation is a very fulfilling process. Watching and being a part of the transplant process for a sick infant or child and caring for that patient through their development into adulthood is an opportunity that is gratifying for transplant professionals. Successful interactions can be achieved by taking the child's developmental stage into consideration and tailoring interactions to that individual child's needs. Fostering independence in child transplant recipients is important for transplant teams, and working with parents to do the same results in a successful long-term outcome for these very special patients.

References

1. Dworetzky 1987:228; Lefrancois 1988: 184 Eight Stages of Life according to Erickson.
2. Berk LE. *Infants, Children, and Adolescents.* Boston, Mass: Allyn and Bacon; 1999.
3. Aley KE. Developmental approach to pediatric transplantation. *Progr Transplant.* 2002;12:86-91.
4. Burns CE, Brady MA, Ardys M. *Pediatric Primary Care: A Handbook for Nursing Practice.* Philadelphia, Pa: W B Saunders; 2004.
5. Stewart SM, Kennard BD. Organ transplantation. In: Brown RT, ed. *Cognitive Aspects of Chronic Illness in Children.* New York, NY: The Guilford Press; 1999:220-237.
6. Simon NB, Smith D. Living with chronic pediatric liver disease: the parents' experience. *Pediatr Nurs.* 1992;18:453-458.
7. Sourkes BM. *Armfuls of Time: The Psychological Experience of the Child With a Life-threatening Illness.* Pittsburgh, Pa: University of Pittsburgh Press; 1995.
8. Kuttner L. *A Child in Pain: How to Help, What to Do.* Point Roberts, Wash: Hartley & Marks Publishing, Inc; 1996.
9. Stilley CS, Lawrence K, Bender A, Olshansky E, Webber SA, Dew MA. Maturity and adherence in adolescent and young adult heart recipients. *Pediatr Transplant.* 2006;10:323-330.
10. Berquist RK, Berquist WE, Esquivel CO, Cox KL, Wayman KI, Litt IF. Adolescent non-adherence: prevalence and consequences in liver transplant recipients. *Pediatr Transplant.* 2006;10:304.
11. Burns JJ, Sadof M, Kamat D. The adolescent with a chronic illness. *Pediatr Ann.* 2006;35:207-216.

Fundamentals of Successful Transplant Administration

Tracy Giacoma, RN, MBA, MSN

History of Transplant Administration

Transplant administration or the act of developing, managing, and directing organ transplant programs has existed since the transplanting of human organs became a medical reality. Initially, roles such as physician directors and transplant nurse coordinators filled every administrative and clinical transplant program need. Over the last 2 decades, however, the increasing complexity of administrating transplant programs has resulted in the creation of a myriad of roles to support all the functions required to operate successful programs. In addition to the physician director and transplant nurse coordinator roles, now there are positions such as transplant administrator, contracting specialist, financial coordinator, database administrator, data coordinator, financial analyst, and operations manager performing the administrative functions within transplant programs. Roles that are traditionally considered clinical roles such as pharmacist and social worker are also being dedicated to support administrative activities required to run a successful program.[1]

Transplant regulatory agencies are acknowledging the value of many new roles that provide administrative support to transplant programs. The Organ Procurement and Transplantation Network (OPTN) is the unified transplant network established by the United States Congress under the National Organ Transplant Act (NOTA) of 1984.[2] The United Network for Organ Sharing (UNOS) administers the OPTN under contract with the Health Resources and Services Administration (HRSA) of the US Department of Health and Human Services (DHHS).[3] The OPTN/UNOS has incorporated several transplant administrative positions into its membership bylaws and guidelines, which are followed by all transplant programs. A Transplant Administrators Committee became one of its standing operational committees in 1998 and is composed of transplant administrator–type roles representing each geographic region in UNOS. This committee addresses administrative issues that affect policy development. The committee also hosts an annual UNOS Transplant Management forum that provides education on current topics influencing the administration of transplant programs and promotes networking among colleagues.

The ability to continually implement new roles, recreate old roles, and adapt to the evolving complexity of transplantation is required to meet future administrative needs of transplant programs.

Unraveling the Mystery of Transplant Administration

Transplant administration has become so complex that comprehending its scope is a daunting task. Disassembling the concept of transplant administration into smaller components assists in clarifying the intricacies of operating a successful transplant program. There are identifiable key administrative roles and responsibilities that should be included in any successful transplant program, as shown in Table 1.

Properly managing these key administrative areas creates a solid foundation to sustain and grow a transplant program. The building of a stable foundation, however, does not happen overnight and it varies by where the transplant program is in its stage of development. Eventually, transplant administration must involve continually addressing the effectiveness in each of these areas in order to achieve thriving transplant programs.

Table 1. KEY ADMINISTRATIVE ROLES IN TRANSPLANT ADMINISTRATION

Organizational	Financial	Clinical	Research	Global
Designing the ideal organizational structure Strategic planning for program growth Creating easy access and a steady referral base	Comprehensive approach to financial management Effective contracting for payment of services	Data management Improvement of program effectiveness Assembling an arsenal for funding of medications Maintaining ethical practices	Supporting research	Promoting organ donation Involvement in the development of health Care policy

Organizational Transplant Administration

Designing the Ideal Organizational Structure

The ideal organizational structure achieves the goals and objectives of transplantation, is efficient and cost-effective, and allows timely decision making to address issues and support growth.[4] These achievements are accomplished by developing departments of transplantation in which as many of the key administrative aspects are managed within the department. The ideal structure contains the personnel with the knowledge and skill that is needed specific to transplantation. These personnel expenses are considered part of the direct costs that are necessary to meet the scientific and technical requirements of running a program.

The personnel typically found in transplant organizational structures include the following:

- Transplant administrators provide leadership and direction to the program, with expertise in business, finance, clinical, and regulatory issues in transplantation.
- Physician program, medical, and surgical directors are responsible for the clinical and administrative duties for their specific organ transplantation program. These roles also serve as primary physician director liaisons to UNOS.
- Transplant clinical coordinators take charge and orchestrate the entire pretransplant, transplantation, and posttransplant processes.
- Clinical operations managers provide clinical personnel oversight.
- Ventricular assist device coordinators educate and support patient and families and coordinate the entire process for managing patients with assist devices.
- Database administrators implement, develop, and maintain a transplant database.
- Data coordinators provide the listing and data reporting functions of UNOS.
- Data analysts enter and extract data from information systems and charts.
- Transplant assistants support the clinical transplant coordinators by performing the nonnursing functions for coordination of care.
- Billing coordinators submit and track payments for medical specialist fees, organ procurement costs, UNOS fees, and other expenses directly paid by the transplant program.
- Administrative assistants facilitate communication with referring physicians, outpatient referrals, and oversee correspondence with UNOS, patients, physicians, and insurers.
- Transplant operations analysts bill and collect all transplant-related patient accounts.
- Research coordinators carry out the clinical trials and ensure compliance with Food and Drug Administration regulations.
- Contracting specialists negotiate contracts with insurance companies and physicians, and implement contracts within the system.

- Financial coordinators help potential recipients understand the costs of transplantation and their level of insurance coverage.
- Nurse practitioners/physician assistants assist physicians with managing patients, coordination of the plan of care, and discharge planning.
- Social workers evaluate the psychosocial needs of transplant recipients. This position also assists with funding of medications, home healthcare, long-term care, and other services after transplantation.
- Dietitians address pretransplant, inpatient, and posttransplant nutritional issues and provide dietary education to recipients and families.
- Pharmacists evaluate use of drugs and therapeutic and cost-effectiveness of drug therapy, provide patient education, and monitor drug therapy.
- A living donor team consisting of a clinical transplant coordinator, donor advocate, social worker, and psychiatrist.

The titles of these roles can vary but the functions performed are necessary for every transplant program. Depending on the transplant program volume, these roles may be combined. These roles are ideally in the transplant department in order to maximize efficiency and decision making.

Other roles such as organ procurement/preservation specialist, clinic support, congestive heart failure coordinator, extracorporeal oxygenation team, hepatobiliary coordinator, nurse manager, housing and transportation supervisor, and HLA supervisor and technologist are needed if the functions of organ procurement, disease management, outpatient clinics, inpatient units, housing and transportation, and HLA laboratory are all part of the transplant structure. These roles vary greatly by program because of differences in the size and internal organizational reporting structures.

A large amount of other facility requirements and additional resources exist outside the department of transplantation and are just as critical to the success of transplant programs but are not typically directly part of the department. Assessing the impact and demands that a transplant program places on these areas is also necessary to ensure effective system wide support.

Strategic Planning for Program Growth

Strategic business planning or strategizing is a powerful tool for growing and sustaining successful transplant programs. A business plan projects the future, defines each step to achieve desired goals, and provides an overview of the business and the resources required to run it. Common contents for any business plan includes (1) executive summary, (2) business overview and description, (3) analysis of industry, market, and competition, (4) strategic and marketing plan development, (5) business objectives, (6) financial analysis, (7) implementation plan, (8) performance targets, (9) monitoring objectives, and (10) appendices.

Even though the **Executive Summary** section appears at the beginning of a business plan, it is actually written after all the research and other components of the plan are completed. The goal of the Executive Summary is to get the readers interested; it provides a succinct overview of the plan and is usually a maximum of 2 pages in length.

The **Business Overview and Description** section details the transplant program operations from the past to the present. This section describes the physician and operational leadership, explains the mission and philosophies, lists the dates personnel were added, explains the rationale for adding personnel, details the history of the program, and describes all current services and how these are operationally provided.

The **Analysis of Industry, Market, and Competition** section profiles the market and validates the need for the existence of the transplant program. The analysis involves detailing the demand for services to be provided, and researching and gathering information to answer key questions about the business of transplantation. Some key information to be addressed is the demographics and expected population growth, disease prevalence and projection of disease in a population, transplantations performed per million population or per volume of access to dialysis patients, statistics and services provided by the competition, referral patterns, and the insurance market.[5] A SWOT (strength, weaknesses, opportunities, and threats) analysis is also performed under this part of the plan. Strengths and weaknesses are internal and identified by internal program review, and opportunities and threats are external to the organization and are completed after the market and competition analysis (Table 2).

The **Strategic and Marketing Plan Development** section details how to reach the targeted transplant population. This is accomplished by defining the strategy and marketing efforts on the basis of objective data in the previous analysis, projecting the volume and areas of growth, and specifying the marketing efforts.[6]

Table 2. SAMPLE SWOT ANALYSIS

	Strengths	Weaknesses
Internal	Advantages Capabilities Resources	Disadvantages Gaps in capabilities Lack of resources
	Opportunities	**Threats**
External	Market developments Competitor's vulnerabilities Technological advances	Market demand Competitors strengths Economy

The **Business Objectives** section explains the aim or intention of the plan. It states the overall objectives such as increasing referrals, patient access, and volumes or to start up a new program. It also narrows or specifies the objectives in order to devise the implementation plan. Examples of specific business objectives are expansion of services, national recognition, differentiation of services from the competition, and increasing participation in insurance networks.

The **Financial Analysis** section provides the details of past and present finances. This section can include information on the program's financial contribution, cash flow, and expected changes in financials or expenses associated with new capital projects. A financial pro forma is included in this section if a new program is being proposed.

The **Implementation Plan** describes what actions to take to accomplish the transplant program business objectives. The actions are identified for the key marketing efforts, program objectives, and responsible person or groups (Table 3).

The 2 sections of **Performance Targets** and **Monitoring of Objectives** specify the timelines and goal attainment measurements in order to monitor progress with plan implementation. One functional tool can be created that combines both areas; it can then be updated with actions completed and adjusted for any unplanned changes on the basis of more current data (Table 3).

The **Appendice(s)** is the last section of the strategic business plan, and includes any specific supporting information that does not fit in the body of the plan.

A well-conceived strategic business plan is required to concentrate efforts and maximize the resources required to grow and sustain a successful transplant program.

Table 3. SAMPLE IMPLEMENTATION AND MONITORING PLAN

Implementation	Person(s) Responsible	Monitoring	Time Lines
1. Visit dialysis centers and provide continuing education (CE at centers)		No. of centers, presentations, and CE offerings No. of referrals	
2. Distribution of new education and contact material		Mailing of newsletter, no. of centers and locations receiving materials	
3. Fund and provide continuing medical education sessions and programs to physicians and other dialysis center staff.		No. of planned and delivered sessions No. of attendees	
4. Outreach efforts by physicians in targeted regional areas.		No. of meetings attended, visits made, events organized, and referrals	

Creating Easy Access and a Steady Referral Base

Patients can access organ transplant services in only a few ways. They are referred by physicians, insurance companies, themselves, or family and friends. Besides effectively contracting with managed-care companies, creating easy access to transplant services is also essential to maintaining and supporting a steady referral base. This is achieved through a variety of processes that include being accessible to referring physicians, patients, and developing hospital processes that support access.

Referring physicians contact the transplant institutions to seek expertise on patient clinical management and to refer patients that only transplant centers should be managing. They desire access to services not available in the community, such as research protocols or the transplant procedure, and creating easy access means responding to referring physicians as they contact the institution.[7] Referring physicians also want prompt notification of patient findings and recommendations for follow-up care, and they always want to be notified when their patient receives a transplant. Transplant centers will develop negative relationships with referring physicians if they lose contact with their patients or the transplant center performs test and procedures the referring physician could perform.

The clinical transplant coordinator often serves as the first contact with a transplant center. The coordinator is able to identify appropriate candidates and can provide education of transplant processes to patients or referring physicians.

The financial coordinator assists patients in gaining access to transplantation by validating and explaining insurance benefits and explaining the costs of transplantation. They assist the patients with understanding their coverage limits, out-of-pocket expenses, and any gaps in coverage. The financial coordinator initiates the process for a letter of agreement to occur if the patient's insurance plan is out of network (does not have an inclusive network agreement with the hospital facility). They also identify patients with financial need and provide them information and assistance with fundraising, completion of charity applications, or application for government programs such as Medicaid or high-risk insurance pools. A long-term financial plan is developed. This process allows the patients and their families to understand the financial impact and responsibilities to receiving an organ transplant.

Several hospital processes need to be in place to support access to transplant services. It is necessary to have timely processes in place for notifying the insurance company of unplanned services, obtaining approval from the primary provider or insurance company for scheduled services, managing direct admissions, and managing transfers from other hospitals for an urgent transplant evaluation.

The transplant program will accomplish lasting referral relationships if the processes that support patient access to services can be executed properly. Programs that cannot consistently perform these processes may lose patients who may seek or be referred for organ transplantation elsewhere. Creating easy access and a steady referral base is necessary for long-term program survival.

Financial Transplant Administration

Comprehensive Approach to Financial Management

A comprehensive approach to financial management is required to capture all opportunities for enhancing revenue and controlling expenses. It is important to determine how each organization performs the functions required to appropriately charge, collect, bill and get paid for transplant services, and track transplant-related revenue. It is also essential to understand the financial contributions or strain that transplant programs place upon an institution.[8]

Within an organization, there can be many different methods of monitoring finances. Areas in which to focus efforts include:
- Charges and payments on patient accounts
- Billing and collection timeframes
- Revenue and expenses in the organ acquisition cost centers
- Pretransplant evaluation expenses on the patient accounts for hospital facility services
- Reimbursement on the Medicare Cost report

- Expenses and reimbursement for immunosuppressant agents
- Charity and bad debt management
- Tracking transplant-related revenue

Separating the expenses for pretransplant, inpatient, outpatient, and prescription services is important to the understanding of how these areas are affecting total revenues.

The charges and payments on patient accounts need to be monitored for accurate charges, denials, and expected payments versus payments received. Transplant centers often have a dedicated operations analyst that monitors charges and bills and posts payments in patient accounts. If there is no dedicated position, then a monthly report for monitoring can be generated from the central business office detailing account activity.

The billing and collection timeframes for hospital services must be known to identify when these processes are held up because of inability to accurately code the medical record or when the insurance information is incorrect. A clinical person may need to assist in resolving the coding errors by clarifying the diagnosis and a financial coordinator may need to revalidate that the correct insurance is being billed.

Each specific organ transplant should have a separate acquisition cost center to account for all the pretransplant income and expenses. The revenue located in the organ acquisition cost centers is typically from the standard organ acquisition fees charged to the patient account at the time of the transplant procedure. This revenue needs to be monitored to ensure that the charge is dropped on the patient's account in a timely manner. The charge is usually entered into the patient's account by the billing coordinator in the transplant department when notified that a transplantation has occurred. The organ acquisition charge is composed of an average of the expenses associated with evaluating and maintaining the listing of the pretransplant recipients and the evaluation and donation procedure for living organ donors. It is important that this charge be evaluated and adjusted annually for increases in organ procurement and evaluation and living donation–associated costs and that it reflects the rates paid by Medicare in the cost report (Table 4).

Table 4. SAMPLE DECEASED DONOR LIVER TRANSPLANT ORGAN ACQUISITION FEE

Organ procurement organization charge	$20,000.00
United Network for Organ Sharing registration fee	450.00
Social work fee	200.00
Clinical transplant coordinator fee	2000.00
Data management and required reporting fee	1,000.00
Nutrition support fee	175.00
Psychological consult fee	500.00
Financial counseling fee	100.00
Physician administrative services fee	1000.00
Clerical, administrative support, management fee	4,000.00
Transportation fee	3000.00
Office space, teaching and office supplies, and equipment fee	2000.00
Total acquisition fee	**$34,425.00**

All expenses in the organ acquisition cost centers need to be monitored for inclusion as an appropriate expense. Only allowable costs should be paid out of the organ-specific cost centers. All expense accounts should be monitored monthly for compliance. If the transplant administrator has questions about the appropriateness of an expense in the acquisition accounts, the cost accountant should be consulted. The cost accountant must be comfortable explaining the expenses to the Medicare cost report auditor; there should be no expenses in the acquisition cost centers that the cost accountant cannot explain. Expenses that are typically found in the organ acquisition cost center are the following:

- donor and recipient evaluation tests and procedures performed outside the hospital facility,
- physician services for evaluation,
- pretransplant staff salaries and expenses,
- pretransplant administrative and operational costs,
- UNOS registration fees,
- surgeon fees for excising the deceased organ, and
- transportation costs of procuring the organ.

Pretransplant accounts must be set up to capture the patient evaluation tests and procedures performed at the hospital facility for inclusion in the cost report. Expenses in the accounts need to be screened to ensure that only transplant-related costs are being included. Any expenses that are not part of the potential recipient or donor standard evaluation protocols should be validated for appropriateness. If a patient is called in for a potential transplantation and the procedure is canceled, the charges are still considered pretransplant expenses and should be on the pretransplant accounts. A report detailing these charges should be generated for routine review of all pretransplant evaluation facility service charges in the accounts.

The reimbursement on the Medicare Cost Report must be monitored for inclusion of all appropriate direct and indirect expenses. It is important that the transplant administrator and cost report accountant communicate regarding the expenses included in the organ acquisition cost centers, what types of disciplines are within the transplant department, and quantification of personnel time spent in pretransplant evaluation. The cost accountant may request data from the transplant department on the following:

- number of transplantations performed,
- Medicare as the primary payor for the transplant procedure,
- Medicare as the secondary payor for the transplant procedure,
- number and type of organs procured at the hospital facility per organ donor,
- revenue received from the organ procurement organization (OPO) for the organ donor expenses,
- the amount that the primary insurer paid toward organ acquisition when Medicare is the secondary payor,
- time studies to document pretransplant time,
- job descriptions,
- space utilization, and
- physician time studies.

The cost report must be completed once a year. The cost report total is compared to what the hospital has already been paid as an interim monthly payment and then reconciled to determine if Medicare owes the hospital money or if the hospital owes Medicare money.

The expenses and reimbursement for immunosuppressant agents and other transplant-related medications can be a major source of financial drain to an otherwise successful transplant program. Long-term management of a transplant population involves ensuring that patients are able to access their medications. These costs should be monitored to ensure copays can be collected and that the payments expected are received. The drug costs must be known in order to identify any financial losses. If the transplant hospital does not supply medications to patients, then this area is not a financial consideration.

The management of charity and bad debt is also important to understand within an organization. There must be processes in place to distinguish between charity versus bad debt or uncompensated care and Medicare bad debt. In order to qualify for charity, a person must complete a charity application and meet the charity criteria established by the institution. If the person qualifies under the charity criteria, then the outstanding patient account can then be written off as charity. A bad debt occurs when the hospital bills and tries to collect an owed amount but the outstanding account goes unpaid. The hospital must go through a normal collection process in order for an account to be considered bad debt. The method of how an outstanding bill is written off to qualify as uncompensated care or as Medicare bad debt requires the capability to document inability to pay versus not being able to collect.

Accounting for all sources of transplant revenue is important to be able to understand the entire picture of financial contributions or losses. Transplant revenue should include all new business with a new program, all business that would go away if transplantation were not available, and all other healthcare services required to serve the needs of the transplant population. Revenue can be tracked by diagnosis codes or diagnostic-related groups, individual patient or population identifiers, or by individual physicians. Tracking physician referrals may be the only method to identify all services for a particular end-stage organ disease.

Comprehensive financial management requires taking the time to learn and interpret the many different areas that affect the funding of transplant programs. Monitoring in this area can mean the difference between the financial success and failure of the transplant programs.

Effective Contracting for Payment of Services

The high costs associated with transplant procedures have led to the development of specialty care service agreements between hospitals and managed-care companies.[9] These carve-out agreements for transplant services can control how patients gain access or are denied access to a specific institution. Effective contracting means understanding where the risks and benefits are in a contract and implementing the contracting procedures within the institution. There are a series of contracting processes that need to be examined to understand the ability of an organization to effectively contract for payment of services. Answering the following list of questions will provide an overview of how effective an institution is at contracting.

A. **Contracting Detail**
   - Can the hospital and physicians contract as one entity, that is, global contracts?
   - How are the phases and timeframes of the transplant process defined in the contracts? Phases are defined as phase 1 for evaluation, phase 2 for maintenance or waiting, phase 3 for transplant procedure and phase 4 and 5 for posttransplant care.
   - What is the methodology for determining costs?
   - How are rates established? Global (everything included for 1 price), case rates (fixed payment for a specific episode), per diem (fixed payment per day), or percentage of discount (off charges)?
   - Is the Standard Request for Information template offered by the UNOS Transplant Administrators Committee used?
   - What quality assurance/performance improvement activities are in place?
   - What standardized protocols and procedures are in place?
   - Is a point person for the contracting department identified?
   - Are the physician curriculum vitas and the descriptions of the team members updated?
   - What services are included or excluded from the contract?

B. **Obtaining Contracts**
   - What contracts do you have?
   - What companies are steering patients away?
   - Are you approaching employers or having patients approach their employers?
   - How many patients still have a choice?
   - Are you able to complete letters of agreement or one-time agreements for out-of-network patients (insurance plans that are not under a network agreement with the facility)?
   - Are you accessing patients from local, regional, or national markets?
   - What are your barriers to contracting?
     a. System issues
     b. Support issues
     c. Position in market

- Do your general service agreements have transplant language or is transplantation a carve-out?

C. Contract Implementation
- How do contracts work through the system?
- What is your intake process?
- How are patients identified as under contract?
- Who alerts everyone a contract patient is in the system?
- Who follows and tracks patients during contracting period?
- Who gathers bills and produces 1 global bill?
- Who ensures that contracts are paid at appropriate rates for hospital and physicians?

D. Contract Evaluation and Marketing
- Do you have a contact database?
- What criteria do you use to evaluate contracts?
- What tracking tool do you use to monitor the insurance carrier number of lives, referral numbers, status of contracting relationships, and marketing efforts?
- Are you making regular contact with VIP list clients?
- Is your marketing material up to date?
- Do you have a complete mailing list with the medical director and insurance company contact names?
- Have you differentiated your product to the insurance company?
   a. Cost
   b. Service
   c. Innovation or uniqueness
   d. Reputation, brand recognition
   e. Product line
   f. Access, transportation, and housing
   g. Research
   h. Experience
- Are you using benchmarking data for comparison or goal attainment?
- Does peer-to-peer contact occur for relationship building?

Managed-care companies contract with hospital and physicians for discounted fees and use case management activities to control and monitor costs and quality of services. Contracting with managed-care companies for transplant services is required to avoid patients being steered away from the program. Effective contracting for payment of services requires negotiating the contract details, gaining access to patients, implementing the contract, monitoring the impact of the contracts, and developing mutually beneficial relationships with managed-care companies.

Clinical Transplant Administration

Data Management

Data management for transplant programs has taken on a life of its own. Time spent meeting regulatory, and research requirements increase exponentially each year with the growth of the programs. Data submission compliance is no longer voluntary but is being mandated by the federal government and OPTN/UNOS. Data submission requirements include reporting of information on all deceased and living donors, potential transplant recipients, and actual transplant recipients. Because transplant program outcomes are being compared actual versus expected, the need to make sure every piece of information is accurate and recorded is critical.

The United States Scientific Registry of Transplant Recipients (SRTR) reports transplant center activity and outcomes. SRTR obtained the contract from HRSA to serve as the scientific registry for organ transplantation. It is administered by the University Renal Research and Education Association (URREA), a nonprofit health research organization, in collaboration with the University of Michigan. SRTR provides the data that are reported to OPTN/UNOS by the transplant programs. The data from all transplant programs with membership in the OPTN/UNOS are accessible on the SRTR Web site.[10]

Every 6 months, transplant programs get the opportunity to validate the data that the SRTR will publish. The accuracy of the reported recipient and donor characteristics, which includes recipient and organ survival, needs to be confirmed. The reported expected outcomes for the transplant programs are statically calculated using the makeup of these characteristics. If the reported characteristics are not accurate, the expected outcomes will not be accurate. The programs actual outcomes are compared to the expected outcomes. If the expected outcomes are not correct, the entire analysis is flawed. It is vital to educate the data coordinators on how to interpret the SRTR reports so it is understood how the accuracy of data entry affects the entire programs publicly reported outcome data.

The workload that transplant data reporting requires is overwhelming and every program is looking toward transplant-specific databases to try and manage the demands on manpower and eliminate human errors. Getting as much data electronically fed into the transplant database from internal and external sources is a solution to minimizing data entry and human error. Most programs are achieving this through a transplant-dedicated information system that includes electronic interfaces, electronically stored data, and scanning of paper documents. Getting all roles that provide services to the transplant patient using and entering data into the same system will eliminate duplication of efforts and increase sharing of the information. Data must be accessible from any location every day of the week and any time of the day. Clinical transplant coordinators and physicians need access to patient clinical and demographic information to ensure that patients and organs can be matched in a timely manner. Transplant research and quality assurance activities also increase data collection requirements. Collection of this data should occur concurrently when feasible, so retrospectively gathering the data can be minimized.

The Health Insurance Portability and Accountability Act of 1996 (HIPAA) requires compliance with the Standards for Privacy of Individually Identifiable Health Information. Protected Health Information (PHI) is known as the privacy rule of HIPPA and holds criminal and civil penalties for not performing due diligence or not providing adequate security of the protected data. Access of PHI is limited to the information needed for performance of services. Guarding and sharing of PHI has added costs and time to the healthcare system. Ensuring all information going out from the transplant center is HIPPA compliant is another obligation that must be met.

The strict and data-intensive requirements of transplant programs continue to increase. Ensuring the clinical and demographic accuracy of the transplant patient and organ donor data is imperative to represent the transplant center population accurately. The main goal of a transplant-specific database is to meet the needs for data accessibility, productivity, and elimination of any potential for human error.

Improvement of Program Effectiveness

Program effectiveness requires perpetual, intensive oversight of regulatory compliance and quality assurance activities. This is achieved through a never-ending effort of short- and long-term accomplishments that address, improve, and avoid problems and attain excellence.

Improvement Through Regulatory Compliance

Regulatory compliance in organ transplantation continues to increase as the government adds more policies and qualifications for transplant programs. The public is also demanding access to more information to make informed choices and be able to compare transplant programs. Currently, regulatory agencies with oversight of organ transplantation includes the OPTN/UNOS, Centers for Medicare and Medicaid (CMS), DHHS, the End Stage Renal Disease Network (ESRD), State Department of Health and Human Services (SDHHS), Joint Commission for the Accreditation of Healthcare Organizations (JCAHO), and the Office of the Inspector General (OIG). In order to maintain regulatory compliance, it is critical to understand and apply the regulations and laws, including keeping up with the continuous changes.

Regulations and interpretations of regulations for transplant programs are found in the OPTN/UNOS bylaws, DHHS federal register, Medicare Intermediary publications, JCAHO hospital survey guidelines, ESRD survey procedures, State Government healthcare laws, Insurance Industry regulations, and SDHHS survey guidelines that include recommendations from the Centers of Disease Control, and the OIG publishes a report on special fraud alerts and areas of focus. Surveys conducted for compliance to the regulations are subject to interpretation, so it is necessary to understand how the regulations may be applied by local review agencies. Surveys and audits of regulatory requirements are considered opportunities for process and practice improvements.[11] It is critically important that any areas found to be deficient by regulatory auditors be corrected and not repeated or found deficient on the next survey. Penalties for repeat offences can have much more severe consequences, including loss of program designation as a transplant center.

Adherence to government billing and cost reporting regulations are areas that have zero tolerance for error and carry financial and legal penalties. The level of punitive consequences for nonadherence to financial regulation depends on whether it is intentional fraud or human error in interpreting or following the guidelines.

Improvement Through Quality Improvement Initiatives

Quality improvement initiatives review the clinical and economic performance of transplant programs. Opportunities for improvement are identified by variances from protocols or internal and external benchmarks and from new advancements in protocols and technology. A formalized process that supports quality improvement activities is vital to ensure ongoing review and continuity.[12]

Forming a transplant quality assurance committee with active working groups can be a formalized method of analyzing all key benchmarks. These quality assurance activities are separate from the physician peer review process of morbidity and mortality case reviews. Typical working group meetings can include protocol review, SRTR data review, educational sessions, and review of benchmarking data.

Protocol review can include the development and reassessment of the following:

- Recipient and donor evaluation protocols
- Immunosuppressant and high-risk protocols
- Acute and antibody-mediated rejection protocols
- Infection protocols
- Patient and living donor selection criteria
- Follow-up protocols
- Preoperative and postoperative orders
- Care pathways detailing daily progress and care requirements
- Acute and long-term care plans
- Patient compliance contracts
- Organ acceptance criteria
- Donor and recipient ABO confirmation procedure
- Informed consents
- Ventricular assist device protocols
- Data entry procedures and auditing standards

SRTR data review occurs at least 4 times per year. Every 6 months the transplant program is notified of when the preliminary data are available for review and a deadline for correcting the data is provided. The transplant program is also notified twice a year when the final data will be published on the SRTR Web site, and at that time the program can add comments that can be published with the final data.

Educational sessions are routinely conducted in order to address knowledge deficits identified during quality assurance activities, remain current in the field, and share knowledge among colleagues. These sessions include grand rounds, tumor conferences, radiology conferences, biopsy conferences, journal clubs, and formal symposiums.

Best practice internal and external benchmarking data should be compared to current practice to identify variances and opportunities for improvement. The data for comparison are often composed of the following:

- utilization of services,
- length of stay,
- cost review,
- volumes,
- readmissions,
- reoperations,
- rejections,
- infections,
- procurement complications,
- operating room time,
- cold and warm ischemic time,
- patient satisfaction,
- patient and graft outcomes,
- organ procurement activity,
- waiting time,
- transplant rates,
- organ acceptance rates, and
- mortality on wait list.

The working groups should meet as often as required to address their areas of focus. A report should be provided to the transplant quality assurance committee summarizing the findings, recommendations, and actions of the working groups. The transplant quality assurance committee reports up through the hospital quality improvement organizational structure.

Improvement Through Recruiting and Retaining Experts

Transplant programs should have clearly defined policies regarding how physicians are recruited. Physician recruitment for growth and succession planning should occur to avoid stagnation or instability in current program services. Remuneration provided by a hospital to recruit a physician is restricted by the Stark law. Stark law, actually 2 separate provisions, generally prohibits physician referrals for certain healthcare services to entities or organizations with which the physician or a member of the physician's immediate family has a financial relationship. The law is named after United States Congressman Pete Stark, who sponsored the initial bill. Stark I and II also prohibit the amount of remuneration paid to physicians to be based on the volume or value of any actual or anticipated referrals by the physician or any other business that would be generated by the relationship.[13] Two examples of a Stark law violation would be payment of a transplant physician's administrative salary at a rate above the documented market value or allowing nonhospital-employed physicians to use hospital-paid clinics without an associated charge. The Stark law is used as the legal guideline by which all physician recruitment and succession strategies are developed.

Recruitment and retention of qualified staff to support the transplant program is critical to maintaining program effectiveness. Transplantation is a specialty that requires professionals to seek extensive continuing education and association with colleagues to maintain expertise. To remain knowledgeable in the field of transplantation and to provide state-of-the-art services, key role staff have educational and self-development requirements such as specialty certification, participation in professional organizations, attendance at professional organizational national meetings, and professional speaking. Transplant programs that do not support or plan for continuing education or participation at a national level of their staff will have difficulty recruiting and retaining qualified people and will not be able to compete in the transplant market for talented individuals.

The ever-changing regulatory environment and clinical advances necessitate a relentless effort to achieve excellence in the practice of organ transplantation. Keeping up to date on regulations and best practices and developing and maintaining program expertise is mandatory for clinical and economic program effectiveness.

Assembling an Arsenal for Funding Medications

The funding of transplant medications for the life of the patient or as long as the patient has a transplanted organ is one of the transplant program's and transplant recipients' greatest challenges. When paying for medications, patients often have limited pharmacy coverage, large out-of-pocket expenses, or no coverage. Before patients receive a transplant, a long-range medication coverage plan must be developed, usually involving social work and financial coordinators working together. Even with the best planning, patients' financial circumstances change rapidly and often.

Developing an extensive list of resources that is available to patients to fund medications prevents patients from being eliminated as candidates or not obtaining the medications needed. Social and charitable programs exist that serve and assist with the financial needs associated with chronic illness and special high-risk populations. Programs are usually designated for short- or long-term support. Financial or medication assistance can be accessed through national programs, state programs, county programs, fundraising organizations, drug industry, and other nonprofit private organizations. The assistance programs vary significantly state by state. Benefits, included in programs such as Medicaid, State DHHS, state high-risk insurance pools, county indigent health services, and community charities, must be identified for each local area.[14]

Back-to-work programs for transplant recipients are also needed to support reentry into the workforce with the opportunity to obtain health insurance benefits. As part of the evaluation process and posttransplant maintenance, the potential to return to work should be determined and any available resources for assistance offered.

Transplant social worker positions are often dedicated to exclusively work with patients to obtain medications or funding for medications after transplantation. Patient and transplanted organ outcomes depend on managing this well. Tapping into every resource available is instrumental to support transplant patients' medication needs.

Maintaining Ethical Practices

Transplant programs are continuously faced with the decision of what is right, proper, or just in the context of values and beliefs in society.[15] The role of transplant administration in maintaining ethical practices involves ensuring access to resources in this area of expertise for transplant physicians and staff. This access is necessary to resolve dilemmas and define ethical business conduct.

Hospital-based ethics committees are routinely used by transplant centers to review informed consents and hospital organ donation policies. As ethical issues continue to expand, ethicists are asked to join patient selection committees that determine acceptable candidates for transplantation. The UNOS ethics committee is also a resource for addressing global transplant-related ethical issues.

Transplant professionals often serve in influential positions in which conflict of interest may exist; for example, determining the purchase or use of products or services, serving on the boards of OPOs and governmental committees, or serving on the UNOS board and committees. Most healthcare employers provide guidelines to their employees on what is expected when conducting business on their behalf and require disclosure of any conflicts of interest. In 2002, the Sarbanes-Oxley Act was passed; this act was designed to prevent financial malpractice and accounting scandals in for-profit entities.[16] This act is also known as the Public Company Accounting Reform and Investor Protection Act. The healthcare industry is also looking at this legislation for application to its institutions. The composition of the board of directors of an organization is defined within this legislation. Board members are also required to declare any potential conflict of interest or remove themselves from being involved in decision making or discussions that influence decision making when a conflict of interest is present. Membership on the board of directors of an organization demands serving the needs of the entity and not serving one's self-interests. The implications of this new legislation and its impact on board operations and membership will need to be followed as the healthcare world is looked at for applicability.

As societal values and beliefs transform, the practice of transplanting human organs will remain entrenched in ethical debate. In order for transplant programs to maintain what is considered by society as ethical practices, the information, tools, and understanding required for making the right decisions will need to be adapted to the ever-changing values and beliefs.

Research Transplant Administration

As long as the need for transplantation exists, the need for research will exist as well. Clinical research offers medical advancements not available in the community, provides recognition as offering cutting-edge healthcare services, generates cash revenue, and offers cost savings to patients and insurers when participation is fully funded.

Clinical research is often supported within the administrative structure of transplant programs. Transplant staff may participate in many forms; activities required to support research can include the following:

- coordination of all phases of a research study,
- data entry for data collection,
- contracting for and negotiating fee rates for physician and technical services,
- billing and collections and payment for hospital and professional services for funded research,
- grant writing,
- designing and writing research proposals,
- designing and managing databases,
- professional writing for publications and presentations, and
- statistical analysis.

Transplant program staff participation at national meetings, presentations at national meetings, and publications in peer-reviewed journals is the result of work in research. Bench research or research performed in a laboratory is also an integral part of transplantation, but is not usually part of a transplant administrative structure.

Global Transplant Administration

Promoting Organ Donation

Hospital organizations with transplant programs carry an even greater responsibility to participate in organ donation activities. Because the biggest problem facing the transplant community is the extreme shortage of organs, collaborative efforts to promote organ donation are an essential part of a transplanting center's activities.

Hospitals must partner with their local OPOs to determine the best practices for organ donation and promote community awareness. Monitoring organ donor death referral rates, rates of conversion of eligible donors to donation, and which professional is asking for donation is part of routine hospital quality assurance activities. Hospitals are reporting significant increases in their conversion rates of organ donation by (1) implementing an early referral process, (2) imbedding the organ procurement team early before the family is approached for donation, and (3) getting the organ procurement and hospital personnel meeting to discuss the case and determine the best approach to asking.[17] Activities, which foster community awareness, may include encouraging transplant recipients to thank their donors, transplant and donor families' volunteerism, and supporting the OPO organ donor awareness programs.

Transplant programs have an obligation to their patients to ensure that processes and efforts are implemented to support organ donation within their hospital organization and community. It is not a conflict of interest. It is a responsibility.

Involvement in the Development of Healthcare Policy

Participation in the development of healthcare policy is important to ensure that transplant patient care issues maintain a position of priority in the public sector of policy making. Transplant healthcare policy is developed within governmental health and human services programs, local and national laws, and the OPTN/UNOS policies.

Centers for Medicare and Medicaid Services is the largest federal government healthcare policy maker providing healthcare coverage for patients that qualify by financial contribution to the system, and either by age, disability, or end-stage renal disease. CMS seeks input into policy making through the hosting of public forums and soliciting public response to proposed rules. Transplant centers must participate as the opportunities for input occur.

Local legislature develops policies on state programs including Medicaid, children's programs, and other special-needs programs such as renal disease and human immunodeficiency virus. Local and national government also pass laws that affect transplant healthcare such as support for organ donation, regulation of the health insurance industry, and creation of insurance pools for high-risk patients. Transplant programs must participate in these law-making opportunities to support issues that affect healthcare of the transplant patient. Suggested activities to get involved in include the following:

- Before an election, meet with the district legislature's potential candidates or their staff.
- Meet with elected representatives before, during, and between legislative sessions to make issues that are important to transplant patients known and to get them on the legislative agenda.
- Conduct phone calls and write letters expressing an opinion on issues and proposing specific bills.
- Attend legislative hearings on specific bills and register or testify for or against bills.
- Participate in coalitions that support mutual concern.

Local legislature will propose or sponsor bills to be considered for law during active sessions on the basis of the ideas, needs, support, and nonsupport of the issues.[18] Getting involved with the national passing of laws requires the same activities and can include getting issues of interest addressed by special lobbyist groups.

The opportunities to influence the development of OPTN/UNOS policies arise through input into policy and bylaws when offered for public comment, participation in OPTN/UNOS committees, or election to the board of UNOS. Input into OPTN/UNOS policies can occur in the form of individual representation as part of the public, transplant institution representation, UNOS regional representation, or professional organization representation.

Healthcare policy greatly affects the services and support of transplant programs and patients. It is important to participate at the local and national level to influence policy development and ensure that transplant patient issues remain at the forefront of any healthcare agenda.

Conclusion

Because the field of organ transplantation is dynamic and evolutionary, the increasing complexity of administrating transplant programs will persist into the future. Successful transplant programs require continuous development and improvement in the fundamental key areas of organizational structure, program planning, patient access, financial management, contracting for services, data management, operational effectiveness, funding for medications, ethical practices, research, organ donation activities, and healthcare policy making. Transplant programs exist to provide lifesaving organ transplant procedures to people who need them. Effectively managing the administrative and business side of transplantation maximizes resources that in turn benefit more patients and make available additional services. Historically, running a transplant program only required physicians and nurse coordinators. Now, and in the future, transplant administrative talent is required within a multitude of roles that provide program support.

References

1. Martin J, Zavala EY. The expanding role of the transplant pharmacist in the multidisciplinary practice of transplantation. *Clin Transplant.* 2004;18:50-54.
2. National Organ Transplant Act. Public Law 98-507. Oct. 19, 1984
3. United Network for Organ Sharing. Analysis, Research, and Dissemination. Available at: http://www.unos.org/data/ar2002/ar02_appendix_H. Accessed April 25, 2005.
4. Sims R. *Managing Organizational Behavior.* West Port, Conn: Quorum Books; 2002.
5. Fraher J, Donnan L. The halo effects of transplant programs. *The Advisory Board.* Feb, 2005;2:1-7.
6. Zavala EY. Transplant center marketing. *Graft.* 2001;4:412-415.
7. Ewel C, Russell M. Strategies to increase liver and kidney/pancreas transplant volumes. *The Advisory Board.* July 2003;7:1-9.
8. Jamieson I, Lipori R, Howard RJ. Financial sustainability in transplant programs. *Graft.* 2001;4:424-426.
9. Dranove D. The economic evolution of American health care: from Marcus Welby to managed care. Princeton, NJ: Princeton University Press; 2000.
10. United States Scientific Registry of Transplant Recipients. Role of SRTR in Organ Transplantation. Available at: http://www.ustransplant.org/explanations/role.php. Accessed April 23, 2005
11. The Joint Commission on Accreditation of Healthcare Organizations. The Joint Commission and Health Care Safety and Quality. Available at: http://jcipatient safety.org/show.asp?durki.9771&site=149&return=9334. Accessed April 26, 2005.
12. National Committee for Quality Assurance. *The State of Healthcare Quality: 2004.* Washington, DC: National Committee for Quality Assurance; 2004.
13. Gosfield AG. The Stark truth about the Stark law: part II. *Family Pract Manage.* 2004;11:41-50.
14. Chisholm M, Tackett L, Kendrich B, DiPiro T. Assistance programs available for medications commonly used in transplant patients. Clin Transplant. 2000;4:269-281.
15. Caplan A, Coelho D. *The Ethics of Organ Transplantation: The Current Debate.* Amherst, NY: Prometheus Books; 1998.
16. One Hundred Seventh Congress. Sarbanes-Oxley Act of 2002. H.R. 3763 1-66. Jan. 23, 2002.
17. United Network for Organ Sharing. Organ Donation in the United States. Available at: http: www.unos.org/data/ar2002/ar02_chapter_three.htm. Accessed April 18, 2005.
18. Gagen J. Being all things to 550,000 everybodies. *Assoc Leadership.* 2004;7:26-28.

Section 3: Organ Donation and Procurement

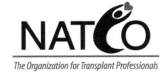

The Organ Donation Breakthrough Collaborative

Teresa Shafer, RN, MSN, CPTC
Virginia McBride, RN, MPH, CPTC
Frank Zampiello, MD
John Chessare, MD, MPH
Dennis Wagner, MPA
Jade Perdue, MPA

Introduction

Organ donation saves lives. Every time a life is saved, a little or a large part of history will be changed, because that individual will create ripples or waves in the sands of time. Organ donation is heroic, although seasoned professionals may minimize it and say it occurs every day. However, even the most seasoned individuals' eyes will fill with tears at the picture and/or poignant story of a donor's family or a grateful recipient. We are drawn to the good work of organ donation because of the good it does for society. We have all come to this point in time, the time of the Organ Donation Breakthrough Collaborative, to make a difference.

The treatment of people with end-stage organ failure through organ transplantation is medically effective and cost-effective, and now constitutes mainstream medicine. Organ transplantation is heroic for a number of reasons (primarily because of the gift of the organ from a living or deceased donor), but nonetheless, it has become commonplace. Even so, more and more people die each year unable to access this treatment. Some individuals cannot access treatment for the same reasons that they cannot access other medical treatment, because of sociological, economic, and educational reasons.

However, most individuals cannot access this treatment because a necessary key ingredient is missing: the *organ*. Waiting lists have grown so large that the waiting time for a kidney transplant exceeds 3 years. The time to transplantation varies among blood types. Blood group O and B registrants wait the longest (median time to transplantation was 1469 and 1815 days, respectively, for those listed in 1999), approximately twice as long as blood group A and 4 times as long as blood group AB (median time to transplantation 740 and 396 days, respectively). The time to transplantation has been increasing steadily in all ethnic groups, but the increase has been greatest among African Americans who, for those listed in 1999, waited more than twice as long as whites.[1] Waiting time for *extrarenal* organs (hearts, lungs, livers) is limited by the one leveling factor that will eventually end the waiting: death.

The United States organ donation system compares favorably to other North American and European countries, as measured in the most common metric used to benchmark organ donation performance in the literature: donors per million (Table 1). The United States compares favorably to other countries using the number of donors, but using the conversion rate, a more appropriate metric, the comparison is not possible because these data have not been historically reported, even in the United States, until recently. However, even though the United States has a "pretty good system," major improvements are necessary. What is *needed* is a *great* system. The United States cannot have a great donation system unless and until the responsibility for donation outcome and system participation includes not only organ donation and transplantation

Chapter 27 THE ORGAN DONATION BREAKTHROUGH COLLABORATIVE

Table 1. INTERNATIONAL ORGAN PROCUREMENT 2003*

Country	Donors	Donors per million
Spain	1443	33.8
United States	6457	23.5†
Ireland	80	21.1
Norway	87	19.1
Portugal	190	19.0
Italy	1402	18.5
Czech Republic	189	18.4
France	1119	18.3
Cuba	194	17.3
Latvia	39	16.9
Finland	85	16.3
Hungary	161	16.1
Uruguay	50	16.1
Puerto Rico	56	14.4
Slovenia	28	14.0
Germany	1140	13.8
Poland	525	13.7
The Netherlands	223	13.7
Canada	428	13.5
Switzerland	93	13.2
Denmark	75	13.0
Sweden	114	12.7
Mexico	1229	11.7
United Kingdom	644	10.9
Australia	179	10.2
Estonia	14	10.0
New Zealand	40	9.9
Chile	136	9.0
Australia	79	9.0
Croatia	39	8.9

*Organs and Tissues. *J Eur Transpl Coord*. 2004; 7(3):159-162.
†Data from the Organ Procurement and Transplantation Network

professionals but also hospital staff such as nurses, physicians, senior leaders, social workers, and chaplains. Critical care nurses are obvious key participants in the system.

In April 2003, Health and Human Services Secretary Tommy G. Thompson joined with key national leaders and practitioners from the nation's transplantation and hospital communities to launch the Organ Donation Breakthrough Collaborative (ODBC), also referred to as the Collaborative. The Collaborative's goal is to dramatically increase access to transplantable organs. The purpose of the initiative was clear, measurable, ambitious, and achievable, "Committed to saving or enhancing thousands of lives a year by spreading known best practices to the nation's largest hospitals, to achieve organ donation rates of 75% or higher in these hospitals."[2]

The participation of hospitals in the donation process must be robust in order for more organs to be recovered in the United States. Until the Collaborative was launched in 2003, responsibility for a hospital's organ donation performance rested solely on the shoulder of the organ procurement organization (OPO) serving that institution. Hospital staff were observers or casual participants. The Collaborative changed that single-participant paradigm. Critical care nurses and physicians partnered with OPO staff in forming teams to participate in the Collaborative to increase organ donation and save lives. The result of this collaboration was a marked increase in the number of organ donors in the United States for the first time in decades.

Identification of Hospital and Organ Procurement Organization Performance

The principal point of interface between organ donors and patients awaiting transplantation is the OPO. OPOs facilitate the organ donation process by developing effective relationships with acute care hospitals, resulting in notification of every in-hospital death; assessment of each death for donation eligibility; consultation with families of eligible donors by trained professionals; and evaluation and placement of every medically suitable organ with a compatible transplant candidate. Less than optimum performance of any of these processes results in denial of a grieving family's opportunity to give the gift of life and the potential death of patients on the waiting list. The measure of how effectively an OPO and hospital are collaborating to provide organ donation services is known as the conversion rate: the ratio of the number of actual donations occurring at the hospital as compared to the number of eligible donors.

In September 2002, OPOs began reporting the number of eligible donors and actual donors to the government each month by hospital, establishing a reasonably sound estimation of the percentage of eligible donors that were being converted to actual donors. A total of 12015 eligible donors were reported in 2002, with 6190 becoming actual donors, a conversion rate of 51.5% (6190 of 12015).[3]

Some hospitals and OPOs had conversion rates higher than 52%, some lower. The conversion rates in hospitals ranged from 0% to 100%. This range, in a hospital with 1 or 2 potential donors per year, was not predictive of overall US donation effectiveness. In addition, this range also existed in the nation's hospitals with the largest number of potential donors. Fifty percent of eligible donors were found in only 206 hospitals of the nation's nearly 6000 acute care hospitals. Seventy-five percent of potential donors are found in 483 hospitals; and 90% of this country's eligible donors are found in only 846 hospitals. There was tremendous variation in conversion rates in the nation's 200 largest donor potential hospitals (Figure 1). Five of the nation's hospitals with the greatest donor potential had conversion rates between 0% and 10%, one hospital had a greater than 90% conversion rate, and most hospitals (n=52) had conversion rates between 40% and 50%.

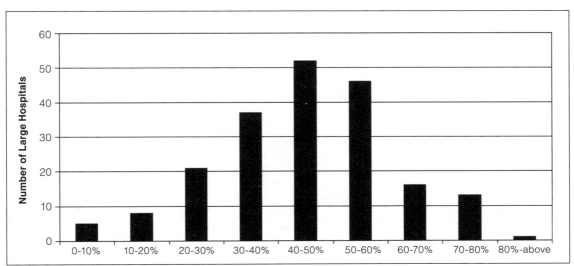

Figure 1. Conversion Rate Distribution Among the Largest 200 Donor-Potential U.S. Hospitals Calendar Year 2002

The concentration of potential donors in the largest hospitals, coupled with the wide variation in their donation rates, creates a situation ripe for rapid, systematic improvements. Questions such as, "Why the variation?" and "What were the high performers doing that caused these results?" needed to be answered and the information shared.

Study of Top-Performing Organizations

A qualitative case study approach was used to identify and describe best practices associated with higher organ donation performance. Six OPOs and 16 affiliated hospitals were selected that were among the higher performers nationally on the basis of rates of consent and organ donation within their communities (Table 2). Background information was gathered and reviewed on selected OPOs and hospitals, and discussions with nearly 300 representatives of OPO and hospital staff, including critical care nurses, were conducted about factors that contribute to high rates of organ donation within the hospital. Data and observations were synthesized and analyzed to formulate overarching principles and best practices.[4]

No "silver bullets" were needed because a very clear set of common principles and best practices emerged from the sites that appeared to contribute to their success (Table 3). The Joint Commission on Accreditation of Healthcare Organizations (JCAHO) had also begun studying organ donation and published many of the same best practices.[5]

Development and Commitment to a Collaborative

The existing crisis of 18 daily deaths of individuals on transplant waiting lists[6] makes it apparent that rapid changes are needed in the donation system. Spreading the knowledge, the *known best practices*, from the OPO and hospital site visits could not be done the way change normally spreads through the healthcare community, including the donation community. The slow process of study, abstract presentation, and publication, all dependent on the right individuals reading, seeing, or hearing the presentation and being motivated to pick up the new knowledge and apply it, was not an option. In the United States, the dilemma was the same that had existed for the previous decade, how to improve a 50% consent rate and 44% conversion rate[7] and how to do it quickly. Tables 4 and 5 present definitions and calculations used in the Collaborative.

Fifteen of the nation's 200 largest hospitals had already achieved organ donation rates of 75% or more in 2002.[8] Many other large hospitals, clustered in certain donation service areas, also had average conversion rates well above the national average. The practices used by OPOs and large hospitals to generate these high rates were increasingly known and could be replicated. Put simply, there was a gap between known best practices and the performance of the existing organ donation system. This Collaborative was conceived to help OPOs and large hospitals rapidly close that gap.

A collaborative is an intensive, full-court-press to facilitate breakthrough transformations in the performance of organizations, on the basis of what already works. It is designed to define, document, and disseminate good ideas, accelerate improvement, achieve results, and build clinical leaders of change. Collaboratives were conceived by the Institute for Healthcare Improvement (IHI), a not-for-profit organization driving the improvement of health by advancing the quality and value of healthcare. Founded in 1991 and based in Cambridge, Mass, IHI helps accelerate change in healthcare by cultivating promising concepts for improving patient care and turning those ideas into action.[9] The IHI had already conducted approximately 45 collaboratives at the time this work started.

Key national leaders, including the Chairman of the Board of IHI, the President of the Association of Organ Procurement Organizations, the Executive Director of the United Network for Organ Sharing, the President of JCAHO, and others joined with the Secretary in committing to this ambitious, but doable Collaborative Aim. The long-range goal of the Collaborative was to create systems that ensured accurate and timely referral, screening, consent, and organ recovery using organ donation best practices. This was to be achieved by implementing OPO- and hospital-specific practices that focused on the needs and strengths of each institution, with the understanding that success is achieved when grieving families find comfort in their decision to donate and end-stage organ failure patients receive the life-sustaining organ they need.[4]

OPOs and large hospitals jointly sent multidisciplinary teams to participate in the intensive series of Collaborative Learning Sessions and Action Periods that took place between September 2003 and September 2004. Drawing from the experience of practitioners with high donation rates, these teams worked together more than 12 months to rapidly learn, adapt, redesign, test, implement, track, and refine

Table 2. HIGH-PERFORMING ORGAN PROCUREMENT ORGANIZATIONS AND HOSPITALS

Organ Procurement Organization	Hospital
Donor Alliance (Denver, Colo)	Denver Health Medical Center (Denver) Memorial Hospital (Colorado Springs) St. Anthony Central Hospital (Denver)
LifeGift Organ Donation Center (Houston, Tex)	Ben Taub General Hospital (Houston) Memorial Hermann Hospital (Houston)
LifeLink of Florida (Tampa, Fla)	Lakeland Regional Medical Center (Lakeland) Tampa General Hospital (Tampa)
Mid-America Transplant Services (St. Louis, Mo)	Barnes Jewish Hospital (St. Louis) St. John's Mercy Medical Center (St. Louis)
New England Organ Bank (Newton, Mass)	Beth Israel Deaconess Hospital (Boston) Boston Medical Center (Boston) Massachusettes General Hospital (Boston)
University of Wisconsin Hospital and Clinics OPO (Madison, Wis)	Gunderson Lutheran Hospital (La Crosse) Theda Clark Regional Medical Center (Neenah) University of Wisconsin Hospital and Clinics (Madison)

Table 3. OVERARCHING PRINCIPLES AND BEST PRACTICES OF SUCCESSFUL ORGAN PROCUREMENT ORGANIZATION (OPO) AND HOSPITAL DONATION SYSTEMS

Overarching Principles

1. Integrate organ donation fully into routine roles and responsibilities.
2. Set high standards for donation performance to reduce the unacceptable shortage of lifesaving organs.
3. Involve OPO and hospital staff in ongoing standards setting and redesign of means to achieve these standards.
4. Hold OPOs, hospitals, and their staff accountable for achieving these standards and recognize the staff accordingly.
5. Establish, maintain, and revitalize a network of interpersonal relationships and trust involving OPO and hospital staff, donor families, and other key agents.
6. Collaborate to meet the range of needs of potential donor families and achieve informed consent to donate.
7. Conduct data collection and feedback to drive decision making toward performance improvement.

Best Practices

1. Orient organizational mission and goals toward increasing organ donation.
2. Do not be satisfied with the status quo; innovate and experiment continuously.
3. Strive to recruit and retain highly motivated and skilled staff.
4. Appoint members to OPO board who can help achieve organ donation goals.
5. Specialize roles to maximize performance.
6. Tailor or adapt the organ donation process to complementary strengths of OPO and individual hospitals.
7. Be there: integrate OPO staff into the fabric of high-potential hospitals.
8. Identify and support organ donation champions at various hospital levels; include leaders who are willing to be called upon to overcome barriers to organ donation in real time.
9. All aboard: secure and maintain buy-in at all levels of hospital staff and across departments/functions that affect organ donation.
10. Educate constantly; tailor and accommodate to staff needs, requests, and constraints.
11. Design, implement, and monitor public education and outreach efforts to achieve informed consent and other donation goals.
12. Referral: anticipate, don't hesitate, call early even when in doubt.
13. Draw on respective OPO and hospital strengths to establish an integrated consent process. One size does not fit all, but getting to an informed "yes" is paramount.
14. Use data to drive decision making.
15. Follow up in a timely and systematic manner. Don't let any issues fester.

Table 4. DEFINITIONS

Eligible donor	Any patient whose age is 70 or less meeting death by neurological criteria, based on the American Academy of Neurology Practice parameters for determining brain death, who does not have any of the following clinical indications: • Tuberculosis • Human immunodeficiency virus (HIV) infection with specified conditions • Creutzfeldt-Jacob disease • Herpetic septicemia • Rabies • Reactive hepatitis B surface antigen • Any retro virus infection • Active malignant neoplasms, except primary central nervous system tumors and skin cancers • Hodgkin's disease, multiple myeloma, leukemia • Miscellaneous carcinomas • Aplastic anemia • Agranulocytosis • Fungal and viral meningitis • Viral encephalitis • Gangrene of bowel • Extreme immaturity • Positive serological or viral culture findings for HIV
Organ donor	Consented donor from whom an organ is recovered for the purpose of transplantation including non-heart-beating donors and donors older than 70 years
No consent	Eligible donor for whom donation consent is denied
No next-of-kin/other	Eligible donor that is not recovered for reasons other than lack of consent (ie, next-of-kin is unavailable)
Medical examiner denial	Denial by medical examiner for organ recovery irrespective of donation consent status
Organ referral	Referral to an organ procurement organization of a patient meeting the criteria for imminent death
Imminent death	A patient with severe, acute brain injury, who (1) requires mechanical ventilation; (2) is in an intensive care unit or emergency department; and (3) has clinical findings consistent with a Glasgow Coma Score that is less than equal to a mutually agreed upon threshold (such as 4 or 5); or • for whom physicians are evaluating a diagnosis of brain death; or • whom a physician has ordered that life-sustaining therapies be withdrawn, pursuant to the family's decision.
Missed eligible referral	An imminent death that was apparently eligible but not referred by the hospital to the OPO. Missed eligible referrals are generally discovered by a death log audit or death record review.

Table 5. MEASUREMENTS/CALCULATIONS

Referral rate	Organ referrals over organ referrals plus missed referrals, expressed as a percentage
Timely notification rate	Number of imminent death notifications made within one hour of a mutually established clinical trigger over the number of imminent deaths, expressed as a percentage
Appropriate requestor rate	Number of cases in which designated requestor met with family over total number of requests made, expressed as a percentage
Conversion rate	Organ donors over eligible donors, expressed as a percentage
Medical examiner denials	Number of medical examiner denials, expressed as a raw number

their organ donation processes with the intention to reach the collaborative goal of a 75% conversion rate or higher. Goals and a timeline for the Collaborative were established (Tables 6 and 7). Leading organizations provided input and support into the development and conduct of the Collaborative (Table 8). The Health Resources and Services Administration managed the Secretarial initiative.

Table 6. GOALS

Conversion rate	75%
Medical examiner denials	Zero
Referral rate	100%
Timely notification rate	100%
Appropriate requestor rate	100%

Table 7. COLLABORATIVE TIMELINE

Study of high-performing organ procurement organizations and hospitals	October 2002 to March 2003
Expert panel to vet study findings	March 2003
HHS secretarial launch of Collaborative	April 2003
Collaborative team formation and prework	Summer 2003
Learning session 1	September 2003
Action period 1	September 2003 to January 2004
Learning session 2	January 2004
Action period 2	January to April 2004
Learning session 3	April 2004
Action period 3	April to September 2004
Team formation and prework for Collaborative 2	Summer 2004
Learning session 4/1 (Collaboratives 1 & 2)	September 2004
Action period 1 of 2nd Collaborative	September 2004 to January 2005
Learning session 2 of 2nd Collaborative	January 2005
Action period 2 of 2nd Collaborative	January to May 2005
National Learning Congress	May 2005

Table 8. KEY LEADERSHIP ORGANIZATIONS

American Association of Critical Care Nurses
American Society of Multicultural Health and Transplantation Professionals
American Society of Transplantation
American Society of Transplant Surgeons
Association of Organ Procurement Organizations
American Hospital Association
Centers for Medicare and Medicaid Services
Institute for Healthcare Improvement
Joint Commission for Accreditation of Healthcare Organizations
National Association of Medical Examiners
National Kidney Foundation
Neurocritical Care Society
North American Transplant Coordinators Organization
Quality Reality Checks, Inc
Society for Critical Care Medicine
United Network for Organ Sharing

Learning Sessions

Learning sessions, face-to-face activities, two days in length, the major integrative events of the Collaborative, were held six times over the course of 20 months. Ninety-five large hospitals and 43 of the 60 OPOs participated in the first collaborative between September 2003 and September 2004; 131 large hospitals and 50 OPOs participated in the second collaborative between September 2004 and May 2005. The first collaborative was such a success that the second collaborative was continued by the Department of Health and Human Services (DHHS) in order to spread the best practices using the collaborative methodology to the next large group (131) of hospitals in the United States. In addition, three and five Canadian hospitals participated in Collaboratives one and two, respectively.

During learning sessions, team participants had the opportunity to learn from faculty and colleagues, receive individual coaching from faculty members, and gather new knowledge on the subject matter and process improvement. They developed organization-specific plans for testing and implementing changes to increase donation. Through their shared experiences, nurses, physicians, and OPO staff collaborated on improvement plans and problem-solved improvement challenges. Participants learned first hand the mantra, "All Teach, All Learn," because it was the participants themselves, critical care nurses, physicians, and OPO staff, who taught one another, sharing their testing of changes and results in building effective donation processes.

The time between learning sessions, termed "action periods," was the period during which collaborative teams tested action items, using the Model for Improvement to achieve breakthrough conversion rates. Participants focused on their own organizations and remained in continuous contact with other teams enrolled in the Collaborative and Collaborative Leadership. This communication took the form of conference calls, e-mail, accessing the extranet, and, occasionally, site visits to other organizations in the Collaborative. In addition, collaborative team members shared the results of their improvement efforts in monthly Senior Leader Reports.

The Model for Improvement and Rapid Spread of Best Practices

The model for the Collaborative combined an iterative, process-improvement approach with fast-paced change brought about through system redesign. The basic premise of the Collaborative's model was that achieving outstanding organ procurement rates required a redesign of the core business and the use of existing knowledge and experience to guide such efforts. Another distinctive feature of the Collaborative was the focus on customer service as a driver of OPO change efforts. This strategy assumed that participating organizations were not bound by the current system, that they could effect changes identified as useful, and that they desired a system that was efficient, effective, and rewarding for both donor families and staff.[4]

The key elements of the success of the Collaborative Model for Improvement are (1) the *will* to do what it takes to change to a new system; (2) the *ideas* on which to base the design of that new system; and (3) the *execution* of those ideas. The *will* began with Secretary Thompson's commitment and charge, and it was embraced by the OPOs and hospitals who joined the Collaborative. The *ideas* came from the high-performing OPOs and hospitals that were already achieving the goal of 75% conversion rates. The *execution* was driven by an improvement model that emphasized rapidly testing changes on a small scale and implementing system-wide improvements on the basis of that learning.

Best practices were identified through site visits to the high-performing OPOs and hospitals, analysis of national data,[4] and the United Network for Organ Sharing Research to Practice National Consensus Conference.[10] They were then vetted by a national expert panel drawn from the organ donation community of successful OPOs and hospitals, and became the ideas upon which collaborative teams built change.

The Model for Improvement provides a methodology to test and implement changes that make a difference and addresses three fundamental questions: What are we trying to accomplish? How will we know that a change is an improvement? What change can we make that will result in improvement? This model is an adaptation of the well-established Plan, Do, Study, Act construct (Nolan-Langley Improvement Model)[11] and is used by collaborative teams to apply the best practice concepts to their systems. It allows for change to be tested quickly on a small scale and provides learning opportunities for rapid implementation (Figure 2).[11] This testing was done between learning sessions and provided the basis for presentations at the subsequent sessions (Figure 3).

Four Overarching Strategies: Change Package Best Practices

The process of organ donation is complex and delicate.[4] To address this nature of organ donation, the Collaborative "Change Package" was identified, consisting of four overarching strategies for success. Within those four strategies were 29 change concepts and 63 action items that could be implemented in OPOs or hospitals. The 4 strategies are discussed below.

Unrelenting Focus on Change, Improvement, and Results. Establishing a strong culture of accountability for results, successful organizations have a laser-like focus on outcome. Their decision making is driven by data in determining organizational priorities and effectiveness of interventions. They seek to improve their organization's performance over its historical experience, constantly changing and adapting processes to achieve results. The focus on outcome results in application of the 80%/20% rule (80% of all potential donors are found in only 20% of hospitals), therefore identifying and targeting hospitals with greatest donor potential and putting resources in those institutions.

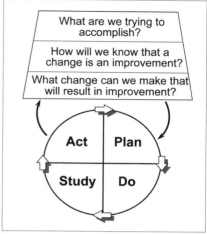

Figure 2. Model for Improvement

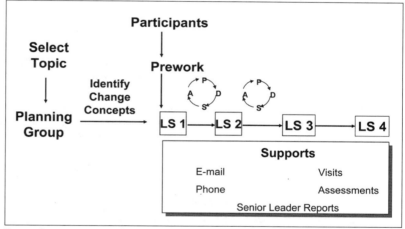

Figure 3. Collaborative Engine. Abbreviations A, act; D, do; LS, learning session; P, plan; S, study.

OPOs and hospitals must maintain a rigorous focus on, and joint accountability for, increasing the number of organ donors by developing and maintaining a seasoned staff and creating a culture of excellence. It is critical to have measurement systems in place, to routinely monitor and report process and outcome data. Performance goals are measured and disseminated, and staff members are held accountable in high-performing organizations.

There is only one point in time to maximize donation during any individual case and therefore, stating what should be obvious, the organization's talent and resources should be applied to each and every case 24/7 in real time. Because these cases occur at any time of the day or night, this means the organization needs to be responsive 24/7 at all levels of management. Successful organizations provide active leadership and management support during donation cases, helping staff overcome obstacles; planning re-approaches for consent after an initial "no" from families, addressing family needs and concerns, and ensuring consistency and quality in their vigorous pursuit of donation.

Creating a culture of excellence also requires defining and maintaining relationships with key stakeholders, including medical examiners, coroners, transplant centers, and hospital physician leadership, and developing a seamless integration with hospital staff. Creating and maintaining a visual presence of OPO staff in hospitals, becoming part of the fabric of high donor potential hospitals to establish, maintain,

Chapter 27 THE ORGAN DONATION BREAKTHROUGH COLLABORATIVE

and activate relationships with all individuals that participate and play a role in the donation process are key to breakthrough levels of performance.

Rapid, Early Referral, and Linkage. Perhaps no other strategy is as critical to success as rapidly referring patients to the OPO as early as possible after injury. Linking key OPO and/or hospital donation staff to potential donor families is a precursor to many of the other best practices. Timely notification to the OPO of potential donors is essential; referral of the potential donor is the first step in the donation process. Hospitals that establish a system-wide commitment to unconditionally identify all opportunities for donation understand the critical nature of starting the process early and collaboratively, with OPO staff present. Creating a visual presence of OPO staff in the hospital either through placement of in-house coordinators directly in the hospital, with office space provided,[12-16] or by having defined family liaisons and hospital development staff who routinely visit the institution is key.

Timely notification to the OPO of potential donors is essential, often preventing a rushed approach to requesting consent from families.[17,18] Establishing the expectation that OPO staff will be called in a systematic manner as soon as it is evident that the patient has a severe injury that may not be survivable (using a clinical trigger for referral, most often a Glasgow Coma Scale score of five or less), the OPO coordinator can more easily interact early and spend more time with families, in large part because the hospital has recognized this early collaboration as critical for donation success. Earlier studies have shown that longer periods spent by OPO staff with families is positively associated with donation.[4,19] In short, early referral leads to more time with the family, which leads to more trust, which leads to higher donation rates.

Research has shown that families who are satisfied with their hospital experience are more predisposed to donate.[20,21] Donation is a process. Obtaining consent does not consist of simply asking the family if they wish to donate, that is, "popping the question." Informed consent takes time, time that is not often available for busy hospital staff. Various needs arise early on in the course of a critical illness or event; as families start receiving information about the condition of their loved one and start asking questions, the donation "process" has begun. OPO staff must be present with hospital and medical staff to begin the collaborative process of obtaining consent. Being notified of a potential donor late in the process, at or near the time of death, prevents any opportunity for collaboration between hospital and OPO staff and prevents OPO staff from spending extended time with families before the actual pronouncement of brain death.[12] Early collaboration between nursing and OPO staff results in a jointly developed consent approach plan.

Successful donation systems result in protocols that personalize the approach to families, allowing nurses and OPO staff to develop a sense of trust with the family and ensuring the family has a positive experience with the donation process. Effective hospital donation systems routinely make every effort to determine a family's willingness to donate, and if consent is denied, recognize that re-approach can provide families with valuable needed time and information that may result in a consent to donate decision.

"Team huddles," with all involved staff before consent approach, are the norm rather than the exception. A team huddle consists of gathering together the health-care professionals involved with the patient's care along with the OPO staff to collaboratively develop the best possible plan for the consent approach. Critical care nurses figure prominently in the team huddle because they have been at the patient's bedside, know the patient's condition, and are likely to have observed family members during visits with the patient (Table 9). An effective team huddle is an "organized" collaboration that allows all participants to be comfortable with the process before it unfolds and be ready to play his or her role.

Integrated Donation Process Management. Among the sample of high performers are OPOs and hospitals that establish and manage an integrated donation process that clearly defines roles and responsibilities and provides feedback. This includes establishing joint OPO- and hospital-designated leadership responsibility and accountability. The OPO provides resources for all donation-related matters and the hospital provides high level support from, at a minimum, the Chief Nursing Officer, Chief Medical Officer, and other administration from the Vice President level. Hospital CEOs should be aware of the donation-related work and outcomes in his or her institution.

Table 9. TEAM HUDDLE

Purpose	☐	To develop an environment for a successful consent outcome
	☐	To involve everyone that was a part of the patient's/family's care and ensure consistent communication between families, hospital staff, and organ procurement organization (OPO) staff
	☐	To create a support system for potential donor families, in order to meet all of their needs • Personal • Cultural • Spiritual
Determine who should be part of huddle	☐	Physicians • Attending • Neurosurgeon • Intensivist
	☐	Family support team • Pastoral care • Case management/social worker
	☐	Nursing staff • Critical care nurses from the intensive care unit taking care of patient (may extend across more than one shift)
	☐	OPO personnel • Organ recovery coordinator • In-house coordinator
Actions during huddle	☐	Discuss family's understanding of situation
	☐	Determine best time for physician to speak with family about death, including which physician has the best relationship and adequate time to spend with family
	☐	Determine who will be in the room with the family during death conversation and depending on family's acceptance of death, if consent conversation will immediately follow or if the family needs time to process information
	☐	Determine how OPO staff will be introduced to family
	☐	Depending on outcome of consent conversation, make plans for reapproach if initial response to donation is "no"

Appropriate material and tools to disseminate the data should be used to provide immediate feedback to hospitals/clinical leadership on donation process, results, and outcomes with specific follow-up requests and action steps. In addition, OPO staff and nursing and physician leaders should analyze data and situational variables to *know what to request* from one another and senior leaders within the institution. Hospital staff are in most instances capable, poised, and ready to provide assistance, but the request must be specific and clear. Regular surveys and other tools are used in effective hospital donation systems to evaluate and monitor the donation process, identifying trends, strengths, and problems.

Achieving an integrated donation process measurement requires building and maintaining collaborative relationships with key hospital staff and physicians at all levels who affect the donation process. Building relationships is not rocket science, but rather results from doing "real work" with hospital clinicians (physicians and nurses), partnering with nurses and physicians, jointly setting stretch goals for the donation outcomes and processes, providing education at regular intervals, and establishing OPO staff consultant responsibilities. Relationships are further developed, as policies are developed clearly defining roles and responsibilities of both OPO and hospital staff; establishing specific policies for brain death and guidelines for brain-death discussion with families, and standards for stabilization of potential donors. To maximize organ recovery, OPO and hospital staff jointly establish expectations, guidelines, and protocols between OPO and hospital operating room management, staff, and anesthesia department. Time is set aside after every donation process to evaluate the outcome and immediately implement modifications. Hospital staff are key participants in this review process. After-action reviews build team relationships and facilitate identification of learning opportunities.

Chapter 27 THE ORGAN DONATION BREAKTHROUGH COLLABORATIVE

An integrated donation management system contains many dynamic processes that, in most cases, begin with the admission of a critically ill patient. The goal of achieving an integrated donation system has been realized when all parties work together seamlessly, across and within one another's "boundaries," while keeping all parties informed and involved as appropriate with their respective work. In other words, an integrated donation system consists of a high degree of communication and collaboration among OPO staff, nurses, physicians, and hospital staff without either party keeping the other at "arms length" at any time during the donation process.

Aggressive Pursuit of Every Donation Opportunity. Aggressive pursuit of every donation opportunity means that every possibility for increased donation is maximized and routinely evaluated through quick deployment of OPO staff, re-approaches for consent when the initial family response is "no," expert donor management, aggressive organ placement efforts, improved organ yield (the number of organs recovered per donor), and real time death record review. Successful systems are those in which do-not-resuscitate and comfort measures only orders are coordinated and planned between nurses, physicians, OPO staff, and other appropriate hospital staff for every potential donor case before talking to the family to avoid conflict with the opportunity for organ donation.

Nursing, medical, and OPO leadership must have a clear expectation of no (zero) medical examiner denials of organ recovery. This can be and is being achieved in most parts of the country.[22-24] The National Association of Medical Examiners has named "zero denials" as an association goal.[25] Their brave and bold statements ushered in the era of OPOs and cities achieving zero rates of denials. Drs Michael Graham, Keith Pinckard, Stephen Nelson, and Micheal Bell, all medical examiners, took early live-saving positions, seizing the stage and changing history.

Successful hospital donation outcomes involve clinicians (nursing, medical, OPO staff) focusing on aggressive pursuit of each case. Successful systems establish, evaluate, and are accountable for a clear donor management process from referral to recovery, with OPO staff in the ICU who obtain assistance from OPO management and/or medical directors as needed. Broad criteria are applied to evaluate every potential organ donor. Organ placement is aggressive; the OPO suspends judgment on rule-out criteria (medical conditions that appear to make the patient unsuitable for donation), instead, leaving such decisions to the transplanting surgeon of listed patients. The hospital staff must understand that the determination of donor suitability is dynamic; what may not be suitable in one instance on any given day, could the next day be life-saving in a similar circumstance. Many organs are lost because of "perception" that they are not suitable. The ultimate test of suitability is one that must be made by the physician caring for a waiting recipient; risks are weighed against the continued risk of waiting. Organ placement efforts are followed to their logical conclusion, that is, the patient is only medically unsuitable if, after disclosure of all donor information, the organ is not accepted by a receiving center for a particular patient.

Although evaluating and addressing every donor case potential may fall slightly more in the realm of the OPO, another opportunity for increasing organ donation falls more squarely in the hospital realm. Perhaps the hallmark of this overarching strategy is that the OPO and the hospital *actively advocate for donation*. Hospitals with consistently high donation rates embrace donation as part of their mission. Indeed, some hospitals have Mission Integration Committees to help focus the institution on community benefit and joint practice with other agencies, in this case, the OPO. Advocating for donation is a responsibility that, before the Collaborative, was largely seen as an OPO responsibility. Although donation is a small part of hospital work in terms of absolute number of cases, enlightened mission-driven CEOs see it as a "huge" part of their work and mission. One such CEO commented during a JCAHO Crossroad symposium, "Donation is a big part of what we do. It's not about the number of cases. We had a four-year-old girl who received a liver from one of our donors come to our hospital and visit. Her life was saved because of a donation in our institution. That is **huge**."[26]

Aggressive pursuit of every donation opportunity requires OPOs to develop, define, and maintain a standard of high-quality service in handling all hospital and physician communications. Increasing the interaction of the OPO medical director with hospital physicians and identifying physician champions, and establishing quality donation processes with hospital staff through one-on-one case reviews contribute to donation system performance.

Finally, there is no more important action item in this overarching strategy than implementing donation after cardiac death (DCD) policy and practice. DCD donation offers the greatest improvement opportunity for significant levels of increased organ recovery in this strategy, because it dramatically increases the size of the potential donor pool. Successful hospitals and OPOs establish policies and protocols for DCD to ensure the referral of all patients with non-recoverable neurological injuries and pursuit of donation options.[27] The Institute of Medicine has endorsed DCD, hospitals across the country are implementing policies and doing their first cases, and families are demanding their right to donate.[28] It is the right thing to do. This emerging practice is fast becoming common practice.

Further Refinements to the Change Package

Don Berwick, MD, founder and CEO of IHI met with the faculty and co-chairs of the Collaborative in March 2004, and challenged the group to "design the new and improved national organ donation system" on the basis of the proven experiences and successes of collaborative teams. Berwick's challenge resulted in two sets of important refinements to the original and rapidly evolving Change Package: First Things First Changes and High Leverage Changes.

First Things First. To take full advantage of the best practices that were the basis for the changes, teams were tested during the first collaborative. The change package was refined and stratified to emphasize those changes that held the greatest promise for immediate improvements in process and outcome. These changes, the necessary building blocks for success, were termed "First Things First." Teams introduced to the collaborative methodology in the second collaborative were encouraged to work on these changes before moving on to more complex strategies (Table 10).

High Leverage Changes. Teams in the second collaborative benefited from experienced collaborative one teams through the refinement of the change package into those action items that had a direct relationship

Table 10. FIRST THINGS FIRST

1	Create organ procurement organization (OPO) hospital presence/in-house coordinator ☐ Create and maintain visual presence of OPO staff in hospitals; become part of the fabric of high-potential hospitals to establish, maintain, and activate relationships with all individuals who participate/play a role in the donation process
2	☐ Establish strong culture of accountability for results: Ensure that OPO and hospital staff know and talk conversion rates and regularly review and respond to data reports of donation key indicators: conversion rates, consent rates, timely notification rates. Use these data to identify where to focus initial efforts and changes in donation system redesign
3	Identify physician/clinician champion ☐ Identify and support organ donation champions at various hospital levels; include leaders who are willing to be called upon to overcome barriers to organ donation in real time
4	Conduct monthly death record reviews ☐ Use death record reviews to establish referral, consent, and donation rates, and automate process to monitor performance in real time
5	Establish clinical trigger ☐ Mutually establish with hospital staff appropriate clinical triggers for referrals
6	Hold donation team huddles ☐ Work as a team with hospital staff to determine the right person(s) to suggest donation and make the request. Establish family communication plan that incorporates all members of patient care team
7	Identify effective requestors (who is your most effective requestor?) ☐ Match requestors appropriately to family, ensuring effective requestors are available; special requestors should be hired and used by the OPO or hospital specific to the ethnicity of the OPO service area population
8	Conduct after action reviews ☐ Maintain a formal process for comprehensive immediate follow-up communication between OPO and hospital on every organ donor referral, regardless of the outcome (after action review); a system to include guidelines for in-person follow-up, debriefing and mutual critique of process as well as written correspondence and email communication to facilitate timely feedback where access is difficult

Table 11. HIGH LEVERAGE CHANGES

Advocate organ donation as the mission	1	Advocate organ donation as the mission 75% conversion rate
	2	Involve senior leadership to get results ☐ Hospital and organ procurement organization (OPO) senior leadership are informed and actively involved as teams press the system redesign to its maximum
	3	Deploy a self-organizing OPO/hospital team ☐ Seamless integration of OPO and hospital roles and responsibilities
Integrated family centered system: ☐ Clinical care services and ☐ Family support services	4	Practice early referral, rapid response ☐ All staff have a clear understanding of what triggers timely referrals, and ensure that the highest donor potential units are using them ☐ Link early referral to rapid response. The entire organization has a commitment to a rapid response to referrals
	5	Master effective requesting ☐ Dedicate most effective requestors to either lead or be part of every hospital referral ☐ Create a reapproach strategy, role-play and test it when the next no consent presents itself ☐ Debrief the entire team involved within 24 hours of each approach to learn what is working and what is making it work ☐ Incorporate this learning into the very next consent opportunity; acknowledge organ donation advocacy as an Appropriate Family Support Objective
	6	Implement donation after cardiac death (DCD) ☐ Vigorously pursue any DCD opportunity, particularly those in which families independently raise the issue; use national DCD experts to support your effort, if your OPO is new to DCD

to outcomes and results. These changes, which often cut across strategies, were observed by collaborative faculty and experienced teams as having a direct relationship to outcomes. They were re-packaged, termed "High Leverage Changes," and represented a synergistic combination of change concepts within or across strategies (Table 11).

The Measurement Strategy

The Collaborative was disciplined in obtaining and tracking data; however, it was always clear that the project was about improvement and increasing the number of organ donors, not about measurement or research. Still, measurement is necessary to evaluate the impact of changes teams made in improving the donation process in their individual institutions. Measurement was designed to accelerate improvement, not slow it down. The focus was on obtaining just enough measurement to determine that the changes being made led to improvement.

The measurement strategy for the Collaborative was intended to identify and track progress in improving key outcome and process measures that are essential to successful organ donation. Teams submitted monthly data on each process and outcome measure. The Collaborative's outcome measures focus on three areas: conversion rate, referral rate, and medical examiner/coroner refusals. In addition, teams tracked two process measures: timely notification and appropriate requester rates (Table 5). The activities of the teams were focused on improvements in each process and outcome measure. Teams were permitted to develop their own additional measures, but the aforementioned measures were *required* measurements for all teams.

An interesting measure added to the measurement strategy early on was the measurement of "Donors Before a Non-donor." Because the numbers of eligible donors are small, even in the largest of potential donor hospitals, eligible donors are a rare event. Therefore, a conversion rate measured month by month is not always useful, because it may be difficult to see an emerging trend. This measurement, developed by IHI, allowed teams to see improvements earlier than they otherwise would have. Figure 4 presents an

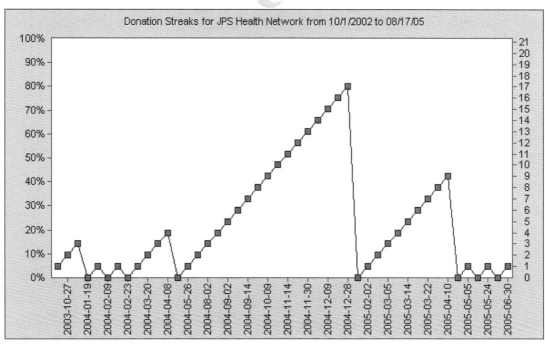

Figure 4. Donors Before Non-Donor Streaks

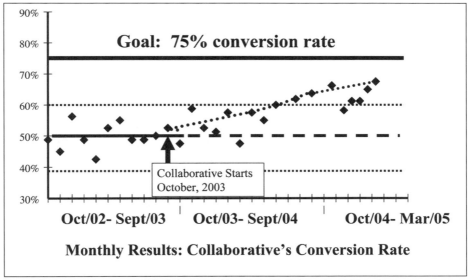

Figure 5. Conversion Rate of Collaborative Hospitals Collaborative 1 Trend

example from one of the hospitals participating in the Collaborative. This measurement, Donors Before a Non-donor, had the added effect of motivating staff before each and every case to continue their streak. Hospital staff were well aware of their lifesaving Donors Before a Non-donor number (Figure 4).

Results

The Organ Donation Breakthrough Collaborative has led to major increases in conversion rates of the collaborative hospitals (Figure 5), as well as national increases in organ donation (Figures 5 and 6). The primary goal of reaching a 75% conversion rate was achieved by 21 of the 95 Collaborative one hospitals

Chapter 27 THE ORGAN DONATION BREAKTHROUGH COLLABORATIVE

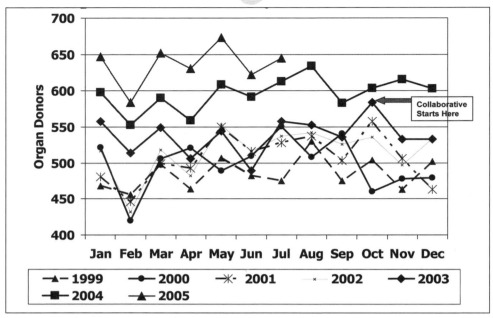

Figure 6. Unprecedented Monthly Donation Records

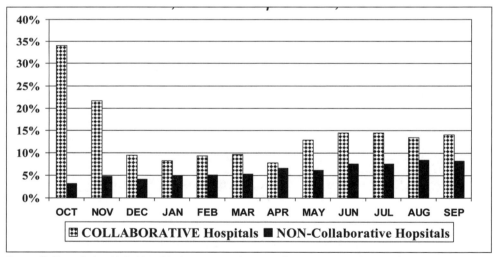

Figure 7. Cumulative U.S. Monthly Increase in Donors: Collaborative VS Non-Collaborative Hospitals *October, 2003 – September, 2004*

by the end of September 2004. Another 15 of the 95 hospitals reached the 75% conversion rate by April 2005. Of the 138 new hospitals participating in Collaborative two that were not also in Collaborative one, 26 reached the goal of a 75% conversion rate. On the final night of Collaborative two, a black tie event was held recognizing all of the Collaborative one and two teams reaching a 75% conversion rate. In addition, 183 hospitals were recognized with a DHHS Medal of Honor, awarded by Dr Elizabeth Duke, Health Resources and Services Administration Administrator, for achieving a 75% conversion rate for any 12-month period from November 2003 to April 2005.

Compared to 2003, total donations in the United States from deceased donors in 2004 increased by 10.8%. The number of deceased donors increased from 6457 in 2003 to 7153 in 2004. Donation increased by 16% in the 95 hospitals participating in the Collaborative, and by 9% in all other US hospitals. The total number of monthly donors in 2004 exceeded the number of donors in the corresponding month of the previous year, every single month. Astoundingly, the total number of monthly donors in 2005 through July exceeded the number of donors in the corresponding month of 2004, every single month, a telling difference from the previous 2 decades (Figure 6). Therefore, in 2005 through July, US organ donation has increased 8.3% over 2004, yet another increase. These increases come on top of a substantial 4.3% increase in 2003. In comparison, the average annual increase in donation over the last 10 years has been 2.9%.[3] Back-to-back annual increases of 4.3%, 10.8%, and 8.3% are unprecedented.

The impressive donation increases, which included an increase in donors recovered from hospitals not participating in the Collaborative, are likely due to the rapid "spread" of effective practices generated by collaborative teams in their donation service areas (Figures 5 through 7). As seen in Figure 7, during the first full year of the Collaborative, collaborative hospitals achieved a 14.1% increase in donation from the previous year as compared to non-collaborative hospitals, which achieved an 8.3% increase in donation. This represents a 70% greater increase in collaborative hospitals over non-collaborative hospitals.

A Transformation in Donation Systems

The Collaborative has truly transformed the hospital and OPO interface and the donation system. Hospital development will never be the same after the Collaborative, which is a terrific achievement. Results are what matters; the numbers matter; the "ones" add up. Vague, poorly directed hospital contact is outdated and out of mode. An OPO's "business" model should be continuous improvement, and a hospital's "business" model should be continuous improvement. The effects of the Collaborative are yet to be fully appreciated. Before the Collaborative started, the core collaborative faculty looked at the high performers and said, "Look at them – lets bring everyone up to where they are." A 75% conversion rate seemed "pie-in-the-sky" to veteran procurement professionals. It was not long before many were revising their goals *upward* from 75% conversion rates. A sea change in the industry was affected by the collaborative faculty, the leadership coordinating council, and, most importantly, the work of the teams.

As OPOs redesign their organizational structures and operations, the targeted work of the Collaborative will surely figure largely in the design. OPOs have re-written hospital development policies (Appendix 1) to fully incorporate the Collaborative's methodology. Such changes are only the beginning of the transformation. National organizations will undoubtedly rework national meetings to continue the work of the Collaborative, the single most effective intervention in increasing organ donation ever implemented.

Conclusions

"Some is not a number – soon is not a time."[29] The single largest impediment to solving the organ shortage is inaction, business as usual, and sticking to old designs and old thinking. Ben Franklin said, "Insanity is doing the same thing over and over again and expecting a different result." The Collaborative has given hospital and OPO staff the courage to believe they can make a difference. More importantly, the Collaborative has demonstrated to healthcare professionals that they can effect change through a systematic application of the Model for Improvement in the implementation of known best practices. Every day, team members share their successes and challenges on the Collaborative listserve, and encourage each other to continue to push and reach for stretch goals.

The underlying practices that led to these increases are now widely known and are systematically replicated by OPOs and hospitals throughout the nation. The Change Package has brought laser-like clarity to the strategies, key concepts, and actions that lead to higher, lifesaving conversion rates. Clinical leaders in hospitals and OPOs now have ready access to the knowledge about what it takes to generate donation rates of 75% or more.

As evidenced by the dramatic improvement in conversion rates, resulting in the largest increase in organ donation in more than a decade, hospital staff, along with their OPO team members, know that outcomes can be improved. The spread of best practices occurred at breakneck speed with the Collaborative. The learning of teams was accelerated by the learning sessions, the Collaborative listserve, and their success was augmented by the active involvement of the leadership organizations earlier mentioned. The

Chapter 27 THE ORGAN DONATION BREAKTHROUGH COLLABORATIVE

Collaborative process – bringing teams together over time to implement change rapidly in healthcare organizations – not only works, but should be seen as the way to drive transformation throughout our healthcare system. Empowered teams across the organ donation community are now ready, willing, and able to apply this methodology to all their improvement efforts.

Finally, the "all teach, all learn" approach of the Collaborative has brought an incredible level of mutual accountability, teamwork, and spirit to the lifesaving interactions between hospitals and OPOs. This spirit of teamwork has made life better for dedicated clinicians involved in this challenging work – work that occurs at the nexus of tragedy and death of patients and loved ones on the one hand, and lifesaving results on the other.

Organ donation can be increased and lives can be saved by hospital and OPO staff remaining in action: making bold requests and offers of assistance, studying what works, testing it in the institution, setting stretch goals, and applying the principles and action items in the change package in collaboration with each other. One of the greatest results of the Collaborative occurred within the participants themselves; they were asked to be bold, to make bold requests, to make bold offers. The abundance created by this new behavior has changed the donation community in many ways, but in the most important way, it has resulted in numerous lives saved. History has been changed.

Acknowledgment:
Adapted in part from an article to be published in Critical Care Nurse *April 2006.*

A CLINICIAN'S GUIDE TO DONATION AND TRANSPLANTATION Chapter 27

ABC ORGAN PROCUREMENT ORGANIZATION   **OFFICIAL PROCEDURE**

SUBJECT:	HOSPITAL DONATION SYSTEM DESIGN
DATE APPROVED:	MARCH 25, 2005
DATE EFFECTIVE:	MARCH 25, 2005
DATE REVISED:	
PROCEDURE NUMBER:	P056

1.0 PURPOSE
    1.1 To create effective, successful, positive organ procurement organization (OPO) hospital donation systems.
    1.2 To test and implement known best donation practices.
    1.3 To designate The Improvement Model as the business model for ABC OPO's staff to use in making changes in their assigned hospital.

2.0 DEFINITIONS

		CALCULATION	DEFINITION
2.1	Aim	Time specific Measurable	An explicit statement summarizing what your team (you and your hospital partners) hope to achieve. The aim helps focus you and the hospital on specific actions to achieve conversion rate goal
2.2	Conversion Rate	Organ donors over eligible donors, expressed as a percentage	Percent of eligible donors that become organ donors (reported monthly)
2.3	Organ Donor		Donor from whom an organ is recovered with the intent and for the purpose of transplantation
2.4	No Consent		Medically suitable potential donor for whom donation consent is denied
2.5	No Next of Kin/Other		Medically suitable potential donor that is not recovered for reasons other than lack of consent (i.e., next of kin is unavailable)
2.6	Medically Suitable Potential Donor		Potential donor that is brain dead, and is medically suitable for donation, as evidenced by a transplant center accepting at least one organ
2.7	Medical Examiner Denial		Denials by medical examiner for organ recovery irrespective of donation consent status, expressed as a raw number
2.8	Organ Referral		Referral to an OPO of a patient meeting the criteria for imminent death
2.9	Imminent Death	A patient with severe, acute brain injury, who (1) requires mechanical ventilation; and, (2) is in an intensive care unit or emergency department; and (3) has clinical findings consistent with a Glasgow Coma Score that is less than or equal to a mutually agreed-upon threshold (such as 4 or 5); **or** (a) for whom physicians are evaluating a diagnosis of brain death; or (b) for whom a physician has ordered that life-sustaining therapies be withdrawn, pursuant to the family's decision	
2.10	Missed Referral		An imminent death that was not referred by the hospital to the OPO. Missed referrals are generally discovered by a death log audit or death record review
2.11	Missed Medically Suitable Referral		An imminent death that was apparently eligible that was not referred by the hospital to the OPO. Missed eligible referrals are generally discovered by a death log audit or death record review
2.12	Referral Rate	Organ referrals over organ referrals plus missed referrals, expressed as a percentage	Percent of imminent deaths referred to the OPO

2.13	Timely Notification	Timely Notification: Prior to the withdrawal of any life-sustaining therapies (i.e., medical or pharmacological support) **and** As soon as it is <u>anticipated</u> a patient will meet the criteria for imminent death (clinical trigger) agreed to by the OPO and hospital **or** As soon as possible <u>after</u> a patient meets the criteria for imminent death (clinical trigger) agreed to by the OPO and the hospital	
2.14	Timely Notification Rate	Number of imminent death notifications made within 1 hour of a mutually established clinical trigger over the number of imminent deaths, expressed as percentage	Percent of cases notification of imminent deaths were made in a timely manner
2.15	Designated Requestor	An individual designated by the hospital to initiate the request to the family (can be an OPO or hospital staff member) who has completed a course offered or approved by the OPO in the methodology for approaching potential donor families and requesting organ donation, and is effective in that role as supported by high consent rates	
2.16	Appropriate Requester	Percent of cases in which designated requestor met with family	Number of cases in which a previously identified effective requestor met with family over total number of requests made, expressed as percentage
2.17	Appropriate Requestor Rate	Consents performed by OPO staff or designated requestor over all consent requests, expressed as a percentage	Percent of consent requests that are made by appropriate requestor
2.18	PDSA	**P**lan **D**o **S**tudy **A**ct	<u>Plan</u>: Plan for Change or Test, Plan for Collection of Data <u>Do</u>: Carry out the Change or Test; begin analysis <u>Study</u>: Complete analysis of the data. Summarize what was learned <u>Act</u>: Are they ready to make a change? Plan for the next cycle

3.0 POLICY

    3.1   The Donation Clinical Specialist (DCS) will read and discuss with their Managing Director: The Improvement Model. The discussion will center around 3 questions:

        3.1.1   What are we trying to accomplish?
        3.1.2   How will we know that a change is an improvement?
        3.1.3   What changes can we make that will result in improvement?

    3.2   The DCS will establish, in collaboration with the hospital, the "aim" for the hospital.

        3.2.1   The aim *must* include:
- Conversion Rate
  - 75% or greater
- Referral Rate
  - 100% goal
- Timely Notification Rate
  - 100% goal
- Appropriate Requestor Rate
  - 100% goal
- Number of Medical Examiner Denials
  - ZERO

        3.2.2   The aim must be stated clearly and with numerical goals.

                3.2.2.1   Teams make better progress when they have unambiguous, specific aims. Setting numeric targets clarifies the aim, helps to focus for change, and directs measurement. For example, an aim to "decrease medical examiner denials by 100%" will be more effective than an aim to "minimize medical examiner denials."

3.2.3 These goals may include other goals from time to time, for example, goals set for measurement purposes for different PDSAs that are being tested in that institution.

3.2.4 The DCS will involve the organization's senior leaders in order to ensure that the aim is aligned with the strategic goals of the hospital and the OPO.

3.2.5 The DCS will examine hospital data in order to relate the aim statement to the hospital and OPO's needs.

3.3 The DCS will use The Change Package, which contains the key elements of high-performing systems, to identify the changes the DCS wants to make to the hospital donation system to achieve the aim.

3.3.1 Best practices are known. Action items that may be tested are included within the Change Package. (Attachment 1)

3.3.1.2 The change package is further stratified into two separate documents, making it more apparent for the DCS, as to where he or she should first focus their efforts.
- First Things First   (Attachment 2)
- High-Leverage Changes   (Attachment 3)

3.3.2 Effective, long-term changes come from:
- An understanding of processes and systems of work
- Creative thinking (a change outside the normal approach)
  - Challenge the boundaries
  - Rearrange the order of steps
  - Look for ways to smooth the flow of activities
  - Visualize the ideal "Wouldn't it be nice if..."
  - Remove "the current way of doing things" as an option
  - Avoid testing "more of the same"
  - Don't get tied up in trying to define the perfect change
  - Evaluate the purpose
- The appropriate use of new or existing technology

3.4 The DCS will use The Improvement Model as a guide in conducting tests (PDSAs) to improve performance. (PDSA Form, Attachment 4; Completed Sample PDSA Attachment 5)

3.5 The DCS will measure hospital results.

3.5.1 A balanced set of five required measures reported each month to ensure that the system is improved. (see 3.2.1)
- Measures are used to guide improvement and test changes.

3.5.2 The DCS will integrate measurement into routine donation processes.

3.5.2.1 Routine reports will be generated to hospital leadership and other key staff.

3.5.2.2 Data will be plotted over time and displayed in graph format in order to demonstrate trends.

3.5.3 The DCS will understand the value and use of data in improving the hospital's donation system.

3.5.3.1 The purpose of measurement is for improvement, not judgment.

3.5.3.2 All measures have limitations, but the limitations do not negate their value.

3.5.3.3 Measures are one voice of the system. Hearing the voice of the system gives us information on how to act within the system.

3.5.3.4 Measures tell a story; goals give a reference point.

Jane Doe, RN, MSN, CPTC
Executive Vice President / Chief Operating Officer

Chapter 27 THE ORGAN DONATION BREAKTHROUGH COLLABORATIVE

PO56: Hospital Donation System Design

Attachment 1

Organ Donation Breakthrough Collaborative Change Package

Strategies to Achieve Joint Accountability for Results	Key Change Concepts for Increased Organ Donation Rates – Experience Indicates That Those in BOLD Are Critical to Success		Suggested Action Items Experience Indicates That Those in BOLD Are Critical to Success	
1. Unrelenting Focus on Change, Improvement, and Results OPO and hospitals maintain a rigorous focus on and joint accountability for increasing the number of organ donors by developing and maintaining a seasoned staff and creating a culture of excellence.	1.01	Establish strong culture of accountability for results: Orient operations toward outcomes rather than processes. Seek to improve each hospital's performance over its historical experience, using collaborative Model for Improvement **HOSPITAL TIERS 1, 2 & 3 TOP CHANGE**	1.01a	Compare performance to other hospitals in region and national benchmarks. H/O
			1.01b	Create policies and guidelines that focus on measurable goals and standard for increasing opportunities for donation, improving consent rates, and establishing feedback for mutual critique and review. O/H
			1.01c	Train OPO staff to know and talk the business (consent rates, conversion rates, timely notification rate, referral rate; OPO response rate). O
			1.01d	**Ensure that hospital staff know and talk conversion rates and regularly review and respond to data reports of donation key indicators (conversion rates, consent rates, timely notification rates). H/O**
			1.01e	Develop annual hospital specific needs assessment and action plans that identify and address barriers to improved donation outcomes.
	1.02	**Apply 80%/20% principle to focus resources; Identify and target hospitals with greatest donor potential.**		
	1.03	Identify Performance Goals; measure, disseminate, and hold staff accountable.	1.03a	Use Week-in-Review Meetings and monthly hospital reviews to dissect missed referrals, "no consents" and "consents" as learning opportunities (analyze the failures as well as the successes). O/H
			1.03b	Establish performance reviews for each staff member with specific individual conversion rate goals; incentivize and/or recognize individuals on the basis of performance. O
	1.04	Provide Active Leadership and Management Support during donation cases, to help staff overcome obstacles, plan reapproaches, address family needs and concerns, and to ensure consistency and quality in their vigorous pursuit of donation.	1.04a	Access and involve hospital and OPO leadership for effective staff support and oversight during donation cases in "real time." O/H
	1.05	Use data-driven decision making to determine priorities and effectiveness.		
	1.06	Define and maintain relationships with key stakeholders, including Medical Examiners, Coroners, Transplant Centers, and Hospital Physician Leadership, and develop a seamless integration with hospital staff.	1.06a	Establish an effective stakeholder Board of Directors by recruiting Board Members with problem-solving capabilities representing key customers, and hold periodic Board Retreats to inform, instruct, and engage in strategic planning. O
			1.06a	Establish an effective working relationship between OPO, CEO and senior leaders of all high potential donor hospitals
	1.07	Create and maintain visual presence of OPO staff in hospitals; become part of the fabric of high potential hospitals in order to establish, maintain, and activate relationships with all individuals that participate/play a role in the donation process.	1.07a	Evaluate customer satisfaction through objective (outside) surveys targeted to attending physicians, hospital nurses, and key staff.

KEY: O = OPO ACTION ITEM; H = HOSPITAL ACTION ITEM; O/H = OPO INITIATED, JOINT ACTION; H/O = HOSPITAL INITIATED, JOINT ACTION
Tier Conversion Rates: Tier 1 = 0-40%; Tier 2 = 41-60%; Tier 3 = 61-100%   OPO = Organ Procurement Organization

PO56: Hospital Donation System Design

Strategies to Achieve Joint Accountability for Results	Key Change Concepts for Increased Organ Donation Rates – Experience Indicates That Those in BOLD Are Critical to Success		Suggested Action Items Experience Indicates That Those in BOLD Are Critical to Success	
1. Unrelenting Focus on Change, Improvement, and Results OPO and hospitals maintain a rigorous focus on and joint accountability for increasing the number of organ donors by developing and maintaining a seasoned staff and creating a culture of excellence.	1.08	Integrate Public Relations, Communications Plan & Community Activities with organizational goals/mission.	1.08a	Design, implement, and monitor public education and outreach efforts to achieve informed consent and other donation goals. O
			1.08b	Promote state registries, if applicable. O/H
			1.08c	Use donor families and transplant recipients to raise awareness and provide opportunities to advance discussions of organ donation. O/H
			1.08d	Target public outreach efforts to specific ethnic groups. O/H
			1.08e	Never lose an opportunity to make a positive, lasting, and communicable impression on donor families and others in the community through public service announcements, media events, news articles, etc. H/O
	1.09	Involve staff in strategic planning, standard setting, and design of the methods to meet organizational goals.		
	1.10	Apply human resource expertise to recruitment, hiring, training, and retention.	1.10a	Integrate role-playing and case scenarios into development of skills for all staff. O/H
	1.11	Provide to hospital CEO, and all nursing staff/medical staff leadership, an OPO/Hospital Annual report that documents donation performance against local and national benchmarks.	1.11a	Assure within OPO Senior Management Team a business model expertise in finance, marketing, account, clinical, and human resource management. O
			1.11b	Emphasize appropriate interpersonal skills in recruitment; use experiential approach in interview process; have potential hires participate in donor process; seek local hospital ICU nurses for key coordinator positions; seek marketing expertise for hospital development positions; seek social work/counseling skills for family support/consent positions. O
			1.11c	For hospital development positions: Develop adult learning skills and "salesmanship" (close the sale; getting to a decision); match individual with appropriate role and hospital culture. O
			1.11d	Cross train key positions. O
			1.11e	Create opportunities for ongoing formal and informal mentoring; develop and measure competencies. O/H
			1.11f	Offer flexible work environments and other benefits. O
			1.11g	Provide opportunities for professional growth and development. O/H
			1.11h	Establish Support Group for peer staff to address potential burnout issues; provide access to psychologist; provide Employee Assistance Program. O/H
	1.12	Provide timely hospital/clinical leadership specific feedback on performance.		

Chapter 27 **THE ORGAN DONATION BREAKTHROUGH COLLABORATIVE**

PO56: Hospital Donation System Design

Strategies to Achieve Joint Accountability for Results	Key Change Concepts for Increased Organ Donation Rates – Experience Indicates That Those in BOLD Are Critical to Success		Suggested Action Items Experience Indicates That Those in BOLD Are Critical to Success	
2. Rapid, Early Referral & Linkage Key OPO and/or hospital donation staff are linked rapidly and early to potential donor families.	2.01	**Establish a system-wide commitment to unconditionally identify all opportunities for donation. Collaboratively control effective consent request steps; anticipate, do not hesitate. Hospital and OPO communicate early – well before brain death is pronounced - in order to jointly develop an approach plan. Establish protocols jointly between hospital and OPO staff to ensure early identification and timely referral of potential donors.** **HOSPITAL TIERS 1 & 2 & 3 TOP CHANGE**	2.01a	Tailor or adapt the organ donation process to complementary strengths of OPO and individual hospitals. O/H OPO and individual hospitals. O/H
			2.01b	Work as a team with hospital staff to determine the right person(s) to suggest donation and make the request. Establish family communication plan that incorporate all members of patient care team. O/H
			2.01c	Teach hospital staff certain clinical triggers for referrals. O/H
			2.01d	Have a "go to" person that is responsible for organ donation on hospital units with high donor potential. H
			2.01e	Track consents rates of all requesters and consistently deploy effective staff accordingly.
			2.01f	Hold an after action review within 24 hours after all successful and/or missed referral or opportunities.
	2.02	Establish customized protocols to standardize the approach to families and ensure that all have a positive experience regardless of consent status. Systematically make every effort to determine a family's willingness to donate, and recognize that reapproach may be necessary. **HOSPITAL TIER 1 & 2 TOP CHANGE**	2.02a	Identify the family support system within each hospital (social work, chaplains, etc) and link these resources with OPO at first point of contact. H
			2.02b	Start early to understand family dynamics. Identify key decision-maker(s), monitor status, and support family needs. O/H
			2.02c	Provide appropriate information and instruction on brain death to families, preferably in writing.
			2.02d	Train staff to ask at the right time and in the right way, and reapproach if needed. O/H
			2.02e	Factor in spiritual and cultural needs of each family; train OPO and hospital staff to increase cultural awareness. Prepare to adapt to particular family needs or requests to facilitate organ donation. O/H
			2.02f	Match requesters appropriately to family, ensuring effective requestors are available; special requestors should be hired and utilized by the OPO or hospital specific to the ethnicity of the OPO service area population. H/O
			2.02g	If OPO staff is not making the request, establish a designated requestor program with training that emphasizes success measured by numbers of families who consent. H/O
			2.02h	Nurses, social workers, hospital-based pastoral care staff may be used as certified organ/tissue requesters. H/O
			2.02i	Closely monitor consent rates, provide feedback to requestors on their rates of success and make changes as indicated by performance. O/H
	2.03	Develop specialized roles keyed to specific skills needed throughout donation process: clinical/technical experience in critical care or trauma settings; family therapy or counseling/social work; business development/ marketing. **HOSPITAL TIER 1 TOP CHANGE**	2.03a	Consider use of in-hospital coordinator with HD [[Spell out.]] responsibility to establish early interaction with family and provide consistent day-to-day management of the organ donation system within the facility. O
			2.03b	Establish a defined family liaison role – use family counselors/specialists as requesters as needed. O/H

PO56: Hospital Donation System Design

Strategies to Achieve Joint Accountability for Results		Key Change Concepts for Increased Organ Donation Rates – Experience Indicates That Those in BOLD Are Critical to Success		Suggested Action Items Experience Indicates That Those in BOLD Are Critical to Success
	2.04	Proactively establish relationships between OPO staff and hospitals to include: key patient care, nursing and medical leadership, family support staff, and administration.	2.04a	**Clarify respective roles of hospital and OPO personnel in the donation process continuum, and educate both regarding complementary roles. O/H**
			2.04b	Dispel the many myths surrounding organ donation for both families and staff. O/H
3. Integrated Donation Process Management OPO and hospitals establish and manage an integrated donation process that clearly defines roles and responsibilities and provides feedback.	3.01	**Establish joint OPO/hospital designated leadership responsibility and accountability. OPO provides resources for all donation-related matters; Hospital provides high level support, with OPO input (at a minimum, CMO, VP level)** **HOSPITAL TIER 2 TOP CHANGE**	3.01a	**Develop action plan to ensure respective roles are known and understood by OPO/hospital leadership and staff. O/H**
			3.01b	**Create expectation that OPO takes responsibility for meeting and maintaining Hospital CMS Regulations requirements by establishing policy defining imminent death, ensuring timely referral, providing education and continual feedback. O/H**
			3.01c	Establish Hospital-Specific Organ Donation Committee with representation from all relevant staff including but not limited to physicians, nurses, hospital administrative leadership, and family support services (social workers, chaplains) to review monthly potential donor data and cases, and address CQI. Ensure strong leadership, hospital sponsorship, significant critical care representation and OPO representation. H/O
	3.02	**Utilize appropriate data and tools to provide immediate feedback to hospitals/clinical leadership on donation process/results/ outcomes with specific follow-up requests and action steps.**	3.02a	**Use Death Record Reviews to establish referral, consent, and donation, rates and automate process in order to monitor performance in real time. O**
			3.02b	Maintain a formal process for comprehensive immediate follow-up communication between OPO and hospital on every organ donor referral regardless of the outcome (After Action Review); system to include guidelines for in-person follow-up, debriefing and mutual critique of process as well as written correspondence and email communication to facilitate timely feedback where access is difficult. O/H
	3.03	**Build and maintain collaborative relationships with key hospital staff/ physicians at all levels that affect the donation process.**	3.03a	Identify and support organ donation champions at various hospital levels; include leaders who are willing to be called upon to overcome barriers to organ donation in real time. H/O
	3.04	Partner, consult with, and provide curriculum to clinical leadership (physicians and nurses) to; establish brain death policy, documentation and guidelines for brain death discussion with family. Establish standards for stabilization of potential donors		
	3.05	Educate appropriate hospital staff/physicians by providing physician and staff in services at regular sessions to create and maintain OPO consultant responsibilities, appropriate awareness, and of understanding policies.	3.05a	Provide hospital unit-based education, and target core curriculum/education to referring staff: donor advocacy, bereavement care, certified (designated) requestor, etc. O/H
			3.05b	Consistently show appreciation to hospital staff for their efforts, and celebrate and communicate successes both internally and externally. O/H

PO56: Hospital Donation System Design

Strategies to Achieve Joint Accountability for Results	Key Change Concepts for Increased Organ Donation Rates – Experience Indicates That Those in BOLD Are Critical to Success		Suggested Action Items Experience Indicates That Those in BOLD Are Critical to Success	
	3.06	Use survey tools to evaluate/monitor donation process, identifying trends/strengths/problems.		
	3.07	In order to maximize better organ recovery, jointly establish expectations, guidelines and protocols between OPO and hospital operating room management, staff and anesthesia department (ie, provide scrub, circulator, anesthesia/CRNA).	3.07a	Create and use standardized mechanisms for feedback, collaboratively identify action steps, if needed and monitor progress. O/H
4. Aggressive Pursuit of Every Donation Opportunity Every possibility for increased donation is maximized and routinely evaluated through death record reviews, quick deployment, re-approaches, donor management and improved organ yield.	4.01	Constantly look for, evaluate, and address every donor potential. Advocate for donation. HOSPITAL TIER 3 TOP CHANGE	4.01a	Use 100% Death Record Reviews and Report of Death Forms to identify missed opportunities, follow-up appropriately with involved staff, and identify and test indicated changes to prevent recurrence. Have death record reviews (as basis for number of eligibles) performed independent of hospital assignments. O/H
			4.01b	Establish hospital policies and procedures to assure (1) timely notification of all brain-injured patients with a Glasgow Scale (GCS) of 5, and (2) maintenance of physiologic function until the OPO has determined suitability and families are offered the option of donation. H/O
			4.01c	Respond on-site by OPO coordinator or designee to every appropriate referral within 1 hour. O
			4.01d	Assess and reevaluate reasons family has declined donation and consider reapproaching if appropriate. O/H
	4.02	Develop, define, and maintain a standard of high quality service in handling all hospital and physician communications.		
	4.03	Establish, evaluate and be accountable for a clear donor management process from referral to recovery with OPO oversight from the Procurement Director and/or Medical Director(s). HOSPITAL TIER 2 TOP CHANGE	4.03a	Manage donors at OPO site. O
			4.03b	Establish OPO-based Recovery Team. O
			4.03c	Create Organ Recovery and Placement Coordinator/Specialist positions. O
			4.03d	Have an Organ Surgery Specialist on OPO Staff. O
			4.03e	Integrate Critical Care Professionals into organ donation process; assure an intensivist is involved in appropriate donor opportunities. O/H
	4.04	Use OPO Procurement Director and/or Medical Director(s) to QA Donor Management and organ placement; Apply broad criteria to evaluate every organ donor for potential; minimize lost recoveries; aggressively pursue organ placement. HOSPITAL TIER 3 TOP CHANGE	4.04a	Aggressively pursue placement efforts beyond the local transplant center determination of "unsuitability" to improve utilization; pursue placement outside of OPO with all appropriate donor information communicated to TC [[Spell out.]] accepting organ. O
			4.04b	Establish system for real-time OPO medical and administrative intervention on all cases of donor turn down or determination of organ "unsuitability." O/H
			4.04c	Require mandatory review of all turndowns and discards. O/H
	4.05	Increase the interaction of OPO Medical Director with hospital physicians by identifying physician champion and establish QI/QA processes with physicians through one-on-one case reviews and education. HOSPITAL TIER 3 TOP CHANGE		

A CLINICIAN'S GUIDE TO DONATION AND TRANSPLANTATION   Chapter 27

PO56: Hospital Donation System Design

Strategies to Achieve Joint Accountability for Results	Key Change Concepts for Increased Organ Donation Rates – Experience Indicates That Those in BOLD Are Critical to Success		Suggested Action Items Experience Indicates That Those in BOLD Are Critical to Success	
	4.06	Have OPO management expectation of no (zero) medical examiner denials	4.06a	Immediately address medical examiner/coroner denials with OPO leadership (medical and administrative) at the time of occurrence. Consider advocating legislation (see Sec. 4.11.a, HHS Secretary's Advisory Committee on Organ Transplantation. Recommendation #10 states that legislative strategies be adopted that will encourage medical examiners and coroners not to withhold life-saving organs and tissues from qualified organ procurement organizations). O/H
	4.07	Coordinate Do Not Resuscitate (DNR) and Comfort Measures Only (CMO) planning process between hospital and OPO staff to avoid conflict with the opportunity for organ donation.	4.07a	Establish hospital protocols that include a provision for maintaining hemodynamic support for potential donors, inclusive of cases where family has requested a DNR order without knowledge of donation options. H
			4.07b	Conduct joint training sessions for hospitals and OPOs on consent, communications, and discussions surrounding end-of-life decision making. Sessions will include skills, practice, and role-playing. O/H
			4.07c	Educate hospital and OPO staff regarding impact of DNR/CMO status on the potential for organ donation. H/O
	4.08	Establish OPO and hospital policies and protocols for donation after cardiac death (DCD) or non-heart beat donation to ensure the referral of all patients with nonrecoverable neurological injuries and pursuit of donation options.	4.08a	Introduce and implement sample policies and procedures based on the Institute of Medicine recommendations. O/H
			4.08b	Establish a comprehensive OPO staff-training program to ensure competency and expertise in guiding hospital through clinical process. O
			4.08c	Integrate DCD routinely into all hospital staff education; develop hospital staff training program to include review o the literature, IOM recommendation, discussion of ethical considerations, case review, and clinical procedures. O/H
			4.08d	Clarify legal hospital specific consent procedure and forms for DCD. O
			4.08e	Aggressively pursue each opportunity for DCD in the instances where it is clinically reasonable and the family wishes to donate regardless of policy status. On a regular basis, measure and report on DCD activity within OPO and Hospital. O/H

PO56: Hospital Donation System Design — Attachment 2

First Things First

To take full advantage of the Best Practices that are the basis for the changes your team will be addressing during the Learning Session, it is important that you concentrate first on the basic building blocks for success. The Collaborative Faculty and experienced teams have learned that success is assured if you do these First Things First. Your Team should come to the learning session with a sense of which of these eight areas your participating hospital need to improve. Before coming to San Diego, collectively determine, for each action, at what level each of your hospitals currently function, and grade accordingly:

1. **Create OPO Hospital Presence/In-House Coordinator**

   Create and maintain visual presence of OPO staff in hospitals; become part of the fabric of high potential hospitals in order to establish, maintain, and activate relationships with all individuals that participate/play a role in the donation process.

2. **Analyze and Apply Current Hospital Specific Data,** (tie the data to current system to identify where to focus initial efforts/changes)

   Establish strong culture of accountability for results: Ensure that OPO and hospital staff know and talk conversion rates and regularly review and respond to data reports of donation key indicators (conversion rates, consent rates, timely notification rates).

3. **Identify Physician/Clinician Champion**

   Identify and support organ donation champions at various hospital levels; include leaders who are willing to be called upon to overcome barriers to organ donation in real time.

4. **Conduct Monthly Death Record Reviews**

   Use Death Record Reviews to establish referral, consent, and donation rates, and automate process in order to monitor performance in real time.

5. **Establish Clinical Triggers**

   Mutually establish with hospital staff appropriate clinical triggers for referrals.

6. **Hold Donation Team Huddles**

   Work as a team with hospital staff to determine the right person(s) to suggest donation and make the request. Establish family communication plan that incorporate all members of patient care team.

7. **Identify Effective Requestors (who is your most effective requester?)**

   Match requestors appropriately to family, ensuring effective requestors are available; special requestors should be hired and utilized by the OPO or hospital specific to the ethnicity of the OPO service area population.

8. **Conduct After Action Reviews**

   Maintain a formal process for comprehensive immediate follow-up communication between OPO and hospital on every organ donor referral regardless of the outcome (After Action Review); system to include guidelines for in-person follow-up, debriefing and mutual critique of process, as well as written correspondence and email communication to facilitate timely feedback where access is difficult.

PO56: Hospital Donation System Design

Attachment 3

Organ Donation Breakthrough Collaborative Change Package

High Leverage Changes

Six steps to install a high performance, organ donation system

1. Advocate Organ Donation as The Mission
2. Involve Senior Management to Get Results
3. Deploy a Self-Organizing OPO/Hospital Team
4. Practice Early Referral, Rapid Response
5. Master Effective Requesting
6. Implement for Donation After Cardiac Death

PO56: Hospital Donation System Design

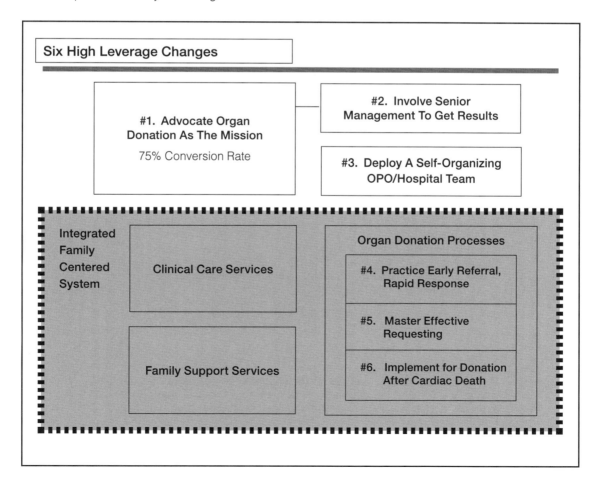

Chapter 27: THE ORGAN DONATION BREAKTHROUGH COLLABORATIVE

PO56: Hospital Donation System Design

#1. **Advocate Organ Donation As The Mission:** build proactive advocacy for organ donation into the mission, business plans, and staff practices of the OPO and hospitals.

Action items

Express Institutional Mission

- with the community take a broad view of the mission: we are responsible for the lives of patients on the wait list; donation is desirable; advocacy is necessary and good
- have OPO and hospital Boards and executive management publicly commit to national organ donation conversion goals (75%)
- put in place high visibility, physical symbols of the institutional commitment to organ donation (statue, photographs, plaques, videos, ...)
- have the community acknowledge the joint OPO/hospital enterprise making itself accountable for high performance in organ donation conversion
- make continuous improvement in organ donation conversion rates and yield part of the mission and business plans of the OPO and hospital
- use organizational missions and business plans as reference points for staff self-initiated action on organ donation

Communicate Mission To The Staff

- present advocacy to the staff as the power to save lives and ask them to be advocates for all the patients on the waiting lists
- build advocacy explicitly into the consent process through staff orientation and training
- align accountability for conversion rates with the staff's passion and responsibility for family support
- present continuous improvement in organ donation conversion rates and yield as a teachable method and core competency of the OPO and hospital staff
- frequently celebrate OPO/hospital team performance in organ donation conversion and yield

Examples Of Simple PDSAs Used To Establish Advocacy

Example A

- Plan: Hold a ceremony to establish advocacy as the practice. OPO and hospital leadership present "mission statement" for organ donation advocacy. All staff sign the commitment board for 75% conversion. Show video designed to guide development of team action agendas
- Study: Survey before and after ceremony to measure staff understanding and commitment to proactive advocacy

#2. **Involve Senior Management To Get Results.** OPO and hospital senior managers actively support each case through a well-defined organ donation process that integrates the roles and responsibilities of the two institutions.

Action items

The commitment

- OPO managers (Executive Director, Medical Director, COO, Procurement Director, ...) and hospital managers (Medical Director, Chief Medical Officer, Chief of Nursing, Pastoral Care Director, Legal Counsel, ...) are prepared to play a constructive, real time role in a case
- OPO staff (Hospital Development Coordinator, Procurement Coordinator, Family Service Coordinator, Transplant Coordinator, ...) and hospital staff (critical care nurse, social worker, chaplain, physicians, ...) know how to engage senior management to facilitate the process

The underlying process

- there is a well-developed and tested system for identifying and running a case that covers all the stages in the Lewin generic process
- everyone knows who does what, everyone acknowledges and respects the roles of others
- possible barriers to donation are identified (e.g. physician reluctance to trigger early referral, medical examiner release not forthcoming, failure to place organ in allocation process) and appropriate senior management action is planned for
- a well-defined communication system in place to make senior management available in real time to any hospital team in action on a case

A CLINICIAN'S GUIDE TO DONATION AND TRANSPLANTATION

PO56: Hospital Donation System Design

Examples Of Simple PDSAs Used To Establish Senior Management Involvement

Example A

- Plan: Test real time response for barrier breakthrough. Develop guidelines, protocol and process for bringing senior management in to facilitate the process
- Study: Track to determine if real time response is realized and effective

#3. **Deploy A Self-Organizing OPO/Hospital Team.** An integrated and flexible "organ donation team" identifies and uses the strengths of all the players in a well-defined organ donation process.

Action items

Team Charter

- OPO/hospital team assumes stewardship of a well-defined organ donation and family support process
- OPO/hospital team assumes responsibility for advocacy and for continuous improvement in conversion rates and yield
- communication systems and agreements in place to get the right people involved at the right time
- OPO Hospital Development Coordinator is available in real time to the hospital team handling a case

Team Practices

- team members decide on roles they will play to ensure best outcomes
- team reorganizes the assets available case by case to make the process work
- team integrates the staff of the organizations involved: run an effective process regardless of affiliation and job definition, account for the strengths and weakness of the organizations
- pre-approach "huddle" is used to decide who will make the request, who needs to be involved
- team leader can change from case to case; members ready to lead
- team knows who are effective requestors and how best to deploy them
- team expects requestor to spend a good amount of time with family, especially when the early responses suggest the family will say no
- team uses a formal "after action review" process to continually improve

Examples Of Simple PDSAs Used To Establish OPO/Hospital Teams

Example A

- Plan: Test the "huddle" concept. Design the team's huddle steps and create an occasion to pilot test it
- Study: use "after action review" to assess the pilot, what works and what can be added to make it better

#4. **Practice Early Referral, Rapid Response**. Follow early referral by the hospital with rapid response by the OPO

Action items

Set it up

- OPO/hospital use a collaborative, evidence-based process to develop "clinical triggers"
- deploy "clinical triggers" for early identification of potential donors
- assure staff access to "clinical trigger" information
- provide training in practice of "clinical triggers"
- OPO establishes in-hospital coordinator where appropriate
- work with the principle: more time with family = more trust = more donation = more lives saved

Make it work

- have OPO staff on-site in early stages, actively interacting with hospital staff and involved in family observation and support
- track referral and response timing
- establish empirical relationship between timing of OPO involvement (first contact with family made, first mention of donation, etc.) and donation process outcomes

PO56: Hospital Donation System Design

Examples of Simple PDSAs Used To Establish Early Referral, Rapid Response

Example A

- Plan: Set and test expectations. Have the team set expectations for early referral and response times in pursuit of organ donation
- Study: Analyze measured outcomes (conversions) relative to early referral and response times. Do we execute early referral and rapid response and does it produce the results we expect?

#5. **Master Effective Requesting.** Establish and manage a well-defined process and set of practices for "effective requesting," regarding the flow of communication with the family

Action items

Set it up

- align effective requesting with the advocacy mission that makes moving to "yes" an imperative
- establish "effective requesting" as a teachable discipline
- develop a well-defined process for "effective requesting" highlighting continuous interaction with family to address concerns and wishes
- benchmark the OPO/hospital requesting process against best practices
- provide training in "effective requesting" using role playing and case studies

Make it work

- involve donor families in the requesting process with the family
- use a formal, tested practice for addressing initial family resistance to donation
- establish culturally appropriate and effective communication with families
- be culturally competent in matching requestors and support staff with families
- track the process and the results of "requesting" (log time spent, action taken, and important events)
- identify effective requestors; celebrate their performance
- track the results of OPO training on "effective requesting"
- do an after action review of "effective requesting" practice
- establish the empirical relationship between time spent with family and conversion rates with initial acceptance, and conversion rates following an initial "no"

Examples Of Simple PDSAs For Effective Requesting

Example A

- Plan: Test a process for dealing with family objections associated with saying "no" to the request. Identify the steps to be taken when re-approach is critical to a successful outcome
- Study: Do an after action review to identify "what worked" and "what to add"

Tools:

- "Key processes" (LS3, Tab 9)
- Videos of effective requestors
- Presumptive Approach

#6. **Prepare For Donation After Cardiac Death.** Establish OPO and hospital policies that promote DCD to assure referral of all patients with non-recoverable neurological injuries

Action items

Set it up

- use sample DCD policies and procedures (IOM recommendations) to initiate OPO/hospital conversations on DCD policy and protocol development
- develop draft OPO policies and hospital policies on DCD that can be adapted for adoption by individual hospitals

Make it work

- regardless of policy status, pursue each DCD opportunity where the family wishes it and use the opportunity to further develop policy
- track and report on DCD activity in the OPO and hospital to show potential and actual impact on donations
- evaluate each DCD experience through "after action review"

A CLINICIAN'S GUIDE TO DONATION AND TRANSPLANTATION   Chapter 27

PO56: Hospital Donation System Design

Examples Of Simple PDSAs Used To Establish DCD Policy And Practice

PDSA: A

- Plan: Establish policy. Introduce DCD to CEO and CMO and request a policy review by the committee. Request that committee put the policy in place
- Study: Track the conversations for progress on adoption

PDSA: B

- Plan: Assess public attitudes and readiness. Develop a survey of hospital volunteers as a surrogate for the lay public
- Study: Assess need for public education, and opportunity for mobilization of public support

PDSA: C

- Plan: Estimate potential impact. Estimate number of potential DCDs in the hospital. Show hospital leadership and staff potential impact of DCD on the organ donation performance of the hospital
- Study: Track understanding and attitude toward DCD

Tools:

- Sample hospital DCD policy statements.

Attachment 4

Model for Improvement   **PDSA Cycle:** _____ **Date:** _____   **Hospital:** _____
Objective for This PDSA Cycle: **P**lan   Questions:
Predictions:
Plan for Change or Test: Who, What, When, Where?
Plan for Collection of Data: Who, What, When, Where?
Do: Carry out the Change or Test; Begin Analysis.
Study: Complete analysis of data; Summarize what was learned.
Act: Are we ready to make a change? Plan for the next cycle.

Chapter 27 THE ORGAN DONATION BREAKTHROUGH COLLABORATIVE

PO56: Hospital Donation System Design *Attachment 5*

Model for Improvement
PDSA Cycle: _____ Date: _____
Hospital: _____

Objective for This PDSA Cycle: Increase Timely Notification

Plan
Questions: Will timely notification increase if IHCs and DCSs make rounds on the units 7 days a week? Will we eliminate missed referrals?

Predictions: Timely notification will increase if IHCs and DCSs make rounds on the units. It will show us that the MICU and CCU are missing clinical triggers to make referrals.

Plan for Change or Test: Who, What, When, Where? The IHCs and DCSs will make rounds daily and when they find a patient that has not been referred that meets the clinical trigger for referral, they will encourage the nurse to make the referral.

Plan for Collection of Data: Who, What, When, Where? The Hospital DCS will review all referrals and determine how many referrals were prompted by the DCS making rounds.

Do: Carry out the Change or Test; Begin Analysis. The DCS will review referrals during the two week period starting 4/23/2004.

Study: Complete analysis of data; Summarize what was learned. Of the 26 referrals made from this hospital during the time period, 30 (68.4%) were made in a timely manner. There were no missed referrals, however, of the 12 referrals that were not made in a timely manner, 8 were prompted by the DCS making rounds.

Act: Are we ready to make a change? Plan for the next cycle. The next phase of the cycle will be inservicing the nurses on clinical triggers in order that all referrals are made in a timely manner and are not prompted or "made" during the "rounding" process. Re-measurement will occur after inservices have been completed.

References

1. Waiting List Removals. Removal Reasons by Years: Removed from the Waiting List, January 1995-October 31, 2005. Richmond, VA: United Network for Organ Sharing. Available at: http://www.optn.org/latestData/rptData.asp. Accessed January 30, 2006.
2. Organ Donation Breakthrough Collaborative. About the Collaborative. Available at: http://www.organdonationnow.org/index.cfm?fuseaction=Page.viewPage&pageId=471. Accessed January 30, 2006.
3. OPTN/SRTR Annual Report. Chapter 3: Organ Donation and Utilization in the U.S., 2004. Table III.1. Eligible, Actual and Additional Donors, 2002-2003. Richmond, VA: United Network for Organ Sharing. Available at: www.optn.org/AR2004/Chapter_III_AR_CD.htm?cp=4. Accessed January 30, 2006. Date accessed: January 30, 2006.
4. The Organ Donation Breakthrough Collaborative: Best Practices Final Report. US Department of Health and Human Services; Health Resources and Services Administration. Office of Special Programs, Division of Transplantation. Contract 240-94-0037. Task Order Number 12, September 2003. Available at: http://www.organdonor.gov/bestpractice.htm. Accessed: January 25, 2006.
5. Joint Commission on Accreditation of Healthcare Organizations. *Health Care at the Crossroads: Strategies for Narrowing the Organ Donation Gap and Protecting Patients.* Joint Commission on Accreditation of Healthcare Organizations; 2004. No. 630-792-5631.
6. Organ Procurement Transplant Network. Available at: http://www.optn.org. Accessed August 8, 2005.
7. Sheehy E, Conrad SL, Brigham LE, et al. Estimating the number of potential donors in the United States. *N Engl J Med.* 2003; 349:667-674.
8. Wagner D. Shared Vision Overview. Secretary Tommy Thompson's Organ Donation Breakthrough Collaborative Learning Session 1. Washington, DC, September 16, 2003.
9. Institute for Health Care Improvement. Available at: http://www.ihi.org. Accessed July 20, 2005.
10. Metzger RA, Taylor GJ, McGaw LJ, Weber PG, Delmonico FL, Prottas JM; UNOS Research to Practice Steering Committee. Research to practice: a national consensus conference.Prog Transplant. 2005 Dec; 15(4):379-84.
11. Langley GJ, Nolan KM, Nolan TW, Norman CL, Provost LP. Methods for improvement. In: *The Improvement Guide. A Practical Approach to Enhancing Organizational Performance.* Jossey-Bass; 1996; 49-138.
12. Shafer TJ, Ehrle RN, Davis KD, et al. Increasing organ recovery from level 1 trauma centers: the in-house coordinator intervention. *Prog Transplant.* 2004; 14:250-263.
13. Shafer TJ, Davis KD, Holtzman SM, Van Buren CT, Crafts NJ, Durand RE. In-house organ procurement organization staff located in level 1 trauma centers increase conversion of potential donors to actual donors. *Transplantation.* 2003; 75:1330-1335.
14. Shafer TJ, Wood RP, Van Buren CT, et al. A success story in minority donation: the LifeGift/BenTaub General Hospital in-house coordinator program. *Transplant Proc.* 1997; 29:3753-3755.
15. Shafer TJ, Wood RP, Van Buren CT, et al. An in-house coordinator program to increase organ donation in public trauma hospitals. *J Transpl Coord* 1998; 8:82-87.
16. Sullivan H, Blakely D, Davis K. An in-house coordinator program to increase organ donation in public teaching hospitals. *J Transpl Coord.* 1998; 8:40-44.
17. Ehrle RN, Shafer TJ, Nelson KR. "Referral, Request, and Consent for Organ Donation: Best Practice – A Blueprint for Success. *Crit Care Nurse.* 1999; 19:21-33.
18. Dickerson J, Valadka AB, Levert T, Davis K, Kuria M, Robertson CS. Organ donation rates in neurosurgical intensive care unit. *J Neurosurg.* 2002; 97:811-814.
19. Siminoff LA, Gordon N, Hewlett J, Arnold RM. Factors influencing families' consent for donation of solid organs for transplantation. JAMA. 2001; 286:71-77.
20. DeJong W, Franz HG, Wolfe SM, et al. Requesting organ donation: an interview study of donor and non-donor families. *Am J Cri Care.* 1998; 7:13-23.
21. Shafer TJ, Van Buren CT, Andrews CE, et al. Program development and routine notification in a large independent OPO: a 12-year review. *J Transpl Coord.* 1999; 9:40-48.
22. Shafer TJ, Schkade LL, Evans RW, O'Connor KJ, Reitsma W. The vital role of medical examiners and coroners in organ transplantation. *Am J Transplant* 2004; 4:160-168.
23. Shafer TJ, Schkade LL, Siminoff LA, Mahoney TA. Ethical analysis of organ recovery denials by medical examiners, coroners and justices of the peace. *J Transplant Coord.* 1999; 9:232-249.
24. Shafer TJ, Schkade LL, Warner HE, et al. The impact of medical examiner/coroner practices on organ recovery in the United States. JAMA. 1994;272:1607-1613.
25. Graham M as President of National Association of Medical Examiners. Bold Offers and Requests. Presented at: Organ Donation Breakthrough Collaborative Learning Session 3; April 27-28, 2004; Detroit, Mich.
26. Romans J. Healthcare at the crossroads: organ donation in the 21st century, a regional program event. Best practices for health care organizations to close the gap: characteristics of effective programs. Presented at: Lessons to date from the HRSA Organ Donation Breakthrough Collaborative; November 17, 2004; Raleigh, NC.

27. Lewis J, Peitier J, Nelson H, et al. Development of the University of Wisconsin Donation after Cardiac Death Evaluation Tool. *Prog Transplant.* 2003; 13:265-73.
28. Institute of Medicine. *Non-Heart-Beating Organ Transplanation: Medical and Ethical Issues in Procurement.* Washington, DC: National Academy Press; 1997.
29. Berwick D. Key note address. Presented at: Secretary Tommy Thompson's Breakthrough Organ Donation Collaborative: Learning Session 1. Department of Health and Human Services, Division of Organ Transplantation; September 16, 2003; Washington, D.C.

Clinical Diagnosis and Confirmatory Testing of Brain Death in Adults

Eelco F. M. Wijdicks, MD

Brain death is anticipated in many cataclysmic neurologic disorders, but it represents only a small proportion of all medical and non-trauma-related surgical intensive care admissions. The incidence of brain death in specialized neurotrauma units is much higher, but again, a severely disabled functional state or death from cardiopulmonary arrest is a far more common outcome than loss of brain function. In our neurologic-neurosurgical intensive care unit, approximately 10 comatose patients per 1,000 acute admissions evolve into brain death. Compression, shift, and neuronal loss of diencephalic structures or brainstem due to an acute mass are common mechanisms, but a more diffuse anoxic-ischemic or overwhelming infection of the central nervous system may rapidly ravage both hemispheres. Precipitous loss of blood pressure and new-onset hypothermia or polyuria are the most characteristic clinical indicators that the brain has been completely destroyed.

This chapter discusses clinical assessment of brain death in adults. It expands on the American Academy of Neurology practice parameter document adopted in 1995.[1,2] A separate discussion concerning infants and children follows in Chapter 5. The determination of brain death in a person precious in the family's memory remains a painful task. Recommendations for family discussion and ways to advocate organ donation are found in Chapter 10.

Clinical Examination

Assessment of brain death in a comatose patient should proceed with a certain set of principles in mind, namely excluding major confounders, establishing the cause of the coma, ascertaining irreversibility, and accurately testing brainstem reflexes at all levels of the brainstem.

Clinical examination should proceed only if certain prerequisites are met (Table 1). In the vast majority of patients, computed tomography (CT) scanning shows a mass with herniation, multiple hemispheric lesions with edema, or edema alone. Obviously, a CT scan abnormality compatible with brain death does not obviate a search for confounders. Conversely, a normal CT scan can be seen early following cardiac or respiratory arrest and in patients with fulminant meningitis or encephalitis. In circumstances of overwhelming infection, examination of cerebrospinal fluid (CSF) should reveal diagnostic findings, such

Table 1. PREREQUISITES BEFORE DETERMINATION OF BRAIN DEATH

Definitive acute catastrophic event involving both hemispheres or brainstem and irreversibility
Exclusion of complicating medical conditions that may confound clinical assessment, particularly severe electrolyte, acid-base, or endocrine disturbances
Core temperature of ≥32°C
No documented evidence of drug intoxication, poisoning, or neuromuscular blocking agents

CLINICAL DIAGNOSIS AND CONFIRMATORY TESTING OF BRAIN DEATH IN ADULTS

as pleocytosis, increased erythrocyte count, or positive Gram stain. Some viruses, parasites, and bacteria can be detected by polymerase chain reaction (PCR), although not in due time. Interpretation of the CT scan in a patient suspected of being brain dead requires knowledge of the patterns that are compatible with brain death (Figure 1). For example, in cases of traumatic brain injury, multiple contusions or a subdural or epidural hematoma should be present which displaces the septum pellucidum from its midline position. Effacement of the basal cistern and sulci is a common finding in patients with diffuse, profound cerebral edema. When major discrepancies exist between the clinical examination and the CT scan, a repeat CT study is warranted and often will document expansion of the mass or an enlarged mass effect. If the CT scan remains incongruent with loss of brain function, other factors should be considered, particularly drugs, poison, or an endocrine or major electrolyte abnormality. Core temperature should be at least 32°C. The potential consequences of these abnormalities for brain death determination are further elaborated on in Chapter 6. In any case, the clinical examination should be methodical and focus on (a) documentation of coma, (b) absence of brainstem reflexes, and (c) demonstration of apnea following maximal stimulation of respiratory centers after induction of acute CSF acidosis.

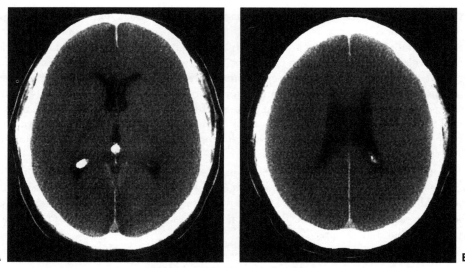

Figure 1. Computed tomography scan patterns commonly seen in patients at time of brain death determination. **A,B:** Cerebral edema following cardiac or respiratory arrest. Note featureless brain with absent sulci and no white matter-gray matter differentiation. *(continued)*

Septum pellucidum - transparent membrane runs down the middle of the brain from the corpus callosum to the area of the fornix.

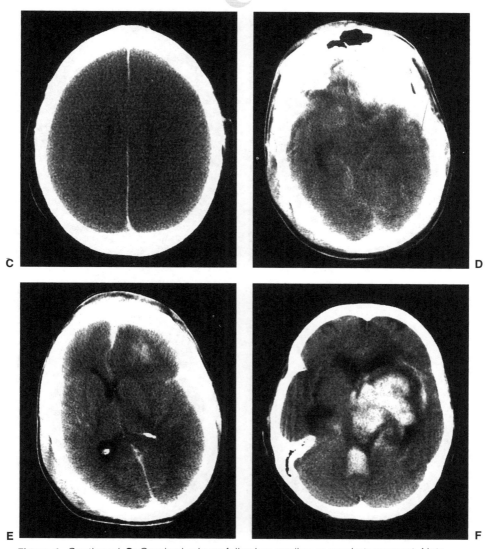

Figure 1. *Continued.* **C:** Cerebral edema following cardiac or respiratory arrest. Note featureless brain with absent sulci and no white matter-gray matter differentiation. **D,E:** Left subdural hematoma and frontal contusion with pronounced shift of the midline structures and septum pellucidum. Early enlargement of the temporal horn and effacement of basal cisterns are seen. **F:** Destructive hemorrhage into the putamen with thalamus extension and hemoventricle. *(continued)*

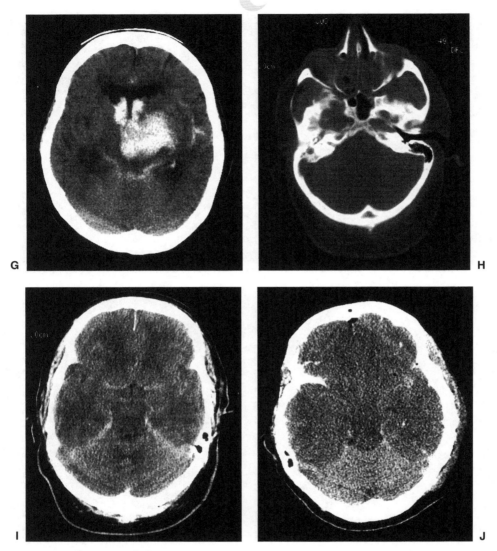

Figure 1. *Continued.* **G:** Destructive putamen hemorrhage with thalamus extension and hemoventricle. **H,I:** Cerebral edema in patient with fulminant pneumococcal meningitis. Note opacification of the right mastoid air cells due to inflammatory disease. *(continued)*

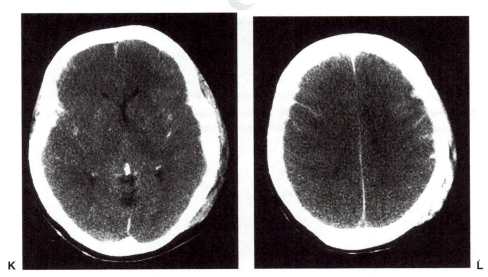

Figure 1. *Continued.* **J-L:** Traumatic brain edema with multiple contusions.

Coma

Patients lack all evidence of responsiveness due to complete loss of consciousness.

Technique

The depth of coma can be assessed by examining eye and motor responses with the use of standard painful stimuli such as pressure on the supraorbital nerve, nail bed pressure, and temporomandibular joint compression.[3] Other pain stimuli, such as sternal rubbing, rubbing knuckles against the ribs in the axilla, twisting the forearm or nipples, and applying pin prick on several body locations, may be equally effective but have not been accepted as the norm. Eye opening and motor responses to voice or pain should be absent on repeated tests (Figure 2).

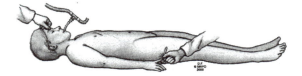

Figure 2. Motor response to pain. (By permission of Mayo Foundation.)

Alerts

Motor responses may occur spontaneously, after painful stimulation, and during apnea testing, particularly when hypoxemia or hypotension intervenes. These responses should be interpreted as spinally generated. They are brief, slow movements in the upper limbs, flexion in the fingers, or arm lifting, and they do not become integrated into truly coordinated decerebrate or decorticate responses. They seldom persist with repeated stimulation. Reproducible eye opening, but with only a minimal eyelid elevation barely showing the beginning of an iris, has been noted in response to twisting of a nipple in patients who fulfilled all clinical criteria of brain death.[4,5] The reflex pathway is not known.

Absence of Brainstem Reflexes

Examination of Pupils

Technique

The response to bright light should be absent in both eyes. Round, oval, or irregularly shaped pupils are compatible with brain death. Most pupils in brain death are in mid position (4 to 6 mm).[6] Dilated pupils are compatible with brain death because intact sympathetic cervical spine pathways connected to the radially arranged fibers of the dilator muscle may remain intact (Figure 3).

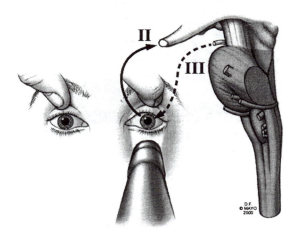

Figure 3. Pupil size and light response. Roman numerals refer to cranial nerves. (By permission of Mayo Foundation.)

Alerts

Many drugs can influence pupil size, but the light response remains intact. In conventional doses, atropine given intravenously has no marked influence on the pupillary response.[7,8] Short-term neuromuscular blocking drugs do not noticeably influence pupil size,[9] but a recent report with escalating doses of atracurium and vecuronium documented reversible mydriasis and ultimately nonreactive light responses.[10] Topical ocular instillation of drugs and trauma to the cornea or bulbus oculi may cause abnormalities in pupil size and can produce nonreactive pupils. Preexisting anatomic abnormalities of the iris or effects of previous surgery should be excluded.

Examination of Ocular Movements

Technique

Ocular movements should be absent, including any type of nystagmus. The oculocephalic reflex, elicited by fast turning of the head from middle position to 90 degrees on both sides, may not be sensitive enough to document the absence of ocular movements.

Ocular movements are also absent after caloric testing with ice water. Caloric testing should preferably be done with the head elevated to 30 degrees during irrigation of the tympanum on each side. With 30 degrees elevation, the horizontal canal becomes vertical. Irrigation of the tympanum can best be accomplished by inserting a small suction catheter into the external auditory canal and connecting it to a 50-mL syringe filled with ice water. A cold stimulus results in sedimentation of the endolymph and stimulation of the hair cells. The normal response in a comatose patient is a slow deviation of the eyes directed to the cold caloric stimulus. The response is absent in brain death. Absent eye movement may be very difficult to appreciate, and placement of pen marks on the lower eyelid at the level of the pupil may be helpful. One should allow up to 1 min of observation after injection, and the time between stimulation on each side should be at least 5 min, to reduce a possible overriding effect from the opposite irrigated ear (Figure 4).

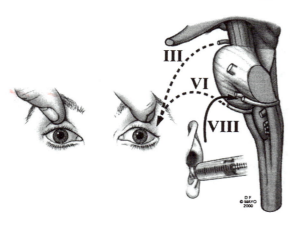

Figure 4. Caloric testing. Roman numerals refer to cranial nerves. (By permission of Mayo Foundation.)

Alerts

Clotted blood or cerumen in the ear may diminish the caloric response, and repeat testing is required. It is prudent to inspect the tympanum directly and to document free access to the cold water injection. Presence of a ruptured eardrum will enhance the caloric response, but such a maneuver can only be allowed when brain death is highly probable. Prior exposure to toxic levels of certain drugs can diminish or completely abolish the caloric response. Some typical examples are aminoglycosides, tricyclic antidepressants, anticholinergics, antiepileptic drugs, and chemotherapeutic agents, among others.[11] After closed head injury or facial trauma, eyelid edema and chemosis of the conjunctiva may limit movement of the globes. Basal fracture of the petrous bone abolishes the caloric response only unilaterally and may be identified by the presence of an ecchymotic mastoid process (Battle's sign).

Examination of Facial Sensation and Facial Motor Response

Technique

Absent corneal reflexes should be confirmed with a throat swab. Blinking requires intact brainstem reflex pathways and is not compatible with brain death. Facial myokymias could be due to muscle contraction from denervation or deafferentation of the facial nucleus and thus are compatible with brain death. Absent grimacing to pain can be documented by applying deep pressure with a blunt object on the nail beds, pressure on the supraorbital nerve, or deep pressure on both condyles at the level of the temporomandibular joint (Figure 5). The jaw reflex should also be absent.

Alerts

Severe facial and ocular trauma may limit or eliminate interpretation of these brainstem reflexes.

Examination of Pharyngeal and Tracheal Reflexes

Technique

Lack of a cough response to bronchial suctioning should be demonstrated by passing a catheter through the endotracheal tube and providing suctioning pressure for several seconds (Figure 6). Although not required as a test, 2 mg of atropine will not produce tachycardia. No change in heart rate after suctioning or atropine is further confirmatory of destruction of the intracranial parasympathetic pathways.

Alerts

In orally intubated patients, the gag response may be difficult to interpret and likely unreliable.

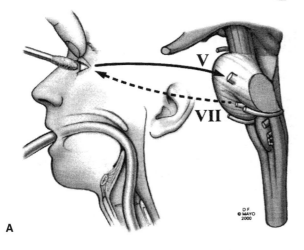

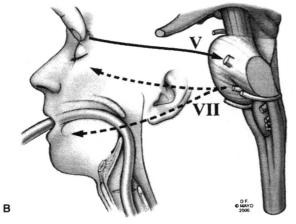

Figure 5. Corneal reflex **(A)** and facial response to pain pressure on the supraorbital nerve **(B)**. Roman numerals refer to cranial nerves. (By permission of Mayo Foundation.)

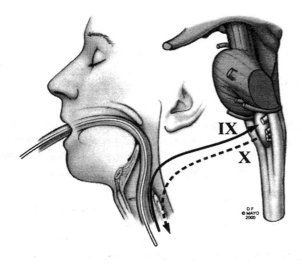

Figure 6. Cough response. Roman numerals refer to cranial nerves. (By permission of Mayo Foundation.)

Apnea

Apneic oxygenation is the most commonly used technique to demonstrate lack of ventilatory drive. This diagnostic tool involves placement of a source of 100% oxygen in the trachea which, through convection, results in oxygen flowing into the lungs.[12-15] Preoxygenation eliminates the nitrogen stores in the respiratory tract and thus facilitates oxygen transport. On the basis of animal experiments and clinical observations, a target $PaCO_2$ of 60 mm Hg has been proposed as a level at which the medullary respiratory centers are maximally stimulated. Traditionally, it has been assumed that the respiratory centers are reset higher due to malfunction from brainstem injury. The target, however, may be much lower, because in the few patients who started to breathe after disconnection of the ventilator, $PaCO_2$ levels were in the low 30's. We have personally seen two patients who started to breathe at $PaCO_2$ levels around 35 mm Hg but lost respiratory drive hours later. However, without detailed documentation on large numbers of patients, a $PaCO_2$ increase to 60 mm Hg or a 20 mm Hg increase from a normal baseline $PaCO_2$ level should remain the recommended target (for an historical overview, see Chapter 1).

The increase in $PaCO_2$ is biphasic, with a steep increase in the first minutes due to equilibration of arterial carbon dioxide with mixed central venous carbon dioxide. In the tracheobronchial phase of the apnea test, oxygen flow ensures uptake of oxygen in pulmonary capillaries, but carbon dioxide exhalation does not take place and therefore there is a rapid rise of $PaCO_2$ due to metabolic production of carbon dioxide. Increase in $PaCO_2$ results in a decrease in CSF pH, which is sensed by the medullary respiratory centers and, when function is present, results in a respiratory drive.[16,17] A rapid increase in $PaCO_2$ to 60 mm Hg or 20 mm Hg above normal baseline maximally stimulates these centers, also because CSF is unable to buffer acidosis with blood bicarbonate owing to its slower diffusion than carbon dioxide.

Many physicians prefer simple disconnection of the ventilator and use of oxygen flow through an endotracheally placed catheter. In addition to monitoring of oxygen saturation, pulse, and blood pressure, visual inspection of thoracic and abdominal movement is required. Disconnecting the patient from the ventilator reduces artifact reading of breathing on the ventilator display often due to continuous positive airway pressure (CPAP) alone. We have noted significant false readings (spontaneous respiratory rates of 20 to 30 per minute) by mechanical ventilator sensors with settings as low as a CPAP of 2.

Lang[18] has suggested a possibly attractive method of carbon dioxide augmentation to reduce observation time, but an overshoot to potentially dangerous hypercarbia is a concern. Monitoring carbon dioxide by using a transcutaneous device may reduce carbon dioxide target overshoot, but discrepancies between transcutaneous and arterial carbon dioxide may be substantial.

Alternatively, manipulating $PaCO_2$ upward by using hypoventilation with end-tidal carbon dioxide monitoring devices has been suggested as a method. It can be cumbersome not only because of the inability to predict $PaCO_2$ but also because the method may lead to gradual CSF buffering and thus failure to produce acute acidosis in the CSF compartment.

Testing for apnea in a patient with otherwise absent brainstem reflexes is standard, and a positive test (no breathing with target $PaCO_2$) confirms brain death. The procedure, however, has generated some debate. The arguments against the apnea test are as follows. First, in the event of preserved respiration, the outcome is similar. No report has been published of an adult patient who, with otherwise absent brainstem reflexes but spontaneous breathing, "recovers" to a persistent vegetative state or better. Second, the procedure may induce hypotension and hypoxemia, which potentially may render organs unsuitable for transplantation. There are no data in the transplant literature to support this contention.[19-21] The apnea test may be very difficult to perform (e.g., because of preservation of adequate oxygenation) in patients with marginal lung function due to contusion or pulmonary edema. Some have argued, and incorrectly so, that hypoxemia or acidosis will result in death of some viable neurons and thus cause brain death. It is one of the reasons behind the Japanese criteria of performing an EEG before an apnea test (see Chapter 1). We believe the apnea test is essential because prolonged preserved medulla oblongata function may occur (see Chapter 6) and its presence can only be detected by a formal apnea test.

The apnea test is generally safe with careful precautions. First, hypothermia should be corrected from 32°C (prerequisite for determination of brain death) to normothermia (36°C to 37°C). In hypothermia, carbon dioxide production may be delayed because of decreased metabolism. Moreover, in hypothermia the oxyhemoglobin dissociation curve shifts to the left, resulting in a decreased oxygen release. Second, persistent hypotension should be corrected and often requires a bolus of 5% albumin or an increase in administration of intravenous dopamine. The presence of a blood pressure of 90 to 100 mm Hg is probably acceptable before an apnea test. Other precautions are shown in Figure 7. If one holds to these strict guidelines, the apnea test is generally safe.[22]

At the start of the apnea test, a $PaCO_2$ within the normal range (35 to 45 mm Hg) is preferred. One can expect the $PaCO_2$ to increase 3 to 6 mm Hg per minute.[23] Therefore, when the $PaCO_2$ is in the normal range, 8 min of disconnection should be sufficient to reach the target level of 60 mm Hg or to produce an increase of 20 mm Hg (Figure 7).[24-27] Apnea can be confirmed with skin sensors from the electrocardiogram leads. On the monitor, these sensors should show only a cardiac artifact and no displacement indicating a breathing effort. Visual inspection of the rib cage and abdomen typically may show minimal movement synchronous with the heartbeat, less frequently some shoulder elevation, and intercostal retraction in the upper thorax.

Hypotension is the most common complication of the apnea test,[22,28-30] and the patient should be reconnected to the ventilator when the blood pressure drops precipitously to 70 mm Hg systolic. Failure to preoxygenate remains an important cause of hypotension during apnea testing. However, when normal oxygen saturation is present, the induced acidosis may reduce myocardial contractility, usually when pH reaches 7.2. Moderate hypercapnia associated with respiratory acidosis does not induce ventricular dysfunction as measured by transesophageal echocardiography.[31] Hypotension without hypoxemia during the apnea test often indicates that the $PaCO_2$ has amply passed 60 mm Hg. Cardiac arrest from the procedure is exceedingly rare; we noted one instance in 145 consecutive procedures.[22] Again, cardiac arrhythmias generally occur in patients whose hypoxemia is not corrected with oxygen supplementation during the apnea test. Patients who have had cardiac arrhythmias during the evolution of the neurologic catastrophe may not have them during the apnea test, and their presence should not preclude apnea testing. When hypoxemia occurs despite adequate preoxygenation and oxygen supply, al Jumah et al.[13] suggested performing the apnea test with the patient connected with zero rate, zero CPAP FIO2 of 1.0, and continuous flow of 40 L/min (15 L/min for pediatric patients; bulk diffusion apnea test). It may still not be an alternative in patients with severe underlying pulmonary disease.[13] Failure to adequately perform the apnea test should be followed by a confirmatory test if organ donation is considered.

Spinal Activity

Body movements after death have been observed, generally during the apnea test but also during nurse preparation for transport, at the time of abdominal incision for organ retrieval, and in the morgue itself. As early as 1971, Goulon et al.[32] supplemented their original paper with additional descriptions of body movements brought on by light stimulation-triple retreat of the legs, adduction or abduction of the arm to the stimulated area, and head rotation. These movements have puzzled the mind and have frightened family members. Evidence that the movements represent only spinal activity is the consistent clinical documentation of brain death with confirmation by an isoelectric electroencephalogram or the absence of intracranial flow. The most impressive body movement is a brief attempt of the body to sit up to 40 to 60 degrees but generally not in a full sitting position. Arms may be raised independently of each other; legs seldom move. Rhythmic flexion of the hip and knee mimicking stepping has occurred at the pontomedullary stage of herniation, but it disappears in brain death.[33] These are slow movements, lasting 10 to 20 s. A painful stimulus rarely produces these complex movements, but we and others have observed them after forceful flexion of the neck or rotation of the body (e.g., when replacing bed linen: Figure 8). A videotape has recently become available.[34] Head turning consistently to one side[35] and back arching may occur. Sometimes a body may partly roll over and dislodge catheters.[36,37] These movements have been named "Lazarus signs," referring to the biblical person said to have been raised by Jesus, but the term is disrespectful to the patient or family and should be avoided in conversation.

Some of this spinal activity may be triggered by the ventilator, synchronous with pulmonary insufflation,[38] and disappear after disconnection of the ventilator. A recent prospective study of 38 patients with brain death, mostly young adults, found a surprisingly high frequency of spinal-generated movements (39%), but included a triple flexion response, facial myokymias, and finger jerks.[36]

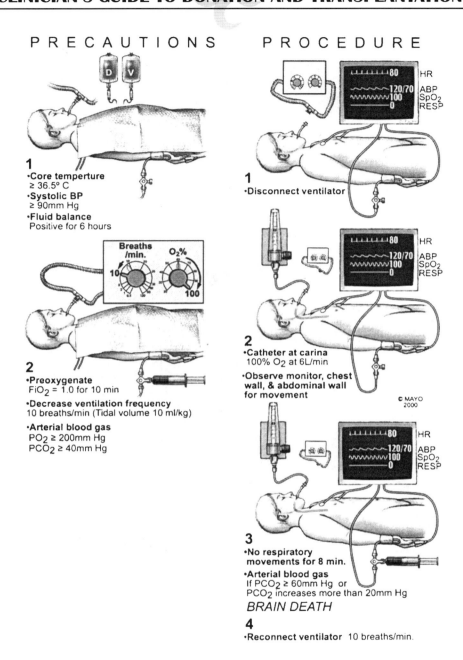

Figure 7. Performance of the apnea test. The apnea test should be optimized by precautionary measures *(above)*. 1. Increasing core temperature to reduce possible effect of hypothermia on CO_2 production; reducing chances of hypotension by stabilizing blood pressure and hemodynamic state. 2. Preoxygenation aiming at PO_2 of at least 200 mm Hg, correcting possible hypocapnea (often due to hyperventilation; caused by high tidal volumes of the mechanical ventilator or possibly due to hypothermia). The apnea test can proceed as follows *(right above)*. 1. Disconnect the ventilator while monitoring heart rate and blood pressure and possible respiratory excursions. 2. Provide adequate oxygen source, preferably with a catheter at the carina. 3. If no respiratory movements are observed, draw new blood gas. If PCO_2 rise fulfills criteria, reconnect ventilator. Any drop in blood pressure (BP ≤70 mm Hg) or cardiac arrhythmia should prompt the physician to abort the procedure and perform a confirmatory test (EEG, TCD, cerebral blood flow study). ABP, arterial blood pressure; BP, blood pressure; D, dopamine; HR, heart rate; RESP, respirations; SpO_2, oxygen saturation by pulse oximetry; V, vasopressin. (By permission of Mayo Foundation.)

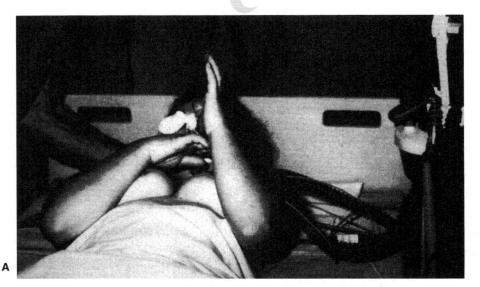
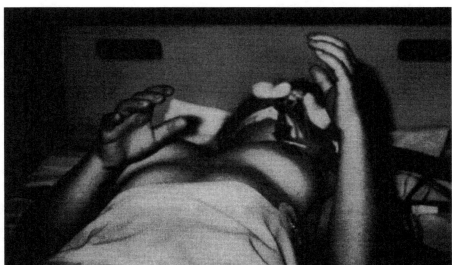

Figure 8. Arm elevation with neck flexion **(A)** and spontaneously **(B)**. (From Turmel A, Roux A, Bojanowski MW. Spinal man after declaration of brain death. *Neurosurgery* 1991;28:298-302, with permission of the Congress of Neurological Surgeons.)

Other manifestations include the undulating toe sign (snapping the big toe leads to an undulating movement of the toes resembling those of a sea anemone),[39] persistent Babinski response, any tendon, abdominal, or cremaster reflex, flushing, shivering, sweating, and myoclonic twitching in limb muscles. The most commonly observed reflexes and movements are shown in Table 2. Usually these movements are single events, but if they are recurrent, paralytic agents should be used to prevent them during organ retrieval.

Primary Brainstem Death

Acute neurologic injury may be confined to the brainstem, but is very uncommon. In many destructive lesions of the brainstem (e.g., ruptured basilar aneurysm), secondary damage to the hemispheres from ischemic injury may have intervened. Conditions associated with isolated brainstem death include

Table 2. SPINAL MOVEMENTS AND REFLEXES IN BRAIN DEATH

Cervical spine
    Tonic neck reflexes (neck flexion)
        Neck-abdominal muscle contraction
        Neck-hip flexion
        Neck-arm flexion
        Neck-shoulder protrusion
    Head turning to side
Upper extremity
    Flexion-withdrawal reflex
    Unilateral extension-pronation
    Isolated finger jerks; finger pinch-finger flexion
    Flexion elevation of arm; joining of hands possible
Trunk
    Asymmetric opisthotonic posturing of trunk
    Flexion of trunk, causing partial sitting movements
    Abdominal reflexes
Lower extremity
    Plantar flexion of toes after percussion
    Triple flexion, Babinski sign

From Goulon M, Nouailhat F, Babinet P. Irreversible coma [French]. *Ann Med Interne* 1971;122:479-486; Hanna JP, Frank JI. Automatic stepping in the pontomedullary stage of central herniation. *Neurology* 1995;45:985-986; Bueri JA, Saposnik G, Maurino J, et al. Lazarus' sign in brain death. *Movement Disorders* 2000;15:583-586; Christie JM, O'Lenic TD, Cane RD. Head turning in brain death. *J Clin Anesth* 1996;8:141-143; Saposnik G, Bueri JA, Maurino J et al. Spontaneous and reflex movements in brain death. Neurology2000;54:221-223; Ropper AH. Unusual spontaneous movements in brain-dead patients. *Neurology* 1984;34:1089-1092; MartiFabregas J, Lopez-Navidad A, Caballero F, et al. Decerebrate-like posturing with mechanical ventilation in brain death. *Neurology* 2000;54:224-227; and Fujimoto K, Yamauchi Y, Yoshida M. Spinal myoclonus in association with brain death [Japanese]. *Rinsho ShinKeigaku* 1989;29:1417-1419.

pontine hemorrhage, basilar artery embolus, and, not uncommonly, gunshot wounds due to a suicide attempt, especially when the barrel of the gun has been placed inside the mouth. The brain hemispheres remain initially untouched until massive hydrocephalus increases intracranial pressure and impedes intracranial flow. This condition is akin to "cerveau isolé." Mature cats with the entire brainstem and cerebellum removed displayed EEG activity with commonly observed sleep spindles.[40] A confirmation test will only confuse the matter, because cerebral blood flow is likely to be present, particularly when the test is performed early. Electroencephalography may show nonreactive alpha or spindle coma patterns. A possible approach is to extend observation time to 24 h, followed by a full repeat neurologic examination (including apnea test). A confirmation test can be considered after this period of long observation but should not be mandatory. In the United States, primary brainstem death does not fit into the concept of whole brain death, but it has been accepted in the United Kingdom and rightly so, because no survivor has been reported when all brainstem function has been lost.

Observation Period

A reasonable effort should be made to allow an observation period after the clinical criteria of brain death have been met. The American Academy of Neurology practice parameters optionally call for 6 h of observation and repeat testing. This is a long way from the original 24-h observation, and Cantu's statement of nearly 30 years ago still carries some truth:

> Today, many potential donor organs are lost from patients with irreversible brain damage because of the required waiting-period of at least 24 h to obtain two flat EEGs. The waiting-period is often longer than 24 h if EEGs are not readily available. The importance of this loss is brought into perspective when we realize that there are now 70 people on dialysis awaiting cadaver-kidney transplantation at one major Boston hospital alone.[41]

Repeat examination should include all brainstem reflexes, but it is not necessary to repeat a formal apnea test. No adult patient is on record in whom breathing resumed after initial adequate documentation of apnea. Many patients may have started to develop labile blood pressure and early neurogenic pulmonary edema, and the observation period can certainly be shortened if a recipient is waiting or when a confirmatory laboratory test has been performed.

Physician Competency in Brain Death Determination

At first sight, it is correctly asserted that the determination of brain death is difficult. Nothing illustrates the complexity of this assessment better than the persistent reports of blatant errors in judgment not only in the medical literature but also in the lay press and on the Internet.[42,43] Unfortunately, even gross misjudgments surface in the neurologic literature.[44] As mentioned, determination of brain death requires not only the proper execution of a series of neurologic tests but also resolution of misleading clinical signs, interpretation of neuroimaging studies, interpretation of possible confounding factors, and determination of a need for confirmatory laboratory tests. Neurologists are often not available on a timely basis, particularly in rural areas. Naturally, any physician should be able to diagnose brain death, but a careful neurologic evaluation requires experience. The clinical examination of patients who are presumed brain dead should be academically precise and fully documented. To avoid any potential conflict, it is common practice to exclude transplant surgeons who are involved in prospective recovery of organs from performing examinations. No one in our practice finds this exclusion denigrating. There are no data to suggest that a second assessment by a different physician reduces errors or avoids neglect of key elements of the neurologic examination. Surprisingly, some states and a large number of hospitals in the United States continue to insist on a second independent examination. This approach not only may delay a declaration of death and thereby potentially jeopardize harvesting of vital organs (as hemodynamic instability and neurogenic pulmonary edema progress) but also may result in examination of a brain-dead patient by a less experienced physician urgently called upon. Even more surprisingly, in Virginia the brain death statute requires that a specialist in the neurosciences make the assessment (see Chapter 8).

So, who does qualify, and are determinations of brain death up to the mark? No formal audits of neurologists and neurosurgeons have been performed recently, but there is no reason to question competence. In our experience with many hundreds of brain death determinations performed by neurologists and neurosurgeons, grossly incomplete examinations were exceptional. Interpretation of unexpected findings, such as retained spinal reflex movements, could lead to a debate but was easily resolved. Intensive care neurologists and neurosurgeons are eminently qualified, but anesthesiologists and medical or surgical intensivists should be considered if they have maintained their clinical skills.[42] A separate team or service would be ideal and would minimize errors and facilitate communication with transplant surgeons and donation agencies. Development of special certificates, as in resuscitation medicine, may need serious consideration.

Confirmatory Test in Adults with Brain Death

Cerebral angiography, electroencephalography, transcranial ultrasonography, and a radionuclide scan can confirm the clinical diagnosis of brain death. Confirmatory tests are recommended in children less than 1 year old and in the occasional situation in which components of clinical testing cannot be reliably evaluated. In several European and Asiatic countries, confirmatory testing is mandated by law. It may be a contradiction of our time not to rely entirely on technologic devices to confirm brain death, but these tests should be performed only to confirm the clinical examination. The ideal practice is to use confirmatory tests after the neurologic examination has unequivocally shown that the patient no longer has any brain function.

Unfortunately, situations arise in which a confirmatory test has been performed before the formal clinical evaluation for possible brain death. In certain circumstances, a confirmatory test may show the presence of blood flow or electroencephalographic activity despite the absence of all brainstem function. This occurs in patients who had their confirmatory tests very early in the determination of brain death and particularly in those in whom the mechanism was other than increased intracranial pressure. It is appropriate not to rely on technical confirmatory tests when they are at odds with a clinical neurologic examination. Confirmatory tests in adults are described in this section, but details are also found in the chapter on brain death in children, where they are more relevant.

A recent disturbing study from Barcelona[45] suggested transcranial Doppler or nuclear scan to "speed up" the diagnosis of brain death in patients with recent administration of barbiturates, benzodiazepines, or opiates. This practice should be strongly rejected. Physicians should not go so far as to place blind faith in machinery and the clinical diagnosis remains a sacrosanct principle.

Cerebral Angiogram

A cerebral angiogram using the Seldinger technique through femoral arteries should document non-filling of intracranial arteries.[41,46-53] Increased intracranial pressure leads to increased cerebral vascular resistance, extreme slowing of flow, and circulatory arrest.[54] Perivascular glial swelling and subintimal bleb formation from ischemia collapse the smaller vessels, leading to increased cerebrovascular resistance, but another mechanism of absent intracranial flow is destruction of the intracerebral vascular tree in conjunction with necrosis of the brain. The common carotid artery commonly bifurcates at C3-C4 into the internal and external portions. The carotid bifurcation to the skull base is called the cervical segment until it enters the carotid canal. The petrous segment ascends 1 cm, then becomes horizontal until it enters the intracranial space at the foramen lacerum. The carotid artery then continues as the cavernous segment. The vertebral artery pierces the dura after traversing the atlanto-occipital membrane and this transition can at times be seen as a smooth band on a normal film. The carotid circulation will demonstrate circulatory arrest first, but the vertebral circulation can still show filling. This can be due to a supratentorial mass that has not transferred pressure to the posterior fossa resulting in cerebellar tonsillar herniation.

Contrast is injected under high pressure in both the anterior and the posterior circulation. With current standardized injection force, it is unlikely that flow can be artificially created by increasing injection pressure. Normally, the intracranial arteries fill first (low-resistance system), followed by the external arteries (high-resistance system). This is reversed with cerebral death. Arch aortography with lateral and anteroposterior views will show the contrast column in the carotids usually arresting abruptly at the level of the skull base at the petrous region of the internal carotid arteries. It should not fill the siphon. The vertebral system will opacify from the aortic arch injection, and a selective vertebral artery injection is not needed. The dye column in the vertebral artery arrests at the atlanto-occipital junction and the contrast level may reach C1 to C2 in 50% of patients. The external carotid circulation remains patent and fills rapidly and early, as opposed to slow filling of the remaining portion of the carotid circulation (Figure 9). Delayed visualization of the superior sagittal sinus results from perfusion through meningeal vessels from the external carotid artery supply or from emissary veins. Some protocols consider at least two injections of contrast medium given with an interval of 20 min to establish persistent absent flow to the brain and thus total neuronal necrosis. Criteria for confirmation of brain death using cerebral angiography have not been developed by neuroradiologic societies.

Electroencephalography

Electroencephalography (EEG) has been used in the determination of brain death in many countries, and it remains an important confirmatory test.[55-60] Usually, a 16- or 18-channel instrument is used, and recordings are obtained for at least 30 min. Typically, electrical activity is absent above 2 μV at a sensitivity of 2 μV/mm with a filter setting at 0.1 or 0.3 s and 70 Hz.[61] There are, however, several examples of abnormal but existing EEG activity that may continue for several hours to days. In one consecutive study of patients who fulfilled the clinical criteria of brain death, 20% of 56 patients had residual EEG activity that lasted up to 168 h. In general, the sensitivity as well as the specificity of EEG is 90%.[62] It should be noted that artifacts are common if a high gain amplification is used in an intensive care environment, with a significant possibility for electrical artifacts. EEG is used in many countries throughout the world, and because of its wide availability it remains a preferred confirmatory test (Figure 10).

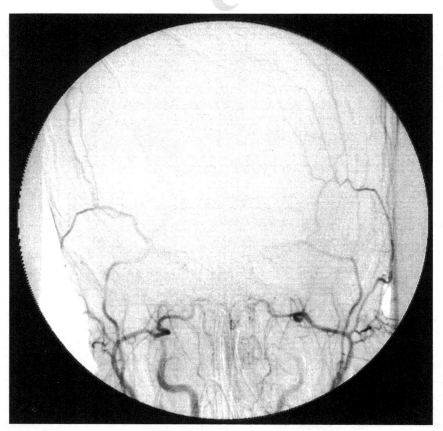

Figure 9. Cerebral angiogram. Arch injection showing absent intracranial flow. The intracranial arteries are not identified, and the vertebral arteries stop below the skull base at C1-C2. Arterial filling involves only the external carotid branches.

Transcranial Doppler Sonography

Transcranial Doppler (TCD) is a validated confirmatory test, with sensitivity varying from 91% to 99% and a specificity of 100%.[63-74] A portable Doppler device is used with insonating of both middle cerebral arteries through the temporal bone above the zygomatic arch. Absent flow intracranially may be due to transmission difficulties and in itself is not a criterion for brain death. In brain death, the typical transcranial Doppler signals, produced by the contractive forces of the arteries, are oscillating flow, defined by signals with forward and reverse flow components in one cardiac cycle.[72] Most of the time, small (less than 50 cm/s) peaks in early systole, indicating very high vascular resistance, are recorded. The pulsatility index is very high (Figure 11). All these TCD patterns indirectly indicate increased intracranial pressure. Thus, TCD may not be diagnostic for brain death in patients with infratentorial lesions and in patients with brain death due to anoxic-ischemic damage. When TCD is done early, hydrocephalus or brain edema (and increased intracranial pressure) may not be present.

A consensus statement by the task force group on cerebral death of the Neurosonology Research Group of the World Federation of Neurology was published in 1998[72] which expanded requirements.

1. Confirmation of cerebral circulatory arrest with extra- and intra-cranial Doppler sonography, bilaterally on two examinations 30 min apart.
2. Systolic spikes or oscillating flow in any cerebral artery (anterior and posterior).
3. Diagnosis established by intracranial examination must be confirmed by the extracranial bilateral recording of the common carotid, internal carotid, and vertebral arteries.

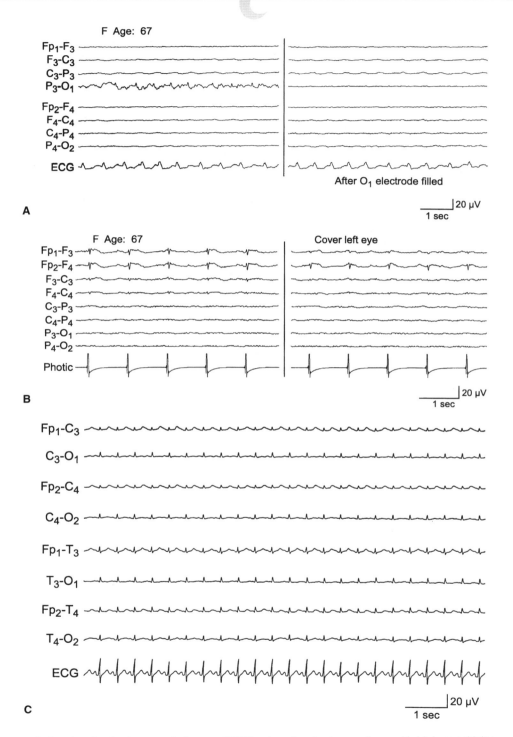

Figure 10. A: Isoelectric electroencephalogram (EEG) using standard recordings with high-sensitivity artifact is seen from a poorly filled electrode and pulse artifact. **B:** Electroretinogram is typically seen with photic stimulation in the frontal leads due to high sensitivity. It is eliminated with covering of each eye. For recommendations for recording electroencephalogram in cases of brain death, see text. **C:** EEG with electrocardiographic artifact. (By permission of the Massachusetts Medical Society.)

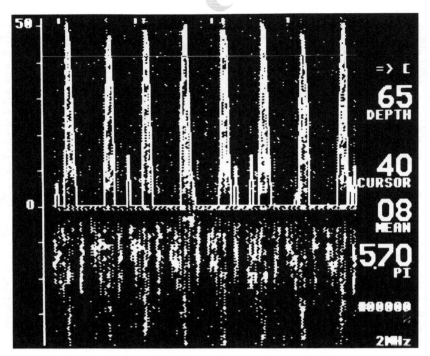

Figure 11. Transcranial Doppler in brain death showing small systolic peaks and significant increase in pulsatility index.

4. Disappearance of intracranial flow signals together with typical extracranial signs can be accepted as proof of circulatory arrest when no intracranial signal is found.
5. Exclusion of patients with ventricular drains or large craniotomy.

The major advantage of this device is its portability and the growing expertise of attending neurointensivists and neurosurgeons who may perform this study without being dependent on other technical resources.

Magnetic Resonance Imaging

Axial T_1-weighted and T_2-weighted images with spin-echo techniques, including three-dimensional time-of-flight fast imaging, have been reported.[75-78] The magnetic resonance (MR) findings are transtentorial or tonsillar herniation, lack of intracranial flow void (Figure 12A), poor gray-white matter differentiation, and marked contrast enhancement of the nose (MR "hot nose") and scalp.[77] Proton density and T_2-weighted MR images can show dissociated intensity changes between gray and white matter.

MR angiography does not show intracranial vessels above the skull base similar to a conventional angiogram (Figure 12B). There is very limited experience with this type of neuroimaging, and often studies have been interpreted retrospectively. Prospective studies in patients with evolving loss of brain function may be useful.

Single Photon Emission Computed Tomography

A single-detector rotating gamma camera is used with capabilities for monitoring and mechanical ventilation.[79-84] A tracer isotope (^{99m}Tc-HMPAO) is injected intravenously 15 to 30 min before scanning. Serial pictures are taken as part of a dynamic study, followed by lateral and anterior static images with a three-dimensional image with good spatial resolution. Arrest of cerebral circulation is found in 96% of cases; in the remaining cases, perfusion may persist in the thalamus and brainstem, particularly in children. Absent uptake produces a highly characteristic "hollow skull" or "empty light bulb" phenomenon.

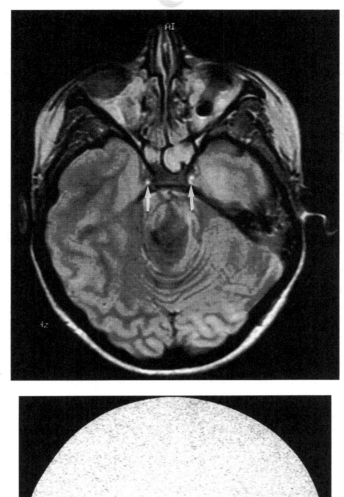
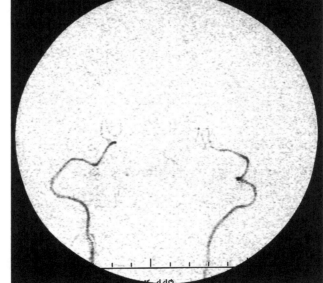

Figure 12. A: Magnetic resonance imaging in a patient fulfilling clinical criteria of brain death (after uncal herniation of a massive infarct) shows high signal in petrous portion of carotids *(arrows)*, indicating stagnation of flow. **B**: Magnetic resonance angiography showing absent intracranial flow at the skull base.

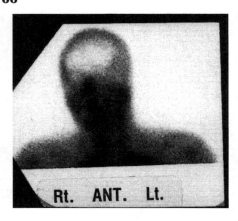

Figure 13. Single photon emission computed tomography scan ("empty light bulb" or "hollow skull phenomenon"). "Hot nose sign" is a consequence of extracerebral blood flow. (By permission of the Massachusetts Medical Society.)

Increased external flow may result in enhancement of the nose ("hot nose sign"; Figure 13). Absent uptake is a reflection of absent intracranial flow due to marked terminal rise in intracranial pressure, which was confirmed in 22 patients with concomitant intracranial pressure recording.[86] Correlation with the cerebral angiogram is excellent.

Tracer injection may be inaccurate but can be checked with imaging of spleen uptake or assessment of the nuclear activity of the carotid arteries. Nuclear scan requires a specialist in nuclear medicine for interpretation and quality control. It is not widely available on an urgent basis.

Evoked Potentials

Both brainstem auditory evoked potentials (BAEP) and somatosensory evoked potentials (SSEP) have been studied as potential confirmatory tests in brain death. Initial enthusiasm was fostered by examples of patients in drug-induced coma, appearing clinically to be brain dead, who had isoelectric EEGs but no change in the individual evoked components.[87] Evoked potentials became a possible indicator of brainstem function in patients with major head trauma and barbiturate use.

BAEP is generated by means of bedside equipment with click intensity set at 65 dB with a 10/s stimulus repetition rate provided by earphones. It is necessary to identify wave I from the ipsilateral ear electrode to prove an intact auditory nerve, which can be destroyed as a result of cochlear trauma. Waves II and III identify the cochlear nucleus and superior olivary complex, and waves IV and V locate the upper pons, therefore, absence of waves II through V indicates profound brainstem dysfunction.[88]

BAEPs are generated within the pons and do not measure tracts in the medulla oblongata. BAEPs do not correlate well with severity of brain injury. Patients with a persistent vegetative state have normal BAEPs,[89] and brain-dead patients may have identifiable wave forms. Patients have been noted to have absent waves II to V after severe head injury or devastating anoxic-ischemic encephalopathy but with intact brainstem reflexes.[90] Another concern is the limited number of studies with detailed clinical and laboratory correlation.

SSEPs are recorded at several sites, including second cervical vertebra and centroparietal areas with stimulation at the median nerve at the wrist at a rate of 5 Hz. Typically, approximately 2,000 responses are averaged, and the evoked potentials are amplified and filtered between 5 and 1,500 Hz. The recorded potentials most likely travel through the proprioceptive pathway in the spinal cord dorsal column to the medial lemniscus and to the primary somatosensory cortex. The cortical wave N20 is typically absent in brain death but is also bilaterally undetectable in approximately 15% to 20% of patients who are comatose but not brain dead. Recent studies suggest that disappearance of the P14 wave (bulbomedullary junction or cuneate nucleus) may be helpful. Distinction from artifacts is difficult, but nasopharyngeal electrode recording of P14 may enhance its detection, only to disappear when brain death occurs. Experience is limited.

Sonoo and co-workers[91] directed attention to the value of the N18 potential possibly generated in the cuneate nucleus, but it was also absent in 3 of 20 comatose patients who were not brain dead. The relatively poor predictive value casts doubt on the use of the BAEP or SSEP as a standard confirmatory test for brain death.[92-102]

Spiral Computed Tomography Scan

Spiral CT scan has the advantage of allowing evaluation of the intracranial circulation through intravenous injection of contrast.[103-105] Circulatory arrest was present in a preliminary study of 14 patients with no flow in the basilar artery, posterior cerebral arteries, pericallosal arteries, and terminal cortical arteries but weak visualization in the M1 segment of the middle cerebral artery and A1 segment of the anterior cerebral artery. There is no other recent published experience.

Conclusion

Clinical neurologic examination in brain death prevails over any technologic investigation. Its reliability has been tested over the years, errors in interpretation are exceptional, and observer agreement is excellent. Change in neurologic examination has not occurred in adults when conducted properly, but observation over time is advised. The apnea test can be performed in a very simplified manner without major complications if oxygenation is guaranteed. The complete determination of this state, however, may best fit in a neurologic or neurosurgical practice.

References

1. The Quality Standards Subcommittee of the American Academy of Neurology. Practice parameters for determining brain death in adults (summary statement). *Neurology*. 1995;45:1012-1014.
2. Wijdicks EFM. Determining brain death in adults. *Neurology*. 1995;45:1003-1011.
3. Wijdicks EFM. Temporomandibular joint compression in coma. *Neurology*. 1996;46:1774.
4. Santamaria J, Orteu N, Iranzo A, et al. Eye opening in brain death [Letter]. *J Neurol*. 1999;246:720-722.
5. Friedman AJ. Sympathetic response and brain death [Letter]. *Arch Neurol*. 1984;41:15.
6. Sims JK, Bickford RG. Non-mydriatic pupils occurring in human brain death. *Bull LA Neurol Soc*. 1973;38:24-32.
7. Greenan J, Prasad J. Comparison of the ocular effects of atropine or glycopyrrolate with two I.V. induction agents. *Br J Anaesth*. 1985;57:180-183.
8. Goetting MG, Contreras E. Systemic atropine administration during cardiac arrest does not cause fixed and dilated pupils. *Ann Emerg Med*. 1991;20:55-57.
9. Gray AT, Krejci ST, Larson MD. Neuromuscular blocking drugs do not alter the pupillary light reflex of anesthetized humans. *Arch Neurol*. 1997;54:579-584.
10. Schmidt JE, Tamburro RF, Hoffman GM. Dilated non-reactive pupils secondary to neuromuscular blockade. *Anesthesiology*. 2000;92:1476-1480.
11. Snavely SR, Hodges GR. The neurotoxicity of antibacterial agents. *Ann Intern Med*. 1984;101:92-104.
12. Draper WB, Whitehead RW. Diffusion respiration in dog anesthetized by pentothal sodium. *Anesthesiology*. 1944;5:262-273.
13. al Jumah M, McLean DR, al Rajeh S, et al. Bulk diffusion apnea test in the diagnosis of brain death. *Crit Care Med*. 1992;20:1564-1567.
14. Feery JJ, Waller GA, Solliday N. The use of apneic-diffusion respiration in the diagnosis of brain death. *Respir Care*. 1985;30:328-333.
15. Ferris EB, Engel GL, Stevens CD, et al. Voluntary breathholding; the relation of the maximum time of breathholding to the oxygen and carbon dioxide tensions of arterial blood, with a note on its clinical and physiological significance. *J Clin Invest*. 1946;25:734-743.
16. Bruce EN, Cherniack NS. Central chemoreceptors. *J Appl Physiol*. 1987;62:389-402.
17. Joels N, Samueloff M. The activity of the medullary centres in diffusion respiration. *J Physiol*. 1956;133:360-372.
18. Lang CJ. Apnea testing by artificial CO_2 augmentation. *Neurology*. 1995;45:966-969.
19. Rohling R, Wagner W, Muhlberg J, et al. Apnea test: pitfalls and correct handling. *Transplant Proc*. 1986;18:388-390.
20. Jeret JS, Benjamin JL. Risk of hypotension during apnea testing. *Arch Neurol*. 1994;51:595-599.
21. Coimbra CG. Implications of ischemic penumbra for the diagnosis of brain death. *Braz J Med Biol Res*. 1999;32:1479-1487.
22. Goudreau JL, Wijdicks EFM, Emery SF. Complications during apnea testing in the determination of brain death: predisposing factors. *Neurology*. 2000;55:1045-1048.

23. Eger EI, Severinghaus JW. The rate of rise of PacCO$_2$ in the apneic anesthetized patient. *Anesthesiology* 1961;22:419-425.
24. Engel GL, Ferris EB, Webb JP, et al. Voluntary breathholding; the relation of the maximum time of breathholding to the oxygen tension of the inspired air. *J Clin Invest.* 1946;25:729-733.
25. Marks SJ, Zisfein J. Apneic oxygenation in apnea tests for brain death. A controlled trial. *Arch Neurol.* 1990;47:1066-1068.
26. Prechter GC, Nelson SB, Hubmayr RD. The ventilatory recruitment threshold for carbon dioxide. *Am Rev Respir Dis.* 1990;141:758-764.
27. Hanks EC, Ngai SH, Fink BR. The respiratory threshold for carbon dioxide in anesthetized man. Determination of carbon dioxide threshold during halothane anesthesia. *Anesthesiology.* 1961;22:393-397.
28. Ropper AH, Kennedy SK, Russel L. Apnea testing in the diagnosis of brain death: clinical and physiological observations. *J Neurosurg.* 1981;55:942-946.
29. Wijdicks EFM. In search of a safe apnea test in brain death: Is the procedure really more dangerous than we think? [Letter]. *Arch Neurol.* 1995;52:338-339.
30. Benzel EC, Mashburn JP, Conrad S, et al. Apnea testing for the determination of brain death: a modified protocol [Technical note]. *J Neurosurg.* 1992;76:1029-1031.
31. Orliaguet GA, Catoire P, Liu N, et al. Transesophageal echocardiographic assessment of left ventricular function during apnea testing for brain death. *Transplantation.* 1994;58:655-658.
32. Goulon M, Nouailhat F, Babinet P. Irreversible coma [French]. *Ann Med Interne (Paris).* 1971;122:479-486.
33. Hanna JP, Frank JI. Automatic stepping in the pontomedullary stage of central herniation. *Neurology.* 1995;45:985-986.
34. Bueri JA, Saposnik G, Maurino J, et al. Lazarus' sign in brain death. *Mov Disord.* 2000;15:583-586.
35. Christie JM, O'Lenic TD, Cane RD. Head turning in brain death. *J Clin Anesth.* 1996;8:141-143.
36. Saposnik G, Bueri JA, Maurino J, et al. Spontaneous and reflex movements in brain death. *Neurology.* 2000;54:221-223.
37. Ropper AH. Unusual spontaneous movements in brain-dead patients. *Neurology.* 1984;34:1089-1092.
38. Marti-Fabregas J, L6pez-Navidad A, Caballero F, et al. Decerebrate-like posturing with mechanical ventilation in brain death. *Neurology.* 2000;54:224-227.
39. McNair NL, Meador KJ. The undulating toe flexion sign in brain death. *Mov Disord.* 1992;7:345-347.
40. Walker AE, Feeney DM, Hovda DA. The electroencephalographic characteristics of the rhomben-cephalectomized cat. *Electroencephalogr Clin Neurophysiol.* 1984;57:156-165.
41. Cantu RC. Brain death as determined by cerebral arteriography [Letter]. *Lancet.* 1973;1:1391-1392.
42. Wijdicks EFM. What anesthesiologists should know about what neurologists should know about declaring brain death [Letter]. *Anesthesiology.* 2000;92:1203-1204.
43. Van Norman GA. A matter of life and death: what every anesthesiologist should know about the medical, legal, and ethical aspects of declaring brain death. *Anesthesiology.* 1999;91:275-287.
44. Koberda JL, Clark WM, Lutsep H, et al. Successful clinical recovery and reversal of mid-basilar occlusion in clinically brain dead patient with intra-arterial urokinase [Abstract]. *Neurology.* 1997;48:A154.
45. Lopez-Navidad A, Caballero F, Domingo P, et al. Early diagnosis of brain death in patients treated with central nervous system depressant drugs. *Transplantation.* 2000;70:131-135.
46. Bergquist E, Bergstrom K. Angiography in cerebral death. *Acta Radiol.* 1972;12:283-288.
47. Korein J, Braunstein P, George A, et al. Brain death: I. Angiographic correlation with the radioisotopic bolus technique for evaluation of critical deficit of cerebral blood flow. *Ann Neurol.* 1977;2:195-205.
48. Korein J, Braunstein P, Kricheff I, et al. Radioisotopic bolus technique as a test to detect circulatory deficit associated with cerebral death. 142 studies on 80 patients demonstrating the bedside use of an innocuous IV procedure as an adjunct in the diagnosis of cerebral death. *Circulation.* 1975;51:924-939.
49. Kricheff II, Pinto RS, George AE, et al. Angiographic findings in brain death. *Ann NY Acad Sci.* 1978;315:168-183.
50. Greitz T, Gordon E, Kolmodin G, et al. Aortocranial and carotid angiography in determination of brain death. *Neuroradiology.* 1973;5:13-19.
51. Hazratji SM, Singh BM, Strobos RJ. Angiography in brain death. *NYS J Med.* 1981;8 t:82-83.
52. Bradac GB, Simon RS. Angiography in brain death. *Neuroradiology.* 1974;7:25-28.
53. Jefferson NR, Ameratunga B, Rajapakse S. Angiographic evidence of brain death. *Australas Radiol.* 1975;19:289-296.
54. Langfitt TW, Kassell NF. Non-filling of cerebral vessels during angiography: correlation with intracranial pressure. *Acta Neurochir.* 1966;14:96-104.
55. Deliyannakis E, Ioannou F, Davaroukas A. Brain stem death with persistence of bioelectric activity of the cerebral hemispheres. *Clin Electroencephalogr.* 1975;6:75-79.
56. Hughes JR. Limitations of the EEG in coma and brain death. *Ann NY Acad Sci.* 1978;315:121-136.
57. Jorgensen EO. Technical contribution. Requirements for recording the EEG at high sensitivity in suspected brain death. *Electrocephalogr Clin Neurophysiol.* 1974;36:65-69.

58. Bennett DR. The EEG in determination of brain death. *Ann NY Acad Sci.* 1978;315:110-120.
59. Grigg MM, Kelly MA, Celesia GG, et al. Electroencephalographic activity after brain death. *Arch Neurol.* 1987;44:948-954.
60. American Electroencephalographic Society. Guideline three: minimum technical standards for EEG recording in suspected cerebral death. *J Clin Neurophysiol.* 1994;11:10-13.
61. Silverman D, Saunders MG, Schwab RS, et al. Cerebral death and the electroencephalogram. Report of the ad hoc committee of the American Electroencephalographic Society on EEG Criteria for Determination of Cerebral Death. *JAMA.* 1969;209:1505-1510.
62. Buchner H, Schuchardt V. Reliability of electroencephalogram in the diagnosis of brain death. *Eur Neurol.* 1990;30:138-141.
63. Hassler W, Steinmetz H, Gawlowski J. Transcranial Doppler ultrasonography in raised intracranial pressure and in intracranial circulatory arrest. *J Neurosurg.* 1988;68:745-751.
64. Klingelhofer J, Conrad B, Benecke R, et al. Evaluation of intracranial pressure from transcranial Doppler studies in cerebral disease. *J Neurol.* 1988;235:159-162.
65. Report of the American Academy of Neurology, Therapeutics and Technology Assessment Subcommittee. Assessment: transcranial Doppler. *Neurology.* 1990;40:680-681.
66. Feri M, Ralli L, Felici M, et al. Transcranial Doppler and brain death diagnosis. *Crit Care Med.* 1994;22:1120-1126.
67. Powers AD, Graeber MC, Smith RR. Transcranial Doppler ultrasonography in the determination of brain death. *Neurosurgery.* 1989;24:884-889.
68. Van Velthoven V, Calliauw L. Diagnosis of brain death. Transcranial Doppler sonography as an additional method. *Acta Neurochir.* 1988;95:57-60.
69. Hadani M, Bruk B, Ram Z, et al. Application of transcranial Doppler ultrasonography for the diagnosis of brain death. *Intensive Care Med.* 1999;25:822-828.
70. Saunders FW, Cledgett P. Intracranial blood velocity in head injury. A transcranial ultrasound Doppler study. *Surg Neurol.* 1988;29:401-409.
71. Ducrocq X, Braun M, Debouverie M, et al. Brain death and transcranial Doppler: experience in 130 cases of brain dead patients. *J Neurol Sci.* 1998;160:41-46.
72. Ducrocq X, Hassler W, Moritake K, et al. Consensus opinion on diagnosis of cerebral circulatory arrest using Doppler-sonography: Task Force Group on Cerebral Death of the Neurosonology Research Group of the World Federation of Neurology. *J Neural Sci.* 1998;159:145-150.
73. Petty GW, Mohr JP, Pedley TA, et al. The role of transcranial Doppler in confirming brain death: sensitivity, specificity, and suggestions for performance and interpretation. *Neurology.* 1990;40:300-303.
74. Ropper AH, Kehne SM, Wechsler L. Transcranial Doppler in brain death. *Neurology.* 1987;37:1733-1735.
75. Ishii K, Onuma T, Kinoshita T, et al. Brain death: MR and MR angiography. *AJNR Am J Neuroradiol.* 1996;17:731-735.
76. Matsumura A, Mequero K, Tsurushima H, et al. Magnetic resonance imaging of brain death. *Neurol Med Clin Chir.* 1996;36:166-171.
77. Orrison WW Jr, Champlin AM, Kesterson OL, et al. MR "hot nose sign" and "intravascular enhancement sign" in brain death. *AJNR Am J Neuroradiol.* 1994;15:913-916.
78. Lee DH, Nathanson JA, Fox AJ, et al. Magnetic resonance imaging of brain death. *Can Assoc Radiol J.* 1995;46a74-178.
79. Rome RO, Launes J, Lindroth L, et al. ^{99m}Tc-hexamethylpropyleneamine oxime scans to confirm brain death [Letter]. *Lancet.* 1986;2:1223-1224.
80. Yatim A, Mercatello A, Caronel B, et al. ^{99m}Tc-HMPAO cerebral scintigraphy in the diagnosis of brain death. *Transplant Proc* 1991;23:2491.
81. George MS. Establishing brain death: the potential role of nuclear medicine in the search for a reliable confirmatory test [Editorial]. *Eur J Nucl Med* 1991;18:75-77.
82. Laurin NR, Driedger AA, Hurwitz GA, et al. Cerebral perfusion imaging with technetium-99m HM-PAO in brain death and severe central nervous system injury. *J Nucl Med* 1989;30:1627-1635.
83. Bonetti MG, Ciritella P, Valle G, et al. ^{99m}Tc HM-PAO brain perfusion SPECT in brain death. *Neuroradiology.* 1995;37:365-369.
84. Facco E, Zucchetta P, Munari M, et al. ^{99m}Tc-HMPAO SPECT in the diagnosis of brain death. *Intensive Care Med.* 1998;24:911-917.
85. Mishkin FS, Dyken ML. Increased early radionuclide activity in the nasopharyngeal area in patients with internal carotid artery obstruction: "hot nose." *Radiology.* 1970;96:77-80.
86. Kurtek RW, Lai KK, Tauxe WN, et al. Tc-99m hexamethylpropylene amine oxime scintigraphy in the diagnosis of brain death and its implications for the harvesting of organs used for transplantation. *Clin Nucl Med.* 2000;25:7-10.
87. Sharbrough FW. Unique contributions of short-latency auditory and somatosensory evoked potentials to neurologic diagnosis. *Prog Clin Neurophysiol.* 1980;7:231-263.
88. Chiappa KH, ed. Evoked potentials in clinical medicine, 3rd ed. Philadelphia: Lippincott-Raven Publishers, 1997.

89. Hansotia PL. Persistent vegetative state. Review and report of electrodiagnostic studies in eight cases. *Arch Neurol.* 1985;42:1048-1052.
90. Brunko E, Delecluse F, Herbaut AG, et al. Unusual pattern of somatosensory and brain-stem auditory evoked potentials after cardiorespiratory arrest. *Electroencephalogr Clin Neurophysiol.* 1985;62:338-342.
91. Sonoo M, Tsai-Shozawa Y, Aoki M, et al. N 18 in median somatosensory evoked potentials: a new indicator of medullary function useful for the diagnosis of brain death. *J Neurol Neurosurg Psychiatry.* 1999;67:374-378.
92. Roncucci P, Lepori P, Mok MS, et al. Nasopharyngeal electrode recording of somatosensory evokedpotentials as an indicator in brain death. *Anaesth Intensive Care.* 1999;27:20-25.
93. Anziska BJ, Cracco RQ. Short latency somatosensory evoked potentials in brain dead patients. *Arch Neural.* 1980;37:222-225.
94. Firsching R. The brain-stem and 40 Hz middle latency auditory evoked potentials in brain death. *Acta Neurochir.* 1989;101:52-55.
95. Garcia-Larrea L, Bertrand 0, Artru F, et al. Brain-stem monitoring II. Preterminal BAEP changes observed until brain death in deeply comatose patients. *Electroencephalogr Clin Neurophysiol.* 1987;68:446-457.
96. Stohr M, Riffel B, Trost E, et al. Short-latency somatosensory evoked potentials in brain death. *J Neurol.* 1987;234:211-214.
97. Starr A. Auditory brain-stem responses in brain death. *Brain.* 1976;99:543-554.
98. Wagner W. SEP testing in deeply comatose and brain dead patients: the role of nasopharyngeal, scalp and earlobe derivations in recording the P14 potential. *Electroencephalogr Clin Neurophysiol.* 1991;80:352-363.
99. Goldie WD, Chiappa KH, Young RR, et al. Brainstem auditory and short-latency somatosensory evoked responses in brain death. *Neurology.* 1981;31:248-256.
100. Chancellor AM, Frith RW, Shaw NA. Somatosensory evoked potentials following severe head injury: loss of the thalamic potential with brain death. *J Neurol Sci.* 1988;87:255-263.
101. Belsh JM, Chokroverty S. Short-latency somatosensory evoked potentials in brain-dead patients. *Electroencephalogr Clin Neurophysiol.* 1987;68:75-78.
102. Machado C, Valdes P, Garcia-Tigera J, et al. Brain-stem auditory evoked potentials and brain death. *Electroencephalogr Clin Neurophysiol.* 1991;80:392-398.
103. Arnold H, Kunhe D, Rohr W, et al. Contrast bolus technique with rapid CT scanning. A reliable diagnostic tool for the determination of brain death. *Neuroradiology.* 1981;22:129-132.
104. Range] RA. Computerized axial tomography in brain death. *Stroke.* 1978;9:597-598.
105. Dupas B. Gayet-Delacroix M, Villers D, et al. Diagnosis of brain death using two-phase spiral CT. *AJNR Am J Neuroradiol.* 1998;19:641-647.

Clinical Diagnosis and Confirmatory Testing of Brain Death in Children

Stephen Ashwal, MD

The diagnosis of brain death in pediatric patients is based on the same principles as in adults. But the neurologic examination is more difficult to perform and interpret because of the smaller size of the patient, immaturity of certain development reflexes being tested, and pathophysiologic differences due to the presence of open sutures and fontanels in the neonate and infant.

Brain death most commonly occurs in children less than 1 year of age and is uncommon in adolescents. Brain death in children is most frequently due to traumatic brain injury from abuse (e.g., shaken baby syndrome) and less often from motor vehicle accidents. Asphyxia is a comparatively common circumstance surrounding brain death in children and occurs after near drowning, from strangulation or suffocation, or from sudden infant death syndrome (SIDS). Brain death secondary to inflammatory diseases such as fulminant encephalitis and meningitis may be complicated by massive cerebral edema with the onset of brain herniation within 1 day of hospitalization. Much less common causes of brain death are metabolic diseases, perioperative central nervous system insults, and acute obstructive hydrocephalus.

Studies from pediatric intensive care units in the past decade have reported that older infants and children with brain death are a very small number of admissions (Table 1). There is a marked variation between institutions and this likely reflects differences in ascertainment. Two Canadian studies have reported mortality data from neonatal and pediatric intensive care units. The mortality rate in the pediatric intensive care unit (PICU) approximated 9%, with 22% of these children declared brain dead.[1] Mortality rate in the neonatal intensive care unit (NICU) was almost 6% with none of the infants declared brain dead.[1] More recently, Parker and co-investigators reported the percentage of brain deaths to overall deaths to be 31% in children over 1 month of age and 6% in neonates.[2] Our data from Loma Linda University Children's Hospital over the past several years found the percentage of brain deaths to overall deaths to be 28% and 2%, respectively, in our pediatric and neonatal units. In some PICUs, the percent of patients diagnosed as brain dead compared to all deaths is even higher (i.e., up to 38%).[3,4]

Declaration and confirmation of brain death in the majority of pediatric patients presenting in coma after a serious central nervous system injury are usually completed within the first 2 days of hospitalization.[5,6] If not referred for organ donation, these children are subsequently removed from life support systems once the diagnosis of brain death is confirmed.[5,6] Rarely, brain-dead pediatric patients have been maintained with ventilator support because cardiac arrest occurred with an average of about 17 days. Longer survival has been claimed by Shewmon after an exhaustive review of the literature and personally examined cases (for detailed discussion, see Chapter 9).

There have been no reports of children recovering neurologic function who met adult brain death criteria on neurologic examination.[7-9] In 1987, guidelines for the determination of brain death in children in the United States were proposed by a Task Force[10] that represented several of the major professional medical and legal societies (Table 2). These guidelines emphasized the importance of the history and

Table 1. INCIDENCE OF BRAIN DEATH IN OLDER CHILDREN AND NEONATES

Study	Patients >1 mo				Neonates (<30 d of age)			
	No. of patients	Mortality rate (%)	Percentage of patients brain dead compared to total	Percentage of patients brain dead compared to death	No. of patients	Mortality rate (%)	Percentage of neonates brain dead compared to total	Percentage of neonates brain dead compared to death
Rowland et al., 1983[7]	2,307	NA	0.65	NA	NA	NA	NA	NA
Vernon et al., 1993	6,000	5.0	1.2	23.3	NA	NA	NA	NA
Ryan et al., 1993[1]	839	8.7	1.2	22	1,333	5.6	0	0
Staworn et al., 1994	14,188	8.5	0.9	11	NA	NA	NA	NA
Parker et al., 1995[2]	2,605	6.5	2.0	31.4	1,455	7.6	0.48	6.3
Loma Linda, 2000*	5,093	5.0	1.3	28.1	2,977	6.2	0.02	2.1

Time period refers to the duration of the study. For several studies, separation of the data by neonates versus older pediatric patients was not possible. In the study by Parker et al. (2), there were seven neonates less than 30 days old, six of whom were less than 7 days old (personal correspondence).

* Ashwal S (personal experience, unpublished data).

Table 2. GUIDELINES FOR BRAIN DEATH DETERMINATION IN CHILDREN

A. History: determine the cause of coma to eliminate reversible conditions
B. Physical examination criteria:
   1. Coma and apnea
   2. Absence of brainstem function
      (a) Midposition or fully dilated pupils
      (b) Absence of spontaneous oculocephalic (doll's eye) and caloric-induced eye movements
      (c) Absence of movement of bulbar musculature, corneal, gag, cough, sucking, and rooting reflexes
      (d) Absence of respiratory effort with standardized testing for apnea
   3. Patient must not be hypothermic or hypotensive
   4. Flaccid tone and absence of spontaneous or induced movements, excluding activity mediated at spinal cord level
   5. Examination should remain consistent for brain death throughout the predetermined period of observation
C. Observation period according to age:
   1. 7 days to 2 months: Two examinations and EEGs 48 h apart
   2. 2 months to 1 year: Two examinations and EEGs 24 h apart or one examination and an initial EEG showing ECS combined with a radionuclide angiogram showing no CBF, or both
   3. More than 1 year: Two examinations 12-24 h apart; EEG and isotope angiography are optional

The Ad Hoc Task Force consisted of representatives from the Academy of Pediatrics, American Academy of Neurology, Child Neurology Society, American Neurological Association, American Bar Association, and the NINCDS.
From Guidelines for the determination of brain death in children. Pediatrics 1987;80:298-300, with permission.

clinical examination in determining the etiology of coma in order to eliminate reversible conditions. In addition, age-related observation periods and the need for specific neurodiagnostic tests were recommended for children below the age of 1 year. In children older than 1 year, it was recommended that the diagnosis of brain death could be made solely on a clinical basis and laboratory studies were optional. Since publication in 1987, these explicit guidelines have been generally accepted.[11,12] At the time these guidelines were developed, criteria for term infants less than 7 days of age and preterm infants were excluded because of the lack of sufficient data. More recent studies have found that criteria used in infants under age 2 months can also be applied to preterm and term infants[13-15] (Figure 1).

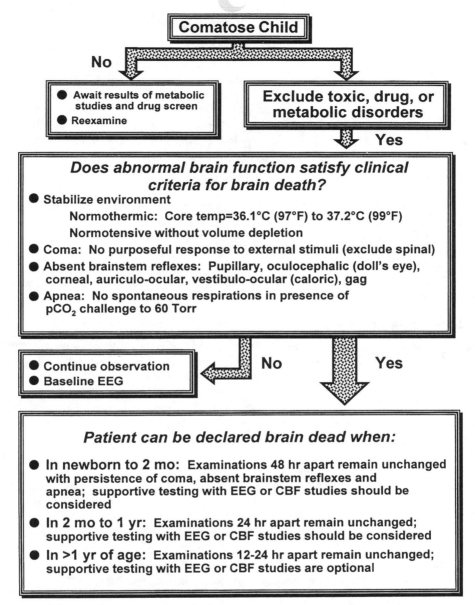

Figure 1. Diagnostic paradigm for the determination of brain death in neonates, infants and children based on the 1987 Pediatric Brain Death Guidelines (Table 2) (10) modified to include newborn infants.

Guideline dissemination remains problematic; that is, many physicians who care for children are not sufficiently aware of the specific diagnostic criteria recommended by the Task Force. For example, in one recent survey using fictional cases, only 36% of pediatric residents and 39% of pediatric attending physicians correctly defined brain death and only 58% of residents or attending physicians recognized that brain death in certain age brackets could be determined without confirmatory testing.[16] Likewise, a survey of pediatric intensivists reported a wide variability in their use of confirmatory laboratory tests.[17] Forty-one percent of respondents to this survey never considered use of the electroencephalogram (EEG) and 33% never considered use of cerebral blood flow (CBF) determinations for confirmation of brain death. Also, although 69% of respondents stated that more than one physician was required to make the diagnosis of brain death, 19% stated that one physician was sufficient and in only 71% of situations was either a neurologist or a neurosurgeon consistently involved.

Clinical Examination

By definition, all children who are declared brain dead are comatose, lack brainstem reflexes, and are apneic. These criteria may not be present on admission in all children who ultimately are declared brain dead,[18] and often are fulfilled after serial examinations. As in adults, reversible conditions associated with hypothermia, altered metabolic states, toxin exposure, severe electrolyte abnormalities, or sedative medication should be excluded. It should be emphasized that hypothermia occurs in about 50% of children who are comatose after catastrophic brain injury, and there is a common need to rewarm the child before neurologic examination and neurodiagnostic tests. It may also prolong the elimination of drugs, if any have been administered soon before assessment.

Coma

Assessment of the lack of consciousness may be difficult in infants and children. Although there is no absolute way to be completely certain that a neonate or young infant has lost all conscious awareness and is "unreceptive and unresponsive" as stated in the original Task Force criteria, testing by tactile, visual, and auditory stimulation is comparable to the older infant. In most instances and irrespective of the age of the child, the bedside clinical examination can satisfactorily accomplish this goal. The absence of any form of repetitive, sustained purposeful activity should be documented.[19] If there is uncertainty that the child is unresponsive, confirmatory neurodiagnostic studies should be performed.

Loss of Brainstem Function

In preterm and term neonates one must take into account that several of the brainstem reflexes are not fully developed[20-22] (Table 3). For example, the pupillary light reflex is absent before 30 weeks gestation and the oculocephalic reflex may not be elicitable prior to 32 weeks. Term and preterm infants are difficult to examine because their small size makes it technically difficult to adequately assess cranial nerve function. The smaller amount of pigmentation and the smaller size of the newborn's pupils can make visualization of changes in the size of the pupil and interpretation of the loss of pupillary reactivity troublesome. In addition, assessment of pupillary reactivity can be compromised at the bedside from difficult access to the infant in an incubator, corneal injury, retinal hemorrhages and other anatomical factors such as swelling with partial fusion of the eyelids. Examination of ocular motility is difficult in the small intubated child and frequently the examiner will need assistance when performing caloric stimulation with ice water. It is more difficult to perform the caloric response in neonates due to small external ear canals; therefore, both the oculocephalic (doll's eye) and the oculovestibular (caloric) reflex should be tested. There are no substantial differences in performing this testing in newborns compared to older children (see Chapter 4).

Table 3. DEVELOPMENT OF REFLEXES IN PRETERM INFANTS

Developmental reflex	Gestational age (weeks) when reflex is elicitable
Suck, root, gag	32-34
Auditory response	30-32
Pupillary response to light	30-32
Oculocephalic response	28-32
Corneal response	28-32
Moro response	28-32
Grasp response	34-36
Breathing response to PCO2 stimulus	33

From Fanaroff A, Martin RJ, Miller MJ. The respiratory system. In: Fanaroff A, Martin RJ, eds. Neonatal-perinatal medicine: diseases of the fetus and newborn. St. Louis: CV Mosby, 1987:617; Hack M. The sensorimotor development of the preterm infant. In: Fanaroff A, Martin RJ, eds. Neonatal-perinatal medicine: diseases of the fetus and newborn. St. Louis: CV Mosby, 1987:473; and Swaiman KF. Neurological examination of the preterm infant. In: Swaiman KF, ed. Pediatric neurology: principles and practice. St. Louis: Mosby, 1994:61, with permission.

The corneal reflex in neonates and infants is potentially the least reliable. Contact irritation, dehydration and maceration of the cornea, use of lubricant drops, and use of eye patches for treatment of hyperbilirubinemia frequently negatively affect tactile surface sensory receptors of the cornea. A noxious stimulus with a soaked Q-tip may be needed.

Assessment of lower cranial nerve function is also limited. There may be a substantial amount of adhesive tape around the face and cheek to secure the endotracheal tube and this impedes the clinician's ability to perform this part of the neurologic assessment, similar to adults. When infants are intubated (either by the oral or nasogastric route), testing their gag and cough reflex is best accomplished with stimulation of the trachea after insertion of a suction catheter through the endotracheal tube.

Apnea

The normal physiologic threshold for apnea (minimum carbon dioxide tension at which respiratory centers are maximally stimulated) can be altered by certain disease states, but the threshold ($PaCO_2 \geq$ 60 mm Hg) for children has been assumed to be the same as that for adults.[2,23,24]

Several studies have examined apnea testing in children with varying techniques. In one study of 10 brain-dead children (10 months to 15 years of age), the $PaCO_2$ was increased from 34.4 mm Hg to 59.5 mm Hg over 5 min while supplying 100% tracheal oxygen, which maintained the arterial Po2 greater than 200 mm Hg during the test period.[24] None of the children had any evidence of respiratory effort. A second study involved 16 apnea tests in nine children ages 4 months to 13 years, four of whom had detectable phenobarbital levels between 10 and 25 mg/dL.[23] These patients were preoxygenated (100% O_2) for 10 min and moderately hyperventilated (mean $PaCO_2$ 28 mm Hg). Oxygen was then delivered at 6 L/min through a catheter into the length of the endotracheal tube with the ventilator turned off during the 15-min study period. The $PaCO_2$ increased 4.4, 3.4, and 2.6 mm Hg per minute at 5, 10, and 15 min, respectively. Arterial $PaCO_2$ at the end of 15 min ranged from 40 to 116 mm Hg, and by 15 min, 14 of 16 patients had $PaCO_2$ levels greater than 60 mm Hg. Two patients had $PaCO_2$ levels of 110 and 116 mm Hg (pH of 6.92 and 6.98, respectively). Arterial PO_2 remained above 100 mm Hg in all patients and in 12 of 16 patients was above 200 mm Hg. Mild alterations of heart rate or blood pressure or both were also observed in six patients but were reversible. A third study in 11 children found that if apnea testing was done when the initial $PaCO_2$ level was between 40 and 50 mm Hg, the rate of $PaCO_2$ increase was linear at 5.1 to 6.7 mm Hg per minute.[25] Parker and colleagues reviewed data on apnea testing in 60 brain-dead children.[2] Nine patients who also had EEGs showed electroencephalographic silence and 26 of 30 patients who had CBF studies had no flow. These children were preoxygenated for 10 min followed by continuous oxygen delivery (6 L/min). The median $PaCO_2$ at the end of testing was 74 mm Hg (range, 55 to 112). None of these patients showed any recovery of respiratory drive.

Recent reports concerning apnea testing in children have raised questions about (a) the effects of brainstem compressive lesions; (b) potential recovery of brainstem respiratory drive; and (c) the $PaCO_2$ threshold in children. Ammar and colleagues in 1993 reported five children, ages 9 months to 7 years. In these patients, severe brainstem dysfunction included loss of pupillary reflexes and apnea and was due to surgically resectable brainstem lesions. Spontaneous respirations and substantial neurologic function returned after surgery.[26] This report suggested that treatment of compressive brainstem lesions might reverse severe neurologic deficits that mimic brain death. However, none of these children were brain dead prior to surgery. Another report is that of a 3-month-old infant who met the 1987 Task Force criteria for pediatric brain death but who on day 43 of hospitalization developed two to three irregular breaths per minute with a normal tidal volume.[27] This infant died 71 days after presentation. At issue is whether this should be considered a return of respiratory function and, if true, whether return of irregular breathing in a single exceptional case in the absence of other brainstem function is an "improvement". An editorial commentary on this study did not accept this as an example of failure of current brain death criteria, and we agree.[28]

The $PaCO_2$ threshold for maximal stimulation of the medullary centers was examined in a case report involving a 4-year-old child with a posterior fossa pilocytic astrocytoma who suffered a cardiac arrest.[29] This child met clinical criteria for brain death but had minimal respiratory effort after 9 min and 23 s into the apnea test. Arterial $PaCO_2$ measured 91 mm Hg and the exhaled tidal volumes of 5 to 7 mL/kg were considered true spontaneous respiratory efforts. He showed "minimal brain stem recovery" and was discharged to a chronic care facility with a gastrostomy and tracheostomy with mechanical ventilation but without return of consciousness. This child's spontaneous breathing was insufficient to maintain life and assisted ventilation was necessary. It was speculated that this child's higher $PaCO_2$ threshold was due to hypoxic-ischemic injury. This example raises questions whether the current standard of a $PaCO_2$ of 60 mm Hg is correct in children. However, no prospective studies have appeared with prolonged apneic oxygenation[6] and, as alluded to earlier, prior examples have not shown appearance of respiratory drive at very high levels of $PaCO_2$.[23] These isolated incidences are of interest but do not seriously challenge the conventional thinking that apnea testing, aiming at acute substantial increase in $PaCO_2$, is the best method in children.

The technique of apnea testing is identical as in adults using apneic oxygenation after disconnecting from the ventilator. Therefore, normalization of the $PaCO_2$, core temperature, and preoxygenation for 5 min before beginning the apnea challenge is recommended. Careful monitoring of the heart rate and blood pressure during the procedure while watching the chest cage for movements is needed. Most studies recommend that $PaCO_2$ levels be determined at 5-min intervals and continue for 15 min if the $PaCO_2$ has not reached 60 mm Hg and if the PO_2 has not fallen below 50 mm Hg. However, calculation of time to target level assuming a $PaCO_2$ rise of 3 mm Hg per minute may reduce blood gas sampling and is preferred. The technique of apnea testing is illustrated in Chapter 4. Prolonged bradycardia or development of hypotension during testing is mostly due to profound acidosis or hypoxemia; and at this juncture, the infant should be placed back on the ventilator.

Confirmatory Tests

EEG documentation of electrocerebral silence (ECS) and measurement of the absence of CBF remain the most widely available and useful methods to confirm the clinical diagnosis of brain death. However, over the past decade, there has been a trend in children to rely more upon repeated clinical examinations than to use confirmatory testing.

Electroencephalography

Guidelines for recordings in brain death have been developed by the American Electroencephalographic Society in 1994[30] and are summarized in Chapter 4. However, certain unique aspects of electroencephalography (EEG) recording must be considered in confirming the diagnosis of brain death in neonates and infants.[8,14,31-35] This includes: shorter interelectrode distances reducing detection of very-low-voltage activity; external artifacts in NICUs and PICUs brought on due to high gain settings; rapid cardiac and respiratory rates of infants and children compared to adults; shorter distances between the heart and the brain making the electrocardiogram contribution disproportionately large in children; reduced amplitude of cortical potentials in preterm and term neonates; and the presence of congenital cerebral nervous system malformations (e.g., hydranencephaly) that can be associated with ECS.[36]

It is well recognized that a certain number of brain-dead infants and children will have persistent EEG activity.[37-39] Most of these EEG patterns depict low-voltage theta or beta activity or intermittent spindle activity. Although electrocortical activity is generated in dying cortical cells, its persistence in otherwise functionally dead brains may continue for days. Moreover, data from several studies have found that the initial EEG in brain-dead children is isoelectric in as low as 48% of patients (Table 4). However, in the majority of children who initially have EEG activity, follow-up studies show ECS.

Conversely, when the initial EEG in children demonstrates ECS, a repeat EEG typically will remain isoelectric.[8,39] However, there have been reported cases of recovery of EEG activity. In some reports, the EEG findings were either inconclusive or the patients had some retained brainstem function and thus did not meet clinical criteria for brain death. It remains unclear in some cases whether the EEGs were not artifactual.[14] Since Green and Lauber's report almost 30 years ago of two infants who had return of some EEG activity after initial ECS, there have been five additional reports in infants in whom EEG activity returned.[14,31,37,40] None of these infants recovered any neurologic function. The ratio of these five infants

Table 4. INITIAL EEG FINDINGS IN CHILDREN WITH BRAIN DEATH

Study	No. of patients	Percentage of patients with ECS
Green and Lauber, 1972[40]	2	100%
Ashwal et al., 1977	11	82%
Holzman et al., 1983[57]	18	61%
McMenamin and Volpe, 1983[64]	3	100%
Furgiuele et al., 1984	10	91%
Coker and Dillehay, 1986[55]	11	100%
Drake et al., 1986[18]	47	70%
Ashwal et al., 1987[5,6]	6	100%
Alvarez et al., 1988[8]	52	100%
LaMancusa et al., 1991[44]	92	100%
Parker et al., 1995[2]	9	100%
Ashwal, 1997[15]	37	51%
Ruiz-Lopez et al. 1999[96]	29	48%
	332 (total)	83% (average)

ECS, electroencephalographic silence.

(i.e., in whom the initial EEG was isoelectric but the second EEG showed activity) to the number of neonatal and pediatric patients diagnosed as brain dead in published reports since 1972 is approximately 5/22,500 or 0.02%.[15] Therefore, concerns about the return of EEG activity have been overemphasized, and the impact of these observations on brain death recommendations is very uncertain and likely inconsequential. None of these five infants recovered and not even to a vegetative or minimally conscious state.

It should be emphasized that electroencephalographic silence may occur soon after a child has had a cardiac arrest.[41] In infants in whom the initial EEG, 8 to 10 h after cardiac arrest, showed an isoelectric recording, a repeat study 12 to 24 h later may show diffuse low-voltage activity. Most of these infants, none fulfilling clinical criteria of brain death, die from associated complications of the acute catastrophic insult; the remaining survivors usually evolve to a permanent vegetative or minimally conscious state.

The Ad Hoc Task Force of the American Academy of Pediatrics recommends two EEGs in children below 1 year of age, but overall, the available data in children may suggest that documentation of isoelectric EEG on the initial recording is probably sufficient to support the clinical diagnosis of brain death.[15] In addition, it is not necessary to obtain an EEG in children over 1 year of age as long as the neurologic examination remains unchanged for the appropriate time period of observation.[10]

Electroencephalography may be confounded by hypothermia and drugs, and recordings in these circumstances unreliable. In children, suppression of EEG activity does not appear until 24°C (75.2°F), and the appearance of an isoelectric EEG does not occur until the temperature is below 18°C (64.4°F).[42,43] Nonetheless due to their smaller body mass compared to the adult, it is easier to control an infant's or child's body temperature with the use of heating lamps or mattresses.

In children, the most common medications causing the reversible loss of brain electrocortical activity include barbiturates, benzodiazepines, narcotics and certain intravenous (thiopental, ketamine, midazolam) and inhalation (halothane and isoflurane) anesthetics. Phenobarbital is the most common drug responsible for reversible isoelectric EEG, as it is widely used for seizure control. In this setting, previous studies have suggested that phenobarbital levels more than 25 µg/mL might suppress EEG activity to the point of isoelectric recordings. Another study in 92 children reported data suggesting that therapeutic levels of phenobarbital (i.e., 15 to 40 µg/mL) do not affect the EEG.[44] Correlation with other antiepileptic agents has not been reported. The exact threshold in children remains difficult to ascertain, but serum levels below 20 to 25 µg/mL are unlikely to cause ECS, affect apnea testing or the examination of brainstem reflexes.[13] (For pentobarbital level in ICP treatment see Chapter 6.)

Cerebral Blood Flow Determination

Neuroimaging techniques can be used to document the absence of CBF and include cerebral angiography, radionuclide scanning, transcranial Doppler (TCD), computed tomography with contrast injection or xenon inhalation, digital subtraction angiography, single photon emission computed tomography (SPECT), and positron emission tomography (PET). Documentation of the absence of CBF is considered confirmatory of brain death, but as shown in Table 5, not all infants and children who are brain dead show absence of CBF or abnormal TCD velocity patterns. In this section, a detailed description of the available literature follows.

Table 5. CEREBRAL BLOOD FLOW OR VELOCITY STUDIES IN CHILDREN WITH BRAIN DEATH

Study	No. of patients	Percentage of patients with no CBF
Radionuclide angiography		
Ashwal et al., 1977	11	91%
Ashwal and Schneider, 1979[37]	5	100%
Holzman et al., 1983[57]	18	56%
Schwartz et al., 1984[54]	9	100%
Coker and Dillehay, 1986[55]	55	96%
Drake et al., 1986[18]	42	64%
Ashwal et al., 1989[45]	9	100%
Singh et al., 1994	26	77%
Parker et al., 1995[2]	30	87%
Ashwal, 1997[15]	18	72%
Transcranial Doppler		
McMenamin and Volpe, 1983[64]	6	100%
Furgiuele et al., 1984	11	100%
Ahmann et al., 1987[65a]	32	59%
Bode et al., 1988[71]	9	89%
Glasier et al., 1989[72]	9	89%
Messer et al., 1990[68]	11	100%
Jalili et al., 1994[70]	7	71%
Qian et al., 1998[66]	17	100%
Cerebral angiography		
Parvey and Gerald, 1976	4	100%
Schwartz et al., 1984[54]	9	100%
Xenon computed tomography		
Ashwal et al., 1989[45]	10	100%
	348 (total)	83% (average)

[a] In the study of Ahmann et al.,[65] 19/23 infants >4 months of age showed characteristic TCD changes seen with brain death; the remaining nine infants were less than 4 months old, and none showed a typical response.

Radionuclide scanning remains the most widely used test in children because it is portable, valid, and convenient to perform. With most methods, circulation is assessed during an early "dynamic" phase and later by examining static images for cerebral uptake of the specific radionuclide (usually technetium-99m pertechnetate, Tc-99m glucoheptonate, or tc-99m DTPA). During the dynamic phase a bolus of the radionuclide is rapidly injected and isotopic cranial images are obtained. During the arterial phase, cerebral activity is detectable within several seconds and, from the time of peak cerebral activity, sagittal sinus activity is observed within 6 to 8s.[49]

If activity is not detectable in this early phase, CBF is considered absent. Most tracers have a half-life of several hours, and therefore, the static phase of a radionuclide imaging study is performed later to image absence or presence of diffuse parenchymal isotopic uptake. Currently, most centers are using SPECT scanning with Tc-99m hexylmethylpropylene aminoexine (HMPAO) as the isotopic agent.[46-56] This agent is more lipophilic, is not dependent on the quality of the bolus injection, and enables more precise static imaging of parenchymatous brain. With this technology, isotope can be injected in the ICU and later images obtained using a mobile camera or after transfer of the patient to the nuclear medicine department.

Multiple studies in adults and children have documented that radionuclide imaging is accurate and reproducible and it has been favorably compared with other methods of detecting the presence or absence of CBF.[2,18,39,45,55-57]

The absence of CBF in brain death is due primarily to very low cerebral perfusion pressure [mean arterial pressure (MAP) – (intracranial pressure (ICP)] and secondarily to release of vasoconstrictors from vascular smooth muscle and brain parenchyma. In the majority of brain-dead children studied at Loma Linda University Children's Hospital, cerebral perfusion pressure has been calculated below 20 to 30 mm Hg when CBF was absent. However, four of 24 brain-dead children with absent CBF and with ICP monitoring had persistently high cerebral perfusion pressures greater than 45 to 50 mm Hg.[56] Holzman et al. observed the same phenomena in four patients, ages 8 months to 3 years.[57] Such findings indicate that, although several mechanisms may be involved in the loss of CBF during brain death, the majority are due to markedly increased ICP.[50]

Some concern about specificity of the radionuclide imaging technique in newborns has been raised. Reduced CBF has been reported in preterm and term infants who survived with relatively intact neurologic function. For example, in one series of preterm infants, xenon cerebral flow values averaged 12 mL/min/100 g in 24 of 42 infants;[58] in another small study of preterm infants using positron emission tomography (PET), flow values ranged from 7 to 11 mL/min/100 g.[59] None of these patients were clinically brain dead.

In a study of eight brain-dead adults using stable xenon computed tomography, cerebral blood flow (XeCTCBF) measured 1.6 ± 2.0 mL/min/100 g.[60] In another study of nine clinically brain-dead children, 1 month to 11 years of age, CBF determined by stable XeCTCBF was compared to radionuclide imaging techniques.[45] All patients showed no flow by radionuclide imaging and had XeCTCBF values of 1.29 ± 1.6 mL/min/100 g. Although none of these patients were preterm infants, three were 1 month, 7 weeks, and 3 months of age. Both the adult and pediatric XeCTCBF investigations showed that CBF at the time of brain death was less than 2 mL/min/100 g and that this value correlated with the absence of flow by radionuclide imaging.[45,60] Therefore, it is likely that radionuclide imaging, available in most hospitals, is valid in newborns as well as older infants and children for determination of CBF.

Clinically brain-dead pediatric patients have been reported who have presence of CBF early after diagnosis (Table 5). In the studies reported by Drake et al., 15 of 47 children who were clinically brain dead had evidence of intact CBF as determined by radionuclide imaging.[18] About two-thirds of the patients who were restudied showed loss of CBF, 2 to 3 days later. This occurred irrespective of whether these patients had an isoelectric EEG or some residual activity recorded at the time the first CBF study was performed. In a more recent report, five of 18 clinically brain-dead preterm and term infants had retained CBF.[14] Greisen and Pryds also reported two suspected brain-dead newborn infants with ECS who had preserved CBF documented by xenon scanning.[61] Even more complicating in these neonates, phenobarbital and diazepam had been administered and a phenobarbital serum level of 42 mg/dL was detected in one of these patients. They were subsequently taken off respiratory support and neuropathologic examination was consistent with diffuse neuronal necrosis and the clinical diagnosis of brain death. Another report of a clinically brain-dead 2month-old child found persistence of CBF and normal glucose metabolism by PET despite an isoelectric EEG. Neuropathologic examination showed extensive necrosis that was believed to be present at the time the PET scan was done.[62] Overall, it is clear that CBF may be present in infants and children who are clinically brain dead. Repeat CBF studies 24 to 48 h later will likely but not uniformly document the loss of CBF. These observations suggest a somehow gradual halting of blood flow due to gradual increase in intracranial pressure finally going beyond the arterial pressure. Moreover, compensatory resources are more substantial in infants who have the ability to expand the skull by separating the sutures.

TCD sonography has been advocated because it is a portable and noninvasive method to ascertain cerebral circulatory arrest.[63-71] Changes noted on TCD in brain death include loss of diastolic flow, appearance of retrograde diastolic flow, and diminution of systolic flow, and in occasional instances, with earlier documentation of a TCD signal, the loss of any detectable flow.

McMenamin and Volpe reported six brain-dead infants, 28 to 40 weeks gestation, who had the characteristic progression of velocity changes as cerebral edema and ICP increased.[64] ICP in four of six infants was elevated and EEGs in three infants showed ECS. Although cerebral angiography or radionuclide imaging were not performed to corroborate the Doppler results, postmortem examination revealed brain necrosis consistent with brain death. In other studies, 19 of 23 brain-dead children older than 4 months showed a characteristic velocity pattern with a single sharp systolic peak followed by a rapid negative deflection below baseline, sharply rebounding to forward flow in early to mid-diastole with gradual tapering at the end of diastole to or below baseline.[65] Eight of the 19 patients with this pattern also demonstrated absent CBF by radionuclide angiography. Infants less than 4 months of age who were studied had atypical waveforms, suggesting that the pulsed Doppler technique in newborns might not be as reliable.

More recent studies found similar Doppler velocity changes in 11 comatose children who progressed to brain death.[68] Other studies, however, have found limitations to this technique. In one report, only five of seven brain-dead patients had bilateral reversal of flow (implying increased cerebrovascular resistance and absent cerebral circulation).[70] Bode and colleagues examined nine brain-dead children and in eight typical findings were reported.[71] However, one newborn showed normal systolic and end-diastolic CBF velocities for 2 days despite clinical and EEG signs of brain death. Others have also encountered individual cases that did not show similar progression as originally described.[72] In one case study of a brain-dead infant due to SIDS, TCD sonography demonstrated nearly normal cerebral perfusion, which even increased day by day, notwithstanding the persistence of other signs of brain death.[73] To complicate matters even further, one case report found similar patterns of reversal of diastolic flow in a 1-month-old infant with status epilepticus who recovered without sequelae.[74] The comparatively poor specificity of TCD in diagnosis of brain death in children may be due to brain injuries not increasing ICP and vascular resistance (e.g., asphyxia).

Digital subtraction angiography (DSA) is another technique that has been used to assess the intracranial circulation. This technique can be performed intravenously[71] or by intraarterial injection.[75] A small amount of nonionic contrast material is injected while digital subtraction imaging of the cerebral vasculature is done, similar to conventional cerebral angiography. This allows visualization of contrast within the major intracranial vessels; lack of such visualization indicates absence of CBF and, beyond question, brain death. There are very few reports of this technique in children and only one recent case report in a brain-dead neonate.[76] A 1989 report using intravenous DSA in 110 patients aged 3 to 83 years with clinical signs of brain death observed absent contrast enhancement in 105 patients.[75] Repeat studies in the remaining five patients within several hours confirmed the cessation of CBF.

Stable xenon and 133-xenon computed tomography are examples of useful, reliable, and well documented tests that are now seldom used due to cost, need for upgraded computer software programs and specially trained personnel.[77] Xenon CT allows quantitative and regional measurement of CBF. In brain-dead adults, CBF values of 1.6 ± 2.0 mL/min/100 g have been reported.[60] Previous studies found an average CBF of 1.3 ± 1.6 mL/min/100 g in 10 brain-dead children, substantially lower than when compared to CBF of 33.5 ± 16.3 mL/min/100 g in 11 profoundly comatose children.[45] In addition, CBF studies were much higher in preterm infants who suffered neurologic injury but who were not brain dead. CBF values in these studies were 12 mL/min/100 g using 133-xenon[58] and 7 to 11 mL/min/100 g using PET scanning,[59] but these values did not approximate those found in comatose infants with retained brainstem function.

The results of PET scanning have been reported in only a few brain-dead pediatric patients.[62,78] Because of its limited availability, cost and lack of comparison studies, it offers no advantages to the more standardized methods previously discussed. Meyer reported an 18-year-old brain-dead adolescent whose dynamic PET study, performed 7 days after a severe traumatic closed-head injury, showed no intracerebral uptake or retention of tracer and was considered consistent with diffuse absence of brain metabolism.[78] Medlock and colleagues reported a 2-month-old brain-dead infant with preserved CBF whose PET scan on the 11th day following injury showed a normal glucose metabolic gradient between gray and white matter.[62] Autopsy revealed widespread necrosis with mononuclear cell infiltrates throughout the cerebral cortex. The persistence of glucose metabolism was thought to be associated with the presence of inflammatory microglial cells and suggested that persistence of CBF and glucose metabolism in brain-dead children might not reflect neuronal survival.

Magnetic resonance imaging (MRI) has been reported in small series of adult brain-dead patients.[79-82] Characteristic features are described and illustrated in Chapter 4, but have not been confirmed in children.

In the past two decades phosphorus (^{31}P) and proton (^{1}H) magnetic resonance spectroscopy (MRS) have been used to noninvasively measure aspects of brain metabolic activity. Recent studies in the neonate and in older infants and children have shown significant abnormalities using these techniques documenting loss of metabolic activity associated with severe acute central nervous system insults.[83,84] Kato et al. reported ^{31}P-MRS in three infants, four children, and 17 adults who were clinically brain dead. Spectra demonstrated the absence of adenosine triphosphate (ATP) and phosphocreatine (PCr) while the inorganic phosphate and phosphodiesterase peaks were still detectable.[85] Another ^{31}P-MRS study involving three brain-dead adults found similar spectral abnormalities.[86] These findings suggest that MRS could provide another technique to objectively assess the complete loss of cerebral function. The advantage of MRS is that it can be done in conjunction with MRI. This allows acquisition of anatomic as well as metabolic data that could further clarify the etiology of the CNS insult and at the same time determine whether there is irreversible neuronal loss. Representative of the often repeated theme of conflicting reports, Terk and coinvestigators reported a term brain-dead infant whose ^{31}P spectra on days 11 and 18 demonstrated three distinct ATP peaks as well as several other peaks that suggested the persistence of metabolic activity.[87] Although no definite reasons could be ascertained for this finding compared to the study of Kato and colleagues,[85] Terk and colleagues suggested that any proposed spectral signature for brain death would need to be modified.[87]

There are no published case reports concerning proton MRS and brain death in children. Recently at Loma Linda University Children's Hospital seven brain-dead children were studied with proton MRS. All spectra were markedly abnormal with severe reductions or loss of the metabolite peaks (N-acetylaspartate, choline, creatine) and a clearly identifiable and elevated lactate peak. Review of these findings compared to other children who were severely brain injured but not brain dead did not demonstrate any obvious differences although it appeared that the reductions in the N-acetylaspartate peak were markedly reduced to absent in the gray matter spectra (Figure 2), whereas it was still discernible in the white matter (Figure 3).

Evoked Responses

Brainstem auditory evoked response (BAER) testing has been extensively studied as an alternative confirmatory method.[88-92] Several studies have raised doubt as to its value in brain death determination, particularly in children less than 6 months of age[88,92-95] but more recent studies claim that BAER is reliable.[96,97] In one report, 90% of 51 brain-dead children had loss of the BAER (complete loss in 27 patients; loss of waveforms III to VII in 18 patients).[96] It was also shown that loss of the BAER preceded flattening of the EEG. This finding suggested that BAER testing might be more useful than the EEG for earlier laboratory confirmation of brain death. However, if BAER testing is performed too "early," a false positive test may result. In one recent report, return of an absent BAER was observed in a 28-month-old infant 18 h after a severe global hypoxic-ischemic insult.[41]

It is doubtful whether somatosensory evoked potentials (SSEPs) have greater discrimination in the confirmation of brain death.[97-102] Recent SSEP studies in children found that only 62.5% of patients had the complete absence of the summated response or only a cervical cord response suggesting limitation of SSEPs as a confirmatory test in children.[92] In addition, absent evoked potentials may be observed in other comatose states.

Brain Death in Newborns

A recent review estimates that each year about 550 newborns out of a total of 4,900,000 live births might be diagnosed as brain dead.[15] Etiologies of brain death based on data from 87 newborns less than 1 month of age included hypoxic-ischemic encephalopathy (61%), birth trauma (8%), malformations (6%), cerebral hemorrhage (6%), infection (7%), SIDS (7%), nonaccidental trauma (4%), and metabolic causes (1%).

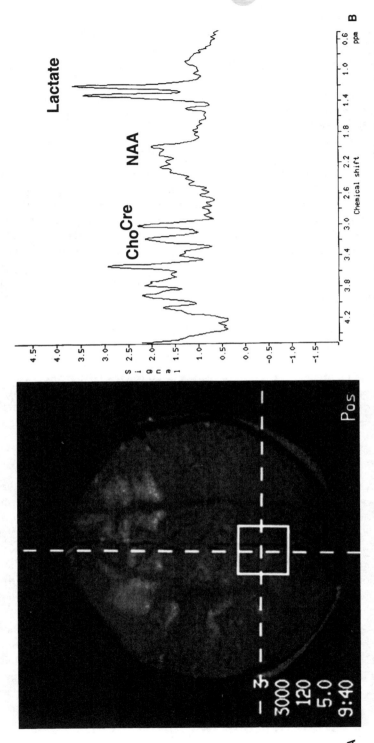

Figure 2. Proton magnetic resonance (MR) spectroscopy in 3-month-old boy who was brain dead after suspected nonaccidental trauma. **A:** Axial T_2-weighted spin-echo image obtained 1 day after admission shows edema and swelling of cortical and subcortical vascular border zones. Increased signal intensity was also noted in the right basal ganglia consistent with a history of acute cerebral anoxia. A highlighted box shows the $2 \times 2 \times 2$ cm^3 volume in occipital gray matter in which the proton spectrum is acquired. **B:** Proton MR spectrum (TR/TE = 3,000/20 ms, stimulated echo acquisition mode) obtained immediately after imaging shows a prominent lactate (Lac) peak. The NAA/Cre ratio is decreased by 75% and the NAA/Cho ratio is decreased by 50% compared to age-matched control values. (Courtesy of Dr. Barbara Hofshouser, Department of Radiology, Loma Linda University Children's Hospital.)

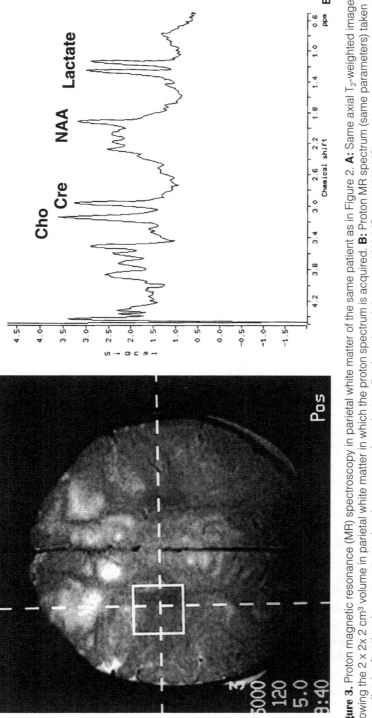

Figure 3. Proton magnetic resonance (MR) spectroscopy in parietal white matter of the same patient as in Figure 2. **A:** Same axial T$_2$-weighted image showing the 2 × 2 × 2 cm^3 volume in parietal white matter in which the proton spectrum is acquired. **B:** Proton MR spectrum (same parameters) taken immediately after the above spectrum also shows a prominent lactate (Lac) peak and decreased NAA/Cre and NAA/Cho ratios. Although significantly decreased compared to normal values, the NAA level in white matter was found to be higher than in the same volume of occipital gray matter. (Courtesy of Dr. Barbara Holshouser, Department of Radiology, Loma Linda University Children's Hospital).

The ability to diagnose brain death in newborns is still viewed with uncertainty.[15] This is due primarily to the small number of brain-dead neonates reported in the literature. Preterm and term neonates less than 7 days of age were excluded from the 1987 pediatric brain death guidelines. It was phrased as follows: "The newborn is difficult to evaluate clinically after perinatal insults. This relates to many factors including difficulties of clinical assessment, determination of proximate cause of coma, and certainty of the validity of laboratory tests. These problems are accentuated in a premature infant".[10] Several years after the publication of these guidelines, data on 18 brain-dead neonates were published and it was suggested that brain death could be diagnosed in term infants and preterm infants greater than 34 weeks gestational age within the first week of life.[14] Because the newborn has patent sutures and an open fontanel, increases in ICP after acute injury are not as significant as in older patients. Thus, the usual cascade of events of herniation that results from increased ICP and reduced cerebral perfusion are less likely to occur in the newborn. Brain death in the newborn can be diagnosed providing the physician is aware of the limitations of the clinical examination and laboratory testing. It is important to carefully and repeatedly examine these infants with particular attention to the examination of brainstem reflexes and apnea testing.

Specific issues regarding certainty of diagnosis, immaturity of the nervous system, and the effects of development on the pathophysiology and diagnosis of brain death in the preterm and term infant have also previously been published.[34,103-105] and recently updated.[15] For the most part, Task Force recommendations concerning the duration of observation of brain death in infants and children of different ages were based on expert opinion and consensus rather than evidence based. Recently collected data from 87 newborns allowed the following estimations: (a) the duration of coma from impact to brain death (37 h); (b) duration of time before brain death confirmation (75 h); and (c) the duration of time to transplantation (20 h).[15] The average duration of brain death in these patients was about 95 h (or almost 4 days). In none of the patients was recovery of brainstem function observed. The duration of brain death was also specifically analyzed in 53 neonates donating organs for transplantation. The total duration of brain death (including time to transplantation) averaged 2.8 days in neonates less than 7 days of age. In the neonates 1 to 3 weeks of age, the duration of brain death was approximately 5.2 days. The data suggest that a 24- to 48-h period of observation in neonates, even in those less than 7 days of age, should be sufficient to establish the diagnosis of brain death.

Because of the significant pathophysiologic differences in the neonatal response to injuries resulting in brain death, previous studies have observed a much higher incidence of newborns with EEG activity or cerebral perfusion.[15] In addition, some newborns with isoelectric EEGs showed preserved CBF and, conversely, others without CBF showed EEG activity. In the neonate, even though CBF and mean arterial blood pressures are much lower, increases in ICP after acute injury are less dramatic. Recent data on 30 newborns who had EEGs and radionuclide perfusion studies found that one-third with isoelectric EEG showed evidence of CBF and 58% of those with absent CBF had evidence of EEG activity.[15]

Data on 37 of 53 brain-dead newborns in whom EEGs were performed revealed the following: isoelectric recording ($n = 21$); very-low-voltage ($n = 13$); burst-suppression ($n = 1$); seizure activity ($n = 1$); normal ($n = 1$).[15] Almost all patients whose first EEG showed ECS had ECS on the second study and most of the patients who initially did not show ECS on their first EEG did so on a repeat study. The data suggest that for confirmation of brain death only one isoelectric EEG is necessary, providing the examination over a fixed time interval remains unchanged.

In a 1989 review on neonatal brain death, CBF data were reported in 29 patients.[14] One infant had contrast cerebral angiography, nine had Doppler and 19 had radionuclide isotopic scans. The outcome of the 11 patients without radionuclide uptake included cardiac arrest ($n = 3$), discontinuation of respiratory support an average of 5 days after diagnosis ($n = 7$), and short-term survival ($n = 1$). Almost one-third of the infants in that study who had radionuclide scans had evidence of cerebral perfusion.

CBF data are now available on an additional 18 patients taken from a larger retrospective review of neonatal brain death reported in 1997.[15] In 72% of these infants CBF was not detected. The median duration of brain death in these 13 patients was 4 days, with four patients showing isoelectric EEG and four patients with low-voltage slow-wave activity. Of the five neonates with CBF, only two had repeat studies and in one CBF was still present. This infant initially had a normal EEG but two followup studies showed isoelectric EEG. No significant differences were noted in the median duration of brain death in those neonates with CBF (4 days) compared to those without CBF (3 days). These findings as well as those described earlier again emphasize the limitations of both CBF determinations and EEG findings for brain death confirmation in neonates. To epitomize, an observation period of 48 h is recommended to confirm the diagnosis. If an EEG is isoelectric or if a CBF study shows no flow, the observation period can be shortened to 24 h. Although there are few cases of preterm infants who are brain dead, it is likely that the same time frame would be applicable. There have been few instances of neonates or older infants who showed minimal transient clinical or EEG recovery but none appear to have regained meaningful neurologic function and all died within brief periods of time.

Brain Death in Infants with Anencephaly

Infants with anencephaly have been considered as possible sources for organ donation but have generated considerable controversy.[106-109] This again drew widespread media attention when the American Medical Association Council report (that was subsequently rescinded) recommended that liveborn anencephalic infants, who did not meet accepted brain death criteria, could be considered for organ donation.[106,108] Because anencephalic infants demonstrate brainstem function, they do not meet the legal requirements of whole brain death as called for by the Uniform Determination of Death Act.

Diagnosis of brain death in anencephalic infants requires careful evaluation because of the severe central nervous system malformations that are present, particularly in the brainstem.[108] However, brain death can be diagnosed by specifically determining the absence or loss of preexisting brainstem function including apnea. Difficulties in performing the examination have been previously reviewed.[108] Serial examinations demonstrating the loss of any previously detectable cranial nerve reflexes and the performance of repeated apnea challenge studies documenting the absence of respiratory effort with a $PaCO_2$ greater than 60 mm Hg over 24 to 48 h should be considered in keeping with previously published guidelines on brain death. It is recommended that the period of observation to confirm the diagnosis of brain death be similar, that is, 24 to 48 h.

Fetal Brain Death

Fetal brain death is recognized by the presence of a prolonged fixed fetal heart rate pattern (even following different types of stress tests); an atonic fetus without breathing and body movement; the appearance of polyhydramnios; and the development of ventriculomegaly.[110,111] The first case, after an uncomplicated pregnancy, was reported in 1977 on the basis of clinical criteria of neonatal brain death with neuropathologic evidence of diffuse central nervous system destruction typical of severe intrauterine anoxia and circulatory failure.[112] Fetal brain death during pregnancy is an extremely rare event with probably less than 20 patients reported.[110,113]

Organ Procurement in Brain-Dead Children

Because brain death is more frequently due to severe asphyxial injury in children than in adults, a risk exists that similar injury to other organs may preclude transplantation. Inotropic agents to support blood pressure and cardiac function are necessary, particularly if the etiology of brain death was related to a preexisting global asphyxial insult which may have caused hypoxic myocardial injury.[114] Organ transplantation can be successfully accomplished from pediatric donors.[115] Brain-dead child abuse victims have infrequently been considered organ donors due to legal issues, but many centers have now tried to obtain surrogate consent and with cooperation from the medical examiner's office have been able to successfully harvest organs.[116] The principles of management of the brain-dead child are comparable to those in adults and discussed in Chapter 10.

Conclusion

It is expected that a certain percentage of infants and children, much like adults, will have neurodiagnostic testing results that do not fit the clinical examination. As is the case in many other areas of pediatrics, serial examinations should allow for the establishment of a definitive diagnosis. Better understanding of the pathophysiology of the evolution of brain death in neonates and infants should help decide whether recommended age-related periods of observation are justified.

References

1. Ryan CA, Byrne P, Kuhn S, et al. No resuscitation and withdrawal of therapy in a neonatal and a pediatric intensive care unit in Canada. *J Pediatr*. 1993;123:534-538.
2. Parker BL, Frewen TC, Levin SD, et al. Declaring pediatric brain death: current practice in a Canadian pediatric critical care unit. *Can Med Assoc J*. 1995;153:909-916.
3. Mejia RE, Pollack MM. Variability in brain death determination practices in children. JAMA. 1995;274:550-553.
4. Martinot A, Lejeune C, Hue V, et al. Modality and causes of 259 deaths in a pediatric intensive care unit. *Arch Pediatr* 1995;2:735-741.
5. Ashwal S, Schneider S. Brain death in children: Part I. *Pediatr Neural*. 1987;3:5-10.
6. Ashwal S, Schneider S. Brain death in children: Part II *Pediatr Neural*. 1987;3:9-77.
7. Rowland RW, Donnelly JH, Jackson AH, et al. Brain death in the pediatric intensive care unit. *Am J Dis Child*. 1983;137:547-550.
8. Alvarez LA, Moshe SL, Belman AL, et al. EEG and brain death determination in children. *Neurology*. 1988;38:227-230.
9. Wijdicks EFM. Determining brain death in adults. *Neurology*. 1995;45:1003-1011.
10. Guidelines for the determination of brain death in children. *Pediatrics*. 1987;80:298-300.
11. Kaufman HH, ed. *Pediatric brain death and organ/tissue retrieval: medical, ethical, and legal aspects*. New York: Plenum, 1989.
12. Farrell MM, Levin DL. Brain death in the pediatric patient: historical, sociological, medical, religious, cultural, legal, and ethical considerations. *Crit Care Med*. 1993;21:1951-1965.
13. Ashwal S. Brain death in early infancy. *J Heart Lung Transplant*. 1993;12:S176-S178.
14. Ashwal S, Schneider S. Brain death in the newborn. Clinical, EEG and blood flow determinations. *Pediatrics*. 1989;84:429-437.
15. Ashwal S. Brain death in the newborn. Current perspectives. *Clin Perinatol*. 1997;24:859-882.
16. Harrison AM, Botkin JR. Can pediatricians define and apply the concept of brain death? *Pediatrics*. 1999;103:e82.
17. Lynch J, Eldadah MK. Brain-death criteria currently used by pediatric intensivists. *Clin Pediatr*. 1992;31:457-1160.
18. Drake B, Ashwal S, Schneider S. Determination of cerebral death in the pediatric intensive care unit. *Pediatrics*. 1986;78:107-112.
19. Ashwal S. The persistent vegetative state in children. *Adv Pediatr*. 1994;41:195-222.
20. Fanaroff A, Martin RJ, Miller MJ. The respiratory system. In: Fanaroff A, Martin RJ, eds. *Neonatal perinatal medicine: diseases of the fetus and newborn*. St. Louis: CV Mosby, 1987:617.
21. Hack M. The sensorimotor development of the preterm infant. In: Fanaroff A, Martin RJ, eds. *Neonatal-perinatal medicine: diseases of the fetus and newborn*. St. Louis: CV Mosby, 1987:473.
22. Swaiman KF. Neurological examination of the preterm infant. In: Swaiman KF, ed. *Pediatric neurology: principles and practice*. St. Louis: Mosby, 1994:61.
23. Rowland TW, Donnelly JH, Jackson AH. Apnea documentation for determination of brain death in children. *Pediatrics*. 1984;74:505-508.
24. Outwater KM, Rockoff MA. Apnea testing to confirm brain death in children. *Crit Care Med*. 1984;12:357-358.
25. Paret G, Barzilay Z. Apnea testing in suspected brain dead children-physiological and mathematical modeling. *Intensive Care Med* .1995;2L247-252.
26. Ammar A, Awada A, Al-Luwami I. Reversibility of severe brain stem dysfunction in children. *Acta Neurochir*. 1993;124:86-91.
27. Okamoto K, Sugimoto T. Return of spontaneous respiration in an infant who fulfilled current criteria to determine brain death. *Pediatrics*. 1995;96:518-520.

28. Fishman MA. Validity of brain death criteria in infants. *Pediatrics*. 1995;96:513-515.
29. Vardis R, Pollack MM. Increased apnea threshold in a pediatric patient with suspected brain death. *Crit Care Med*. 1998;26:1917-1919.
30. American Electroencephalographic Society. Guideline three: minimum technical standards for EEG recording in suspected cerebral death. *J Clin Neurophysiol*. 1994;11:10-13.
31. Kohrman MH, Spivack BS. Brain death in infants: sensitivity and specificity of current criteria. *Pedieter Neurol*. 1990;6:47-50.
32. Moshe S. Usefulness of EEG in the evaluation of brain death in children: the pros. *Electroencephalogr Clin Neurophysiol*. 1989;73:272-275.
33. Schneider S. Usefulness of EEG in the evaluation of brain death in children: the cons. *Electroencephalogr Clin Neurophysiol*. 1989;73:276-278.
34. Ashwal S. Brain death in the newborn. *Clin Perinatol*. 1989;16:501-518.
35. Volpe JJ. Commentary-brain death determination in the newborn. *Pediatrics* .1987;80:293-297.
36. Ashwal S, Schneider S. Pediatric brain death: current perspectives. In: Barness LA, ed. *Advances in pediatrics*. Volume 38. Chicago: Mosby Year Book, 1991:181-202.
37. Ashwal S, Schneider S. Failure of electroencephalography to diagnose brain death in comatose patients. *Ann Neurol*. 1979;6:512-517.
38. Grigg G, Kelly M, Celesia G, et al. Electroencephalographic activity after brain death. *Arch Neurol*. 1987;44:948-954.
39. Ruiz-Garcia M, Gonzalez-Astiazaran A, Collado-Corona MA, et al. Brain death in children: clinical, neurophysiological and radioisotopic angiography findings in 125 patients. *Childs Nerv Syst*. 2000;16:40-46.
40. Green JR, Lauber A. Recovery of activity in young children after ECS. *J Neurol Neurosurg Psychiatry*. 1972;35:103-107.
41. Schmitt B, Simma B, Burger R, et al. Resuscitation after severe hypoxia in a young child: temporary isoelectric EEG and loss of BAEP components. *Intensive Care Med*. 1993;19:420-422.
42. Hicks RC, Poole JL. Electroencephalographic changes with hypothermia and cardiopulmonary by pass in children. *J Thorac Cardiovasc Surg*. 1981;81:781-786.
43. Jorgensen EO, Malchow-Moller A. Cerebral prognostic signs during cardiopulmonary resuscitation. *Resuscitation*. 1978;6:217-225.
44. LaMancusa J, Cooper R, Vieth R, et al. The effects of the falling therapeutic and subtherapeutic barbiturate blood levels on electrocerebral silence in clinically brain-dead children. *Clin Electroencephalogr*. 1991;22:112-117.
45. Ashwal S, Schneider S, Thompson J. Xenon computed tomography measuring cerebral blood flow in the determination of brain death in children. *Ann Neurol*. 1989;25:539-546.
46. Mrhac L, Zakko S, Parikh Y. Brain death: the evaluation of semi-quantitative parameters and other signs in HMPAO scintigraphy. *Nucl Med Commun*. 1995;16:1016-1020.
47. Wilson K, Gormon L, Seeby JB. The diagnosis of brain death with Tc-99m HmPAO. *Clin Nucl Med*. 1993;18:428-434.
48. Bonetti MG, Ciritella P, Valle G, et al. ^{99m}Tc HM-PAO brain perfusion SPECT in brain death. *Neuroradiology*. 1995;37:365-369.
49. Wieler H, March K, Kaisar KP, et al. Tc-99m HMPAO cerebral scintigraphy: a reliable, noninvasive method for determination of brain death. *Clin Nucl Med*. 1993;18:104-109.
50. Villani A, Onofri A, Bianchi R, et al. Determination of brain death in intensive pediatric therapy. *Pediatr Med Chir*. 1998;20:19-23.
51. Valle G, Ciritella P, Bonetti MG, et al. Considerations of brain death on a SPECT cerebral perfusion study. *Clin Nucl Med*. 1993;18:953-954.
52. Abdel Dayem HM, Bahar RH, Sigurdsson GH, et al. The hollow skull: a sign of brain death in Tc99m HM-PAO brain scintigraphy. *Clin Nucl Med*. 1989;14:912-916.
53. Galaske RG, Schober 0, Heyer R. ^{99m}Tc-HM-PAO and ^{123}I-amphetamine cerebral scintigraphy: a new, non-invasive method in determination of brain death in children. *Eur J Nucl Med*. 1988;14:446-452.
54. Schwartz JA, Baxter J, Brill DR. Diagnosis of brain death in children by radionuclide cerebral imaging. *Pediatrics*. 1984;73:14-18.
55. Coker SB, Dillehay GL. Radionuclide cerebral imaging for confirmation of brain death in children: the significance of dural sinus activity. *Pediatr Neurol*. 1986;2:43-46.

56. Goodman JM, Heck LL, Moore BD. Confirmation of brain death with portable isotope angiography: a review of 204 consecutive cases. *Neurosurgery.* 1985;16:492-497.
57. Holzman BH, Curless RG, Sfakianakis GN, et al. Radionuclide cerebral perfusion scintigraphy in determination of brain death in children. *Neurology.* 1983;33:1027-1031.
58. Greisen G. Cerebral blood flow in preterm infants during the first week of life. *Acta Paediatr Scand.* 1986;75:43-51.
59. Altman DL, Powers WJ, Perlman JM, et al. Cerebral blood flow requirements for brain viability in newborn infants is lower than in adults. *Ann Neurol.* 1988;24:218-226.
60. Darby JM, Yonas H, Gur D, et al. Xenon-enhanced computed tomography in brain death. *Arch Neurol.* 1987;44:551-554.
61. Greisen G, Pryds 0, Low CBF. Discontinuous EEG activity, and periventricular brain injury in ill, preterm neonates. *Brain Dev.* 1989;11:164-168
62. Medlock MD, Hanigan WC, Cruse RP. Dissociation of cerebral blood flow, glucose metabolism, and electrical activity in pediatric brain death. *J Neurosurg.* 1993;79:752-775.
63. Ducrocq X, Hassler W, Moritake K, et al. Consensus opinion on diagnosis of cerebral circulatory arrest using Doppler-sonography: Task Force Group on Cerebral Death of the Neurosonology Research Group of the World Federation of Neurology. *J Neurol Sci.* 1998;159:145-150.
64. McMenamin JB, Volpe JJ. Doppler ultrasonography in the determination of neonatal brain death. *Ann Neurol.* 1983;14:302-307.
65. Ahmann PA, Carrigan TA, Carlton D, et al. Brain death in children. Characteristic common carotid arterial velocity patterns measured with pulsed Doppler ultrasound. *J Pediatr.* 1987;110:723-728.
66. Qian SY, Fan XM, Yin HH. Transcranial Doppler assessment of brain death in children. *Singapore Med J.* 1998;39:247-250.
67. Feri M, Ralli L, Felici M, et al. Transcranial Doppler and brain death diagnosis. *Crit Care Med.* 1994;22:1120-1126.
68. Messer J, Burtscher A, Haddad J, et al. Contribution of transcranial Doppler sonography to the diagnosis of brain death in children. *Arch Fr Pediatr.* 1990;47:647-65 1.
69. Manno EM. Transcranial Doppler ultrasonography in the neurocritical care unit. *Crit Care Clin* 1997;13:79-104.
70. Jalili M, Crade M, Davis AL. Carotid blood-flow velocity changes detected by Doppler ultrasound in determination of brain death in children. A preliminary report. *Clin Pediatr Phila.* 1994;3:669-674.
71. Bode H, Sauer M, Pringsheim W. Diagnosis of brain death by transcranial Doppler sonography. *Arch Dis Child.* 1988;63:1474-1478.
72. Glasier CM, Seibert JJ, Chadduck WM, et al. Brain death in infants: evaluation with Doppler US. *Radiology.* 1989;172:377-380.
73. Sanker P, Roth B, Frowein RA, et al. Cerebral reperfusion in brain death of a newborn. Case report. *Neurosurg Rev.* 1992;15:315-317.
74. Chin NC, Shen EY, Lee BS. Reversal of diastolic cerebral blood flow in infants without brain death. *Pediatr Neurol.* 1994;11:337-340.
75. Van Bunnen Y, Delcour C, Wery D, et al. Intravenous digital subtraction angiography. A criteria of brain death. *Ann Radiol (Paris).* 1989;32:279-281.
76. Albertini A, Schonfeld S, Hiatt M, et al. Digital subtraction angiography-a new approach to brain death determination in the newborn. *Pediatr Radiol.* 1993;23:195-197.
77. Pistoia F, Johnson DW, Darby JM, et al. The role of xenon CT measurements of cerebral blood flow in the clinical determination of brain death. *AJNR Am J Neuroradiol.* 1991;12:97-103.
78. Meyer MA. Evaluating brain death with positron emission tomography: case report on dynamic imaging of ^{18}F-fluorodeoxyglucose activity after intravenous bolus injection. *J Neuroimaging.* 1996;6:117-119.
79. Orrison WW Jr, Champlin AM, Kesterson OL, et al. MR "hot nose sign" and "intravascular enhancement sign" in brain death. *AJNR Am J Neuroradiol.* 1994;15:913-916.
80. Lee DH, Nathanson JA, Fox AJ, et al. Magnetic resonance imaging of brain death. *Can Assoc. Radiol J.* 1995;46:174-178.
81. Matsumura A, Meguro K, Tsurushima H, et al. Magnetic resonance imaging of brain death. *Neurol Med Chir (Tokyo).* 1996;36:166-171.
82. Ishii K, Onuma T, Kinoshita T, et al. Brain death: MR and MR angiography. *AJNR Am J Neuroradiol.* 1996;17:731-735.
83. Holshouser BA, Ashwal S, Luh GY, et al. Proton MR spectroscopy after acute central nervous system injury: outcome prediction in neonates, infants and children. *Radiology.* 1997;202:487-496.

84. Martin E, Buchli R, Ritter S, et al. Diagnostic and prognostic value of cerebral ^{31}P magnetic resonance spectroscopy in neonates with perinatal asphyxia. *Pediatr Res.* 1996;40:749-758.
85. Kato T, Tokumaru A, O'uchi T, et al. Assessment of brain death in children by means of P-31 MR spectroscopy: preliminary note. *Radiology.* 1991;179:95-99.
86. Aichner F, Felber S, Birbamer G, et al: Magnetic resonance: a noninvasive approach to metabolism, circulation, and morphology in human brain death. *Ann Neurol.* 1992;32:507-511.
87. Terk MR, Gober JR, DeGiorgio C, et al. Brain death in the neonate: assessment with P-31 MR spectroscopy. *Radiology.* 1992;182:582-583.
88. Guerit JM. Evoked potentials: a safe brain-death confirmatory tool? *Eur J Med.* 1992;1:233-243.
89. Machado C, Valdes P, Garcia Tigera J, et al. Brain-stem auditory evoked potentials and brain death. *Electroencephalogr Clin Neurophysiol.* 1991;80:392-398.
90. Lutschg J, Pfenninger J, Ludin HP, et al. Brain-stem auditory evoked potentials and early somatosensory evoked potentials in neurointensively treated comatose children. *Am J Dis Child.* 1983;137:421-426.
91. Litscher G, Schwartz G, Kleinert R. Brainstem auditory evoked potential monitoring. Variations of stimulus artifact in brain death. *Electroencephalogr Clin Neurophysiol.* 1995;96:413-419.
92. Steinhart CM, Weiss IP. Use of brainstem auditory evoked potentials in pediatric brain death. *Crit Care Med.* 1985;13:560-562.
93. Taylor MJ, Houston BD, Lowry NJ. Recovery of auditory brainstem responses after a severe hypoxic ischemic insult. *N Engl J Med.* 1983;309:1169-1170.
94. Dear PRF, Godfrey DL Neonatal auditory brainstem response cannot reliably diagnose brainstem death. *Arch Dis Child.* 1985;60:17-19.
95. De Meirleir LJ, Taylor MJ. Evoked potentials in comatose children. Auditory brain stem responses. *Pediatr Neurol.* 1986;2:31-34.
96. Ruiz-Lopez MJ, Martinez de Azagra A, Serrano A, et al. Brain death and evoked potentials in pediatric patients. *Crit Care Med.* 1999;27:412-416.
97. Butinar D, Gostisa A. Brainstem auditory evoked potentials and somatosensory evoked potentials in prediction of posttraumatic coma in children. *Pflugers Arch.* 1996;431:R289-R290.
98. Beca J, Cox PN, Taylor MJ, et al. Somatosensory evoked potentials for prediction of outcome in acute severe brain injury. *J Pediatr.* 1995;126:44 49.
99. Wagner W. Scalp, earlobe and nasopharyngeal recordings of the median nerve somatosensory evoked p14 potential in coma and brain death. Detailed latency and amplitude analysis in 181 patients. *Brain.* 1996;119:1507-1521.
100. Machado C. Multimodality evoked potentials and electroretinography in a test battery for an early diagnosis of brain death. *J Neurosurg Sci.* 1993;37:125-131.
101. Goldie WD, Chiappa KH, Young RR, et al. Brainstem auditory and short-latency somatosensory evoked responses in brain death. *Neurology.* 1981;31:248-256.
102. Facco E, Casartelli Liviero M, Munari M, et al. Short latency evoked potentials: new criteria for brain death? *J Neurol Neurosurg Psychiatry.* 1990;53:351-353.
103. Kohrman MH. Brain death in neonates. *Semin Neurol.* 1993;13:116-122.
104. Freeman JM, Ferry PC. New brain death guidelines in children: further confusion. *Pediatrics.* 1988;81:301-303.
105. Coulter DL. Neurologic uncertainty in newborn intensive care. *N Engl J Med.* 1987;316:840-844.
106. American Medical Association. Council on Ethical and Judicial Affairs. The use of anencephalic neonates as organ donors. *JAMA.* 1995;273:1614-1618.
107. The Medical Task Force on Anencephaly: the infant with anencephaly. *N Engl J Med.* 1990;22:669-674.
108. Walters J, Ashwal S, Masek T. Anencephaly: where do we now stand? *Semin Neurol.* 1997;17:249-255.
109. Ashwal S, Peabody JL, Schneider S, et al. Anencephaly: clinical determination of brain death and neuropathologic studies. *Pediatr Neurol.* 1990;6:233-239.
110. Zimmer EZ, Jakobi P, Goldstein 1, et al. Cardiotocographic and sonographic findings in two cases of antenatally diagnosed intrauterine fetal brain death. *Prenat Diagn.* 1992;12:271-276.
111. Nijhuis JG, Crevels AJ, van Dongen PW. Fetal brain death: the definition of a fetal heart rate pattern and its clinical consequences. *Obstet Gynecol Surv.* 1990;45:229-232.
112. Adams RD, Prod'hom LS, Rabinowicz T. Intrauterine brain death. Neuraxial reticular core necrosis. *Acta Neuropathol (Berl).* 1977;40:41-49.
113. James SL Fetal brain death syndrome-a case report and literature review. *Aust N Z J Obstet Gynaecol.* 1998;38:217-220.

114. Goldstein B, DeKing D, DeLong DJ, et al. Autonomic cardiovascular state after severe brain injury and brain death in children. *Crit Care Med.* 1993;21:228-233.
115. Doroshow RW, Ashwal S, Saukel GW. Availability and selection of donors for pediatric heart transplantation. *J Heart Lung Transplant.* 1995;14:52-58.
116. Duthie SE, Peterson BM, Cutler J, et al. Successful organ donation in victims of child abuse. *Clin Transplant.* 1995;9:415-418.

Requesting Organ Donation: Effective Communication

Laura A. Siminoff, PhD
Anne Kean
Teresa Shafer, RN, MSN, CPTC
Rebecca Teagarden, BS, MA
Stacey Wertlieb, MBe
Meredith Wylie, BA, MA
Sheldon Zink, PhD

What Is Effective Communication?

To be successful, organ procurement organizations (OPOs) must be able to obtain consent for organ donation. Despite donor registries, first person consent, and the sharp rise in living donation, transplantation medicine continues to rely on the donation of organs from deceased individuals. Most of these requests are made to the deceased's next-of-kin. Of all the activities performed by OPOs, obtaining consent to donation is *the* most important activity because it facilitates all other aspects of the organ procurement and transplantation process.

Successful requests for organ donation involve communicating with families about the option to donate, providing them with sufficient information to make an informed decision, and maximizing their ability to consider the request. Although it is the goal of each approach to obtain consent from families to donate some or all of the potential donor's organs, research has shown that families frequently refuse these requests.[1-3] Thus, requesters have to determine how to approach donation discussions in a manner that is supportive of the grieving family but still achieves the goal of obtaining consent to donation. In other words, requests must be persuasive but not coercive.

Making a request for organ donation requires communication of information and intent between requester and family. Effective communication is therefore at the heart of the donation request process. Basic communication theory and research conducted over the past decade into the communication and decision-making process for organ donation allows us to identify effective practices in the black community as well.

Communication research suggests that certain types of messages are more effective than others. Early work found that refutational messages (those dispelling false beliefs) were more persuasive than 1-sided (positive) messages in creating behavioral change – for example, signing an organ donor card.[4] Ford and Smith[5] also found that refutational messages appear to be more persuasive than 1-sided messages. Another study reported that although refutational messages are not well processed, they result in greater belief and behavioral change.[6] Finally, Siminoff et al[1] have demonstrated that provision of specific information about the benefits of donation is important to dispelling (refuting) false beliefs and persuading families to donate. Other researchers have investigated the cognitive and affective responses to statistical and narrative persuasive messages.[7-9] Statistical messages have been found to have a greater impact over time, whereas narrative messages were found to produce more affective (emotional) reactions. Indeed, a large study[1] of family attitudes and knowledge about donation found that providing specific information about organ donation, its need, and its process, to potential donor families increased the likelihood of donation 5-fold.

Similar to many healthcare communications, individuals' own beliefs, attitudes, and values act as a filter in interpreting information. Therefore, requesters need to engage families in a discussion of key donation-related issues and use active listening skills for communication to be effective. For example,

Chapter 30 REQUESTING ORGAN DONATION: EFFECTIVE COMMUNICATION

research has demonstrated that families are often concerned about whether donation will add to the hospital bill; worry about funeral expenses and funeral arrangements; and are unclear if they have a choice as to what to donate.[1] Discussing these issues with the family, even if the family has not raised these issues, provides an opportunity for several things to happen. First, important information is conveyed to the family. Second, requesters give permission to families to engage in discussions about potentially important topics. Finally, requesters increase a sense of relationship and trust between themselves and the family during a stressful and emotional time.[10] The goal, then, is to build rapport, reduce uncertainty, and exchange information.[11] These relational messages, sent and received by both members of the interaction, influence how the interaction unfolds.[12] Using effective communication, requesters are mindful of these relational aspects, present messages in ways that are generally effective but cognizant of families' different sociodemographic traits and personalities, and are aware of the emotional climate in which the exchange takes place.

The remainder of this chapter provides evidence compiled from over a decade of research, and explores ways in which to effectively communicate with families about organ donation.

The Consent Environment

An effective donation environment is established well before the potential donor admission. It is aided by the hospital's system-wide commitment to unconditionally identify all opportunities for donation. The consent environment includes not only the entire milieu of the critical care unit at the time of the patient's hospitalization, such as nursing, medical, and other hospital staff roles and attitudes, behaviors, and practice, but also the senior and executive level administrative support for donation. The organ recovery coordinator should be an integral *member* (not an invited guest) of the hospital healthcare team. Recently, hospitals have given offices in the unit or in close proximity to the unit, allowing the OPO to place an in-house coordinator (IHC) in the hospital. Such scenarios signal to hospital staff the importance hospital leadership gives organ donation and contribute to staff trust of the OPO staff member. Dickerson et al[13] noted the importance of healthcare attitudes toward donation and commented on the presence of the IHC making the process less "onerous for the physicians." However, even in the absence of a structured OPO presence within the 4 hospital walls, the hospital can make commitments to organ donation that provide strong executive, medical, and nursing support for organ donation and create an environment that is designed to achieve high (75% or greater) organ donation conversion rates.

The hi-tech intensive care unit environment can be intimidating to families who are coping with grief and extreme stress. Donor families have identified the most stressful aspects of this situation as: (1) the threat of losing a loved one, (2) adjusting to the loss, and (3) confirmation of brain death.[14] High levels of anxiety also surround the decision of whether to continue maintaining a family member on life support.[15,16] Heightened emotions and extreme stress make information processing more difficult, especially when it is delivered in medical jargon.[16]

Several factors may mitigate this stress and enhance the climate in which organ donation is discussed, including the support of family and friends,[17] being able to spend time with the patient, and receiving information and emotional support.[18,19] Another important factor is to provide families with adequate time to understand the patient's condition. Thus, it is important that families be made aware of the patient's condition and that they be allowed to confirm their understanding to the healthcare professional.[20] Families also need to be prepared to hear a request about organ donation. Families who are surprised by the donation request or who feel harassed or pressured to make a decision are less likely to donate than families who did not feel surprised or pressured (66% vs 34% and 66% vs 34%, respectively).[1] Once the request is made, families need to have time to discuss the request, consider it, and ask as many questions as needed.

Displays of empathy can contribute to the family's perception of the request.[21] Families who believe that the healthcare providers involved are not caring or concerned are somewhat less likely to donate.[1] Poor communication with the family about the patient and lack of trust between the family members and the healthcare staff can contribute to a perception of poor quality of care for the patient.[15] Dissatisfaction with hospital care can have ramifications for donation rates, because donor families tend to be more satisfied with the quality of care in the hospital than nondonor families.[18]

A major barrier to the creation of a donation-friendly environment that is sensitive to the psychosocial needs of families is the lack of time OPO staff often have with the family. One solution is for the OPO staff person to have a daily presence within the hospital, or, at the very least, for the OPO to have a significant presence in the hospital. This way, the staff person may more easily interact early and spend more time with families. If not, an effective introduction by hospital staff achieved at an appropriate time, and as early as possible, can maximize interaction between the OPO staff and the family. Obtaining consent does not consist of simply asking the family if they wish to donate, in essence, "popping the question." The consent environment should also consist of providing a steady stream of information to families about the condition of the patient and the purpose of all tests and treatments. Previous research has revealed that families who are satisfied with their hospital experience are more predisposed to donate.[18,22] Receiving timely information is critical to families' satisfaction with their hospital experience.

The coordinator and hospital staff collaboratively control effective consent requests. Together they can anticipate and avoid hesitation when positively framing the request.[23] Hospital-based interventions, such as the IHC and family support coordinators, have been implemented in efforts to provide a more supportive donation environment for families. These interventions have focused on several aspects of the request process: bereavement and emotional support services,[24,25] clarification of roles of the support team, and streamlining referral protocols.[26,27] In another study by DeJong et al,[18] responses from donor and nondonor families could be differentiated on the basis of reactions to requesters' attitudes. During interviews with family members who participated in the donation request process, the researchers found that 97% (n=102) of families involved in donor cases compared with only 59% (n=62) of those in nondonor cases agreed that the person who initiated the request did so in a way that was sensitive to the needs and concerns of the family members. Similarly, 97% of donors agreed that the person who approached the family with consent forms was sensitive, whereas only 62% of nondonors supported that claim. Therefore, displays of sensitivity and support can influence donation decisions.

It should be noted that donor families report that organ donation helped with their grief process and can be part of the effort to create meaning from a tragic and senseless loss.[14,28] In addition, the opportunity to decide about organ donation is often the first time during the hospitalization of the patient that family members feel a sense of control.[29] The chance to make a decision about organ donation is therefore an opportunity that family members should be offered, even if healthcare providers feel hesitant about offering donation to a particular family.[1]

Recent work from the US Department of Health and Human Services Organ Donation Breakthrough Collaborative has also introduced the practice of a "team huddle" before staff-family interaction. On the basis of the concept that collective knowledge is powerful, planning the approach and anticipating roadblocks or objections, the organ procurement coordinator along with the entire healthcare team is prepared to assume any role he or she might need to assume on the basis of the family's reaction to the request. Put simply, all members of the team are prepared, knowledgeable, and pulling in the same direction. During the huddle, a plan is developed with input from every member of the healthcare team present, with the end goal of obtaining family consent for donation. As self-evident as it may seem, a plan and clear knowledge of how each member of the team will respond if called upon will result in a successful outcome more often than "winging it." The number of families who consent to donate determines success of the process.

For the actual consent request, the OPO staff person should identify an area and structure the physical and emotional environment so that it is private, accepting, caring, and conducive to communication and comfortable for the family who will be asked to donate. A private family waiting room is desirable, but circumstances may require greater flexibility such as locating an empty patient room, office, or conference room. A private area will allow the coordinator to control environmental stimuli, which can affect a family's ability to function, cope, and understand detailed information. In advance, the OPO coordinator can provide for comfort for the family by furnishing an adequate number of chairs, and having water, tissues, and a phone with access to outside lines available.

The Table presents a summary of items that effectively establish a positive consent environment. Many of the items on the checklist are accomplished before any particular donor event, but all contribute to a positive environment for the donation process within the hospital and to a successful donation program.

Chapter 30 REQUESTING ORGAN DONATION: EFFECTIVE COMMUNICATION

Structuring the Consent Environment – Checklist

1. Educate hospital staff who work with potential donor families (medical, nursing, social workers, pastoral care) about organ donation issues and processes and provide ongoing opportunities for their questions and concerns to be addressed. Dispel the many myths surrounding organ donation.
   - Clarify respective roles of hospital and OPO personnel in the donation process continuum, and educate both regarding complementary roles
2. Create as much family support continuity of care as possible during the potential donor's hospitalization. When the family needs to be notified of the patient's presence at hospital, a social worker or chaplain who can meet them on arrival should call them initially. When emergency department family support staff differs from intensive care unit family support staff, provide an opportunity to pass the case off, and directly introduce the family to the new staff.
3. Start early to understand family dynamics, identify key decision maker(s), monitor status, and support family needs.
   - Meet with the family as soon as possible after arrival in a private space to provide honest and compassionate communication about what is known about the patient's illness/injury, establishing trust that team will be forthright and sensitive throughout process.
   - Orient family to hospital setting, available resources, intensive care unit guidelines and expectations, and means of contacting team. Provide this information in writing when possible.
   - Assess whether there is a difference between next-of-kin (or healthcare proxy) and actual family decision maker/leader. Share information about family dynamics, needs, and decision makers between hospital and OPO staff.
   - Begin assessment of family dynamics and spiritual and cultural needs. Involve spiritual and cultural leaders in family support as appropriate.
   - Communicate in the family's primary language and at a level at which they can understand.
4. OPO and hospital staff jointly develop plan for providing family support. If OPO is going to interact with the family before potential request, try to use relationship with hospital team to transfer trust to OPO.
5. Assess the family's understanding of the gravity of the situation and provide information about the patient's condition. Encourage the family to write down questions if this is helpful to them and use appropriate team members to address their questions and concerns as they arise.
6. Create and implement joint OPO/hospital plan for brain-death explanation; continually assess the family's understanding of brain death and continue to provide and reinforce information as case progresses.
7. Create and implement joint OPO/hospital plan for effective donation request at appropriate time. Designate an effective request leader who can manage process whether he or she will be directly approaching the family for consent.
8. Choose the most effective person to initiate discussion with family regarding donation.
   - Match requesters appropriately to family, ensuring effective requesters are available (effective determined by actual documented consent rate of requester)
   - Special requesters specific to the ethnicity of the OPO service area population may be provided by the OPO.
   - Because of donation expertise and *time availability*, OPO staff are normally the dominant presence in the consent process. If, however, a hospital staff member is determined to be the most effective requester and the one who will make the request, the OPO staff must be present with the requester to set the stage for reapproach if necessary.
9. Give the family the time they need to discuss donation, ask questions, and surface their concerns and fears. Dispel the many myths the family may have heard about organ donation. If the family is opposed to donation, explore whether their concerns can be addressed and reapproach whenever possible.
10. Continue to meet with the family regardless of their consent decision, to provide emotional and logistical support. Provide written information when possible about grief, funeral issues, community resources, and, if the patient is a donor, about donation process and follow-up support resources.
11. Include hospital family support staff in post-donor OPO/hospital case review to explore areas for future improvement.
12. Closely monitor consent rates, provide feedback to requesters on their rates of success, and make changes as indicated by performance.

Abbreviation: OPO, organ procurement organization.

Introducing the OPO Staff

Research has unequivocally demonstrated that OPO staff members are the best individuals to discuss organ donation with families. Hospital staff are often reluctant to introduce organ donation as an option at the end of life and cannot spend the time needed with families. OPO staff members are generally better trained and more comfortable with discussing organ donation with families.[1,2,30,31]

For example, Gortmaker and colleagues[2] found in an examination of cases involving 707 potential donors that the highest consent rates occurred when OPO staff were present to make requests. Similar results were demonstrated in a study by Siminoff et al.[1] Healthcare provider endorsement can be helpful and optimally OPO staff should be introduced by the patient's nurse or physician to the family. The continued positive presence of the hospital healthcare provider can also make a positive contribution.[2,30,31]

Early Referral and Timing of the Request

Effective requests for donation require adequate time for the OPO requesters to assess each family's situation and adequate time to spend with the family. Current regulations mandate that hospitals notify the local OPO of all deaths and imminent deaths, and that hospital and OPO staff collaborate to ensure that all families of potential donors be approached about donation.[32] Unfortunately, many referrals are made too late to support effective consent. Referrals made after the patient has been declared brain dead, taken off mechanical supports, or the decision has been made to withdraw supports, are unlikely to result in a successful request. In fact, premature removal of mechanical supports is a major barrier to organ donation.[33]

Thus, no other single intervention to a successful consent environment and outcome is more important than timely notification.[23] Families start receiving information about the condition of their loved one, start asking questions, and various needs arise early on in the course of a critical illness or event. The donation "process," therefore, begins long before the formal discussion of organ donation begins.[34] If the referral is made in a timely manner, within 1 hour of meeting a clinical trigger for referral, such as achieving a Glasgow Coma Scale of 5 or less, a rushed approach to requesting consent from families can be avoided.[34] Hospital and OPO staff must communicate early – well before brain death is pronounced – to develop an approach plan. Protocols should be jointly established between hospital and OPO staff to ensure early identification and timely referral of potential donors.[35] The ability of OPO staff to interact early with potential donor families allows them time to establish a relationship with families and hopefully establish trust, a critical element in families consenting to donation.

Initial concerns about timing of organ donation requests focused on when the request was made vis a vis the pronouncement of death. The concept of "decoupling," that is, separating requests for organs from informing the family that the patient has died, has been promoted as an important factor since the early 1990s.[36] However, a closer look at the concept reveals that decoupling, per se, is not influential on consent rates. One early retrospective review of 155 consecutive donor referrals reported that decoupling resulted in higher consent rates.[36] Unfortunately, the study only included cases in which the OPO had been called, which skewed study results through selection bias. Another retrospective review[30] demonstrated a nonsignificant trend toward consent being more likely if the donation request was made subsequent to notification of death. On the other hand, a similar study[37] indicated that timing made no difference. In a more comprehensive study, Niles et al[38] retrospectively analyzed all calls to an OPO over 23 months. They found that asking at the time of death was associated with a lower consent rate (25%; 3 of 12 cases donated), but there was no difference between requests before (62%; 32 of 52) and after death (57%; 36 of 63).[38] Finally, Siminoff et al[33] failed to find support for decoupling in a large prospective study. Instead, this study found that asking *before* notification of brain death was associated with higher consent rates (63.0% vs 56.6%). Rather, timing is important not to decouple requests, but to allow OPO staff to spend significant time with the family.

Early referral of potential donors to OPOs is paramount to facilitating effective consent, but is not the entire picture. For example, Beasley and colleagues[39] developed a 2-year intervention to increase consent rates.[2] The intervention, implemented and evaluated in 50 hospitals, included education of healthcare professionals and 3 process elements: (1) decoupling--separating the request for organ donation from the declaration of death; (2) privacy; and (3) OPO participation. Although the intervention increased referrals by 25% and requests to families by 17%, the rate of consent remained at 51%. In other studies,[27,40] these practices have been found to have similar results. Thus, hospital development programs are necessary prerequisites, but not sufficient in and of themselves to increase organ donation consent rates. Successful hospital development programs alone have led to an increase in the number of donors identified, but not to an increase in organ donation conversion rates.

Data suggest that early and consistent involvement of OPO staff increases organ donation when it is coupled with effective communication. In a small study[41] of a single hospital in Texas, use of early notification and an IHC was associated with an increase in donation rates from 25% (n=15 of the 60 medically suitable referrals in 1994) to 72% (n=39 of the 54 of medically eligible potential donors in 1996). Other studies of IHCs by this same group have replicated these results.[41] In another study, Burris et al[42] found that consent rates were higher when OPO coordinators spoke to families before physicians or nurses. In a recent large, descriptive study of the donor request process, Siminoff et al[1,33] reported that the most important extrinsic factor to obtaining consent to organ donation was time spent by family decision makers with OPO staff requesters and discussing specific donation-related issues.

In sum, early referral allows OPO requesters to coordinate the donation request process and spend significant time with the potential donor family. Successful procurement involves (1) developing a functional and working relationship with hospitals to facilitate time-sensitive referrals of potential donor patients, and (2) communicating with families about the donation option in a way that provides them with sufficient information to make an informed decision within an environment that optimizes their ability to consider the request.

Being an Advocate for Organ Donation

Favorable attitudes of healthcare providers and OPO requesters have been demonstrated to have a positive impact on donation consent rates. In one study,[43] it was shown that requesters who had confidence in their abilities to obtain consent, in addition to those who believed that donation could be beneficial to families, tended to have higher consent rates. For instance, in cases in which requesters believed that families would consent if asked, 56% of families agreed to donate, whereas only 29% of families consented to the requests of those who did not. Further, when requesters believed that organ donation would help families grieve, 44% of families consented, compared to 32% for those who did not.[43] Finally, when requesters specifically endorsed organ donation by making positive statements to families about organ donation, consent rates were higher.[43]

Explaining Brain Death

For families to make an informed decision about organ donation, they need to understand the concept of brain death, which is often misunderstood. Results of a word-association experiment suggest that people interpret the term "brain dead" differently than "dead."[44] In another study,[45] using an experimental simulation method, researchers found that only 30% of subjects correctly interpreted the meaning of brain death. Both studies revealed that brain death is perceived as less than terminal. This finding was affirmed by a 1993 Gallup poll,[46] in which 21% of respondents thought it possible for a brain-dead person to recover from his or her injury. A more recent study[47] reported similar misunderstandings. For the potential donor families who actually see the patient who has been declared brain dead, the concept has proven no easier to understand. Part of the difficulty is that brain-dead patients show signs of viability–they are "breathing" and warm to the touch.

Many studies of families who have made a donation decision report that even after receiving an explanation of brain death from a physician, families fail to grasp the concept. Nonetheless, many of these families consent to donation even when they do not understand that their loved one is dead. A study[25] of 99 families who consented to donation found that the explanations provided were too vague to comprehend and led many families to consent to donation before an understanding of this concept. In a small study[14] of donor family members, 5 of 9 families felt that the explanation of brain death was insufficient to come to terms with the patient's death.

The issue, therefore, is not whether brain death is explained to families, but how it is explained. One of the larger studies[20] of families who were asked to donate found that those families who had received an explanation of brain death did not show significantly greater knowledge than those who did not receive an explanation. Twenty-eight percent of donors and 45% of nondonors associated brain death with coma; 12% of donor and 27% of nondonors disagreed with the statement that brain death is death even though the heart is still beating; and 20% of donors and 52% of nondonors thought that recovery is possible when a person is brain dead. Brain death explanations must provide clear and simple explanations with as little use of medical jargon as possible.[48]

In a large survey of the general public (n=1351), 28% thought "brain dead" people can hear. Only 40% classified someone who is brain dead as "dead," whereas 43% classified brain dead as "as good as dead," and 16% stated that brain-dead persons are "alive." Nonetheless, almost 80% of respondents who defined brain death as "as good as dead," and 66% who defined it as "alive," were willing to donate.[47]

In a 1987 study, Batten and Prottas[28] reported that 39% of donor families found the concept of brain death difficult to understand but still donated. Another study[49] found that willingness to donate in a hypothetical situation was correlated with certainty of death but not understanding of brain death. Siminoff and colleagues[50] have also examined this issue and explored its impact on consent to donation. Their findings reveal that although brain death is not effectively explained to families, almost all (96%) families were told about brain death. In this study, only 28% were able to provide a completely correct definition of brain death. Despite lack of comprehension, no association was found between the families' understanding of brain death and willingness to donate. Rather, an association was found between the families' consent to donation and the families' acceptance that the patient's condition was hopeless; 60% families who had given up hope for a recovery donated compared to 48% who had not. Moreover, in this same study, 57% of families who were unsure when their loved one's death had occurred donated.[51] The evidence, therefore, points to the conclusion that *understanding brain death does not determine a family's willingness to consent to donation.*

Ensuring that families understand the concept of brain death is important to guarantee that consent is informed. To ensure understanding, requesters must provide an explanation that is simple and eschews medical jargon. Studies have shown that explanations of brain death provided to families are often inconsistent and obscured by medical jargon. Families expect to see visible signs of death and will be confused when the patients appear, to their eyes, alive. Thus, care must be taken to explain that these signs of life are artificial and a result of machines. Requesters should avoid the use of the term "life support."

Discussing Funeral Arrangements, Mutilation, and Costs of Donation

Many Americans still have fears and beliefs that are impediments to consent to organ donation. The following have been identified as issues that are of concern to many donor-eligible families as they consider whether to donate: (1) concern over funeral arrangements; (2) fear of disfigurement; and (3) confusion about the costs of donation to the family. Families have been found to have concerns about funeral arrangements after organ donation. Batten and Prottas[28] reported that 19% of the 242 donor families surveyed had unanswered questions about funeral arrangements. Another study reported that less than half of families asked to donate had been provided with information about funeral arrangements.[50] Numerous studies have also examined families' concerns about mutilation or disfigurement of the body.[52,53] Maintaining the integrity of the body after death is important to many cultures and religions where biological death must be acknowledged as the social death of the person. For many individuals, part of that process is viewing the body of the deceased during the funeral.[54,55] Fear of mutilation is especially pronounced in the African-American community.[56,57]

Finally, 2 studies[1,50] have explored the issue of costs of donation to the donor family. The most recent study[1] found a significant impact with families who refused donation having had fewer discussions about this issue compared to donor families. Overall, most families stated that this was an issue they would have wanted to discuss.

In conclusion, families hold misconceptions about donation-related issues. Moreover, they often do not share their concerns with OPO personnel or healthcare providers. It is important to be aware that such concerns may exist even if families do not bring them up. Reassurances that donation will not have an effect on funeral arrangements and information about the costs of donation are crucial pieces of information for families. Families also need to be reassured that the donor's body will be treated respectfully.

Patient Donation Wishes and First Person Consent

Families' knowledge of the wishes of the deceased is one of the most important factors when deciding whether to donate.[1,16,29,58] Two major reasons for not consenting to donation are knowledge of the deceased's wish not to donate and being unsure of the deceased's wishes.[45,52,53,59] Conversely, knowing that the patient had a donor card, having had an explicit discussion about donation with the patient, and a belief the patient would have wanted to donate, even exclusive of an explicit discussion, are strongly associated with consent to organ donation.[1,18,45,60] Few families actually refuse donation if presented with evidence of the patient's wishes to donate. Unfortunately, only a minority of people discusses donation with their families or has a donor card.[2,18,56]

Requesters should assume that in cases in which the wishes of the patient are not known, families attempt to use what they know about the attributes of the deceased, hoping to honor what the patient would have wanted.[16,61] It is a less frequent scenario that a family's wishes conflict with the explicit wishes of the patient.[18]

When definitive documentation of wishes is available, attitudes toward decision making are more uniform. Surveys of both the lay public and of transplant professionals indicate that the majority believes that the family's objections should not overrule a signed donor card.[62,63] An early telephone survey of the general public (n=2056) found that 58% of respondents felt that if a person signs a donor card, his or her decision should not be subjected to familial approval. Moreover, 71% believed that displays of disapproval by family members should not override the potential donor's wishes as expressed on a donor card, whereas 17% felt that family members' wishes should take precedence, and 12% were undecided.[64] In a more recent survey of 739 transplant-related professionals, Oz and colleagues[63] found that 84% felt that patients' next-of-kin should be asked for consent, but 77% further stipulated that consultation should not be required if the potential donor had a signed donor card.

OPOs are now confronted with how to proceed when presented with evidence that the patient wanted to donate. A survey[65] of 61 OPOs conducted in 2001 indicates that 12% of OPOs would move ahead with organ donation in the presence of definitive documentation of the patient's wishes. In cases in which the deceased wanted to donate, but next-of-kin cannot be located, 77% of OPOs indicated they would procure based on documentation. Overall, 31% of OPOs said that they would follow the wishes of the deceased, 31% would follow the next-of-kin's wishes, 21% would procure if neither party objects, and 13% would procure if either party consents or if neither objects.

Presently, all but 9 states have legislation in place that recognizes the primacy of the deceased documented wish to donate (known as first person consent).[66] In Pennsylvania, for example, the standard request procedure consists of OPO coordinators either reaffirming the donor's wishes with family members (in lieu of asking for permission) or making a request for donation in the event that wishes were not documented by the implementation of first person consent laws now in their first stages. Although the vast majority of states has employed or is in the process of drafting legislation, the lack of standardization concerning the scope of legal practices has, for instance, hindered the potential of state-to-state transfer.[67] Given the importance families place on following patients' wishes, implementation of first person consent should increase donation. Furthermore, unlike in the past, donor cards and license registry take on renewed importance. Donor registries that are accessible to OPO requesters are key to optimizing the potential of first person consent laws.

The Divided/Dysfunctional Family

Conflicts within families over donation make the process of decision making difficult and tend to result in refusing consent. Unfortunately, little except anecdotal information is available to confirm or disconfirm its impact on consent rates. One study concluded that when hostile family dynamics exist, such as parents who are divorced, the conflict will result in a refusal to donate. Moreover, in certain cultural communities, consultation with extended family members before making important decisions is deemed to be an essential practice. In many Hispanic and Asian communities, the legal next-of-kin will defer to family elders. Any expression of skepticism by the elder about donation is likely to result in refusal to donate.[68] Other groups who rely on opinions of elders or group leaders include the Amish and certain evangelical Christian groups. Increasing the number of opinions being considered has been shown to complicate efforts to arrive at the resolution to donate.[59] In a study of 68 cases involving potential donors in Spain, Martinez et al[59] documented that 4 of the 18 refusals involved family conflicts. In the coordinator's opinion, families that maintained "regular or poor relations" were disproportionately represented among the instances of refusal[59].

Organ Donation and Minorities

Minority groups have a pressing need for transplantable organs, especially kidneys. Yet most minorities have rates of donation that are half that of white Americans. A 1993 Gallup Poll found that expressed support of organ donation for whites, blacks, and Hispanic Americans were 87%, 69%, and 75%, respectively.[36] A similar finding was reported in a 1998 study by Yuen et al.[69] Minorities are also less likely to have made a decision about organ donation for themselves. Forty-five percent of white respondents indicated that they had made a decision about the donation of their own organs, and 27% had considered the donation of relatives' organs. In contrast, only 21% of blacks stated that they would donate their own organs and only 12% had considered donating a relative's organs. Forty percent of Hispanic Americans reported they had made a decision for themselves and 19% had made a decision about a family member.[46]

Studies have explored the reasons for these differences. Lack of communication between family members has been described as 1 barrier to increasing consent rates among minorities.[56,70,71] A survey by Siminoff and Arnold[71] found that 58% of white respondents had discussed their wishes with family members, compared to 42% of blacks. The 1993 Gallup Poll reported that 28% of blacks and 29% of Hispanic Americans were hesitant to discuss organ donation with their families compared to only 17% of white respondents.[36] Twenty-one percent of the Hispanic respondents attributed their lack of familial communication to the fact that they do not discuss death.[46] Other studies report similar findings.[72,73]

Other contributing factors to the lack of donations among minorities have been frequently cited in the literature and include a lack of awareness about the need;[56,70,73-76] lack of referrals;[74] distrust of the medical community;[56,73-76] fear that a loved one will be declared dead prematurely;[56,71,74-76] fear of bodily mutilation;[56,70,71,73] religious myths;[71,73-76] and reluctance to discuss death.[56,70] Blacks in particular are concerned that organs will not be given to other blacks[73-76] and are affected by their experiences of institutional racism.[56] Language barriers[70,74] and the role of the extended family[70,74] are particularly salient barriers for Hispanic Americans.

There are some data that indicate minority donation rates can be increased through the use of ethnically sensitive IHCs or like-like requesters. In 1997, Shafer and colleagues[77] demonstrated that through the use of black IHCs at a hospital that served a large proportion of indigent and minority populations, black consent rates rose from 34% (1993-1995) to 73% in 1996, and rates among Hispanic Americans increased during the same period from 50% to 74%. Similarly, another study[78] found that when a black OPO coordinator handled request discussions with black families, referral rates rose from 8% to 15%, and consent rates increased from 0% to 60% in 1994 and to 80% in 1995. Kappel et al[79] reported an increase in consent rates by employing a black health educator to request donation from black families. Although these results appear to be rather convincing, not all studies have supported the use of race-specific requesters. In its Consent Analysis Summary, the Indiana Organ Procurement Organization[80] found that higher consent rates across all races were obtained when nonlike requesters carried out conversations with families of potential donors.

Two major problems affecting the request process with minorities have been found in the hospital setting. First, patients who are members of ethnic minorities are less likely to be identified by the healthcare team as potential donors. Hartwig et al[81] found that white patients were significantly more likely to be identified as potential donors than black patients. Second, families of white patients were approached for donation more frequently (69%) than families of black patients (46%).[81] Reluctance to identify and approach minority families about donation may be related to stereotyping of minorities as unwilling to donate and lack of experience with nonmajority cultures.[75,82]

In a study[82] that compared black and white families' donation request experiences, blacks were uniformly viewed as less likely to want to donate, and their views on organ donation were more frequently misconstrued when compared to white families. Black families also were less likely to meet with an OPO requester, spent less time with the OPO requester, and had less complete discussions about organ donation when compared to white families.[82]

Organ donation efforts for minority communities must also work to promote public education to dispel some of the deeply embedded myths and fears through culturally sensitive methods. Additionally, appropriate training of healthcare professionals and OPO staff members in terms of communication with families of minority patients is crucial toward establishing trust in the healthcare system. Finally, those requesting donation must shed their stereotypes of who will or will not consent to organ donation and provide complete and comprehensive information about donation to all families.

Presumptive Consent

The presumptive approach is based on the premise that families want to donate and given the opportunity to save a life, most people will. Organ donation is believed to be "the right thing to do." Thus, the presumptive approach takes a positive, affirmative stance toward donation. The presumptive approach is a shift in language, which reflects a sensitive yet positive view of donation, presenting it as the correct and natural decision, while continuing to address concerns as they arise. This is a change from the current consent discussion, which is often an approach focused on obtaining permission and overcoming family objections while presenting donation in a neutral manner. In either approach, the family makes the final, fully informed decision.

Presumptivity is simply an alteration in the way the coordinator presents the information. The hallmark of this approach is offering a family the "opportunity to donate" rather than the "option of donation." This subtle shift embodies the philosophy that donation is a good thing, and that families want to donate whenever possible as opposed to something that families are forced to consider. In this way, the presumptive approach lessens what some perceive as an unnecessary burden on families in grief, the decision to donate, by affirming decedent wishes and ensuring families that donation is the right thing to do.

The presumptive approach was developed and is being tested through a 4-year Health Resources and Services Administration-funded research study, "A Study of the Presumptive Approach to Consent for Organ Donation.[83] To quantify the success of a presumptive approach, the approach was defined by the use of 6 key elements: (1) intention to be presumptive; (2) introducing the OPO requester as part of the medical team or donation expert; (3) use of a presumptive transition from discussion of brain death to organ donation; (4) explicit references to recipients during the donation conversation (e.g., referencing the number of people on the transplant waiting list); (5) use of presumptive statements about donation, such as, "Based on what I am hearing about your daughter, donating organs to help so many others is a fitting way to commemorate your daughter's legacy"; and (6) use of a presumptive ask (e.g., assuming the person will donate). Preliminary data analysis shows an increase of 10% in consent rates among transplant coordinators using the presumptive approach over a 6-month period.

Reapproach After a Refusal to Donate

OPO requesters must often reapproach a family about organ donation. This should always occur if the expression of disinterest was to a hospital healthcare provider. The reason for this is that hospital healthcare providers are poor judges of families' openness to donation. In one study[1] of 420 cases, hospital healthcare providers were correct in their assessment of families' initial response to donation requests only 47% of the time. Thus, the hospital's initial assessment of a refusal to donate always merits reapproach. Reapproach should also be considered even when the families' initial refusal was to an OPO staff person.

Several studies have demonstrated the potential of family members to alter their original position when making a final donation decision. For example, Frutos et al[53], in a study of 248 potential donors, found that 13 of 64 families that initially refused donation, in addition to 25 of 38 families who were undecided, eventually consented when reapproached. Another study found that when donation was first discussed with donor-eligible families, 38% were initially favorable, 17% were undecided, and 45% were opposed to donation. Those that expressed an initial willingness to donate were provided with significantly more information on donation than those who were undecided or unfavorable. The mean number of items pertaining to donation that were discussed with favorable families was 11. Means for families that were unsure and those that initially refused dropped to 6.[50] This indicates that families who do not express an initial willingness to donate may not receive an appropriate or thoughtful request process.

Conclusions

The role of the OPO requester is to obtain consent to organ donation. This may be the most difficult and complex task in the process of providing lifesaving transplantation medicine to the thousands of Americans in need each year. Success is dependent on several factors including the creation of an appropriate "donor culture" within hospitals, timely referral of potential donor patients to the OPO, and communicating effectively with family decision makers.

The evidence to date suggests that the following constitute effective communication practices:

- Create a supportive environment in which to discuss organ donation with the family.
- Work with hospital staff ahead of time so that they are comfortable introducing the OPO requester to the family. Welcome supportive hospital staff as request partners, but be aware that the OPO requester is trained to play the central role in discussing donation with the family.
- It is not necessary to "decouple" the request from the declaration of death. Although families' understanding of brain death is an ethical requirement, it does not affect consent rates. Discussions of brain death should be simple, jargon-free, and unequivocal that brain death means the patient has died.
- Earlier rather than later discussions about organ donation are more likely to be successful.
- Consent to organ donation is higher when families have understood that the patients' injuries are fatal. Honest communication about the patient's condition is crucial.
- Spend as much time as necessary with the family. Increased time with OPO staff is strongly associated with increased consent rates. Building a relationship is critical.
- The OPO staff person must be an advocate for organ donation. Positive messages and endorsement of organ donation, use of statistics to support the need for donation, and information that refutes the most common myths about donation must be conveyed to the family.
- Engage all families in discussions about organ donation. Remember to reassure families about disfigurement, funeral arrangements and that donation will not cost the family anything. Actively listen to the families' concerns.
- Discuss what the patient wanted. If the family is unsure, discuss the patient's values and appeal to their knowledge about how organ donation can fulfill those values. Note how few people can actually donate upon death and that most Americans support organ donation.

- In complex family situations, make sure all parties are heard and acknowledged.
- Assume that every family wants to donate, no matter their religion, race or ethnicity.
- Always reapproach families who have not had a discussion with an OPO staff person. Consider reapproaching any family who has not had adequate time to discuss donation with a knowledgeable requester.

Comprehensive request models such as the dual advocate model and presumptivity seem to be effective. These models essentially combine many of the elements reviewed in this chapter. These approaches should be combined with programs that train requesters in basic health communication skills and outstanding hospital development programs.

References

1. Siminoff LA, Gordon N, Hewlett J, Arnold RM. Factors influencing families' consent for donation of solid organs for transplantation. *JAMA*. 2001; 286:71-77.
2. Gortmaker SL, Beasley CL, Sheehy E, et al. Improving the request process to increase family consent for organ donation. *J Transplant Coord*. 1998; 8:210-217.
3. Siminoff LA, Arnold RM, Caplan AL, Virnig BA, Seltzer DL. Public policy governing organ and tissue procurement in the United States: results from the National Organ and Tissue Procurement Study. *Ann Intern Med*. 1995; 123:10-17.
4. Winkel FW. Public communication on donor cards: a comparison of persuasive styles. *Soc Sci Med*. 1984; 19:957-963.
5. Ford LA, Smith SW. Memorability and persuasiveness of organ donation message strategies. *Am Behav Sci*. 1991; 34:695-711.
6. Smith SW, Morrison K, Kopfman JE. The influence of prior thought and intent on the memorability and persuasiveness of organ donation message strategies. *Health Commun*. 1994; 6(1):1-20.
7. Kopfman JE, Smith SW. Understanding the audiences of a health communication campaign: a discriminant analysis of potential organ donors based on intent to donate. *J Appl Commun Res*. 1996; 24:33-49.
8. Kopfman JE, Smith SW, Ah Yun JK, Hodges A. Affective and cognitive reactions to narrative versus statistical evidence organ donation messages. *J Appl Commun Res*. 1998; 26:279-300.
9. Allen M, Preiss RW. Comparing the persuasiveness of narrative and statistical evidence using meta-analysis. *Commun Res Rep*. 1997; 14:125-131.
10. Ratzan SC. Effective decision-making: a negotiation perspective for health psychology and health communication. *J Health Psychol*. 1996; 1:323-333.
11. Watzlawick P, Beavin JH, Jackson DD. *Pragmatics of Human Communication*. New York, NY: Norton; 1967.
12. Burgoon JK, Hale JL. Validation and measurement of the fundamental themes of relational communication. *Commun Monographs*. 1987; 54:19-41.
13. Dickerson J, Valadka AB, LeVert T, Davis KD, Kurian M, Robertson CS. Organ donation rates in a neurosurgical intensive care unit. *J Neurosurg*. 2002; 97:811-814.
14. Pelletier M. The organ donor family members' perception of stressful situations during the organ donation experience. *J AdvNurs*. 1992; 17:90-97.
15. Haddow G. Donor and nondonor families' accounts of communication and relations with healthcare professionals. *Prog Transplant*. 2004; 14:41-48.
16. Sque M, Payne SA. Dissonant loss: the experiences of donor relatives. *Soc Sci Med*. 1996; 43:1359-1370.
17. Gordon AK, Herzog A, Lichtenfeld D. Surveying donor families: a comparison of two organ procurement organizations. *Clin Transplant*. 1995; 9(3 pt 1):141-145.
18. DeJong W, Franz HG, Wolfe SM, et al. Requesting organ donation: an interview of donor and nondonor families. *Am J Crit Care*. 1998; 7:13-23.
19. Pelletier ML. The needs of family members of organ and tissue donors. *Heart Lung*. 1993; 22:151-157.
20. Franz HG, DeJong W, Wolfe SM, et al. Explaining brain death: a critical feature of the donation process. *J Transplant Coord*. 1997; 7:14-21.
21. Pearson A, Robertson-Malt S, Walsh K, Fitzgerald M. Intensive care nurses' experiences of caring for brain dead organ donor patients. *J Clin Nurs*. 2001; 10:132-139.
22. Issues in Transplantation review. Study reveals satisfaction with hospital experience major factor in decision to donate. *Nephrol News Issues*. June 1998; 12:64-66.
23. Shafer TJ, Ehrle RN, Davis KD, et al. Increasing organ recovery from level 1 trauma centers: the in-house coordinator intervention. *Prog Transplant*. 2004; 14:250-263.
24. Duckworth RM, Sproat GW, Morien M, Jeffrey TB. Acute bereavement services and routine referral as a mechanism to increase donation. *J Transplant Coord*. 1998; 8:16-18.

25. Savaria DT, Rovell MA, Schweizer RT. Donor family surveys provide useful information for organ procurement. *Transplant Proc.* 1990; 22:316-317.
26. Thall CR, Jensen G, Wright C, Baker S, Meade R. The role of hospital-based family support teams in improving the quality of the organ donation process. *Transplant Proc.* 1997; 29:3252-3253.
27. Linyear AS, Tartaglia A. Family communication coordination: a program to increase organ donation. *J Transplant Coord.* 1999; 9:165-174.
28. Batten HL, Prottas JM. Kind strangers: the families of organ donors. *Health Aff.* 1987; 6(2):35-47.
29. Sque M, Long T, Payne SA. Organ donation: key factors influencing families' decision-making. *Transplant Proc.* 2005; 37:543-546.
30. Cutler JA, David SD, Kress CJ, et al. Increasing the availability of cadaveric organs for transplantation maximizing the consent rate. *Transplantation.* 1993; 56:225-228.
31. Noah P, Morgan SE. Organ/tissue donation request: a multidisciplinary approach. *Crit Care Nurs Clin North Am.* 1999; 22(3):30-38.
32. HCFA Department of Health and Human Services. Medicare and Medicaid Programs; Hospital Conditions of Participation: Identification of potential organ, tissue, and eye donors and transplant hospitals' provisions of transplant-related data. Final rule. *Federal Register.* 119 (1998) (codified at 42 CFR § 482.45).
33. Siminoff LA, Lawrence RH, Zhang A. Decoupling: what is it and does it really help increase consent to organ donation? *Prog Transplant.* 2002; 12:52-60.
34. Ehrle RN, Shafer TJ, Nelson KR. Referral, request, and consent for organ donation: best practice -- a blueprint for success. *Crit Care Nurse.* April 1999; 19:21-30, 32-33.
35. US Department of Health and Human Services, Health Resources and Services Administration. The Organ Donation Breakthrough Collaborative: The Change Package. In: Do T, ed. Office of Special Programs. Vol Contract 240-94-0037; 2003.
36. Garrison RN, Bentley FR, Raque GH. There is an answer to the shortage of organ donors. *Surg Gynecol Obstet.* 1991; 173:391-396.
37. Morris JA, Slaton J, Gibbs D. Vascular organ procurement in the trauma population. *J Trauma.* 1989; 29:782-788.
38. Niles PA, Mattice BJ. The timing factor in the consent process. *J Transplant Coord.* June 1996; 6:84-87.
39. Beasley CL, Capossela CL, Brigham LE, Gunderson S, Weber P, Gortmaker SL. The impact of a comprehensive, hospital-focused intervention to increase organ donation. *J Transplant Coord.* March 1997; 7:6-13.
40. French E. Communication coordinators boost organ donation rate. *Crit Care Nurs.* August 1999; 19:96.
41. Sullivan H, Blakely D, Davis K. An in-house coordinator program to increase organ donation in public teaching hospitals. *J Transplant Coord.* March 1998; 8:40-42.
42. Burris GW, Jacobs AJ. A continuous quality improvement process to increase organ and tissue donation. *J Transplant Coord.* June 1996; 6:88-92.
43. Siminoff LA, Saunders Sturm CM. Nursing and the procurement of organs and tissues in the acute care hospital setting. *Nurs Clin North Am.* 1998; 33:239-249.
44. Shanteau J, Linin KA. Subjective meaning of terms used in organ donation: analysis of word associations. In: Shanteau J, Harris RJ, eds. *Organ Donation and Transplantation: Psychological and Behavioral Factors.* Washington, DC: American Psychological Association; 1990:37-49.
45. Jasper JD, Harris RJ, Lee BC, Miller KE. Organ donation terminology: are we communicating life or death? *Health Psychol.* 1991; 10(1):34-41. Health Psychol. 1991; 10(1):34-41.
46. The Gallup Organization I. *The American Public's Attitude Toward Organ Donation and Transplantation.* Boston, Mass: The Partnership for Organ Donation; 1993.
47. Siminoff LA, Burant CJ, Youngner SJ. Death and organ procurement: public beliefs and attitudes. *Kennedy Inst Ethics J.* 2004; 14:217-234.
48. Cleiren MP, Van Zoelen AA. Post-mortem organ donation and grief: a study of consent, refusal and well-being in bereavement. *Death Studies.* 2002; 26:837-849.
49. Walker JA, McGrath PJ, Mac Donald NE, Wells G, Petrusic W, Nolan BE. Parental attitudes toward pediatric organ donation: a survey. *Can Med Assoc J.* 1990; 142:1383-1387.
50. Siminoff LA, Arnold RM, Hewlett J. The process of organ donation and its effects on consent. *Clin Transplant.* February 2001; 15:39-47.
51. Siminoff LA, Mercer MB, Arnold RM. Families' understanding of brain death. *Prog Transplant.* 2003; 13:218-224.
52. Chapman G, Elstein AS, Hughes K. Effects of patient education on decisions about breast cancer treatments: a preliminary report. *Med Decision Making.* 1995; 15:231-239.
53. Frutos MA, Ruiz P, Requena MV, Daga D. Family refusal in organ donation: analysis of three patterns. *Transplant Proc.* 2002; 34:2513-2514.
54. Kometsi K, Louw J. Deciding on cadaveric organ donation in Black African families. *Clin Transplant.* 1999; 13:473-478.
55. Ohnuki-Tierney E. Brain death and organ transplantation: cultural bases of medical technology. *Curr Anthropol.* 1994; 35:233-253.

56. Atkins L, Davis KD, Holtzman SM, Durand R, Decker PJ. Family discussion about organ donation among African Americans. *Prog Transplant.* 2003; 13:28-32.
57. Jacob-Arriola KR, Perryman JP, Doldren M. Moving beyond attitudinal barriers: understanding African Americans' support for organ and tissue donation. *J Nat Med Assoc.* 2005; 97:339-350.
58. Tymstra TJ, Heyink JW, Pruim J, Slooff MJH. Experience of bereaved relatives who granted or refused permission of organ donation. *Fam Pract.* 1992; 9:141-144.
59. Martinez JM, Lopez JS, Martin A, Martin MJ, Scandroglio B, Martin JM. Organ donation and family decision-making within the Spanish donation system. *Soc Sci Med.* 2001; 53:405-421.
60. Burroughs TE, Hong BA, Kapel DF, Freedman BK. The stability of family decisions to consent or refuse organ donation: would you do it again? *Psychosom Med.* 1998; 60:156-162.
61. Radecki CM, Jaccard J. Psychological aspects of organ donation: a critical review and synthesis of individual and next-of-kin donation decisions. *Health Psychol.* 1997; 16:183-195.
62. May T, Aulisio MP, DeVita MA. Patients, families, and organ donation: who should decide? *Milbank Q.* 2000; 78:323-336.
63. Oz MC, Kherani AR, Rowe A, et al. How to improve organ donation: results of the ISHLT/FACT poll. *J Heart Lung Transplant.* 2003; 22:389-410.
64. Manninen DL, Evans RW. Public attitudes and behavior regarding organ donation. *JAMA.* 1985; 253:3111-3115.
65. Wendler D, Dickert N. The consent process for cadaveric organ procurement: how does it work? How can it be improved? *JAMA.* 2001; 285:329-333.
66. Sharing UNFO. UNOS Newsroom Factsheet: Donor Designation (First Person Consent) Status by State. Available at: http://www.unos.org/inTheNews/faxtsheets.asp?fs=6. Accessed June 28, 2005.
67. Sokohl K. First person consent: OPOs across the country are adapting to the change. UNOS Update. 2002 Sep-Oct;:1, 3.
68. Fernandez M, Zayas E, Gonzalez ZA, Morales-Otero LA, Santiago-Delpin EA. Factors in a meager organ donation pattern of a Hispanic population. *Transplant Proc.* 1991; 23:1799-1801.
69. Yuen CC, Burton W, Chiraseveenuprapund P, et al. Attitudes and beliefs about organ donation among different racial groups. *J Natl Med Assoc.* January, 1998; 90(1):13-18. 70. Pietz CA, Mayes T, Naclerio A, Taylor RJ. Pediatric organ transplantation and the Hispanic population: approaching families and obtaining their consent. *Transplant Proc.* 2004; 36:1237-1240.
71. Siminoff LA, Arnold RM. Increasing organ donation in the African-American community: altruism in the face of an untrustworthy system. *Ann Intern Med.* 1999; 130:607-609.
72. Morgan SE, Miller JK. Beyond the organ donor card: the effect of knowledge, attitudes, and values on willingness to communicate about organ donation to family members. *Health Commun.* 2002; 14:121-134.
73. Morgan SE, Cannon T. African Americans' knowledge about organ donation: closing the gap with more effective persuasive message strategies. *Natl Med Assoc.* 2003; 95:1066-1071.
74. Perez LM, Schulman B, Davis F, Olson L, Tellis VA, Matas AJ. Organ donation in three major American cities with large Latino and Black populations. *Transplantation.* 1988; 46:553-557.
75. Guadagnoli E, Christiansen CL, DeJong W, et al. The public's willingness to discuss their preference for organ donation with family members. *Clin Transplant.* 1999; 13:342-348.
76. Callender CO, Miles P. Obstacles to organ donation in ethnic minorities: a national stratagem. *Pediatr Transplant.* 2001; 5:383-385.
77. Shafer T, Wood RP, Van Buren CT, et al. A Success story in minority donation: the LifeGift/Ben Taub General Hospital in-house coordinator program. *Transplant Proc.* 1997; 29:3753-3755.
78. Gentry D, Brown-Holbert J, Andrews C. Racial impact: increasing minority consent rate by altering the racial mix of an organ procurement organization. *Transplant Proc.* 1997; 29:3758-3759.
79. Kappel DF, Whitlock ME, Parks-Thomas TD, Hong BA, Freedman BK. Increasing African American organ donation: the St. Louis experience. *Transplant Proc.* 1993; 25:2489-2490.
80. Indiana Organ Procurement Organization (IOPO). *6 Month Consent Analysis Summary.* Indiana Organ Procurement Organization; 2004.
81. Hartwig MS, Hall G, Hathaway D, Gaber O. Effect of organ donor race on health care team procurement efforts. *Arch Surg.* 1993; 128:1331-1335.
82. Siminoff LA, Lawrence RH, Arnold RM. Comparison of black and white families' experiences and perceptions regarding organ donation requests. *Crit Care Med.* 2003; 31:146-151.
83. Zink S. Grant No. H39 OT 00073 from Health Resources and Services Administration (HRSA), Office of Special Programs, Division of Transplantation.

Evaluation and Assessment of Organ Donors

Rebecca Menza, RN, MS, CPTC
P J Geraghty, REMT-P, BS, CPTC, CTBS

Introduction

Although transplantation has been studied rather intensely in the past 20 years, the science of organ *donation* is truly in its nascent phase. Only recently have concepts of the physiological changes associated with brain death begun to be developed and the effects of these derangements on end organ function described; still less is known about the relationship between individual donor characteristics and utilization or graft survival. Important outcome-based research is starkly needed, and it is with this in mind that the following recommendations are made.

What is certain is that several hurdles must be overcome on the way to any transplant. Referrals must be identified by the host hospital, families must give consent, and before any organs are offered for transplantation, the organ procurement organization (OPO) must first determine that the donor (or the potential graft) meets medical suitability. It is in this stage of the process where many organs may be lost. In the past 10 years, the boundaries of acceptability have shifted dramatically. Whereas lungs were once considered to be unsuitable if the potential donor's smoking history was greater than 15 pack-years, or if the chest radiograph showed infiltrate, nowadays long-term smokers and donors with purulence are successfully included in the potential pool for lungs. Preliminary results for 30-day and 1-year graft survival are encouraging for the use of so called "marginal" grafts. Until more is understood about individual organ suitability, it is recommended that all consented organs be critically evaluated from the vantage point of assumed suitability.

Well-timed and skilled evaluation of potential organ donors will lead to increased yield in individual organs for transplantation. Many donors present initially in a shock state and with compromised organ function requiring appropriate interventions to stabilize the cells. Targeted interventions have been developed to help guide donors back to aerobic metabolism (see section on donor management), and it is recommended that evaluation of the organ donor be postponed until these resuscitative efforts have been implemented.

Some medical histories raise serious questions about medical suitability and the potential safety of a transplant. Individual examples are discussed in each organ-specific section of this chapter; however, one overarching philosophy can be applied to all organs: increased diagnostic testing may provide important answers about suitability, and the associated costs are offset by the benefit of producing even one more organ for transplant. Computed tomography (CT) scans, magnetic resonance imaging (MRI), early bronchoscopy, and cardiac catheterizations are often seen as adding expense to the already costly donor process. These important aspects of donor evaluation should not be forsaken because of concerns about timing and cost; they yield valuable information that contributes to increased utilization.

Medical and Social History

A critical part of any donor workup is the physical assessment of the donor as well as the gathering of a complete medical, and social (or behavioral) history. The 2 facets of the assessment go hand in hand, as clues from one may assist in the completion of the other.

If possible, it is advisable for the organ recovery coordinator (ORC) to perform a brief physical assessment of the donor before starting the interview with the historian. An assessment such as this may provide clues to help direct the interview. Findings such as old scars, piercings, and tattoos can often be overlooked or forgotten by family members but may be important in providing a proper history. As well, a historian's lack of awareness of a particular aspect of the assessment may indicate that he/she is not a reliable historian, and the ORC may ask for assistance from other potential historians. Tattoos, especially, can provide an insight into the donor's participation in gangs or drug use.

Each OPO is required by United Network for Organ Sharing (UNOS) policy to identify and assess donor history, including behavioral risk factors for infectious disease.[1] As well, the Food and Drug Administration (FDA) requires that histories be obtained on all tissue donors. It is incumbent upon the OPO to develop an interview tool that meets both regulatory guidelines and the needs of local practitioners.

A history interview should be conducted with sensitivity and discretion. The ORC should identify the best historians (usually family members or close friends of the donor), explain the purpose of the interview and give a brief description of the type of questions that will be asked. This process will allow the presumed historian the opportunity to decide if he or she is the best historian for these types of questions or if another person should be included. Likewise, when given notice of the sensitive nature of some of the questions, the historian may opt to continue the interview in a more private setting.

ORCs should be very comfortable with the history instrument designed by the OPO. ORCs should ask the questions in an appropriately sensitive manner. When given an affirmative answer, the ORC should strive to gather as much information as possible about the answer. As an example, when the historian answers affirmatively to a question regarding drug use, the ORC should attempt to elicit information about the type of drug use, the route of administration, as well as the frequency and duration of use. Similarly, a historian who confirms that the donor was hypertensive should be asked how the hypertension was controlled or treated, if the donor was compliant with the treatment regimen, how long ago the hypertension had been diagnosed, and other pertinent information. ORCs should be aware of nonverbal cues such as looking away, coughing, and fidgeting, which may indicate that a historian is being less than forthcoming, or that another person present has additional information that he is uncomfortable sharing with the group at this time. In some cases, it may be obvious that the historian cannot provide enough information about the donor; in these situations, it may be helpful to ask the historian to recommend another individual who might be able to provide more information.

Along with the interview, a review of available medical records may prove useful in assessing donor suitability. ORCs should review the record of the entire hospitalization beginning at admission as well as all available old records. (Here, too, the historian may be able to provide the name of the donor's physician who might also be able to provide additional historical information.) The ORC should be especially sensitive to any operative procedures and the findings from those procedures, including biopsy results, anatomical abnormality, damage, or other significant findings mentioned in the operative report. The ORC should review any available radiological studies for clues about the donor's clinical status. Radiographs and CT scans can provide a wealth of information about the donor that may not appear in the progress notes. With the movement to electronic charting systems in many hospitals, ORCs may not be able to review paper records as easily as in the past; OPOs should be aware of this trend and should work with hospitals to provide ORCs the appropriate level of access to electronic medical records.

A more detailed physical assessment should include assessment and documentation of injuries, tattoos, track marks, fractures, or other pertinent findings on the donor. ORCs should assess heart tones, lung sounds, and bowel sounds and should document the quantity and appearance of urine. ORCs should also document any procedures performed on the donor, including placement of arterial and central venous catheters, peripheral intravenous catheters, chest tubes, and urinary catheters as well as casting, bandaging, and other therapies. In some cases, the medical examiner may review these notes to determine which injuries are the result of the initial accident and which are the result of hospitalization.

The history interview and physical examination of the donor are critical aspects of the assessment of donor suitability. Both are useful to transplant center staff as they decide about the suitability of the organs for their recipients, and both can give clues about the donor that might not otherwise be evident. ORCs must be diligent in performing these critical functions in order to ensure the safety and efficacy of the transplanted organs.

Serological Tests

All potential organ donors undergo serological testing to determine previous exposure to infections.[2] Deceased donor testing is required by UNOS.[3] Three infectious diseases are of primary interest: hepatitis B virus (HBV), hepatitis C virus (HCV), and human immunodeficiency virus (HIV).[2]

Three different markers for HBV can be detected in the bloodstream. Hepatitis B surface antigen (HBsAg) typically appears at 4 weeks after exposure and remains detectable during the entire phase of acute illness. Antibody to hepatitis B core antigen (HBcAb) is detectable 1 to 2 weeks after the appearance of HBsAg. Hepatitis B surface antibody appears weeks or months later.[4] In general, HBcAb and HBsAb remain detectable after an individual has recovered from HBV infection. HBsAg persists in those who cannot clear the virus and develop chronic hepatitis B. Isolated HBsAb is generally indicative of previous immunization against HBV.[4] Organs from HBsAg-positive donors generally carry a high risk of HBV transmission,[3] although 1 study [5] demonstrated that the use of HBsAg-positive hearts in immunized (HBsAb-positive) recipients did not transmit HBV and suggested that the use of these grafts was acceptable for critically ill candidates. Another center described the use of HBcAb-positive kidneys in recipients who had varied HBcAb and HBsAb statuses; only the HBV-naïve patients received lamivudine prophylaxis and neither group suffered HBV infection.[6]

HCV infection is the most common indication for liver transplantation.[7] No vaccination exists for the prevention of HCV infection. There can be as much as an 8- to 10-week "window" period between infection with HCV and seropositivity. During this interval, the donor may be able to transmit the disease, as happened in one case in 2002.[8] In an effort to reduce this window and the associated risks of accidental transmission of HCV, some OPOs perform HCV-RNA testing. Such testing, however, is not yet required by UNOS. Many centers accept livers and kidneys from HCV-positive donors who do not demonstrate histological evidence of acute disease, especially if the candidates are themselves HCV-positive. However, one center reports an increased risk of post-transplant coronary artery disease in recipients of hearts from HCV-positive donors.[9]

HIV infection is still considered a contraindication to donation. While some centers have had success in transplanting organs from patients who are HIV-positive, most centers and UNOS still prohibit the recovery of organs from HIV-positive donors.

Human T-cell leukemia-lymphoma virus (HTLV I and II) is often considered a contraindication to donation. HTLV was confirmed in 0.015% of 8.9 million blood donations in 1989.[10] However, given the high rate of falsely positive screening tests,[11] some centers will consider using organs from these donors if the donor is not a member of an identified risk group.[10]

All serology testing should be done with specimens deemed appropriate by the test kit manufacturer. Although the Food and Drug Administration requires that testing be done on pretransfusion/preinfusion samples for potential tissue donors,[12] no such requirement exists for organ donors. HIV transmission has been documented from an organ donor who tested negative for HIV antibodies after receiving more than 50 units of blood, but whose pretransfusion specimen tested positive for HIV antibodies.[13] In the event that serological testing is done on a posttransfusion sample, the ORC should notify the transplant center of the quantity and types of infusions and transfusions the donor received before the serology sample was obtained.

Liver

Evaluation of a potential liver graft includes (but is not limited to) assessment of cause of death, serological status and medical social history, potential cold ischemic time, use of inotropic agents, and results of liver function tests.[14,15] Feng et al[16] describe 7 characteristics of donors that are independent predictors of increased risk of hepatic graft failure: donor age (>40 years, and especially >60 years), split/segmented grafts, donation after cardiac death (DCD), cerebral vascular accident as cause of death, African American race, and short stature. Assessment of liver function by means of the international normalized ratio (INR) and platelet count can be complicated by consumption coagulopathies associated with massive brain injuries; especially in cases of fulminant disseminated intravascular coagulation (DIC), admission laboratory values may be most revealing.

When exposed to ischemia, cells lining the bile invaginations of the liver can become congested, in turn leading to a transient increase in the conjugated bilirubin. These states of poor perfusion can be the result of the initial injury (anoxia), or of a low-flow state following herniation due either to hypotension or to poor cardiac output because of a stunned myocardium. Simultaneous increases may also be seen in transaminases after ischemia; however, if the creatinine clearance is normal, these levels should begin to stabilize and decrease during the subsequent 24-hour period. Measurement Gamma-glutamyltransferase (GGT) level may be a more specific test to assess for current liver damage when the creatinine is elevated or in the setting of massive tissue injury (i.e., rhabdomyolysis).

As body mass index increases (especially >29), so too does concern for the presence of nonalcoholic fatty liver disease.[17] Unfortunately, radiographic imaging, either via CT or ultrasound, is specific but not sensitive for detection of fat overall.[18] Further, and perhaps more significantly, this means of assessment also does not allow for the differentiation of macrovesicular and microvesicular fat content, an important distinction when considering the overall suitability of a potential graft.[19] Though grafts with higher fat content have been successfully used,[20] there is evidence which shows that the combination of higher fat content and longer ischemic time can lead to compromised results.[21] Macrovesicular fat content less than 30% is desirable; microvesicular fat content seems to be less important (with levels >50% acceptable).[22,23]

The best means to assess potentially fatty livers is via biopsy. While a biopsy can be done directly during the procurement, these results are typically limited to a frozen-section interpretation, which can prove difficult to interpret accurately. Permanent section is preferable, and if possible the sample should be obtained at the earliest time to ensure appropriate allocation with minimal cold ischemic time.

Alcoholism is difficult to quantify, and its effects on the liver are harder still to predict. Calculation of the ratio of aspartate aminotransferase (AST) to alanine aminotransferase (ALT) at admission can sometimes cue the coordinator to investigate alcohol history; findings on physical exam such as spider angiomas, a fluid wave on percussion of the abdomen, and varices should be noted. If there are concerns about the potential for alcoholic cirrhosis in the organ donor, a biopsy is recommended to quantify the level of disease. Positive results of serological tests were addressed earlier in this section, and many would suggest that a biopsy be performed in cases in which HCV is detected in order to assess for degree of inflammation and manifestation of cirrhosis.

Donors who present with fulminant liver failure (often due to acetaminophen overdose) can successfully donate their thoracic organs for transplantation and should not be ruled out as potential organ donors.

Kidney

Kidney transplantation is well established as a successful therapy for end-stage renal disease. Historically, many donors were managed as kidney-only donors because of the scarcity of extrarenal transplant programs. As such, the management goals were simple: maintain urine output and proceed to surgical recovery of the organs. As transplantation and donation have advanced, however, the process has become a bit more complex.

A CLINICIAN'S GUIDE TO DONATION AND TRANSPLANTATION Chapter 31

The kidney is perhaps the most resilient of the organs transplanted. Kidneys remain fairly refractory to donor ischemia; patients with cardiopulmonary arrest times of as much as an hour or more can still be suitable kidney donors. Donors are susceptible to diabetes insipidus, which, though potentially detrimental to other organs, can demonstrate good pre-recovery kidney function. A common acute change found in donor kidneys is the presence of microthrombi related to the presence of disseminated intravascular coagulation (DIC). These microthrombi can cause the kidneys to cease functioning entirely during the management phase in the intensive care unit. However, if properly controlled, DIC is not a contraindication to kidney donation.[24]

Because of the relative ease of kidney transplantation, the kidney waiting list is the longest of the candidate lists. In some areas of the country, wait times for deceased donor kidneys exceed 5 years. For this reason, some programs are exploring avenues to increase the number of kidneys recovered and transplanted. Pediatric donors and so-called expanded donors are receiving increased attention as a source of donor kidneys.

Kidney function is assessed preoperatively by reviewing trends in serum creatinine level, urinalysis, and urine output. In older donors, assessment of creatinine clearance may prove useful as an evaluation of the kidney's function over a period of time. In many hospitals, the creatinine clearance is a 24-hour test; often this interval is shortened for donor evaluations. A creatinine clearance of 60 mL/min is considered acceptable.[25]

Although serum creatinine level, urinalysis, and urine output remain the standard pre-recovery assessments of potential kidney donors, intraoperative assessment remains the final hurdle. Kidneys recovered from donors with severe atherosclerotic disease in the aorta and/or renal arteries may be technically difficult or impossible to transplant. Pretransplant biopsy has become the standard for elderly donor kidneys or kidneys with other risk factors (DCD, diabetes, hypertension, abnormal urinalysis). Biopsies allow evaluation for interstitial fibrosis, glomerulosclerosis, and other histological changes within the kidneys. Wedge biopsy specimens are usually taken intraoperatively and evaluated via frozen section, which allows for rapid assessment of these conditions. Even in the face of histological changes, however, some centers may elect to transplant both kidneys into a single recipient.[26]

UNOS has defined specific criteria for expanded-criteria kidney donors (ECD). These criteria (Table 1) are based on reviews of centers' experiences with these types of donors and the demonstrated relative risk of graft failure or delayed function. The definition of ECD criteria has allowed transplant centers to identify the type of donors they would accept for a particular patient, and UNOS has modified allocation algorithms to promote rapid allocation and transplantation of these ECD kidneys into recipients for whom they are considered most appropriate.

Table 1. UNOS DEFINED SPECIFIC CRITERIA FOR EXPANDED-CRITERIA KIDNEY DONORS (ECD)

Donor Condition	Donor Age Categories				
	< 10	10 – 39	40 – 49	50 – 59	≥ 60
CVA + HTN + Creat > 1.5				X	X
CVA + HTN				X	X
CVA + Creat > 1.5				X	X
HTN + Creat > 1.5				X	X
CVA					X
HTN					X
Creatinine > 1.5					X
None of the above					X

X=Expanded Criteria Donor
CVA=CVA was cause of death
HTN=history of hypertension at any time
Creat > 1.5 = creatinine > 1.5 mg/dl
Source: United Network for Organ Sharing Policy 3.0 Organ Distribution. http://www.unos.org/PoliciesandBylaws2/policies/docs/policy_70.doc, accessed July 2, 2006

Other relative contraindications to renal transplantation include polycystic disease, atrophic kidney (usually unilateral), or increasing creatinine level with concomitant decreased urine output. Some centers have experienced success with donors with increasing creatinine but normal urine output.

Many centers use pulsatile machine preservation for kidneys. Pulsatile preservation has been associated with decreased rates of delayed graft function (DGF) even in the face of increased cold ischemic times. Pulsatile preservation is especially encouraged in the case of donors after cardiac death or expanded criteria donors.

Pancreas

Pancreas transplantation is a recognized therapy for the treatment of type 1 diabetes and can control the secondary effects of this disease. Simultaneous kidney-pancreas transplantation is commonly performed in type 1 diabetics with end-stage renal disease because it has a better patient- and graft-survival rate than does pancreas-after-kidney transplantation.[27]

In general, pancreas donors are patients between the ages of 6 and 55 years, with a body mass index (BMI) less than 30 kg/m^2, with no history of pancreatic disease or diabetes.[28] Serum glucose levels should be normal or, if elevated by use of glucose-rich intravenous fluids, should be well-controlled with insulin, but hyperglycemia itself is not a contraindication to pancreas donation.[29] Many programs will evaluate trends in serum amylase[30] and lipase, but these may not be entirely reliable predictors of pancreatic injury in a trauma patient[31] or a patient who has had a cerebrovascular accident.[32] If possible, the serum hemoglobin A_{1c} should be obtained and shared with the transplant center, but few hospitals have this test available in a time frame suitable for organ recovery.[33]

Excessive fluid resuscitation and massive transfusion can lead to pancreatic edema, a relative contraindication to transplantation. As well, if the donor liver biopsy reveals greater than 25% to 30% macrovascular steatosis, this can be associated with a fatty pancreas, which has an increased risk of early graft loss.[28]

Some donors who do not meet the BMI criteria for pancreas donation may be candidates for islet cell donation, especially to recipients with a lower BMI.[34] Although the process is still in development, results are promising, and islet cell transplantation could become the therapy of choice for insulin independence over whole pancreas transplantation.

Small Bowel

Small-bowel donation is one of the newest areas of donor management. Practiced for several years in a few isolated centers, the number of candidates continues to increase and more centers are beginning these programs. Small bowels are often transplanted with other organs (liver, pancreas, and/or kidney) and are most frequently performed on children with short-gut syndrome.[35]

Different centers have different criteria for what constitutes an acceptable small-bowel donor, but in general the donor should be cytomegalovirus (CMV)-negative, have little or no period of hypotension or cardiac arrest, and should be free of any preexisting liver or pancreatic disease. Because so many of the candidates are children, size matching of donor and recipient is often an issue; an OPO may have a clinically suitable small-bowel donor but there may not be a suitably sized potential recipient listed.

Frequently, transplant centers will inquire about results of hepatic function tests, bowel sounds, nutrition history (especially for longer premortem hospitalizations), and blood transfusions. Transfusion of the donor with CMV-negative blood, always a consideration, is especially important in small-bowel transplantation as so many of the candidates are CMV-naïve children.

Small-bowel candidates requiring multiple organs (multivisceral candidates) are often at a disadvantage because of the high number of isolated liver candidates.[36] Different OPOs have different policies regarding the decision to allocate livers to isolated liver candidates or to multivisceral candidates. As the number of small-bowel candidates increases, this issue will become more contentious.

Heart

One of the presumed tenets of heart transplantation was that if grafts were healthy and free of disease, they would function well in recipients. It was with this in mind that the standard criteria for heart donors were established in the 1970s. Shumway and DeBakey, arguably the fathers of cardiac transplantation, described the "ideal" cardiac donor as being young (no older than 40) and without structural or functional deficit.[37,38] As recently as 1995, clinical experts advocated for a restrictive pool of donors which included only those less than 50 years old, with an ejection fraction (EF) greater than 50 %, echocardiogram without important segmental abnormalities, cold ischemic time less than 4 hours, and no evidence of donor infection.[39] These and other demographic, functional, and structural assignments quickly became a fixed set of standards that are only now being reexamined.

In 1994, Young et al[40] advocated for appropriate matching of the donor heart to the recipient. This pairing was designed to account for not only age and size but also some structural changes and injury to the potential graft; with careful recipient selection tailored to the findings in the donor, risk could be reduced, and more grafts were deemed usable. Although some of the examples described by Young have evolved over the past decade, the principle of intensive donor evaluation remains the key to successful matching of donor and recipient.

Several researchers have demonstrated excellent outcomes from the use of older donor hearts,[41,42] and former donor age limits have been lifted in current practice. Correlated with increased donor age, however, is an increase in the prevalence of both coronary artery disease (CAD) and the development of post-transplant coronary artery disease.[43,44] In light of this, current conservative recommendations for the evaluation of donor hearts suggest angiography for all women more than 50 years of age and males more than 45 years. If the donor is more than 35 years old and used cocaine or had 3 or more risk factors for CAD (hypertension, dyslipidemia, smoking history, diabetes, or early family history), then prospective catheterization is recommended.[45]

The use of hearts with CAD has been described in small retrospective analyses that show only a small decrease in short-term graft survival (as compared with non-diseased grafts) and no difference in long-term survival.[44,46,47] Post-recovery, ex-vivo coronary artery grafting of the diseased donor heart has also been performed by several groups with acceptable outcomes.[48-50]

Transplanters at Papworth demonstrated effective functional assessment of cardiac donors using only pulmonary artery catheters.[51] However, echo is still considered the gold standard as it allows evaluation of the valves and assessment of wall thickness.

Poor ejection fraction is one of the most common barriers to utilization of a donor heart.[52] Although some hearts have wall-motion abnormalities after severe brain injury, most will regain their functional status and can ultimately be used successfully. Zaroff et al[53] have shown reversibility of these wall-motion abnormalities in organ donors and demonstrated excellent 30-day and 1-year survival of the recipients of hearts with transiently compromised ejection fraction. Consequently, it is recommended that a donor be managed aggressively and reevaluated if the echo shows poor function initially (EF <45%).

Left ventricular hypertrophy (LVH) in a potential donor heart should not automatically preclude use for transplantation as these grafts have been used successfully in several programs.[54-56] Instead, LVH shown by echocardiography should be defined quantitatively to include thickness of the septal wall and left ventricular posterior wall. The Crystal City Consensus Group has suggested that septal wall thickness of 13 mm or less should not preclude utilization.[45] Voltage criteria for LVH should be evaluated on electrocardiograms (ECG), and the results shall be paired with wall measurements, age, and history of hypertension to assess the severity of the LVH.

As with grafts that have CAD, hypertrophied donor hearts may be associated with a slightly lower short-term survival (but no difference in long-term survival). This pattern suggests that neither tolerate preservation as well as hearts that are free from structural defect. Consequently, care should be taken to minimize the cold ischemic time for both.

All potential cardiac donors should receive a 12-lead ECG. Many will have diffuse nonspecific changes in the ST-T segments associated with brain injury. This pattern should not be mistaken for cardiac injury.

Donors with Wolff-Parkinson-White syndrome can be identified through this means and the donor heart may be treated with ablation before implantation.[41]

Ideally cardiac donors will not have elevated cardiac enzymes. Some evidence suggests that elevated levels of troponin T or I in the donor is predictive of increased inotropic support requirements in the recipient, rejection rates, and early graft dysfunction.[57-59] However, others have reported no difference in the outcomes of recipients of grafts with troponin leak.[60] Additionally, many donors have troponin leak with no evidence of left ventricular dysfunction or pressor dependence, and it remains unclear what real use these markers have in the evaluation of cardiac donors.

Lung

In the early years of lung transplantation, criteria for acceptability for lung donors were based largely on single-center experiences and presumed functional standards. Potential lung donors were required to have a terminal PaO_2 greater than 300 mm Hg at a fraction of inspired oxygen (FIO_2) of 100%, a clear chest radiograph, smoking history less than 20 pack-years, no inhaled drug use, age less than 55 years, absence of purulent secretions on bronchoscopy, no evidence of aspiration, a Gram stain free of organisms, and without significant increases in white blood cell count. Owing largely to a lack of evidence in the field, these criteria came to be known as the "standard" for suitability of lung donors.[61] In the past 5 years, these criteria have been challenged in registry analysis, review pieces, and single-center publications, and it has been shown that adherence to these standard criteria exclude transplantable lungs from the donor pool.[62]

Increased donor age (i.e. >55 years) does not appear to carry increased risk for potential lung recipients unless combined with increased cold ischemic time.[63,64] There remain the same concerns as for other organ systems of the increased risks of generalized disease process (i.e. cancer) and cumulative disease (i.e. emphysema), but as long as these are independently assessed, older donors may be suitable candidates for lung donation.[65]

Arterial blood gas analysis is an important aspect of the evaluation of a potential lung donor. Although ongoing assessments of oxygenation are made throughout the management phase of the donor workup, evaluation as a potential lung donor should not be finally assessed until the donor has been managed to meet the hemodynamic guidelines established by the OPO. When the central venous pressure is greater than 8 mm Hg, the arterial oxygen gradient is greater,[66] and transplantable lungs may be overlooked because of treatable pulmonary edema, atelectasis, and resultant poor function.

A recent arterial blood gas analysis (no more than 2 hours before the organ offer) with a calculated $Pao_2:FIO_2$ ratio or a challenge gas (drawn on a sample obtained after 20 minutes of 100% FIO_2) is considered essential.[67] The terminal ABG (obtained just prior to organ recovery) is the sample that should be used to finally determine organ suitability,[68] not samples obtained during the earlier phases of management. Recommendations that the $Pao_2:FIO_2$ ratio must exceed 300 mm Hg are not evidence based, and centers report acceptable outcomes with lower oxygenation.[63,64] Lungs with initially poor function ($Pao_2:FIO_2$ < 150 mm Hg) can be successfully managed to show improvements in gas exchange and have been safely used for single and double lung transplants.[69] When one lung has suffered profound injury (eg contusion), some centers have successfully employed pulmonary vein gas analysis and/or single lung ventilation in the operating room to evaluate the other solitary viable donor lung.[70]

Donor smoking history should be quantified in pack-years as part of the organ offer. Histories of greater than 20 pack years should not exclude the donor as a candidate for lung donation, and ORCs are encouraged to offer these lungs to transplant centers. Barring evidence of chronic obstructive pulmonary disease or pulmonary fibrosis on chest radiographs, lungs from a donor with any smoking history may be acceptable for transplantation.[61,64,65,71] If the donor has risk factors for emphysema (eg, long-term smoking history, smoking crack cocaine, and pack-years greater than 25 with age greater than 50 years), it is recommended that the OPO obtain a CT scan of the chest to complete the evaluation.

Positive results on a Gram stain are no longer considered to be exclusionary criteria for lung donation. Most studies show no correlation between donor Gram stain results (both from endotracheal aspirate and from bronchoalveolar lavage) and recipient's outcome (eg, pneumonia, duration of mechanical ventilation, or oxygenation difficulties).[63,72,73] Although the role of the donor's Gram stain when determining organ suitability has been diminished, recipients are still treated prophylactically for organisms that culture out of donor lungs; pulmonary cultures should be obtained by the OPO and the results reported to the transplant center as soon as they are available.[73]

Ideally a lung donor's chest radiograph will be clear; however, small abnormalities on the donor's chest radiographs are no longer considered exclusionary. Attempts should be made to quantify the findings and to pair them with results of the clinical examination such as bronchoscopy findings and volume status. Evidence of unilateral infection or infiltrate in the donor are acceptable and safe,[74,75] and atelectasis in the setting of a normal bronchoscopy has also been shown to be safe.[76]

Newly described correlations between levels of potent cytokines such as interleukin-8 and interleukin-6 in donor bronchoalveolar lavage and incidence of primary graft failure in lung transplant recipients [77] may shape the evaluation process and donor management in the future.

Extended Criteria Donors

Non Central Nervous System Neoplasm

Immunosupression renders transplant recipients especially vulnerable to donor transmitted malignancy. Several neoplasms carry a high rate of transmission from donor to recipient. Sample transmission rates include 41% for lung cancer, 19% for colon cancer, 29% for breast cancer, and 29% for prostate cancer, according to the Israel Penn International Transplant Tumor Registry (IPITTR).[2]

Discovery of accidental transplantation of grafts from donors with cancer necessitates urgent relisting, retransplantation, or, (when possible) removal of the donor graft (eg, kidney).[78] Despite rapid retransplantation (7 days), deaths due to donor-transmitted metastatic disease (eg, pulmonary adenocarcinoma in a liver recipient) have been reported.[79]

Grafts from older donors are associated with increased risk for cancer transmission, and consequently any donors who have specific risk factors for malignancy should be assessed for current undiagnosed disease.[80] Metastasis to the central nervous system may be a cause for primary intracranial hemorrhage; the IPITTR reports misdiagnosis of 29 donors thought to have benign intracranial hemorrhage (ICH) and later discovered to have melanoma, choriocarcinoma, sarcoma, and other metastatic solid tumors, with resultant transmission to recipients of these organs.[81] Chest radiographs from older smokers should be interpreted carefully for potential malignant neoplasms even when an abdominal-only procurement is planned. Intraoperatively, the abdominal procurement team should examine the entire length of bowel, the thoracic cavity, and all accessible lymph tissue for insidious disease.[82]

Use of prostate-specific antigen (PSA) for evaluation of potential prostate cancer in older men should be limited to those donors who have a history of prostate disease. PSA is not sensitive or specific in donors, and reliance on this test may eliminate a valid candidate for donation. Instead it is recommended that donors with a high PSA undergo urgent pathological studies.[83]

Renal cell carcinoma is not only a risk to the potential kidney recipients but also to recipients of thoracic and hepatic organs from these donors. IPITTR registry data suggest a 63% transmission rate.[2] Vascular invasion of the renal mass results in early transmission of cancer to recipients of all organs. Despite the relatively high rate of reported transmission, some renal cell carcinomas may be safe— specifically those without capsular invasion.[84] In fact, these donors may even donate kidneys under specific circumstances. Some report that kidneys with small (<4 cm), unifocal, subcapsular tumors have been safely used for transplantation. These lesions must be resected during the procurement, and the negativity of the surgical margins must be verified as well. Because of the potential transmissibility of renal cell carcinomas to all recipients, all kidneys shall be thoroughly assessed during the procurement and prior to packaging for any unsuspected lesions. Biopsies of any lesions should be performed urgently so as to prevent transplantation of the other, potentially problematic, organs.[85]

By contrast, transmission of tumors from donors with thyroid, head and neck, or testicular cancers, lymphoma-leukemia, or hepatobiliary malignant neoplasms has not been reported to date.[2] Additionally, many donors with a *history* of skin and solid tumor cancer (but without active disease) have successfully donated, and the recipients of these organs do not demonstrate an increased incidence of malignancy when compared with the cohort of "non–cancer history donors," and no cases of cancer transmission were reported in this group.[2] When assessing the suitability of a donor with a history of solid-organ neoplasm, careful consideration should be given to the staging and histology of the tumor at the time of diagnosis, likely behavior of the tumor, and length of time the donor has been in "remission". Some tumors (eg, breast cancer, lung cancer, and lymphoma) have unpredictable recurrence patterns, and consequently donors with these histories should be avoided.[2]

Due to the high rate of transmission (77%)[2] and early death,[84,86] any history of donor melanoma should preclude organ donation. Choriocarcinoma has a similar risk profile (93% transmission)[2] and is also considered a finding that precludes donation.[84] Some authors have suggested testing serum of female donors for levels of β-human chorionic gonadotropin to evaluate for choriocarcinoma,[2] especially those whose cause of death is determined to be nontraumatic ICH,[87] but this has not yet become a recommendation because of concerns for specificity.

Neoplasms of the Central Nervous System

Use of organs from donors with primary malignant neoplasms of the central nervous system (CNS) remains controversial. Cardiac grafts have been successfully transplanted from donors with astrocytoma, glioblastoma, meningioma, medulloblastoma, ependymoma, pinealoma, acoustic neuroma, and pituitary gland adenoma.[88] Others have reported "low" rates of transmission (to both abdominal and cardiothoracic organ recipients) from primary CNS tumors and advocate for the use of these donors, justifying the added risk by comparing it with the risk of dying while waiting for a transplant.[89] Registry data show donor transmission of glioblastoma multiforme and medulloblastoma.[88] High-grade glioblastoma histology, history of craniotomy, and ventricular shunting are associated risk factors for transmission of disease.[90] Consequently some advocate that the use of organs from donors with malignant brain tumors who have undergone ventricular shunting should be avoided.[88] In fact, transmission of donor disease was assessed at approximately 7% in the absence of important risk factors, but increased to 53% when at least 1 of these risk factors (high-grade tumor, prior chemotherapy, prior radiation therapy, or craniotomy) was present.[91] At the very least, caution should be exercised with the use of high-grade tumors of the central nervous system, and relative risk should be weighed against the urgency of the recipient's need.

Conclusion

Evaluation of the potential organ donor must include thoughtful and complete history taking and a systematic approach to all positive findings. Many more organs may be deemed suitable if risk factors for disease are addressed in the workup of the donor. Once assessed, this information should be shared with transplant centers. Given the ongoing shortage of available organs for transplantation, transplant centers have begun to use grafts previously deemed unsuitable. Transplant centers will weigh any potential relative risk against the potential recipient's risk of death while on the waiting list. The aim of all donor evaluation must be to increase utilization of consented organs while minimizing risk to recipients; this goal can be accomplished through collaboration between OPOs and transplant centers and through ongoing research and publications related to donor suitability.

References

1. United Network for Organ Sharing Policies. Available at: http://www.unos.org/PoliciesandBylaws2/policies/pdfs/policy_2.pdf. Accessed April 16, 2006.
2. Feng S, Buell JF, Cherikh WS, et al. Organ donors with positive viral serology or malignancy: risk of disease transmission by transplantation. *Transplantation*. 2002;74:1657-1663.
3. United Network for Organ Sharing. Policies. Available at: http://www.unos.org/PoliciesandBylaws2/policies/pdfs/policy_2.pdf. Accessed April 16, 2006.
4. Chung RT, Feng S, Delmonico FL. Approach to the management of allograft recipients following the detection of hepatitis B virus on the prospective organ donor. *Am J Transplant*. 2001;1:185-191.
5. Wang SS, Chou NK, Ko WJ, et al. Heart transplantation using donors positive for hepatitis. *Transplant Proc*. 2004;36:2371-2373.
6. Akalin E, Ames S, Sehgal V, Murphy B, Bromberg JS. Safety of using hepatitis B virus core antibody or surface antigen-positive donors in kidney or pancreas transplantation. *Clin Transplant*. 2005;19:364-366.
7. Condron SL, Heneghan MA, Patel K, Dev A, McHutchison JG, Muir AJ. Effect of donor age on survival of liver transplant recipients with hepatitis C virus infection. *Transplantation*. 2005;80:145-148.
8. Centers for Disease Control. Hepatitis C virus transmission from an antibody-negative organ and tissue donor: United States, 2000-2002. 2003. Available at: http://www.cdc.gov/mmwr/preview/mmwrhtml/mm5213a2.htm. Accessed April 16, 2006.
9. Haji SA, Starling RC, Avery RK, et al. Donor hepatitis-C seropositivity is an independent risk factor for the development of accelerated coronary vasculopathy and predicts outcome after cardiac transplantation. *J Heart Lung Transplant*. 2004;23:277-283.
10. Chamberland M, Khabbaz RF. Emerging issues in blood safety. *Infect Dis Clin North Am*. 1998;12:217-229.
11. Downes KA, Yomtovian R. Advances in pretransfusion infectious disease testing: ensuring the safety of transfusion therapy. *Clin Lab Med*. 2002;22:475-490.
12. Determination of donor suitability for human tissue intended for transplantation. 21 CFR §1270.21. Available at: http://frwebgate3.access.gpo.gov/cgi-bin/waisgate.cgi?WAISdocID=2359444772+1+0+0&WAISaction=retrieve. Accessed April 1, 2006.
13. Centers for Disease Control. Epidemiologic Notes and Reports. 1987. Human immunodeficiency virus infection transmitted from on organ donor screened for HIV antibody: North Carolina. Available at: http://www.cdc.gov/mmwr/preview/mmwrhtml/00019010.htm. Accessed April 16, 2006.
14. Fernandez-Merino FJ, Nuno-Garza J, Lopez-Hervas P, et al. Impact of donor, recipient, and graft features on the development of primary dysfunction in liver transplants. *Transplant Proc*. 2003;35:1793-1794.
15. Vidal RR, Momblan D, Gonzalez FX, et al. Evaluation of potential liver donors: limits imposed by donor variables in liver transplantation. *Liver Transplant*. 2003;9:389-393.
16. Feng S, Goodrich NP, Brag-Gresham JL, et al. Characteristics associated with liver graft failure: the concept of a donor risk index. *Am J Transplant*. 2006;6:783-790.
17. Rinella ME, Alonso E, Rao S, et al. Body mass index as a predictor of hepatic steatosis in living liver donors. *Liver Transplant*. 2001;7:409-414.
18. Saadeh S, Younossi ZM, Remer EM, et al. The utility of radiological imaging in nonalcoholic fatty liver disease. *Gastroenterology*. 2002;123:745-750.
19. Limanond P, Raman SS, Lassman C, et al. Macrovesicular hepatic steatosis in living related liver donors: correlation between CT and histologic findings. *Radiology*. 2004;230:276-280.
20. Urena MA, Moreno Gonzalez E, Romero CJ, Ruiz-Delgado FC, Moreno C. An approach to the rational use of steatotic donor livers in liver transplantation. *Hepatogastroenterology*. 1999;46:1164-1173.
21. Zamboni F, Franchello A, Davi, E, et al. Effect of macrovesicular steatosis and other donor and recipient characteristics on the outcome of liver transplantation. *Clin Transplant*. 2001;15:53-57.
22. Verran D, Kusyk T, Painter D, et al. Clinical experience gained from the use of 120 steatotic donor livers for orthotopic liver transplantation. *Liver Transplant*. 2003;9:500-505.
23. Salizzoni M, Franchello A, Zamboni F, et al. Marginal grafts: finding the correct treatment for fatty livers. *Transplant Int*. 2003;16:486-493.
24. Bunnapradist S, Gritsch HA, Peng A, Jordan SC, Cho YW. Dual kidneys from marginal adult donors as a source for cadaveric renal transplantation in the United States. *J Am Soc Nephrol*. 2003;14:1031-1036.
25. Ramos E, Aoun S, Harmon WE. Expanding the donor pool: effect on graft outcome. *J Am Soc Nephrol*. 2002;13:2590-2599.

26. Modlin CS, Goldfarb DA, Novick AC. The use of expanded criteria cadaver and live donor kidneys for transplantation. *Urol Clin North Am.* 2001;28:687-707.
27. Reddy KS, Stablein D, Taranto S, et al. Long-term survival following simultaneous kidney-pancreas transplantation versus kidney transplantation alone in patients with type 1 diabetes mellitus and renal failure. *Am J Kidney Dis.* 2003;41:464-470.
28. Hariharan S, Pirsch JD, Lu CY, et al. Pancreas after kidney transplantation. *J Am Soc Nephrol.* 2002;13:1109-1118.
29. Lutz-Dettinger N, de Jaeger A, Kerremans I. Care of the potential pediatric organ donor. *Pediatr Clin North Am.* 2001;48:715-749.
30. Michalak G, Kwiatkowski A, Czerwi ski J Simultaneous pancreas-kidney transplantation: analysis of donor factors. *Transplant Proc.* 2003;35:2337-2338.
31. Keller MS, Coln CE, Trimble JA, Green MC, Weber TR. The utility of routine trauma laboratories in pediatric trauma resuscitations. *Am J Surg.* 2004;188:671-678.
32. Justice AD, DiBenedetto RJ, Stanford E. Significance of elevated pancreatic enzymes in intracranial bleeding. *South Med J.* 1994;87:889-893.
33. Powner DJ. Donor care before pancreatic tissue transplantation. *Progr Transplant.* 2005;15:129-137.
34. Larson-Wadd K, Belani KG. Pancreas and islet cell transplantation. *Anesthesiol Clin North Am.* 2004;22:663-674.
35. Mittal NK, Tzakis AG, Kato T, Thompson JF. Current status of small bowel transplantation in children: update 2003. *Pediatr Clin North Am.* 2003;50:1419-1433.
36. Saggi BH, Farmer DG, Yersiz H, Busuttil RW. Surgical advances in liver and bowel transplantation. *Anesthesiol Clin North Am.* 2004;22:713-740.
37. DeBakey ME, Deitrich EB, Glick G, et al. Human cardiac transplantation: clinical experience. *J Thorac Cardiovasc Surg.* 1969;58:303-317.
38. Griepp RB, Stinson EB, Clark DA, Shumway NE. The cardiac donor. *Surg Gynecol Obstet.* 1971;133:792-798.
39. Copeland JG. Only optimal donors should be accepted for heart transplantation: protagonist. *J Heart Lung Transplant.* 1995;14:1038-1042.
40. Young J, Naftel D, Bourge R, et al. Matching the heart donor and the heart recipient. *J Heart Lung Transplant.* 1994;13:353-365.
41. Jeevanandam V, Satoshi F, Prendergrast TW, Todd B, Eisen HJ, McClurken JB. Standard Criteria for an Acceptable Donor Heart Are Restricting Heart Transplantation. *Annals of Thoracic Surgery*, 1996:62-1268-73
42. El Oakley RM, Yonan NA, Simpson BM, Deiraniya AK. Extended criteria for cardiac allograft donors: a consensus study. *J Heart Lung Transplant.* 1996;15:255-259.
43. Lietz K, John R, Mancini DM, Edwards NM. Outcomes in cardiac transplant recipients using allografts from older donors versus mortality on the transplant waiting list: implications for selection criteria. *J Am Cardiol.* 2004;43:1553-1561.
44. Shao-Zhou G, Hunt SA, Alderman EL, Liang D, Yeung AC, Schroeder JS. Relation of donor age and preexisting coronary artery disease on angiography and intracoronary ultrasound to later development of accelerated allograft coronary artery disease. *J Am Coll Cardiol.* 1997;29:623-629.
45. Zaroff J, Rosengard BR, Armstrong WF, et al. Consensus Conference Report: Maximizing use of organs recovered from the cadaver donor: cardiac recommendations. *Circulation.* 2002;106:836-841.
46. Grauhan O, Patzurek MH, Lehmkuhl H, et al. Donor transmitted coronary atherosclerosis. *J Heart Lung Transplant.* 2003;22:568-573.
47. Grauhan O, Hetzer R. Impact of donor-transmitted coronary atherosclerosis. *J Heart Lung Transplant.* 2003;23(suppl 9):S260-S262.
48. Marelli D, Laks H, Bresson S, et al. Results after transplantation using donor hearts with preexisting coronary artery disease. *J Thorac Cardiovasc Surg.* 2003;126:821-825.
49. Musci M, Pasic M, Grauhan O, et al. Orthotopic heart transplantation with concurrent coronary artery bypass grafting or previous stent implantation. *Kardiologie.* 2004;93:971-974.
50. Abid Q, Parry G, Forty J, Dark JH. Concurrent coronary grafting of the donor heart with left internal mammary artery: 10 year experience. *J Heart Lung Transplant.* 2002;21:812-814.
51. Wheeldon DR, Potter CD, Oduro A. Transforming the "unacceptable" donor: outcomes from the adoption of a standardized donor management technique. *J Heart Lung Transplant.* 1995;14:734-742.
52. Zaroff JG, Babcock WD, Shiboski SC. The impact of left ventricular dysfunction on cardiac donor transplant rates. *J Heart Lung Transplant.* 2003;22:334-337.
53. Zaroff JG, Babcock WD, Shiboski SC, Solinger LL, Rosengard BR. Temporal changes in left ventricular systolic function in heart donors: results of serial echocardiography. *J Heart Lung Transplant.* 2003;22:383-388.

54. Marelli D, Laks H, Fazio D, Moore S, Moriguchi J, Kobashigawa J. The use of donor hearts with left ventricular hypertrophy. *J Heart Lung Transplant.* 2000;19:496-503.
55. Laks H, Marelli D, Fonarow G, et al. Use of two recipient lists for adults requiring heart transplantation. *J Thorac Cardiovasc Surg.* 2003;125:49-59.
56. Aziz S, Soine LA, Lewis SL, et al. Donor left ventricular hypertrophy increases risk for early graft failure. *Transplant Int.* 1997;10:446-450.
57. Anderson JR, Hossein-Nia M, Brown P, et al. Donor cardiac troponin T predicts subsequent inotrope requirements following cardiac transplantation. *Transplantation.* 1994;58:1056-1057.
58. Vijay P, Scavo VA, Morelock RJ, et al. Donor cardiac troponin T: a marker to predict heart transplant rejection. *Ann Thorac Surg.* 1998;66:1934-1939.
59. Popatov EV, Ivanitskaia EA, Loebe M, et al. Value of cardiac troponin I and T for selection of heart donors and as predictors of early graft failure. Transplantation. 2001;71:1394-1400.
60. Menza RL, Babcock WD, Zaroff JG. Does donor cardiac troponin I predict 30 day survival after cardiac transplantation? Abstract presented at: American Transplant Congress (ATC), May 3-5, 2003; Washington, DC.
61. Weill D. Donor criteria in lung transplantation: an issue revisited. *Chest.* 2002;121:2029-2031.
62. Fisher AJ, Donnelly SC, Pritchard G, Dark JH, Corris P. Objective assessment of criterion for selection of donor lungs suitable for transplantation. *Thorax.* 2004;59:434-437.
63. Orens JB, Boehler A, de Perrot M, et al. A review of lung transplant donor acceptability criteria. *J Heart Lung Transplant.* 2003;22:1183-1200.
64. Lardinois D, Banysch M, Korom S, et al. Extended donor lungs: eleven years experience in a consecutive series. *Eur J Cardiothorac Surg.* 2005;27:762-767.
65. Aigner C, Winkler G, Jaksch P, et al. Extended donor criteria for lung transplantation: a clinical reality. *Eur J Cardiothorac Surg.* 2005;27:757-761.
66. Pennefather SH, Bullock RE, Dark JH. The effect of fluid therapy on alveolar arterial oxygen gradient in brain dead organ donors. *Transplantation.* 1993;56:1418-1422.
67. United Network for Organ Sharing. *Policies and Procedures: Minimum Information for Thoracic Offers (policy 3.7.12).* Richmond, VA: UNOS; 2005.
68. Gabbay E, Williams TJ, Griffiths AP, et al. Maximizing the utilization of donor organs offered for lung transplantation. *Am J Respir Crit Care Med.* 1999;56:1418-1422.
69. Straznicka M, Follette DM, Eisner MD, Roberts PF, Menza RL, Babcock WD. Aggressive management of lung donors classified as unacceptable: excellent recipient survival one year after transplantation. *J Thorac Cardiovasc Surg.* 2002;124:250-258.
70. el-Gamel AL, Egan L, Rahman A, Deiraniya AK, Yonan N. Application of pulmonary vein gas analysis: a novel approach which may increase the pool of potential lung transplant donors. *J Heart Lung Transplant.* 1996;15:315-316.
71. Shumway SJ, Hertz MI, Petty MG, Bolman RM III. Liberalization of donor criteria in lung and heart-lung transplantation. *Ann Thorac Surg.* 1994;57:92-95.
72. Weil D, Dey GC, Hicks A, et al. A positive donor gram stain does not predict outcome following lung transplantation. *J Heart Lung Transplant.* 2003;12:555-558.
73. Low DE, Kaiser LR, Haydock DA, Trulock E, Cooper JD. The donor lung: infectious and pathologic factors affecting outcome in lung transplantation. *J Thorac Cardiovasc Surg.* 1993;106:614-621.
74. Pierre AF, Sekine Y, Hutcheon M, Wadedell TK, Keshavjee S. Marginal donor lungs: a reassessment. *J Thorac Cardiovasc Surg.* 2002;123:421-428.
75. Puskas JD, Winton TL, Miller JD, Scavuzzo M, Paterson GA. Unilateral donor lung dysfunction does not preclude successful contralateral single lung transplantation. *J Thorac Cardiovasc Surg.* 1992;103:1015-1017.
76. Bhorade SM, Vigneswaran W, McCabe Garrity ER. Liberalization of the door criteria may expand the donor pool without adverse consequence in lung transplantation. *J Heart Lung Transplant.* 2000;19:1199-1204.
77. Fisher AJ, Donnelly SC, Hirani N et al., Enhanced pulmonary inflammation in organ donors following fatal non-traumatic brain injury, *Lancet* 353 (1999), pp. 1412–1413.
78. Kriesel D, Engels F, Krupnick A, et al. Emergent lung retransplantation after discovery of two primary malignancies in the donor. *Transplantation.* 2001;71:1859-1862.
79. Lipshutz GS, Baxter-Lowe LA, Ngyue T, Jones KD, Ascher NL, Feng S. Death from donor-transmitted malignancy despite emergency liver retransplantation. *Liver Transplant.* 2003;10:1102-1107.
80. Buell JF, Beebe TM, Trofe J, et al. Donor transmitted malignancies. *Ann Transplant.* 2004;9:53-56.
81. Buell JF, Gross RR, Alloway JT, Woodle ES. Central nervous system tumors in donors: misdiagnosis carries a high morbidity and mortality. *Transplant Proc.* 2005;37:583-584.

82. Kauffman HM, McBride MA, Cherikh WS, Spain PC, Marks WH, Roza AM. Transplant tumor registry: donor related malignancies. *Transplantation*. 2002;74:358-362.
83. Frutos MA, Daga D, Ruiz P, Mansilla J, Requena M. Prostate specific antigen in the assessment of organ donors. *Transplant Proc*. 2003;35:1644-1646.
84. Buell JF, Trofe J, Hanaway MJ, et al. Transmission of donor cancer into cardiothoracic recipients. *Surgery*. 2001;130:660-668.
85. Wunderlich H, Wilhelm S, Reichelt O, Zermann DH, Borner R, Schubert J. Renal cell carcinoma in renal graft recipients and donors: incidence and consequences. *Urology*. 2001; 67:24-27.
86. Morris-Stiff G, Steel A, Savage P, et al. Transmission of donor melanoma to multiple organ transplant recipients. *Am J Transplant*. 2004:4:444-446.
87. Kauffman HM, McBride MA, Cerikh WS, Spain PC, Marks WH, Roza AM. Transplant tumor registry: donor related malignancies. *Transplantation*. 2002;74:358-362.
88. Hornik L, Tenderich G, Wlost S, Zittermann K, Minami K, Koefer R. Organs from donors with primary brain malignancy: the fate of cardiac allograft recipients. *Transplant Proc*. 2004;36:3133-3137.
89. Pokorna E, Stefan V. The fate of recipients of organs from donors with diagnosis of primary brain tumor. *Transplant Int*. 2001;14:346-347.
90. Collignon FP, Holland EC, Feng S. Organ donors with malignant gliomas: an update. *Am J Transplant*. 2004;4:15-21.
91. Buell JF, Trofe J, Sethuraman G, et al. Donors with central nervous system malignancies: are they truly safe? *Transplantation*. 2003;76:340-343.

Adult Clinical Donor Care

David J. Powner, MD, FCCP, FCCM
Kevin J. O'Connor, PA, MS, CPTC

Introduction

Effective organ donor care, defined as optimizing the function and viability of all transplantable organs, is the cornerstone of successful transplantation. With the total pool of potential brain-dead organ donors in the United States estimated to be only 10500 to 13800 per year,[1] expert clinical care of every potential organ donor is essential to maximize the supply of organs for transplantation. There is currently wide variation in recovery fractions of specific organs from standard criteria donors.[2] Moreover, in 2004, more than 6300 patients with end-organ failure died while waiting for a lifesaving organ transplant.[3] These findings serve as clear evidence for an opportunity, and a responsibility, to improve the overall rate of organ recovery and utilization through improved care of the organ donor.

Critically injured brain-dead patients often present with complex clinical management challenges, including hemodynamic instability, hypoxemia, electrolyte abnormalities, coagulopathies, and neurogenic diabetes insipidus. The alteration in neuroendocrine function that accompanies brain death further complicates the care of these patients.[4] Without prompt, aggressive, and effective recognition, management, and correction, these disorders may result in progressive end-organ deterioration leading to irretrievable organ failure and consequent loss of otherwise suitable organs for transplantation.

Clinicians involved in the care of potential organ donors must be familiar with these challenges and their proper treatment, as well as sensitive to the competing interests and preferences of specific organ transplant programs. For example, preferred fluid management for lung donation (central venous pressure <6) may be perceived as inadequate by kidney programs that favor a higher renal blood flow rate and a brisk diuresis (3-4 mL/kg/h).

Effective donor care requires clinical expertise, vigilance, flexibility, and the ability to address multiple complex clinical issues simultaneously and effectively. Collaboration among organ procurement organization (OPO) staff, donor hospital critical care staff and consultants, and transplant program staff is of paramount importance in optimizing care of organ donors and maximizing the supply of organs suitable for transplantation.

The focus of this chapter is on care of the brain-dead potential organ donor. Donation after cardiac death is fully discussed in another chapter. The following sections describe recommended approaches to the brain-dead organ donor, and provide a foundation for maximizing organ recovery and transplantation by reducing the loss of suitable organs because of suboptimal clinical donor support.

Care of the organ donor should be guided by evidence-based clinical studies that identify optimal, or at least tolerable, hemodynamic, laboratory, and physiologic parameters to be maintained before organ explantation. Presently, it is not, because no such database currently exists to guide the organ procurement coordinator (OPC). Studies that attempt to correlate donor selection with recipient or graft outcome are largely uncontrolled retrospective analyses that often highlight factors such as age, cause of death, and gender, which cannot be altered during donor care. Although these variables remain important during allocation of organs, little investigational emphasis has been placed on correlating donor characteristics that could be altered after brain death with optimal organ or recipient outcomes. Such studies would also serve to expand the concept of "marginal organs" by identifying "acceptable" ranges for parameters that are associated with successful transplantation. Donor care provides limitless opportunities for important research in these areas.

At present, donor care is usually provided using guidelines adopted by each OPO. These often reflect priorities of the OPO medical advisors or referral transplant centers. "Authoritative" consensus groups or experienced practitioners have also provided detailed sets of guidelines, as shown in Table 1.[5-12]

Table 1. PUBLISHED GUIDELINES FOR DONOR CARE

Indiana University/State University of New York – (1989)[5]
Addenbrookes Hospital, Cambridge UK – (1989)[6]
University of Pittsburgh – (1989)[7]
Alfred Hospital, Melbourne – (1995)[8]
UNOS Critical Pathway – (1999)[9]
Crystal City Consensus Conference – (2002)[10]
University of Texas/University of Pittsburgh – (2004)[11]
University of Wisconsin – (2004)[12]

Most guidelines advise how to maintain donor physiology and organ function within "normal limits." These boundaries are appropriate, but it is largely unknown if satisfactory, or perhaps even superior, organ function would occur if laboratory or physiological parameters were extended outside such normal boundaries. Similarly, it is unknown if various combinations of nonnormative values, such as low intravascular hydrostatic pressure but high serum oncotic forces might improve organ availability and/or function in the recipient.

One set of published guidelines[11] has been selected for presentation in this chapter and was developed through a series of publications in *Progress in Transplantation*.[13-20] Concepts and references defending these recommendations are cited in those primary publications. Principles of donor care will be reviewed below, but specific interventions are provided in this chapter's Appendix. These guidelines are offered as recommendations based on current critical care practices and the limited literature cited in those primary publications. However, treatment specified by an OPO would, of course, supersede the recommendations offered here. It is suggested, however, that final OPO treatment plans be of similar precision and detail.

Overview

Although the OPC may be present as imminent death evolves through brain-death certification, responsibility for donor care is not usually assumed until after consent for donation has been obtained. Advice to care providers beforehand, however, may be appropriate and appreciated and should be offered as accepted by local practice.

Transfer of continuing donor care to the OPO via its medical designees should be documented in the medical record as soon as appropriate. Revision of existing orders or placement of new medical orders is intended to: (1) discontinue medications no longer needed or appropriate, e.g., anticonvulsants, mannitol, sedatives, and analgesics; (2) continue needed medications, or therapy, e.g., vasoactive drug infusions, intravenous fluids, and mechanical ventilator settings; (3) create "call-orders" that inform bedside personnel of goals for physiologic parameters and alert the OPC of changes in donor status, e.g., urine output, body temperature, and intravascular pressures (central venous, pulmonary artery, or arterial); (4) initiate immediate and repetitive laboratory testing to monitor electrolyte, hematological, coagulation, or acid base status—in general, repeated testing of routine variables (sodium, potassium, chloride, bicarbonate, arterial blood gas values, hematocrit, glucose) every 4 hours is useful, but suggested treatment guidelines (see Appendix) often recommend more frequent testing; (5) modify or establish the donor's "code status" as directed by OPO guidelines; and (6) initiate organ assessment or allocation decisions, e.g., echocardiogram, arterial blood gas values, and chest radiograph.

The new order set solidifies communication between the OPC and other bedside personnel and refocuses treatment toward organ transplantation. Similarly, a physician resource(s) must be identified, who can be available to the OPC for discussion and/or provision of needed procedures. This may either be physicians at the hospital or an OPO medical consultant(s). This resource is critical and is frequently referenced in the suggested guidelines.

See Rx Guideline – Fundamental Donor Care, page 11.

A CLINICIAN'S GUIDE TO DONATION AND TRANSPLANTATION

Clinical Considerations

Cardiovascular[14,19-21]

Brain injury or ischemia produces extensive hormonal effects throughout other organ systems, especially in the heart and vasculature. Catecholamines (epinephrine, norepinephrine, and dopamine) are released from the brain after injury or ischemia, and increase further during final evolution of brain death.[4] As discussed elsewhere in this text, a powerful discharge of the sympathetic nervous system also appears to occur, followed by a generalized loss of sympathetic nervous system tone. In addition, cytokines are produced centrally in the brain and distally in organs being readied for removal and exert profound effects in the donor and recipient.

The clinical manifestations of this catastrophic physiologic process during the evolution of brain death in about 50% of donors is a period of severe hypertension, followed, usually within minutes or a few hours, by hypotension. Cardiac arrhythmias are more frequent during this time and may include ectopic ventricular and/or supraventricular depolarizations, bradycardia, tachycardias of sinus or atrial origin, and atrial fibrillation. On the basis of animal data, this hyper-hypotension cycle most commonly occurs when progression from injury to brain death evolves rapidly.[22] If intracerebral hypertension develops slowly, although still culminating in brain death, less severe hypertension, hypotension, and cardiac instability are noted. Although the OPC may not provide primary care during this period, it is important to be aware of these changes.

Although subsequent donor hypertension is often not treated, it increases cardiac work and may contribute to poor cardiac performance. OPO guidelines should specify at what systolic and mean arterial blood pressures treatment should be initiated and when therapy should be stopped before explantation. A short-acting ß-receptor antagonist, for example, esmolol, small doses of an intermediate ß-blocker, for example, labetalol, or a short-acting calcium channel blocker, for example, nicardipine, will likely be effective.

Preexisting or concomitant conditions may cause donor hypotension. Hemorrhagic, obstructive, and distributive forms of shock should be considered, as well as those cardiogenic causes of hypotension most often associated with brain death. Monitoring blood pressure via an arterial catheter during assessment and subsequent treatment is preferred. Central venous and/or pulmonary artery pressure monitoring may also be indicated to better assess the determinants of cardiac output, preload, afterload, contractility, and heart rate. Data measured or derived from vascular pressure monitoring, especially systemic vascular resistance index and left ventricular stroke work index, are extensively discussed in a reference publication.[20] The reliability of central venous and pulmonary artery "wedge" pressures as estimates of intravascular volume has been questioned in several patient groups,[23] but has not been investigated among donors. Despite these concerns, the Rx Guidelines for Hypotension (see Appendix) uses vascular pressure (central venous pressure and pulmonary artery occlusion pressure) in treatment algorithms to ensure a mean arterial pressure of >65 mm Hg. Initial therapy ensures adequate intravascular volume, preload. Thereafter, selection of a vasoactive drug is most appropriately guided by the systemic vascular resistance and left ventricular stroke work derived from cardiopulmonary "profiling." If volume expansion and titrated inotropic or vasopressor medications are unable to maintain mean arterial pressure, thyroid hormone, corticosteroid, vasopressin, and insulin may be indicated, but remain controversial.[24]

See Rx Guidelines – Hypertension, page 11 and Hypotension, page 12.

Mechanical Ventilation[13,18]

Because all donors are apneic, a controlled mode of mechanical ventilation, either volume or pressure limited, is used. Most commonly volume-controlled mechanical ventilation is selected during which a present tidal volume (6-10 mL/kg/breath) is delivered at a preset flow rate and frequency (rate) and is supported by positive end-expiratory pressure (PEEP) and an inspired oxygen concentration (fraction of inspired oxygen [FIO_2]). In this mode of ventilation, peak and plateau airway pressures may vary as lung or thoracic compliance ("stiffness") and/or airway resistance change, and must be carefully monitored. High airway pressure may cause lung rupture (barotrauma) or decreased venous return (preload), causing hypotension.

By adjusting ventilator settings or changing to pressure-limited (PL) ventilation, airway pressure may be kept within safe limits (plateau airway pressure <35 cm H_2O). Interrelationships among ventilator settings must be understood by the OPC as inappropriate settings may quickly lead to adverse consequences. The interactions of tidal volume, flow rate, cycle time, inspiration:expiration ratio, and airway/intrathoracic pressure are discussed in the primary reference[13] and summarized in Table 2.

PL ventilation may be in use as the OPC begins donor care or may be initiated if airway pressure remains high. The advantage of the PL mode is control of peak airway pressure. However, variations in tidal volume, and hence carbon dioxide elimination, may occur because of changes in lung/thoracic compliance or airway resistance, and is the primary variable to be monitored during PL ventilation. Ventilator settings differ between these 2 modes and are compared in Table 3 for treatment of hypoxemia and managing $PaCO_2$. Other modes of ventilation, airway pressure release ventilation, and high-frequency oscillatory or percussive ventilation[25-27] have been recently reviewed and may become common during donor care.

In all modes of ventilation, the 2 determinants of oxygenation remain FIO_2 and mean airway pressure. Increasing FIO_2 to 100% is appropriate for short-term treatment of hypoxemia but rapidly "washes-out" nitrogen from the lung and possibly causes resorption atelectasis, leading to increased shunt-effect and worse hypoxemia. Ventilator adjustments to elevate mean airway pressure must be orchestrated carefully to avoid high peak airway pressures (volume controlled ventilation), loss of tidal volume (PL ventilation), or creation of auto-PEEP (both modes).

Carbon dioxide elimination or retention is determined by minute alveolar ventilation (V_{ALV} = rate (tidal volume − dead space). Pulmonary dead space represents areas of the lung or ventilator tubing circuit where carbon dioxide elimination does not occur and may include mechanical, anatomic, and physiological components. Of particular clinical importance is avoiding creation of physiological dead space described as West's Zone 1[28] wherein high airway pressure, low cardiac output, or low pulmonary capillary blood flow allows compression of capillaries and decreases carbon dioxide elimination. Adjustments in tidal volume or rate usually suffice to control $PaCO_2$ but reduction in dead space may be necessary. As discussed below, carbon dioxide elimination is the primary technique to ensure that arterial pH remains normal.

See Rx Guideline – Mechanical Ventilation, page 16.

Table 2. INTERRELATIONSHIPS OF PARAMETERS DURING VOLUME CONTROLLED MECHANICAL VENTILATION

Parameter Increase*	Effect
V_T	↑ Peak AWP
	↑ Mean AWP
	↑ Ti
	↓ Te (beware of auto-PEEP)
Set PEEP	↑ Peak AWP
	↑ Mean AWP
	No effect on Ti or Te
Flow rate†	↑ Peak AWP
	↓ Mean AWP
	↓ Ti
	↑ Te
Frequency (or rate)	No change in AWP unless auto-PEEP occurs
	No change in Ti
	↓ Te (beware of auto-PEEP)
Pause time	↑ Ti
	↓ Te (beware of auto-PEEP)
	↑ Mean AWP
	No change in peak AWP unless auto-PEEP occurs

Abbreviations: AWP, airway pressure; PEEP, positive end-expiratory pressure; T_I, inspiratory time; Te, expiratory time; V_T, tidal volume; ↑, increased; ↓, decreased.

*A decrease in these parameters will have the opposite effect from that shown here.

† Effect on mean AWP may be variable, but increased flow rate shortens TI, causing the lung to be gas filled for less time during 1 minute; hence mean AWP usually falls.

Reprinted with permission from Progress in Transplantation.

Fluid and Electrolytes[15]

The OPC will likely encounter electrolyte abnormalities as donor care begins. Thereafter, frequent laboratory assessment and intravenous administration of fluid or electrolytes as quickly as permitted by local hospital pharmacy rules are usually necessary.

Table 3. COMPARISON BETWEEN VOLUME CONTROLLED (VC) AND PRESSURE LIMITED (PL) MECHANICAL VENTILATION

Goal	VC	PL
Treat hypoxemia	1. Increase FIO_2 2. Increase mean AWP without increasing plateau AWP* • Decrease flow rate† • Add inspiratory pause 3. Increase PEEP‡	1. Increase FIO_2 2. Increase inspiratory time by change in I:E ratio† 3. Increase PEEP§
Increase ventilation (decrease $PaCO_2$)	1. Increase ventilator rate† 2. Increase V_T (will increase peak AWP and inspiratory time†) 3. Minimize V_D by ensuring intravascular volume and cardiac output are optimal	1. Increase ventilator rate† 2. Increase pressure limit (will increase V_T and peak AWP) 3. Same 4. Increase inspiratory time (may increase V_T)

Abbreviations: AWP, airway pressure; PL, pressure-limited mechanical ventilation; VC, volume controlled mechanical ventilation; FIO_2, fraction of inspired oxygen; I:E, inspiratory-expiratory ratio; PEEP, positive end-expiratory pressure; V_D, volume of dead space; V_T, tidal volume.

* Assumes peak and plateau AWPs are already elevated and of concern.
† Will change inspiratory and expiratory times. Beware of auto-PEEP.
‡ May increase peak and plateau AWPs.
§ Will reduce V_T.

Reprinted with permission from Progress in Transplantation.

Laboratory measurements are always in units of electrolyte (or other substance) per unit of plasma volume, often milliequivalents or millimoles per liter (mEq/L or mmol/L). These "concentration" units emphasize the importance of both the solute (electrolyte or other substance) and the solvent (mostly plasma water) in assessing physiological availability of the ion/substance. In general, a low concentration is treated by administering the ion or substance, whereas a high concentration is treated by administering water and withholding the ion or substance. Relocation of water from the interstitial to the intravascular compartment of the extracellular fluid space may be affected by administration of colloid fluids (hetastarch or albumin). Although such therapy remains controversial,[29] it may assist in reducing lung edema or other morbidity.[30,31]

Some electrolytes (sodium, chloride, bicarbonate) are distributed almost exclusively in the extracellular fluid compartment (plasma and interstitial spaces). Blood specimens, therefore, reflect total body reserves for those ions. Others, such as potassium, magnesium, phosphorous, and calcium, are distributed mostly within cells, and serum measurements do not reflect their total body stores. Replacement of both extracellular and intracellular ions, however, depends greatly upon frequent laboratory testing, as redistribution of ions is common. Only ionized calcium, as the unbound and biologically active form of calcium, should be measured and replaced.

Electrolytes function in many cellular processes that may not be clinically apparent. Their role in maintaining transmembrane "bioelectrical" gradients and creation or propagation of action potentials, however, may cause dysrhythmias (arrhythmias) as a common sign of imbalance.[21]

The presence of donor hypernatremia (>155 mEq/L) was shown to worsen recipient graft function.[32] If the serum sodium concentration was reduced to less than 155 mEq/L, however, improved graft function was observed. This is the only specific electrolyte abnormality shown to directly influence recipient outcome, but others have not been well investigated.

Diabetes insipidus, producing excessive renal free water loss and hypernatremia, is common after brain death, but other causes of polyuria (ie, residual effects of osmotic agents or diuretics, hyperglycemia, or physiological fluid loss) must also be considered. Diabetes insipidus may rapidly produce dehydration, hypovolemia, and hypotension. Hourly replacement of urine output with hypotonic intravenous fluids and administration of desmopressin (DDAVP) or aqueous vasopressin may be required.

See Rx Guidelines – Fluid and Electrolyte Treatment, page 18 and Polyuria, page 19.

Glucose[15,34]

The serum concentration at which blood sugar should be maintained remains controversial. Accumulated medical literature indicates harmful effects of hyperglycemia (increased infection, accentuated inflammatory response, decreased white blood cell function, and renal failure) among intensive care unit patients.[33] How these data apply to donors is not known. However, hyperglycemia (> ~200 mg/dL) may produce an osmotic diuresis, contributing to donor polyuria, free water loss, hypovolemia, and hypotension.

Other published data and surgeon preference, support some level of hyperglycemia to stimulate islet cells before pancreatic or islet cell transplantation.[34] Similarly, providing adequate glycogen stores in the liver before its removal improves tolerance to cold ischemia and preserves function in the recipient.[35]

Therefore, OPO protocols should define specific blood glucose goals and methods to administer insulin. Recommendations in the Appendix combine subcutaneous and intravenous bolus insulin therapy. Most intensive care units have adopted similar protocols and/or continuous intravenous insulin infusion procedures. Although the OPC may prescribe specific glucose ranges, use of local hospital protocols with which bedside nursing staff is most familiar with best ensures achieving glucose goals.

See Rx Guideline – Glucose Management, page 13.

Acid-Base[16]

An imbalance in donor acid-base status may cause dysrhythmias, abnormal serum electrolytes, altered oxygen binding to hemoglobin, and lower cardiac output. Abnormal blood pH (acidemia, alkalemia) may not reflect abnormalities in organs/tissues (acidosis or alkalosis).

The primary tool to assess acid-base status is testing arterial blood gas (ABG) values, which provides pH, $PaCO_2$, PaO_2, HCO_3, and usually base excess (BE). The BE is a useful tool to estimate the metabolic (vs respiratory) component of the acid-base derangement. It is the amount of acid or base that should be added to the blood to normalize the pH, assuming a normal $PaCO_2$. Normal BE is zero, a larger number reflects a greater abnormality, a negative sign (-BE) indicates metabolic acidosis, and a positive BE (+BE) indicates metabolic alkalosis. "Respiratory" alkalemia or academia is always iatrogenic as the donor is apneic and respirations are controlled by the OPC.

Metabolic alkalemia is unusual during donor care but may be seen if the donor is dehydrated as may have occurred during treatment of intracranial hypertension. Most often this "contraction alkalosis" can be reversed with fluid expansion of the intravascular space. Acetazolamide (Diamox) should not be used during donor care as its effect on the kidney will extend beyond transplantation.

Metabolic acidosis is more common especially when severe hypotension is present. The anion gap (sodium – (chloride + HCO_3) is used to identify diagnostic categories of metabolic acidosis. Acidosis with a normal gap (<12) most often is secondary to hyperchloremia after administration of 0.9% (normal) or hypertonic saline (3% or greater) during previous resuscitation or treatment of head injury. Other less common causes include early renal failure, parenteral nutrition, chronic hyperventilation during mechanical ventilation (low $PaCO_2$), or extensive use of acetazolamide (Diamox). Increased anion gap (>12) acidosis associated with increased serum lactic acid may be of physiological significance. During donor care, increased gap metabolic acidosis with hyperlactemia should prompt an aggressive search for any cause of shock.

The guidelines in the Appendix focus on initial treatment to correct the pH by adjusting the mechanical ventilator tidal volume or rate to change the $PaCO_2$. The $PaCO_2$ may be changed over a wide range because an excess or deficit of carbon dioxide itself produces few physiological consequences. If such respiratory adjustments are not sufficient, sodium bicarbonate in metabolic acidosis or, rarely, a metabolic acid in metabolic alkalosis may be necessary. It is important to recall that sodium bicarbonate administration may induce intracellular acidosis, as carbon dioxide generated from bicarbonate freely diffuses into cells and lowers intracellular pH.

See Rx Guideline – Acid-Base Treatment, page 20.

Coagulation Abnormalities[17]

Abnormal coagulation may occur because of the following:
1. "consumption" or dilution of serum proteins (coagulation factors) responsible for a portion of the coagulation process;
2. previous use of medications intended to provide anticoagulation, e.g., warfarin, heparin, and thrombolytics;
3. abnormal platelet function after aspirin, clopidogrel (Plavix), ticlopidine (Ticlid™), or glycoprotein IIbIIIa platelet receptor blockers, abciximab (ReoPro), eptifibatide (Integrilin™), and tirofiban (Aggrastat™);
4. low platelet counts (thrombocytopenia); and
5. accelerated function of the plasminogin/fibrinolysis plasma system of proteins responsible for normal clot dissolution.

Any of these causes or medications may have contributed to intracerebral hemorrhage/brain death, and may still be present as the OPC assumes donor care.

Laboratory evaluation includes a platelet count, prothrombin time, partial thromboplastin time, and fibrinogen. Abnormal platelet function may be evaluated by thromboelastography, commercially available platelet function assay machines, and a bleeding time, although these devices are not commonly in use and the bleeding time may not be offered by all laboratories. Other tests, d-dimer or fibrin "split" products, used to diagnose disseminated intravascular coagulation are often abnormal if previous trauma or clotting has occurred.

Severe hemorrhage may accompany a coagulopathy. Treatment with packed red blood cell transfusions and frequent monitoring of hemoglobin and hematocrit may be necessary. Platelet transfusions should correct thrombocytopenia to a "safe" level as specified by OPO guidelines (recommended >80 000 plts/mm^3). Each platelet donor unit provided by the blood bank may elevate the platelet count by 10 000, but this effect may be less during continuing consumption or dilution. Cryoprecipitate is only used to increase serum fibrinogen to above 100 mg/dL. (2.9 micromoles/L). Fresh frozen plasma (15 mL/kg) (~200 mL/U) is given to replace a coagulation factor deficit (elevated prothrombin time and partial thromboplastin time). Vitamin K requires 4 to 6 hours to begin its effect and is not recommended here.

Drugs prescribed to provide anticoagulation have become more common. Counteracting their effects may have already been done as part of patient care. However, if brain death has evolved quickly or no therapy was given, some treatment may be indicated. Aspirin, clopidogrel, and ticlopidine cause irreversible loss of function to all affected platelets. Therefore, unaltered platelets are infused (usually ~12 single donor units; 1 donor unit/10 kg donor weight) to replace defective platelets. Other categories of drugs, glycoprotein IIbIIIa receptor antagonists and direct thrombolytics, require a combination of agents to counteract their effect.[36] As more data accumulates, recombinant factor VII may become important in donor care.[36-38]

The general process in treating bleeding complicated by abnormal coagulation is to assess and treat blood loss, administer appropriate agents to correct the coagulation derangement, and repeat the laboratory assessment and treatment as necessary until the clinical status is stabilized. In addition, plans for organ retrieval are expedited.

See Rx Guideline – Coagulopathy and Thrombocytopenia, page 15.

Temperature[17]

After loss of hypothalamic temperature regulating centers following brain death, the body temperature of most donors falls toward ambient environmental temperature (poikilothermia). Hypothermia, therefore, is common and may be worsened by administration of cold blood bank products or room temperature intravenous fluids. Temperature measurements using core (pulmonary artery, esophageal) or urinary thermistors and rectal thermometers are more accurate than oral or tympanic measurements.

Hypothermia may interfere with blood coagulation; decrease cardiac contractility; increase polyuria; or cause dysrhythmias, vasoconstriction, or decreased oxygen availability to tissues. Hypovolemia, reduced regional blood flow, tissue hypoxia, and organ loss may result.

Prompt interventions to rewarm the donor or prevent further cooling should begin early. Heated humidified gas via the ventilator and heated air or water "mattresses" are usually sufficient to maintain body temperature above 36ºC.

Hyperthermia may occur during donor care from endogenous pyrogens during infection. It is rarely severe and nonaspirin antipyretics (e.g., acetaminophen) are usually sufficient. Treatment of any known infections should, of course, continue or be initiated.

See Rx Guideline – Temperature, page 14.

Anemia

Blood loss as a consequence of primary injuries or complicated by a coagulopathy or hypothermia may endanger organ donation. Primary sites of bleeding should be treated to ensure hemostasis. Serial measurements of hemoglobin and hematocrit will guide the need for transfusion.

Blood transfusion therapy has been shown to be potentially harmful to intensive care unit patients,[39,40] but has not been separately evaluated among donors. OPO guidelines should identify an appropriate minimal hemoglobin or hematocrit at which optimal oxygen-carrying capacity will provide sufficient oxygen delivery to organs.

See Rx Guideline – Anemia, page 15.

Conclusion

The OPC has been empowered by federal regulation, the OPO and its medical advisors and directors, the donor, the donor's family, and the recipient to provide the best possible organs for transplantation. This profound responsibility must be taken seriously and implemented with all the professionalism demanded by the lifesaving outcomes of transplantation. The complex physiology surrounding brain death makes the care of organ donors one of the most difficult clinical challenges in critical care. It must be done correctly to maximize outcome potentials. The OPO carries a similarly important responsibility, to make resources, education, and expertise available to its coordinators to fulfill that mission. These or similar guidelines are intended to assist in those important goals.

References

1. Sheehy E, Conrad SL, Brigham LE, et al. Estimating the number of potential organ donors in the United States. *N Eng J Med.* 2003;349:667-674.
2. Delmonico FL, Sheehy E, Marks SH, Baliga P, McGowan JJ, Magee JC. Organ donation and utilization in the United States, 2004. *Am J Transplant.* 2005;5:862-873.
3. United Network for Organ Sharing. Removal reasons by year. Available at: http://www.unos.org. Accessed May16, 2005.
4. Powner DJ, Hendrich A, Lagler RG, Ng RH, Madden RL. Hormonal changes in brain dead patients. *Crit Care Med.*1990;18:702-798.
5. Powner DJ, Jastremski M, Lagler RG. Continuing care of multiorgan donor patients. *J Intensive Care Med.* 1989;4:75-83.
6. Bodenham A, Park GR. Care of the multiple organ donor. *Intensive Care Med.* 1989;15:340-348.
7. Darby JM, Stein K, Grenvik A, Stuart SA. Approach to management of the heartbeating 'brain dead' organ donor. *JAMA.* 1989;261:2222-2228.
8. Scheinkestel CD, Tuxen DV, Cooper DJ, Butt W. Medical management of the (potential) organ donor. *Anaesth Intens Care.* 1995;23:51-59.
9. Holmquist M, Chabalewski F, Blount T, et al. A critical pathway: guiding care for organ donors. *Crit Care Nurse.* April 1999;19:84-98.
10. Zaroff JG, Rosengard BR, Armstrong WF, et al. Consensus Conference Report. Maximizing use of organs recovered from the cadaver donor: cardiac recommendations. *J Heart Lung Transplant.* 2002;21:1153-1160.
11. Powner DJ, Darby JM, Kellum JA. Proposed treatment guidelines for donor care. *Prog Transplant.* 2004;14:16-28.
12. Wood KE, Becker BN, McCartney JG, D'Alessandro AM, Coursin DB. Care of the potential organ donor. *N Engl J Med.* 2004;351:2730-2739.
13. Powner DJ, Darby JM, Stuart SA. Recommendations for mechanical ventilation during donor care. *Prog Transplant.* 2000;10:33-40.
14. Powner DJ, Darby JM. Management of variations in blood pressure during care of organ donors. *Prog Transplant.* 2000;10:25-32.
15. Powner DJ, Kellum JA, Darby JM. Abnormalities in fluids, electrolytes, and metabolism of organ donors. *Prog Transplant.* 2000;10:88-96.
16. Powner DJ, Kellum JA. Maintaining acid-base balance in organ donors. *Prog Transplant.* 2000;10:98-105.
17. Powner DJ, Reich HS. Regulation of coagulation abnormalities and temperature in organ donors. *Prog Transplant.* 2000;10:146-153.
18. Powner DJ, Delgado E. Using pressure-limited mechanical ventilation in caring for organ donors. *Prog Transplant.* 2001;11:174-181.
19. Powner DJ. Effects of gene induction and cytokine production in donor care. *Prog Transplant.* 2003;13:9-16.
20. Powner DJ, Crommett JW. Advanced assessment of hemodynamic parameters during donor care. *Prog Transplant.* 2003;13:249-257.
21. Powner DJ, Allison TA. Cardiac dysrhythmias during donor care. *Prog Transplant.* 2006;16:74-81.
22. Shivalker B, Van Loon J, Wieland W, et al. Variable effects of explosive or gradual increase of intracranial pressure on myocardial structure and function. *Circulation.* 1993;87-230-239.
23. Powner DJ, Miller ER, Levine RL. CVP and PAoP measurements are discordant during fluid therapy after traumatic brain injury. *J Intensive Care Med.* 2005;2 0:28-33.
24. Powner DJ, Hernandez MS. A review of thyroid hormone administration during donor care. *Prog Transplant.* 2005;15:202-207.
25. Habashi NM. Other approaches to open-lung ventilation: airway pressure release ventilation. *Crit Care Med.* 2005;33(suppl):S228-S240.
26. Chan KPW, Stewart TE. Clinical use of high-frequency oscillatory ventilation in adult patients with acute respiratory distress syndrome. *Crit Care Med.* 2005;33(suppl):S170-S174.
27. Salim A, Martin M. High-frequency percussive ventilation. *Crit Care Med.* 2005;33(suppl):S241-S245.
28. West JB. Regional differences in the lung. *Chest.* 1978;74:426-437.
29. Finfer S, Bellomo R, Boyce N, et al. A comparison of albumin and saline for fluid resuscitation in the intensive care unit. *N Engl J Med.* 2004;350:2247-2256.
30. Vincent JL, Navickis RJ, Wilkes MM. Morbidity in hospitalized patients receiving human albumin: A meta-analysis of randomized, controlled trials. *Crit Care Med.* 2004;32:2029-2038.
31. Martin GS, Mangialardi RJ, Wheeler AP, Dupont WD, Morris JA, Bernard GR. Albumin and furosemide therapy in hypoproteinemic patients with acute lung injury. *Crit Care Med.* 2002;30:2175-2182.

32. Totsuka E, Dodson F, Urakami A, et al. Influence of high donor serum sodium levels on early postoperative graft function in human liver transplantation: effect of correction of donor hypernatremia. *Liver Transplant Surg.* 1999;5:421-428.
33. van den Berghe G, Wouters PJ, Bouillon R, et al. Outcome benefits of intensive insulin therapy in the critically ill: insulin dose versus glycemic control. *Crit Care Med.* 2003;31:359-366.
34. Powner DJ. Donor care before pancreatic tissue transplantation. *Prog Transplant.* 2005;15:129-137.
35. Powner DJ. Factors during donor care that may affect liver transplantation outcome. *Prog Transplant.* 2004;14:241-249.
36. Powner DJ, Hartwell EA, Hoots WK. Counteracting the effects of anticoagulants and anti-platelet agents during neurosurgical emergencies. *Neurosurgery.* In press. [[AU: Has this manuscript been published?]]
37. Levi M, Peters M, Büller HR. Efficacy and safety of recombinant factor VIIa for treatment of severe bleeding: a systemic review. *Crit Care Med.* 2005;33:883-890.
38. Mayer SA, Brun NC, Begtrup K, et al. Recombinant activated factor VII for acute intracerebral hemorrhage. *N Engl J Med.* 2005;352:777-785.
39. Toy P, Popovsky MA, Abraham E, et al. Transfusion-related acute lung injury: definition and review. *Crit Care Med.* 2005;33:721-726.
40. Robinson WP, Ahn J, Stiffler A, et al. Blood transfusion is an independent predictor of increased mortality in nonoperatively managed blunt hepatic and splenic injuries. *J Trauma.* 2005;58:437-445.

A CLINICIAN'S GUIDE TO DONATION AND TRANSPLANTATION

Appendix – Recommended Treatment Guidelines for Donor Care

Rx Guideline – Fundamental Donor Care

Introduction: As the procurement coordinator assumes responsibility for continuing donor care, priorities for assessment and treatment change to ensure that the best physiological support will be given to maximize the potential for successful organ transplantation. That transition is facilitated by policies that allow ongoing care orders be written by the coordinator and supported by the organ procurement organization's (OPO's) medical staff. Some previous treatment may no longer be appropriate for organ procurement, but many aspects of fundamental patient care should be continued.

The coordinator should write orders to initiate standard donor care:

1. Transfer care to [Name of OPO]
2. Vital signs – blood pressure, heart rate, temperature, urine output, central venous pressure (CVP) [if central venous catheter present], pulmonary artery occlusion pressure (PAOP) [if pulmonary artery (PA) catheter is present] every 1 hour
3. Reorder mechanical ventilator parameters as previously set
4. Maintain head of bed at 30 to 40° elevation
5. Continue routine pulmonary suctioning and side-to-side body positioning
6. Warming blanket to maintain body temperature above 36.5°C
7. Maintain sequential compression devices (SCDs)
8. [If present] Continue chest tube suction or water seal as previously ordered
9. [If present] Nasogastric (orogastric) tube to low intermittent suction
10. Intravenous fluid—D5 0.45% saline plus 20 mEq KCl per liter at 75 mL/h
11. Call OPO coordinator if: mean arterial pressure (MAP) <70 mm Hg; systolic pressure >170 mm Hg; heart rate <60 >130 beats/min; temperature <36.5°C or >37.8°C; urine output <75 >250 mL/h; CVP or PAOP <8 >18 mm Hg
12. Medications: intravenous (IV) pantoprazole 40 mg every 24 hours, first dose now (or other medication for prophylaxis against gastrointestinal bleeding)

    Artificial tears every 1 hour and as required to prevent corneal drying

    Albuteral and Atrovent unit dose per aerosol every 4 hours

    Continue antibiotics previously ordered at same dose and frequency. Review all medications previously ordered. Most (anticonvulsants, pain medications, laxatives, gastrointestinal motility agents, eye drops, antihypertensives, antinausea agents, subcutaneous heparin, osmotic agents [mannitol], and diuretics) are unnecessary during donor care and may be discontinued.

    Continue vasoactive drug infusions (dopamine, norepinephrine, etc) at previously ordered concentrations and infusion rates

    Review any other medications in question with physician
13. Send electrolytes, magnesium, ionized calcium, complete blood cell count (CBC), platelets, glucose, blood urea nitrogen, creatinine, phosphorous, arterial blood gas, prothrombin time (PT), partial thromboplastin time (PTT), STAT and repeat every 4 hours.
14. [If not previously done] Send blood for type and screen
15. Finger stick glucose every 2 hours – call glucose <90 >180 mg/dL
16. Electrocardiogram STAT
17. Chest radiograph STAT—Indication: initial donor evaluation.
18. [Add other orders for specific organ evaluation as indicated]

The above order set provides a "safety net" of call orders so that the coordinator is alerted to significant changes in donor status. It also prescribes the foundation for ongoing monitoring of physiological and laboratory variables.

Donor care is subsequently directed and "fine-tuned" through the **Rx Guidelines** that follow. Each may be referenced as that circumstance/problem arises. Although the guidelines are not intended to compartmentalize the complex process of overall donor care, they may be helpful in providing useful resources in methods of treatment, precautions, and points at which physician consultation is appropriate.

Rx Guideline – Hypertension

Introduction: It is unusual for hypertension to occur after brain death, although it is common during the evolution of brain death. Because donor organs are likely at more risk from hypotension than hypertension, a conservative treatment plan is recommended. The goal for MAP is <90 mm Hg when the donor is hypertensive, but always above 65 to 70 mm Hg. The MAP is measured via an intra-arterial catheter, noninvasive blood pressure device or calculated by: diastolic pressure + 1/3(systolic – diastolic pressures) + 5. Placement of the arterial catheter in an upper extremity is preferred.

Treatment:
- A. Reduce or discontinue inotropic or vasopressor medications or infusions
- B. If the **difference** between the MAP recorded via an arterial catheter and noninvasive machine is >20 mm Hg, discuss which blood pressure to follow with the physician consultant. Differences in measurements taken from an automatic oscillometric noninvasive device and an arterial catheter may be due to several technical factors.
- C. Labetalol 10 to 20 mg IV bolus every 20 minutes up to 2 doses
- D. If ineffective, nicardipine IV infusion at 5 mg/h may be titrated up to 15 mg/h.
- E. If the above are ineffective in lowering blood pressure to <90 mm Hg, consult physician.

Rx Guideline – Hypotension

Introduction: Hypotension commonly follows brain death and may be caused by ongoing or preexisting conditions leading to hemorrhagic, cardiogenic, distributive, or obstructive types of "shock." In the absence of these preexisting conditions causing shock, hypotension commonly occurs after brain death because of loss of vasomotor centers in the brain causing vasodilation, decreased contractility of the heart, or hypovolemia due to ongoing fluid loss due to diabetes insipidus. Hypotension will be defined as a MAP of < 60 mm Hg, as measured from an indwelling arterial catheter, noninvasive blood pressure machine, or calculated by: diastolic pressure + 1/3 (systolic – diastolic pressure) + 5. Placement of an arterial catheter for monitoring is desirable, and insertion in an upper extremity is preferred. The treatment goal for MAP is 65 to 75 mm Hg.

I. Assessment:
- A. Review medical record for evidence of recent blood loss. Confirm that the most recent hematocrit level is >0.28 and reaffirm with an immediate repeat hematocrit. (Refer to Rx Guidelines – Anemia and Coagulopathy and treat as indicated if the hematocrit level is <0.28 or a coagulation disorder is present.)
- B. Review medical record for evidence of concomitant myocardial ischemia/infarction during this admission. Repeat electrocardiogram (ECG) and maintain at bedside. Consult physician for ECG interpretation.
- C. Review medical record for evidence of excessive fluid losses above intake (output > intake by > 1500 mL in the last 24 hours) during current hospitalization. If polyuria is present, refer to Rx Guideline – Polyuria.
- D. Review current patient status for a central venous catheter and evaluate CVP or PA catheter and evaluate PAOP. The goal is to maintain both at 12 to 15 mm Hg. If PA catheter present, obtain information regarding cardiac output, cardiac index, systemic vascular resistance index, and left ventricular stroke work index.
- E. Review the medical record for evidence of ongoing severe infection, drug or other allergic reactions (e.g., due to transfusion), pericardial effusion, or pneumothorax. Obtain a chest radiograph and consult physician for its interpretation.

II. Treatment Algorithm
- A. Ensure any signs of continuing hemorrhage (external, gastrointestinal (GI), urinary, abdominal, etc.) have been evaluated and interventions initiated.
- B. Discontinue medications that may contribute to hypotension (e.g., antihypertensives, β-blockers).
- C. The general principle of treatment is to first ensure that adequate intravascular volume (preload) is present as evidenced by a CVP and/or PAOP greater than 12 mm Hg.
- D. Begin treatment with a crystalloid solution such as 0.9% saline (normal saline) or Ringer's lactate. Colloid solutions may be added and may be preferable for repeated fluid challenges (5% albumin- 250 or 500 mL). Thereafter, either inotropic or vasopressor medications will be infused and titrated to the MAP goal or other hemodynamic parameters. If a PA catheter is available or at any time is inserted, a cardiac/hemodynamic profile should be obtained. If the donor demonstrates a low systemic vascular resistance index (SVRI) (< 1400 $dyne.sec.m^2/cm^5$) a vasopressor (e.g., norepinephrine, phenylephrine) is the vasoactive drug of choice and subsequently titrated to maintain the MAP >60 mm Hg. If the left ventricular stroke work index (LVSWI) is low (<35 $g.m/m^2$), a positive inotropic agent (e.g., dopamine, dobutamine) should be used. The algorithm below assumes that if the MAP, CVP, heart rate, and PAOP goals are reached, vital signs will continue to be monitored. Vasoactive medications should be weaned and removed as soon as possible, while maintaining the MAP goal. Subsequent deviations from goal values may require return to the guidelines.

A CLINICIAN'S GUIDE TO DONATION AND TRANSPLANTATION   Chapter 32

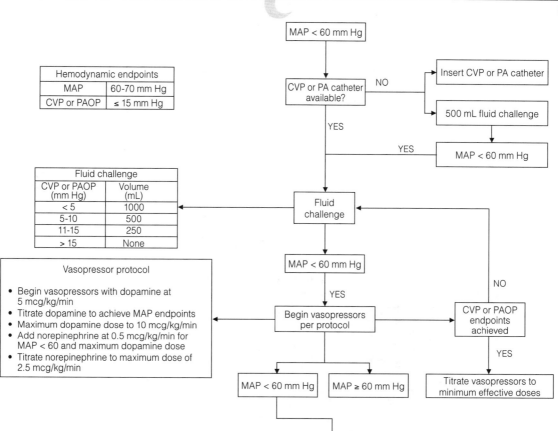

Rx Guideline – Glucose Management

Introduction: Both hypoglycemia and hyperglycemia may harm donor organs. Measure serum glucose every 4 hours and obtain finger stick glucose (FSG) per glucometer every 2 hours unless as described below.

I. **Hypoglycemia:** Treat <75 mg/dL
   A. Give 1 premixed syringe of 50% dextrose (D50).
   B. Repeat glucose or obtain FSG in 30 minutes and repeat 50% dextrose if glucose <75 mg/dL
   C. If laboratory or FSG remains <75 mg/dL after 2 doses of D50, consult physician.

II. **Hyperglycemia:** Treat serum glucose > 150 mg/dL
   A. Ensure glucose removed from all IV fluids/infusions unless required by pharmacy.
   B. Current intensive care unit (ICU) protocols may exist for glucose control. Bedside nursing personnel may be most familiar with and prefer to use them. Initiate treatment as indicated therein.
   C. The algorithms below show a subcutaneous insulin sliding scale and a supplemental IV insulin regimen.
      Note: Give subcutaneous insulin no more often than every 4 hours. When supplemental IV insulin is also needed, give the IV insulin bolus prescribed by the IV sliding scale every hour after the hourly FSG. Stop IV insulin when the blood sugar drops below 250 mg/dL.
   D. In summary, hyperglycemia is treated by first removing sources of exogenous glucose, followed by subcutaneous insulin per the above sliding scale every 4 hours. Supplemental IV insulin is given each hour and thereafter **only if** the blood glucose remains above 225 mg/dL.

E. Subcutaneous insulin sliding scale:

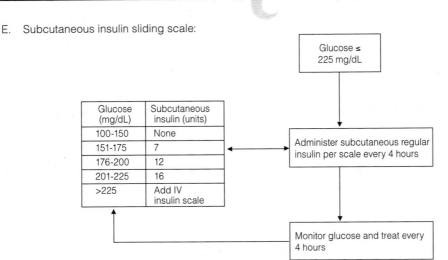

F. Supplemental IV insulin sliding scale. Give the subcutaneous insulin every 4 hours as prescribed above plus the hourly IV bolus prescribed below when the blood glucose or FSG is >225 mg/dL.

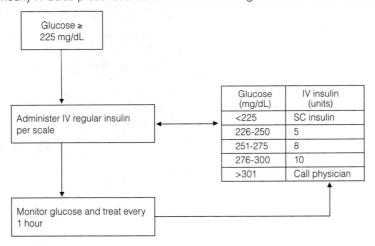

G. If glucose remains >250 mg/dL 4 hours after the initial subcutaneous insulin and subsequent IV insulin therapy, consult physician to discuss an insulin infusion.

Rx Guideline – Temperature

Introduction: Brain death usually causes loss of thermal regulation in the donor, commonly resulting in hypothermia. The temperature goal is 36°C to 37.5°C (97°F-99.5°F).

I. **Hypothermia:** Treat <36°C (97°F)
   A. The preferred method of body temperature measurement is from a core site, such as a PA catheter or bladder (specialized catheter). Axillary temperatures should not be used, and oral temperatures are less accurate in hypothermia. Rectal temperatures can be used if hypothermia is not severe (>35°C).
   B. Use active surface warming with a heated-liquid or hot air warming blanket plus insulating thermal blankets.
   C. Warm the inspired gas from the ventilator to 38.5°C (101.3°F).
   D. Minimize the amount of body surface and time of exposure to environmental temperatures.
   E. If temperature remains <36°C after 3 hours of attempted rewarming, consult physician.

A CLINICIAN'S GUIDE TO DONATION AND TRANSPLANTATION Chapter 32

II. Hyperthermia: (Unusual after brain death) Treat >37.8°C (100.1°F)
   A. Remove unnecessary blankets.
   B. Do NOT cool inspired gas.
   C. Acetaminophen 650 mg per suppository or per gastric tube every 3 hours.
   D. Use automated fluid-filled cooling blanket.
   E. If temperature remains >101°F after 3 hours of cooling, consult physician.

Rx Guideline – Anemia

Introduction: Although the differential diagnosis for anemia may be extensive, during donor care the most likely causes are continuing blood loss or excessive blood draws for laboratory testing. Hemolysis may rarely occur. The goal is to maintain the hematocrit above 0.30 (30%).

I. Assessment
   A. Review medical record for evidence of bleeding sites, previous blood transfusions and their frequencies, or other information about blood loss or hemolysis.
   B. Observe for signs of ongoing bleeding from:
      1. External wounds, IV sites, etc.
      2. GI tract via gastric tube or bowel movements; observe for abdominal distension and/or firmness and changes during repeat abdominal assessment
      3. Urinary tract by observation or laboratory assessment for blood in urine.
   B. Refer to Rx Guideline – Coagulopathy. Obtain PT, PTT, fibrinogen and platelet count and treat as indicated.
   C. If hematocrit 0.28 to –0.30 and no signs of bleeding are present begin every 4 hour hematocrit measurements.
   D. If hematocrit 0.28 –to 0.30 and no gastric tube is in place, insert orogastric tube and lavage stomach to assess for upper GI blood.

II. Treatment
   A. If previous transfusions have been required, submit blood bank order to maintain 2 to 4 units of packed red blood cells (PRBC) available. Otherwise write order to type and cross-match and maintain 2 units PRBC available.
   B. If hematocrit <0.30, transfuse 2 units PRBC rapidly.
   C. Reassess hematocrit 1 hour after last unit PRBC infused and repeat transfusion if hematocrit <0.30.
   D. Reassess hematocrit 1 hour after 4th unit PRBC and reconsider above assessment items. If hematocrit <0.30 after 4 units PRBC, consult physician.

Rx Guideline – Coagulopathy and Thrombocytopenia

Introduction: Blood loss from any cause may endanger continued perfusion to donor organs. Disseminated intravascular coagulation or a "dilutional" coagulopathy may occur after severe trauma and resuscitation. The treatment goal is to correct a clinically important coagulopathy and thrombocytopenia. Because ongoing hemorrhage may worsen coagulation abnormalities and/or thrombocytopenia, refer to Rx Guideline – Anemia, and correct disorders noted.

It is recognized that commonly performed laboratory tests of coagulation, ie, PTT, PT, fibrinogen, and the platelet count may be abnormal but treatment may not be required. Treatment is reserved for donors who appear to have continuing significant blood loss evidenced by physical assessment, hemodynamic instability, and changes in coagulation parameters.

I. Assessment
   A. The donor's medical record should be reviewed for any possible injury that may account for bleeding. If found, discuss with physician.
   B. Review medical record to ensure that no drugs that might interfere with coagulation or platelet function have recently been given, e.g., warfarin, aspirin, heparin, clopidogrel, ticlopidine, glycoprotein IIbIIIa inhibitors, thrombolytics, dypyridamole, etc. Notify physician if recent administration is documented.
   C. Laboratory assessment: PT, PTT, fibrinogen, platelet count – repeat coagulation tests should be done 30 minutes after any administration of blood products.
   Normal values: PT <14.5 seconds, platelet count >150,000/mL^3
   PTT <35.6 seconds, fibrinogen 150 to 350 mg/dL

D. Measure ionized calcium – refer to Rx Guideline – Fluid/Electrolytes and treat hypoionized calcemia at < 2.3 mEq/L (<1.2 mmol/L).

II. **Treatment of continued signs of significant blood loss and associated abnormal coagulation results or platelet count:**
   A. Consult physician for external bleeding or further assessment of possible GI or urinary injury. Treat anemia as per Rx Guideline – Anemia.
   B. Platelets: Platelet dysfunction because of previous aspirin intake can be overcome by infusing a platelet 5-pack dose even though the platelet count is normal. Discuss with physician. Otherwise, treat for platelet count <80,000/mm³
      1. Transfuse 1 platelet pack (usually 5 or 6 individual units of platelets) intravenously as rapid infusion.
      2. Recheck platelet count 1 hour after first platelet pack and transfuse second platelet pack if platelet count remains <80,000/mm³. Obtain follow up platelet count exactly 1 hour after second platelet infusion completed.
      3. If platelet count remains < 80,000/mm³ after second platelet infusion, consult physician.
   C. Coagulopathy **(Increased PT, PTT):** Treat PT >15 seconds, PTT >38 seconds
      1. If donor had been receiving intravenous heparin and PTT is > 75 seconds, discuss administration of protamine with physician.
      2. Rapidly infuse 4 units fresh frozen plasma (FFP).
      3. Repeat PT, PTT measurements 30 minutes after initial FFP – repeat FFP if PT and PTT remain above treatment ranges.
      4. Repeat PT and PTT measurements 30 minutes after second FFP infusion – if PTT and PT remain elevated above treatment ranges, consult physician.
   D. Coagulopathy **(Decreased fibrinogen):** Treat fibrinogen <100 mg/dL
      1. Infuse 6 units of cryoprecipitate, rapidly
      2. Repeat fibrinogen 1 hour after initial cryoprecipitate infusion – repeat infusion of cryoprecipitate if fibrinogen remains <100 mg/dL
      3. Repeat fibrinogen 1 hour after second infusion of cryoprecipitate. If concentration remains <100 mg/dL, consult physician.

Rx Guideline – Mechanical Ventilation

Introduction: Under most circumstances, volume-controlled mechanical ventilation will be used during donor care. Pressure-limited mechanical ventilation is indicated when peak and plateau airway pressures are elevated, indicating high airway resistance or poor lung compliance (see below). The goals during mechanical ventilation are the following:
   A. Peak airway pressure (AWP) <40 cm H_2O
   B. Plateau AWP <35 cm H_2O
   C. Fraction of inspired oxygen (FIO_2) lowest possible to maintain SpO_2 > 92% and PaO_2 >70 mm Hg
   D. Positive end-expiratory pressure (PEEP) minimum 5 cm H_2O, adjust to maintain PaO_2 >70 mm Hg
   E. Auto-PEEP <5 cm H_2O
   F. Arterial blood gas (ABG) values: pH 7.35 to 7.45; $PaCO_2$ > 16 mm Hg, < 60 mm Hg to maintain pH within goal range; PaO_2 > 70 mm Hg; HCO_3 not independently adjusted.

I. **Assessment**
   A. Evaluate the medical record for cardiopulmonary diseases before or during this admission. Assess related issues such as chronic oxygen use at home, ongoing pneumonia, chest radiograph results, culture results, antibiotics ordered, respiratory treatments given, etc.
   B. Ensure recent ABG results available or obtain sample for testing. Compare results to the above treatment goals.
   C. Perform a physical examination with attention to abnormalities such as wheezing, rhonchi, sputum appearance/thickness/tenacity, etc.
   D. Repeat ABGs at least every 4 hours or more frequently to assess changes in respiratory status or after adjustments in ventilator settings.
   E. Consult with a respiratory care practitioner to identify if above mechanical ventilation goals are being met, i.e., auto-PEEP, airway pressures, etc.

II. General Ventilator Settings

A. Volume-controlled ventilation
1. Tidal volume (V_T) – 10 mL/kg ideal body weight (kg). If high peak AWP is present, reduce V_T to 6 to 8 mL/kg ideal body weight (kg).
   Ideal body weight:
   a. Male – 50 kg + 2.3 kg per inch > 60 inches
   b. Female – 45 kg + 2.3 kg per inch > 60 inches
2. Rate (f) – adjusted to maintain minute ventilation (V_T x f)(V_E) of approximately 8 to 10 L/min or to maintain $PaCO_2$ >16 mm Hg <60 mm Hg, so as to maintain arterial pH at 7.35 to 7.45. Downward adjustment in rate may be needed to minimize auto-PEEP.
3. Flow rate – usually about 60 L/min; adjust to minimize peak AWP; beware of auto-PEEP as flow rate is slowed; higher flow rate may be needed to minimize auto-PEEP.
4. PEEP – minimum 5 cm H_2O – adjusted to assist in maintaining PaO_2 >70 mm Hg.
5. FIO_2 – adjust to maintain PaO_2 >70 mm Hg.
6. Use decelerating (ramp) pattern for flow delivery, when available.

B. Pressure- limited ventilation
1. Inspiratory pressure setting – to limit peak AWP at 35 to 40 cm H_2O, consult with respiratory care practitioner for final pressure limit setting due to various ventilator types.
2. Rate – same as A(2) above.
3. PEEP – same as A(4) above. However, recall PEEP adjustments may change delivered V_T and V_E during pressure-limited ventilation, ie, increased PEEP will generally decrease V_T and V_E causing $PaCO_2$ to rise (reverse with decreased PEEP).
4. FIO_2 – same as A(5) above.

III. General Respiratory Treatments

A. Assure adequate suctioning of excessive sputum.
B. Ensure bronchodilators are ordered as indicated by wheezing or a peak AWP– plateau AWP gradient of >10 cm H_2O.
C. Other forms of chest physiotherapy or related devices are optional but should be considered.

IV. Ventilator Adjustments – Volume-controlled ventilation

Note: Repeat ABGs 30 minutes after any change of ventilator settings to assess effects
Note: Combinations of adjustments listed below may be necessary as guided by
ABG results and AWPs.

A. Acidemic pH – arterial pH <7.35
1. Increase V_T to maximum 12 mL/kg ideal weight as long as plateau AWP remains <35 cm H_2O, or
2. Increase rate to maximum 22 breaths/min as long as auto-PEEP remains <5 cm H_2O.
3. If pH remains <7.32 after above changes, refer to Rx Guideline- Acid-Base Treatment.

B. Alkalemic pH – arterial pH >7.45
1. Decrease ventilator rate sequentially to minimum of 6 breaths/min to achieve pH goal.
2. Decrease V_T to minimum of 6 mL/kg ideal body weight.
3. If pH remains >7.45, consult physician.

C. High plateau AWP >35 cm H_2O
1. Reduce flow rate to minimum 50 L/min – as long as auto-PEEP remains <5 cm H_2O.
2. Reduce V_T to minimum of 6 mL/kg ideal body weight – assess effect on arterial pH.
3. Reduce PEEP to minimum 5 cm H_2O – assess effect on PaO_2.
4. If plateau AWP remains > 35 cm H_2O, consult physician.

D. Auto PEEP >5 cm H_2O
1. Increase flow rate to maximum of 90 L/min – as long as plateau AWP remains <35cm H_2O.
2. Decrease V_T to minimum 6 mL/kg ideal body weight – assess effect on arterial pH.
3. Decrease ventilator rate sequentially to minimum of 8 breaths/min to minimize auto-PEEP – assess effect on arterial pH.
4. If auto-PEEP remains >5 cm H_2O, consult physician.

E. Low PaO_2 – PaO_2 < 70 mm Hg
1. Increase FIO_2 to maximum 1.0 (100%).
2. Increase PEEP to maximum 15 cm H_2O – as long as plateau AWP remains <35 cm H_2O.

3. Add inspiratory pause (hold) to maximum 1.0 seconds as long as auto-PEEP remains <5 cm H_2O.
4. If PaO_2 remains <70 mm Hg, consult physician.

V. **Ventilator Adjustments – Pressure-limited mechanical ventilation**
   A. Acidemic pH – arterial pH <7.35
      1. Increase ventilator rate to maximum 22 breaths/min as long as auto-PEEP <5 cm H_2O
         Note: Auto-PEEP will decrease V_T delivered and may worsen acidemia.
      2. Increase inspiratory pressure setting to maximum peak AWP of 45 cm H_2O.
      3. If arterial pH remains <7.32, consult physician.
   B. Alkalemic pH – arterial pH >7.45
      1. Decrease ventilator rate sequentially to minimum of 6 breaths/min to achieve pH goals.
      2. Decrease inspiratory pressure setting but maintain V_T above 6 mL/kg ideal body weight.
      3. If arterial pH remains >7.45, consult physician.
   C. Auto-PEEP – auto-PEEP >5 cm H_2O
      1. Decrease ventilator rate sequentially to minimum 8 breaths/min – assess effect on arterial pH.
      2. If >5 cm H_2O auto-PEEP persists, consult physician.
   D. Low PaO_2 – PaO_2 <70 mm Hg
      1. Increase FIO_2 to maximum 1.0 (100%).
      2. Increase ventilator PEEP to maximum of 15 cm H_2O as long as pH remains >7.35. (increased PEEP will decrease tidal volume delivered in pressure-limited ventilation.
      3. If PaO_2 remains <70 mm Hg, consult physician.

Rx Guideline – Fluid Electrolyte Treatment

Introduction: The treatment goal is to maintain electrolytes within the normal limits established by the clinical laboratory in each hospital. To achieve that goal, laboratory testing of sodium (Na), potassium (K), chloride (Cl), bicarbonate (HCO_3), magnesium (Mg), phosphorous (P), and ionized calcium (Ca^{++}), should be completed every 4 hours. More frequent testing may be needed to monitor and treat critical levels. Any testing should be delayed for 30 minutes after the last dose of the electrolyte being treated. All electrolyte replacement should be administered by the IV route.

I. **General Table of Normal Values:**
   Na 136-142 mEq/L (mmol/L)   Mg 1.5-2.3 mg/L (0.65-1.05 mmol/L)
   K 3.5-5.0 mEq/L (mmol/L)   Phos 2.3-4.7 mg/dL (0.74-1.52 mmol/L)
   Cl 96-106 mEq/L (mmol/L) Ca^{++} 2.3-2.54 mEq/L (1.15-1.27 mmol/L)
   HCO_3 21-28 mEq/L (mmol/L)

II. **Electrolyte Therapy**
   A. Sodium (Na)
      1. Hypernatremia – treat Na >150 mEq/L
         a. With polyuria (>250 mL of urine above intake per hour) – see Rx Guideline – Polyuria.
         b. Without polyuria – give 1 liter 0.2% saline (1/4 normal saline) as rapid infusion and replace urine output cc/cc/hr with 0.2% saline. Assure that all medications are mixed in 0.45% (1/2 normal saline) or 0.2% saline if pharmaceutically possible and that any maintenance IV is D5% 0.2% saline. Avoid use of diuretics.
      2. Hyponatremia: Treat for serum Na <133 mEq/L
         a. Mix all medications in 0.9% saline (normal saline) if pharmaceutically possible. Change maintenance IV to D5 0.9% saline.
         b. If hyperglycemia is present, the serum Na may be low because of the high blood glucose. If blood sugar >300, a "corrected" serum Na may be calculated by adding to the measured Na – 1.6 mEq for each 100 g/dL of blood glucose above 100. See Rx Guideline – Hyperglycemia and treat.
         c. If Na <128 mEq/L give 3% NaCl per infusion (central catheter preferred) at 40 mL/h for 3 hours.
         d. If Na remains <133 mEq/h after 3% NaCl infusion, consult physician.
   B. Potassium (K)
      1. Hyperkalemia: Treat serum K ≥ 5.8 mEq/L
         a. Note: do not treat K if laboratory reports specimen "hemolyzed" – send a new specimen for testing.
         b. Enssure all K removed from current infusions.

c. Repeat serum K every 1 hour
d. Give IV:
1. 50 mL of 50% dextrose (D50) (1 prefilled syringe)
2. 15 units regular humulin insulin
3. 1 amp $NaHCO_3$ (44 or 50 mEq via prefilled syringe)
e. If K > 5.8 mEq/L after above intervention, consult physician.
2. Hypokalemia: Treat ≤ 3.4 mEq/L
a. Delay administration of any diuretic.
b. Give 20 mEq KCL over 1 hour (central catheter preferred) as:
1. Serum K <3.4 mEq/L – 2 doses
2. Serum K <3.1 mEq/L – 3 doses
3. Serum K <2.9 mEq/L – 4 doses
c. If K remains >2.9 or <3.8 mEq/L – repeat above
d. If K remains <3.2 mEq/L thereafter, consult physician.
C. Chloride (Cl): Not independently treated
D. Bicarbonate (HCO_3): Not independently treated
E. Magnesium (Mg)
1. Hypermagnesemia: Not independently treated
2. Hypomagnesemia: Treat Mg <1.5 mg/dL (0.62 mmol/L)
a. Administer 4 grams magnesium sulfate ($MgSO_4$) over 2 hours – repeat as indicated by subsequent laboratory assessments to maintain above goal levels.
b. If Mg remains <1.5 mg/dL after 8 g $MgSO_4$, consult physician.
F. Phosphorus (P)
1. Hyperphosphatemia: Not independently treated
2. Hypophosphatemia: Treat serum P <2.2 mg/dL (0.71 mmol/L)
a. Give 30 mmol potassium or sodium phosphate over 3 hours and repeat (total of 2 doses).
b. If P remains <2.2 mg/dL (0.71 mmol/L) after 60 mmol sodium or potassium phosphate given, consult physician.
G. Calcium (Ca): Measure and treat only the ionized calcium value
1. Hyperionized calcemia: Not separately treated; withhold additional calcium
2. Hypoionized calcemia: Treat <4.4 mg/dL or <2.1 mEq/L or <1.1 mmol/L
a. Give 10 mLc 10% solution of calcium gluconate slow IV push.
b. Remeasure ionized Ca in 1 hour
c. Repeat above dose if ionized Ca remains low
d. If the ionized Ca remains low after 20 mL, 10% calcium gluconate is given, consult physician.

Rx Guideline – Polyuria

Introduction: Polyuria may quickly lead to hypovolemia and hypoperfusion of donor organs. The causes of polyuria may be (1) physiological diuresis after previous fluid administration, (2) osmotic diuresis because of previous mannitol therapy or continuing hyperglycemia, (3) diuresis from prescribed diuretics, or (4) diabetes insipidus. Physiological diuresis does not lead to hypotension, but all other forms may. If the donor demonstrates hypotension and polyuria, continue in this guideline, but refer also to Rx Guideline – Hypotension. The urine output goal is 75-150 mL/h.

I. Initial Assessment
A. Evaluate blood sugar per laboratory or FSG measurement. Glucose values >200 mg/dL may contribute to polyuria. Refer to Rx Guideline – Glucose Management.
B. Stop any prescribed diuretic therapy.
C. Calculate recent fluid intake/output balance and adjust intake to be 100 mL/h less than total output. Example: The urine output over the last 3 hours averaged about 400 mL/h; adjust total IV fluid intake to equal about 300 mL/h.
D. Follow every 2 hour with measurements of serum Na and glucose.
E. If Na >148 mEq/L, assume excessive free H_2O loss has occurred, and proceed with treatment plan below.
F. If serum Na 135 to 147 mEq/L when last measured, observe urine output and repeated serum Na measurements. Maintain fluid intake 100 mL less than urine output each hour.

II. Treatment

A. Stop excessive intake (maintain intake 100 mL less than output until intake and output are equal and then maintain intake = output).
B. If urine output >250 mL above IV intake for the last 2 hours and serum Na >145 mEq/L when last measured, give 1 microgram desmopressin (DDAVP) intravenously.
C. Begin replacement of urine output each hour mL/mL with 0.2% saline (1/4 normal saline; no dextrose).
D. If urine output has not declined below 200 mL above intake (urine out >200 mL above fluid intake) in the next hour, give an additional 1 microgram of DDAVP intravenously.
E. If urine output has not decreased to <200 mL above IV intake (urine output >200 mL above fluid intake) and Na has not fallen to <146 mEq/L in 2 additional hours, consult physician.

Rx Guideline – Acid-Base Treatment

Introduction: During donor care, monitoring and treating the arterial pH becomes the primary acid-base goal. Because there are few primary effects of hypocarbia or hypercarbia, the PaCO$_2$ will be adjusted to normalize the arterial pH (pH 7.35-7.45). Modifications of the mechanical ventilator to alter the PCO$_2$, and hence pH, are reviewed in the Rx Guideline – Mechanical Ventilation.

I. Assessment (Because hospitals may report either the base excess (BE) or base deficit (BD) with ABG results, both are included here.)

A. **Acidosis:** Review the ABG measurement obtained before manipulation of the mechanical ventilator recommended in the Rx Guideline – Mechanical Ventilation. Assess the BE or BD provided as part of the ABG results. If the BE is more negative than -6 or the BD is more positive than +6, metabolic acidosis is likely present.
B. **Alkalosis:** Review the ABG before adjustment of the mechanical ventilator as above. If the BE is more positive than +6 or BD is more negative than -6, metabolic alkalosis is likely present, although very unusual during donor care.

II. Treatment

A. **Metabolic Acidosis:** If the arterial pH remains <7.32 after the changes recommended in the Rx Guideline – Mechanical Ventilation (section IVA), administer 1 premixed syringe (44 or 50 mEq) NaHCO$_3$ slow IV push. However, if the Na is concurrently >150 mEq/L, consult physician before giving NaHCO$_3$. If the arterial pH remains <7.32 after retesting in 30 minutes, repeat the NaHCO$_3$ administration. If the arterial pH remains <7.32 thereafter, consult physician.
B. **Metabolic Alkalosis:** If the arterial pH remains >7.45 after the changes recommended in the Rx Guideline – Mechanical Ventilation (Section IVB), consult physician.

Management of the Pediatric Organ Donor

Thomas A. Nakagawa, MD
Steven S. Mou, MD

Introduction

The demand for organs and tissues continues to increase despite efforts to increase the donor pool. Historically, patients in need of organs and tissues have died from their organ failure, but these patients are now living longer because of advancements in pharmacologic and medical technology. Advancements in physiologic support mechanisms such as mechanical ventilation, cardiac assist devices, and renal and liver dialysis have extended these patients' lives, increasing the need for donors. Furthermore, the use and refinement of passenger safety restraint systems,[1] helmets, and other safety measures, as well as increased awareness of such precautions and technology,[2,3] have led to a reduction in accident-related fatalities, dramatically reducing the numbers of potential donors; obviously, these advancements are very important in the human condition, but they impose significant pressure to offset the discrepancy between supply and demand in the field of organ donation. The Organ Donation Breakthrough Collaborative efforts to increase organ donation has resulted in a 10.8% increase in the United States during 2004. However, despite these efforts, a large gap continues to exist between the number of donors and recipients.[4]

The ability to recover appropriate and viable organs for the pediatric population comes with a unique set of limitations, making the acquisition of these organs difficult. Size and weight constraints are a major limiting factor, most notably for small children and infants. Furthermore, a greater proportion of potential pediatric organ donors suffer brain injury as result of anoxia and ischemia, making the certainty of the diagnosis of irreversible brain injury more difficult. Therefore, an age-related variation in the timing associated with the confirmation of neurologic death in pediatric donors is suggested. The duration of the waiting period to pronounce neurologic death in children may affect the viability of suitable organs for transplantation by delaying their acquisition. Lastly, the specialized care required for aggressive management of the pediatric organ donor following neurologic death may be lacking at institutions that have limited expertise and support for children.

The management of potential pediatric organ donors requires knowledge of the physiologic derangements associated with this specific patient population. Typical derangements include metabolic and endocrine abnormalities, aberrations in ventilation and oxygenation, hemodynamic instability, and coagulation disturbances. In addition to meticulous management of physiologic derangements, care of the family provided by a team of social workers, chaplains, and other support staff is integral.[5,6] This chapter focuses on the management of potential pediatric organ donors who have progressed to neurologic death. Meticulous care of pediatric organ donors is essential to ensure successful recovery of organs in this selected group of patients.

Donor Suitability

Trauma is the leading cause of neurologic death in both children and adults, although asphyxia and hypoxic-ischemic insults are also significant causes of neurologic devastation and death in children.[7,8] Unique conditions in which nonaccidental trauma has resulted in the death of a child require close cooperation between forensic investigators, treating physicians, the transplant team, and the organ procurement organization to allow for successful procurement of organs.[9-14] Protocols to facilitate organ recovery in child abuse victims can decrease denials for organ donation from medical examiners.[15,16] In addition, involvement of the district attorney during protocol development should be a consideration.

Pediatric donors become eligible for organ procurement after the determination of neurologic death has been made. Although the vast majority of pediatric donors will be standard criteria donors, donation after cardiac death (DCD), or non-heart-beating organ donors, has the potential to increase organ donation in children.[17] An in-depth discussion about pediatric DCD is beyond the scope of this chapter; however, any child in which a "do not resuscitate" or "withdrawal of care" occurs in the course of management, or any child who expires a nonneurologic death should be considered as a potential DCD donor. The reevaluation of this common means of recovering organs before the development of brain death criteria continues to intensify as attempts are made to meet the demands of a growing national transplant list. In addition, DCD focuses on recovery of the two most commonly needed organs for children, liver and kidney. The most important point is that organ donation should be considered in any patient where end-of-life issues are being discussed.

The Determination of Brain Death

The determination of neurologic death in children remains a clinical diagnosis and is no different than in adults. No unique legal issues exist differentiating declaration of neurologic death in children. However, age-related issues can make confirmation of irreversible injury and declaration of neurologic death more difficult, resulting in age-based recommendations.[18]

The cause of coma and brain injury must be determined to ensure that an irreversible condition has occurred. Duration of observation and the need for ancillary tests should be based on history and clinical examination. Physical examination criteria for neurologic death rely on the coexistence of coma and apnea in a child that is not significantly hypothermic, hypotensive for age, and has not received recent doses of sedative or neuromuscular blocking agents. Absence of brainstem function is defined by the manifestation of all of the following features on physical examination: mid-position or fully dilated nonreactive pupils; absence of spontaneous eye movements induced by oculocephalic or oculovestibular testing; absence of cough, corneal, gag, and rooting reflexes; and absent respiratory effort off ventilator support. The examination results should remain consistent with brain death throughout the observation and testing period.[18]

The apnea test is essential for the confirmation of neurologic death. Testing for apnea must allow adequate time for $PaCO_2$ to increase to levels that would normally stimulate respiration. Apnea testing must be performed while maintaining normal oxygenation and stable hemodynamics.[19-21] Patients should be preoxygenated with 100% oxygen to prevent hypoxia, and mechanical ventilation should be discontinued or changed to continuous positive pressure ventilation while observing the patient for any spontaneous

Table 1. RECOMMENDED OBSERVATION PERIOD AND ANCILLARY TESTING ON THE BASIS OF THE AGE OF THE PATIENT[18]

7 days to 2 months
- Two examinations and EEGs separated by at least 48 hours

2 months to 1 year
- Two examinations and EEGs separated by at least 24 hours; a repeat EEG is not necessary if a cerebral radionuclide scan or cerebral angiography demonstrates no flow or visualization of the cerebral arteries

Older than 1 year
- When an irreversible cause exists, ancillary testing is not required and an observation period of 12 hours is recommended.
- The observation period may be decreased if the EEG demonstrates electrocerebral silence or the cerebral radionuclide or cerebral angiography study demonstrates no flow or visualization of the cerebral vessels.

Abbreviation: EEG, electroencephalogram

respiratory movements over a 5- to 10-minute period. The $PaCO_2$ should be measured and allowed to rise to 60 torr or greater. If no respiratory effort is noted during this time, documentation of the apnea test consistent with neurologic death is noted, and the patient is placed back on mechanical ventilation support until death is confirmed with a repeat clinical examination, or ancillary testing.[22,23] The recommended clinical observation period in children differs from adults, with a greater duration between examinations suggested for younger children. Table 1 lists guidelines recommended from the Special Task Force for Brain Death Guidelines in Children.[18] Observation periods have never been validated and should be used as recommendations only. Many authors agree that except in very immature, preterm newborns, the same criteria to declare brain death can be applied to full-term newborns, infants older than 7 days of age, children, and adults.[8,23-27] The special taskforce guidelines for the determination of brain death provide no guidelines to diagnose cerebral death in infants younger than 7 days of age.[18] Guidelines for this age group were not published in 1987, because there was limited experience, and establishing irreversibility and neurologic death was more difficult to confirm at that time.[19,28] This does not infer that neurologic death does not occur in this patient population. Diagnosing neurologic death can occur in the term infant, even those younger than 7 days of age; however, an observation period of 48 hours has been recommended to confirm the diagnosis.[29] The observation period can be shortened to 24 hours if ancillary studies demonstrate no cerebral blood flow or an isoelectric electroencephalogram (EEG).[28,29] The younger the child, the more cautious determination of neurologic death should be.

Ancillary testing can provide data to confirm neurologic death when the clinical examination and apnea test are not feasible or cannot be completed because of undue circumstances. Ancillary tests are not mandatory if clinical brain death determination is feasible; however, they can provide another layer of comfort to the physician who is uncomfortable declaring neurologic death on the basis of clinical examination alone. Ancillary tests may also be used to expedite the diagnosis of brain death by reducing the clinical observation period, potentially increasing viability of transplant tissue. However, if ancillary tests are equivocal or demonstrate blood flow or electrical activity, the patient should be observed according to proposed age-specific guidelines until another clinical examination is performed to confirm neurologic death.

A 4-vessel angiogram evaluating anterior and posterior cerebral circulation remains the gold standard in ancillary testing[30]; however, this test is difficult to perform in small children and requires technical expertise that may not be available in every facility. Furthermore, the requirement for transportation of a potentially unstable patient to the angiography suite complicates this process. Radionuclide flow scan using a portable gamma camera is more easily accomplished at the bedside, without the need for extraordinary technical expertise; therefore, this is one of the most frequently used tests in children.[30,31] In addition, improved radiotracer agents such as Tc-99m hexamethylpropylene-amine oxime have improved the ability to evaluate greater segments of the intracerebral circulation, most notably the posterior fossa.

EEG combined with a neurologic examination remains an accepted means to determine neurologic death in children. EEG testing should not be used alone to determine neurologic death because it does not assess brainstem function, a key in the final determination of brain death. In addition, EEG is influenced by factors such as hypothermia and sedative medications, which can complicate declaration of neurologic death and affect potential organ donation.[32] Doppler ultrasonography and brainstem audio evoked potentials have been used,[33] but have not been validated in children and cannot be relied on as a dependable ancillary study.[24,34] The clinical diagnosis of brain death is highly reliable when made by experienced examiners using established criteria.[35,36] Each state and institution has guidelines for determination of death, but the diagnosis of brain death still requires the thoughtful, mature judgment of a knowledgeable physician who takes all the facts into careful deliberation in each case.[25]

Brain Death Physiology

As neurologic death occurs, multiple physiologic changes become manifest. These derangements develop as a result of the loss of normal central nervous system (CNS) regulation. Endocrine dysfunction occurs because of inhibition or lack of hormonal stimulation from the hypothalamus. This neuroendocrine dysfunction can result in fluid and electrolyte disturbances and cardiovascular instability. Hypothermia should be an anticipated derangement as a result of hypothalamic dysfunction and increased heat loss from systemic vasodilation as loss of vascular tone occurs. Hypothermia requires aggressive treatment to avoid aggravation of coagulation disturbances and reduction in cardiac output. The brain normally consumes 20% of the cardiac output. Without the metabolic contribution of the brain, glucose needs are reduced and the patient is prone to hyperglycemia that may necessitate the use of an insulin infusion. Furthermore, with such a significant reduction in cerebral metabolism, carbon dioxide production falls and can be observed by a reduction in $PaCO_2$ on serial blood gas sampling.

Once a decision has been made by the family to proceed with organ donation following determination of neurologic death, the focus of care shifts toward the preservation of vital organs. The subsequent care may vary from the management that has occurred up to that point. Previous efforts to reduce intracranial pressure using interventions such as moderate hyperventilation, hypothermia, and sedatives are abandoned and attention moves toward providing ample blood flow and oxygen delivery to prospective transplantable organs. The principles in management are largely the same, including maintenance of adequate oxygen delivery to the tissues through the optimization of cardiac output and oxygen content. Hemodynamics are managed to maintain normal blood pressure for age (Table 2). Reduction in cerebral edema treated with volume restriction and diuretic agents that result in decreased intravascular volume must be corrected. Attention to intravascular volume loss from derangements such as diabetes insipidus (DI) must be anticipated and appropriately addressed. Excessive volume depletion can lead to hemodynamic compromise and end-organ failure secondary to inadequate perfusion if left untreated. Additional management goals include the normalization of $PaCO_2$ via adjustments of mechanical ventilation, normalization of temperature, and addressing neuroendocrine dysfunction with correction of metabolic disturbances. Progression of organ failure following neurologic death results in the loss of 10% to 20% of potential donors; therefore, timely and definitive treatment of the donor is critical.[38,39]

Table 2. NORMAL VITAL SIGNS FOR CHILDREN

Vital signs	Respiratory rate (breaths/min)	Pulse (beats/min)	Systolic blood pressure (mm Hg)*[37]
Infant	30-60	120-160	60-70
Toddler	25-40	90-140	75-90
School age	22-34	80-120	80-100
Adolescent	12-20	60-90	90-120

*Lowest acceptable systolic blood pressure is (2 × age in years) + 70.

General Considerations for Potential Pediatric Organ Donors

Pediatric donor management requires an understanding of the anatomic and physiologic differences in children. The respiratory system of children is much different from that of an adult. The trachea is shorter, which can predispose to misplacement of the endotracheal tube. Smaller airways have increased airway resistance, the chest wall is more compliant, and respiratory muscles are less developed. Cardiovascular dynamics require a higher resting heart rate to maintain cardiac output because the smaller heart of children cannot generate large stroke volumes. Drastic decreases in heart rate result in decreased cardiac output leading to problems with end-organ perfusion. The child also has a larger body surface area and is more prone to develop hypothermia. Radiant warmers, warm blankets and pads, warm intravenous (IV) fluids or a blood warmer for infusion of blood products, increasing the temperature of inspired gas through the humidified ventilator circuit, and environmental warming can be used to maintain the patient in a normothermic state. Limited glycogen stores place infants at greater risk for hypoglycemia and limited catecholamine stores can be depleted leading to hypotension and altered cardiac output. Understanding these anatomic and physiologic differences is important when managing pediatric organ donors.

Vascular access can be challenging in small children. Unlike adults, multilumen pulmonary artery catheters are rarely used in children because of size constraints and potential technical challenges during catheter placement. Double and triple lumen central venous catheters are most commonly used in children.

Small lumen size, predisposing to obstruction, and limiting large volume administration, and compatibility of multiple IV infusions, may require additional vascular access. Although a logical solution would be placement of another multilumen central venous catheter, this is not always possible in a small infant or child. Peripheral IVs are frequently used, but must be checked frequently to ensure patency and infusion of agents into the vascular system. Placement of a peripheral IV in a potential donor can be difficult because of tissue edema, hypothermia, and small, fragile vessels that can be difficult to cannulate.

Donor management goals for children are the same as for adult donors; however, it is important to remember that children are not small adults. There are special considerations when dealing with pediatric donors that require a specialized team of physicians, nurses, respiratory therapists, and social workers, who are all trained in pediatric physiology and the unique needs of the child and the family. The transplant professional should use this team of pediatric specialists as a resource for planning management and intervention of pediatric donors.

Management of Pulmonary Issues for Potential Pediatric Organ Donors

Every donor should be considered and managed as a potential lung donor; therefore, in addition to meticulous care to ensure ventilation and oxygenation, attention should be afforded to prevent barotrauma and any potential further lung injury. This strategy will improve the chances and quality of all potential organs recovered.

Impairments in oxygenation and ventilation can result from lung disease and injury such as pulmonary hemorrhage or contusion, and inhalation or thermal injury. Furthermore, management of pulmonary physiology may be complicated by the development of pulmonary edema either from the progression of brain injury and associated neurogenic pulmonary edema,[40] acute respiratory distress syndrome, or because of volume administration used to correct hemodynamic instability. Infectious etiologies can compound the effects of existing lung disease or injury leading to further impairment in ventilation and oxygenation. In addition, impaired cardiac output, anemia, and inadequate ventilatory support can all contribute to further impairment in oxygen delivery to the tissues. Because of the importance of maintaining oxygenation and ventilation in the potential donor and the myriad of pathologic states that can complicate management, a basic understanding of airway management and oxygenation and ventilation is necessary. This knowledge will equip those caring for these patients to be better able to deal with, and anticipate potential pulmonary problems that may be encountered.

Maintenance and protection of the airway is essential to provide adequate oxygenation and ventilation to potential pediatric organ donors. The endotracheal tube (ETT) used to secure the airway can be cuffed or uncuffed. Cuffed ETTs are used when higher airway pressures are anticipated, for example, in patients with pulmonary edema or underlying respiratory pathology. The appropriate-sized ETT is imperative to providing adequate care for these patients. The size can be estimated on the basis of age ([age in years + 16]/4).[37] Dislodgement of the ETT can easily occur because of the shorter trachea in children. It is important to check the placement of the ETT using radiographic studies. The tip of the ETT should reside between the third and forth vertebral body visualized on an anterior-posterior chest radiograph. A useful formula to assist with the depth of ETT placement is 3 times the size of the ETT,[37] thus, a 4.0 ETT should be approximately 12 cm at the lip. An ETT that is too large will be deeper, and an ETT that is too small will reside higher using this formula. For children 1 to 12 years of age, the formula, "10 + the age in years" can be used to check proper depth of the ETT.[41] Appropriate placement of the ETT is crucial as a 1-cm difference in the depth of the ETT can result in right mainstem bronchus placement or extubation. To prevent the ETT from slipping through the tape from excessive secretions, it should be securely wrapped in a spiral fashion. Maintaining pulmonary toilet is essential in an effort to maintain adequate oxygenation and ventilation.

Basic continuous noninvasive monitoring and serial laboratory testing play a crucial part in the appropriate management of these patients and in detecting physiologic derangements in oxygenation and ventilation. Continuous pulse oximetry and capnography allow monitoring of a patient's oxygen saturation and exhaled carbon dioxide tension, providing measurements of oxygenation and ventilation. Arterial blood gas analysis provides a direct measure of dissolved oxygen and carbon dioxide concentration, showing efforts at oxygenation and ventilation. Attention to such noninvasive monitoring and blood gas analysis is a cornerstone in patient management.

Acute changes in physiology frequently occur in the management of pediatric organ donors. Acute changes that result in oxygen desaturation require prompt evaluation and intervention that must precede investigation because of the potential consequences to organ viability. Oxygen desaturation must be avoided at all costs. Manual ventilation using a bag valve mask with 100% oxygen should ensue and the cause of the desaturation episode investigated.

Oxygen desaturation can be a result of a dislodged, kinked, or obstructed ETT; bronchospasm; or pneumothorax. A dislodged ETT must be replaced immediately. If the ETT is kinked, examining and repositioning the ETT will restore patency of the airway. Regular pulmonary toilet is essential to clear secretions and alleviate any mucous plugging that can result in obstruction of the airway. This is particularly important with younger children who require a smaller ETT. Bronchospasm can be detected by wheezing or a prolonged expiratory phase and can be more common in predisposed individuals, individuals with pulmonary edema, or those treated with β-blockers for hypertension. The first line therapy for management of bronchospasm is inhaled beta-agonist such as albuterol. Albuterol has also been shown *ex vivo* and in animal studies to augment the clearance of pulmonary edema and may be considered, along with diuretics should this problem occur or contribute to bronchospasm.[42] Corticosteroids can be administered by inhalation or IV for persistent bronchospasm. In addition, corticosteroids may have the added benefit of stabilizing lung function in potential organ donors.[43] In situations in which bronchospasm is unresponsive to inhaled adjunctive agents, IV beta-agonists or IV methylxanthines can be considered.

Sudden oxygen desaturation can also occur from a pneumothorax as a result of high airway pressures used during manual or mechanical ventilation. Needle aspiration of the chest or placement of a chest tube to evacuate the pressurized air in the thorax is imperative to avoid cardiopulmonary collapse.

Understanding oxygenation and ventilation as two separate entities will assist in the treatment of specific pulmonary problems commonly encountered in pediatric organ donors. Oxygen delivery is dependent on hemoglobin concentration, the fraction of inspired oxygen (FiO_2), PaO_2, and cardiac output. Cardiac output is determined by stroke volume and heart rate. Correction of derangements in oxygenation begins with treatment of the underlying cause and in the majority of cases, measures to improve oxygenation require manipulation of the determinants of oxygen delivery, as previously mentioned. The ability to oxygenate can be improved by such maneuvers as increasing the FiO_2, improving cardiac output using volume expansion and/or inotropic support, and increasing the hemoglobin concentration by transfusing red blood cells. Maneuvers to improve PaO_2 can be pursued as well, but discussion of such interventions will be reserved for the portion of this chapter dedicated to mechanical ventilation.

Oxygen saturation is the percentage of hemoglobin that binds oxygen. Although a major determinant of oxygen delivery, it is important to remember that oxygen saturation is not always a reliable indicator of adequate oxygen delivery to the tissues. A child can be well saturated, but still have inadequate oxygen delivery; therefore, the means to detect the adequacy of oxygen delivery is crucial in guiding therapy. Measurements such as PaO_2, lactate, and mixed venous oxygen saturation can be used as additional measures of oxygen delivery.

Oxygen saturation can also be improved by altering pulmonary blood flow, which can affect ventilation/perfusion matching. Increasing pulmonary blood flow can be achieved by altering pH and using mechanical ventilation and pharmacologic agents.

The use of alkalosis, either by respiratory or metabolic therapies, can reduce pulmonary vascular resistance (PVR), thereby increasing pulmonary blood flow. Alkalosis can reduce the ability of oxygen unloading from hemoglobin at the tissue level as the hemoglobin/oxygen dissociation curve shifts leftward, thus potentially reducing tissue levels of oxygen. In contrast, a respiratory or metabolic acidosis will increase PVR, thus decreasing blood flow to the lungs. Acidosis enhances the unloading of oxygen to the tissues. The manipulation of PVR by altering pH to improve oxygenation, although appealing, does not come without consequence; therefore, if manipulation of PVR is desired, use of a selective pulmonary vasodilator such as inhaled nitric oxide is worthy of consideration.[44-47] Maintaining arterial pH in the normal range, between 7.35 and 7.45, in addition to keeping the $PaCO_2$ between 35 and 40 mm Hg, thereby maximizing oxygen unloading to the tissues to maintain end organ viability, is preferable. In addition, the PaO_2 should be kept greater than 100 mm Hg.

Ventilatory requirements may become minimal in the organ donor as neurologic death occurs with loss of respiratory regulation. Decreased glucose metabolism, oxygen consumption, and a respiratory alkalosis occur as metabolic production of carbon dioxide from the brain ceases and compliance of the chest wall changes. The attainment of normocarbia is important because of previously discussed effects on the unloading characteristics of oxygen from hemoglobin, with obvious implications on availability of oxygen to the tissues. Decreasing ventilation parameters is not uncommon to restore normocarbia with a goal of 35 to 40 mm Hg in the child who is progressing or has achieved neurologic death. Minute ventilation, which affects $PaCO_2$, is determined by respiratory rate and tidal volume. Adjusting either of these parameters will alter exchange of carbon dioxide. Further discussion regarding adjustment of ventilation parameters is discussed in the next section.

Mechanical Ventilation

Ventilator parameters should be adjusted on an individual basis. Variables that require adjustment for mechanical ventilation in children include tidal volume, peak inspiratory pressure, positive end-expiratory pressure (PEEP), inspiratory time, rate, and FiO_2. Although manipulation of ventilator parameters is required to control oxygenation and ventilation, decisions regarding ventilation strategies are best left to the pediatric intensivist or anesthesiologist, who routinely provides assisted ventilation to children. PEEP should be provided for all children who are receiving mechanical ventilation to maintain alveolar inflation. Inspiratory time is typically set to provide an inspiratory-expiratory ratio of 1:3. Normal inspiratory time is 0.6 to 0.75 seconds for infants and smaller children respectively; an inspiratory time of 1 second is appropriate for older children. Improvement in oxygenation can be achieved by increasing the inspiratory time with a net effect of increasing mean airway pressure. When adjusting inspiratory time, it is important to consider the effect on the expiratory time. If the inspiratory time is increased, there will be an obligatory decrease in the expiratory time. To avoid stacking of breaths leading to carbon dioxide retention, the inspiratory-expiratory ratio should not exceed 1:1.

To maintain adequate oxygen saturation in children receiving mechanical ventilation, the FiO_2 can be increased. High concentrations of oxygen should be used only as needed. Hyperoxia can result in toxicity to the pneumocytes and interfere with surfactant production predisposing to altered physiology and pathology such as atelectasis and scar formation. Although the lowest concentration of inspired oxygen that results in appropriate oxygen delivery and saturations should be used, 0.4 FiO_2 for the patient requiring less oxygen provides a buffer should the ETT become obstructed or dislodged, leading to desaturation. If further improvement in oxygenation is needed beyond that which can be achieved by raising FiO_2, increasing the inspiratory time or increasing PEEP, to recruit and maintain alveolar inflation resulting in an improvement in functional residual capacity, are reasonable considerations. PEEP can also assist in decreasing pulmonary edema. The benefit associated with the use of PEEP must be balanced against the risk of potential barotrauma and effects on preload, which can potentially decrease cardiac output in donors with cardiac dysfunction. Cardiovascular effects can be minimized if adequate preload is ensured before the escalation of PEEP.

Minute ventilation is determined by respiratory rate and tidal volume. Adjustment of tidal volume can be made either by direct manipulation of measured volume if ventilating in a volume-based ventilation mode or adjusting peak inspiratory pressure when ventilating in a pressure-based ventilation mode. The magnitude of an adequate tidal breath, which can be determined by the volume of air required to expand the chest adequately by direct observation, usually corresponds to 8 to 10 mL/kg. This value allows for compensation of the ventilator circuit, tubing compliance, and gas compressibility. The lowest possible tidal volume that promotes chest rise is recommended to avoid excessive hyperventilation. Evidence suggests that high volumes potentiate barotrauma.[48] Synchronous modes of ventilation are not indicated in this particular patient population, because neurologic death has occurred and spontaneous respiratory effort is absent.

Treatment of Hemodynamic Instability

Cardiac dysfunction is the greatest limiting factor to successful organ procurement. Of all the physiologic derangements encountered in prospective organ donors, the cardiovascular system is fraught with the greatest complexity and variation. This variation is a reflection of the powerful neuroendocrine changes that occur during progression to neurologic death. The efforts to regulate cerebral perfusion pressure, hemodynamic manifestations of herniation, and, ultimately, the physiology of an absent CNS, all contribute to the unstable physiology that commonly occurs in the prospective organ donor.

Management goals for pediatric organ donors is directed at achieving and maintaining adequate circulating blood volume, optimizing cardiac output and oxygen delivery to the tissues, and maintaining normal blood pressure for age. Inotropic agents such as dopamine, dobutamine, and epinephrine can be titrated to effect; however, establishing appropriate circulating volume is essential before using inotropic support. Central venous pressure (CVP) monitoring, and clinical indicators such as perfusion and urine output are used in determining adequate intravascular volume, but must be evaluated in the context of the child with profound CNS alterations. Serial lactate levels serve as a guide of tissue perfusion. Elevations in serum lactate and the development of a metabolic acidosis provide evidence of tissue ischemia and should prompt immediate attention. As the patient with severe intracranial pathology progresses toward cerebral death, the associated neuroendocrine dysfunction will result in tremendous variations in physiology that require the application and adjustment of specific interventions to restore normal physiologic parameters.

Intracranial hypertension with cerebral ischemia leads to massive sympathetic discharge, "sympathetic or autonomic storm." Organs are exposed to extreme sympathetic stimulation either from direct neural stimulation or from endogenous catecholamines, resulting in systemic hypertension and tachycardia.[49] The local effects of sympathetic stimulation result in increased vascular tone, effectively reducing blood flow and potentially causing ischemia to end organs. This autonomic storm also has direct effects to the myocardium, as the surge of catecholamines increases systemic vascular resistance, thus increasing myocardial work and oxygen consumption. Myocardial injury can occur as the left ventricle is exposed to a significant increase in afterload, which reduces cardiac output. Ischemic changes have been reported as a result of this imbalance between myocardial oxygen supply and demand.[49,50]

As left ventricular afterload increases, impairment of cardiac output may result with consequential dysfunction to organ systems. Left ventricular end diastolic pressure rises, which results in increased left atrial pressure. As left atrial pressure exceeds pulmonary artery pressure, a hydrostatically induced extrusion of fluid into the interstitial space of the lungs occurs, resulting in pulmonary edema. This condition is further exacerbated by the increase in venous return as a result of catecholamine-mediated systemic vasoconstriction. The increased volume load to the right heart not only exacerbates the hydrostatic pressure in the pulmonary vasculature, but also displaces the ventricular septum into the left ventricle, further impairing left ventricular preload and, therefore, cardiac output through a mechanism called ventricular interdependence.[51]

The sympathetic storm with associated hypertension is a predictably transient phenomenon. Although end-organ ischemia can transiently occur, treatment with antihypertensive agents may not be warranted and could create additional problems with perfusion when this phase of sympathetic outflow has passed. If hypertension is severe and treatment is felt to be indicated, IV infusions of ultra short-acting antihypertensive agents such as nitroprusside sodium (Nipride) or esmolol hydrochloride (Brevibloc) can be titrated to effect. β-Blockers may aggravate a low cardiac output state, in addition to promoting bronchospasm in predisposed individuals, and should be used with caution. Longer-acting agents require close observation to avoid hypotension. Intermittent doses of IV hydralazine hydrochloride (Apresoline) or labetalol (Trandate, Normodyne) can also be used to control hypertension.

As neurologic death occurs, sympathetic outflow is reduced. This results in a loss of autonomic tone, leading to vasodilation with potential impairment in cardiac output and hypotension. Vasodilation results in decreased circulating volume, which can be compounded by excessive urine output because of hormonal imbalances leading to DI and hyperglycemia. These derangements warrant the use of volume as the intervention of choice. Inadequate intravascular volume will be signified by a drop in CVP and narrowed pulse pressure with a reduction in blood pressure and perfusion. Urine output may not be a good clinical indicator if DI is present or being aggressively managed using pharmacologic agents. Loss of beat-to-beat variation and a fixed heart rate are also common as brainstem death occurs; therefore, heart rate will also not be a reliable sign of intravascular volume status. In addition, perfusion may be altered if the child is hypothermic. The goal during this phase of patient management is restoration of circulating volume using blood pressure, perfusion, and CVP monitoring as a guide. Aggressive volume resuscitation must occur to restore and maintain adequate perfusion to vital tissues for possible transplantation.

The use of isotonic fluids for volume resuscitation is principle, and fluids containing dextrose should never be used as a volume expander. Bolus infusions of 10 to 20 mL/kg of crystalloid, such as isotonic sodium chloride solution or lactated Ringer's solution, or colloid such as 5% albumin should be used and repeated as needed to support the blood pressure with a goal appropriate for the age of the child. Table 2 shows normal vital signs on the basis of the age of the child. The normal blood pressure for any child older than 1 year of age is 2 times the age in years plus 80, with the lowest acceptable blood pressure equaling 2 times the age in years plus 70.[37] For infants younger than 30 days of age, a systolic blood pressure of 60 mm Hg is acceptable, and for children 1 month to 1 year of age, a systolic blood pressure of 70 mm Hg is appropriate.[37] Infants are proportionately more dependent on circulating free calcium for cardiac function, which must be considered when administering 5% albumin in this age group. The sarcoplasmic reticulum of the infant myocardium is underdeveloped and therefore cannot store reserves of calcium as effectively as older children and adults; therefore, infants are particularly vulnerable to administration of large amounts of albumin solution, which can bind free calcium resulting in hypocalcemia and hypotension.[52,53] Intermittent or continuous IV administration of calcium chloride or calcium gluconate to maintain the ionized calcium levels greater than 1.0 mmol/dL can reverse this effect. Artificial plasma expanders such as Hespan or Dextran should be avoided because large volumes can alter coagulation parameters.[54,55] Blood products such as packed red blood cells for significant blood loss or anemia can be administered in aliquots of 10 to 15 mL/kg administered over 2 to 4 hours, or faster, if hemodynamic instability with ongoing blood loss requires more aggressive resuscitative measures. Blood can be warmed to help maintain or restore thermoregulatory stability in potential donors, if needed.

If volume loading with 60 to 80 mL/kg of IV fluids does not restore normal blood pressure, the use of inotropic agents such as dopamine or dobutamine, administered through a central venous catheter, should be considered. Both these agents help improve cardiac function and increase blood pressure. Patients who have an inadequate response to these inotropic agents may require additional vasopressors such as epinephrine, norepinephrine, or phenylephrine to help support their blood pressure. Although necessary, the administration of vasoactive agents can be associated with reduced perfusion to donor organs, potentially jeopardizing their viability upon acquisition. Hormonal replacement therapy using thyroid hormone and steroids should be considered in children who are refractory to high-dose inotropic infusions. Ideally, a management strategy to maintain blood pressure, normovolemia, and optimization of cardiac output, with the least amount of vasoactive agents, has been adopted in many centers that are involved in donor management and organ procurement.

Arrhythmias can occur for many reasons during the progression toward and following the achievement of neurologic death. The catecholamine storm resulting in increased adrenergic stimulation can promote rhythm disturbances and myocardial ischemia. Hypotension secondary to hypovolemia with resultant myocardial ischemia; acidosis secondary to poor cardiac output; hypoxemia secondary to pulmonary insufficiency; hypothermia; cardiac trauma; proarrhythmic properties of inotropes; and electrolyte and metabolic disturbances such as hypomagnesemia, hypocalcemia, and hypokalemia that occur with DI can also precipitate rhythm disturbances. Identification and correction of the underlying cause for the arrhythmia are essential to minimize or eradicate rhythm disturbances. Replacement of deficient electrolytes such as potassium, calcium, or magnesium can reduce or eliminate ventricular rhythm disturbances and improve blood pressure.[56] Hypotension should be treated with volume resuscitation and inotropic support. Reducing the amount of inotrope, provided that the blood pressure will tolerate this maneuver, may be beneficial in decreasing or eliminating rhythm abnormalities. Sodium bicarbonate or tromethamine (THAM) can be used to correct metabolic acidosis and ventilator adjustments to improve minute ventilation may be used to correct a respiratory acidosis. Hypoxemia can be corrected by adjusting ventilator parameters, and cardiac output and oxygen delivery can be improved by achieving volume and/

or inotropic support, and transfusion of red blood cells. Hypothermia can be corrected by active warming measures. Intravenous lidocaine or amiodarone (Cordarone) can be used to treat ventricular arrhythmias once metabolic disturbances have been corrected, whereas IV adenosine (Adenocard IV) can be used to treat supraventricular arrhythmias such as supraventricular tachycardia (SVT). IV amiodarone can be used as well, if recurrent SVT becomes problematic. For hemodynamically unstable SVT, synchronized electrical cardioversion is considered first-line therapy.[37]

Hormonal Replacement Therapy

The use of hormonal replacement therapy has been controversial in the adult literature.[43,50,51] Thyroid and cortisol depletion may contribute to the hemodynamic instability encountered in patients who have progressed to neurologic death, although no studies have firmly established this fact. Furthermore, correlations between hormone usage, cardiac function, and clinical outcome measures have been disappointing.[57-61] However, hormonal replacement therapy has shown promise in reducing requirements for vasoactive agents in 100% of unstable donors and abolished the need in 53% of such donors in 1 adult series,[62] whereas other retrospective series have demonstrated that hormone replacement therapy was associated with a significant increase in the number of organs transplanted from donors.[63] This benefit has been noted by Zuppa and associates,[64] who observed decreased inotropic requirements in children who received levothyroxine. Given these observations, many organ procurement teams have adopted the use of hormone replacement therapy as a routine part of organ donor management. Furthermore, it is reasonable to consider these agents in situations in which the hemodynamic status of the child is refractory to conventional therapy with fluid and inotropic administration.[51,64,65] Thyroid hormone has also been associated with an increase in transplanted organs from donors receiving hormone replacement therapy.[63,66,67] Commonly used agents and doses for hormonal resuscitation in children are listed in Table 3.

Levothyroxine (Synthroid) and triiodothyronine (T3) are the two IV thyroid agents available for administration. Dosing of thyroid hormone for pediatric organ donors is not well established. Levothroxine dosing, like many other pharmacologic agents used for this patient population, is based on the weight of the child. One retrospective study[64] provided younger children with a larger bolus and infusion dose compared with older children, and demonstrated an ability to wean inotropic support in children who progressed to neurologic death. Administration of T3 is used in some centers for hormonal replacement therapy; however, its cost may be prohibitive and the benefits in this patient population are controversial. Novitsky et al[61] has reported beneficial hemodynamic effects in brain-dead patients receiving T3 administration,

Table 3. PHARMACOLOGIC AGENTS USED FOR HORMONAL RESUSCITATION IN CHILDREN[68]

Drug	Dose	Route	Comments
Desmopressin (DDAVP)	0.5 mcg/h	IV	Terminal half life, 75 minutes (range 0.4-4 hours) Titrate to effect to control urine
Vasopressin (Pitressin)	0.5 mU/kg/h	IV	Half life, 10-35 minutes Titrate to effect to control urine output Hypertension can occur
Levothyroxine (Synthroid)	0.8-1.4 mcg/kg/h	IV	Titrate to effect Bolus dose 1-5 mcg/kg can be administered; smaller infants and children require a higher bolus and infusion dose
Triiodothyronine (T3)	0.05-0.2 mcg/kg/h	IV	Titrate to effect
Hydrocortisone (Solucortef)	1 mg/kg	IV	Fluid retention and glucose intolerance
Insulin	0.05-0.1 U/kg/h	IV	Titrate to effect to control blood glucose levels Monitor for hypoglycemia

Abbreviations: IV, intravenous

whereas others studies[69,70] have shown no benefit with this agent. The effects of thyroid hormone on myocardial contractility are complex and can be immediate or delayed. The acute inotropic properties of T3 may occur as a result of β-adrenoreceptor sensitization or may be completely independent of β-adrenergic receptors.[68-72] Furthermore, T3 administration may play an important role in maintaining aerobic metabolism at the tissue level after brain death has occurred.[73]

Steroids, such as hydrocortisone, are another adjunct used by many centers to assist with hemodynamic support; however, there is even less data attesting to its benefits in potential pediatric donors.[51] The potential benefit of hydrocortisone and other steroids may lie in its ability to alter adrenergic receptors and regulate vascular tone by increasing sensitivity to catecholamines; but to date the clinical benefit remains untested in this population.[74-76]

Application of hormonal replacement therapy in potential pediatric organ donors has generated some support through scientific studies.[60,61,64] Although hormonal replacement therapy is controversial; it is widely practiced despite lack of convincing evidence. The combination of thyroid hormone and steroids may be used as pharmacologic adjuncts to reduce dosing of vasoactive agents in children requiring high-dose inotropic support and this application may indeed improve success in organ procurement for children; however, further studies are clearly warranted.

Fluid and Electrolyte Disturbances

The disturbances in the management of fluids and electrolytes in pediatric donors are the result of physiologic derangements, as well as iatrogenesis. Derangements commonly encountered include dehydration, hyperglycemia, sodium and potassium derangements, and hypocalcemia. Meticulous management of fluids and electrolytes is necessary because metabolic swings associated with neurologic death can adversely affect organ viability.

Addressing basic fluid management in pediatric patients requires an understanding of the normal physiologic needs of these patients. Fluid requirements can be determined on the basis of weight for infants and small children who require a proportionately greater amount of fluids compared to their older counterparts, in whom fluids can also be calculated on the basis of body surface area (m^2). Standard calculations for estimated maintenance fluids can be found in Table 4. Another important consideration in children is their reduced need for sodium and greater glucose requirement. Because of their standard daily sodium needs, infants up to 1 year of age require one fourth or one third normal saline solution as their maintenance IV fluids. For a child older than 1 year, one third to one half normal saline solution is appropriate because of their greater maintenance sodium requirement. Limited glycogen stores in young infants make them particularly vulnerable to hypoglycemia. For these infants, fluids containing a 10% dextrose concentration and frequent reassessment of their blood glucose levels are imperative to prevent hypoglycemia. After 6 months to 1 year of age, glycogen storage matures and solutions containing 5% dextrose can be used. Age-appropriate fluid management remains important for children who become candidates for organ donation.

In children with traumatic brain injury that has progressed to neurologic death, intravascular volume depletion is frequently encountered because of fluid restriction and treatment with hypertonic solutions and osmotic diuretics used in the management of cerebral edema. Additional contributors to intravascular volume depletion are hyperglycemia, as a result of steroid and catecholamine use, and the increased availability of glucose because of loss of cerebral metabolism. Furthermore, DI compounds sodium and

Table 4. STANDARD CALCULATIONS FOR MAINTENANCE INTRAVENOUS FLUIDS

Patient weight (kg)	Hourly fluid rate (mL/h)
1st 10 kg	4 mL/kg
2nd 10 kg	2 mL/kg
>20 kg	Weight (kg) + 40

Example: 16 kg child: 1st 10 kg x 4 mL/kg = 40 mL + 6 kg x 2 mL/kg = 12 mL: Total hourly fluids = 52 mL

water balance if left untreated. As previously discussed, potential pediatric organ donors must be adequately volume resuscitated, guided by CVP, perfusion, and potentially serial lactate measurements. The choice of fluid for volume resuscitation is isotonic crystalloid in doses of 10 to 20 mL/kg. Restoring intravascular volume is the mainstay of securing organ viability.

Diabetes Insipidus

In potential pediatric donors who develop DI, there is excessive free water loss resulting in fluid and electrolyte disturbances. DI is characterized by hypernatremia and polyuria, with elevated serum osmolarity and urine specific gravity of <1.002. In this condition, loss of antidiuretic hormone produced in the CNS allows unrestricted free water loss without regard to intravascular volume. Hypernatremia, with a serum sodium level greater than 150 mg/dL, is commonly encountered in DI and can be detrimental to end organs. Hypernatremia has been associated with graft failure after liver transplantation[77,78]; thus meticulous and definitive management is imperative to preserve organ function.

The management of DI requires supplementation of antidiuretic hormone to restrict free water loss, while replacing free water to avoid significant dehydration. Hormonal replacement therapy with pharmacologic agents such as vasopressin or desmopressin (DDAVP) can be used to control urine output. Each agent has specific indications and side effects that must be considered when contemplating its use in pediatric patients.

Vasopressin is a polypeptide hormone secreted by the hypothalamus and stored in the posterior pituitary. Vasopressin acts on the V_1 and V_2 vasopressin receptors and stimulates contraction of vascular smooth muscle resulting in vasoconstriction. It has a short half life of 10 to 20 minutes, and unlike Desmopressin has no effect upon platelets.[79] Vasopressin can be administered by bolus or continuous IV infusion. The most desirable features of this agent are its titratability to control urine output and, when no longer required, its effects are short lived. Vasopressin is administered at doses of 0.5 milliunits/kg/h and can be titrated to control urine output to 2 to 4 mL/kg/h.[79] By titrating to this degree, renal function can continue to be preserved, and volume overload and metabolic derangements such as hyperkalemia can be avoided. Vasoconstrictive effects of vasopressin in high doses may reduce splanchnic perfusion, which can be detrimental to hepatic and pancreatic blood flow, and increased smooth muscle contractility may affect coronary and pulmonary blood flow.[50] Excessive dosing of vasopressin should be avoided to preserve end-organ function. Vasoconstriction may result in hypertension, which may facilitate weaning of other inotropic agents for blood pressure support.

Desmopressin is a synthetic polypeptide structurally related to vasopressin and has a more potent antidiuretic effect. This agent lacks smooth muscle contractile properties and is more specific for the V_2-vasopressin receptor.[80] Desmopressin enhances platelet aggregation and it has a longer half life of 6 to 20 hours when administered as a single IV dose.[81-83] The lack of hemodynamic side effects may make Desmopressin a better agent for the correction of hypernatremia in the hemodynamically stable donor. It may also be preferred because of its ability to enhance platelet function in potential donors with an existing coagulopathy. Desmopressin can be administered by continuous infusion at 0.5 mcg/h and titrated to control urine output. Intramuscular and intranasal administration can result in erratic absorption and should be avoided. The terminal half life of Desmopressin administered by continuous IV infusion is 75 minutes, with a range of 0.4 to 4 hours.[84] The longer half life makes Desmopressin a less desirable agent to some transplant surgeons who prefer the shorter half life of vasopressin. One approach in dealing with this situation is to discontinue Desmopressin therapy 4 to 5 hours before organ recovery and administer fluid replacement for excessive urine output as needed over the following hours.

The replacement of ongoing volume loss in DI is imperative to preserve organ function for transplantation. The use of hypotonic solutions such as one half or one fourth normal saline solution to provide more free water will help correct hypernatremia and maintain euvolemia. Excessive uncontrolled urine output can result in dehydration and hypovolemic shock. Urine output over 3 to 4 mL/kg/h should be aggressively replaced 1:1 or milliliter for milliliter with one fourth or one half normal saline solution on an hourly basis to prevent intravascular volume depletion. Measuring the urine sodium concentration can be used as a guide to facilitate sodium replacement in patients with DI. The concentration of isotonic sodium chloride solution is 154 mEq/dL; therefore, if the measured urine sodium content were approximately 70 mEq/dL, one half normal saline solution would be an appropriate replacement fluid. If urine sodium were closer to 40 mEq/dL, one fourth normal saline solution would be a reasonable choice for fluid replacement. Lastly, the use of enteral water supplementation administered through a nasogastric tube can be considered for the correction of severe hypernatremia. Rapid osmolar shifts during correction of hypernatremia are inconsequential because the child has already progressed to neurologic death.

Oliguria

Oliguria, although less common, can be secondary to volume depletion, acute renal insufficiency or failure, and iatrogenesis from overly aggressive DI management. If urine output falls to less than 1 mL/kg/h and iatrogenesis has been ruled out, the patient's intravascular volume status must be evaluated. If the patient's intravascular volume appears depleted, a bolus of 10 to 20 mL/kg of isotonic sodium chloride or lactated Ringer's solution, or colloid is indicated. If urine output remains low, additional administration of isotonic IV fluids may be repeated. The patency of the Foley catheter must be checked to ensure that obstruction of the catheter is not the primary cause for decreased urine output. If several boluses of crystalloid result in no improvement in urine output, colloid for volume expansion or vasopressor support, if poor perfusion is present, may assist in improving urine output. Furosemide (Lasix) or mannitol can be used to stimulate urine output in patients with adequate intravascular volume status.

Glucose Derangements

Hyperglycemia, as a result of steroid and catecholamine use and the increased availability of glucose because of the loss of cerebral metabolism, can lead to an osmolar diuresis, exacerbating an already depleted volume status. Hyperglycemia can be avoided by frequently assessing blood glucose levels and making appropriate adjustments in the dextrose concentration in the maintenance fluids. If these maneuvers are unsuccessful in controlling blood glucose levels, an insulin infusion should be instituted to maintain glucose levels between 80 to 150 mg/dL. Insulin infusion at a starting dose of 0.05 to 0.1 U/kg/h can be titrated to effect. It is important to follow serum glucose levels closely to avoid hypoglycemia.

Neonates and infants have a continuously high glucose need with limited glycogen stores, as previously noted. Hypoglycemia, although less common, can develop rapidly and result in end-organ damage if left untreated. In addition, hypoglycemia can present with poor cardiac output and signs of decreased perfusion. Furthermore, hypoglycemia may also be an indication of sepsis. If glucose levels fall below 60 mg/dL, a bolus of 2 to 4 mL/kg of 10% dextrose IV should be administered to increase the serum glucose level. Tight glycemic control may help restore normal energy metabolism to tissues and enhance energy delivery, thus acting as a positive inotrope.[85]

Potassium Derangements

Potassium derangements can result from diuresis, renal insufficiency or failure, and steroid administration. Potassium can be supplemented if hypokalemia becomes a significant problem. However, the adverse effects of hyperkalemia are clearly more detrimental than hypokalemia. If treatment of hypokalemia is pursued, potassium replacement should be undertaken in the face of a normal serum pH, because serum potassium levels may be falsely reduced in the presence of an alkaline pH. The opposite is true if the patient is acidotic.

Potassium supplementation can be administered using potassium chloride or potassium acetate. Potassium acetate can be used to buffer a metabolic acidosis secondary to renal disease, increased lactate production, or hyperchloremia. The adverse effects of hypokalemia most likely to affect potential donors are arrhythmias.

Calcium Derangements

Hypocalcemia typically occurs secondary to large volume replacement with colloids such as albumin,[53] massive blood transfusions that result in large amounts of citrate reducing free calcium concentrations, and sepsis. Calcium is important for muscle contraction and acts as an inotrope to support blood pressure. The use of calcium chloride is preferred because this agent is not dependent on hepatic activation unlike calcium gluconate. Calcium chloride should be administered through a central venous catheter because extravasation of this agent into the skin and soft tissues can cause profound tissue necrosis. A continuous infusion of calcium chloride or calcium gluconate can be used to treat hypocalcemia or augment blood pressure support in donors with persistent hypocalcemia. The use of calcium supplementation should be guided by ionized calcium levels.

Metabolic Acidosis

There are several causes for metabolic acidosis. Decreased cardiac output results in impaired oxygen delivery to the tissues resulting in a lactic acidosis. Excessive bicarbonate losses from the gastrointestinal tract, renal wasting of bicarbonate secondary to renal insufficiency or failure, and increased chloride in IV fluids can result in a hyperchloremic metabolic acidosis. It is important to define and treat the underlying cause of the metabolic acidosis, such as increased chloride, ongoing bicarbonate losses, or restoration of normal cardiac output to improve oxygen delivery to the tissues. Agents such as sodium bicarbonate or buffers such as tromethamine can be used to correct a metabolic acidosis. Excessive doses of sodium bicarbonate may exacerbate an existing hyperosmolar state and increase production of carbon dioxide, which must be compensated for by increasing minute ventilation to avoid carbon dioxide retention and a resultant respiratory acidosis. Tromethamine should be avoided in patients with renal insufficiency. Tromethamine administered in high doses may cause hypoglycemia, and can exacerbate an existing coagulopathy.[86]

Coagulation Abnormalities

Coagulation abnormalities can occur secondary to the release of tissue thromboplastin and cerebral gangliosides from injured brain.[87,88] Thrombocytopenia and platelet dysfunction can be induced by common drugs such as heparin, antibiotics, β-blockers, calcium channel blockers, and hespan.[89] Patients with liver disease can have reduced synthesis of vitamin K-dependent clotting factors. Interestingly, coagulopathy may be related to the catecholamine surge associated with traumatic brain injury as well.[51,90] A dilutional coagulopathy can also occur from massive transfusions without replenishing coagulation factors. Correction of the coagulopathy can be treated using fresh frozen plasma, platelets, and cryoprecipitate. The goal of blood product replacement for coagulopathy should be tailored on the basis of the derangements encountered.

Platelets should be used for inadequate circulating platelets and clinically significant bleeding, with a reasonable goal being greater than 50 000/mm³. If surgery is anticipated, a platelet count greater than 75 000/mm³ is preferable. Fresh frozen plasma is a rich source of coagulation factors and can be used to keep the prothrombin time less than 25 and partial thromboplastin time less than 40 seconds. Hypofibrinogenemia can be treated with cryoprecipitate for fibrinogen levels less than 100 mg/dL.

Vitamin K is another adjunct in the management of coagulopathy, which can be administered intramuscularly or intravenously. IV administration of vitamin K is preferred because intramuscular injections can result in a depot effect with erratic uptake into the systemic circulation. The effects of vitamin K are slower compared to fresh frozen plasma, platelet, and cryoprecipitate administration. The use of aminocaproic acid (Amicar), an antifibrinolytic agent, and other similar hemostatic agents is not recommended because microvascular thrombosis may be induced in donor organs.[50]

Coagulation abnormalities can also be influenced by hypothermia; therefore, it is essential to keep pediatric organ donors normothermic. Vasodilation with an inability to compensate for heat loss by shivering or vasoconstriction is a common cause of thermoregulatory instability following neurologic death. In addition, infusion of large volumes of IV fluids at room temperature to treat DI and volume depletion can contribute to hypothermia. Hypothermia can promote cardiac dysfunction, arrhythmias, coagulopathy, a cold-induced diuresis secondary to decreased renal tubular concentration gradient, and a leftward shift of the oxyhemoglobin dissociation curve resulting in decreased oxygen delivery to the tissues.[91] Radiant warmers, warm blankets, thermal mattresses, warm IV fluids or a blood warmer for infusion of blood products, and environmental warming will help maintain body temperature. In addition, the temperature of the heated inspired gases can be adjusted to help control body temperature. Prevention of hypothermia is essential to prevent deterioration of potential organ donors.

Summary

Care of pediatric organ donors requires a skilled team of specialists who deal not only with the deceased child, but also the family, and multiple potential recipients. Early involvement of the organ procurement organization and coordination with physicians, social workers, chaplains, and family support services enhances the chance for the family to understand and agree to organ donation. The option to donate should be available to every family and it should be the expectation that the family will be approached in a professional, compassionate manner that allows for open discussion during the most difficult, agonizing time in their lives. Care of pediatric organ donors is a natural extension of care for a critically ill and injured child. Early recognition of brain death and shifting the focus of care to preservation of organs for transplantation is essential for positive outcomes and can greatly facilitate the management of this selected group of patients. This continuum of care and anticipation and timely intervention are essential in well-managed pediatric donors to preserve organ function. Meticulous care of potential donors, combined with teamwork, will result in more transplantable organs with better function that can mean the difference between life and death for another person waiting for a needed organ. The best outcomes occur as pediatric intensive care specialists work together with a dedicated team of professionals to provide specialized care to a very limited group of potential donors.[92]

References

1. Centers for Disease Control. Seat belt use-United States. *MMWR Morb Mortal Wkly Rep.* 1986;35:301-304.
2. Centers for Disease Control and Prevention. Child passenger deaths involving drinking drivers-United States, 1997-2002. *MMWR Morb Mortal Wkly Rep.* 2004;53:77-79.
3. Campbell BJ. Safety belt injury reduction related to crash severity and front seated position. *J Trauma.* 1987;27:733-739.
4. OPTN: Organ Procurement and Transplantation Network. Available at: http://www.optn.org/data. Accessed June 30, 2006.
5. Powers KS, Goldstein B, Merriam C, Chiafery M, Tornabene L, Paprocki S. A multi-disciplinary approach to families of brain dead children. *Clin Intensive Care.* 1994;5:191-196.
6. Tsai E, Shemie SD, Cox PN, Furst S, McCarthy L, Hebert D. Organ donation in children: role of the pediatric intensive care unit. *Pediatr Crit Care Med.* 2000;1:156-160.
7. Wijdicks EF. Determining brain death in adults. *Neurology.* 1995;45:1003-1011.
8. Ashwal S, Schneider S. Brain death in children: part II. *Pediatr Neurol.* 1987;3:69-77.
9. American Academy of Pediatrics: Committee on Hospital Care and Section on Surgery. Pediatric organ donation and transplantation: policy statement. Organizational principles to guide and define the child health care system and/or improve the health of all children. *Pediatrics.* 2002;109:982-984.
10. Graham M. The role of the medical examiner in fatal child abuse: organ and tissue transplantation issues. In: Monteleone JA, Brodeur AE, eds. *Child Maltreatment: A Clinical Guide and Reference.* St Louis, Mo: GW Medical Publishing Inc; 1994:453-454.
11. Kirschner RH, Wilson HL. Fatal child abuse-the pathologist's perspective. In: Reece RM, ed. *Child Abuse: Medical Diagnosis and Management.* Philadelphia, Pa: Lea and Febiger. 1994;325-357.
12. Wick L, Mickell J, Barnes T, Allen J. Pediatric organ donation: impact of medical examiner refusal. *Transplant Proc.* 1995;27:2539-2544.
13. Miracle KL, Broznick BA, Stuart SA. Coroner/medical examiner cooperation with the donation process: one OPO's experience. *J Transpl Coord.* 1993;3:23-26.
14. Shafer TJ, Schkade LL, Siminoff LA, Mahoney TA. Ethical analysis of organ recovery denials by medical examiners, coroners, and justices of the peace. *J Transpl Coord.* 1999;9:232-249.
15. Duthie SE, Peterson BM, Cutler J, Blackbourne B. Successful organ donation in victims of child abuse. *Clin Transplant.* 1995;9:415-418.
16. Sheridan F. Pediatric death rates and donor yield: a medical examiner's view. *J Heart Lung Transplant.* 1993;12:S179-S185.
17. Koogler T, Costarino AT Jr. The potential benefits of the pediatric nonheartbeating organ donor. *Pediatrics.* 1998;101:1049-1052.
18. American Academy of Pediatrics Task Force on Brain Death in Children. Guidelines for the determination of brain death in children. *Pediatrics.* 1987;80:298-300.
19. Ashwal S, Schneider S. Pediatric brain death: current perspectives. *Adv Pediatr.* 1991;38:181-202.
20. The Quality Standards Subcommittee of the American Academy of Neurology. Practice parameters for determining brain death in adults: summary statement. *Neurology.* 1995;45:1012-1014.
21. Van Norman GA. A matter of life and death: what every anesthesiologist should know about the medical, legal, and ethical aspects of declaring brain death. *Anesthesiology.* 1999;91:275-287.
22. Outwater KM, Rockoff MA. Apnea testing to confirm brain death in children. *Crit Care Med.* 1984;12:357-358.
23. Vernon DD, Holzman BH. Brain death: considerations for pediatrics. *J Clin Neurophysiol.* 1986;3:251-265.
24. Farrell MM, Levin DL. Brain death in the pediatric patient: historical, sociological, medical, religious, cultural, legal, and ethical considerations. *Crit Care Med* 1993;21:1951-1965.
25. Freeman JM, Ferry PC. New brain death guidelines in children: further confusion. *Pediatrics.* 1988;81:301-303.
26. Ashwal S, Schneider S. Brain death in children: part I. *Pediatr Neurol.* 1987;3:5-11.
27. Fackler JC, Troncoso JC, Gioia FR. Age-specific characteristics of brain death in children. *Am J Dis Child.* 1988;142:999-1003.
28. Ashwal S. Brain death in the newborn. *Clin Perinatol.* 1989;16:501-518.
29. Ashwal S. Brain death in the newborn. Current perspectives. *Clin Perinatol.* 1997;24:859-882.
30. Flowers WM Jr, Patel BR. Radionuclide angiography as a confirmatory test for brain death: a review of 229 studies in 219 patients. *South Med J.* 1997;90:1091-1096.
31. Schwartz JA, Baxter J, Brill DR. Diagnosis of brain death in children by radionuclide cerebral imaging. *Pediatrics.* 1984;73:14-18.
32. Shaheen FA, al-Khader A, Souqiyyeh MZ, et al. Medical causes of failure to obtain consent for organ retrieval from brain-dead donors. *Transplant Proc.* 1996;28:167-168
33. Ruiz-Lopez MJ, Martinez de Azagra A, Serrano A, Casado-Flores J. Brain death and evoked potentials in pediatric patients. *Crit Care Med.* 1999;27:412-416.

34. Canadian Neurocritical Care Group. Guidelines for the diagnosis of brain death. *Can J Neurol Sci.* 1999;26:64-66.
35. Flowers WM Jr, Patel BR. Accuracy of clinical evaluation in the determination of brain death. *South Med J.* 2000;93:203-206.
36. Harrison AM, Botkin JR. Can pediatricians define and apply the concept of brain death? *Pediatrics.* June 1999;103:e82.
37. The American Heart Association in collaboration with the International Liaison Committee on Resuscitation. Guidelines 2000 for Cardiopulmonary Resuscitation and Emergency Cardiovascular Care. Part 10: pediatric advanced life support. *Circulation.* 2000;102(8 suppl):I291-I342.
38. Lopez-Navidad A, Domingo P, Viedma MA. Professional characteristics of the transplant coordinator. *Transplant Proc.* 1997;29:1607-1613.
39. Grossman MD, Reilly PM, McMahon DJ. Loss of potential organ donors due to medical failure. *Crit Care Med.* 1996;24:A76.
40. Novitzky D. Donor management: state of the art. *Transplant Proc.* 1997;29:3773-3775.
41. Nakagawa TA, Tellez DW. Emergency airway management and critical care issues for the child with a difficult airway. In: Josephson DG, Wohl DL, eds. *Complications in Pediatric Otolaryngology.* Boca Raton, Fla: Taylor & Francis Group. 2005;79-103.
42. Sakuma T, Folkesson HG, Suzuki S, Okaniwa G, Fujimura S, Matthay MA. Beta-adrenergic agonist stimulated alveolar fluid clearance in ex vivo human and rat lungs. *Am J Respir Crit Care Med.* 1997;155:506-512.
43. Wood KE, Becker BN, McCartney JG, D'Alessandro AM, Coursin DB. Care of the potential organ donor. *N Engl J Med.* 2004;351:2730-2739.
44. Nakagawa TA, Morris A, Gomez RJ, Johnston SJ, Sharkey PT, Zaritsky AL. Dose response to inhaled nitric oxide in pediatric patients with pulmonary hypertension and acute respiratory distress syndrome. *J Pediatr.* 1997;131:63-69.
45. Abman SH, Griebel JL, Parker DK, Schmidt JM, Swanton D, Kinsella JP. Acute effects of inhaled nitric oxide in children with severe hypoxemic respiratory failure. *J Pediatr.* 1994;124:881-888.
46. Dobyns EL, Cornfield DN, Anas NG, et al. Multicenter randomized controlled trial of the effects of inhaled nitric oxide therapy on gas exchange in children with acute hypoxemic respiratory failure. *J Pediatr.* 1999;134:406-412.
47. Ream RS, Hauver JF, Lynch RE, Kountzman B, Gale GB, Mink RB. Low-dose inhaled nitric oxide improves the oxygenation and ventilation of infants and children with acute, hypoxemic respiratory failure. *Crit Care Med.* 1999;27:989-996.
48. Marini JJ. New options for the ventilatory management of acute lung injury. *New Horiz.* 1993;1:489-503.
49. Power BM, Van Heerden PV. The physiological changes associated with brain death-current concepts and implications for treatment of the brain dead organ donor. *Anaesth Intensive Care.* 1995;23:26-36.
50. Scheinkestel CD, Tuxen DV, Cooper DJ, Butt W. Medical management of the (potential) organ donor. *Anaesth Intensive Care.* 1995;23:51-59.
51. Lutz-Dettinger N, de Jaeger A, Kerremans I. Care of the potential pediatric organ donor. *Pediatr Clin North Am.* 2001;48:715-749.
52. Klitzner TS, Friedman WF. A diminished role for the sarcoplasmic reticulum in newborn myocardial contraction: effects of ryanodine. *Pediatr Res.* 1989;26:98-101.
53. Mimouni A, Mimouni F, Mimouni C, Mou S, Ho M. Effects of albumin on ionized calcium in vitro. *Pediatr Emerg Care.* 1991;7:149-151.
54. Barron ME, Wilkes MM, Navickis RJ. A systematic review of the comparative safety of colloids. *Arch Surg.* 2004;139:552-563.
55. Cittanova ML, Leblanc I, Legendre C, Mouquet C, Riou B, Coriat P. Effect of hydroxyethylstarch in brain-dead kidney donors on renal function in kidney-transplant recipients. *Lancet.* 1996;348:1620-1622.
56. Satur CMR. Magnesium and its role in cardiac surgical practice: a review. *J Clin Basic Cardiol.* 2002;3:67-73.
57. Powner DJ, Snyder JV, Grenvik A. Brain death certification. A review. *Crit Care Med.* 1977;5:230-233.
58. Koller J, Wieser C, Gottardis M, et al. Thyroid hormones and their impact on the hemodynamic and metabolic stability of organ donors and on kidney graft function after transplantation. *Transplant Proc.* 1990;22:355-357.
59. Robertson KM, Hramiak IM, Gelb AW. Endocrine changes and haemodynamic stability after brain death. *Transplant Proc.* 1989;21:1197-1198.
60. Taniguchi S, Kitamura S, Kawachi K, Doi Y, Aoyama N. Effects of hormonal supplements on the maintenance of cardiac function in potential donor patients after cerebral death. *Eur J Cardiothorac Surg.* 1992;6:96-102.
61. Novitzky D, Cooper DK, Reichart B. Hemodynamic and metabolic responses to hormonal therapy in brain-dead potential organ donors. *Transplantation.* 1987;43:852-854.
62. Salim A, Vassiliu P, Velmahos GC, et al. The role of thyroid hormone administration in potential organ donors. *Arch Surg.* 2001;136:1377-1380.
63. Rosendale JD, Kauffman HM, McBride MA, et al. Aggressive pharmacologic donor management results in more transplanted organs. *Transplantation.* 2003;75:482-487.
64. Zuppa AF, Nadkarni V, Davis L, et al. The effect of a thyroid hormone infusion on vasopressor support in critically ill children with cessation of neurologic function. *Crit Care Med.* 2004;32:2318-2322.

65. Finfer S, Bohn D, Colpitts D, Cox P, Fleming F, Barker G. Intensive care management of paediatric organ donors and its effect on post-transplant organ function. *Intensive Care Med.* 1996;22:1424-1432.
66. Orlowski JP. Evidence that thyroxine (T-4) is effective as a hemodynamic rescue agent in management of organ donors. *Transplantation.* 1993;55:959-960.
67. Orlowski JP, Spees EK. Improved cardiac transplant survival with thyroxine treatment of hemodynamically unstable donors: 95.2% graft survival at 6 and 30 months. *Transplant Proc.* 1993;25:1535.
68. Nakagawa TA. Pediatric Donor Management Guidelines. North American Transplant Coordinators Organization. 2005
69. Randell TT, Hockerstedt KA. Triiodothyronine treatment in brain-dead multiorgan donors-a controlled study. *Transplantation.* 1992;54:736-738.
70. Goarin JP, Cohen S, Riou B, et al. The effects of triiodothyronine on hemodynamic status and cardiac function in potential heart donors. *Anesth Analg.* 1996;83:41-47.
71. Polikar R, Burger AG, Scherrer U, Nicod P. The thyroid and the heart. *Circulation.* 1993;87:1435-1441.
72. Ririe DG, Butterworth JF IV, Royster RL, MacGregor DA, Zaloga GP. Triiodothyronine increases contractility independent of beta-adrenergic receptors or stimulation of cyclic-3',5'-adenosine monophosphate. *Anesthesiology.* 1995;82:1004-1012.
73. Novitzky D, Cooper DK, Morrell D, Isaacs S. Change from aerobic to anaerobic metabolism after brain death, and reversal following triiodothyronine therapy. *Transplantation.* 1988;45:32-36.
74. Marik PE, Zaloga GP. Adrenal insufficiency in the critically ill: a new look at an old problem. *Chest.* 2002;122:1784-1796.
75. Ullian ME. The role of corticosteriods in the regulation of vascular tone. *Cardiovasc Res.* 1999;41:55-64.
76. Pirpiris M, Sudhir K, Yeung S, Jennings G, Whitworth JA. Pressor responsiveness in corticosteroid-induced hypertension in humans. *Hypertension.* 1992;19:567-574.
77. Totsuka E, Fung U, Hakamada K, et al. Analysis of clinical variables of donors and recipients with respect to short-term graft outcome in human liver transplantation. *Transplant Proc.* 2004;36:2215-2218.
78. Totsuka E, Dodson F, Urakami A, et al. Influence of high donor serum sodium levels on early postoperative graft function in human liver transplantation: effect of correction of donor hypernatremia. *Liver Transpl Surg.* 1999;5:421-428.
79. Takemoto CK, Hodding JH, Kraus DM. *Pediatric Dosage Handbook.* 12th ed. Hudson, Ohio: Lexi-Comp;2005:1287-1288.
80. Pennefather SH, Bullock RE, Mantle D, Dark JH. Use of low dose arginine vasopressin to support brain-dead organ donors. *Transplantation.* 1995;59:58-62.
81. Brink LW, Ballew A. Care of the pediatric organ donor. *Am J Dis Child.* 1992;146:1045-1050.
82. Agerso H, Seiding Larsen L, Riis A, Lovgren U, Karlsson MO, Senderovitz T. Pharmacokinetics and renal excretion of desmopressin after intravenous administration to healthy subjects and renally impaired patients. *Br J Clin Pharmacol.* 2004;58:352-358.
83. Kohler M, Harris A. Pharmacokinetics and haematological effects of desmopressin. *Eur J Clin Pharmacol.* 1988;35:281-285.
84. Takemoto CK, Hodding JH, Kraus DM. *Pediatric Dosage Handbook.* 12th ed. Hudson, Ohio: Lexi-Comp;2005:387-389.
85. Srinivasan V, Spinella PC, Drott HR, Roth CL, Helfaer MA, Nadkarni V. Association of timing, duration, and intensity of hyperglycemia with intensive care unit mortality in critically ill children. *Pediatr Crit Care Med.* 2004;5:329-336.
86. Nahas GG, Sutin KM, Fermon C, et al. Guidelines for the treatment of acidaemia with THAM. *Drugs.* 1998;55:191-224.
87. Miner ME, Kaufman HH, Graham SH, Haar FH, Gildenberg PL. Disseminated intravascular coagulation fibrinolytic syndrome following head injury in children: frequency and prognostic implications. *J Pediatr.* 1982;100:687-691.
88. Hulka F, Mullins RJ, Frank EH. Blunt brain injury activates the coagulation process. *Arch Surg.* 1996;131:923-928.
89. Ansell JE. Acquired bleeding disorders. In: Rippe JM, Alper JS, Irwin RS. *Intensive Care Medicine.* 2nd ed. Boston, Mass: Little, Brown & Co; 1991:1013-1023.
90. Kearney TJ, Bentt L, Grode M, Lee S, Hiatt JR, Shabot MM. Coagulopathy and catecholamines in severe head injury. *J Trauma.* 1992;32:608-612.
91. Danzl DF, Pozos RS. Accidental hypothermia. *N Engl J Med.* 1994;331:1756-1760.
92. Organ Transplantation Breakthrough Collaborative: Best Practices Evaluation. Final Report. US Department of Health and Human Services Health Resources and Services Administration Healthcare System Bureau, Division of Transplantation. September 2005.

Surgical Recovery of Organs

Tammie Peterson, RN, BSN, CPTC
Jennifer Johnson, RN, BSN, CPTC
Amy Fleming, RN, BSN, CPTC
Mark Smith, CST
Marlon F. Levy, MD

Introduction

Surgical recovery of the organs is the conclusion of the organ procurement process but just the beginning of the journey of transplantation. The goal of the surgical recovery process is to provide optimal organs for transplantation and to fulfill the wishes of the donor and the donor's family. The surgical recovery continues a cascade of events that affects the lives of a great number of people, including transplant recipients, hospital personnel, physicians, nurses, and all of those touched by the world of transplantation.

Since transplantation became a reality in the 1960s, the need for organs for transplantation has continued to increase, yet the availability of organs has not been able to keep up with the demand. Because of the need for transplantable organs and the development of transplantation of multiple types of solid organs, an overall goal in the organ procurement process is to maximize the number of organs recovered and transplanted. Techniques and specific protocols vary among organ procurement organizations (OPOs) and transplant centers, but the goal remains the same—the facilitation of a process that maximizes the number of transplantable organs recovered. Every organ for which consent for donation is given by the donor's family is considered and evaluated for multiorgan recovery, unless contraindications exist. Although technicalities and style are different among OPOs and transplant centers, the chain of events that occur during the surgical procedure are the same.

Setting the Operating Room Time

The surgical recovery phase of organ procurement begins to unfold while the donor is still in the intensive care unit (ICU). The busy schedules of the operating room and transplantation personnel make careful planning and effective communication essential skills for the organ recovery coordinator (ORC), who must set an operating room time. The ORC should inform the operating room at the beginning of the ICU phase of donor management that a potential organ donor is in the ICU and that an operating room time may need to be coordinated at the completion of organ placement. Depending on the system in place at the donor hospital, the charge nurse in the operating room and/or the house supervisor should be the point of contact for setting an operating room time. The ORC must not only coordinate an operating room time that accommodates the schedule of the donor operating room, but must also work with all of the transplant centers that have accepted organs and the recovery personnel who will be involved in the procurement. The ORC must also be prepared for the transition to the operating room and must set an operating room time that will allow the ORC to complete his or her responsibilities before proceeding to the operating room. The ORC should ensure that all needed documentation is completed, the donor's medical record is copied for each organ being recovered and each tissue recovery agency involved in the case, and documents are ready for the medical examiner and/or justice of the peace if the potential donor will be going to one of them (rather than the funeral home) after donation . Once all of these details are in place, the transition can be made from the ICU to the operating room. The ORC must remain the donor's primary advocate. ORCs must do their best to accommodate recovery/transplant personnel as well as the staff at the donor hospital, but it is their overall decision to set the most appropriate and reasonable operating room time. The ORC must consider the needs and wishes of the donor family as well as the needs of the hospital and transplant center, but the ORC makes the final decision on an operating room time.

Personnel Requirements

A smooth transition to the operating room not only requires that a reasonable operating room time be set by the ORC but also requires the presence of the right team of personnel. Certain personnel are required in the surgical recovery to ensure that the process is smooth and effective. This team makeup may vary slightly in different OPOs and hospitals throughout the country, but overall the team members involved in the recovery remain consistent. The donor hospital personnel used during the organ recovery are a circulating nurse and scrub technician/scrub nurse. The OPO personnel include 1 or 2 ORCs and in many OPOs a surgical services coordinator, who often has a background as a surgical technician in the operating room. There must also be recovery personnel, who consist mainly of transplant physicians, fellow, and residents from transplant centers.

Anesthesia Duties

Anesthesia personnel are also required during the surgical recovery of organs. The primary role of the anesthesia personnel in the operating room is to manage the donor hemodynamically during the surgical recovery process. This role includes management of the ventilator to optimize oxygenation and administering any fluids or medications to maintain the hemodynamic stability of the donor in the operating room. Agents administered can include, but are not limited to, crystalloids, colloids, blood products, vasopressors, diuretics, and medications to maintain hemodynamic stability.

According to the standards of the Association of Organ Procurement Associations, the anesthesiologist should be instructed by the OPO personnel about the key items that should be monitored and the interventions that may need to occur. Before the start of the case, the anesthesiologist must assess the current hemodynamic state of the donor, get a short history of the patient and the patient's hospital course, determine which organs are going to be recovered, and take note of any special needs of the surgical teams coming to recover the organs. The anesthesia personnel also should assess the vascular access present and what may be required during the case to administer any needed fluids or medications. The anesthesia personnel should insert any additional venous or arterial access devices that they deem necessary to maintain hemodynamic stability during the surgical recovery. The ORC should explain the surgical recovery process and what to expect throughout the case to the anesthesia personnel. The anesthesia personnel should be informed of the timeline of the recovery of organs and should be given an overview of the medications that may be required during the case. The ORC makes sure that the anesthesia personnel understand the purpose of giving heparin before cross-clamping and should ensure the availability of heparin in the operating room.

The anesthesia personnel should also understand their role in maintaining the overall hemodynamic stability of the donor in the operating room. They should be informed to maintain communication with the operating room staff and surgeons about any significant changes in the donor's hemodynamic status. During the case, the donor is maintained on a fraction of inspired oxygen of 100% to maximize oxygenation. In addition, oxygen saturation is monitored and should be greater than 90%. The donor's body temperature also must be maintained at greater than 36ºC.

Continuous monitoring of blood pressure is necessary, and the systolic pressure should be maintained at greater than 90 mm Hg. The first line of treatment in blood pressure management is administration of crystalloids and colloids. If the pressure cannot be maintained with fluid management alone, vasopressors are instituted to maintain the blood pressure. The vasopressor of choice is dopamine. Vasopressors such as neosynephrine, norepinephrine, and epinephrine may be instituted as a last resort if other treatment measures are not successful. Treatment measures should always be discussed with the recovery team to decide in advance the best form of treatment for hemodynamic instability not responding to conventional donor management protocols. Urine output should be to maintained at greater than 1mL/kg per hour and if a significant increase or decrease occurs, the recovery team should be notified.

A CLINICIAN'S GUIDE TO DONATION AND TRANSPLANTATION   Chapter 34

Although it is the primary responsibility of the anesthesia personnel to maintain the hemodynamic stability of the organ donor, the ORC should also remain aware of the hemodynamic status of the patient throughout the case.

The role of the anesthesia personnel may also include obtaining blood samples to accompany the organ as well as for laboratory tests during the surgical recovery to assess the organ's function and oxygenation. Toward the end of the case and before cross-clamping, the surgeon will ask that heparin be given. The dose of heparin given is generally 20,000 to 30,000 units or 300 units per kilogram in children. The timing of heparinization is coordinated between the recovery surgeons. Approximately 3 to 5 minutes after heparinization, cross-clamping occurs. After cross-clamping has occurred, the anesthesiologist turns off the mechanical ventilator and ceases all infusions of fluids and/or medications. At this point, the anesthesia personnel's job is complete. The only exception is in the case of lung recovery, where the anesthesia personnel should remain approximately 1 hour longer in order to oxygenate the lungs through mechanical ventilation until they are removed.

The anesthesia personnel can consist of anesthesiologists, anesthesia residents, and/or certified registered nurse anaesthesists. In some OPOs, organs are recovered in the OPO's own facility instead of the hospital. In this case, the ORC may be responsible for the duties of the anesthesia personnel; however, the principles remain the same.

Operating Room Setup

Approximately 1 hour before the beginning of surgery, the ORC and/or the surgical services coordinator should arrive at the operating room. This period before the case allows the coordinator time to interact with the operating room staff and provide any necessary information about the donation process and address any questions or concerns that the hospital personnel may have. This time is also used to help facilitate the room setup and prepare the organ recovery back tables for each organ being recovered. In addition, setup of equipment and supplies needed for recovery teams can be completed. Allowing adequate time to set up for the surgical recovery is crucial in developing a good relationship with the surgical team and for a successful recovery. Figure 1 shows the overall setup of a typical donor operating room. It may be beneficial to provide the hospital staff with a guide such as Figure 1 so that they can have a clear picture of how to set up the room for the recovery.

The following equipment is needed during the surgical recovery of organs:

- 2 electrocautery units
- 2 tandem or large suction units
- 2 slush machines (if available)
- 3 back tables
- 3 intravenous poles
- nonsterile ice
- bronchoscopy supplies (if lungs are to be recovered)
- Oxygen tank (necessary for 2-layer preservation method for pancreatic islet cells)

Some OPOs obtain most necessary supplies from the donor's operating room; some bring many of their own supplies for use during the case. Who provides which supplies is coordinated between the OPO personnel and hospital's operating room staff before the start of the case. The supplies needed for the case include, but are not limited to the following:

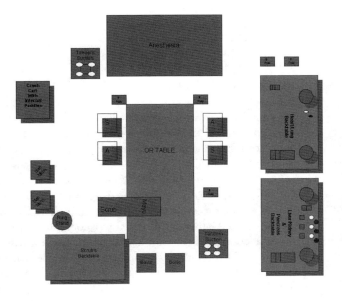

Preferred Surgical Setup Suggested by the Southwest Transplant Alliance, Dallas, Texas.

- major abdominal set
- assortment of vascular clamps
- sternal saw and blade (Lebsche knife is not available)
- medium and large clips
- light handle covers
- Bovie extension
- sterile gloves
- preparation kit
- drapes for patient and table
- plastic or metal basins
- staplers (various types, will be at the discretion of the recovery surgeons)
  - surgical towels
  - umbilical tape
  - skin stapler
  - Tru-Cut needles (if biopsies are to be performed)
  - specimen cups
  - sterile ruler
  - sterile marker
  - 10 L cold isotonic sodium chloride solution

Instrumentation and Suture

- 2 mosquito clamps
- 6 hemostats
- 2 peon forceps
- 4-6 tonsil clamps (for dissection and passing ties)
- 2 right angle clamps
- 2 Oschner clamps
- 4 Allis clamps (for securing Bovie extensions and suctions to drapes)
- 2 long Debakey forceps
- 2 medium Debakey forceps
- 1 long Metzenbaum scissors
- 1 medium Metzenbaum scissors
- 1 curved Mayo scissors
- 1 suture scissors
- 1 Cooley scissors (if available)
- 1 knife 15 blade #3 handle
- 1 knife 11 blade #7 handle
- 0, 2-0, 3-0 silk ties (all on passers)
- Umbilical tapes (all on passers)
- 2-0, 3-0 silk sutures on SH needles
- 4-0, 5-0, 6-0 prolene sutures on SH and RB needles
- #2 Ethilon (on large cutting needle to close)

Sterile slush will be needed during the recovery procedure to cool the organs after cross-clamping. This slush is very important during the preservation process and cooling of the organs during the recovery. In most hospitals, a slush machine is the optimal way to prepare sterile slush. If a slush machine is not available, coordinators can make their own simply by placing numerous bottles of isotonic sodium chloride solution or lactated Ringer's solution into a cooler filled with ice. Alcohol is then poured on top of the ice, and in some cases rock salt can also be used. Mixing this together and shaking the bottles periodically should allow a slush solution to form inside the bottles within approximately 1 hour. Care should be taken to periodically shake the bottles so that the ice does not freeze solid inside the bottles. The slush solution can then be poured onto the sterile field by the OPO or hospital staff.

Before the start of the case, the OPO staff should ensure that suction will be adequate during the recovery. Because suction is crucial in keeping the surgical field free of fluid, the coordinator must make certain that the circulating nurse has provided a large number of suction canisters in the room. During the recovery or organs, all of the blood will be drained from the body, and preservation solutions will be perfused through the organs, so monitoring the canisters is crucial in keeping the surgical recovery smooth and free from excess fluid in the sterile field. The canisters may have to be changed 5 to 10 times depending on the volume that each canister holds. The circulating nurse must be aware of this before the start of the case so the nurse can ensure that enough suction canisters are available.

Once the room is set up and the teams are ready, the donor is brought to the operating room. The operating room team, OPO staff, and anesthesia personnel should work together to ensure a smooth transition from the ICU to the operating room. The donor should be transported from the ICU to the operating room by using a transport monitor so that the hemodynamic status of the patient can be monitored during transport. Once the donor arrives in the operating room, the donor should be transferred from the bed to the operating room table and positioned on the table supine with the arms tucked.

Surgical preparation of the operative site can be done with any solutions approved by the Association of Operating Room Nurses. The surgical preparation should be done from the chin to mid thigh at about an 8-in (20 cm) width. If needed, the donor's chest, abdomen, and pubic areas should be shaved.

Once the donor is prepared, the donor is draped with towels exposing the prepared area, making sure that the extent from the sternal notch to the pubic area is exposed. The towels are secured in place with a skin stapler. After the towels are secured, the universal drape is applied, beginning with the bottom drape, top drape, and then the 2 side drapes. Folds of the side drapes are created in order hold the Bovie extensions and suctions as they are passed off and secured to the drapes with Allis clamps. The Bovie extensions are connected to the electrocautery units and set at 80 coag, 0 cut, and the suctions are connected to the tandem or large suction units. The sternal saw is then passed off the field and connected to the power source. Depending on the donor packs used or the operating room supplies, the draping procedure may be slightly different.

After the donor is prepared and draped and the surgical recovery teams are present, the surgical recovery process can officially begin. An incision is made from the suprasternal notch to the pubis by using electrocautery. The chest is opened by using a sternal saw or Lebsche knife. Between electrocautery and use of bone wax, hemostasis is obtained. This type of incision is done in all recoveries except for a kidney-only recovery. In a kidney-only recovery, it is not necessary to open the chest to allow full exposure of organs and prevent injuries to vessels. A self-retaining retractor is used to hold open both the thoracic and abdominal cavities. Upon opening, careful attention is given when exploring the abdominal cavity for incidental discovery of malignant neoplasms, peritonitis, and ischemic bowel, or any other contraindications that may be present upon opening.

Technical procedures of organ recovery are somewhat varied between recovery surgeons, but the overall principles remain the same. After the incision is made and the organs are exposed, initial dissection of the organs to be recovered begins. The organs to be recovered are isolated in addition to their vascular structures, and cannulas are placed for in situ perfusion of the organs after cross-clamping. Once all of the organs are isolated and the recovery surgeons are finished with their initial dissection, the anesthesia personnel are instructed to give the heparin. The team waits 3 to 5 minutes and then cross-clamps the aorta. At this point slush is added to the abdominal and thoracic cavities to cool the organs, and the infusion of preservation solutions begins. The types of preservation solutions used are determined by the policies and procedures set up by the OPO and transplant centers. Further dissection may need to occur before the removal of the organs. The organs are removed in order according to their sensitivity to ischemia time and anatomical placement. The order of recovery in a multiple organ recovery is as follows:

1. Heart
2. Lungs
3. Liver
4. Pancreas
5. Small intestine
6. Kidneys

The technical aspects of recovery of each type of organ are discussed in detail in the following sections.

Kidney Procurement

Historically, kidneys were the only organ to be recovered, but today, one rarely goes to the operating room for kidneys only. If other abdominal organs are going to be recovered, it is ideal to consider using the same recovery team for all of the abdominal organs. Use of the same recovery team decreases the number of personnel in the room and makes for a smoother recovery.

After heart, lungs, liver, and pancreas have been removed, the kidneys are procured. Most kidneys are removed en bloc with a segment of aorta and inferior vena cava to allow for adequate reanastomosis in the recipient. First, the ureters are identified and dissected free in the deep pelvis close to the bladder. If the liver has been procured, the right kidney is already exposed. To expose the left kidney, the left colon is retracted and the splenic and diaphragmatic attachments are released. After the division of the left mesenteric colon, the left kidney is completely dissected. Once the inferior vena cava and aorta are transected, the kidneys are lifted out and placed in a cold slush solution. Once on the back table, the perinephric fat is removed, the kidneys are divided, and the vasculature (i.e., arteries, veins) along with the ureters are identified, measured, and documented for the recipient surgeon. The coordinator records all of this information in the donor's medical record.

The left kidney is the one with the longer vein and is generally the preferred kidney for transplantation. When the surgeon refers to a cuff, it means that the renal artery is still connected to a piece of the aorta. If the surgeon states that there is a patch of the cava, this means that the renal vein remains connected to a section of the vena cava. Also, the kidneys are inspected for arterial/aortic plaque, cysts, hematomas, and damage to the capsule, and a biopsy may be done because of the patient's age, medical social history, or increasing creatinine level or at the request of the recipient surgeon. The kidneys are then placed in a cold preservation solution, packaged and labeled according to the policy of the OPO or the United Network for Organ Sharing (UNOS), and transported with tissue typing and a copy of the donor's record to the receiving transplant center.

Kidney-Alone Procurement

The kidney procurement begins after preliminary dissection of the right colon, the small bowel, and the pancreas, which allows the right kidney, aorta, vena cava, and superior mesenteric artery to be visualized. Two umbilical tapes are used to encircle the aorta. The superior mesenteric artery is then prepared for ligation with heavy ties. A last umbilical tape is placed around the supraceliac aorta. After heparinization, the distal aorta is cannulated and then the supraceliac aorta is cross-clamped. Cold perfusion is started and the vena cava is incised to allow exsanguination. The abdominal cavity is filled with slush and the dissection and removal ensues.

Liver Procurement

The method for recovering the liver depends on the surgeon's training, preference, and experience. The liver is visually assessed for color, size, or injury and is palpated for consistency. Normally, small lacerations or hematomas do not affect the use of the organ for transplantation. Dissection begins with the mobilization of the round ligament, which is tied and cut. Electrocautery is used to divide the falciform and left triangular ligaments. Aortic dissection is performed early so that in the event of hemodynamic instability, the aorta can be quickly cannulated and preservation solution can be immediately infused.

Next, the cecum, the right colon, and the small intestines are freed to expose the inferior vena cava and left renal vein. Umbilical ties are placed around the abdominal aorta, then the inferior mesenteric artery is ligated. An incision is made along the surface of the gallbladder to enable the removal of bile, preventing mucosal necrosis from bile stasis once the liver is removed. The portal vein is found, typically under the gastroduodenal artery. After dissection, cannulas are placed in the aorta and portal vein in preparation for cross-clamping. Once dissection and cannulation are complete, heparin is given to the donor. The aorta is then ligated below the level of the cannula, and a second umbilical tape is used to secure the cannula in place within the aorta.

Once the thoracic and abdominal teams are ready, a large vascular clamp is placed across the supraceliac aorta and cardiopulmonary circulation ceases. Cold preservation solutions are infused through the aorta and portal vein. The vena cava is cut at the level of the right atrium to allow exsanguination. The abdominal and thoracic cavities are filled with a frozen slush solution. After the onset of cold perfusion, the superior mesenteric artery and vein are ligated.

Before the liver is removed, the inferior vena cava is removed at the level of the pericardium. Care should be taken not to exert force on the liver or kidney that could cause capsular tears. The inferior vena cava is then transected above the left renal vein. The liver is gently lifted and retroperitoneal attachments are divided along with the aorta. The liver is then gently lifted out of the cavity and placed in a container for a second flushing. At this time, vasculature that may need to be relayed to the transplanting surgeon can be identified. Once all organs are recovered, the iliac vessels are taken for possible use in the vascular reconstruction of the recipient. Some programs prefer to reflush the liver on the back table. The liver is then packaged and labeled according to UNOS policy and delivered with tissue typing and a copy of the donor's chart to the transplant center.[1]

Heart Procurement

If possible, the heart procurement team should be present at the beginning of the surgical recovery process. The innominate vein is exposed and the thymus is divided. The pericardium is opened in a vertical direction, and the incision is extended laterally at the level of the diaphragm. Pericardial sutures are then placed. Intraoperative assessment of the heart is performed for any contraindications to organ donation. Umbilical tapes are placed around the aorta, the superior vena cava, and the inferior vena cava. A purse string suture is placed in the ascending aorta for the administration of cardioplegia solution. Once the abdominal team has finished the dissection, heparin is given. A cardioplegia needle is placed in the purse string and secured. The heart is allowed to beat empty for 5 beats, then aortic cross-clamping is applied and the cardioplegia solution is administered. Once the cardioplegia solution has been given, the cardioplegia needle is removed, and the aortic purse string is secured. The inferior vena cava transection is now complete.

The heart is elevated anteriorly and superiorly to reveal the 4 pulmonary veins, which are divided flush with the pericardium. The right and left pulmonary arteries and aorta are then divided. The heart is again lifted from the chest, and any remaining attachments are divided. Heavy Mayo scissors are used for this division. Care is taken to avoid the trachea and the main stem bronchi. The heart, once removed from the chest, is inspected and then placed in a basin of cold slush solution. The heart is then placed in a sterile jar with a liter of cold solution. The lid is secured. The heart is then placed in 2 additional sterile bags, labeled according to UNOS policy, and placed in an ice chest for transport.[2]

Lung Procurement

Because of the propensity for donor lungs to deteriorate, recovery should not be delayed unnecessarily. If possible, the lung team should be present at the beginning of the surgical recovery. The lung team often performs a bronchoscopy by using a flexible bronchoscope in the operating room. Bronchoscopy can be done before, after, or even while the donor is being prepared and draped. If no contraindications to organ donation are found during the bronchoscopic examination, the team proceeds with the recovery.

Through a median sternotomy incision, the pericardial cavity is opened and cut edges are secured with sutures. The heart and lungs are examined visually and palpated, then a final decision is made to proceed. The superior vena cava is mobilized up to the innominate vein and the azygos vein is identified, tied off, and divided. The aorta is then entirely mobilized and separated off the pulmonary artery. The innominate vein is ligated and divided. Both pleural cavities are opened, and the inferior pulmonary ligaments are mobilized on both sides. The pulmonary artery cannula is placed in the purse string suture and connected to a lung preservation solution infusion line. The trachea is mobilized to the level of the larynx.

At this point, the organs are ready to be removed, and the superior vena cava is tied down between ligatures and then divided. The donor is heparinized and the aorta is cannulated. The donor should be ventilated on 100% inspired oxygen with lungs fully inflated to avoid perfusion with areas of atelectasis. Prostin (500 μg in 10 mL of sterile water) is injected into the superior vena cava followed by ligation of this vessel and the transection of the inferior vena cava. When the heart is decompressed, the ascending aorta is cross-clamped. The heart is perfused with preservation solution. The tip of the left atrial appendage is amputated to vent the left side of the heart. During perfusion, the lungs are gently ventilated on 100%

oxygen. After the completion of perfusion, the apex of the heart is lifted, allowing access to the pulmonary veins.

The left atrial cuff is fashioned by making an incision in the left atrial wall midway between the confluence of the left pulmonary veins and the atrioventricular groove and then continuing circumferentially around the orifices of the veins. On the right side, a similar venous cuff is created. The superior vena cava is divided, the main pulmonary artery and the ascending aorta are transected, and the heart is removed following division of the pericardial reflection. The pericardium anterior to the hilum of each lung is excised and the pulmonary ligaments are divided. The lung block is then excised by dividing mediastinal soft tissue and pleura anterior to the esophagus or stapling the esophagus and removing the entire mediastinal contents anterior to the vertebral column. The trachea is clamped and divided, with the lungs inflated with 100% oxygen. On the back table, if lungs are separated, there is a division at the pulmonary artery bifurcation, and mediastinal soft tissue by stapling the trachea, and then dividing the left main bronchus *with a stapler*. Both lungs are packed either separately or together in preservation solution and in 3 sterile bags and labeled accordance with UNOS policy. The lungs are placed in the ice chest with labels to indicate left or right or both.[2]

Pancreas Procurement

A pancreas recovery is generally part of a multiorgan procurement. When both the liver and the pancreas are to be recovered, great care must be taken during the recovery because of shared anatomy. Such is also the case when the small bowel is involved. One must preserve the arterial blood supply and make certain that the length of portal vein is adequate for both organs. In addition, the pancreas has a dual arterial supply. The head of the pancreas and the duodenum are supplied by the pancreaticoduodenal arcades, which arise from the superior or mesenteric artery and the gastroduodenal artery. Because the gastroduodenal artery is a branch of the common hepatic artery, it is usually ligated to preserve the arterial supply to the liver. The tail of the pancreas is supplied by the splenic artery, which arises from the celiac axis. The venous drainage of the pancreas is the superior mesenteric vein and splenic vein, which join to form the portal vein and drain the liver. Because of shared anatomy and the possibility of a difficult recovery or abnormalities, good communication must occur between all surgeons involved in this recovery.

To begin the procedure, the arterial supply to the liver must be identified. The right colon and small bowel are mobilized to visualize the retroperitoneum. The omentum should be divided and the pancreas examined. The spleen should also be examined for any signs of trauma. The inferior mesenteric artery is divided between ligatures, and the distal aorta is encircled. The supraceliac aorta is encircled after division of diaphragmatic muscle fibers. The bile duct is divided close to the duodenum. The hepatic artery is identified and isolated as already described. The gastroduodenal, right gastric, and left gastric arteries are divided between ligatures. The splenic artery is preserved. The portal vein is dissected free. The inferior mesenteric vein is dissected and cannulated for portal perfusion. The cannula is advanced into the portal vein. The splenic vein is preserved and should not be used for cannulation.

The greater omentum is divided between ligatures along its entire length. The short gastric vessels between the stomach and spleen are ligated and divided. The spleen is mobilized by dividing the splenocolic and splenorenal ligaments and diaphragmatic attachments. The spleen is used as a handle to minimize trauma to the pancreas. However, the spleen and tail of the pancreas are left undisturbed to minimize trauma and decrease the risk of pancreatitis after transplantation. The stomach is retracted upward and to the right, exposing the lesser sac and the anterior surface of the pancreas. The peritoneum at the superior and inferior borders of the pancreas is incised. Ligation of identifiable blood vessels prevents pancreatic injury that may happen during the control of bleeding from these vessels. Ligation also prevents bleeding after implantation. The spleen is retracted medially, and the tail of the pancreas is dissected free of the retroperitoneum. Care should be taken to carry out the dissection away from the surface of the pancreas. Mobilization of the pancreatic head with duodenum is next. The ligament of Treitz is divided. The duodenum and pancreas are retracted to the left until the aorta is exposed.

The stomach and duodenum are irrigated with a povidone-iodine solution through a nasogastric tube. The duodenum is transected just distal to the pylorus with a gastrointestinal anastomosis (GIA) stapler. The proximal jejunum just distal to the ligament of Treitz is cleared circumferentially and divided in the same way. Spillage of intestinal content is avoided to prevent contamination of the abdominal cavity. Next, the root of small-bowel mesentery is divided after ligation of mesenteric vessels. After preliminary dissection of the pancreas, it is ready for perfusion. After preservation solution has been instilled through the aortic and portal cannulas, the portal vein is ligated over the previously placed cannula, leaving 2 cm of portal vein on the pancreas side. The portal vein is incised just below the ligature for venous decompression of the pancreas. Topical cooling is performed with slushed ice.

After completion of preservation, the liver is recovered first. During the liver retrieval, the splenic artery is ligated close to the celiac axis and divided, leaving as much length of the splenic artery with the pancreas as possible. The free end of the splenic artery is marked for identification. The portal vein is divided between the liver and pancreas. Nerve bundles and lymphatic tissue around the superior mesenteric artery are divided, and the superior mesenteric artery is dissected free down to the aorta. The superior mesenteric artery with a narrow cuff of aorta is excised. If the patient has an aberrant right hepatic artery, the surgeon can divide the superior mesenteric artery up to the takeoff of the right hepatic artery. If the right hepatic artery passes through the head of the pancreas, the pancreas cannot be recovered.[1]

After removal, the pancreas is irrigated with a povidone-iodine and amphotericin solution (this may differ between programs) and the effluent is drained outside the basin. The pancreas is then packaged and labeled according to UNOS policy.

If the liver is not going to be recovered, the gastroduodenal artery is preserved and the portal vein can be transected high in the hilum of the liver, leaving a long portal vein with the pancreas.

If the pancreas is going to be recovered for the purpose of islet cell transplant, then surgical recovery is the same. However, during the operating room period, the coordinator must bubble the mixture of University of Wisconsin solution and perfluorocarbon with oxygen if a 2-layer method of pancreas preservation is being used. This technique is used in an effort to extend the preservation time of the pancreas until islets can be isolated and also to increase the yield of islets during the isolation.

Small-Bowel Procurement

The intestine was the first organ to be used on an experimental basis; however, it was the last organ to actually be transplanted. Small-bowel recovery can be a part of a multivisceral procurement or stand alone. When opening up the donor, extreme care is taken to avoid inadvertently burning the small bowel. If an accidental burn occurs, it should be identified with a suture. The entire small and large bowel are inspected carefully, specifically looking for tears, hematomas, and so on. A good bowel is pink and shows good mesenteric pulsation. If dusky areas are apparent, the bowel should be wrapped in a warm lap sponge and reevaluated. An Atgam infusion may be used in the donor when dissection begins. Whether or not Atgam is used is determined by the center that is accepting the organ for transplant.

If the small bowel is recovered in a multivisceral recovery, it is removed in a cluster with a double central stem consisting of the celiac axis and superior mesenteric artery. If only the small bowel is to be recovered, then only the superior mesenteric artery is preserved. The recovery begins by the falciform ligament being divided. The aorta is exposed to the level of the superior mesenteric artery, and the inferior vena cava is exposed to the lower aspect of the liver. The inferior mesenteric vein is exposed, and a cannula is inserted for flushing. Ties are placed around the distal aorta after ligation of any lumbar branches. If the intestines are recovered without the liver, the venous drainage of the graft is by the portal vein.

The procedure proceeds similarly to a liver recovery. The duodenum is cauterized. The distal and supraceliac aorta are encircled in the usual manner. The portal vein is cannulated through the inferior mesenteric vein. The hepatoduodenal ligament is dissected out. The gastroduodenal, splenic, and left gastric arteries are ligated and divided to isolate the celiac axis. If a left hepatic artery arising from left gastric artery is found, it is preserved. The common bile duct is encircled and transected distally. The gallbladder fundus is incised and the bile is washed out by irrigating with isotonic sodium chloride solution. The gastrocolic omentum is divided between ligatures. The right and middle colic vessels are divided, sparing ileal branches of the ileocolic artery. The right and transverse colon are mobilized completely. The jejunum is divided with a GIA stapler just distal to the ligament of Treitz. The peritoneum at the inferior border of the pancreas is incised. The neck of the pancreas is encircled with blunt dissection and divided between heavy ligatures.

The pancreas and duodenum are dissected from the intestinal graft with ligation of potentially numerous small branches of the superior mesenteric artery and vein at this location. The distal part of the small bowel is transected with a GIA stapler at the ileocecal valve. The distal aorta is cannulated after systemic heparinization. After cross-clamping, the diaphragm is divided around the inferior vena cava, the ligaments are freed, the infrahepatic inferior vena cava is divided, and the spleen and the pancreas are mobilized from the retroperitoneum. The aorta is recovered from the left subclavian artery to the inferior border of the superior mesenteric artery. Care should be taken to divide the lower end of the aorta 2 to 3 mm below the origin of the superior mesenteric artery so that this can be closed on the back table without narrowing the lumen of the origin of the superior mesenteric artery. In child donors, the renal arteries may rise very close to the superior mesenteric arteries and the kidneys may not receive an aortic cuff. This problem should be discussed with the kidney transplant surgeon. The duodenum is stapled at the level distal to the pylorus. The liver, pancreas, and small bowel are removed en bloc. The distal small bowel at the ileocecal junction is taken for biopsy.

Once the cluster is removed, then the back table work begins. The thoracic and abdominal aorta of the periadventitial tissue are dissected with individual ligation of the intercostal arteries. Mass ligation of the intercostal arteries should not be done because this may cause kinking of the aorta and an increased risk of thrombosis in the recipient. The distal aorta is closed. The celiac axis is not dissected in a child donor but it is dissected in an adult. The splenic and left gastric arteries may be dissected and ligated. The gastroduodenal artery is not to be ligated. The splenic vein is dissected from the tail of the pancreas toward the confluence with the superior mesenteric vein. The pancreas is divided to the right of the portal vein. The splenic vein is left long in continuity for the possible anastomoses with the recipient portal vein. The cut surface of the pancreas is oversewn. The pancreatic duct is identified on the cut surface and ligated.[1]

After the organs are recovered, lymph nodes are obtained by the recovery surgeons for tissue typing. The recovery surgeon must ensure that enough lymph nodes are recovered to be able to send a set of tissue typing with each recovered organ. The ORC will be primarily responsible for packaging the tissue typing specimens and ensuring that they are sent with each organ. The spleen can also be used for tissue typing purposes, in addition to lymph nodes if the pancreas is not being recovered, because most of the time the spleen is recovered with the pancreas. There will also be further recovery of vessels to be sent with the liver and pancreas in order to supply sufficient vasculature for the transplant surgeon if artery conduits may be necessary during the transplantation. Documentation must be completed prior to and during the surgical recovery process. The ORC is responsible for ensuring that this documentation is complete before the end of the case.

After all organs, vessels, and tissue typing materials have been recovered, the incision is closed with suture by the recovery personnel. The donor is cleaned and prepared for transport to its next location, whether it be for tissue donation, the funeral home, medical examiner or justice of the peace, or morgue. Operating room staff are often not accustomed to death, and the presence of a dead body at the end of a case can be somewhat overwhelming and unfamiliar. The OPO staff stays to help the staff in cleaning up the body and to address any questions and concerns that the hospital staff may have. At the completion of the case, the OPO personnel stay to help the hospital staff clean the body and the room. The OPO coordinator should always ensure that the donor has an identification bracelet on before the body leaves the operating room.

Suggested Reading

Klintmalm GB, Levy MF. *Organ Procurement and Preservation.* Austin, Tex: R.G. Landes Co; 1999.
Phillips M. *UNOS Organ Procurement, Preservation and Distribution in Transplantation.* Richmond, Va: United Network for Organ Sharing; 1996.
Southwest Transplant Alliance, Operative/Medical Examiner Report. Dallas, Tex: Southwest Transplant Alliance
Southwest Transplant Alliance, Organ Recovery Phase Training Manual. Dallas, Tex: Southwest Transplant Alliance
Baylor University Medical Center, Procedure for Small-Bowel Recovery. Dallas, Tex: Baylor University

Developing a Policy for Donation After Cardiac Death

Danielle L. Cornell, RN, BSN, CPTC
Charlie Alexander, RN, MSN, MBA, CPTC
Karen Kennedy, RN, CPTC

Organ procurement organizations (OPOs) vary tremendously in their development and implementation of policies for donation after cardiac death (DCD). Some OPOs have specific and individualized DCD policies in place for each hospital where organs are recovered from DCD donors. Others use an OPO-specific DCD policy that guides practice at their donor hospitals when DCD organs are being recovered. As the practice of DCD donation continues to evolve and become more widely adopted throughout the United States, hospital policies specific to the recovery of DCD organs will be necessary. Both the Centers for Medicare and Medicaid Services and the Joint Commission on Accreditation of Healthcare Organizations strongly encourage the implementation of DCD policies for every acute care hospital and donation service area (DSA) in the country.[1]

The development of a DCD program within a DSA is typically accomplished through the evaluation and implementation of DCD policies from peer programs. Most DSAs begin this process with the development of an OPO policy for the process of DCD organ recovery.[2] Crucial components of a DCD policy are shown in Table 1. Although a policy should be tailored to suit the needs of a community, a sample policy is provided for readers to review (Table 2).

Table 1. CRUCIAL COMPONENTS OF POLICIES FOR DONATION AFTER CARDIAC DEATH (DCD)

- Donor selection criteria
    - Acceptable donor age ranges
    - Assessment of likelihood that the patient will die within defined time parameters
    - Comorbid diseases that may preclude donation
- Specific delineation of the roles of the various care teams
    - Hospital
    - Transplant service (if applicable)
    - Organ procurement organization
    - Family support
    - Ethics (if indicated/required)
    - Risk management (if indicated)
- Clinical processes for the recovery of donor organs
    - Determination of death
    - Location of withdrawal of life-sustaining measures (typically family driven)
    - Operating room staff—orientation to recoveries from DCD donors (as distinguished from the recovery process from brain-dead donors)
- Provision for family care before, during, and after the withdrawal of life-sustaining measures
- Statement of the hospital's responsibility for normal and customary comfort measures for the DCD donors
- Logistical guidelines for the recovery of organs from a DCD donor, and provision for palliative care if the patient does not die and become a donor

Chapter 35 DEVELOPING A POLICY FOR DONATION AFTER CARDIAC DEATH

Table 2. SAMPLE POLICY FOR DONATION AFTER CARDIAC DEATH

Title of SOP: ORGAN DONATION PROCESS AFTER CARDIAC DEATH

SOP # 7-304.01	Effective Date:	Total # of Pages: 4

Originated by: Jane Doe **Department:** Clinical Services
Revised by: John Doe here **Department:** Quality
Scope: All Departments Quality Consent Donor Services Organ Recovery Tissue Recovery Skin Communications: Hospital Public Administration: ADM HR IT FIN

Approved by: _____ Title: Director, Clinical Services Date: _____
Approved by: _____ Title: Chief Executive Officer Date: _____
Approved by: _____ Title: Director, Quality Systems Date: _____
Approved by: _____ Title: Medical Director Date: _____
Approved by: _____ Title: _____ Date: _____

I PURPOSE
  To describe the process by which organ donation after cardiac death (DCD) is facilitated, adhering to both TRC clinical and donor hospital policies.

II MATERIALS/EQUIPMENT REQUIRED
  A. Indelible pen, black or blue ink

III RECORDS REQUIRED
  A. AOPO Donor Work-up Form
  B. Donor specific hospital DCD policy
  C. Patient's hospital medical record
  D. Operating Room Requirements for Organ Donation After Cardiac Death, QA Form 742, Attachment I
  E. TRC DCD Worksheet, QA Form 744, Attachment II

IV DEFINITIONS
  AOPO Work-up Form - A set of forms designed to document organ donor referral, management, and recovery data and information. The forms include all aspects of the organ donor case to include, but not limited to, donor demographics, hemodynamics, vital signs, fluid intake and output, lab values and organ recovery information.

  Organ Donation After Cardiac Death (DCD) - Process in which organs are recovered, with proper consent and declaration of death, after the declaration of death by cardiac criteria.

  TRC DCD Worksheet - A form designed to document the declaration of death process, including vital signs such as heart rate, blood pressure, and oxygen saturation.

V POLICY
  A. All patients will be declared cardiac dead by the appropriate treating or attending physician in accordance with standard medical practice, Maryland State Law, and the established policies of the donor hospital.
  B. No member of a hospital transplant service should be involved with any part of the informed consent or declaration of death process for organ and tissue donation.
  C. No procedures related to the donor process shall be initiated until informed consent has been obtained from the legal next of kin.
  D. Standards for Organ Donation After Cardiac Death (DCD)
    1. The standard process for the identification, referral and evaluation of potential organ donors will be followed according to TRC SOP # 7-300, Response to Potential Organ Referrals.
    2. Hospital and TRC DCD protocols will be initiated in those cases where the patient meets initial suitability criteria for donation according to SOP # 7-301, Initial Suitability Determination of a Potential Organ Donor and either:

Reprinted with Permission from Transplant Resource Center of Maryland

Table 2. SAMPLE POLICY FOR DONATION AFTER CARDIAC DEATH (continued)

      a. The patient does not meet brain death criteria and the family wishes to donate; or
      b. The family has chosen to withdraw mechanical, ventilator, and medical support.
    3. Unless the topic of donation has been brought up by the family, a discussion about donation should not occur until after the family has made a decision to change the patient's status to "Do Not Resuscitate" or if they decide to withdraw ventilator and medical support.
    4. Documentation by the healthcare team regarding the above information should be reviewed in the patient's medical record and a copy made for the TRC record.

E. Initiation of DCD Protocols
    1. Once the patient meets the items listed in Step D2, the Organ Recovery Coordinator (ORC) should contact the Administrator On-Call (AOC) to review the case.
    2. The ORC and the AOC will review the donor hospital's DCD policy to ensure that all hospital protocols are followed. If the hospital does not have a DCD policy, the ORC should contact the Hospital Services Coordinator to discuss the specifics of the case and ascertain next steps for moving forward with the DCD process.
    3. Patient's whose injuries are deemed "not survivable" and who are predicted to suffer a cardiac arrest and cardiac death within the timeframes established in their individual hospital policy, are potential DCD donors. Those parameters shall be discussed among the healthcare team caring for the patient, the ORC, and the AOC. For those hospitals without a DCD policy, the established timeframe for cardiac death is up to 2 hours from withdrawal.
    4. The family of potential candidates for DCD must be informed of the imminent status of the patient by the hospital healthcare team. In addition, they must have a good understanding of the patient's irreversible medical condition and a discussion has to have taken place about the options available to them in this circumstance.
    5. Once the family has made their decision, the TRC Family Advocate or designee, in collaboration with the patient's physician will present donation options to the family. The family shall be provided information about the donation process and what can be expected during the process according to SOP # 5-001, Obtaining Informed Consent.
    6. If consent is given, all paperwork should be completed following SOP # 5-001, Obtaining Informed Consent, and a medical/social history should be obtained following SOP # 5-002, Obtaining a Medical/Social History.

F. Initiation of Process of Organ Donation After Cardiac Death
    1. Once consent has been obtained, the ORC will draw blood for serological testing and tissue typing following SOP # 7-305, Obtaining Blood and Tissue Typing Material from an Organ Donor.
    2. The ORC will obtain release from the Office of the Chief Medical Examiner (OCME), following SOP # 7-101, Medical Examiner Notification for Organ and Tissue Donation.
    3. The Operating Room (OR) staff at the hospital shall be apprised of the pending recovery. The ORC will collaborate with the unit charge nurse, the OR charge nurse, and the nurse and physician caring for the patient to prepare for the withdrawal and recovery process, adhering to the donor hospital's policies. A copy of the Operating Room Requirements for Organ Recovery After Cardiac Death, QA Form 742, will be given to the hospital staff.
    4. Once all evaluation, allocation, and recovery arrangements have been made, the withdrawal of care will take place in accordance with the hospital's policies and the plan developed with the staff and family. For those hospitals without a DCD policy, the withdrawal of care will take place in the Operating Room.
NOTE: It is TRC's preference that the withdrawal of care take place in the Operating Room.
    5. The physician caring for the patient may order, in accordance with his/her usual and customary practice, ongoing pain relief if it is the physician's belief that it is medically and ethically necessary.
    6. No member of TRC or the transplant team shall be present or involved during this phase of the process.
    7. The patient's vital signs shall be documented by the nurse every 5 minutes from the time the ventilator and any medical support are withdrawn. This may be documented in the patient's medical record or on the TRC DCD Worksheet, QA Form 744.
    8. The patient will be pronounced dead by the physician of record after 5 minutes (or as designated in hospital policy) as measured by:
      a. Absence of conducting electrical activity;
      b. Absence of arterial pulse waveform; and
      c. Absence of ventilator support.
    9. After the declaration of death has been documented and the death certificate completed, the surgical recovery of organs shall proceed, in accordance with SOP # 7-401, Surgical Recovery of Organs from Brain Dead Donors.
    10. If the cardiac death does not occur within the designated time frame, the patient will be transferred to the designated patient care area for palliative care in accordance with the plan established by the hospital staff and family.

VI. REFERENCES
    A. Association of Organ Procurement Organization Standards and Requirements, current version
    B. United Network for Organ Sharing Policies and Procedures, current version
    C. The Annotated Code of Maryland, Health- General Section 5-502
    D. Donation After Cardiac Death Tool, QA Form 745
    E. Guidelines for Evaluating a Patient for Donation after Cardiac Death, QA Form 746

Diligence and careful consideration in the development of OPO-based DCD policies are imperative to the success of a DSA's efforts to recover and transplant DCD organs. With sound operational understanding of the established DCD policies and protocols among all of the DSA team members, the OPO can serve as the educational resource throughout the DCD process. A clear understanding of the ethical, operational, and logistical issues relevant to the process should be carefully addressed within the OPO and articulated clearly to the DSA's constituency. This constituency includes donor hospital staff and administration, donor families, the medical examiner's office, the legislative community, and the public.

Delineation of Roles of Team Members

Collaboration with donor hospitals regarding implementation of the DCD policy is vital to the success of any DCD program. Whether a DSA-wide policy is adopted or individualized hospital policies are developed, those policies must be adapted to the culture and administrative structure of each hospital. DCD cases require the support and cooperation of staff from multiple hospital departments (Table 3): critical care, surgery, social work, risk management, and nursing and physician administration. Engaging the input and support of key personnel representing these departments is essential to the success of the process. An additional area of consideration in policy development is the inclusion of the hospital's ethics committee to protect the patient and the patient's family during the process.

Table 3. KEY HOSPITAL DEPARTMENTS FOR SUCCESSFUL DEVELOPMENT OF A POLICY FOR DONATION AFTER CARDIAC DEATH

- Intensive care unit
- Operating room
- Social work
- Nursing and physician administration
- Risk management
- Ethics committee

The DCD process is family driven. Policy development should include protocols that allow patients' families to be involved in the decision-making process. These protocols should include provisions for family care and support, as well as the inclusion of the patient's family in the withdrawal process, for those families requesting to be present during withdrawal of life support.

The OPO typically coordinates all of the required communication between the medical examiner or coroner and the donor hospital to ensure that all of the necessary approval steps are addressed. The DCD process varies from the process for brain-dead donors in that the medical examiner or coroner must be contacted before death because there will not be time for a lengthy decision-making process on the medical examiner's part after death is pronounced. Any preliminary investigations by the medical examiner or his staff into the circumstances of the case must be done before termination of life support if these investigations must be accomplished before the medical examiner or coroner releases the body.

Community Involvement in Development of DCD Policies

The goal of effective community involvement in the implementation of DCD policies throughout DSAs should focus on educating the public about the importance of organ and tissue donation. It provides an opportunity to share with the community the 2 types of circumstances in which individuals can donate their organs after their death, in language that can be understood by a public audience. The need for media and legislative outreach largely serves as a proactive educational step in the event that a DCD donor case should be questioned by a member of the public or professional community. If education is done proactively, the risk of unintended misinterpretation of the process is minimized, and the preservation of public trust in the donation and transplantation process is maintained.

Developing Policy for Clinical Processes

Developing a Policy for Determination of Death

One of the key considerations in policy development surrounds the creation of the framework for the determination of death. Clinical, ethical, and legal considerations must be addressed and explicitly defined in any DCD policy.

The following excerpt summarizes the intent and scope of the DCD Consensus Conference, held in April 2005, for recommendations for the determination of death[3]:

> The ethical axiom of organ donation is adherence to the dead donor rule: the retrieval of organs for transplantation should not cause the death of a donor. A prospective organ donor's death may be determined by either circulatory or brain criteria as prescribed by the President's Commission provided in their proposed death statute, the Uniform Determination of Death Act, which stated that an individual satisfying *either* the cardiopulmonary or neurological criteria is dead. The circulatory criterion of death (used in DCD) is employed when the donor does not fulfill brain death criteria, ventilatory support is not used or has been withdrawn, and circulation and respiration have ceased.
>
> In clinical situations that fulfill either brain death criteria or the circulatory criterion of death, the President's Commission stipulated that the diagnosis of death requires the determination of both *cessation of functions* and *irreversibility*.

A review of the policies of 58 OPOs in the United States today shows that, of the 51 programs with active DCD policies in place, 92% of them use a 5-minute waiting period between cessation of cardiopulmonary function and the initiation of organ recovery.[3] This waiting period is thought to be in response to the recommendations mentioned above. Of the remaining 4 OPOs with active DCD policies, the practice varies from waiting times of 4 minutes (at 1 OPO) to 2 minutes (at 3 OPOs). The Society of Critical Care Medicine concluded that "at least 2 minutes of observation is required, and more than 5 minutes is not recommended."[3] The effect of this recommendation is not yet clear with regard to its effect on the practice of OPOs and donor hospitals throughout the country.

As noted, decisions regarding time intervals for the declaration of death should be made with attention to all applicable ethical and legal standards, as well as with consideration of the recommendations from the Institute of Medicine.[4] As policies are constructed, it is also vital that attention be paid to the implications of those decisions on the successful recovery and transplantation of DCD organs. It is essential that the time interval between the time of death and the recovery of DCD organs be minimized. Warm ischemia time (WIT) plays an important role in the viability of DCD organs for transplantation. The definitions used to describe the time intervals associated with measuring the phases of WIT are not uniformly recognized throughout the organ donation or transplantation community. The DCD Consensus Conference of 2005 formulated a work group that was specifically tasked with proposing such definitions that DSAs must consider when developing a policy.

Adoption of a uniform reporting process for measuring WIT intervals will be beneficial to the determination of suitability of DCD donor organs currently recovered and will serve as a framework for future research.

Location for Withdrawal of Support

Another equally important consideration in policy development is the place in which the withdrawal will occur. These decisions have clinical implications as well as implications for the patient's family. The locations for withdrawal might include the intensive care unit (ICU) where the patient is being treated, a location adjacent to the operating room (e.g., a holding area), or the operating room itself. As a matter of policy development, imparting a level of autonomy in decision making to the donor's family is very important.

Although the process is designed to be as therapeutic as possible for the donor family, these clinical considerations should be presented to the donor's family as they consider donation. This discussion with the donor's family is held in the context of informed consent and in no way should be construed or approached in a coercive manner.

Family Considerations

DCD donation is a family-driven process, and it is for this reason that the logistics of the withdrawal of life-sustaining measures is discussed with them. Many DCD donor families choose to be present with the donor at the time of death. In these cases, the ability to meet the family's need to be present, while minimizing WIT, can be jointly achieved through a family-sensitive discussion of the options available.

Meeting the donor family's needs while ensuring the viability of the donated organs from DCD donors can only be accomplished through effective working relationships between donor hospitals and OPOs, supported by well-developed policies. Surgical staff are traditionally reticent to allow a patient's family to be present in the operating room during the withdrawal processes. This reluctance is typically based on the infrequency of patients dying in the operating room, the atypical event of bringing patients' family members into the surgical suite, and a concern to maintain sterility in the room. The process by which OPOs and hospitals manage this challenge is specific to each clinical setting and should be addressed in hospital policies.

Collaborative OPO and Hospital Processes

Once an OPO implements a DCD program and it becomes well established, the number of referrals and subsequent on-site OPO responses to such referrals typically increases. In some cases, the increase in potential donor referral activity can double or triple when DCD clinical triggers are implemented throughout a DSA. OPOs have traditionally focused on a key clinical trigger: referring any patient in the ICU or emergency department for whom life-sustaining measures are to be withdrawn. The most frequent mechanism of death (nearly 90% of ICU deaths) is a result of deceleration and/or withdrawal of care due to the nonsurvivable nature of the patient's injury.[2] In these cases, the focus shifts from life-saving care to palliative care. It is at this time that the donor hospital is typically in communication with the OPO for determination of DCD donor potential.

An additional clinical trigger for the referral of a potential DCD donor may be a planned family meeting where discussions of options regarding ongoing treatment will occur. When the OPO is aware of family meetings in which withdrawal of life-sustaining measures may be decided, the assessment of DCD donor suitability may be done in advance. Such advance assessment helps to ensure that donation options are understood and clearly presented, if appropriate, in the event the patient's family desires to withdraw care. Careful assessment is needed by the hospital care team, the OPO, and the OPO's medical director to determine if the patient will meet the OPO's criteria for DCD donation.

The concept of a "donation huddle" has been developed and refined through the work of the Department of Health and Human Services Organ Donation Breakthrough Collaborative. OPOs vary widely in their use of huddles. Huddles may be used during the referral and evaluation process, before presenting donation options to patients' families, or at the start of a consented donor case to frame the objectives of donor management. One of the key goals of any of these huddle interventions is to formally bring together each of the members of the hospital's multidisciplinary team responsible for the continuum of care for the potential donor patient. The huddle serves as a forum to discuss the potential donors' medical and social history, hospital course, current medical status, and family support systems. When used during the referral and evaluation process, this huddle sets a framework for the determination of donor suitability inclusive of the OPO (typically in consultation with the OPO's medical director or administrator on call) and the hospital's medical team. Additionally, the huddle allows a more complete understanding of the potential donor family's dynamics. In this manner, an effective family care plan can be developed that both supports the patient's family and supports an effective request for consent for donation inclusive of the medical staff, hospital family support systems, and OPO family support services.

Using the Ethics Committee for Successful DCD Policy

Patients' families are often well aware of potential end-of-life options because of the more widespread use of advance directives and other documents outlining an individual's wishes at the time of death. In many cases, patients' family members may inquire about donation options before the decision to withdraw support is made, or, they may ask other questions that lead hospital staff to believe that they are moving forward in considering what the future holds, what their options may be. In these situations, it is imperative that the healthcare team be prepared to answer questions about organ and tissue donation effectively, while avoiding any perceived conflict of interest in discussing withdrawal of support options.

These scenarios are examples that have served as the impetus for the inclusion of ethics committee reviews in many DCD policies, providing a forum for both the patient's family and the hospital staff to discuss and clarify the steps in the DCD process, especially the medications that may be used during the withdrawal process. Ethics committees typically outline appropriate hospital guidelines that serve to ensure that the option of the withdrawal of life-sustaining measures is independent of the expressed wish to donate organs and tissues, while ensuring that patients' families are fully informed of their options *before* care is de-escalated. Earlier rather than later contact with OPO staff and at least an initial mention of donation have empirically been shown to be the best approach. Collaboration between hospital and OPO staff will allow the patient's family to be appropriately apprised of their options in order to make an informed and *timely* decision. Numerous family interviews (brain death cases) reveal that families "told us they thought they had donated but did not. They did not donate because they were unaware that removal from mechanical supports before donation would preclude solid-organ donation—no one told them! They went on to donate tissue believing that they had also donated organs. This same scenario is applicable to families of potential DCD donors" (personal written communication, L. Siminoff, PhD July 8, 2006).

The ethics committee may provide a third-party institutional consultation during actual DCD cases to include: a review of the hospital course, the independent nature of the decision to withdraw life-sustaining measures, the decision to donate organs, documentation of medical futility, and the factors that have contributed to the discussion of withdrawal of life-sustaining measures. The ethics committee can also serve as an integral part of a hospital's DCD donor program by participating in the development of hospital policies and the determination of how these policies and protocols should be best used within the institution.

Presenting donation options to families of potential DCD donors is similar to the discussion held with the families of brain-dead donors; although in most DCD cases fewer organs can be donated. Several key elements are different in DCD cases, though, and must be fully explored with donor families. The process steps and timing logistics for DCD donation differ in many ways from those for organ donation after brain death declaration. The elements of informed consent for DCD donation focus not only on the donation processes, but also on the administration of end-of-life comfort and care measures.

Policy Surrounding the Medical Management of Potential DCD

The medical management of DCD donors in the preoperative phases of donation is the responsibility of the donor hospital's care team. Although medical interventions that maintain organ perfusion may be in the best interest of the donation process, they are not typically incongruent with the normal and customary ICU management of the patient. In this manner, not only the best care of the patient occurs but the opportunity for donation is present. Most OPOs have explicit policy statements that preclude any OPO-based donor management of the DCD donor before the recovery of organs in the operating room.

Education of the Donor Hospital Staff

One of the most important components of a successful and effective DCD donor program is clinical education for the donor hospital staff involved in the process. The staff in the ICU or other clinical settings where the DCD patient may be should receive comprehensive education on the process of DCD donation. Although both the DCD and brain-dead donor process have many similarities in the prerecovery phases, several key process elements are unique to DCD cases. As noted, prior treatments and orders remain the responsibility of the treating healthcare team. Certain diagnostic tests, such as echocardiograms, are not indicated in DCD cases. A key consideration in the facilitation of DCD cases involves the need for the ICU physician and nurse to accompany the donor to the location of the withdrawal of life-sustaining measures. Although the clinical processes for the provision of palliative and end-of-life care are relatively commonplace for ICU physicians and nurses, the need for this staff to leave the ICU to potentially tend to these activities in an operating room or postanesthesia care unit are unique. Provisions must be made to accommodate the absence of this staff from their clinical setting for 1 to 2 hours for this process.

As noted, education of the operating room staff about the process is vital to its success and effectiveness. This education should include specific details about the clinical aspects of the DCD organ recovery. An important part of the planning process for the operating room staff will be determined by where the withdrawal of care will take place. For example, if the withdrawal of care takes place outside of the operating room, the staff must be ready to receive the DCD donor patient within minutes of the patient's time of death and should be ready to immediately initiate the recovery of donated organs. If the withdrawal of care is to take place in the operating room, the preparation for the patient and the family must be well planned and coordinated among the OPO, ICU, and operating room personnel.

In addition to the logistical issues that are unique to the DCD recovery process, there are many process steps that reinforce the dignity of the donation process and the protection of the rights of the donor and the donor family during the process. It is the OPO's responsibility to ensure that the process occurs in a dignified manner, always respectful of the gracious gift of organ and tissue donation. Further, the OPO staff are the stewards of conveying the message that it is the family's wish that their loved one be provided with a compassionate withdrawal of care and not be maintained through continued medical intervention, and it is also their wish that organ donation take place if possible. Operating room staff are not accustomed to participating in end-of-life care and reinforcing this idea to them is very important.

Conclusion

OPOs and hospitals should have policies in place that facilitate DCD and clearly delineate roles of responsibilities of hospital and OPO staff. Involvement of OPO and hospital leaders as well as medical and nursing staff is key to successful development and implementation of policy. The hospital's ethics committee may review and facilitate adoption of the hospital's DCD policy.

Ultimately, the DCD process depends on expert clinicians from both the hospital and the OPO. Policy adoption should vary little from policy adoption for other procedures performed in the hospital. Because DCD has become mainstream, it should be viewed as simply another service provided by the hospital and OPO for patients and their families and performed in the spirit of community benefit.

References

1. JCAHO: Organ Donation Proposed Regulations. Available at: http://www.jointcommission.org/PublicPolicy/organ_donation.htm. Accessed June 16, 2006.
2. Edwards J, Mulvania P, Robertson V, et al. Maximizing organ donation opportunities through donation after cardiac death. *Crit Care Nurse*. April 2006;26:101-115.
3. Bernat JL, D'Alessandro AM. Report of a national conference on donation after cardiac death. *Am J Transplant*. 2006;6:281-291.
4. Childress JF, Liverman CT, eds. *Institute of Medicine: Organ Donation Opportunities for Action*. Washington, DC: The National Academies Press; 2006.

Maximizing Organ Donation Opportunities Through Donation After Cardiac Death

John Edwards, RN, RRT, CPTC
Patti Mulvania, RN, CEN, CPTC
Virginia Robertson
Gweneth George
Richard Hasz, MFS, CPTC
Howard Nathan, CPTC
Anthony D'Alessandro, MD

Organ transplantation is established therapy for many patients with a variety of end-stage diseases. The survival benefits are remarkable, as are the improvements in quality of life. Unfortunately, the supply of donor organs remains insufficient to meet the need.

Recently, through participation in the breakthrough collaboratives of the Health and Human Resources Administration, organ procurement organizations (OPOs) have become engaged in systems change through application of the principles of continuous improvement. So-called best practices are being shared by OPOs. This sharing, in turn, has created a level of synergy among OPO professionals and hospitals alike that is having a positive impact on the donor supply (Table 1).

Clearly, reasons for optimism exist, but a stark reality must be confronted: there will never be a single solution to the donor dilemma. Organ donation is multifactorial, a fact that often eludes people who are consumed by the search for a "magic bullet." Predictably, frustration eventually gives way to disillusionment. Thus, it should come as no surprise that aggressive efforts are being made to better use existing donors by expanding the traditional criteria

Table 1 Number of deceased organ donors and DCD donors from 1994 through 2004*

Year	No. of deceased donors	DCD donors No.	DCD donors %	No. of OPOs recovering organs from at least 1 DCD donor
1994	5099	57	1.1	22
1995	5362	64	1.2	22
1996	5416	71	1.3	21
1997	5478	78	1.4	19
1998	5794	75	1.3	16
1999	5824	87	1.5	20
2000	5985	118	2.0	30
2001	6079	169	2.8	33
2002	6190	189	3.1	30
2003	6427	270	4.2	35
2004	7151	395	5.5	41

Abbreviations: DCD, donation after cardiac death; OPO, organ procurement organization.

*Data from the United Network for Organ Sharing and the Organ Procurement and Transplantation Network.

for organ donation. In addition, concerted attempts are being made to redefine what constitutes a potential donor.

In this article, we provide a general introduction to donation after cardiac death (DCD) relative to end-of-life care, distinguish among various concepts critical to understanding DCD, discuss a widely accepted critical pathway for managing donors after cardiac death, and quantify the outcomes of patients who have received organs from donors after cardiac death. Most important, our premise is that organ donation should be considered what it actually is: a pressing national public health crisis and an often-neglected aspect of end-of-life care.

The Paradox of Transplantation and the Relevance of End-of-Life Care

Since its inception, transplantation has raised many highly controversial public policy issues. Strangely, yet tragically, it takes a death to save a life. While one family grieves, another family rejoices. By its nature, organ donation is a complex socio-cultural phenomenon that is largely shaped by clinical considerations, many of which laypersons do not understand. In this regard, approach-avoidance behavior is the rule, not the exception. For most people, life is to be embraced, and death is to be avoided.

Organ donation typically and unfortunately follows a tragic event for which families are unprepared. The circumstances surrounding conventional organ donation can be daunting for members of the care giving team but are even more disconcerting if DCD is introduced without previous education or experience. Regardless, the introduction of organ donation to the grieving family of a patient translates into the need for additional resources for the care giving team, resources that are both emotional and clinical.

Fortunately, critical care medicine has evolved to a point where practitioners increasingly recognize their changing obligations to patients in life, dying, and death. From this perspective, the practitioners not only are responsible for treating disease and trauma but also are committed to managing a dying process that results in a dignified death.

Currently, approximately 90% of patients who die in intensive care units (ICUs) do so after a decision to limit therapy.[1] As a result, the treatment objective shifts from a curative to a palliative model of care, a shift that is directly relevant to DCD.

DCD creates unfamiliar challenges for many critical care nurses. In DCD, organ donation is considered before an unequivocal pronouncement of death. Thus, when DCD is an option, critical care staff must have an in-depth knowledge of end-of-life decision making and must be committed to the goal of providing compassionate care.

Communications between care-givers and patients' families are already complex without introducing the possibility of DCD. Fortunately, the focus of a growing body of work is the provision of high-quality, compassionate, interdisciplinary care in these circumstances.

Under the conditions described here, organ procurement professionals are most effective when they are "partnered in" as integral members of the end-of-life care team and are highly skilled in counseling patients' families about opportunities for organ donation. In this role, organ procurement professionals serve as "dual advocates," striking a delicate balance between their commitment to patients awaiting transplantation and their concern and care for patients' families who are faced with the important end-of-life decision about organ donation. This dual advocacy is possible only if the procurement professional is sensitive to the needs of each donor patient, the donor patient's family, and prospective transplant recipients.

As a dual advocate, an organ procurement professional should make certain that grieving families are given the empowering opportunity of sparing other families from a similar grief. Through their gift of life, a patient's family members can make the tragic death of their loved one meaningful and allow their loved one to leave behind a life-long legacy.

Understanding DCD

DCD, also known as non-heart-beating organ donation, is not a novel concept; it is the very foundation of modern transplantation. Before the Harvard Committee report in 1968, which established acceptable criteria for the determination of death based on neurological findings, all deceased or cadaveric donors were pronounced dead on the basis of cessation of cardiopulmonary function.[2]

Criteria for brain death gained acceptance in the 1970s. By the 1980s, every state had passed legislation enabling the recovery of organs from "brain-dead" patients maintained by using mechanical ventilation.

Because of concerns about the quality of organs obtained after cardiac death and about the outcome of transplantation of these organs, interest in DCD diminished in the United States and elsewhere. However, in some countries, including Japan, which has continued to struggle with the concept of brain death, and some European countries, interest in the use of DCD has been sustained.

The early 1990s saw a renewed interest among OPOs in pursuing DCD more routinely. This interest was the result of both dramatic increases in the number of patients on the transplant waiting list and recurring requests from patients' family members who had made the decision to withdraw life support from their loved ones. Recognizing that withdrawal of life support meant imminent death, family members were requesting the opportunity to donate their loved ones' organs as a way to bring meaning to the families' losses and to help others.

During the resurgence of DCD, a number of misinformed media reports created fear and trepidation in the donation and transplant community as well as in the general public. These reports led many healthcare professionals to question the practice of recovering organs after cardiac death. As a result of these concerns, the US Department of Health and Human Services asked the Institute of Medicine to review DCD procedures to ensure that interventions taken were in the best interest of the donor patient. The Institute of Medicine concluded that DCD is an ethically proper approach for recovering organs from a deceased patient for the purposes of transplantation.[3,4] In addition, the ethics committee of the American College of Critical Care Medicine, Society of Critical Care Medicine published a position paper that not only indicated the ethical soundness of DCD but also offered a series of recommendations, including that donation of organs from infants and children after cardiac death should be offered routinely to patients' families.[5]

Organ Donation After Brain Death

Approximately 95% of organ donations occur after the determination of brain death, which is defined as complete and irreversible loss of all brain and brain stem function. Upon determination of brain death, a patient is pronounced dead, and the time of death is established and recorded in the medical record. If the patient appears to be medically suitable for organ donation, hemodynamic and ventilatory support is continued until the patient's family can be counseled about potential opportunities for organ donation. If the patient's legal next-of-kin agrees to organ donation, these physiological support systems remain in place throughout organ evaluation and allocation and the surgical recovery of organs in the operating room.

Organ Donation After Cardiac Death

In contrast to organ donation after brain death, DCD is defined as the surgical recovery of organs after the pronouncement of death based on cessation of cardiopulmonary function. Patients considered for DCD most often have sustained a devastating and nonrecoverable neurological injury that does not culminate in brain death, and the patients' family members have elected to withdraw life-sustaining therapies. Any patient who has sustained a nonrecoverable injury and for whom life support is being withdrawn can be considered for DCD; however, most often only those patients who have sustained a nonrecoverable neurological injury are eligible.

After the decision to withdraw life support has been made, the patient is evaluated to determine whether death most likely will occur within a predetermined period (generally 1 hour) after withdrawal of life support; this period is considered the maximum acceptable interval between withdrawal of support and recovery of organs for minimizing ischemic organ injury. If cessation of cardiorespiratory effort most likely will occur within this period and the patient otherwise seems to be medically suitable as an organ donor, then the patient's family is counseled about the possibility of organ donation. In order to safeguard against conflicts of interest, the decision to withdraw life support must not be intertwined with the discussion of opportunities for organ donation.

If the patient's legal next-of-kin agrees to donation, physiological support is continued through the evaluation-and-allocation phase, similar to the procedure in organ donation after brain death. Once the transplant teams arrive at the hospital, the patient is transferred to the operating room or a room close to the operating room for the withdrawal of life support. Life support is withdrawn in the presence of the caregiving team in the same fashion as it would be in the critical care unit. Once cardiorespiratory function has ceased, the patient is pronounced dead on the basis of cardiopulmonary criteria by the attending physician or the physician's designee. After death is determined, the time of death is recorded in the medical record. The transplant team then waits for a preestablished time (5 minutes, according to Institute of Medicine guidelines, or up to 10 minutes, according to individual hospital protocols) and begins the surgical recovery of the organ or organs to be donated.

Procedures in DCD Controlled Versus Uncontrolled DCD

In the United States, organ donations after cardiac death can be divided into 2 categories on the basis of the process and timing of the organ recovery: controlled and uncontrolled. Controlled donation most closely simulates the ideal conditions for organ recovery and therefore is the preferred scenario of most OPOs.

Although both controlled and uncontrolled situations are ethically appropriate, in this article, we primarily focus on controlled DCD, which is the preference covered in the critical pathway for DCD of the Organ Procurement and Transplantation Network/United Network for Organ Sharing. Table 2 compares and contrasts key elements of both controlled and uncontrolled DCD.

Critical Pathway for DCD

In 2001, the critical care advisory council of the Organ Procurement and Transplantation Network/United Network for Organ Sharing developed a critical pathway for DCD. The council consists of representatives not only from OPOs but also from the American Association of Critical-Care Nurses, American Association of Neuroscience Nurses, Society of Critical Care Medicine, National Medical Association, American Society of Transplant Surgeons, North American Transplant Coordinators Organization, and the Association of Organ Procurement Organizations. The pathway delineates roles and identifies courses of action to be taken in a brief, understandable format. It also encourages collaboration between the caregiving team and the OPO (Figure 1).

Preliminary Evaluation of Candidates for DCD

Potential organ donors after cardiac death, like potential donors after brain death, should be referred to an OPO when established clinical criteria or triggers are met. Also, as in donation after brain death, referral to an OPO is not synonymous with the request for donation; rather it is an opportunity to enter into dialog with the referring nursing and medical staff about the clinical situation of the potential donor. The established clinical trigger for referral to an OPO in neurologically injured patients is a score of 5 or less on the Glasgow Coma Scale. Because DCD is possible for patients with nonneurological injuries, all patients should be referred to an OPO when the patients' families and physicians have decided that life-sustaining therapies will be withdrawn. Examples of potential DCD donors are patients with progressive neuromuscular degeneration such as amyotrophiclateral sclerosis and patients who have high spinal cord injuries (involving upper cervical cord segments C1 through C4) and are ventilator dependent. Other potential DCD donors are patients with significant cardiopulmonary diseases, such as patients who have

Table 2 Differentiation of controlled and uncontrolled donation after cardiac death (DCD)

Variable	Controlled	Uncontrolled
Case characteristics	Patient sustains nonrecoverable injury	Patient sustains nonrecoverable injury
	Family elects to withdraw support in collaboration with hospital care team	Patient has sudden cardiac arrest or condition becomes profoundly unstable
	If organ procurement organization (OPO) not previously notified, patient referral is made	If OPO not previously notified, urgent patient referral is made
	Overall stability of patient's condition is aggressively maintained	Resuscitation measures, including cardiopulmonary resuscitation, are aggressively continued
Withdrawal decision/family approach	Once the family has communicated its decision to withdraw life support, the OPO presents the opportunity for DCD in a supportive environment.	Once resuscitation efforts are determined to be futile or instability of patient's condition is determined to be irreversible, by necessity the family may be presented with the opportunity to donate during a crisis situation
	Withdrawal typically occurs in a progressive, controlled fashion	
	Time to discuss all aspects of the process may be unlimited	Opportunity to consider DCD must be presented to the family urgently and succinctly, emphasizing that extending resuscitation times may decrease the chance for successful transplantation of recovered organs
Withdrawal of support/recovery process	All aspects of withdrawal and organ recovery are collaboratively planned among the family, caregiving team, and OPO	Collaboration between OPO and caregiving team must occur quickly, with minimal time for discussion
	Possibility for coordination of ideal circumstances exists	No possibility exists for coordination of ideal circumstances; everyone is committed to working within the constraints of the situation
	Withdrawal is done in the operating room	
	Caregiving staff are in attendance	Formal withdrawal does not occur because the patient most often is undergoing cardiac massage up until time of organ recovery
	Recovery teams are present, and organ preservation process is ready	
	Family has adequate time for closure and rituals	Operating suite is rapidly secured
		Recovery teams are emergently transported
		Organ preservation may be delayed

cystic fibrosis or who use left ventricular assist devices, for whom the decision to withdraw life-sustaining therapies has been made. Referral of these potential donors allows the OPO, in collaboration with the referring ICU team, to determine medical suitability and enables better counsel for the potential donors' family members when the decision is made to discuss organ donation. Medical suitability of potential donors after cardiac death is determined by the OPO in the same manner as for potential donors after brain death.

Of note, discussion of organ donation does not occur until a patient's physician and family have made a determination to forgo life-sustaining therapies. As with organ donation after brain death, organ donation in the DCD setting should be offered only after the patient's family has processed the gravity of the clinical situation involving their family member. The conversation about organ donation should not be initiated by the family; it should, in all instances, be initiated by a certified requestor. However, sometimes the family members of a patient inquire about organ donation before the discussion of withdrawing life-

MAXIMIZING ORGAN DONATION OPPORTUNITIES THROUGH DONATION AFTER CARDIAC DEATH

AOPO — Association of Organ Procurement Organizations | AST — American Society of Transplantation | ASTS | NATCO | UNOS

Collaborative practice	Phase I Identification & referral	Phase II Preliminary evaluation	Phase III Family discussion & consent	Phase IV Comprehensive evaluation & donor management	Phase V Withdrawal of support /pronouncement of death/organ recovery
The following health care professionals may be involved in the Donation After Cardiac Death (DCD) donation process: Check all that apply: ○ Physician (MD) ○ Critical Care RN ○ Nurse Supervisor ○ Medical Examiner /Coroner ○ Respiratory Therapy (RT) ○ Laboratory ○ Pharmacy ○ Radiology ○ Anesthesiology ○ OR/Surgery Staff ○ Clergy ○ Social Worker ○ Organ Procurement Coordinator (OPC) ○ Organ Procurement Organization (OPO)	Prior to withdrawing life support, contact local OPO for any patient who fulfills the following criteria: ○ Devastating neurologic injury and/or other organ failure requiring mechanical ventilatory or circulatory support ○ Family and/or care giving team initiate conversation about withdrawal of support Following referral, additional evaluation is done collaboratively to determine if death is likely to occur within one hour (or within a specified timeframe as determined by caregiving team and OPO) following withdrawal of support Patient conditions might include the following: ○ **Ventilator dependent for respiratory insufficiency:** apneic or severe hypopneic; tachypnea ≥ 30 breaths /min after DC ventilator ○ **Dependent on mechanical circulatory support** (LVAD; RVAD; V-A ECMO; Pacemaker with unassisted rhythm < 30 beats per minute. **Severe disruption in oxygenation:** PEEP ≥ 10 and SaO_2 ≤ 92%; FiO_2 ≥ .50 and SaO_2 ≤ 92%; V-V ECMO requirement ○ **Dependent upon pharmacologic circulatory assist**: Norephinephrine, epinephrine, or phenylephrine ≥ 0.2 ug/kg/min; Dopamine ≥ 15 ug/kg/min ○ **IABP and inotropic support:** IABP 1:1 and dobutamine or dopamine ≥10 ug/kg/min and CI ≤ 2.2 L/min/M2; IABP 1:1 & CI ≤ 1.5 L/min/M^2	Physician ○ Supportive of withdrawal of care and has communicated grave prognosis to family ○ Review DCD procedure with OPC ○ Will be involved in withdrawal/ pronouncement ○ Will designate a person to be involved with withdrawal and/or pronouncement Family ○ Has received grave prognosis ○ Understands prognosis ○ In conjunction with care giving team, decide to withdraw support Patient ○ Age ____ ○ Weight ____ ○ Height ____ ○ ABO ____ ○ Medical Hx ____ ○ Surgical Hx ____ ○ Social Hx ____ ○ Death likely < 1 hour following withdrawal (determined collaboratively by evaluating: injury, level of support, respiratory drive assessment)	○ Support services offered to family ○ OPC/Hospital staff approach family about donation options ○ Legal next-of-kin (NOK) fully informed of donation options and recovery procedures ○ Legal NOK grants consent for DCD following withdrawal of support ○ Family offered opportunity to be present during withdrawal of support ○ OPC obtains ____ Witnessed consent from legal NOK for DCD ____ Signed consent Time ____ Date ____ ____ Detailed med/soc history Notification of donation ○ Hospital supervisor ○ ME/Coroner notified ____ ME/Coroner & releases for donation ____ ME/Coroner has restrictions *Stop Pathway if –* ○ *Family, ME/Coroner denies consent* ○ *Patient determined to be unsuitable candidate for DCD* ○ *Patient progresses to brain death during evaluation – refer to brain dead pathway*	○ MD, in collaboration with OPO, implements management guidelines. ○ Establish location and time of withdrawal of support. ○ Review plan for withdrawal to include: - Pronouncing MD (should be in attendance for duration of withdrawal of support, determination of death, and may not be a member of the transplant team) - Comfort Care - Extubation and discontinuation of ventilator support - Establish plan for continued supportive care if pt survives > one hour or predetermined time interval after withdrawal of support ○ Notify OR/Anesthesia ____ Review patient's clinical course, withdrawal plan and potential organ recovery procedures ____ Schedule OR time ○ Notify recovery teams ○ Prepare patient for transport to prearranged area for withdrawal of support ○ Patient transported to prearranged area ○ Note: Should the clinical situation require pre-mortem femoral cannulation, the following should be reviewed: - family consent or understanding - MD inserting cannula - Time and location of cannula insertion - If death does not occur, determine if cannula should be removed	○ Withdrawal occurs in ____ OR ____ ICU ____ Other ○ Family present for withdrawal of support ____ yes ____ no ○ OR/Room prepared and equipment set up ○ Transplant team in the OR (not in attendance during withdrawal) ○ Care giving team present ○ Administration of pre-approved medication (e.g. Heparin/Regitine) ○ Withdrawal of support according to hospital/ MD practice guidelines Time ____ Date ____ ○ Vital signs are monitored and recorded every minute (see attached sheet) ○ Pt pronounced dead and appropriate documentation completed Time ____ Date ____ MD ____ ○ Transplant Team initiates surgical recovery at prescribed time following pronouncement of death ○ Allocation of organs per OPTN/UNOS policy ○ *If cardiac death not established within 1 hour or predetermined time interval after withdrawal of support – Stop Pathway. Patient moved to predetermined area for continuation of supportive care.* ○ Post mortem care administered *Continued*

sustaining treatment. Each situation is different, and the physician caring for the patient may elect to defer the discussion of organ donation or may call the OPO to provide additional information to the family. Also, when a referral is made in the DCD setting, a discussion of the stability of the patient's hemodynamic

A CLINICIAN'S GUIDE TO DONATION AND TRANSPLANTATION Chapter 36

Collaborative practice	Phase I Identification & referral	Phase II Preliminary evaluation	Phase III Family discussion & consent	Phase IV Comprehensive evaluation & donor management	Phase V Withdrawal of support /pronouncement of death/organ recovery
Labs / diagnostics		○ ABO ○ Electrolytes ○ LFTs ○ PT/PTT ○ CBC with Diff ○ Beta HCG (female pts) ○ ABG		Repeat full panel of labs additionally: ○ Serology Testing infectious disease profile ○ Blood cultures X 2 ○ UA & urine culture ○ Sputum culture ○ Tissue typing	
Respiratory	○ Maintain ventilator support ○ Pulmonary toilet PRN	○ Respiratory drive assessment RR _____ VT _____ VE _____ NIF _____ Minutes off ventilator _____ ○ Hemodynamics while off ventilator HR _____ BP _____ SaO_2 _____	○ ABGs as requested ○ Notify RT of location and time of withdrawal of support	○ Transport with mechanical ventilation using lowest FiO_2 possible while maintaining the SaO_2 >90%	
Treatments / ongoing care	Maintain standard nursing care to include: ○ Vital signs q 1 hour ○ I & O q 1 hour				○ Post mortem care at conclusion of case
Medications				○ Provide medications as directed by MD in consult with OPC	○ Heparin and other medications prior to withdrawal of support
Optimal outcomes	The potential DCD donor is identified & a referral is made to the OPO.	The donor is evaluated & found to be a suitable candidate for donation.	The family is offered the option of donation & their decision is supported.	Optimal organ function is maintained, withdrawal of support plan is established, and personnel prepared for potential organ recovery.	Death occurs within one hour of withdrawal of support and all suitable organs and tissues are recovered for transplant.

This work supported by HRSA contract 231-00-0115.

Figure 1 Critical pathway for donation after cardiac death.

Abbreviations: ABG, arterial blood gases; BP, blood pressure; CBC with Diff, complete blood cell count with differential; CI, cardiac index; DC, disconnect; FiO_2, fraction of inspired oxygen; HCG, human chorionic gonadotropin; HR, heart rate; Hx, history; I & O, intake and output; IABP, intra-aortic balloon pump; ICU, intensive care unit; LFTs, liver function tests; LVAD, left ventricular assist device; ME, medical examiner; MD, doctor of medicine; NIF, negative inspiratory force; OPTN, Organ Procurement and Transplantation Network; OR, operating room; PEEP, positive end-expiratory pressure; PRN, as needed; pt or Pt, patient; PT, prothrombin time; PTT, partial thromboplastin time; q, every; RR, respiratory rate; RVAD, right ventricular assist device; SaO_2, oxygen saturation; UA, urinalysis; UNOS, United Network for Organ Sharing; V-A ECMO, venoatrial extracorporeal membrane oxygenation; VE, expired volume per unit time; VT, tidal volume; V-V ECMO, venovenous extracorporeal membrane oxygenation.

Reprinted with permission from United Network for Organ Sharing/Organ Procurement and Transplantation Network, Richmond, Va, 2005.

condition is important. With potential donors after cardiac death, in contrast to potential donors after brain death, a do-not-resuscitate order has often been entered before any discussion has occurred about withdrawal of life support or organ donation. In these instances, adequate physiological support must be maintained for organ preservation in the event that organ donation is ultimately the choice of the patient or the patient's family.

Prediction of Death

After the decision has been made to withdraw life-sustaining therapy and the OPO has determined the medical suitability of a patient for organ donation, a determination must be made about whether the patient will die within a time frame consistent with donation. Hypoxia and hypotension develop with invariable periods after a patient is extubated and all other life-sustaining therapies (eg, use of vasopressors) are withdrawn, a situation that results in some ischemic damage to vital organs. A period of 1 hour from extubation and withdrawal of support to pronouncement of death is usually considered consistent with organ donation; this time frame may also be increased depending on the stability of the patient's condition after withdrawal of life support. If the patient does not experience circulatory arrest within the designated time frame, organ recovery does not proceed because of the high likelihood that the organs will not function after transplantation.

When the option of DCD is discussed with a patient's family, the requestor for donation must accurately convey that additional time will be necessary to get a surgical team on site, run the necessary serological tests required for organ donation, and allocate recovered organs to appropriate recipients.

Because many patients referred as potential DCD donors are not suitable candidates, the question of how suitability is determined is of paramount importance. Information about the clinical situation of a patient may be helpful but is often not predictive. In an effort to develop objective criteria for determining whether a patient is a suitable candidate for DCD, a scoring tool was developed by the University of Wisconsin.[6] This tool is essentially an assessment of respiratory drive that is used to predict the likelihood of continued spontaneous respirations beyond 1 and 2 hours after extubation. Figures 2 and 3 depict the information collected and the scoring system used to make the prediction. Because this assessment requires that mechanical ventilation be stopped for a brief time, the procedure should be clearly explained to the patient's family, and consent should be obtained.

In 2003 and 2004, the University of Wisconsin OPO had 83 referrals for DCD in which the evaluation tool was used. On the basis of the findings with the tool, 27 patients were not considered potential candidates for DCD. For the remaining 56 patients, the scores provided an accurate prediction that 53 (94.6%) would die within 1 to 2 hours. When the option of DCD is discussed with patients' families, as well as with medical and nursing staff, it is important to communicate that 5% to 10% of patients will not have circulatory arrest in a time frame consistent with organ donation, and in such instances, the primary team responsible for the patient will continue end-of-life care.

The scores on the tool were also predictive, but at a somewhat lower rate, of those patients who would have spontaneous respirations beyond 2 hours after extubation. The scores were accurate in 22 (81.5%) of 27 cases; 5 potential donations were missed. The current policy of the University of Wisconsin OPO is to send a team for patients with scores greater than 12 on the evaluation tool, because scores of 12 or less are less predictive. At the request of the patients' families, the OPO sent recovery teams in 6 instances in which the score was 12 or less, and although organs were not recovered, each family was appreciative of the OPO's efforts and support, and each instance was an educational opportunity for the nursing and medical staff of the referring hospital.

Medical Management

Medical management of potential donors after cardiac death is similar to that for potential donors after brain death. However, because patients suitable for DCD have not progressed to brain death and therefore have not experienced the catecholamine release induced by brain death, their hemodynamic status tends to be more stable. In one study,[7] 76.9% of patients who donated organs after brain death required vasopressor support, whereas only 33% of those who donated after cardiac death required such support. As previously mentioned, even if a do-not-resuscitate order is in place, physiological support of the major organ systems should be maintained in potential donors after cardiac death to preserve the option for donation. Once a patient has been determined to be a suitable candidate for DCD and the patient's family has consented to donation, the do-not-resuscitate status should be discussed. The family should be informed that physiological support must continue until the team arrives for the withdrawal of support and recovery of organs. Consideration should be given to suspending the do-not-resuscitate order during this period.

The following evaluation should not occur until after the decision has been made by the patient's family and patient's physician to withdraw support. The patient's physician must be consulted prior to the evaluation.

Step one: Place a checkmark in the box next to the appropriate category in each table.

Type of intubation	
Endotracheal	
Tracheostomy	

Vasopressor status	
None	
Single vasopressor	
Two or more vasopressors	

Step two: Record the patient's vital signs prior to beginning the test.

Vital signs	
Blood pressure	
Pulse	
Oxygen saturation	

Height & weight	
Height (in)	
Weight (kg)	

Step three: Disconnect the patient from the ventilator. ***After 10 minutes**** record the information in each of the tables below.

Respiratory effort?	
Yes	
No	

If yes:

Respiratory rate

Negative Inspiratory Force (NIF)*

*RT can do this mearurement using a manometer

Vital signs	
Blood pressure	
Pulse	
Oxygen saturation	

Tidal volume

**If at any time the patient becomes unstable (pulse ox <70%, systolic BP <80), it is expected that the evaluation will stop and the above parameters will be recorded.*

Figure 2 Information collected from referring hospitals for evaluation of a patient's suitability for organ donation after cardiac death.

Abbreviations: BP, blood pressure; pulse ox, pulse oximetry; RT, respiratory therapist.

Reprinted with permission from the University of Wisconsin Hospitals and Clinics Authority.

Because potential candidates for DCD cannot be declared brain dead, the primary treating team, not the OPO, is responsible for medical management of these patients. Medical management consists of maintaining good oxygenation, a systolic blood pressure greater than 90 mm Hg, adequate urine output, a normal electrolyte balance, and hematological and coagulation profiles with in normal reference ranges. Assessment of individual organ function for kidney, pancreas, liver, and lung donation is similar to that for patients who donate organs after brain death.

Withdrawal of Physiological Support and Determination of Death

Once a patient is determined to be a suitable candidate for DCD, a number of logistic issues must be considered. Unlike donation after brain death, in which death is declared on the basis of neurological criteria and all donors are conveyed to the operating room, withdrawal of support and declaration of death in DCD may occur in a number of locations before the donor is conveyed to the operating room

Criteria	Assigned points	Pt. score
Spontaneous respirations after 10 min.	-	
Rate >12	1	
Rate <12	3	
TV >200 cc	1	
TV <200 cc	3	
NIF >20	1	
NIF <20	3	
No spontaneous respirations	9	
BMI		
<25	1	
25-29	2	
>30	3	
Vasopressors		
No vasopressors	1	
Single vasopressor	2	
Multiple vasopressors	3	
Patient age		
0-30	1	
31-50	2	
51+	3	
Intubation		
Endotracheal tube	3	
Tracheostomy	1	
Oxygenation after 10 minutes		
O_2 sat >90%	1	
O_2 sat 80-89%	2	
O_2 sat <79%	3	
	Final score	
Date of extubation	Time of extubation	
Date of expiration	Time of expiration	
	Total time	

Scoring:
8-12 High risk for continuing to breath after extubation
13-18 Moderate risk for continuing to breath after extubation
19-24 Low risk for continuing to breath after extubation

Figure 3 Scoring system for Donation After Cardiac Death Evaluation Tool.

Abbreviations: BMI, body mass index; NIF, negative inspiratory force; O_2 sat, oxygen saturation; Pt, patient; TV, tidal volume.

Reprinted with permission from the University of Wisconsin Hospitals and Clinics Authority.

for organ recovery. The decision about where support will be withdrawn should always be based on the needs of the patient's family. Support may be withdrawn in the operating room, with or without the family in attendance; in the ICU; or in a room near or adjacent to the operating room. All options should be discussed with the family, including which organs may or may not be recovered.

If support is withdrawn in the ICU and additional warm ischemia occurs during transport to the operating room after the patient dies, organ viability may be affected. Generally, kidneys can be recovered in all cases, but because use of extrarenal organs from DCD donors is fairly new, most extrarenal organs are recovered from patients who have had support withdrawn in the operating room. Because medical and nursing personnel in the operating room may not be familiar with the potential organ donor and may not know why life-sustaining therapies are being withdrawn, it is important for the OPO staff to discuss this information, in addition to the actual logistics of withdrawal of life support and surgical recovery, with operating room personnel.

If withdrawal of support occurs in the operating room with the patient's family in attendance, additional logistical considerations must be addressed. In this setting, the nursing and surgical organ recovery teams should not be in the operating room, and only a limited number of people should be present, namely, the physician responsible for withdrawing life support, the patient's family, an OPO staff member, and the ICU nurse who was caring for the patient. The patient may or may not be draped, depending on the family's wishes; the family members should wear operating room suits over street clothes, usually with surgical hats and masks.

Before withdrawal of support, a clear plan should be devised to determine who will withdraw support and declare death. The physician who withdraws support should be experienced in end-of-life care and cannot be a member of the OPO team or the transplant team. This physician may be the patient's primary physician or an intensivist, an on-call physician, or an ICU fellow with end-of-life training. Physicians inexperienced in end-of-life care, as well as residents and interns, should not be called on in DCD.

In addition, before withdrawal of life support and during the discussions with a patient's family about the process of DCD, separate consent should be obtained for any medications or invasive procedures that are required before withdrawal. The administration of any medications that are not usually given in the care of a dying patient but may improve the likelihood of a successful transplant should be discussed with the patient's family. This discussion should include a disclosure of potential risks to the donor. The most common medications administered before withdrawal of support are heparin, an anticoagulant, and phentolamine, an α-adrenergic blocker. Heparin prevents thrombosis of small blood vessels, and phentolamine prevents vasospasm, allowing improved flushing of the solution used to preserve organs. The patient's family as well as medical and nursing staff must understand that the intent of the administration of these medications and procedures is to improve organ function after recovery and not to hasten the death of the potential donor.

Although the majority of patients who donate organs after cardiac death are adults, both the University of Wisconsin and the Gift of Life Donor Program have successfully coordinated DCD in children; infants and children have accounted for approximately 30% of all donations after cardiac death in the combined experience of the 2 organizations. The logistic considerations in children in DCD are similar to those in adults; however, most parents and family members choose to be with their child when life support is withdrawn, and some choose to be with the child after organ recovery. Also, the DCD evaluation tool is not applicable to small children and infants and, as a result, is currently being modified for use in such patients. The potential for DCD in children is significant. In an analysis of deaths in a children's hospital, Koogler and Costarino[8] found that routine use of DCD had the potential to increase organ donation by 42% in a single center.

Once consent is obtained and logistic considerations are addressed, life support is withdrawn by discontinuing any medications (eg, vasopressors) and extubating the patient. During the withdrawal phase of the process, the patient's oxygen saturation, blood pressure, and urine output are recorded. These data will help determine the amount of warm ischemic injury to the recovered organs. Because circulatory arrest is essential in the determination of death, an arterial catheter and monitor are necessary to determine the time of circulatory arrest. If use of an arterial catheter is not possible, bedside cardiac echocardiography maybe used.

Once circulatory arrest occurs and respiration ceases, a period of observation is required before organ recovery can begin. For most OPOs, this period is 5 minutes, as recommended by the Institute of Medicine,[3,4] and is used to observe the patient for autoresuscitation. However, because no recorded cases of autoresuscitation have occurred after 65 seconds, a few OPOs use 2 minutes as the observation period. (Autoresuscitation refers to the return of any cardiac mechanical activity; if this rare event occurs, the observation period is reset to zero and begins again after loss of circulatory activity.) Of note, the observation period begins with documentation of circulatory arrest and not with electrocardiographic silence.

After the observation period and declaration of death by the physician who is withdrawing life support, the surgical recovery team can immediately begin flushing preservation solutions and then start the surgical procedure, if withdrawal occurred in the operating room. If withdrawal of support occurred in the ICU or in a room near the operating room, transport to the operating room may begin during or after the observation period, in accordance with the family's wishes, with organ recovery beginning after the conclusion of the observation period and the declaration of death.

Perfusion of the organs with cold preservation solutions is achieved via aortic cannulation. The time from extubation to the start of perfusion of the organs with cold solution is also recorded as the warm ischemic time and is used to help guide the determination as to which organs are suitable for transplantation.

The organs recovered after cardiac death may be kidneys only or kidney sand extrarenal organs such as the liver, pancreas, and lungs. Patients 50 years and older are considered for kidney donation only; patients less than 50 years old are considered for both kidney and extrarenal donation. However, no absolute age cutoff exists, and extrarenal organs from patients more than 50 years old have been successfully transplanted. The recovery of extrarenal organs also depends on the time from withdrawal of support to the start of perfusion with cold solutions. If that time exceeds 30 minutes, the liver may not be recovered, and if it exceeds 45 minutes, the pancreas may not be recovered. In the majority of donors, this time does not exceed 1 hour. However, a small number of donors may have a period of relative stability after withdrawal of life support, and in such cases, this time may be extended beyond 1 hour without additional warm injury to the organs.

If kidneys are the only organs being recovered, the surgical procedure is similar to kidney recovery in donation after brain death and occurs after the kidneys are flushed with preservation solution (predominantly the conventional solution developed by the University of Wisconsin or, as done recently in a few cases, histidinetryptophan-ketoglutarate solution). Machine preservation of kidneys appears to substantially reduce the rate of delayed graft function, especially in DCD.[9]

If extrarenal organs are being recovered in addition to the kidneys, the procedure differs substantially from that used in donation after brain death. Because warm ischemia may injure organs obtained after cardiac death, the organs must be flushed and removed rapidly by using enbloc techniques of recovery. This procedure differs from procedures in donation after brain death, in which individual organs are dissected in situ. In DCD, the organs are dissected ex vivo after they are removed en bloc.

The University of Wisconsin has developed the en bloc technique depicted in Figure 4.[10] Briefly, after the chest and abdomen are opened, the thoracic aorta is clamped, and all abdominal organs are removed, beginning at the diaphragm. The distal ureters, aorta, and vena cava are divided, and the distal esophagus and sigmoid colon undergo gastrointestinal anastomotic stapling. Additional preservation solution is infused ex vivo into the renal, superior mesenteric, and celiac arteries and into the superior mesenteric vein. If lungs are being recovered, after the surgical procedure has begun, the physician replaces the endotracheal tube to oxygenate and inflate the lungs before stapling the bronchus so that the lungs can be preserved and transported while they are inflated.

Transplant Outcomes in DCD Kidney Transplantation

The results of transplantation of kidneys from DCD donors have been similar to results with kidneys obtained after brain death. In an analysis in 2002 of data from the Scientific Registry of Transplant Recipients, Rudich et al[11] compared 97990 recipients of kidneys from heart-beating deceased donors with 708 recipients of kidneys from non–heart-beating donors (ie, DCD donors). The results showed no differences between the 2 groups in 6-year death-censored survival of recipients (cases in which the recipient died with functioning kidneys were not treated as graft failures) and grafts.[11] However, recipients of kidneys from DCD donors had higher rates of delayed graft function and primary nonfunction, whereas recipients of kidneys from living donors had higher rates of thrombosis and graft loss from rejection. Cooper et al[12] compared 382 recipients of kidneys obtained after cardiac death with 1089 recipients of kidneys obtained after brain death. Although recipients of kidneys from DCD donors had a higher rate of delayed graft function (27.5% vs 21.3%, $P=.02$) and a higher creatinine

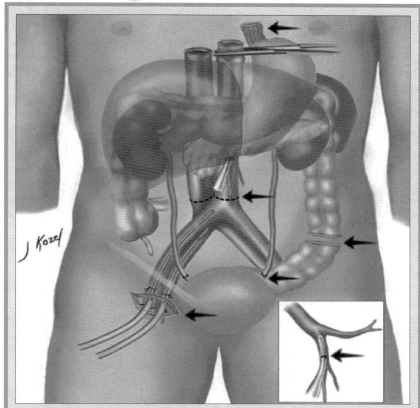

Figure 4 En bloc technique of abdominal organ recovery in organ donation after cardiac death.

Reprinted from D'Alessandro et al,[10] with permission from Lippincott Williams & Wilkins.

level at discharge (1.9 vs 1.7 mg/dL, $P=.001$), the 2 groups of recipients did not differ in primary graft nonfunction, rate of complications, or 5- and 10-year graft survival (65% and 45%, respectively, vs 71% and 48% for kidneys obtained after brain death). Weber et al[13] likewise found no difference in 1-, 5-, and 10-year graft survival but did detect a higher rate of delayed graft function and higher creatinine levels at 7 days in recipients of kidneys from nonliving donors. In a more recent analysis,[14] the Scientific Registry of Transplant Recipients found no difference in the relative rate of graft failure when 35290 kidneys from non-DCD donors were compared with 1258 kidneys from DCD donors (hazards ratio 1.00 vs 1.05, $P=.48$); 3-year adjusted graft survival also did not differ between the groups. Clearly, on the basis of these studies as well as others,[11-13] all OPOs and donor hospitals should be offering the option of DCD to patients' families and all transplant centers should be using organs obtained after cardiac death for transplantation. Because the largest number of patients on national waiting lists are potential kidney recipients, DCD renal donation could have a major impact on reducing the number of patients in need of a kidney transplant.

Pancreas Transplantation

The first series of simultaneous pancreas-kidney transplants from DCD donors was reported by D'Alessandro et al[15] in 2000. This series was followed by a comparison of 31 recipients who received transplants obtained after cardiac death with 45 who received transplants obtained after brain death.[16] The University of Wisconsin has subsequently performed an additional 16 simultaneous pancreas-kidney transplants for a total of 47 transplantations of these organs from DCD donors. As in renal transplantation, the rate of delayed graft function was higher for transplants from DCD donors (25.8% vs 5.3%, $P=.001$); however, no differences were detected in pancreatic function as measured by postoperative serum levels of amylase, glucose, and hemoglobin A_{1C}.

Except for a higher rate of urinary tract infections in recipients of organs from DCD donors, the 2 groups of recipients had no differences in post-operative complications. Serum levels of glucose and hemoglobin A_{1C} 6 months after transplantation also did not differ between the 2 groups. In addition, 5-year graft survival rates did not differ; pancreas and kidney survival rates were 79.1% and 79.2%, respectively, for organs obtained after cardiac death and 79.2% and 81.8%, respectively, for organs obtained after brain death.

In this study,[16] the mean warm ischemic time (ie, time from extubation until the start of perfusion with cold solution) for organs from DCD donors was 15.3 minutes; the cold ischemic time (ie, time from the cross clamping of the aorta to reperfusion) was similar for both groups (approximately 16 hours for the pancreas and 17 hours for the kidney).

These results indicate that transplantation of pancreases from DCD donors yields results that are no different from those for pancreases from donors with brain death. Although pancreases from donors with brain death currently may be underused in the United States, pancreases from DCD donors have the potential to markedly decrease the size of the waiting list for pancreas transplantation, particularly if DCD donors are also considered as a source for islet cell transplants.[17]

Liver Transplantation

Transplantation of livers from DCD donors is more complex because of the susceptibility of the liver parenchyma and biliary epithelia to warm ischemia and the severity of illness in patients in need of a liver transplant. In an early study[15] from the University of Wisconsin on 19 liver transplants from non–heart-beating donors, no difference was noted in recipient and graft survival or rate of biliary complications between recipients of livers from non–heart-beating donors and recipients of livers from heart-beating donors. Other early single-center reports were similar,[18-21] although Abt et al[22] found an increased incidence of biliary tract complications in recipients of livers from non–heart-beating donors.

Subsequently, Foley et al[7] compared 36 liver transplants from DCD donors with 553 liver transplants from donors with brain death and found that as the number of liver transplants from DCD donors increased, certain patterns began to emerge. On the first postoperative day after transplantation, as well as the day of discharge, levels of hepatocellular enzymes and canalicular enzymes (eg, γ-glutamyl transferase and alkaline phosphatase) were higher in recipients of livers from DCD donors, as was use of blood products in the operating room. In this analysis, the incidence of hepatic artery stenosis was higher in livers from DCD donors (16.6% vs 5.4%, $P=.001$), and biliary strictures developed in 5 of 6 patients with hepatic artery stenosis. Likewise, the overall rate of biliary stricture rate was increased in recipients of livers from DCD donors (27.8% vs 10.3%, $P=.001$), and there transplantation rate was higher (19.4% vs 7.1%, $P=.01$). However, the rate of primary graft nonfunction did not differ between the 2 groups of recipients (5.5% vs 1.3%). Also, 3-year recipient and graft survival rates were lower in recipients of livers from DCD donors (68% vs 84%, $P=.002$, and 56% vs 80%, $P=.006$, respectively), but when results from recipients of livers from DCD donors less than 40 years old were compared with those in recipients of livers from DCD donors more than 40 years old, the rates of recipient and graft survival were higher and the rate of biliary complications decreased. Abt et al[23] had similar results in a study in which they compared 144 liver transplants obtained after cardiac death with 26856 liver transplants obtained after brain death. Rates of primary nonfunction and retransplantation were higher and 3-year graft survival was significantly lower in recipients of livers from DCD donors, but 3-year recipient survival did not differ between the 2 groups.

In a more recent analysis[14] by the Scientific Registry of Transplant Recipients in which 277 liver transplants from DCD donors were compared with 17533 liver transplants from non-DCD donors for transplants done from January 1, 2000, through October 31, 2003, the hazards ratios were 1.45 for recipient survival and 1.85 for graft survival for recipients of livers from DCD donors. Likewise, DCD donor age of 50 years or more was associated with a higher hazards ratio for graft loss than was donor age less than 50 years.

Recommendations for improving the results of liver transplantation for livers from DCD donors include using livers from donors aged less than 50 years, limiting warm ischemic time to 30 minutes or less and cold ischemic time to less than 8 hours (preferably <6 hours), and avoiding use of livers from DCD donors in technically challenging recipients, such as recipients who have had previous multiple abdominal procedures or retransplants.

In addition, when livers from DCD donors are transplanted, consideration should be given to the benefit a recipient will receive from the transplant compared with the risk of dying while on the waiting list. The system currently used to prioritize patients who are waiting for liver transplantation is based on statistical formulas used to predict death inpatients with liver disease. In this system, the model for end-stage liver disease, scores range from 6 (less ill) to 40 (gravely ill). Patients with scores greater than 17 may be more appropriate candidates for transplantation of livers from DCD donors, because patients with lower scores can wait longer and have lower risk of mortality while on the waiting list.

Lung Transplantation

The first successful lung transplants from non-heart-beating donors were reported by Love et al[24] and Steen et al.[25] Little has been published since these studies, but surgeons at the University of Wisconsin have done 16 transplantations of lungs from DCD donors, 6 single and 5 double, in 11 recipients (unpublished data). All recipients were critically ill in the ICU; 1 recipient was receiving extracorporeal membrane oxygenation at the time of transplantation. The 1-year patient survival rate is 71%; 1 patient was alive 8 years after transplantation of lungs from a DCD donor.

Heart Transplantation

One transplantation of a heart obtained after cardiac death has been performed in a child at the University of Colorado, and although the patient is currently alive after transplantation, few details about this case are known.

Summary

Current results of transplantation of kidneys from DCD donors indicate an increased rate of delayed graft function but a long-term graft survival rate similar to that in recipients of kidneys from donors with brain death. This similarity in rates also appears to be true for pancreas transplantation, but the number of transplants performed is substantially smaller than for kidney transplantation. The results of transplantation of livers from DCD donors are less favorable than those of transplantation of livers from donors with brain death, but with reductions in donor age and both warm and cold ischemia times and improvements in the selection of donors and recipients, these results should improve. Also, improvements in preservation and in methods used to abrogate warm ischemia injury may result in fewer biliary complications. Finally, the outcomes of lung transplantation in a few critically ill patients have been surprisingly good and may be applicable to less critically ill patients.

Conclusions

Transplantation is remarkably successful for many patients with a variety of end-stage diseases. Unfortunately, the supply of donor organs remains insufficient to meet demand. Although impressive steps have been taken to address this issue, more work remains to be done.

DCD is an option that can help narrow the gap between need and supply. The concept is not novel; it has served as the clinical basis for modern transplantation. Unfortunately, however, recovering organs from DCD donors is particularly challenging, resource intensive, and ethically debatable. Despite considerable controversy, DCD is considered ethically defensible, but if this approach to organ donation is to be successful on a large scale, it must be fully integrated into the decision-making processes for end-of-life care.

From the evidence we have presented, 2 conclusions can be clearly stated. First, all OPOs and donor hospitals should be offering the option of DCD to patients' families, and all transplant centers should be using organs obtained after cardiac death for transplantation. Second, clinical practices and public policies will inevitably evolve on the basis of further experience with DCD.

References

1. Prendergrast TJ, Luce JM. Increasing incidences of withholding and withdrawal of life support from the critically ill. *Am J Respir Crit Care Med.* 1997;155:15-20.
2. Edwards JM, Hasz RD Jr, Robertson VM. Non-heart-beating organ donation: process and review. *AACN Clin Issues*. 1999;10:293-300.
3. Institute of Medicine, National Academy of Sciences. Non-Heart-Beating Organ Transplantation: Medical and Ethical Issues in Procurement. Washington, DC: National Academy Press; 1997.
4. Institute of Medicine, National Academy of Sciences. Non-Heart-Beating Organ Transplantation: Practice and Protocols. Washington, DC: National Academy Press; 2000.
5. Ethics Committee, American College of Critical Care Medicine; Society of Critical Care Medicine. Recommendations for non-heartbeating organ donation: a position paper by the Ethics Committee, American College of Critical Care Medicine, Society of Critical Care Medicine. *Crit Care Med.* 2001;29:1826-1831.
6. Lewis J, Peltier J, Nelson H, et al. Development of the University of Wisconsin Donation After Cardiac Death Evaluation Tool. *Prog Transplant.* 2003;13:265-273.
7. Foley DP, Fernandez LA, Leverson G, et al. Donation after cardiac death: the University of Wisconsin experience with liver transplantation. *Ann Surg.* 2005;242:724-731.
8. Koogler T, Costarino AT Jr. The potential benefits of the pediatric nonheartbeating organ donor. *Pediatrics.* 1998;101:1049-1052.
9. Wight J, Chilcott J, Holmes M, Brewer N. The clinical and cost-effectiveness of pulsatile machine perfusion versus cold storage of kidneys for transplantation retrieved from heart-beating and non-heart-beating donors. *Health Technol Assess.* 2003;7:1-94.
10. D'Alessandro AM, Hoffmann RM, Knechtle SJ, et al. Successful extrarenal transplantation from non-heart-beating donors. *Transplantation.* 1995;59:977-982.
11. Rudich SM, Kaplan B, Magee JC, et al. Renal transplantations performed using non-heart-beating organ donors: going back to the future? *Transplantation.* 2002;74:1715-1720.
12. Cooper JT, Chin LT, Krieger NR, et al. Donation after cardiac death: the University of Wisconsin experience with renal transplantation. *Am J Transplant.* 2004;4:1490-1494.
13. Weber M, Dindo D, Demartines N, et al. Kidney transplantation from donors without a heartbeat. *N Engl J Med.* 2002;347:248-255.
14. Scientific Registry of Transplant Recipients. National reports page. Available at: http://www.ustransplant.org/csr/current/nats.aspx. Accessed February 25, 2006.
15. D'Alessandro AM, Odorico JS, Knechtle SJ, et al. Simultaneous pancreas-kidney transplantation from controlled non-heart-beating donors. *Cell Transplant.* 2000;9:889-893.
16. Fernandez LA, Di Carlo A, Odorico JS, et al. Simultaneous pancreas-kidney transplantation from donation after cardiac death: successful long-term outcomes. *Ann Surg.* 2005;242:716-723.
17. Markmann JF, Deng S, Desai NM, et al. The use of non-heart-beating donors for isolated pancreatic islet transplantation. *Transplantation.* 2003;75:1423-1429.
18. Casavilla A, Ramirez C, Shapiro R, et al. Experience with liver and kidney allografts from non-heart-beating donors. *Transplantation.* 1995;59:197-203.
19. Reich DJ, Munoz SJ, Rothstein KD, et al. Controlled non-heart-beating donor liver transplantation: a successful single center experience, with topic update. *Transplantation.* 2000;70:1159-1166.
20. Fukumori T, Kato T, Levi D, et al. Use of older controlled non-heart-beating donors for liver transplantation. *Transplantation.* 2003;75:1171-1174.
21. Manzarbeitia CY, Ortiz JA, Jeon H, et al. Long-term outcome of controlled, non-heart-beating donor liver transplantation. *Transplantation.* 2004;78:211-215.
22. Abt P, Crawford M, Desai N, et al. Liver transplantation from controlled non-heart-beating donors: an increased incidence of biliary complications. *Transplantation.* 2003;75:1659-1663.
23. Abt PL, Desai NM, Crawford MD, et al. Survival following liver transplantation from non-heart-beating donors. *Ann Surg.* 2004;239:87-92. 24. Love RB, Stringham J, Chomiak PN, et al. First successful lung transplantation using a nonheart-beating donor [abstract]. *J Heart Lung Transplant.* 1995;14(1 pt 2):S88. 25. Steen S, Sjoberg T, Pierre L, et al. Transplantation of lungs from a non-heart-beating donor. *Lancet.* 2001;357:825-829.

Organ Preservation

Louise M. Jacobbi, CCTC, CPTC
Mitchell L. Henry, MD

If one could substitute for the heart a kind of injection, of arterial blood, either natural or artificially made, one would succeed easily in maintaining alive indefinitely part of the body.

Julien Jean Cesar Le Gallois[1] (1770-1819)

Introduction

The continuing development of organ preservation technology has helped make transplantation of solid organs a clinical reality for thousands of patients. In reviewing its progress, the evolution of organ preservation during its first 50 years was greatly influenced by 3 distinct and simultaneous tracks, which complemented its journey from bench to bedside: first, new technology in both pharmacological and mechanical engineering; second, medical/surgical advancements that virtually made all types of organs transplantable; and third, society's acceptance of transplantation as a treatment of end-stage organ failure, which was initiated by enabling legislation and community participation in the donor process.

Historical Perspective

In the late 1960s and early 1970s, after the first kidney transplant by Dr Joseph Murray, the need for a constant supply of organs became apparent, compelling the transplant community to identify new sources of donor organs as well as a way to preserve them. The cascade of events from the recognition of this need to current practice patterns in preservation was a journey with interesting paths, encounters, and relationships.

The need was the initiating raison d'être the 1972 Social Security amendment Public Law 92-603 legislation for End Stage Renal Disease (ESRD) was enacted. This legislation enabled more patients to have access to transplantation, causing a drastic escalation of waitlisted patients for transplantation. Second, the development and acceptance of the 1968 Harvard Medical School ad hoc committee on brain-death criteria opened the door to obtaining all vital organs from deceased patients in a medically controlled fashion. The third was enactment of the 1968 Uniform Anatomical Gift Act (UAGA), which gave individuals the right to donate their organs at the time of their death. Lastly, the acceptance of transplantation was greatly advanced by improved graft and patient survival rates in grafts from living related donors (LRD). Each of these drove the need to find ways of preserving organs from deceased donors in a way that would, (1) protect organ viability and function; (2) provide comparable outcomes to LRD grafts; (3) provide sufficient time to identify and prepare potential recipients for surgery; and (4) subsequently, increase the pool of organs for transplantation.

In the early years of clinical transplantation, living donors were usually the single source of donors and all but a few were close family members of patients in end-stage renal failure. Preservation of organs from living donors was of little concern, as in most cases side-by-side donor and recipient procedures were performed with organ revascularization occurring within less than 60 minutes of recovery. Organs were simply flushed with a cold solution (Ringers lactate) and immediately transplanted, imparting little if any impact to the integrity of the organ. This practice continues to be employed[2] and works extremely well for living donor grafts, as they experience no real ischemia time or insults from outside sources.

ORGAN PRESERVATION

The use of organs from deceased patients', although documented in early scientific journals as intriguing were ideas for researchers only because preservation of organs was not yet available. The concept of preserving organs from deceased donors was first described by Dr Alexis Carrel, who, with Charles Lindberg[3], in the early 1930s designed an *ex vivo* preservation system for hearts and kidneys. They described a device that mimicked the body by pumping a solution through the organ and oxygenating it at the same temperature, pressure, and flow as in the body.

Almost 30 years after Carrel and Lindberg had described an organ preservation system, their ideas were implemented by researchers who understood and appreciated that donor sources other than living donors had to be pursued, and a reliable organ preservation methodology was fundamental to making it happen. Researchers began by examining each step in the process of obtaining a usable organ from a deceased donor and documenting the critical events that would influence or more specifically compromise organ function (Table 1). Of particular importance were the time and the conditions needed to keep an organ viable once recovered and the methodology to store it until transplantation.

In the early 1960s, Belzer and colleagues[4] developed a machine perfusion (MP) device that pumped a blood component through an organ at a set pressure and flow rate that could be monitored and modulated as needed. The device continued to be modified over the next several years, with subsequent incorporation of a pulsatile pump and membrane oxygenator.

The first solutions used were a whole blood mixture, a buffered plasma, and cryo-precipitated plasma. This later version contained a concentrated albumin component, which was believed to be necessary to sustain organ viability. Other researchers reported that colloid and/or crystalloid solutions, with unique buffering agents, had fewer side effects than the blood-based solutions and were cheaper and easier to make and in some form have been modified and continue to be used today. These solutions, developed by Collins et al[5-7] Ross and Marshall,[8-10] and Bretschneider et al,[11,12] were usually phosphate buffered with additional agents such as histidine, tryptophan, HEPES [(4-(2-Hydroxyethyl)-1 piperazineethanene sulfonic acid), dextran, glucose, citrate, sucrose, and mannitol. The additives were incorporated into the solutions to assist in maintaining pH and to stabilize cell permeability.

Hoffmann and Southard et al[13] subsequently developed a synthetic perfusate for kidney preservation. The use of this perfusate in 72-hour preservation of dog kidneys demonstrated that albumin could effectively be replaced with hydroxyethyl starch (HES), which gave superior results. This solution became the one of choice when using MP and continues to be used when employing MP today. The MP method of preserving kidneys from deceased donors became popular because it was relatively simple and the solution was easy to acquire. It also provided a safe longer storage time, and outcomes were good and results consistent.

In these early years, every solution was developed to support organ preservation under hypothermic conditions known as static cold storage (CS). In the ensuing years, acceptance and advancements in transplantation were attributed to improved immunosuppressive therapy, improved kidney graft outcomes, and the pursuit of transplanter's to make transplantation of all vital organs a clinical reality. These initiatives made the development of new preservation models a necessity in order to increase the pool

Table 1. INSULTS DECEASED DONOR ORGANS ENDURE

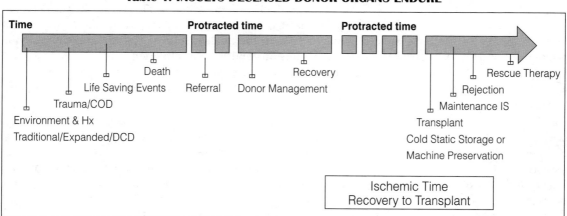

of organs available for transplantation. The challenge was to design a method to preserve and care for all organs from deceased donors until they could be transplanted. Researchers also recognized that each organ type has different requirements when it is MP versus preservation in CS, and that each solution and device configuration would need to be tailored to individual organ requirements.[14,15] Using the kidney perfusion pump as a model, researchers tried to produce devices for other organs, which could be used clinically, and this remains a work in progress.

The interest in transplanting other organs led Belzer et al[17-19] to modify their machine preservation solution (MPS), and in the early 1970s, these researchers designed a broad-spectrum intracellular static solution that would support preservation of other organs [20, 21] in CS. The solution, known as the University of Wisconsin Solution (UW), had the same basic composition of the Belzer MPS with modifications to support an organ in the static state. In Table 2 the composition of the 2 UW solutions are depicted, showing how MPS is modified from an extra cellular solution to an intracellular solution. Other MP and CS solutions were developed and used during this time, but most of these solutions were variations of those listed with minor modifications, and these solutions, or a variation, continue to survive in today's practice.

The early researchers concluded that a hypothermic environment was best for organ preservation because it would reduce the metabolic rate, thereby requiring less nutrients and oxygen, but could induce endothelial injury and subsequent reperfusion injury. Although this potential was concerning, it could be controlled with careful attention to temperature and pressure.

Table 2. BELZER – UNIVERSITY OF WISCONSIN SOLUTIONS (UW)

Machine Perfusion (MPS)	Cold Storage (CS)
Na gluconate	Lactobionic acid
K gluconate	KOH
Mg gluconate	NaOH
Adenine	Adenosine
Mannitol (USP)	Allopurinol
KH2PO4	KH2PO4
HES	HES
Ribose	Glutathione
Glucose	Raffinose
CaC12	MgSo4
HEPES	

Modification and additives alter the machine perfusion extracellular solution to a static cold storage intracellular solution.

This cohort of pioneers implemented hypothermic organ preservation as an integral component of transplantation. Their legacy has allowed organs to be shared over a greater time and distance. In current organ allocation strategies, preservation is the process enabler. The devices and solutions, or modified versions, developed by these early researchers are the foundation of organ preservation today and their legacy has helped make organ transplantation a clinical reality.

Principles and Goals of Graft (Solid Organ) Preservation

The continuing development of preservation technology[22] is guided by the need to either modify or prevent conditions that influence organ stability, viability, and/or function. The crucial periods in preservation of deceased donor organs are donor management both before and after death, surgical organ recovery, and warm ischemic time (WIT) as well as cold ischemic time (CIT). Each of these preservation periods has the potential to influence and compromise initial graft function and ultimate graft outcome (Table 1). The search for the best method of preserving organs, once surgical recovery has occurred, was and still is motivated by the initial observations of the early researchers.

The aim of optimal preservation is to preserve organ viability, ameliorate any insult to the organ that may have occurred during the crucial preservation periods, and evaluate organ function. The goals, therefore, of *ex vivo* organ preservation are to suppress and/or minimize cellular swelling; minimize the metabolic process; provide adequate hydration and oxygenation; minimize ischemia and reperfusion injury by stabilizing cell permeability; and, if possible, remove any accumulation of metabolic waste incurred during the recovery and preservation period.

Concurrent with the early development of preservation solutions and an important advancement in organ preservation was the development of clinical MP devices that incorporated most of the principles described by Carrel and Lindbergh in their 1935 patent. The most commonly used MP device, in early studies, was the Waters MOX-100; others included the Belzer LI-400, Travenol, Gambro, and most recently the Organ Recovery Systems LifePort. All these devices used hypothermia as their platform and all except the LifePort use external manual reading and calculation of pressure and flow and most require regular if not constant monitoring.

After almost 5 decades of development, several solutions and 2 methodologies emerged as the most useful in today's practice. All the solutions developed for human organ preservation have certain common components that are added to protect the organ. The optimization of pH and electrolytes to ensure a stable physiological environment is paramount in normalizing the effects of pre mortem and post mortem donor conditions and sets the environment of *ex vivo* preservation of an organ. The current clinical treatments are either hypothermic MP or CS, and both meet most of the goals of preservation. Hypothermia is used because the metabolic rate is reduced by half for every 10°C decrease in temperature. Because of this decrease, metabolic activities slow down, lowering the need for oxygenation, which result in decreased ATP (adenosine triphosphate) consumption, and a decreased function of the sodium/potassium ATPase pump, which prevents cellular swelling. Additives to the various solutions are intended to mediate reperfusion injury, preserve the pH, stabilize cell membrane permeability, and suppress cell swelling. Comparison of the solutions demonstrates they share many of the same components, with slight variations in additives and their amounts. Table 3 provides a summary of the composition of the most common preservation solutions which survived into current practice. The variations in the solutions account for formulation design for specific organs and the desired preservation path of action (intracellular or extra cellular) of the solution. The preservation process has become even more important as donor and recipient criteria continue to expand and new immunosuppressive therapies are designed.

Table 3. COMPOSITION OF HYPOTHERMIC PRESERVATION SOLUTIONS

MPS Belzer	UW-Belzer	HTK	Cel	EC	LPD-glucose
80 Na gluconate	100 Lactobionic acid	15 NaCl	80 Lactobionic Acid	10 Na	134 Na
Na OH	20 KOH(5M)	9 KCl	15 KCl	115 K+	6 K+
5 Mg Gluconate	5 NaOH(5M)	1 Potassium-ketoglutarate	100 NaOH	57.5 Phosphate	0.8 Phosphate
5 Adenine	5 Adenosine	4 MgCl	13 MgCl	0 Sulfate	0.8 Sulfate
30 Mannitol	3 Allopurinol	18 Histidine HCl H_2O	20 Glutamic Acid	10 Bicarbonate	0 Bicarbonate
25 KH_2PO_4	25 KH_2PO_4	180 Histidine	30 Histidine		
5g% HES		2 Tryptophan	3 Glutathione	0 Dextran	5.0 g/L Dextran
3 Gluathione	3 Glutathione	30 Mannitol	60 Mannitol	15 g/L Glucose	0.9 g/L Glucose
5 Ribose	30 Raffinose	0.015 CaCl	0.025 CaCl	15 Cl⁻	142 Cl⁻
10 Glucose					
0.5 $CaCl_2$	5 $MgSO_4$				
10 HEPES					

Amounts are mM/1000ml quantity per package insert
Commerical solutions: MPS & KPS-1 (Belzer formula machine perfusion solutions)
ViaSpan (Belzer static storage University of Wisconsin solution)
HTK – Custodial (Brettschneider solution)
Cel – Celsior
EC – Euro-Collins (modified Collins solution)
LPD – Perfadex (Steen cold storage solution)

Preservation Modalities and Solutions

Hypothermic preservation (4-8°C) is a simple way to control metabolism and diminishes the need to find a way of eliminating metabolic waste. The formulated solutions controlled swelling and the need for continuous oxygenation.

Static cold storage is the most widely used method of preservation. This treatment mode is easy to use, the solutions could be used for multiple organ types, the solutions used are relatively inexpensive, and commercially available. The limiting factors of CS (1) it does not eliminate metabolic waste, (2) it does not allow for organ function evaluation during preservation, and (3) it does not add nutrients during storage. These factors are of particular importance when extended times are required to prepare a potential recipient for surgery, transport an organ to a waiting patient location, and/or if the organ is compromised during pre mortem or post mortem care.

The CS solutions designed specifically for human organ preservation that have been cleared by the Food and Drug Administration (in the United States) or are CE marked (in Europe, "Conformité Européene") for clinical use for both *in situ* flush and abdominal organ storage are UW and the Bretschneider Solution/Histidine, Tryptophan, Ketoglutarate solution (HTK). HTK is also used clinically for hearts, as are Celsior, Perfadex, and EuroCollins solutions. These solutions and UW are also used for lungs. The evolution of this group of solutions is attributed to specific organ requirements while stored in hypothermic conditions that protect it and allow it to resume immediate function once normal physiologic conditions are met. In Table 4, the most common solutions and preservation modalities for each organ type are presented.

Table 4. ORGAN SPECIFIC SOLUTIONS WITH MODALITY

Organ	Preservation Modality	Solution
Heart	CS	HTK/Cel
Lung	CS	Cel/LPD/EC/UW
Liver	CS	UW/HTK
Kidney	CS	UW/HTK
Kidney	MP	MPS
Pancreas	CS	UW/HTK/LPD
Sm Intestine	CS	UW/HTK

Commercial solutions:
Perfadex-LPD-glucose; Custodial-HTK; UW-ViaSpan; MPS- KPS-1; Cel-Celsior

Today, hypothermic MP at 4 to 8°C is limited clinically to kidney preservation. It is used in about 16% of the procedures performed. The Belzer MPS is the solution used in this modality because of its lower viscosity and cell protection components. This type of preservation is generally accepted as superior[23, 21] to CS for kidneys, but because several studies[24,25] in the 1980s reported no difference between the 2 methodologies, it was abandoned by many centers. In addition, it appeared to be more cumbersome and more expensive than CS. In the past decade, however, these early evaluation studies are being reevaluated because of the availability, stability, and modification of the original formulated solution; the increasing use of extended criteria donors (ECDs)[26-28] and donors after cardiac death (DCD);[29-31] and outcome analysis demonstrating better graft survival rates. Therefore, the use of MP is again becoming the preservation modality of choice for kidneys. This method offers the ability to evaluate organs from all deceased donors, allows for longer CITs, can provide oxygen and nutrients, and may be a way of eliminating metabolic waste.

Recent retrospective reports from individual investigators[32,33] and the Organ Procurement and Transplantation Network /United Network for Organ Sharing (OPTN/UNOS) comparing outcomes of MP and CS kidneys have shown better outcomes in initial function and long-term graft survival of those preserved with MP. This is particularly evident when the donor source is categorized and the data sorted by preservation modality before being analyzed. Table 5 shows the Scientific Registry for Transplant Recipients (SRTR) analyzed kidney graft outcomes between 2000 and 2004 which shows significantly less delayed graft function (DGF) in MP grafts from both the DCD and BDD donors. Using the same cohort of patients, sorted by organ preservation modality, Table 6 shows the relative risk of graft failure was found to be significantly lower in patients when their grafts were preserved using MP.

Table 5. PERCENT AND ADJUSTED *ODDS RATIO (OR) OF DELAYED GRAFT FUNCTION (DGF) BY *BRAIN DEATH (BDD) & DONATION AFTER *CARDIAC DEATH DONORS (DCD)

Preservation Modality: CS vs. MP

2000-2004

DCD & BDD MP vs. CS	% DGF	OR*	P value	
BDD/ CS	23.9	1.00	ref	} Significance
BDD/ MP	17.0	0.54	<0.0001	
DCD/ CS	42.3	2.52	<0.0001	} P = 0.15
DCD/ MP	40.2	2.04	<0.001	

*Adjusted for recipient age, race, PRA, ESRD cause, years of ESRD, HLA mismatch, year of transplant, previous transplant, transfusions and donor age, sex, race, hypertension, diabetes, cause of death, creatinine, and cold ischemia time.

*BDD depicts combine standard and extended criteria donor outcomes.

OPTN/SRTR 2005 June

Table 6. RELATIVE RATE (RR)* OF GRAFT FAILURE (GF) IN BRAIN DEATH (BDD)* & DONATION AFTER CARDIAC DEATH (DCD)* DONORS: COLD STORAGE (CS) VS. MACHINE PRESERVATION (MP)

2000-2004

DCD & BDD CS vs. MP	RR* GF	P value	
BDD/ CS	1.00	ref	
BDD/ MP	0.88	0.003	
DCD/ CS	0.85	0.15	} P = 0.03
DCD/ MP	1.23	0.03	

*Adjusted for recipient age, race, PRA, ESRD cause, years of ESRD, HLA mismatch, year of transplant, previous transplant, transfusions and donor age, sex, race, hypertension, diabetes, cause of death, creatinine, and cold ischemia time.

*BDD depicts combine standard and extended criteria donor outcomes.

OPTN/SRTR 2005 June

Relationship of Preservation Time to Graft Outcome

In literature reviews of graft outcomes, the preservation method is always mentioned as one of the key risk factors to be considered when evaluating outcome. The optimal accepted CIT and the CIT range for each organ is unique and varies with solutions and modality (Table 4). Current practice suggests that minimizing CIT is optimal for all organs, particularly when CS preservation is used (Table 7).

The relationship of preservation to outcome is not always apparent, as found by Ojo et al[34]; in particular, when delayed graft function (DGF) was identified as a key risk factor in kidney graft survival. In later reviews when all the influencing factors had been identified and the organs were sorted by preservation method, it became apparent that DGF and graft survival could be reduced by changing the preservation modality.

Numerous reports[35,36] in the literature provide evidence that minimizing ischemia time, both WIT and CIT, provide better graft outcomes. WIT[37] is the period after death when there is no blood flowing through the organ, both before and after the organ has been flushed with a cold solution. WIT can occur at the time of graft removal and at implantation. CIT is the period when the cold (usually 4-8°C) preservation solution is flushed through or in which the organ is stored. Accepted WIT in DCD donors is currently less than 60 minutes (Table 8). Most of the organs recovered from DCD donors are abdominal organs, although there have also been reports of successful lung recovery. The term DCD donors was defined in the mid-1990s at a clinical meeting of practitioners. Their definitions are referred to as the Maastricht donor classifications l-V (Table 9).[38]

Table 7. ORGAN SPECIFIC CIT WITH PRESERVATION MODALITY

Organ/ Modality	Accepted CIT Hours	CIT Range
Heart/ CS	4	8
Lung/ CS	8	12+
Liver/ CS	12	21
Kidney/ CS	<24	31
Kidney/ MP	24	31+
Pancreas/ CS	17	31
Small Intestine/ CS	6	10

OPTN/SRTR June 2005

Table 8. DONATION AFTER CARDIAC DEATH DONOR (DCD)

Reported Acceptable Ischemia Times

Organ	WIT	CIT
Liver	60 min	< 24 hours
*Kidney	30 min	< 8 hours
Pancreas	60 min	< 18 hours

OPTN/SRTR 2005 Report

*this report does not separate MPS and CS
++ Lung   30min WIT   < 12hours

Table 9. MAASTRICHT DONOR CLASSIFICATION

- Type I: dead on arrival (irreversible cardiac arrest on the street)
- Type II: unsuccessful resuscitation (this includes patients brought into the ER while being resuscitated by the ambulance crew
- Type III: imminent cardiac arrest in intensive care (ventilator switch-off)
- Type IV: cardiac arrest during or after the brain death diagnostic procedure
- Type V: unexpected cardiac arrest in intensive care

When comparing MP to CS the incidence of DGF in kidney transplantation has been shown in nearly all studies to increase with increasing CIT. Also the use of MP appears to extend the optimal accepted CIT, and can abrogate the increased incidence of DGF in standard donors (SD), ECD, and DCD donors. In Table 10 is an analysis of the OPTN/UNOS data in which the author's sorted and categorized all deceased donor kidney transplants by donor type and preservation modality and demonstrated that CIT impacted DGF and MP lessened the incidence of DGF in both BDD and DCD patient transplants.

Relationship of Preservation Modality to Graft Outcome

The current preservation modality for all non-renal organs is CS. The development of MP for other organs continues to both intrigue and plague transplant researchers as each organ has its own specific needs and requirements. Although MP continues to provide better outcomes in initial and long-term kidney graft function, it remains the least used method of preservation.[39]

For organs for which CS is the preservation modality there is a relationship between preservation and/or ischemia time and graft survival. Outcome studies comparing one solution to another are equivocal and therefore several no one solution is being used (See Table 4). Several of these agents were developed with specific requirements and they only have approval for certain organs, although there are studies being conducted to expand their use in other organ systems.

Relationship of Donor Source and Preservation to Graft Outcome

Emerging evidence suggests that the length of WIT and CIT, directly related to donor source, may cause DCD criteria to be redefined into ECD's and standard categories as in deceased brain-dead donors (BDD).

The long-term outcome for grafts from either DCD or ECDs is related to donor source, organ function at death, and preservation time. The greatest amount of data available on preservation-related outcomes is from patients who received kidney transplants. Numerous studies[40,41] have found that transplanted kidneys that have experienced DGF have a greater risk of graft loss. Burdick et al[42] reported that kidneys, which were preserved using MP, experienced significantly less DGF than those maintained in CS. Jacobbi et al[43,44] reported that depending on the donor source, MP could reduce DGF by as much as 40% (Table 10).

In recent years, the pursuit and utilization of ECDs and DCD donors have increased the use of MP for kidneys, and preliminary reports indicate that the short-term benefits of reducing DGF are evident.

There are conflicting data between the US[42] and European[29,45] experiences in regard to DCD kidney graft outcomes. In the United States, early reports indicate a high incidence of DGF (>40%) in DCD kidneys preserved using both cold storage and MP. The study emanating from Belgium[45] however, reports an incidence of 30% DGF concomitant with good graft survival for the same period (See Table 11). Also, in a recent early report from this same group of investigators for 2005, they continue to show a decrease in DGF for type III and IV DCD donors. In addition, reports from the United Kingdom[46] are indicating similar results. Because these are still early studies, it will take some time to properly evaluate outcomes. One explanation for the significant differences could be that the European centers were using MP in defined controlled protocols, which has not been the experience in the United States.

The utilization of heart, lung, liver, pancreas, and small bowel from ECDs is beginning to emerge and evaluation of long-term outcomes is optimistic. The use of organs from these donors is primarily based on donor history, organ-specific function studies, and biopsy results. With heart and lungs, additional functional testing is always performed, along with the usual visual examination at the time of at recovery. In DCD donors, the abdominal organs are usually recovered on the basis of history and function at death.

Table 10. OUTCOME ANALYSIS: 57, 217 OPTN
KIDNEYS TRANSPLANTED 1995-2002
Odds Ratio (OR) of DGF ... MP vs. CS

	OR	P value	Conclusion
SD	0.557	<.0001	DGF with MP is significantly reduced
ECD	0.572	0.0268	DGF with MP is reduced
All kidneys	0.561	<.0001	DGF with MP is significantly reduced
ECD	1.898	<.0001	DGF is increased with ECD
>24 hrs CIT	1.108	<.0001	DGF increases with increased CIT >24 hrs.

OR Adjusted for:
Donor... sex, race
Recipient... sex, age, race, ethnicity, PRA, HLA mm, < & > 24 hours CIT, cause of ESRD, previous transplant, previous transfusion
Data analysis SRTR 2003 All donors: Less than 2% of donors were reported as DCD.

Jacobbi et al. ITS Miami 2003

Table 11. EXPÉRIENCE BELGE

RÉSULTATS

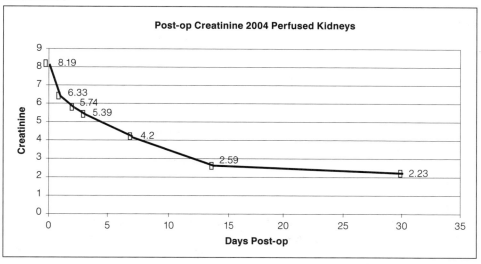

Non Fonction primaire:	0%
Fonction Retardée:	30%
Survie greffon / patient:	100%

Chart courtesy of Authors

Table 12. OUTCOME BY ORGAN TYPE: 1995-2002 PRIMARY TRANSPLANTS

	1 year (%)	3 year (%)	5 year (%)
Kidney	91	82	70
Kidney/Pancreas	92	84	75
Liver	82	74	67
Heart	86	78	56
Lung	89	59	44

Organ Procurement and Transplant Network (OPTN)   http://www.unos.org June 2005
All Kaplan-Meier Graft Survival Rates

Except for kidneys, CS is the only preservation modality for organs recovered from DCD donors and ECDs, and the primary discriminating elements in the decision to transplant these organs are function and ischemic time. In addition, WIT and CIT are major determining factors influencing outcome. Because of new donor sources and escalating waiting lists, there continues to be an opportunity for taking advantage of technological advances to improve preservation methodology to help increase the number of transplantable organs and to improve graft survival (Table 12).

Future of Preservation Solutions and Preservation Modalities

Current technology available for most organs is CS with 3 solutions for abdominal organs and 3 for thoracic organs. This method of preservation offers no dynamic evaluation (i.e., perfusion characteristics), and reported outcomes using varying solutions have been equivalent.[21]. Kidney preservation does have the second option of MP, which also offers an evaluation element (dynamic perfusion characteristics) and well-documented reports of reduced risk of DGF when compared to the more common CS methodology. The newest MP device is truly portable and offers computer-driven data reports without the human variability

Table 13. INCORPORATING MP INTO CLINICAL SETTING

Product Consideration
Solution & Device

• Cleared	by FDA or has CE mark as an *in-situ* flush and preservation solution
• Cost	Reasonable and reimbursable
• Availability	Readily

Device

• Organ chamber	single use, single chamber provides environment for monitoring individual organ function and secures sterile environment with a sealed chamber
• Perfusion regulation	automatically controls constant pressure to the organ
• Temperature control	1-8°C, maintained for minimum of 24 hours, ice slush for portability
• Instrumented sensors	pressure, flow, temperature, battery status
• Portability/weight	required and user friendly
• Commercial flight	accepted in running condition by most commercial airlines, preferable unattended
• Intervention & analysis	safe port for injecting intervention agents and sampling
• Fail safe	device valves close to protect against air entering vascular circuit and continues to maintain organ in hypothermic state if pump system fails
• Filter system	in-line filter system for perfusate
• Pulsatility	selectable: continuous or pulsatile 30bpm
• Power system	Batteries last 24hours on single charge/ 100V or 240V electrical outlet
• Bubble traps	Preferred redundant system
• Computer	On board microprocessor onboard to give real time monitoring of organ and minimize manual calculation and readings

of pump measures, as well as the availability of Web-based data transfer of organ parameters in real time. Determination of the best device and solution must be based on how it best fits with local practice; but there are several underlying components that should influence this decision (Table 13).

Today, researchers and clinicians involved in organ preservation are revisiting methodologies previously discarded with a better understanding of organ physiology and chemistry, and are armed with state of the art engineering and pharmacologic agents previously not available. Rather than continuing with hypothermic solutions, clinicians are now considering using either mid- or normo thermic solutions and MP, which would offer the ability to better evaluate each organ function, as well as provide nutrients and oxygen. With newer, more controllable devices and warmer temperature MP could also provide a means to eliminate metabolic waste. New engineering, pharmaceuticals, and immunomodulation agents also offer a host of therapies, which could now be developed for *ex vivo* treatment of organs.

Several groups are using the kidney MP model and are working toward the development of devices for all organs, which would offer longer optimal CIT and the ability to evaluate and treat organs during their preservation time. There are reports of heart, liver, lung, and pancreas solutions and MP devices being tested on animals, which have very promising results.

Preservation continues to be a frontier in transplantation because there is no real understanding of how or why one methodology, when applied, has a superior outcome. Possibly, the first step would be a multicenter prospective study of the 2 modalities, incorporating a study to better examine and determine the mechanism by which MP functions.

Organ preservation remains a frontier within transplantation and an exciting venue for investigators to explore the potential of *ex vivo* organ therapies to resuscitate organs that may have been previously damaged during the (1) agonal phase of death, (2) attempts at patient resuscitation, (3) donor management, and (4) organ recovery. Information about these events or organ-specific resuscitation therapies could then be applied to all organs, as new devices and solutions are developed and the preservation process is better understood. The next logical step would be to design immune modulation therapies that could be administered to the organ during preservation or, conversely, preserving the organ until a recipient could be conditioned to specific donor antigens.

Table 14. POTENTIAL OF MACHINE PRESERVATION OF HUMAN ORGANS
In vitro organ therapy...

Mechanical Present	Chemical Present Potential	Immune Future
Pressure	Electrolytes	Unique chemical agents
Flow	Enzymes	Enzymes
pH	Vasopressors	Gene
Visualization	Cytokines	Monoclonal Antibodies
Surgical intervention Designed to evaluate and preserve organ function	Mechanical and chemical protocols designed to better evaluate, improve & restore organ function	Therapies designed to increase & improve graft survival
Hypothermic	*Hypothermic*	*Hypothermic-, midthermic, & normothermic*

Chart courtesy of Organ Recovery Systems

As transplantation further explores the expansion of donor sources and new immunosuppressive therapies, the next generation of preservation technology can continue to be the enabler that provides more transplantable organs through *in vitro* preservation with resuscitation therapies and an enabler of better graft survival through application of *in vitro* immune modulation therapies (Table 14). The future of preservation is limited only by the insight and imagination of researchers and clinicians working toward the common goal of more transplantable organs and better and longer graft survival.

References

1. Le Gallois JJC. Experiences sur le Principede de la Vie. *Classics of Neurology & Neurosurgery Library*. Nancrede NC, Nancrede JN, trans. New York, NY 1994.
2. Starzl TE, Shapiro R, Simmons RI. *The Atlas of Organ Transplantation*. New York, NY: Gower Medical Publishing; 1992.
3. Carrel A, Lindbergh CA. *The Culture of Organs*. New York, NY: Paul B Hoeber, IN, Harper Bothers; 1935
4. Belzer FO, Ashby BS, Gulyassy PF, Powell M. Successful seventeen-hour preservation and transplantation of human-cadaver kidney. *N Engl J Med*. 1968; 278:608-610.
5. Collins GM, Bravo-Shugarman M, Teraski PI. Kidney preservation for transportation. Initial perfusion and 30 hours' ice storage. *Lancet*. 1969; 2:1219-1222.
6. Collins GM, Hartley LC, Clunie GJA. Kidney preservation for transportation. Experimental analysis of optimal perfusate composition. *Br J Surg*. 1972; 59:187-189
7. Collins GM, Green RD, Halasz NA. Importance of anion content and osmolarity in flush solutions for 48 to 72 hr hypothermic kidney storage. *Cryobiology*. 1979; 11:309-313.
8. Marshall VC, Ross H, Scott DF, et al. Preservation of cadaver renal allografts: comparison of ice storage and machine perfusion. *Med J Aust*. 1977; 2:353-356.
9. Ross H, Marshall VC, Escott ML. 72-hr canine kidney preservation without continuous perfusion. *Transplantation*. 1976; 21:498-501.
10. Marshall VC, Howden BO, Jablonski P, et al. Sucrose-containing solutions for kidney preservation. *Cryobiology*. 1985; 22:622.
11. Brettschneider L, Daloze PM, Huguet C. The use of combined preservation techniques for extended storage of orthotopic liver homografts. *Surg Gynecol Obstet*. 1968; 126:263.
12. Erhard J, Lange R, Scherer R, et al. Comparison of histidine-tryptophane-ketoglutarate (HTK) solution vs. University of Wisconsin Solution (UW) for organ preservation in human liver Transplantation: a prospective, randomized study. *Transplantation*. 1994; 7:177-181.
13. Hoffman RM, Southard JH, Lutz MF, et al. Synthetic perfusate for kidney preservation. Its use in 72-hour preservation of dog kidneys. *Arch Surg*. 1983; 118:919-921.
14. Wicomb WN, Cooper DKC, Barnard CN. Twenty-four hour preservation of the pig heart by a portable hypothermic perfusion system. *Transplantation*. 1982; 34:246-250.
15. Levy MN. Oxygen consumption and blood flow in the hypothermic, perfused kidney. *Am J Physiol*. 1959; 197:11
16. Belzer FO, Glass NR, Sollinger HW, et al. A new perfusate for kidney preservation. *Transplantation*. 1982; 33:322.
17. Belzer FO. Evaluation of preservation of the intra-abdominal organs. *Transplant Proc*. 1989; 25:2527-2530.

18. Belzer FO. D'Alessandro AM, Hoffman RM, et al. The use of UW solution in clinical transplantation. A 4-year experience. *Ann Surg.* 1992; 215:579-583.
19. Ploeg RJ, Goossens D, McAnulty JM, et al. Successful 72-hour cold storage of dog kidneys with UW solution. *Transplantation.* 1988; 46:191-196.
20. D'Alessandro AM, Reed A, Hoffman RM, et al. Results of combined hepatic, pancreatic duodenal and renal procurements. *Transplant Proc.* 1991; 23:2309-2311.
21. Henry ML. Pulsatile preservation in renal transplantation. In: Collins GM, Dubernard JM, Perin GG, Land W, eds. *Land Procurement, Preservation, and Allocation of Vascularized Organs.* The Netherlands: Kluwer Academic Publishers; 1997:131-135.
22. Toledo-Pereyra LH, Condie RM, Callender CO, et al. Hypothermic pulsatile kidney preservation. *Arch Surg.* 1974; 109:816.
23. Jacobbi LM, Gage F, Montgomery RA, Sonnenday CJ. Machine preservation improves functional outcomes in cadaveric renal transplantation. *Am J Transplant.* 2003; 428(suppl 5):S1080.
24. Merion RM, Oh HK, Port FK, et al. A prospective controlled trial of cold-storage versus machine-perfusion preservation in cadaveric renal transplantation. Transplantation 1990; 50:230-233.
25. Halloran P, Aprile M. A randomized prospective trial of cold storage versus pulsatile perfusion for cadaver kidney preservation. *Transplantation.* 1987; 43:827-832.
26. Jacobbi LM, McBride VA, Etheredge EE, et al. The risks, benefits, and costs of expanding donor criteria. *Transplantation.* 1995; 60:1491-1496.
27. Jacobbi LM, McBride VA, Etheredge EE, et al. Costs associated with expanding donor criteria: a collaborative statewide prospective study. *Transplant Proc.* 1997; 29:1550-1556.
28. Kauffman HM, Bennett LE, McBride MA. Ellison MD. The expanded donor. *Transplant Rev.* 1997; 11:165-190.
29. Van Renterghem Y. Cautious approach to use of NHBD. *Lancet.* 2000; 356:528.
30. Light JA, Sasaki TM, Aquino AO, et al. Excellent long-term graft survival with kidneys from the uncontrolled non-heart-beating donor. *Transplant Proc.* 2000; 32:186-187.
31. Cho YW, Terasaki PI, Cecka JM, Gjertson DW. Transplantation of kidneys from donors whose heart have stopped beating. *N Engl J Med.* 1998; 338:221-225.
32. Matsino N, Sakurai E, Tamaki I, et al. The effect of machine perfusion preservation versus cold storage on the function of kidneys from non-heart-beating donors. *Transplantation.* 1994; 57:293-294.
33. Wright J, Chilcott J, Holmes M, Brewer N. The clinical and cost effectiveness of pulsatile machine perfusion versus cold storage of kidneys for transplantation retrieved from heart beating and non-heart beating donors. *Health Technol Assess.* 2003; 7:1-94.
34. Ojo A, Wolfe RA, Held PJ, Port FK, Schmoider RL. Delayed graft function: risk factors and implication for renal allograft survival. *Transplantation.* 1997; 63:968-974.
35. Gjertson G. DGF by cold ischemia time and donor age. *Clin Transplant.* 2000; 467-480.
36. Wright JP, Chilcott JB, Holmes, MW, Brewer N. Pulsatile machine perfusion vs. cold storage of kidneys for transplantation: a rapid and systematic review. *Clin Transplant.* 2003; 17:293-307.
37. Olson L, Davi R, Barnhart J, et al. Non-heart beating cadaver donor hepatectomy: the operative procedure. *Clin Transplant.* 1999; 13(1 pt 2):98-103.
38. Sanchez-Fructuoso AL, Prats D, Torrente J, et al. Renal transplantation from non-heart beating donors: a promising alternative to enlarge the donor pool. *J Am Soc Nephrol.* 2000; 11:350-358.
39. Polyak MM, Arrington BO, Stubenbord WT, et al. The influence of pulsatile preservation on renal transplantation the 1990's. *Transplantation.* 2000; 69:249-258.
40. Light JA, Kowalski AR, Gage F, Callender CO, Sasaki TM. Immediate function and cost comparison between ice storage and pulsatile preservation in kidney recipients at one hospital. *Transplant Proc.* 1995; 27:2962-2964.
41. Organ Procurement and Transplantation Network. Annual Report, 2003. Reviewed August 2005. www.unos.org June 2005
42. Burdick JF, Rosendale JD, McBride MA, et al. National impact of pulsatile perfusion on cadaveric kidney transplantation. *Transplantation.* 1997; 64:1730-1733.
43. Jacobbi L, et at. Novel Machine Preservation Protocol Improves Outcome of Expanded Criteria Kidneys, ITS, Rome 2003
44. Jacobbi L, et al. Machine Preservation Improves Functional Outcomes in Cadaveric Renal Transplantation, American Transplant Congress, Miami 2003
45. Van Deynse D, Squifflet J-P, Van Gelder F, et al. Expanding the kidney transplant pool: a cooperative Belgian pilot study in NHBD using machine perfusion. Presented at British Transplant Society Meeting; London, March 2004.
46. Begsarani D, Muthusamy A, et al. Oxford Experience of Non-Heart of Renal Transplantation; British Society of Transplantation; Edinburgh UK, 2006

The Vital Role of Medical Examiners and Coroners in Organ Transplantation

Teresa J. Shafer, RN, MSN, CPTC
Lawrence L. Schkade, PhD, CCP
Roger W. Evans, PhD
Kevin J. O'Connor, MS, PA, CPTC
William Reitsma, RN, BSN, CPTC

Forward

Organ transplantation saves lives and medical examiners contribute to saving lives through release of 100% of all cases brought before them for death investigation. This chapter shall include the most recently published paper about these issues, "The Vital Role of Medical Examiners and Coroners in Organ Transplantation," published in the February 2004 issue of the American Journal of Transplantation, and reprinted with permission herein. This article thoroughly explored and updated the data and thinking about medical examiner release of organs from previously published reports, many from the same authors. However, this forward will bring news of the progress and recent developments since its publication.

Health and Human Services Secretary Tommy G. Thompson joined with key national leaders and practitioners from the nation's transplantation and hospital communities in April 2003 to launch the Organ Donation Breakthrough Collaborative (ODBC). The Collaborative was designed to dramatically increase access to transplantable organs. The purpose of the initiative was clear, measurable, ambitious and achievable: "Committed to saving or enhancing thousands of lives a year by spreading known best practices to the nation's largest hospitals, to achieve organ donation rates of 75% or higher in these hospitals." One of the five stated goals of the collaborative was: ***zero medical examiner/coroner denials of organ recovery***. Key national leaders, including the Chairman of the Board of the Institute for Healthcare Improvement (IHI), the President of the Association of Organ Procurement Organizations (AOPO), the Executive Director of the United Network for Organ Sharing (UNOS), the President of the Joint Commission on the Accreditation of Healthcare Organizations (JCAHO) and others joined with the Secretary in committing to this ambitious, but do-able Collaborative Aim. The Department of Health and Human Services teamed up with the Institute for Health Care Improvement and launched Secretary Tommy Thompson's ODBC. Two hundred fifty large hospitals and 48 OPOs participated in either Collaborative I and/or II. The success of this intiative has been heralded elsewhere.

One of the key ingredients of the ODBC success was the Leadership Coordinating Council, a council comprised of presidents, executive directors, and key leaders from national organizations who have an important stake or involvement in the donation and transplantation processes. The Leadership Coordinating Council included the Presidents or key leaders from the following organizations: JCAHO, UNOS, AOPO, National Association of Medical Examiners (NAME), Society for Critical Care Medicine (SCCM), American Hospital Association (AHA), American Association of Critical Care Nurses (AACN), North American Transplant Coordinators Organizations (NATCO), the Centers for Medicare & Medicaid Services (CMS), American College of Healthcare Executives (ACHE) and many others. NAME played a bold role early in the first collaborative, fielding bold requests from transplant leaders and making bold offers of assistance in real time to teams on donors in which a denial was being made by a local medical examiner. Further, when asked to provide a faculty member to the collaborative, NAME nominated Dr. Keith Pinckard, Dallas County Medical Examiner, Southwestern Institute of Forensic Sciences. As a member of the Collaborative faculty, Dr. Pinckard attended all learning sessions and faculty meetings, providing direction and assistance to teams experiencing difficulty with medical examiners and achieving the goal of zero denials.

Notably and publicly, however, Dr. Michael Graham, President of NAME, made the following statement in response to a challenge by DHHS Secretary Tommy Thompson in Detroit, Michigan: **"It is now the official policy of the National Association of Medical Examiners to support not only the concept of zero denials, but to make it a reality."** Dr. Graham offered that NAME "is willing to review all denials, to see why organs were denied, to see if anything could have been done differently and, if so, what. There will be useful information coming out of that in the individual cases. However, I think what we will also see are the patterns, and who is denying, not as a person, but what kind of offices are denying and why are they denying. And by recognizing that, we then can work together to circumvent those denials, yet still fulfill our responsibilities in the medical/legal world." He finished his extraordinary statements with a bold offer: "On a personal level, I am willing to help any of you address issues, either individual issues or systemic issues, with any groups to see what we can do to make this work better." (Department of Health and Human Services Organ Donation Breakthrough Collaborative. Learning Session 3. *Powerful Offers & Requests*. Detroit, Michigan, April, 2004)

Finally, in addition to the complete review of the medical examiner role in transplantation which follows this introduction, I would advise readers to complete their understanding of this complex issue by understanding not only the numbers and the life-saving work of medical examiners, but also why it is 'wrong' for denials to occur. Please see: Shafer TJ, Schkade LL, Siminoff LA, Mahoney TA. Ethical analysis of organ recovery denials by medical examiners, coroners and justices of the peace. *Journal of Transplant Coordination*, Vol. 9, No. 4, December 1999: pp.[2] 232-249. Among other things, this article concludes, "Medical examiners could turn their attention to including within their professional code of ethics an explicit obligation to contribute to the health and welfare of the community they serve by routinely releasing organs for transplantation, after appropriate review. They could assume a leadership role, working on public policy together with other medical, social, and legal groups, spearheading protective state legislation to require such release of organs." The ODBC gave medical examiners their stage, their opportunity to seize the moment and change history by making such bold offers. They have already done so as evidenced by their public actions and pronouncements. The future challenge will be to actually reach the goal of zero denials; to fall 100% of the time on the side of life and love. The graph below demonstrates what the concentrated efforts of all previously mentioned have been able to accomplish through the Organ Donation Breakthrough Collaborative. Zero denials is achievable.

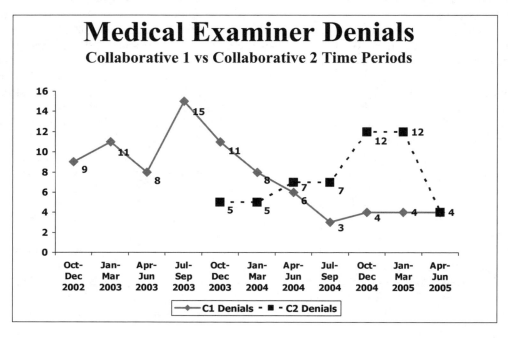

A CLINICIAN'S GUIDE TO DONATION AND TRANSPLANTATION

Abstract

Many people die due to the shortage of donor organs. Medical examiners and coroners (ME/Cs) play a vital role in making organs available for potential recipients. ME/C case data were collected using a structured confirmatory-recorded methodology for calendar years 2000-01 and were linked and analyzed with donor and transplant data from the United Network for Organ Sharing, predicting the nature and extent of the loss of donor organs. Nearly seven percent of ME/C cases were denied recovery during 2000-01. Because 353 and likely, 411 potential organ donors (PODS) were denied, as many as 1,400 persons on transplant waiting lists did not receive organs due to ME/C denials. Problematically for pediatric patients awaiting transplantation, nearly half of all ME/C denials occurred in pediatric patients. Eighteen percent of PODs age five or less and 44.2% of child abuse PODs were denied recovery by the ME/C. There were no (zero) denials in three of the five largest U.S. cities and in four states. Since 1994, two states have enacted legislation restricting the circumstances of ME/C denials, resulting in an 83% decrease in ME/C denials. Release of *all* organs from ME/C cases is needed urgently to protect the lives of those persons awaiting transplantation. ME/Cs deserve recognition for their efforts in advocating methods and/or regulation/legislation designed to achieve 100% release of life saving organs for transplantation.

Introduction

The demand for organs for transplantation remains unmet. While nearly 100,000 persons could have benefited from a solid organ transplant in 2001, fewer than 20,000 did so.[1] Regrettably, thousands of people needlessly die each year due to a chronic shortage of organ donors. Medical examiners and coroners (ME/Cs) have the ability to ease, to some degree, what has become a public health crisis. They directly determine whether or not organs will be recovered from potential donors who die from circumstances within the jurisdiction of the ME/C. Their permission to recover organs is vital.[2] Due to the sheer size of the recipient waiting list and the lack of organs, such decisions directly impact the fate of terminally ill transplant candidates.

The focus of this study was to determine the number of organs currently not recovered because of ME/C denials of organ recovery in ME/C cases. Second, the study compares the current state of ME/C denials with a previous study in order to determine the progress or lack of progress in achieving 100% ME/C organ release. Finally, the study explores measures implemented to achieve 100% release of organs from ME/C cases.

As the donor organ shortage has worsened, reports in the literature and in the media of non-recovery of organs as a result of ME/C denials have continued to surface.[3-15] When death investigation and organ donation cannot be accomplished simultaneously, the consequences are serious, as one organ procurement organization (OPO) reported that greater than 40% of potential organ donors were lost in one year due to ME/C denials.[16-19]

There is no empirical evidence to support non-recovery of organs in ME/C cases, including child abuse and homicide cases. An exhaustive case law review revealed no instance in which a state was unable to adequately investigate a crime or to prosecute a criminal defendant because necessary evidence had been altered by organ donation. Moreover, in no instance did the removal of organs for transplantation compromise autopsy proceedings to the point where cause of death could not be determined.[3,20]

More than a decade has passed since the landmark study by Shafer et al.[3] Since then, awareness of the need for complete cooperation between death investigation and organ recovery activities with the goal of 100% organ release has resulted in improved public policy, either in the form of actual practice, regulation, or legislation. Many medical examiners have spoken in favor of organ donation and have advocated policies for zero denials.[21-23]

Methods

The concepts critical to this study are defined in Table 1. Data collection procedures adhered to the concepts and definitions included in the table. Data were not obtained that could have enabled a comparison of actions by ME/Cs who were physicians versus those who were not.

Table 1. CONCEPTUAL FRAMEWORK AND DEFINITIONS FOR THE STUDY

Concept	Definition	Calculations
Coroner	For purposes of this study, coroner shall also mean justice of the peace as the terms are used interchangeably between different geographical areas, as those individuals charged with conducting death investigations for a particular geographic area, usually county.	None Required
Medical Examiner / Coroner Jurisdiction (ME/C Case)	Deaths falling within the jurisdiction of a ME/C generally include deaths from homicide, unnatural causes, unknown cause, suicide, deaths occurring within 24 hours of admission to the hospital and deaths of unidentified persons.	Percent of Potential Organ Donors that are ME/C Cases = (ME/C Case Organ Donors + ME/C Denials) / (ME/C Case Organ Donors + ME/C Denials + Non-ME/C Case Organ Donors)
Medical Examiner or Coroner Denial (ME/C Denial)	Refusal for organ recovery by the ME/C of any potential organ donor, regardless of what stage during the donation process that the denial occurred (i.e., whether the refusal came during the pre-referral, referral, evaluation, management or procurement stage of the donation process.	Percent of ME/C Cases that are Denied Recovery = ME/C Denials / (ME/C Case Organ Donors + ME/C Denials)
ME/C Denial Extended	The data obtained from the study OPOs accounted for 85.8% of the U.S. donor population during the survey periods. For that population, 353 ME/C denials were reported. "ME/C Denials Extended" estimates the denial experience of 100% of the U.S. potential donor population.	ME/C Denials Extended = ME/C Denials x [1 + (1-.858)]
Potential Organ Donor (POD)	A patient (1) who is brain dead or has an injury or disease capable of resulting in brain death (2) who is medically suitable for donation and (3) for whom family consent for donation has not been denied. *(This definition, for the purposes of this study, does not examine PODs that do not become donors for reasons of medical unsuitability, or family refusal, or ME/C denial.)*	None Required
Organ Donor	A patient from whom one or more organs are recovered for purposes of transplantation. (In 2000-2001, an average of 3.6 organs were recovered from each organ donor.)	Organs not recovered due to ME/C Denials = ME/C Denials x 3.6 Organs not recovered due to ME/C Denials Extended = ME/C Denials Extended x 3.6

Following extensive pre-testing, in February 2002, a data collection instrument was distributed to U.S. OPOs certified and designated by the Centers for Medicare and Medicaid Services to coordinate organ recovery in all 50 states and the territory of Puerto Rico. ME/C case data were collected using a structured confirmatory-recorded methodology for calendar years 2000 and 2001. ME/C denials were categorized according to the United Network for Organ Sharing (UNOS) classification system – a system applied routinely and uniformly to all potential organ donors.

Data were reported by 49 of 59 (83.1%) OPOs. For the study period, these OPOs recovered 85.8% of all organ donors in the U.S. There was no evidence of significant bias in the reported data, except for the following circumstance. The reported number of ME/C denials of PODs is included in the study, but it was not possible to report cases in which OPOs were never notified. Thus, the number and type of deaths for these cases remain indeterminate, and the data reported in this study may understate the total number of ME/C case denials. Data for the 1990-1993 period were obtained from a previous publication[3] and were compared to the 2000-2001 data collected in this study.

Results

The study results are reported for two time periods – 2000-01 and the previously published 1990-92 time period.[3] This approach enables direct comparisons to document changes during the past decade.

2000-01 Study Period Findings

As shown in Table 2, during 2000-01, there were 12,066 organ donors in the U.S. The 49 OPOs participating in the study were responsible for 10,356 donors; therefore, the study accounts for 85.8% of the U.S. donor population. Of these donors, 4,874 (47.1%) died from circumstances within the jurisdiction of ME/Cs, another 4,125 donors (39.8%) were not ME/C cases, and 1,357 (13.1%) were reported as unknown. A total of 353 PODs were denied recovery of ME/Cs. In total, ME/C cases represented 56% of U.S. potential organ donors, with denials in 6.8% of donor eligible cases.

Most donors are the source of multiple organs. The national mean organ yield per donor for 2000-01 was 3.6 organs.[24] Therefore, it is estimated that as many as 1,271 donor organs, approximately 636 organs per year, were not recovered due to ME/C denials.

Cause, circumstance, and mechanism of death. As shown in Table 3, head trauma was the cause of death most often associated with ME/C denial (53.8%). The circumstance of death with the greatest frequency of denial was child abuse (25.2%), followed by homicide (24.9%). Blunt injury was the most often stated mechanism of death (34.6%). When child abuse cases are grouped with homicide cases, half of all ME/C denials concern homicide. While child abuse victims constituted only 1.1% of organ donors, these cases amount to 25.2% of all ME/C denials. Overall, 44.2% of child abuse and 57.6% of all Sudden Infant Death Syndrome (SIDS) cases that were PODs were denied recovery by an ME/C.

Table 2. OVERALL SUMMARY DATA

Variable	2000		2001		Total (2000-01)	
	Number	%	Number	%	Number	%
Organ Procurement Organizations (OPOs)						
Universe † (U.S. Total)	59	100.0	59	100.0	59	100.0
Study Participants	48	81.3	49	83.0	49	83.0
Organ Donors						
Universe † (U.S. Total)	5,985	100.0	6,081	100.0	12,066	100.0
Study Total	5,029	84.0	5,327	87.6	10,356	85.8
Study Organ Donors: ME/C Case versus Non-ME/C Cases						
ME/C Case Organ Donors	2,335	46.4	2,539	47.7	4,874	47.1
Non-MC/E Case Organ Donors	2,084	41.4	2,041	38.3	4,125	39.8
Unknown Type Organ Donors	610	12.1	747	14.0	1,357	13.1
Total	5,029	100.0	5,327	100.0	10,356	100.0
Organ Donors That Are ME/C Cases ‡						
Percent of Organ Donors	N/A	54.6	N/A	57.1	N/A	55.9
ME/C Denials of Potential Organ Donors						
Number of ME/C Denials	170	N/A	183	N/A	353	N/A
Number of ME/C Denials Extended‡	197	N/A	206	N/A	403	N/A
Percent of ME/C Cases that are Denied Recovery‡	N/A	6.8	N/A	6.7	N/A	6.8
Organs Not Recovered						
Organs Not Recovered Owing to ME/C Denials	612	N/A	659	N/A	1,271	N/A
Organs Not Recovered Owing to ME/C Denials – Extended‡	710	N/A	740	N/A	1,451	N/A

N/A = not applicable; ME = Medical Examiner; C = Coroner.

† see reference 24.

‡ For a description of calculations, see Table 1.

Age. The largest percentage of denials occurred in pediatric PODs. During the study period, 20.1% of all ME/C denials involved children less than 1 year of age increasing to 41% of all denials involving children age 10 and less. There were only 183 organ donors less than 1 year of age, therefore, nearly one-third (31.1%) of PODs less than 1 year of age were denied recovery. (Table 3)

During the study period, there were 412 donors between the ages of 1 and 5 years. An additional 61 PODs (14.7% of the potential donors in this age category) were denied recovery by a ME/C. Individuals aged 17 and less comprised 16.6% of all donors, but almost half (47.6%) of all denials. In sum, pediatric patients (age 17 and less) comprised almost half of all ME/C denials (47.6%); and the percentage of pediatric PODs denied, 9.8%, (196/2003 from Table 3) was 4.7 times greater than the 2.1% (215/10,064) seen in the adult population.

Race and ethnicity. African-American PODs were more than three times as likely to be denied as Caucasians (7.0 % vs. 2.3%). Similarly, Hispanic PODs were twice as likely to be denied by ME/Cs (4.6% vs. 2.3%) as Caucasians.

Geographic region. ME/C denials vary by geographic area, as well as by regions of the United Network for Organ Sharing (UNOS), as is apparent in Tables 3-6. Table 4 shows that, during the study period, in New York, NY, Houston, TX, and Philadelphia, PA – three of the five largest cities in the U.S. – there were no (0) potential organ donor denials by ME/Cs. Table 5 summarizes state-level ME/C denials. Data was not obtained for seven states, and incomplete data was reported for five states owing to the sample size of 83% (49 of 59) OPOs. Several states for which complete data were available had no (0) potential organ donors denied by ME/Cs. These states include New Jersey, New Hampshire, Delaware, and Vermont. (Tables 4 and 5).

Discussion

As shown in Table 2, it is possible that more than 1,400 persons on transplant waiting lists did not receive donor organs due to ME/C denials in 2000-01. Denials in pediatric PODs remain a serious issue due to the inability of many children to receive organs from adult donors. As noted previously, denials of pediatric PODs constituted nearly half of all denials in 2000-01. During 1990-92, 22% of all ME/C denials were from child abuse cases,[2] compared with 44% in 2000-01 (Table 3).

The foregoing results are important findings that are both significant and troublesome. During 2000-01, there were, on average, 1,131 children, age 5 and less, that were added to the waiting list each year. Approximately 697 children in this age group were transplanted each year, but tragically 277 organs from children in this age category were denied each year. On average, 182 children in this age group died while waiting per year (Table 7). Some ME/Cs remain reluctant to consider the release of organs from child abuse and/or SIDS PODs.[12,25]

Comparison Study Periods: 2000-01 vs. 1990-92

More than a decade has passed since the first published study documented the magnitude of PODs lost in the U.S. due to denial of organ recovery by ME/Cs.[3] The percentage of ME/C denials appears to have remained virtually unchanged: 7.2% in 1990, and 6.7% in 2001; a modest decline of 6.9% (Table 7).

These results are fairly consistent with those reported elsewhere, using less rigorous data collection techniques. For example, Sopher recently contacted 64 city, county, and state medical examiner offices. Forty-four offices responded to the survey, corresponding to approximately 29% of the U.S. population. The offices reported that, overall, 7% of the requests were denied, 70% were granted unconditionally, and the remainder were granted, but with restrictions.[4]

In light of the continued status quo in parts of the country, this situation must be addressed with urgency and effectiveness. As is apparent from the data, some states and localities have taken important steps to assure all potential donors are released. Such efforts have included a mixture of local protocol, regulatory and/or legislative approaches.

Table 3. MEDICAL EXAMINER/CORONER DENIALS ACCORDING TO VARIOUS CHARACTERISTICS OF U.S. ORGAN DONORS

Variable	Total for 2000-01		Total Number of U.S. Organ Donors †	% of Denials	% of U.S. Organ Donors	% of U.S. Potential Organ Donors Denied by MC/E
	ME/C Denials	MC/E Denials Extended				
Cause of Death						
Anoxia	75	87	1,314	21.2	10.9	6.2
Cerebrovascular/Stroke	53	62	5,203	15.0	43.1	1.2
Head Trauma	190	221	5,037	53.8	41.7	4.2
CNS Tumor	2	2	114	0.6	0.9	2.0
Other	28	33	316	7.9	2.6	9.4
Unknown	5	6	83	1.4	0.7	6.6
Total	**353**	**411**	**12,067**	**100.0**	**100.0**	**3.3**
Circumstance of Death						
Motor Vehicle Accident	31	36	2,800	8.8	23.2	1.3
Suicide	10	12	908	2.8	7.5	1.3
Homicide	88	103	685	24.9	5.7	13.0
Child Abuse	89	104	131	25.2	1.1	44.2
Non-Motor Vehicle Accident	26	30	986	7.4	8.2	3.0
None of the Above	58	68	3,645	16.4	30.2	1.8
Other Specify or Natural Causes	32	37	2,823	9.1	23.4	1.3
Unknown	19	22	89	5.4	0.7	19.9
Total	**353**	**411**	**12,067**	**100.0**	**100.0**	**3.3**
Mechanism of Death						
Drowning	1	1	96	0.3	0.8	1.2
Sudden Infant Death Syndrome (SIDS)	14	16	12	4.0	0.1	57.6
Intracranial Hemorrhage/Stroke	53	62	5,537	15.0	45.9	1.1
Seizure	5	6	82	1.4	0.7	6.6
Drug Intoxication	7	8	149	2.0	1.2	5.2
Asphyxiation	18	21	285	5.1	2.4	6.9
Cardiovascular	35	41	713	9.9	5.9	5.4
Gunshot Wound/Stab	53	62	1,235	15.0	10.2	4.8
Blunt Injury	122	142	3,454	34.6	28.6	4.0
None of the Above/Natural Causes	18	21	412	5.1	3.4	4.8
Other, Specify	6	7	6	1.7	0.0	53.8
Unknown	21	24	86	5.9	0.7	22.2
Total	**353**	**411**	**12,067**	**100.0**	**100.0**	**3.3**

Table 3. MEDICAL EXAMINER/CORONER DENIALS ACCORDING TO VARIOUS CHARACTERISTICS OF U.S. ORGAN DONORS

Variable	Total for 2000-01			% of Denials	% of U.S. Organ Donors	% of U.S. Potential Organ Donors Denied by MC/E
	ME/C Denials	MC/E Denials Extended	Total Number of U.S. Organ Donors †			
Age Group						
<1 Year	71	83	183	20.1	1.5	31.1
1-5 Years	61	71	412	17.3	3.4	14.7
6-10 Years	14	16	328	4.0	2.7	4.7
11-17 Years	22	26	1,080	6.2	9.0	2.3
18-34 Years	79	92	3,088	22.4	25.6	2.9
35-49 Years	60	70	3,192	17.0	26.5	2.1
50-64 Years	35	41	2,788	9.9	23.1	1.4
65+ Years	7	8	996	2.0	8.3	0.8
Unknown	4	5	0	1.1	0.0	100.0
Total	353	411	12,067	100.0	100.0	3.3
Race/Ethnicity						
Caucasian	181	211	8,891	51.3	73.7	2.3
Black	92	107	1,429	26.1	11.8	7.0
Hispanic	57	66	1,376	16.1	11.4	4.6
Asian	13	15	261	3.7	2.2	5.5
Other	5	6	110	1.4	0.9	5.0
Unknown	5	6	0	1.4	0.0	100.0
Total	353	411	12,067	100.0	100.0	3.3
UNOS Region						
Region 1	9	10	480	2.5	4.0	2.1
Region 2	11	13	1,515	3.1	12.6	0.8
Region 3	95	111	2,017	26.9	16.7	5.2
Region 4	12	14	1,083	3.4	9.0	1.3
Region 5	107	125	1,573	30.3	13.0	7.3
Region 6	9	10	515	2.5	4.3	2.0
Region 7	27	31	1,141	7.6	9.5	2.7
Region 8	38	44	783	10.8	6.5	5.4
Region 9	1	1	681	0.3	5.6	0.2
Region 10	23	27	1,091	6.5	9.0	2.4
Region 11	21	24	1,188	5.9	9.8	2.0
Total	353	411	12,067	100.0	100.0	3.3

† United Network for Organ Sharing, Richmond, VA.

Table 4. STATES AND LARGE CITIES WITH NO (ZERO) MEDICAL EXAMINER DENIALS, RANKED IN ORDER OF POPULATION

States	Cities†
New Jersey	New York, NY
New Hampshire	Houston, TX
Delaware	Philadelphia, PA
Vermont	San Antonio, TX
	Memphis, TN
	Washington, D.C.
	Boston, MA
	Austin, TX
	Fort Worth, TX
	Fresno, CA

† Cities among the top 50 cities in U.S. with zero ME/C denials

Table 5. MEDICAL EXAMINER DENIALS BY STATE

State	2000	2001	Total (2000-01)	State	2000	2001	Total (2000-01)
Alabama	8	7	15	Nevada	1	5	6
Alaska	N/A	N/A	N/A	New Hampshire	0	0	0
Arizona	N/A	N/A	N/A	New Jersey	0	0	0
Arkansas	2	8	10	New Mexico	0	1	1
California	51	48	99	New York †	0	1	1
Colorado	2	3	5	North Carolina †	0	0	0
Connecticut	2	3	5	North Dakota	4	3	7
Delaware	0	0	0	Ohio †	4	8	12
Florida †	18	16	34	Oklahoma	4	2	6
Georgia	1	3	4	Oregon	0	1	1
Hawaii	3	5	8	Pennsylvania †	2	4	6
Illinois	6	8	14	Puerto Rico	0	2	2
Indiana	5	1	6	Rhode Island	3	2	5
Iowa	0	1	1	South Carolina	11	1	12
Kansas	3	8	11	South Dakota	1	0	1
Kentucky	N/A	N/A	N/A	Tennessee	0	2	2
Louisiana	18	12	30	Texas	0	6	6
Maine	0	1	1	Utah	1	0	1
Maryland	1	1	2	Vermont	0	0	0
Massachusetts	0	1	1	Virginia	5	2	7
Michigan	1	4	5	Washington, D.C.	0	0	0
Minnesota	1	2	3	Washington	N/A	N/A	N/A
Mississippi	N/A	N/A	N/A	West Virginia	N/A	N/A	N/A
Missouri	2	3	5	Wisconsin	0	2	2
Montana	N/A	N/A	N/A	Wyoming	N/A	N/A	N/A
Nebraska	10	6	16	**Totals**	**170**	**183**	**353**

N/A = Data not available. OPO in the state did not participate.
† Incomplete reporting for this area. Some OPOs in the state did not participate.

THE VITAL ROLE OF MEDICAL EXAMINERS AND CORONERS IN ORGAN TRANSPLANTATION

Table 6. COMPARISON OF MEDICAL EXAMINER AND CORONER DENIALS AND DONOR POPULATION CHARACTERISTICS FOR TWO TIME PERIODS: 1990-92 (STUDY 1) AND 2000-01 (STUDY 2)

Characteristic	Study 1[†]			Study 2	
	1990	1991	1992	2000	2001
ME/C Potential Organ Donors Denied – Extended (Number)	219	302	363	198	207
ME/C Potential Organ Donors Denied (%)	7.2	9.6	11.4	6.8	6.7
Decrease in Percent of ME/C Potential Organ Donors Denied from 1990 to 2001 (%)	N/A	N/A	N/A	N/A	6.9
Total U.S. Organ Donors (Number)	4,533	4,530	4,548	5,985	6,081
Percent of Organ Donors that are ME/C Cases (%)	66.9	69.1	69.9	54.6	57.1
U.S. Estimate of Number of Organ Donors that are ME/C Cases (Number)[‡]	3,033	3,130	3,179	3,268	3,472
Increase in ME/C Organ Donors from 1990 through 2001 (%)	N/A	N/A	N/A	N/A	14.5
U.S. Estimate of Number of Organ Donors that are not ME/C Cases (Number)[‡]	1500	1400	1369	2717	2609
Increase in non-ME/C Organ Donors from 1990 through 2001 (%)	N/A	N/A	N/A	N/A	73.9

N/A = Not applicable.
[†] See reference number 3.
[‡] Calculated by taking the percentage of donors that are ME/C cases times the actual number of U.S. organ donors.

Table 7. PEDIATRIC PATIENTS (AGE ≤5 YEARS): WAITING LIST, TRANSPLANT, DEATHS ON THE WAITING LIST, AND ME/C DENIALS[‡]

Characteristic	Average per Year 2000-2001
Patients Added to List Each Year	1131
Patients Transplanted	697
Deaths on the Waiting List	182
ME/C Organs Denied[†]	277

[†] From Table 3. In 2000-2002, the average ME/C Denials Extended per year (154/2=77) times mean national organ yield of 3.6 equals 277.
[‡] See reference 35.

Legislation

Prior to 1994, two states, New York and Tennessee, had laws requiring the release of organs from PODs in ME/C cases.[26-27] Since 1994, two other states, New Jersey and Texas, have enacted legislation that severely restricts the ability of ME/Cs to deny organ recovery. The New Jersey law directs MEs to release organs if they are not present at the time of recovery, viewing the organ in question, and determining at that time, that the organ cannot be released for transplantation.[28] Following enactment of this legislation, MEs released all organs for recovery during the survey period in New Jersey. The Texas legislation is nearly identical to that of New Jersey. The law stipulates that if the ME decides that any specific organ may not be recovered for organ transplantation, because that organ may be relevant in determining cause of death, the ME has the obligation to make that determination when present in the operating room during the organ recovery surgery. The ME may request a biopsy of the recovered organ or deny its removal, but if removal is denied, the ME must explain the reason for denial in writing.[29]

Although the above legislation was recently enacted, the historical background and legislative history of these laws are rooted firmly in the Uniform Anatomical Gift Act (UAGA), finalized in 1968. The Act offers the following stipulation:

> Subsection (d) is necessary to preclude the frustration of the important medical examiners' duties in cases of death by suspected crime or violence. However, since such cases often can provide transplants of value to living persons, it may prove desirable in many if not most states to reexamine and amend the medical examiner statutes to authorize and direct medical examiners to expedite their autopsy procedures in cases in which the public interest will not suffer.[26]

The New Jersey and Texas legislatures effectively implemented the original intent of the UAGA when revising medical examiner statutes. These legislatures defined statutory procedures that would accommodate the legitimate interest of ME/Cs in death investigation and furthered the public policy of encouraging organ donations. The legislation was unanimously passed in both states. The New Jersey and Texas laws represent a reasoned balance between the societal needs for increased donor organs, and the legitimate law enforcement needs necessary to determine the cause and manner of death in suspicious cases. Since the passage of legislation by these two states, a comparative analysis reveals that ME/C denials decreased 83% in these two states from 1990-93 to 2000-01. If the percent of ME/C denials had remained at their "pre-legislative" level in the 2000-01-study period, then 37, not six, PODs would have been lost, and as many as 136 people would have been denied life-saving transplants in Texas and New Jersey alone.

On November 19, 2002, the Advisory Committee on Organ Transplantation, appointed by Tommy G. Thompson, Department of Health and Human Services, unanimously agreed on a series of recommendations concerning various aspects of organ donation and transplantation. One of the recommendations directs the Secretary to use his good standing with the National Governor's Association, the National Association of State Legislatures, the Uniform Commissioners of State Laws, and/or with individual states to amend the Uniform Anatomical Gift Act (UAGA) to add a new subsection that mirrors the Texas and New Jersey laws. The amendment, which would appear at the end of Section 4 of the Act, would insert language nearly identical to that of the Texas medical examiner law. Further, the Secretary has been asked to encourage individual states to adopt state laws to the same or similar effect.[30] Colorado attempted unsuccessfully in 2000 to pass the Texas and New Jersey medical examiner laws while California, in 2003, passed the legislation through both houses.[14,31]

Regulations and Protocols

While legislation is being increasingly considered when other efforts fail, some localities and states have variously tried regulation and/or policy and protocol development. Localities such as Boston, MA and others have established protocols and achieved cooperation resulting in ME release of 100% of PODs. The state of Florida recently adopted regulations that include: "When permission is requested to proceed with a vascular organ donation, the paramount concern of the medical examiner must be to save the life of the intended recipient(s)." The Florida regulations further list specific reasons that are generally not regarded as sufficient to deny permission for vascular organ explantation.[32] Therefore it is important for all involved to carefully look at the structure, current practice and, above all, the single life or lives that could be saved in deciding how to achieve 100% release in all ME/C cases.

Clearly, vital steps have been taken to remedy situations in parts of the country where successful death investigations and organ recovery do not occur in tandem with one another each and every time such opportunities arise. However, serious concerns remain. For example, many ME/Cs fear the possibility that even one case of miscarried justice may result, despite the admonitions of their colleagues. The Chief Medical Examiner in Chicago, Illinois has repeatedly noted: "There has never been a homicide prosecution endangered by organ transplantation."[33] Chicago had a single denial in the two-year study period. Nonetheless, for some medical examiners, the improbable still appears to underscore the significance of the unacceptable – a botched death investigation. Because of this fear, it is a foregone conclusion in some ME/C jurisdictions that, in certain cases, such as homicides, or deaths involving child abuse, PODs will not be released.

Non-physician Coroners and Justices of the Peace

More concerning are the denials from *non-physician* elected officials, (coroners or justices of the peace, JP), individuals with little or no medical background, in essence, making life and death decisions. Texas specifically addressed this possible occurrence during the 2003 legislative session with SB 1225, providing that the decision for release or non-release of organs in JP cases rests with the ME performing the autopsy. In those unusual cases in which a ME is not performing the autopsy, then the JP or his designee is required to attend the organ recovery surgery and view the organ in question if he is considering denying organ recovery.[34]

As noted previously, denial data was not gathered in a manner to determine whether a medical examiner or a non-medical coroner or justice of the peace made the denial. Hanzlick, in a 1998 review of ME/C systems, documented that only 48% of the U.S. is served by medical examiner systems, and that the type of system in place to perform medico-legal review of deaths varies from state-to-state, as well as from county-to-county.[35]

Coroners and justices of the peace are often elected officials who serve a single county for one or more specified terms and need not be physicians. At any given time, there are approximately 2,759 individuals serving as coroners. Nationwide, the number of newly elected or annually appointed coroners (and justices of the peace) ranges from 159 to 1,546.[36]

Summary

Given the large number, diverse educational backgrounds, variation in levels of training, and generally autonomous practice of the individuals who serve as coroners, justices of the peace, pathologists, and MEs, it is unlikely that a "cooperative" system to reach the goal of 100% release of PODs nationwide will be achieved. With few exceptions, when the issue of legislation is raised or proposed, ME/Cs voice concerns about intrusions into individual practice patterns, having their practice "legislated." As in all fields, practice patterns may be allowed to vary when the resulting differences are inconsequential relative to the public good. However, individual practice patterns that result in the non-recovery of organs, given the dire consequences of the organ shortage, are harmful and outdated. ME/Cs are already advocating and/or achieving 100% release of organs in many parts of the country and should receive more credit for their life saving role than they have in the past. Clearly, successful death investigations and lifesaving organ transplantations can, and do, occur every day in this country.

Potential recipients currently depend on good working relationships between ME/Cs and OPOs. While such coordination should be the operational expectation of every OPO and every ME/C, the lack of it should not harm potential recipients. Instead, the public should expect definitive public policy – policy that makes certain that life-saving organs are recovered in all cases, while ensuring that death investigation is conducted competently and without untoward consequences for organ donation. Persons on organ transplant waiting lists, as well as the transplant professionals, are most grateful to ME/Cs who achieve 100% release, and thereby assist in making the gift of life available to individuals in dire need. Such ME/Cs demonstrate the leadership qualities that others should emulate in both word and deed. Whether the 100% release is achieved by policy, regulation, or by legislation, recognition for these life saving efforts should be properly credited to medical examiners and coroners, whose role is vital to organ transplantation.

While death investigation remains their first priority, ultimately, ME/Cs assume a critical role in improving the health and welfare of communities. In the case of *physician* MEs, they in effect fulfill an ethical and a moral obligation every time they release an organ for transplantation.[37] Investigating deaths can have a noble purpose for both the deceased, as well as living persons whose lives could be saved. The obvious is clear–in death there can be life.

Acknowledgements:

The authors would like to thank the Association of Organ Procurement Organizations (AOPO) and the United Network for Organ Sharing (UNOS) for their support in data collection.

References

1. Evans RW. Coming to terms with reality: why xenotransplantation is a necessity. Xenotransplantation Platt JL, ed. Washington, D.C. ASM Press, Inc., 2001:29-51.
2. Jason D. The role of the medical examiner/coroner in organ and tissue procurement for transplantation. *Am J Forensic Med Pathol.* 1994; 15(3):192-202.
3. Shafer TJ, Schkade LL, Warner HE, Eakin M, O'Connor K, Springer J, Jankiewicz,T, Reitsma W, Steele J, Keen-Denton K. The Impact of Medical Examiner/Coroner Practices on Organ Recovery in the United States. JAMA. 1994; 272:1607-1613.
4. Voelker R. Can forensic medicine and organ donation coexist for the public good? JAMA. 1994; 271:891-892.
5. Warren J. D.C. medical examiner, WRTC dispute may trigger federal investigation. *Transplant News.* 1993; 3:1-2.
6. Carter JM. Letter to the Editor. Reform organ-tissue transplantation. *J Natl Med Assoc.* 1994; 86:647,666,685.
7. Hanzlick R. Letter to the Editor. JAMA. 1995; 273:1578.
8. Shafer T. In Reply. JAMA. 1995; 273:1579.
9. Chinnock RE, Bailey LL. Letter to the Editor. JAMA. 1995; 273:1578.
10. Medical examiners limiting organ use. Pittsburgh Post Gazette. 1994, Nov 23.
11. Some organs withheld for no good reason. New Orleans Times Picayune, New Orleans Edition 1994, Nov 24.
12. Sturner WQ. Can baby organs be donated in all forensic cases? Proposed guidelines for organ donation from infants under medical examiner jurisdiction. *Am J Forensic Med Pathol.* 1995; 16:215-218.
13. Associated Press (Peoria, Illinois). Doctors seek to harvest organs of crime victims. Mattoon Journal Gazzette. 1999 Feb 20.
14. Zugibe FT, Costello J, Breithaupt M, Segelbacher J. Model organ description protocols for completion by transplant surgeons using organs procured from medical examiner cases. *J Transpl Coord.* 1999; 9:73-80.
15. Vaughn K. Battle looms over organ donations. Rocky Mountain News. 2000, April 17.
16. Jaynes C, Springer JW. Evaluating a successful coroner protocol. J Transpl Coord. 1996; 6:28-31.
17. Kramer JL. Letter to the Editor. *Am J Forensic Med Pathol.* 1995; 16(3):257.
18. Lantz PE, Jason D, Davis GJ. Letter to the Editor. *Am J Forensic Med Pathol.* 1995; 16:257-259.
19. Jaynes C. In reply. *Am J Forensic Med Pathol.* 1995; 16(3):259-260.
20. Strama BT, Burling-Hatcher S, and Shafer TJ. Criminal Investigations and Prosecutions Not Adversely Affected by Organ Donation. A Case Law Review. Newsletter of Medicine and Law Committee. Tort and Insurance Practice Section, American Bar Association Summer. 1994;15-21.
21. Community Cable Television. Tarrant Topics: Dr. Nizam Peerwani, Chief Medical Examiner, Tarrant County, TX. 1993, Dec 8.
22. Donoghue ER, Lifschultz BD. Every Organ, Every Time. Could We Do It? Special Session – Organ and Tissue Donation and Effective Death Investigations: Tensions and Resolutions. Proceedings of the Annual Meeting of the National Association of Medical Examiners; 1998, Oct 30-Nov 4; Albuquerque, New Mexico.
23. Dixon DS, Blackbourne BD. Letter to the Editor. Clinical forensic medicine and organ transplantation. *Am J Forensic Med Pathol.* 1987; 8:88-91.
24. 2001 Annual Report of the U.S. Organ Procurement and Transplantation Network and the Scientific Registry for Transplant Recipients: Transplant Data 1991-2000. Department of Health and Human Services, Health Resources and Services Administration, Office of Sepcial Programs, Division of Transplanation, Rockville, MD; United Network for Organ Sharing, Richmond, VA; University Renal Research and Education Association, Ann Arbor, MI.
25. Goldstein B, Shafer TJ, Greer D, Stephens BG. Medical examiner/coroner denial for organ donation in brain-dead victims of child abuse: controversies and solutions. Clin Intensive Care. 1997; 8:136-141.
26. N.Y. County Law §674-a (McKinney 1977).
27. Tenn. Code Ann. § 38-7-108 (2002).
28. N.J. Stat. Ann. § 52:17B-88.8 (2002).
29. Tex. Health & Safety Code Ann. § 693.002 (Vernon Supp. 2003).
30. Interim report, Recommendations and Appendices 2003. DHHS Secretary's Advisory Committee on Organ Transplantation (ACOT). ACOT authorized by section 121.12 of the Amended Final Rule of the Organ Procurement and Transplantation Network (OPTN) (42 CFR Part 121).
31. California State Legislature Concurrence in Senate Amendments AB 777 (Dutton). As amended July 15, 2003 As passed ASM Floor 5/29/2003, Senate 7/21/2003.
32. Adams V, Beaver T, Coburn M Rao V, Bedore L, Bailey R, Mittlemean R. Practice Guidelines for Florida Medical Examiners; Section 1: Jurisdiction and Anatomical Gifts. Draft. 2003 May 15; Ocala, Florida:

33. Donoghue ER. Organ and Tissue Problem and Solutions. Every Organ, Every Time. Could We Do It? Annual Meeting of the North American Transplant Coordinators Organization, 2000 Aug. 6-9; Orlando, FL
34. Texas State Legislature, 78th Regular Session SB 1225 (Nelson). As passed by Senate 4/25/2003, House 5/28/2003
35. Hanzlick R, Combs D. Medical examiner and coroner systems. JAMA. 1998; 279:870-874.
36. Hanzlick R. Coroner training needs: a numerical and geographic analysis. JAMA. 1996; 276:1775-1778.
37. Shafer TJ, Schkade LL, Siminoff LA, Mahoney TA. Ethical analysis of organ recovery denials by medical examiners, coroners, and justices of the peace. *J Transpl Coord*. 1999; 9:232-249.
38. Organ Procurement Transplant Network Death removals by age group by year. Waiting list additions age by listing year. Transplants in the U.S. by recipient age. Available at: http://www.optn.org. Accessed February 16, 2003.

General NATCO Resources

Core Competencies for the Clinical and Procurement Transplant Coordinator

Core Competencies for the Requestor

Progress in Transplantation

Donor Management Compendium Volume 1

Donor Management Compendium Volume 2

These can all be obtained by contacting the NATCO Executive Office at natco-info@goamp.com or visiting the NATCO web site at www.natco1.org.

Index

Abciximab (ReoPro), 825
Abdomen, trauma to, 483
Abel, John Jacob, 131
ABG status. *See* Arterial blood gas status
ABO typing, 325
ABTC. *See* American Board of Transplant Coordinators
ACAD. *See* Allograft coronary artery disease
Access, 699
    issues, 345-346
ACE inhibitors. *See* Angiotensin-converting enzyme inhibitors
Acetaminophen, 635
ACHE. *See* American College of Healthcare Executives
Acid-base balance, 824-825
    assessment of, 838
    care guidelines for, 838
Acidosis, 422, 824
    in pediatric donors, 852
    treatment of, 838
ACOT. *See* Advisory Committee on Organ Transplantation
Acquired immunodeficiency syndrome (AIDS), 464-465
Acquisition fees, deceased donor liver transplant, 700
Actinomycin C., 140
Acute ischemia, 610
Ad Hoc Task Force, 777, 784
ADA. *See* American Diabetes Association
Adenocard IV. *See* IV adenosine
IV adenosine (Adenocard IV), 848
Adenovirus, 592-593
    clinical manifestations of, 592
    diagnosis and monitoring of, 593
    prevention and treatment of, 593
Adherence, 555-556
    factors effecting, 556
Adjusted graft survival, 358
Administrators, economics and, 366
Adolescence
    development, 692
    interventions, 692-693
    transplantation issues during, 692
Advisory Committee on Organ Transplantation (ACOT), 535, 537
AFP. *See* α-Fetoprotein
African Americans, 799-800
Aggressive pursuit, 722, 736-737
AHA. *See* American Hospital Association
AIDS. *See* Acquired immunodeficiency syndrome
Airway ischemia, 448

Akagi, Don, 297
Alanine aminotransferase (ALT), 656, 808
Albumin, 656
Alcohol abuse, 475
Alemtuzumab, 616
    adverse reactions to, 616
    dosing, 616
    mechanism of action of, 616
Alendronate, 570
Alexander, Charles E., 124, 181, 299, 300, 301, 302, 304
Alexandre, Guy, 14-15, 140, 143, 145
Alkaline phosphatase, 656
Alkalosis, 844
    treatment of, 838
Allocation. *See* Organ allocation
Allograft, 372, 378
    benefits and disadvantages of, heart valves, 383
    heart valves/conduits, 381-382
    musculoskeletal, 376-379
    skin, 379-380
    surgical specialties that use, 378
    vein and arteries, 380-381
Allograft coronary artery disease (ACAD), 437
ALT. *See* Alanine aminotransferase
American Academy of Pediatrics, 777
American Association of Tissue Banks, 342, 372, 373, 389-390
    banks accredited by, 373
    contamination control guidelines, 378
    Guidance Document, 387
    standards, 377
    Standards for Tissue Banking, 385, 387
    tests required by, 376
American Bar Association, 16
American Board of Transplant Coordinators (ABTC), 75, 76-77, 163, 165, 253-254
    goals of, 254
American Burn Association, 379-380
American College of Cardiology, 428
American College of Healthcare Executives (ACHE), 903
American Council on Transplantation, 162
American Diabetes Association (ADA), 564
American Electroencephalographic Society, 776
American Hospital Association (AHA), 903
American Registry of Transplant Coordinators (ARTC), 77
American Society of Multicultural Health and Transplant Professionals (ASMHTP), 352
American Society of Transplantation, 400

American Transplant Society (ATS), 44
Amiodarone (Cordarone), 848
Amlodipine, 562
Amos, Bernard, 149
AMP. See Applied Management Professionals
Amphotericin B, 579
Amyloidosis, 560
ANA. See Antinuclear antibodies
Analgesics, 635
Ancillary testing, 840, 841
Anderson, Billy G., 34, 88-89, 276, 356
Anemia, 826
    assessment of, 833
    care guidelines, 833
    treatment of, 833
Anencephaly, 785
Anesthesia, in organ recovery, 858-859
Angiotensin-converting enzyme (ACE) inhibitors, 562, 631, 633
Angiotensin-receptor blockers (ARBs), 633-634
Anidulafungin, 585
Anion gap, 657-658
Ankle transplantation, 179
Anti-basement membrane nephritis, 560
Antibiotics, 627
Anticoagulation medications, 825
Antifungals, 628-629
Antigenic testing, 670
Antigen-presenting cells, 608
Antigens, 606
Antihistamines, 638
Antihypertensive medications, 562, 630, 631-632
Anti-infectives, 626-629
Antinuclear antibodies (ANA), 658
Antiproliferatives, 617, 620-621
Anti-smooth muscle antibody, 658
Antithymocyte globulin rabbit (RATG)
    adverse reactions to, 615
    dosing, 615
    mechanism of action of, 615
Antithymoglobulin equine (ATG), 615
    adverse reactions to, 615
    dosing, 615
    mechanism of action of, 615
α_1-antitrypsin deficiency, 560
Antivirals, 627-628
AOPO. See Association of Organ Procurement Organizations
Aortic valve, 382
Apnea, 755-756
    in children, 775-776
    performance of, 757
    testing for, 755
Applied Management Professionals (AMP), 166
Appropriate requestor rates, 716, 730
    goals, 717
Apresoline. See Hydralazine hydrochloride
ARBs. See Angiotensin-receptor blockers
Arm elevation, 758
Armstrong, Greg, 85, 87, 166, 172, 173, 297, 298

Arnott, Lindsay, 304
Arrhythmia, 847
ARTC. See American Registry of Transplant Coordinators
Arterial blood gas (ABG) status, 824
Arterial grafts, 380-381
ASMHTP. See American Society of Multicultural Health and Transplant Professionals
Aspartate aminotransferase (AST), 656, 808
Aspergillus, 450, 573, 578
Aspirin, 825
Assessment for Transplant Candidacy, 344
Association of Operating Room Nurses, 861
Association of Organ Procurement Organizations (AOPO), 91, 110, 114, 342, 352, 362, 387, 858, 903
    Task Force on Multicultural Issues, 352
AST. See Aspartate aminotransferase
ATCA. See Australasian Transplant Coordinators Association
Atenolol, 562
ATG. See Antithymoglobulin equine
Atkins, Carolyn, 28, 30-31, 294, 303
Atkins, Jim, 303
Atorvastatin, 568
Atrial arrhythmias, 448
ATS. See American Transplant Society
Australasian Transplant Coordinators Association (ATCA), 78, 165, 166
Autonomy, 337
    living donor, 511-512
Azathioprine, 20, 24, 140, 620-621
    adverse reactions to, 621
    dosing, 621
    drug-drug interactions, 626
    mechanism of action of, 620
Azoles, 580
Azotemia, 655

B cells, 609
Babinski response, 758
Bacterial infections, 573-577
    in heart transplantation, 576
    in kidney transplantations, 574-575
    in liver transplantations, 575-576
    in lung transplantation, 576-577
    in pancreas transplantations, 574-575
BAEP. See Brainstem auditory evoked potentials
BAER. See Brainstem auditory evoked responses
Bailey, Leonard, 16-17, 161
Ballinger, Walter F., 150
Banting, Frederick G., 132
Barber, Patricia L., 155, 279
Barnard, Christian, 22, 23, 146, 427
Barnes, Benjamin, 148
Barratt-Boyes, Brian, 372
Bartucci, Marilyn R., 33, 296, 298
Basiliximab
    adverse reactions to, 615
    dosing, 614

mechanism of action of, 614
BDD. *See* Brain-dead donors
Bearden, Charles, 302
Behavior, 343–344
    change, 791
Behavioral risk assessment, 385–386
Belzer, Folkert O., 25, 53–54, 146, 165, 277
    with Kidney Preservation machine, 275
Belzer LI-400, 894
Benazepril, 562
Beneficence, 337
Beraprost, 446
Berwick, Don, 723
Best, Charles H., 132
Bicarbonate, 837
Bile acid sequestrants, 568
Biliary leaks, 544
Biliary tract, 474
Bilirubin, 656
Billing timeframes, 700
Billingham, Margaret, 435
Billingham, Rupert E., 136
Bismuth subsalicylate, 637
Bisphosphates, 570
BIVAD. *See* Bi-ventricular assist devices
Bi-ventricular assist devices (BIVAD), 431
Bladder
    drainage, 417, 422–423
    leaks, 423
Blazek, Jamie, 298
Bleeding, postoperative, 418–419, 448
Bleifuss, John, 41, 152
α-blockers, 563, 632, 634
β-blockers, 562, 631, 632–633, 846
Blood gas analysis, 812
Blood group compatibility, 329
Blood pressure, 858
    immunosuppression and, 561
Blood transfusion, 128, 826
Blood vessel connection, 129
Blundell, James, 128
Bocchino, Carmella, 169
Bogardus, G.M., 136
Bone Bank, 134
Bone marrow transplantation, 137, 147, 151
Bone transplant, 128
Borel, Jean-Francois, 152
BOS. *See* Bronchitis obliterans syndrome
Boyle, Nancy, 300
Brain death, 13–16, 137, 147, 150, 201
    CBF in, 778–781
    in children, 771–786
    clinical examination of, 747–756, 774–776
    confirmatory tests for, 760–761, 776–781
    definition of, 16
    determination of, 747
    diagnostic paradigm for, 773
    electroencephalography for, 761–767, 776–777
    explaining, 796–797
    fetal, 785
    guidelines for, in children, 772, 841
    incidence of, in children, 772
    in infants with anencephaly, 785
    MRI for, 764
    in newborns, 781–785
    observation period, 759–760
    organ donation after, 877
    in pediatric donors, 840–841
    physician competency in determining, 760
    physiology of, 841–842
    primary brainstem, 758–759
    single photon emission computed tomography for, 764
    spinal movements and reflexes in, 759
Brain ischemia, 821
Brain-dead donors (BDD), 898
Brainstem auditory evoked potentials (BAEP), 766
Brainstem auditory evoked responses (BAER), 781
Breidenback, Warren C., 176
Brent, Leslie, 136
Bretschnieder Solution, 895
Brevibloc. *See* Esmolol hydrochloride
Brigham, Lori E., 179
Brittain, Robert, 140
Brock, Ross M., 427
Bromberg, Sandy, 10
Bronchial dehiscence, 23
Bronchioalveolar carcinoma, 560
Bronchitis obliterans syndrome (BOS), 452
    grading system for, 453
Bronchoscopy supplies, 859
Brown, Marguerite, 10, 28
Broznick, Brian, 10, 36, 68, 70, 90–91, 159, 162, 292
Brunius, U., 136
Budd-Chiari syndrome, 560
Bumetanide, 562
Burden of disease, 322
Bush, Barbara, 295

CAD. *See* Coronary artery disease
Cadaveric donations, 13, 14
Calcineurin inhibitors, 564, 617, 618–6618
    adverse effects of, 619–620
    mechanism of action of, 618
Calcitonin, 570
Calcium, 570, 655, 837
    in pediatric donors, 852
Calcium channel blockers (CCB), 562, 632, 633–634
Callahan, Mike, 10
Calne, Roy, 14, 20, 21, 81, 136, 139, 140, 153
Caloric testing, 753
CAM. *See* Complementary and alternative medicine
Cameron, Beth, 30, 141
Canadian Association of Transplantation, 154
Candesartan, 562
Candida albicans, 375, 450, 578, 583, 584
Candidate selection, for pancreas transplantation, 414–416
Cannon, Jack A., 137
Capsofungin, 583–584

Captain's Announcement, 63
Captopril, 562
Carbon dioxide, 654, 822
Carcinoembryonic antigen (CEA), 467
Cardiac transplantation, 12
Cardiopulmonary bypass (CPB), 447
Cardiovascular considerations, 821
Cardiovascular disease, 406-407, 444
Carnot, Sadi, 11-12
Carotid artery, 761
Carrel, Alexis, 11-12, 21-22, 129, 130, 132, 892
Casuistry, 337
Catecholamines, 847
CAV. *See* Coronary artery vasculopathy
CBC. *See* Complete blood cell count
CBF. *See* Cerebral blood flow
CCB. *See* Calcium channel blockers
CEA. *See* Carcinoembryonic antigen
Celsior, 895
Center for Organ Recovery and Education (CORE), 90
Centers for Medicare and Medicaid Services (CMS), 903
Central venous pressure (CVP), 846
Cephalosporins, 575
Cerebral angiography, 760, 762
    in brain death determination, 761
Cerebral blood flow (CBF), 773
    determination of, 778-781
Cerebral edema, 749, 750, 751
Cerebrospinal fluid (CSF), 747
Cerivastatin, 568
Certification, 74-75
Ceruloplasmin, 658-659
Cerveau isole, 759
CF. *See* Cystic Fibrosis
Chablewski, Franki, 176, 181
Change Package, 731
Chari, Ravi S., 170
Chessare, John, 178, 180, 301
Children. *See also* Infants; Neonates; Preschoolers; School age children; Toddlers
    apnea in, 775-776
    brain death in, 771-786
    in coma, 774
Childs-Turcotte-Pugh score, 465
Chilnick, Lawrence, 279
Chinnock, Richard, 16-17
Chlamydia trachomatis, 386
Chloride, 654, 837
Chlorothiazide, 562
Chlorthalidone, 562
Cholangiocarcinoma, 560
Cholesterol absorption inhibitors, 568
Cholestyramine, 568
Choose Life, 44-45
Chronic allograft nephropathy, 405-406
Chronic intestinal pseudo-obstruction, 484
Chronic liver disease, 457-458
    causes of, 458, 459
    complications of, 460
Chronic renal disease, heart transplantation and, 439

Chrysler, Gayl, 67, 296
Churchill, Winston, 11
Ciba Symposium on Transplantation, 15
Cidofovir, 590
Cigarette smoking, 444, 812
CIT. *See* Cold ischemic time
CJD. *See* Creutzfeldt-Jakob disease
CLAS. *See* Culturally and Linguistically Appropriate Services in Health Care
Clindamycin, 627
Clinical Laboratory Improvement Act, 388
Clinical Training Courses, 288
Clofibrate, 568
Clopidogrel, 825
Clostridium difficile, 450
CMS. *See* Centers for Medicare and Medicaid Services
CMV. *See* Cytomegalovirus
Coagulation abnormalities, 825-826
    care guideline, 833-834
    in pediatric donors, 852-853
Coagulation factors, 653
Coccidioides, 451
Cochran, Larry, 285
Codeine, 638
Cohen, Bernard, 157, 162
Cold ischemic time (CIT), 893, 896
Cold storage (CS), 892, 893, 895
Coleman, Lori, 304
Colesevelam, 568
Colestipol, 568
Collaborative Learning Sessions and Action Periods, 714
Collins, Geoffrey, 149
Collins, William, 14
Colpart, Jean-Jacques, 169
Coma, 751
    alerts, 751
    children in, 774
    technique for assessing, 751
Comellas, Carrie, 300, 304
Committee reports, 65-66
Communitarianism, 336
Comorbidities, 413
Complementary and alternative medicine (CAM), 639-641
    drug-drug interactions with, 639-640
    hepatotoxicity of, 640
    immunomodulating effects of, 641
    immunosuppresion and, 639
    nephrotoxicity of, 640
Complete blood cell count (CBC), 461, 651-653
Compliance, 555-556
Comprehensive metabolic panel, 653-657
Computed tomography (CT), 462, 747, 748, 805
    scan patterns, 748
    xenon, 779
Condie, Richard, 139
Conflicts of interest, 512-513
Connective tissue, 377
Conrad, Suzanne Lane, 114-115, 179
Consent environment, 792-794

structuring, 794
Continuous positive airway pressure (CPAP), 755
Contraception, 674
Contracting, 702–703
   detail, 702
   evaluation and marketing, 703
   implementation, 703
   obtaining, 702–703
Converse, John Marquis, 96, 136
Conversion rates, 713, 716, 725, 729
   goals, 717
Cooley, Denton, 23, 147
Coon, Ann Christin, 158
Cooper, Joel, 24, 159, 164
Cordarone. See Amiodarone
CORE. See Center for Organ Recovery and Education
Corneal reflex, 754
Corneal transplantation, 373
Coronary artery disease (CAD), 462, 811
Coronary artery vasculopathy (CAV), 437
   invasive diagnostic tests for, 437
   management of, 437
Coroners. See Medical examiners/coroners
Corry, Robert, 107
Corticosteroids, 617, 622, 624–625
   adverse drug reactions, 622
   dosing, 622
   mechanism of action of, 622
Cosimi, A. Benedict, 156
Cosmos, Saint, 11, 127
Cost accounts for IOPOs, 361–362
Cough
   response, 754
   suppressants, 638–639
CPAP. See Continuous positive airway pressure
CPB. See Cardiopulmonary bypass
Crandall, Betty C., 37
Creatinine, 655, 809
   clearance of, 657
Cremaster reflex, 758
Creutzfeldt-Jakob disease (CJD), 375
Critical Care Nurse, 176, 181
Crohn's disease, 483
Cross contamination, 377
Crossmatch, 607
Cryoprecipitate, 275
Cryopreservation, 381
   heart valve, 382
   vessel allograft, 381
Cryptococcus, 451
Cryptogenic cirrhosis, 560
CS. See Cold storage
CSF. See Cerebrospinal fluid
CT. See Computed tomography
Cultural competency, 351–353
Cultural distinctions, 339
Culturally and Linguistically Appropriate Services in Health Care (CLAS), 353
Cultures, 669–670
CVP. See Central venous pressure

Cyclosporine, 20, 21, 24–25, 45–46, 152, 153, 567, 624–625, 630, 677
   dosing, 618
   drug-drug interactions, 624
CYP3A4, 582, 584, 638
CYP450 system, 582, 583, 624
Cystic Fibrosis (CF), 521
Cytokines, 609
Cytomegalovirus (CMV), 461, 468, 496, 523, 573, 586–588, 810
   clinical manifestations of, 586
   diagnosis and monitoring of, 586, 667
   immune globulin, 589
   prevention of, 586–586
   treatment of, 588, 589

Daclizumab (Zenapax), 25, 614–615
   adverse reactions to, 615
   dosing, 614
   mechanism of action of, 614
Dameshek, William, 139
Damien, Saint, 11, 127
Darvall, Denise, 22, 146
Data management, 703–704
Dausset, Jean G.P.J., 138, 149
Davis, Faye D., 35, 156, 158, 161, 280, 289, 290, 291, 293
   certificate of merit given to, 265
Day, Claire, 28, 30, 141, 155, 286, 290, 295
DCCT. See Diabetes Control and Complications Trial
DCD. See Donation after cardiac death
DCS. See Donation Clinical Specialist
Death Committees, 13
Death Record Reviews, 738
DeBakey, Michael E., 148
Decastello, Alfred von, 129
Deceased donors
   kidney, 395
   liver, 700
Dehydration, 422
Delaware Valley Transplant Program, 202
Delayed graft function (DGF), 395, 810, 895, 896
DeMayo, Eileen, 291
Demeester, Wivina, 163
Demikhov, Vladimir, 12, 22, 23, 133
Demske, Amy, 301
Demsopressin, 850
Denny, Donald, 10, 33, 46, 47, 70, 158, 159, 162, 290, 291
   prepared statement of, 197–208
   questioning of, 208–223
   statement of, 192–197
Denys, Jean-Baptiste, 127
Department of Health and Human Services (DHHS), 321, 695
Department of Health, Education, and Welfare, 360
Derom, Frits, 149
Descotes, J., 137, 138
Designated requestors, 730
Desmoid tumors, abdominal, 483
"The Desperate Hunt for Life" (article), 68–69

Deutsche Stiftung Organtransplantation, 160
Devauchelle, Bernard, 180
DeVries, William C., 156
Dextromethorphan, 638
DGF. See Delayed graft function
DHHS. See Department of Health and Human Services
Diabetes Control and Complications Trial (DCCT), 501
Diabetes insipidus, 832, 842
  in pediatric donors, 850-851
Diabetes mellitus, 564-565. See also Posttransplant Diabetes Mellitus
  risk factors, 565
  transplant options for, 415
Diabetic nephropathy, 560
Diagnostic related groups (DRGs), 368-369
Dialysis, 12-13, 131, 132, 133, 135
  long-term, 139
  survival rates of patients receiving, 394
DIC. See Disseminated intravascular coagulation
Diffuse panbronchiolitis, 560
Digital subtraction angiography (DSA), 780
Diltiazem, 562
Discharge planning
  education on, 555
  lung transplantation, 451-452
Disseminated intravascular coagulation (DIC), 809
Distribution, musculoskeletal donation, 378
Diuretics, 562, 632
Division of Organization Transplantation, 47
Dobutamine, 847
Donahue, Phil, 291
Donation after cardiac death (DCD), 723, 742-743, 808, 840, 877-878, 895, 897, 898
  candidates for, 883
  collaborative OPO and hospital processes, 872
  community involvement in policy-making, 870
  controlled v. uncontrolled, 878, 879
  critical pathway for, 878
  determination of death, 871
  education of staff, 873-874
  ethics committee and, 873
  family considerations in, 872
  heart transplantation, 889
  key hospital departments for, 870
  kidney transplantation, 886-887
  lung transplantation, 889
  medical management of, 873, 882-883
  pancreas transplantation, 887-888
  phases of, 880, 881
  policy for, 867-874
  prediction of death in, 882
  preliminary evaluation of candidates for, 878-881
  sample policy for, 868-869
  scoring system for, 884
  team member roles, 870
  transplantation and end-of-life care and, 876
  understanding, 876
  withdrawal of support, 871-872, 883-886
Donation and transplantation continuum, 340
Donation Clinical Specialist (DCS), 730-731
  Change Package, 731
  Improvement Model, 731
Donation huddles, 872
Donation rates, in multicultural communities, 354
Donation service area (DSA), 867
Donor Action Foundation, 175
Donor age, 199
Donor cards, 200
Donor criteria
  for heart transplantation, 432-433
  for lung transplantation, 447
Donor designation, 384
Donor information forms, 522
Donor reconstruction, 389
Donor registries, 342
Donors Before Non-Donor numbers, 725
Dopamine, 847
Drangstveit, Mary Beth, 299
Dreffer, Ronald L., 34, 103, 161, 162, 282, 289, 290, 291, 294, 302
DRGs. See Diagnostic related groups
Driver, Lynne, 292, 304
Drug-induced immunological tolerance, 139
DSA. See Digital subtraction angiography; Donation service area
Dubernard, Jean-Michel, 175, 177, 180
Dubost, Charles, 135
Duckworth, Bob, 10, 32-33, 56, 71-72, 163, 282, 284, 302
Dunne-Smith, Gina, 300, 304
Dutton, Sue, 289, 291
Dyslipidemia, 567
  treatment of, 568

E. coli, 575
Eakin, Mark, 171, 179
EBV. See Epstein-Barr virus
ECD. See Expanded criteria donors
ECG. See Electrocardiograms
Echinocandins, 582
Economics, 359
  global contracting, 367-368
  implications of, for administrators, 366
  Medicaid and, 368
  medicare beneficiaries, 366-367
  Medicare physician fee schedule, 369
  OPO overview of, 359-360
  reimbursement, 360-361
  transplant center, 363-365
ECS. See Electrocerebral silence
Edmonton Protocol, 175
Education. See also Learning; Public education
  on adherence and compliance, 555-556
  DCD, 873-874
  on discharge planning, 555
  for end-stage organ disease patients, 552-553
  on expanded criteria donation, 554
  on living donation, 553
  on long-term health promotion, 557
  medication-related factors, 556-557

on medications, 555
methods of, 551
on multiple listing, 554
organ allocation, 552
patient, 550-551
patient-specific factors, 556
posttransplant, 555-557
pretransplant teaching, 551
on risks and benefits, 554
on standard criteria donation, 553
tools, 550
transplant team in, 552
transplantation options, 553-554
transplant-related factors, 557
on when to call transplant team, 557
Education Committee, 65-66
EEG. See Electroencephalography
EF. See Ejection fraction
Effective communication, 791-792
800-DONORALERT, 55, 193
Eisenmenger's syndrome, 441
Ejection fraction (EF), 811
Electrocardiograms (ECG), 811
Electrocautery units, 859
Electrocerebral silence (ECS), 776
Electroencephalography (EEG), 760, 773
    in brain death determination, 761-767, 776-777
    initial findings, 777
    isoelectric, 763
Electrolyte balance, 470, 580, 822-824
    care guidelines for, 836-837
    in pediatric donors, 849-850
Elick, Barbara, 10, 17, 37, 67, 109, 168, 169, 288, 295, 303
Eligible donors, 716
Emmit, Lea, 289
En bloc techniques, 887
Enalapril, 562
End stage renal disease (ESRD), 197, 364, 393, 414, 891
    regulation follow-up, 272
End Stage Renal Disease Medicare Amendment, 13
Endocrine function, 421
End-of-life care, 876
Endomyocardial biopsy, 434
    grading system, 435
Endotracheal tube (ETT), 843, 844
Enteric conversion, 423
Enteric drainage, 417
Enterobacteriaceae, 575
Epoprostenol (Flolan), 446
Epstein-Barr virus (EBV), 451, 496, 523, 573, 591-592, 665-666
    clinical manifestations of, 592
    diagnosis and monitoring of, 592
    infection, 666
    prevention of, 592
    treatment of, 592
Eptifibatide (Integrilin), 825
Equity, 322
Esmolol hydrochloride (Brevibloc), 846
ESRD. See End stage renal disease
Estrogen, 570
ETCO. See European Transplant Coordinators Organization
Ethacrynic acid, 562
Ethics. See Medical ethics
Ethics Committee, 65-66
    on criminals, 344
    DCD and, 873
Ethics of care, 337
Ethnicity, 799-800
Etidronate, 570
ETT. See Endotracheal tube
EuroCollins, 895
European Beat Practice Guidelines, 677
European Transplant Coordinators Organization (ETCO), 25, 78-79, 157, 162, 164, 167, 170, 173, 174
Eurotransplant, 145
Evoked potentials, 766-767, 781
    brainstem auditory, 766-767
    somatosensory, 766-767, 781
Exocrine secretion drainage, in pancreas transplantation, 416-417
Expanded criteria donors (ECD), 396-397, 809, 813-814, 895, 898
    education on, 554
Expectorants, 638-639
Eye Bank Association of America, 342, 373
Ezetimibe, 568

Facial motor response, examination of, 753
    alerts, 753
    technique for, 753
Factor V Leiden, 659-660
Fageeh, Wafa, 177
Falvey, Sue, 85, 297
Family, 371
    DCD and, 872
    divided/dysfunctional, 799
    support, 389
Famulari, Antonio, 157
FDA. See Food and Drug Administration
Fee schedules, 369
Felodipine, 562
Femoral arteries, 761
Fenofibrate, 568
Fertility, 673
β-Fetoprotein (AFP), 658
Fibrates, 568
Fibrinogen, 834
Financial incentives, for living donors, 517
Fine, Richard, 44
Fine, Shawney, 34, 41, 152
Finn, Jan, 300, 304
First person consent, 798
Fish oil, 562
Fiske, Charles, 47
Fiske, Jamie, 47
Fiske, Marilyn, 47

FK506, 21
Flolan. *See* Epoprostenol
Fluconazole, 580–581
Flucystine, 580
Fluid balance, 496–497, 822–824
    care guidelines for, 836–837
    in pediatric donors, 849–850
Fluoroquinolones, 575
Fluvastatin, 568
Focal segmental glomerulosclerosis, 560
Food and Drug Administration (FDA), 372, 375–376, 388, 806
    tests required by, 376
Foscarnet, 589
Fosinopril, 562
Foster, Tabatha, 164
Friedman, Barry S., 121, 296, 298, 300, 302
Fulminant hepatic failure, 459–460
    causes of, 459
Fundamental donor care, 829
Funeral arrangements, 797–798
Fungal infections, 450, 577–585
    heart transplantation, 578–585
    in intestinal transplantation, 577–578
    in kidney transplantation, 577
    in liver transplantation, 577–578
    lung transplantation, 578
    in pancreas transplantation, 577
    treatment of, 579–585
Furosemide, 562

Gabel, Haken, 85
Gaines, Paul, 287
Gale, Pam, 118
Gamberg, Patricia, 32
Gambro, 894
Ganciclovir, 589, 591
Garvey, Cathy, 304
Gastrointestinal anastamosis (GIA) stapler, 864
Gastrointestinal complications
    heart transplantation and, 438
    lung transplantation and, 449
Gastroschisis, 483
Gemfibrozil, 568
Genitourinary evaluation, 398
Geographic distribution, 667–668
GF. *See* Graft failure
GIA stapler. *See* Gastrointestinal anastamosis stapler
Giannini, Sandro, 179
Giant cell interstitial pneumonitis, 560
Gibbon, John Heysham, 136
Gift of Life Donor Program, 885
Gift-specific donation, 376–383
"The Gift of Life" (article), 70
Gilman, Cy, 155
Gilmore, Christine J., 113–114, 172, 173, 293, 298
Global contracting, 367–368
Glucose, 655, 810, 824. *See also* Hyperglycemia; Hypoglycemia
    care guidelines for management of, 831
    in pediatric donors, 851
Glucose regulation, 421–422
Glycemic control, postoperative, 419
Glycosylated hemoglobin, 657
Gohke, Mary, 23–24
Goldman, Mitch, 292
Good, Robert A., 147
Goodwin, William E., 17
Gore, Albert, 46, 158
    in National Organ Transplant Act hearings, 208–223
Gorer, Peter, 134, 140
Gosnell, Robert, 29, 43, 45, 65, 100, 141, 153, 156, 280, 286, 302, 303
Goulet, Olivier, 167
Goulon, M., 137
Graft failure (GF), 896
Graft pancreatitis, 420–421
Graham, Judy S., 120, 178, 299
Graham, Michael, 904
Graham, Thomas, 128
Graham, Walter, 296
Gram stains, 668
Gram-negative bacteria, 668
Gram-positive bacteria, 668
Grant, David R., 166
Green, Nicholas, 171
Guaifenesin, 638–639
Guthrie, Charles, 21–22
Gutkind, Lee, 10

Haas, Georg, 132
Haemophilus influenzae, 450
Haid, Steve, 66, 104, 164, 291, 294
Hakala, Thomas R., 202
Hall, Brandon, 47, 264
Hall, Gary, 26, 46, 92, 158, 285
Hall, Julie, 44, 153
Hamburger, Jean, 14, 18, 135, 136, 137, 138, 139, 143
Hammond, Alesha, 294
Hand transplantation, 144, 176
Hardwick, Ben, 81
Hardy, James, 22, 142, 143
Harrell, Jason, 285
Harrington, Nancy, 304
Harrison, Hartwell, 19, 136
Harvey, William, 127
Hasskamp, Bill, 304
HAT. *See* Hepatic artery thrombosis
Hatch, Orrin G., 160
HBcAg. *See* Hepatitis B core antigen
HBV. *See* Hepatitis B
HCC. *See* Hepatocellular carcinoma
HCV. *See* Hepatitis C
Health care, 203
    policy development, 709
Health Care Financing Administration, 208
Health Insurance Portability and Accountability Act of 1996, 704
Health Resources and Services Administration (HRSA), 108, 695

Hearings, National Organ Transplant, 184-191
Heart allocation, 324-325
    blood type Z designation and, 325
    pediatric, 324
    prioritization, 324
    sensitized, 325
    status code for, 324
Heart transplantation, 21-23, 129, 137, 143
    bacterial infections in, 576
    biatrial techniques, 433
    bicaval techniques, 433
    causes of death after, 428
    CAV and, 437
    chronic renal disease and, 439
    contraindications for, 428-429
    DCD and, 889
    donor management, 432-433
    early reports of, 21-22
    evaluation of donors, 811-812
    evaluation of recipients, 429, 430
    expected outcomes, 427
    first human to human, 22-23
    fungal infections in, 578-585
    gastrointestinal complications of, 438
    hyperlipidemia and, 439
    hypertension and, 438-439
    indications for, 428-429
    infection and, 437
    long-term complications of, 437-440
    malignancy and, 438
    mechanical bridging to, 431-432
    organ recovery, 863
    osteoporosis and, 439
    pharmacological bridging to, 431-432
    pig, 147
    posttransplant considerations, 434-439
    pregnancy and, 682
    rejection, 434-437
    risk factors for mortality during, 428
    selection and listing of recipients, 430
    surgical problems, 433
    transplantation surgery, 433-434
    waiting period, 430-432
Heart valve transplantations, 381-382
Heart-lung allocation, 327
Heart-lung transplant, 147, 155, 448
    programs, 207
Heckler, Margaret, 47
Heigel, Bernd, 151, 153, 157
Hematocrit, 652
Hematopoietic abnormalities, kidney transplantation and, 408
Hematuria, 422
Hemochromatosis, 560
Hemodynamic instability, in pediatric donors, 846-848
Hemoglobin, 651
    glycosylated, 657
    in plasma, 653
Hemolytic uremic syndrome, 560
Henoch-Schönlein purpura, 560

HEPA. *See* High-efficiency particulate air
Hepatectomy, 542
    left, 542
    left lateral, 542
    right, 542
Hepatic artery thrombosis (HAT), 459
Hepatitis A, 464
Hepatitis B (HBV), 386, 464, 471, 475, 476, 560, 573, 595, 807
    diagnosis and monitoring of, 595
    interpretation of panel, 661
    prevention and treatment of, 595
    serological tests for, 660-661
Hepatitis B core antigen (HBcAg), 661
Hepatitis C (HCV), 375, 386, 471, 475, 560, 573, 595-596, 680, 807
    diagnosis and monitoring of, 596, 663
    infection with, 662-663
    long-term effects of, 662
    prevention and treatment of, 596, 663
    transmission of, 662
Hepatobiliary evaluation, 398
Hepatocellular carcinoma (HCC), 458, 460, 463, 476, 560
    recurrent, 475
Hernandez, Nelva Lou, 148
Herpes simplex virus (HSV), 451, 461, 590-591
    clinical manifestations of, 590-591
    diagnosis and monitoring of, 591, 666
    prevention and treatment of, 591
HES. *See* Hydroxyethyl starch
Heterograft, 144
Hexylmethylpropylene amineoxine (HMPAO), 778
High-efficiency particulate air (HEPA), 377
Hiraga, Seigo, 81-82, 85, 86, 87, 172, 297
Hirschsprung's disease, 484
Hispanic Americans, 799
Histoplasma capsulatum, 451
Hitchings, Claude, 142
HIV, 344, 372, 375, 385, 386, 388, 461, 573, 807
    diagnostic testing of, 664
HLA system. *See* Human leucocyte antigen
HMG-CoA reductase inhibitors, 568
HMPAO. *See* Hexylmethylpropylene amineoxine
Hoffmann, Frances M., 115
Hoffmann, Robert, 25, 28, 29, 54, 141, 156, 277, 292
    with Kidney Preservation machine, 275
HOPOs. *See* Hospital based OPOs
Hormone replacement therapy, 673, 683
    in pediatric donors, 848-849
Horns, Gloria, 34-35
Hospital based OPOs (HOPOs), 360
Hospital donation system design, 739-744
    DCD and, 742-743
    early referral, rapid response, 741-742
    effective requesting, 742
    institutional mission, 740
    self-organizing OPOs, 741
    senior management in, 740-741
House, Mary Ann, 157, 284, 289

HRSA. *See* Health Resources and Services Administration
HSV. *See* Herpes simplex virus
HTK. *See* Ketoglutarate solution
HTLV. *See* Human T-cell leukemia-lymphoma virus
Hudson, Alan R., 166
Hufnagel, Charles, 134
Human leucocyte antigen (HLA) system, 134, 138, 329, 522, 605
   class I molecules, 606
   class II molecules, 606
   crossmatch, 607
   discrepant, 330
   preformed antibodies and, 607
   typing, 606
Human papilloma virus, 593–594
   clinical manifestations of, 593
   diagnosis and monitoring of, 594
   prevention of, 594
   treatment of, 594
Human parvovirus B19, 593
   clinical manifestations of, 593
   diagnosis and monitoring of, 593
   prevention and treatment of, 593
Human T-cell leukemia-lymphoma virus (HTLV), 807
Human transmissible spongiform encephalopathy, 386
Hume, David, 14, 17, 20, 134, 135, 139, 141, 149
Hume, Kate, 34, 35, 43, 44, 100, 153, 155, 279, 280, 294
Humphries, Arthur, 145
Hunsicker, Larry L., 179
Hunter, John, 127
Hydralazine hydrochloride (Apresoline), 846
Hydrocortisone, 849
Hydroxyethyl starch (HES), 892
Hyperglycemia, 421–422, 851
   management of, 831
Hyperkalemia, 836–837
Hyperlipidemia, 407, 565–567
   heart transplantation and, 439
Hypernatremia, 823, 836
Hypertension, 560–561, 563, 629–634, 821
   care guidelines, 829–830
   epidemiology of, 630
   heart transplantation and, 438–439
   intracranial, 846
   pathophysiology of, 630
   risk factors for, 561
   treatment of, 630–634, 830
Hyperthermia, 826
Hypoglycemia, 421, 851
   management of, 831
Hypokalemia, 837
Hyponatremia, 836
   euvolemic, 653
   hypervolemic, 653
   hypovolemic, 653
Hypotension, 756, 821
   assessment of, 830
   care guidelines, 830
   treatment algorithms, 830

Hypothermia, 777, 826

Ibandronate, 570
ICOP. *See* International Congress on Organ Procurement
ICP. *See* Intracranial pressure
ICUs. *See* Intensive care units
IDAT. *See* Independent donor advocates team
Idiopathic pulmonary hemosiderosis, 560
IgA nephropathy, 560
IHC. *See* In-house coordinators
IHI. *See* Institute for Healthcare Improvement
Iloprost, 446
Imminent death, 716
Immune origin of rejection, 133
Immunofluorescence, 670
Immunological evaluation, 398
Immunology
   immune responses, 608–610
   immune system cells, 605
   of rejection, 610
   upregulation of immune response, 610–611
Immunomodulation, 641
Immunosuppression, 137, 139, 140, 467
   acute rejection treatment, 623
   blood pressure and, 561
   CAM and, 639
   chemical, 139
   complications of, 453
   drug-drug interactions, 623–626
   expenses of, 701
   induction of, 402, 613–616
   in kidney transplant recipients, 402–405
   lung transplantation and, 450
   maintenance of, 402, 617–622
   metabolic pathways of, 624
   renal disease and, 563
   withdrawal and conversion, 404
Improvement Model, 731
Independent donor advocates, 513
Independent donor advocates team (IDAT), 535
   role of, 537
Independent organ procurement organizations (IOPO), 361
   cost account for, 361–362
Induction therapies, 402, 613–616
Infants, 687–688. *See also* Sudden infant death syndrome
   brain death in, 785
   development of, 688
   interventions, 688
   reflex development in, 774
   transplantation issues, 688
Infections. *See also* Bacterial infections; Fungal infections; Viral infections
   after lung transplantation, 450–451
   heart transplantation and, 437
   intestinal transplantation, 495–496
   intra-abdominal, 419
   kidney transplantation and, 406
   urinary tract, 422–423

Infectious disease status, 344–345
   testing for, 376, 388
Informed consent, 341–342
   basic elements of, 348
   living donor, 346–347, 514
   model elements of, 348–349
Infusion-related reactions, 580
In-house coordinators (IHC), 738, 792, 796
INR. *See* International normalized ratio
Institute for Healthcare Improvement (IHI), 714, 903
Institutional mission, 740
Integrated donation process management, 720–723, 735–736
   achieving, 721–722
Integrilin. *See* Eptifibatide
Intensive care management, after liver transplant, 470–471
Intensive care units (ICUs), 857, 876
Interferon-γ, 609
Interim Rule for Donors of Human Tissues for Transplantation, 385
Internal Revenue Service (IRS), 361
International Congress on Organ Procurement (ICOP), 84
International distribution, 374–375
International normalized ratio (INR), 808
International Transplant Coordinators Meeting (ITCM), 255–256
   invitation to, 273
International Transplant Coordinators Society (ITCS), 84–87, 122, 172, 176, 178, 180, 297
   welcome address, 87
International Transplant Registry, 492
Inter-regional collaboration, 207
Intestinal allocation, 328
Intestinal atresia, 483
Intestinal failure, 483
   irreversibility of, 487
Intestinal transplantation, 164
   causes of death from, 495
   consultations required for, 489
   evaluation for, 485–490
   fluid balance, 496
   fungal infections in, 577–578
   graft removal, 495
   immediate postoperative care, 494
   indications for, 481–484
   infections, 495–496
   initial referral for, 486
   laboratory testing for evaluation of, 488
   listing for, 490
   living donor, 492
   long-term management, 497
   nursing considerations, 494
   nutrition and, 496–497
   patient survival, 498
   radiology tests for, 489
   recipient operations, 491–492
   rejection, 494–495
   surgical, 491
   surgical complications, 493
   waiting times for, 490
Intestinal-liver allocation, 328
Intra-abdominal infection, 419
Intracranial pressure (ICP), 779, 784
IOPO. *See* Independent organ procurement organizations
Irbesartan, 562
IRS. *See* Internal Revenue Service
Ischemic heart disease, 560
Islet administration, 506
   procedural care after, 506
Islet allocation, 332
Islet cell transplantation, 150, 179, 332
   candidates for, 504
   common screening eligibility questions, 502
   common tests performed during evaluation, 503
   contraindications for, 501–502
   evaluation process, 502
   indications for, 501
   medications, 506–507, 507
   procedural risks of, 505
   procedure for, 505–506
   product release testing, 505
   rejection, 507
   risks and benefits of, 504–505
Isotonic fluids, 847
Isradipine, 562
Israel Penn International Transplant Tumor Registry, 813
ITCM. *See* International Transplant Coordinators Meeting
ITCS. *See* International Transplant Coordinators Society
Itraconazole, 581

Jaboulay, Mathieu, 18
Jacobbi, Louise M., 108, 161, 163, 281, 303
Jankiewicz, Timothy, 171
Japanese Transplant Coordinators Organization (JATCO), 81–84, 93, 168
JATCO. *See* Japanese Transplant Coordinators Organization
JCAHO. *See* Joint Commission on Accreditation of Healthcare Organizations
Johnson, Keith, 61, 161
Joint Commission on Accreditation of Healthcare Organizations (JCAHO), 352, 379, 714, 903
Jones, Linda, 28, 30, 41, 66, 110, 153, 170, 279, 302
Jos, Philip, 279
Journal of Transplant Coordination. See Progress in Transplantation
Jouvet, Michel, 137, 138
Justice, 337

Kantianism, 336
Kantrowitz, Adrian, 146
Karbe, Tom, 85, 293
Kato, Osamu, 82, 85, 297
Kean, Anne, 791
Keen-Denton, Karyn, 171

Kelleher, Mary Dunston, 134
Kelley, Stephen, 28, 31, 141, 278
Kelly, William, 24, 145, 149
Kemp, Charles B., 150
Kermer, Christian, 178
Ketoglutarate solution (HTK), 895
Kidney allocation, 328–330
    blood group compatibility, 329
    double, 330
    expanded criteria donor, 330
    pediatric, 330
    previous living donors and, 330
    standard, 329–330
    wait time, 329
Kidney donors, deceased v. living, 395
Kidney Preservation machine, 275, 276
    first working, 277
Kidney transplant alone (KTA), 411
Kidney transplantation, 18–20, 130, 131, 133, 134, 135, 136, 137, 138, 200. *See also* Living kidney donors
    adjusted graft survival, 358
    animal to human, 131
    bacterial infections in, 574–575
    cadaveric, 140, 141
    contraindications to, 399
    DCD and, 886–887
    diagram of diseases and transplanted kidney, 401
    donors for, 135
    evaluation of donors, 808–810
    evaluation of recipients, 398–399
    first recorded animal to human, 18
    first recorded human to human, 18
    fungal infections in, 577
    graft survival in, 393
    hematopoietic abnormalities and, 408
    immunosuppression in, 402–405
    infectious complications of, 406
    long-term complications, 406–408
    malignancy and, 407–408
    operative procedure, 401–402
    organ recovery, 862
    postoperative management of, 402–409
    preemptive, 398
    pregnancy and, 677–678
    preoperative management, 400–401
    recipient selection criteria, 397–400
    rejection, 405–406
    short-term complications of, 402
    skeletal disorders and, 408
    successful, 136
    types of donors, 395–397
    waiting list, 394, 400
Kidneys, transplantation of, 17
Kitagawa, Sadayoshi, 82
Klintmalm, Goran, 82
Kluyskens, Paul, 149
Kneteman, Norman, 169
Kochik, Rob, 294
Kolff, Willem J., 12, 133

Kong, Sally, 162, 172, 176, 297
Koop, C. Everett, 101
Kootstra, Gauke, 173
Kory, Lisa, 111, 301
Kountz, Samuel, 53, 279
KTA. *See* Kidney transplant alone
Küss, René, 135, 139

Labetalol (Trandate, Normodyne), 846
Laboratory blood tests, 461
Lactobacillus, 637
Lacy, Paul E., 150
Lakey, Jonathan, 24–25, 175
Landsteiner, Ernest, 134
Landsteiner, Karl, 129
Language barriers, 357, 799
Laparoscopic nephrectomy, 532
LaPointe Rudow, Dianne, 123, 180, 181, 182, 299, 300, 301, 304
Larynx transplantation, 149
Lawler, Richard H., 134
Laxatives, 635–637
    bulk-forming, 635–636
    emollient, 636
    lubricant, 636
    osmotic, 636
    saline, 636
    stimulant, 636–637
LCMV. *See* Lymphocytic choriomeningitis virus
LDLT. *See* Living donor liver transplantation; Living donor lung transplantation
Leacock, John Henry, 128
Learning. *See also* Education
    needs, 549
    sessions, 718
    styles, 357
Leavitt, Michael, 301
Lee, HM, 139
Left ventricular assist devices (LVAD), 431
Left ventricular hypertrophy (LVH), 811
Legal Committee, 65–66
Legionella, 450
Length of stay (LOS), 368
Leslie-Bottenfield, Helen, 89
Leukocytes, 610
Levothyroxine (Synthroid), 848
Lexer, Enrich, 131
Liberal individualism, 336
Life on the Cutting Edge of Medicine (Duckworth), 71–73
LifeLine, 119
LifeNet, 88, 89
Lillehei, Richard, 23, 24, 145, 146, 149
Lindbergh, Charles, 132, 892
Linkage, 720, 734–735
Lipcaman, Gerda, 41, 153, 279
Lisinopril, 562
Listeria monocytogenes, 450, 573
Liver allocation, 327–328
    considerations for, 328
    MELD/PELD scores and, 327–328

for segmental transplantation, 328
Liver transplantation, 21, 137, 146, 167
    acquisition fees, 700
    allograft rejection, 474–475
    bacterial infections in, 575–576
    biliary tract complications of, 474
    care management of recipients, 470–471
    cause of complications of, 473
    causes of, 457–460
    complexities of, 470
    complications after, 472–476
    consultations for, 463–464
    contraindications to, 464–465
    DCD and, 888–889
    diagnosis of complications of, 473
    donor characteristics, 469
    evaluation, 460–464, 808
    evaluation of dysfunction after, 471
    first, 21
    fungal infections in, 577–578
    initial assessment, 461
    laboratory testing, 461–462
    liver function after, 470
    minimal listing criteria, 465–466
    organ recovery, 862–863
    organ source, 468
    pregnancy and, 680, 681
    presentation of complications of, 473
    primary graft dysfunction, 472
    recurrent disease after, 475–476
    split, 166
    surgery, 469–470
    timing of, 466
    treatment of complications of, 473
    vascular complications of, 472–473
    waiting list management, 467–468
Liver-bowl transplantation, 166
Liver-intestine enbloc graft, 492
Living donor liver transplantation (LDLT), 457, 469
    adult, 535
    cancer screening of donors, 538–540
    consultations, 540
    contraindications to, 536–537
    donor complications, 544
    educational needs of donor, 541–542
    evaluation of donors, 538–541
    financial effects of, 545–546
    follow-up care, 542–543
    history of, 535–536
    IDAT in, 537
    infectious disease screening in donors, 540
    initial screening of donors, 538
    laboratory evaluation of donors, 538
    liver-related complications, 544–545
    long-term complications of, 546
    medical evaluation of donors, 538
    outcomes for donors in, 543
    psychological effects of, 545
    psychosocial evaluation of donors, 540
    pulmonary complications, 545
    quality of life after, 546
    radiological evaluation of donors, 540
    selection criteria, 536
    short-term complications of, 544–545
    surgical considerations of donors, 540
    surgical procedure, 542
    wound complications, 545
Living donor lung transplantation (LDLT), 521
    evaluation phase, 523–524
    follow-up care, 525
    outcomes for donors in, 525
    selection criteria/screening phase for, 521–523
    surgical procedure, 524
Living donors, 346–347
    autonomous decision making, 511–512
    consent, 346–347
    differences, 510–511
    educating, 523, 553
    ethics of, 509–518
    financial incentives for, 517
    independent advocates, 513
    informed consent, 514
    intestinal transplantation, 492
    nondirected, 515
    psychosocial evaluations, 515–516
    relationship, 346
    risks and benefits, 514–515
    selection of, 493
    solicitation, 516–517
Living kidney donors, 396–397, 527
    activities of, 532–533
    complications of, 533
    consultations, 529–530
    contraindications to, 528
    diagnostic testing of, 529
    educational needs of, 531
    evaluation of, 528–529
    exclusion criteria, 528
    hospitalization of, 532–533
    laboratory testing of, 529
    medical evaluation of, 529
    outcomes of, 533–534
    psychosocial evaluation of, 531
    restrictions of, 532–533
    selection criteria, 527
    surgical considerations, 532
Living related donors (LRD), 891
Long-term complications, 559–571
Loperamide, 637
Loring, Louise, 65
LOS. *See* Length of stay
Losartan, 562
Lovastatin, 568
Lower, Richard, 22, 140, 144, 427
LRD. *See* Living related donors
Lung allocation, 325–326
    calculating score, 445
    score, 326
    sequence of adult donor, 326
Lung rupture, 821

Lung transplantation, 23–24, 142, 149
    bacterial infections in, 576–577
    bridges to, 446
    cardiovascular management after, 450
    contraindications to, 444–445
    criteria for recipient selection, 441–442
    DCD and, 889
    diagnostic tests for recipient evaluation, 443
    discharge planning, 451–452
    donor criteria for, 447
    double, 448
    evaluation process, 442–444, 812–813
    fungal infections in, 578
    gastrointestinal complications, 449
    immediate postoperative care, 449
    indications for, 441, 442
    long term management, 453
    maintenance immunosuppression, 450
    nutrition after, 450
    organ recovery, 863–864
    pediatric donors and, 843–845
    posttransplant care, 449–450
    pregnancy and, 682
    recurrent disease, 453–454
    reevaluation while waiting for, 446
    rejection, 452–453
    respiratory management, 449–450
    risks and benefits of, 445
    single, 447
    surgery, 447–449
    surgical complications, 448–449
    waiting period for, 445–446
Luskin, Richard, 179
LVAD. *See* Left ventricular assist devices
LVH. *See* Left ventricular hypertrophy
Lymphangioleiomyomatosis, 560
Lymphocytic choriomeningitis virus (LCMV), 596
Lymphoid depletion, 21

Maastricht donor classification, 897
MacEwan, William, 371–372
Machine perfusion (MP), 892, 901
    in clinical setting, 900
Machine perfusion solution (MPS), 893
Mack, Winifred B., 35, 43, 46, 47, 101, 158, 280, 289, 290, 294
Magnesium, 837
Magnetic resonance imaging (MRI), 462, 764, 765, 805
    in brain death determination, 764
Magnetic resonance spectroscopy (MRS), 781
    proton, 782, 783
Mainous, Dave, 65
Maintenance therapy, 617–622
Malignancy
    heart transplantation and, 438
    kidney transplantation and, 407–408
Many Sleepless Nights (Gutkind), 10
MAP. *See* Mean arterial pressure
Martyn, Bet, 165
Masteller, Meredith A., 35, 44, 153

Mathe, Georges, 142
Matrice, Burton J., 159, 280, 304
Mayes, Gwen, 284
McAtee, Robert K., 65, 67
McCabe, Jim, 300
McDonald, John, 161
McGiffin, David, 287
Mean arterial pressure (MAP), 779
Mean corpuscular volume, 651
ME/C. *See* Medical examiners/coroners
Mechanical bridging, 431
Mechanical ventilation, 821–822
    adjustments, 835–836
    assessment of, 834–835
    care guidelines, 834–836
    parameters during, 822
    in pediatric donors, 845
    respiratory treatments in, 835
    settings, 835
Medawar, Peter Brian, 12, 136
Medicaid, 368
Medical ethics, 335
    access issues, 345–346
    code of, for transplant practitioner, 349
    conflicts, 341
    donation and transplantation continuum, 340
    ethically acceptable options, 338
    ethically relevant considerations, 338–340
    informed consent models and, 341–342
    living donor, 346–347, 509–518
    maintenance of, 707–708
    morality v., 335–336
    organ acceptability and, 345
    postconsent, 343
    in potential donation hospital environments, 342–343
    prehospital, 341
    theories, 336–37
    transplant candidate and recipient issues, 343–345
    working towards solutions, 338–340
Medical examiners/coroners (ME/C), 905
    comparison of study periods, 908–914
    denials, 716, 717, 722, 729, 904, 909, 911
        denials, 911
    legislation, 912–913
    methods, 905–906
    non-physician, 914
    regulations and protocol, 913–914
    study findings, 907–908
Medical history, 384, 385–386, 806–807
    interview, 385–386
Medical records, review of, 386–387
Medically suitable potential donors, 729
Medicare, 363–364
    beneficiaries, 366–367
    cost reports, 701
    Intermediary publications, 705
    physician fee schedule, 369
Medicare as secondary payor (MSP), 359
Meeker, William, 139

Meeneren, Job van, 127
Meier, Eileen, 169
MELD scores. *See* Model for End Stage Liver Disease scores
Membership Committee for Procurement Personnel, 65–66
Membership Committee for Transplant Nursing professional, 65–66
Membranoproliferative glomerulonephritis, 560
Membranous nephropathy, 560
Merrill, John P., 135, 139
Merriman, Michael L., 66
Metastatic hepatic malignant neoplasms, 560
Metoprolol, 562
Métras, Henry, 134
Metz, Richard, 299
Meyer, Jayne, 294
MIC. *See* Minimal inhibitory concentration
Micafungin, 584
Michon, Louis, 18, 136
Mickey, M. Ray, 150
Microvillous inclusion, 484
Mid-South Transplant Foundation, 92
Miller, Donald, 19
Miller, Joan, 10, 28, 32, 294
Millez, P., 135
Minimal inhibitory concentration (MIC), 669
Minorities, 799–800
Missed eligible referral, 716
Missed medically suitable referrals, 729
Missed referrals, 729
Mitoff, Jeffrey S., 119, 177
MMF. *See* Mycophenolate mofetil
Model Elements of Informed Consent for Organ and Tissue Donation, 342, 374
Model for End Stage Liver Disease (MELD) scores, 466, 468
  liver allocation and, 327–328
Modern organ transplantation, advent of, 17–25
Mollaret, P., 137
Moncure, Michael, 181
Monoclonal antibodies, 156, 452
Montgomery, Robert, 45
Monthly donation records, 726
Moore, Francis D., 14
Morality, ethics v., 335–336
Morelle, Jean, 143
Morgan, Rudy, 292, 302
Moritsugu, Kenneth, 301
Morris, Peter J., 153
MP. *See* Machine perfusion
MPS. *See* Machine perfusion solution
MRI. *See* Magnetic resonance imaging
MRS. *See* Magnetic resonance spectroscopy
MSP. *See* Medicare as secondary payor
Multicultural communities, donation rates in, 354–355
Multi-Organ Committee, 266
Multiple listing, education, 554
Muromonab-CD3 (OKT3), 616
  adverse reactions to, 616
  dosing, 616
  mechanism of action of, 616
Murphy, Raymond, 134
Murray, Gordon, 137
Murray, Joseph, 15, 19, 20, 48, 136, 137, 138, 139, 141
Musculoskeletal donation, 376–379
  distribution, 378
Mutilation, 797–798
Mycophenolate mofetil (MMF), 675, 676
Mycophenolic acid derivatives, 621
  adverse effects of, 621
  dosing, 621
  drug-drug interactions, 626
  mechanism of action of, 621
Myoclonic twitching, 758

Nadalol, 562
Najarian, John, 24, 145
NAME. *See* National Association of Medical Examiners
NAT. *See* Nucleic acid testing
NATCO. *See* North American Transplant Coordinator's Organization
Nathan, Howard, 10, 36, 162, 168, 282, 286, 289, 290, 302
National Association of Medical Examiners (NAME), 903, 904
National Institutes of Health (NIH), 108
National Kidney Foundation, 108
National Kidney Recipient Pool List, 278
National Organ Donor Awareness Week, 262
National Organ Transplant Act (NOTA), 102, 158, 160, 321, 353, 552, 695
  hearings, 184–191
National Organ Transplant Hearings
  Denny, Donald, in, 192–223
  notice of, 263
National Transplant Waiting List, 323
National Transplantation Pregnancy Registry (NTPR), 675, 676, 677, 678
NDLDs. *See* Nondirected living donors
Neck flexion, 758
Necrotizing enterocolitis, 483
Neisseria gonorrhea, 386
Neonates, 687–688
  development of, 688
  interventions, 688
  transplantation issues, 688
Neoplasms
  central nervous system, 813–814
  non-central nervous system, 813–814
Nephrectomy, 173
Neuhof, Harold, 132
Neumann, Ernst, 128
Neurological evaluation, 398
Neurosonology Research Group, 762
New England Organ Bank, 148
New Waters Preservation machine, 277
Niacin, 568
Nicardipine, 562
Nicely, Bruce, 118, 296

Nifedipine, 562
NIH. *See* National Institutes of Health
Nipride. *See* Nitroprusside sodium
Nisoldipine, 562
Nitroprusside sodium (Nipride), 846
No consent, 716, 729
No next of kin, 716, 729
Nocardia asteroides, 450, 573
Nolan, Shirley, 150
Non central nervous system neoplasm, 813–814
Nondirected living donors (NDLDs), 515
Nonmaleficence, 337
Nonprescription medications, 634–639
    antidiarrheals, 637–638
    antihistamines, 638
    cough suppressants and expectorants, 638–639
    laxatives, 635–637
Nonresident aliens, 344
Nonsteroidal anti-inflammatory drugs (NSAIDs), 635
Normodyne. *See* Labetalol
North American Transplant Coordinator's Organization (NATCO), 10, 194, 205–206, 903
    annual meetings, 48
    birth of, 41, 42
    Code of Ethics for the Transplant Practitioner, 347
    committee reports, 65–66
    committee roster, 259, 260, 261
    on donor registries, 342
    eighteenth annual meeting, 170
    eighth annual meeting, 158
    eleventh annual meeting, 163
    fifteenth annual meeting of, 167
    fifth annual meeting of, 154
    first class of training course, 281
    fourteenth annual meeting of, 167
    newsletters, 64–67, 266
    nineteenth annual meeting, 171
    ninth annual meeting, 159
    officers of, 42–43
    presidents, 99–126
    seventeenth annual meeting, 170
    seventh annual meeting, 156
    sixth annual meeting, 155
    subcommittee for training, 274
    tenth annual meeting, 161
    thirteenth annual meeting, 165
    thirtieth annual meeting, 180
    thirty-first annual meeting, 181
    thirty-second annual meeting, 182
    training courses, 48–53
    twelfth annual meeting, 164
    twentieth annual meeting, 173
    twenty-eighth annual meeting, 178
    twenty-fifth annual meeting, 177
    twenty-first annual meeting, 173
    twenty-fourth annual meeting, 175
    twenty-ninth annual meeting, 179
    twenty-second annual meeting, 174
    twenty-seventh annual meeting, 178
    twenty-sixth annual meeting, 177
    twenty-third annual meeting, 174
    UNOS and, 267, 268–269
NOTA. *See* National Organ Transplant Act
Not-for-profit agencies, 374
NSAIDs. *See* Nonsteroidal anti-inflammatory drugs
NTPR. *See* National Transplantation Pregnancy Registry
Nucleic acid testing (NAT), 375
Nuesse, Barbara, 300, 304
Nutrition
    after lung transplantation, 450
    intestinal transplantation and, 496–497
Nystatin, 579

OACC. *See* Organ acquisition cost centers
O'Connor, Kevin, 171, 181
Ocular movements, examination of, 752–753
    alerts, 753
    technique for, 752
ODBC. *See* Organ Donation Breakthrough Collaborative
Oeconomos, Nicolas, 18, 135, 136
Ohler, Linda, 68, 171, 176, 182, 300
OKT3. *See* Muronomab-CD3
Oliguria, 851
Olmesartan, 562
Olsen, Les, 28, 30, 141, 275
Omega-3 fatty acids, 562
Omnell-Persson, Marie, 158
Omphalocele, 483
OPCs. *See* Organ procurement coodinators
OPOs. *See* Organ procurement organizations
ORC. *See* Organ recovery coordinator
Organ acceptability, 345
Organ acquisition cost centers (OACC), 364–365
    donor suitability determination costs, 365
    patient maintenance costs, 365
    program operating costs, 365
Organ allocation, 321–324
    alternative, 333
    balancing, 322
    education and, 552
    equitable, 322
    geography and, 322–323
    heart, 324–325
    heart-lung, 327
    intestinal, 328
    intestinal-liver, 328
    islet, 332
    kidney, 328–330
    liver, 327–328
    lung, 325–326
    medical benefit, 322
    to multiple organ transplant patients, 333
    objectives of, 323
    pancreas, 330–332
    policies, 333
    policy-making, 333–334
Organ and Tissue Donation for Transplantation (Elick), 17
Organ Center, 323
Organ costs, 362–363

Organ Donation Breakthrough Collaborative (ODBC), 46-47, 712, 903, 904
    Change Package, 732-737
    collaborative engine, 719
    development of, 714-717
    donation system transformations due to, 727
    donor increases due to, 726
    improvement model, 718-719
    learning sessions, 718
    measurement strategy of, 724-725
    overarching strategies, 719-723
    refinements to, 723-724
    results of, 725-727
    timeline, 717
Organ Donors, 324
Organ perfusion machine, 132
Organ preservation
    composition of solutions, 894
    donor source and graft outcome, 898-899
    future of, 899-901
    historical perspective on, 891-893
    modalities and solutions, 894-896
    preservation modality and graft outcome, 897-898
    preservation time and graft outcome, 896-897
    principles and goals of, 893-894
Organ Procurement and Transplant Network (OTPN), 160, 163, 321, 323, 343, 396, 457, 490, 521, 552, 695, 709
    input from minorities during public comment period, 353-354
    policy development, 333-334
Organ procurement coordinators (OPCs), 819
Organ procurement organizations (OPOs), 26, 163, 321, 359, 360, 373, 502, 708, 729-730
    advocating donation, 796
    collaborative processes, 872
    consent environment in, 792-794
    as donor advocates, 513
    on economics of organ donation, 359-360
    goals of, 717
    high-performance, 715
    hospital-based, 360
    identification of, 713
    in-house coordinators, 738
    international, 712
    overarching principles of, 715
    self-organizing, 741
    staff, 795
    strategies for running, 719-723
    top-performing, 714
    transformations in, 727
Organ recovery
    anesthesia duties, 858-859
    heart, 863
    instrumentation and suture, 860-861
    kidney, 862
    liver, 862-863
    lung, 863-864
    operating room setup, 859-861
    operating room time setting, 857-858
    pancreas, 864-865
    personnel requirements, 858
    small bowel, 865-866
Organ recovery coordinator (ORC), 806-807
Organ Recovery Systems LifePort, 894
Organ referral, 716, 729
Organ sharing, 53-55
Organ Transplant Breakthrough Collaborative, 180
"Organ Transplantation: The Practical Possibilities" (Murray), 15
Organizational structure, 696-697
O'Rourke, Marian, 125, 182, 299, 300, 304
Osteonecrosis, 408
Osteopenia, drug therapy for, 570
Osteoporosis, 444, 567-571
    detection of, 569
    drug therapy for, 570
    heart transplantation and, 439
    risk factors, 569
OTC products. See Over-the-counter products
OTPN. See Organ Procurement and Transplant Network
Over-the-counter (OTC) products, 634
Oxalosis, 560
Oxygen saturation, 844, 845
Oxygen tank, 859

$PaCO_2$, 755, 775, 776, 842
PAH. See Pulmonary arterial hypertension
Pain, motor response to, 751
PAK. See Pancreas after kidney transplant
Palumbi, Mary Ann, 117, 172, 303
Pamidronate, 570
Pancreas after kidney transplant (PAK), 411
    advantages to, 415
Pancreas allocation, 330-332
    facilitated, 332
    zero antigen mismatch, 331-332
Pancreas transplant alone (PTA), 411
Pancreas transplantation, 24-25, 129, 132, 145, 149, 152, 154, 411-414k
    bacterial infections in, 574-575
    bladder drainage and, 417, 422-423
    bleeding and, 418-419
    candidate selection, 414-416
    contraindications for, 416
    DCD and, 887-888
    evaluation for, 413, 810
    exocrine secretion drainage, 416-417
    fungal infections in, 577
    glucose regulation and, 421-422
    glycemic control, 419
    graft function, 412
    indications for, 411
    infection and, 419
    long-term management of, 423-424
    organ procurement and bench preparation in, 416
    organ recovery, 864-865
    patient survival, 412
    postoperative management, 417-423
    rejection, 419-421

surgery, 416–418
    thrombosis and, 418
    transplant evaluation, 411–414
    transplant surgical procedure, 416
    waiting list for, 417–418
Pancreas-kidney transplant (SPK), 411, 417
    advantages of, 414
    pregnancy and, 679–680
Panel reactive antibody (PRA), 329, 607
Panjeda, Deidre Gish, 166, 293, 301
P.AP. *See* Pulmonary artery pressure
Parathyroid hormones, 570
Park, Mary Anne, 37
Partial face transplantation, 180
Partial thromboplastin time, 653
Patient curriculum, 550
Patient donation wishes, 798
Patient referral, 485
Patient services, 272
Paton, R. Townley, 133
PBC. *See* Primary biliary cirrhosis
PCR, 669, 748
PDSA (Plan Do Study Act), 730, 731, 738, 740, 743, 744
Pearson, Griffith, 24
Pediatric donors
    acidosis in, 852
    ancillary testing based on age of, 840
    brain death in, 840–841
    calcium derangements in, 852
    coagulation abnormalities in, 852–853
    diabetes insipidus in, 851
    fluid and electrolyte balance in, 849–850
    general considerations for, 842–843
    glucose derangements in, 851
    hemodynamic instability in, 846–848
    hormone replacement therapy in, 848–849
    normal vital signs for, 842
    potassium derangements in, 851
    pulmonary issues, 843–845
    suitability of, 839–840
Pediatric End-Stage Liver Disease (PELD) scores, 466, 468
    liver allocation and, 327–328
Peele, Amy, 25, 36, 37, 46, 47, 79, 102, 157, 158, 159, 270, 286, 289, 291, 303
PEEP. *See* Positive end expiratory pressure
Pegg, D.E., 136
PELD scores. *See* Pediatric End-Stage Liver Disease scores
Penicilins, 575, 627
Penke, Hans, 154
Percutaneous biopsy, 405
Perfadex, 895
Perindopril, 562
Perper, Robert J., 145
PET. *See* Positron emission tomography
Peterson, Corbin, 292
PFT. *See* Pulmonary function test
Phagocytosis, 609–610
Pharmacodynamic interactions, 623

Pharmacokinetic interactions, 623
Pharmacological bridging, 431
Pharyngeal reflex, examination of, 753–756
    technique for, 753
Phenobarbital, 777
PHI. *See* Protected Health Information
Phillips, Michael G., 34, 278, 292
Phosphorus, 837
Phrenic nerve damage, 449
Pichlmayr, Rudolf, 166
Pierce, Gene, 157
PL ventilation. *See* Pressure-limited ventilation
Plan Do Study Act. *See* PDSA
Platelets, 653
Ploeg, Rutger Jan, 157
Pneumocystis carinii, 451, 573
Pneumocystis jiroveci, 625
Pneumonia, 576
Polycarbophil, 637
Polyclonal antibodies, 452
Polyenes, 579–580
Polyomavirus, 594–595
    clinical manifestations of, 594–595
    treatment of, 595
Polyuria, 837–838
    assessment, 837
    treatment, 837
Portal vein access, 506
Portal vein thrombosis (PVT), 459
Portal venous circulation, 421
Portopulmonary hypertension (PPH), 462
Positive end expiratory pressure (PEEP), 821, 845
Positron emission tomography (PET), 778, 779, 780
Posttransplant Diabetes Mellitus (PTDM), 407, 564–565
Posttransplant lymphoproliferative disease (PTLD), 407, 451, 496
Potassium, 654, 836–837
    in pediatric donors, 851
Potential donation hospitals, 342–343
PPH. *See* Portopulmonary hypertension
PRA. *See* Panel reactive antibody
Pravastatin, 568
Prednisone, 21
Pregnancy, 674–683
    fathered by male transplant recipients, 675
    heart transplantation and, 682
    kidney transplantation and, 677–678
    liver transplantation and, 680, 681
    lung transplantation and, 682
    pancreas-kidney transplants and, 679–680
    thoracic organ transplant recipients and, 680–682
Preprocessing cultures, 377
Preschoolers
    development of, 689–690
    interventions, 690
    transplantation issues, 690
Preservation. *See* Organ preservation
Preservation injury, 474
Pressure-limited (PL) ventilation, 822
    VC ventilation v., 823

Presumptive consent, 800
Pre-transplant issues, 355
Primary biliary cirrhosis (PBC), 458, 475, 560
Primary brainstem death, 758-759
Primary graft dysfunction, 472
Primary sclerosing cholangitis (PSC), 458, 560
Princeteau, M., 130
Principe, Anita L., 35, 67, 106, 290, 294
Principles, 337
Prisoners, 344
Procurement, 272
    in pancreas transplant surgery, 416
    training course, 51-53
Procurement Team, 324
Profit agencies, 374
Progress in Transplantation, 67-68, 112, 118, 820
Propranolol, 562
Prostate-specific antigen (PSA), 813
Protected Health Information (PHI), 704
Protein, 656, 825
Protein C, 660
Protein S, 660
Prothrombin, 653
PSA. See Prostate-specific antigen
PSC. See Primary sclerosing cholangitis
Pseudomonas aeruginosa, 445, 575
Psychosocial evaluation, 399
    in LDLT donors, 540
    of living donors, 515-516
    of living kidney donors, 531
PTA. See Pancreas transplant alone
PTDM. See Posttransplant Diabetes Mellitus
PTLD. See Posttransplant lymphoproliferative disease
Public education, 200, 201, 371
Public Health Improvement Act, 360
Pulmonary alveolar proteinosis, 560
Pulmonary arterial hypertension (PAH), 441, 446
Pulmonary artery pressure (PAP), 462
Pulmonary function test (PFT), 523, 524
Pulmonary valve, 382
Pulmonary vascular resistance (PVR), 844
Pupils, examination of, 752
    alerts, 752
    technique for, 752
Puzzle People (Starzl), 11, 17, 71
PVR. See Pulmonary vascular resistance
PVT. See Portal vein thrombosis
Pybus, Charles, 132

QOL. See Quality of life
Quality improvement initiatives, 705-706
Quality of life (QOL), 482
    after LDLT, 546
Quinapril, 562

Race, 799-800
Radiation enteritis, 484
Radionuclide scan, 760, 778
Rajotte, Ray, 169
Ramipril, 562

Rapamune. See Sirolimus
Rapamycin inhibitors, 617, 621-622
Rapaport, Felix, 96
Rapid plasma regain (RPR), 523
Rasmussen, Geraldine M., 33, 41, 152, 279
RATG. See Antithymocyte globulin rabbit
Ratner, Lloyd, 45, 173
RCDAD. See Relevant communicable disease agent or disease
Reams, Bernard, 46
Recipient selection criteria
    heart transplant, 430
    kidney transplant, 397-400
    lung transplant, 441-442
Recruitment, staff, 706-707
Recurrent diseases, 408, 560
    rates, 409
Red blood cell count, 651
Reemtsma, Keith, 142, 144
Referral process, 383-384, 699
    early, 795-796
    rapid, 720, 734-735, 741-742
    rates, 716, 729
Refutational messages, 791
Regional Organ Procurement Agency (ROPA), 44, 84, 99, 151
Regulatory compliance, 704-705
Reimbursement, 360-361
Reimplantation, 448
Reiner, Mark R., 35, 104, 155, 163, 294, 302
Reitsma, William, 171
Reitz, Bruce, 23, 155
Rejection, 405-406
    acute, 405, 419-420
    cellular, 436
    chronic, 405, 420, 452
    clinical history and, 434
    diagnosis of, 434-437
    grading system for, 452
    graft pancreatitis v., 420-421
    heart transplantation, 434-437
    humoral, 435, 436-437
    hyperacute, 405, 436
    immunology of, 610
    intestinal transplantation, 494-495
    islet cell, 507
    liver transplantation, 474-475
    lung transplantation, 452-453
    pancreas transplant, 419-421
    physical examination for, 434
Relevant communicable disease agent or disease (RCDAD), 386
Religious beliefs, 339, 344, 356
    defining, 356
    stances of various, on transplantation, 356
Reloxifene, 570
Renal disease, 561-564
    immunosuppression and, 563
    risk factors, 563
Renard, Marius, 18

ReoPro. *See* Abciximab
Reperfusion injury, 610
"Replaceable Body: How Transplants Save Lives" (article), 69–70
Requests, 384
Respiratory management, 449–450
Reticulocyte count, 652
Revascularization, 401
Richardson, Ken, 60–661
Richet, Gabriel, 19
Right ventricular assist devices (RVAD), 431
Ringoir, Severin, 149
Risedronate, 570
Riteris, John, 137
Roels, Leo, 32, 82, 85, 151, 170, 172, 173, 174, 296, 297, 298, 299
Rolling Ridge, 281, 282, 284, 286
    Procurement Class Courses, 282
ROPA. *See* Regional Organ Procurement Agency
Ross, Donald N., 147, 372
Rosuvastatin, 568
Rougeulle, J., 135
Rowntree, Leonard C., 131
RPR. *See* Rapid plasma regain
Rudy, Laura, 287
Russell, John, 142
RVAD. *See* Right ventricular assist devices

SAC. *See* Standard acquisition charge
Salicylates, 635
Sampson, John, 276
Sarcoidosis, 560
SBS. *See* Short-bowel syndrome
SCCM. *See* Society for Critical Care Medicine
Schanbacher, Barbara, 33, 43, 66, 107, 153, 163, 280, 287, 288, 289, 294
Scharp, David W., 150, 168
Schkade, Lawrence L., 171, 179
Schlosser, R.J., 136
Schonstadt, 131
School age children, 690–691
    development of, 690
    interventions, 691
    transplantation issues, 691
Schulman, Barbara, 33, 41, 42–43, 43, 99, 152, 153, 154, 280, 290, 294, 295
Schulz, Christl, 151, 154
Schwartz, Robert, 139
Sciatic nerve transplantations, 166
Scientific Committee, 65–66
Scientific Registry of Transplant Recipients (SRTR), 357, 552, 705, 895
Sclerosing cholangitis, 475
Scola, James V., 135
Scribner, Belding, 12, 139
Second European Congress for Transplant Coordinators, 79
Selby, Rick, 45
Seldinger technique, 761
Selective estrogen receptor modulators, 570

Senst, Nancy L., 122, 299, 300, 301
SEOPF. *See* South-Eastern Organ Procurement Foundation
Sepsis, 445
Serial transverse enteroplasty (S.T.E.P), 487
Serological tests, 807
Servelle, Marceau, 135
Seven Springs, 288
Shafer, Teresa, 16, 68, 85, 112, 171, 172, 178, 180, 182, 284, 297, 299, 301, 791
Shapiro, James, 24–25, 175
Sheedy, Ellen, 179
Shelley, Mary Wollstonecraft, 128
Sheppeck, Rick, 57, 159
Sherlock, Joel, 101
Shields, Clyde, 13
Short-bowel syndrome (SBS), 481
Shumway, Norman, 16, 22, 23, 140, 144, 147, 155, 427
SIDS. *See* Sudden infant death syndrome
Siminoff, Laura A., 791
Simple Cold Storage of Organs, 136, 149
Simvastatin, 568
Single photon emission computed tomography (SPECT), 778
    in brain death determination, 764–766
Sirolimus (Rapamune), 25, 621–622, 624–625
    adverse drug reactions, 622
    dosing, 622
    drug-drug interactions, 624
    mechanism of action of, 622
Skeletal disorders, kidney transplantation and, 408
Skin cancer, 408
Skin donation, 379–380
Skin grafts, 129
    first reported use of, 11
Slaton, Jolie, 293
Slush machines, 859, 860
Small bowel donation, 810
    procurement, 865–866
Smit, Heiner, 153
Smith, Allison, 285
Smith, Kathleen, 169
Smith, Roger, 28, 31, 41, 66, 141, 152, 287, 289
Snell, George D., 134
Social history, 806–807
Society for Critical Care Medicine (SCCM), 903
Society for Organ Sharing (SOS), 86
Sodium, 653–654, 836
Soft tissue, 377
Solicitation, living donor, 516–517
Solis, Bennie, 21
Somatosensory evoked potentials (SSEP), 766, 781
Sophie, Laura, 79, 155, 157
SOS. *See* Society for Organ Sharing
South-Eastern Organ Procurement Foundation (SEOPF), 152, 157, 164, 204
SPECT. *See* Single photon emission computed tomography
Spinal activity, 756–758
Spiral computed tomography scan, in brain death

determination, 767
Spiritual distinctions, 339
SPK. *See* Pancreas-kidney transplant
Springer, James W., 34, 60, 61, 171, 282, 302, 303
SRTR. *See* Scientific Registry of Transplant Recipients
SSEP. *See* Somatosensory evoked potentials
Staff recruitment, 706–707
Stakeholders, 338, 340
Standard acquisition charge (SAC), 360
    renal, 363
Standard criteria donation, education on, 553
Standards for Tissue Banking, 385
Standards of practice, 75, 76
Staphylococcus aureus, 445, 450
Stark law, 706
Starnes, Vaughn A., 167, 171
Starzl, Thomas, 9, 11, 15, 17, 21, 28, 61, 69, 71, 140, 141, 142, 145, 146, 150, 154, 161, 164, 170, 301
Staschak, Sandra, 10, 74, 295
Status, 343–344
STATUS NINE, 266
STATUS ONE, 266
STATUS THREE, 266
STATUS TWO, 266
Steele, Janet, 171
Stenotrophomas maltiphilia, 450
S.T.E.P. *See* Serial transverse enteroplasty
Stephens, Laura, 299
Steroids, 565, 567, 849
Stevens, Keith, 299
Stonington, Oliver, 140
Streptococcus pneumoniae, 450
Strome, Marshall, 175
Strong, Russell W., 167
Subcommittee on Public Education and Outreach Initiatives, 354
Subdural hematoma, 749
Substance abuse, 444–445
Sudden infant death syndrome (SIDS), 771
Sulfamethoxazole, 574
Sulfamethoxazole-trimethoprim, 627
Superior mesenteric thrombosis, 483
Supplemental IV insulin sliding scale, 832
Supplemental oxygen therapy, 446
Supraventricular tachycardia (SVT), 848
Sutherland, David E.R., 151, 152, 154, 170
SVT. *See* Supraventricular tachycardia
SWOT analysis, 698
Syllabus, meeting, 243–244, 245–247, 248–252
Synthroid. *See* Levothyroxine
Syphilis, 664

T cells, 608
T3. *See* Triiodothyronine
Tabor, Sally, 79–80, 151, 157
Tacrolimus, 25, 171, 565, 567, 618–619, 624–625, 630
    adverse reactions to, 619
    drug-drug interactions, 624
Takagi, Hiroshi, 164, 168
Tamaki, Isao, 81, 82, 93–94, 168, 297

Tamoxifen, 570
Tan, Sally, 85
Taylor, Paul, 28, 29, 43, 61, 70, 71, 85, 141, 153, 159, 275, 280, 295, 296, 297
Taylor, Ross, 81
TCD. *See* Transcranial Doppler sonography
Teachey, Herbert E., 35, 70, 156, 159, 162, 280, 292
Teagarden, Rebecca, 791
Team huddles, 720, 723, 738
Teinturier, J., 135
Temperature regulation, 825–826
    care guidelines, 832–833
Terasaki, Paul, 41, 44, 144, 150, 278
Teriparatide, 570
Test kit packages, 388
Testosterone, 570
THAM. *See* Tromethamine
The Transplantation Society (TTS), 86
Thiazide diuretics, 631
Thiel, B., 149
Thompson, Tommy G., 712
Thoracotomy lobectomy, 524
Thrombocytopenia, 825
    care guidelines, 833–834
Thrombosis, 482
    postoperative, 418
Thyroid function studies, 659
Thyroid-stimulating hormone (TSH), 659
Ticlid. *See* Ticlopidine
Ticlopidine (Ticlid), 825
Tidal volume, 845
Tilney, Nicholas, 11, 15, 17
Timely notification rate, 716, 730
    goals, 717
Timolol, 562
Ting, Alan, 153
TIPS. *See* Transjugular intrahepatic portosystemic shunt
Tissue banks, accredited, 373
Tissue recovery, 386–387
    sites of, 389
    technical practices, 387–388
    time restrictions for, 387
Tissue recovery agencies, 384
Tissue typing, 140
Toddlers, 688–689
    development of, 688
    interventions, 689
    transplantation issues, 689
Toledo, Louis, 275
TOPF. *See* Transplant Organ Procurement Foundation
Toronto Lung Transplant Group, 24
Torsemide, 562
Total aganglionosis, 484
Total parenteral nutrition (TPN), 481, 482
Toxoplasmosis, 573, 664
    algorithm, 665
TPN. *See* Total parenteral nutrition
Tracheal reflex, examination of, 753–756
    technique for, 753
Training courses, 48–53

on clinical care, 50-51
on procurement, 49-50, 51-53
Trandate. *See* Labetalol
Trandolapril, 562
Transcranial Doppler sonography (TCD), 762-764, 778, 779-780
Transcranial ultrasonography, 760
Transjugular intrahepatic portosystemic shunt (TIPS), 467
Transplant administration
   clinical, 703-704
   contracting, 702-703
   creating access and referral bases, 699
   data management, 703-704
   ethical practice maintenance, 707-708
   explaining, 695
   financial, 699-702
   funding medications, 707
   global, 708-709
   healthcare policy development and, 709
   history of, 695
   implementation and monitoring plan, 698
   key roles in, 696
   organizational, 696-699
   program effectiveness, 704-707
   program growth planning, 697-698
   promoting organ donation, 708-709
   research, 708
   SWOT analysis, 698
Transplant candidates, behavior or status as factor for, 343-344
Transplant center economics, 363-365
Transplant Chronicles, 116
Transplant coordinators
   American v. European, 9
   birth of, 25-40
   certification of, 74-75
   certification statistics, 77
   clinical, 27-28, 73
   dedication of, 70-74
   early, 28-38
   evolution of titles for, 240
   first annual meeting of, 152
   fourth meeting of, 153
   future of, 95-98
   international organizations, 78-87
   meeting syllabus, 243-244, 245-247, 248-252
   need for, 9
   organ sharing and, 53-55
   philosophy of, 241-242
   in press, 68-70
   procurement, 26-27
   recertification, 77-78
   research, 64-70
   role of, 9-10
   second annual meeting of, 152, 258
   societies, 254
   steps of, 272
   third meeting of, 153
   training courses for, 48-53

   typical, 271
Transplant Foundation, 202, 205
Transplant: From Myth to Reality (Tilney), 11, 17
Transplant Organ Procurement Foundation (TOPF), 57
Transplant Patient, 324
Transplant Recipient, 324
Transplant Recipients International Organization (TRIO), 111
Transplant Team, 324
Transplantation
   events leading to modern era of, 11-13
   growth and development of, 371-373
   national hearings on, 45-47
Travel, 667-668
Travenol, 894
Travitzky, Virginia, 294
Treatment guidelines, 829-838
Triiodothyronine (T3), 848
Trimethoprim, 574
TRIO. *See* Transplant Recipients International Organization
Tromethamine (THAM), 847
Truman, Chester, 53
Tryptophan, 895
Tsang, Victor, 181
TSH. *See* Thyroid-stimulating hormone
TTS. *See* The Transplantation Society
Tuberculosis, diagnosis of, 667
Tufting enteropathy, 484
Turner, Benjamin B., 131
Tuskegee Experiment, 356
24-ALERT System, 55-64, 194, 206
   articles about, 56
   how it works, 58-59
   NATCO newsletter article on, 266
Tzakis, Andreas G., 172
Tzanck test, 670

UAGA. *See* Uniform Anatomical Gift Act
UKT. *See* United Kingdom Transplant
UKTCA. *See* United Kingdom Transplant Coordinators Association
Ullman, Emerich, 18, 129
UNet[SM], 324
Unger, Ernst, 18, 131
Uniform Anatomical Gift Act (UAGA), 16, 148, 341, 345, 517, 891
United Kingdom Transplant (UKT), 169
United Kingdom Transplant Coordinators Association (UKTCA), 79-81, 157
United Kingdom Transplant Service, 154
United Network for Organ Sharing (UNOS), 58, 106, 110, 111, 112, 121, 157, 160, 161, 164, 168, 204, 206, 323, 400, 427, 430, 445, 457, 490, 552, 695, 705, 709, 862, 903, 906
   Ethics Committee, 344
   input from minorities during public comment period, 353-354
   NATCO and, 267, 268-269
   policy development, 333-334

specific criteria of, 809
United States, 711-712
University of Wisconsin Solution (UW), 893, 895
UNOS. *See* United Network for Organ Sharing
Urea nitrogen, 654-655
Ureteroneocystostomy, 401
Urethritis, 423
Urinary protein, 657
Urinary tract infections, 422-423
Ursodeoxycholic acid, 467
Utilitarianism, 336
UW. *See* University of Wisconsin Solution

Vaccination, 597, 598, 629
VAD. *See* Ventricular assist device
Valacyclovir, 589
Valganciclovir, 587, 589
Valsartan, 562
Van Hook, Jane, 158, 282
van Wyk, Jonathan, 23
Vancomycin, 627
Vanhaelewijck, Betty, 151
VanRood, Jon J., 145
Varicella zoster virus (VZV), 451, 573, 588-590, 588-591, 667
    clinical manifestations of, 590
    diagnosis and monitoring of, 590
    prevention of, 590
    treatment of, 590
Vascular access, 842-843
Vascular anastomosis, 12
Vascular thrombus, 544
Vasopressin, 850
Vaughn, Bill, 285
Vaysse, Jean, 18, 136
VC ventilation. *See* Volume controlled ventilation
Vein grafts, 380-381
Venezuelan National Transplant Organization, 174
Ventricular assist device (VAD), 431
Verapamil, 562
Viral infections, 585-598
Viral laboratory diagnosis, 670
    immunological studies of sera, 670
    microscopic methods, 670
Virtue, 336
Vitamin D, 570
Vitamin K, 825, 852
Vliet, Daan van der, 154
Volume controlled (VC) ventilation, 822
    PL ventilation v., 823
Volume criteria, 364
Volvulus, 483
Voriconazole, 581-582
Voronoff, Serge, 131
Voronoy, Yu Yu, 133
VOTAN, 58
Vuyosevich, Elaine, 304
VZV. *See* Varicella zoster virus

Waddell, Bill, 140
Wagner, Dennis, 178, 180, 181
Wagner, Karl, 154
Waiting list/waiting times, 467-468
    for heart transplantation, 430-432
    for intestinal transplantation, 415-490
    for kidney transplantation, 394, 400
    liver transplantation, 468
    for lung transplantation, 445-446
    for pancreas transplantation, 415-416
Walters MOX-100, 894
Warm ischemic time (WIT), 871, 888, 893, 896
Warmbrodt, Jane A., 36-37, 162
Warner, Howell E., 171
Warnock, Garth, 169
Warren, Holly, 298, 300
Warren, Jim, 302
Washkansky, Louis, 22, 23
Watkins, Cozzie, 299
Watzinger, Franz, 178
Weber, Phyllis, 16, 28, 31, 141, 179
Wegener granulomatosis, 560
Welch, Stuart C., 137
Wertheimer, Pierre, 137, 138
Wertlieb, Stacey, 791
West, James, 134
West Nile Virus (WNV), 596
    clinical manifestations of, 596
    diagnosis and monitoring of, 596
    prevention and treatment of, 596
White blood cell count, 652
White, Celia, 85
Wight, Celia, 10, 37-38, 157, 164, 167, 296, 297
Williams, G. Melville, 13, 54, 58, 95-96, 97, 164, 293
Williams, Laura, 116, 303
Williams, Watson, 129
Wilmert, Justine, 28, 29-30, 41, 43, 107, 141, 152, 153, 280, 281
Wishes, patient donor, 798
WIT. *See* Warm ischemic time
WNV. *See* West Nile Virus
Wolff-Parkinson-White syndrome, 812
Womb transplantation, 177
Women's health, 673-683
Woolley, Scott, 285
World Federation of Neurology, 762
Wylie, Meredith, 791

XeCTCBF. *See* Xenon computed tomography, cerebral blood flow
Xenograft, 144
Xenon computed tomography, cerebral blood flow (XeCTCBF), 779
Xenotransplantation experiments, 128, 132, 140, 142
    testicular, 131

Yacoub, Magdi, 181
Yeager, Curtis, 41, 153, 279
Yeo, Elizabeth, 156, 165

Zenapax. *See* Daclizumab
Zero antigen mismatch pancreas, 331–332
Zimmerman, David, 300
Zink, Sheldon, 791
Zirm, Eduard, 130
Zukoski, Charles, 20, 139